MJ

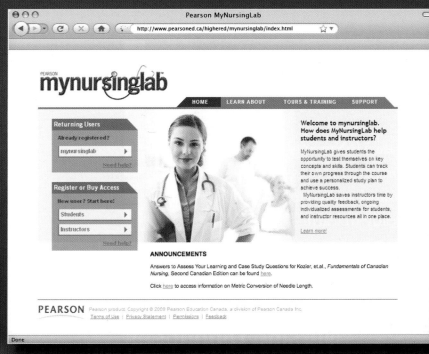

Save Time!

In MyNursingLab you are treated as an individual with specific learning needs.

Chapter Pre-Test

Using CRNE-type questions, this quiz measures your understanding of the chapter material and the expected learning outcomes for that chapter.

Customized Study Plan

Based on the results of the chapter pre-test, you receive a plan to help you practise important concepts and applications where you need improvement.

eText

The study plan links to the online page discussing the very concept being applied.

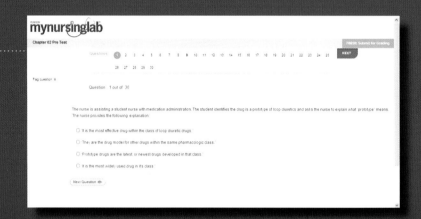

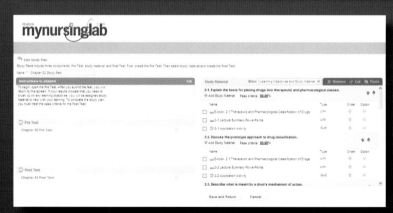

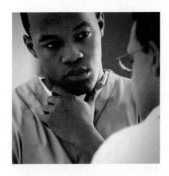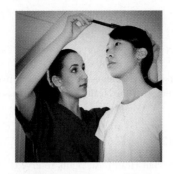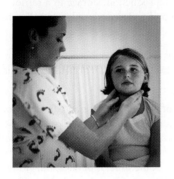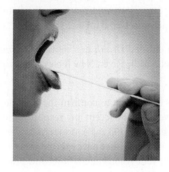

HEALTH & PHYSICAL ASSESSMENT IN NURSING

CANADIAN EDITION

DONITA **D'AMICO**
William Paterson University

COLLEEN **BARBARITO**
William Paterson University

CREINA **TWOMEY**
Memorial University

NICOLE **HARDER**
University of Manitoba

Pearson Canada
Toronto

Library and Archives Canada Cataloguing in Publication

Health & physical assessment in nursing / Donita D'Amico ... [et al.].
— Canadian ed.

Includes index.
ISBN 978-0-13-515860-9

1. Nursing assessment—Textbooks. 2. Physical diagnosis—Textbooks.
I. D'Amico, Donita II. Title: Health and physical assessment in nursing.

RT48.H42 2012   616.07'5   C2010-902228-9

Notice: Care has been taken to confirm the accuracy of information presented in this book. The authors, editors, and the publisher, however, cannot accept any responsibility for errors or omissions or for consequences from application of the information in this book and make no warranty, express or implied, with respect to its contents.

The authors and publisher have exerted every effort to ensure that drug selections and dosages set forth in this text are in accord with current recommendations and practice at the time of publication. However, in view of ongoing research, changes in government regulations, and the constant flow of information relating to drug therapy and drug reactions, the reader is urged to check the package inserts of all drugs for any change in indications of dosage and for added warnings and precautions. This is particularly important when the recommended agent is a new and/or infrequently employed drug.

ISBN-13: 978-0-13-515860-9
ISBN-10: 0-13-515860-5

Vice President, Editorial Director: Gary Bennett
Executive Editor: Michelle Sartor
Marketing Manager: Julia Jevmenova
Senior Developmental Editor: Madhu Ranadive
Production Editor: Leanne Rancourt
Copy Editor: Dawn Hunter
Proofreader: Susan Broadhurst
Technical Checker: Sandra Carter
Assistant Production/Editorial Manager: Patricia Ciardullo
Composition: Hermia Chung
Photo and Permissions Research: Karen Hunter
Art Director: Julia Hall
Cover and Interior Design: Anthony Leung
Cover Images (clockwise from top left): Masterfile, Masterfile, Masterfile, Stockbyte/Getty

For permission to reproduce copyrighted material, the publisher gratefully acknowledges the copyright holders listed on pages CR-1–CR-2, which are considered an extension of this copyright page.

Statistics Canada information is used with the permission of Statistics Canada. Users are forbidden to copy the data and redisseminate them, in an original or modified form, for commercial purposes, without permission from Statistics Canada. Information on the availability of the wide range of data from Statistics Canada can be obtained from Statistics Canada's Regional Offices, its World Wide Web site at http://www.statcan.gc.ca, and its toll-free access number 1-800-263-1136.

1 2 3 4 5   16 15 14 13 12

Printed and bound in the U.S.A.

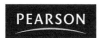

ABOUT THE AUTHORS

Donita D'Amico, MEd, RN

Donita D'Amico, a diploma nursing school graduate, earned her baccalaureate degree in nursing from William Paterson College. She earned a master's degree in Nursing Education at Teacher's College, Columbia University, with a specialization in Adult Health. Donita has been a faculty member at William Paterson University for more than 25 years. Her teaching responsibilities include physical assessment, medical-surgical nursing, nursing theory, and fundamentals in the classroom, skills laboratory, and clinical settings.

Donita co-authored several textbooks, including *Health Assessment in Nursing* and its companion clinical handbook by Sims, D'Amico, Stiesmeyer, and Webster; as well as *Comprehensive Health Assessment: A Student Workbook* and *Modules for Medication Administration* with Dr. Colleen Barbarito.

Donita is active in the community. Within the university, she is a charter member of the Iota Alpha Chapter of Sigma Theta Tau International. She continues to serve at the chapter and state levels. She also serves as a consultant and contributor to local organizations.

Colleen Barbarito, EdD, RN

Colleen Barbarito received a nursing diploma from Orange Memorial Hospital School of Nursing, graduated with a baccalaureate degree from William Paterson College, and earned a master's degree from Seton Hall University, all in New Jersey. She received her Doctor of Education from Teacher's College, Columbia University. Prior to a position in education, Colleen's clinical experiences included medical-surgical, critical care, and emergency nursing. Colleen has been a faculty member at William Paterson University since 1984, where she has taught physical assessment and a variety of clinical laboratory courses for undergraduate nursing students and curriculum development at the graduate level.

Colleen co-authored two books with Donita D'Amico—*Modules for Medication Administration* and *Comprehensive Health Assessment: A Student Workbook*. She published articles on anaphylaxis in *American Journal of Nursing* and *Coping with Allergies and Asthma*. Her research includes physical assessment and collaboration on revising a physical assessment project with results published as a brief in *Nurse Educator*. As a faculty member, Colleen participated in committees to explore curricular change and to develop multimedia learning modules for critical thinking.

Colleen is a member of Sigma Theta Tau International Honor Society of Nursing. She was an officer and serves as Faculty Advisor for the Iota Alpha Chapter at William Paterson University.

Creina Twomey, RN, MN, PhD(c)

Creina Twomey is a 1988 graduate of the General Hospital School of Nursing in St. John's, Newfoundland. She then attended Memorial University where she completed a Bachelor of Nursing degree in 1993 and a Master of Nursing degree in 1996. Creina is currently enrolled in a PhD program in clinical epidemiology. She has been employed by Memorial University for the past 15 years and teaches health assessment in the BN and post RN BN programs. In 2002 Creina developed the first online distance education health assessment course offered by Memorial's School of Nursing for post RN BNs. Her main areas of teaching are health assessment, medicine/surgery, clinical practice, complex care, and nursing research.

Creina's research topics include psychosocial adaptation to chronic illness, quality of life, psychometrics, men in nursing, clinical epidemiology, and community health assessment. Her PhD dissertation focus is twofold: first she is assessing adaptation to life on hemodialysis, and second she is developing and refining an instrument that measures adjustment to chronic kidney disease and its treatment. She has also developed a questionnaire that assesses men's reasons for choosing nursing, the barriers they experience in practice, and their level of job satisfaction. She has been co-lead investigator on three funded research projects and published her findings on male nurses in *Canadian Nurse* and the *Canadian Journal of Career Development*. Her research in the area of community assessment has resulted in five research grants, five unpublished research reports, and one publication in *Canadian Nurse*. In 2008, the research team Creina works with was awarded Primary Care Researcher of the Year by the Scientific Assembly of the Newfoundland Chapter of the College of Family Physicians of Canada. This award was for the team's 12 years of work in assessing the community health needs of the people of Newfoundland and Labrador.

Nicole Harder, RN, MPA, PhD(c)

Nicole has been with the University of Manitoba, Faculty of Nursing, for the past 11 years and was the Coordinator of the Learning Laboratories for eight years before becoming the Coordinator of the Simulation Learning Centre in 2010. Nicole has taught health assessment in the undergraduate nursing program and graduate nurse practitioner program and continues to look for new ways to help students understand and apply the concepts being taught. In addition to teaching health assessment, Nicole has taught medical/surgical nursing courses, as well as courses related to providing care in diverse societies. She is currently a committee member involved with curriculum development at the undergraduate nursing level at the University of Manitoba. Nicole has written and published articles in the *Journal of Nursing Education* and *Clinical Simulation in Nursing* related to high-fidelity simulation in nursing education and has co-authored articles based on teaching excellence in the *Journal of Professional Nursing*. Her current research areas include teaching and learning with technology and factors that affect student learning in high-fidelity simulation.

Nicole is a doctoral candidate in the Faculty of Nursing at the University of Alberta. Her research interest is in the area of simulations, and her thesis is titled 'Perceptions and Experiences of Nursing Students: Learning in High-Fidelity Simulation.' She has also created a DVD titled *How to Facilitate a Successful Simulation*, which was released in the fall of 2008. Nicole was recently elected as Vice-President for Membership of the International Nursing Association Clinical Simulation and Learning.

CONTRIBUTORS

Canadian Chapter Authors

Chapter 2: Health Promotion and the *Health Promotion Assessment Tool*

Candace Lind, RN, PhD
University of Calgary

Sylvia Loewen, RN, MN
University of Calgary

Aliyah Mawji, RN, PhD(c)
University of Calgary

Dr. Candace Lind is an assistant professor in the Faculty of Nursing at the University of Calgary. Candace is an RN who completed doctoral studies in nursing at the University of Calgary in 2005 and a postdoctoral research fellowship at the University of Ottawa in 2007. She teaches community health theory and practice. Candace's program of research is in community and population-based adolescent health promotion and encompasses research that is relationship-based, builds research capacity in non-academic researchers, informs nursing practice and policy development, and addresses the ways in which adolescents are conceptualized in society. Informed by the attributes of social justice and the social determinants of health, the goal of her program of research is to improve health outcomes for adolescents through individual, community, and social change. Candace is a member of the College & Association of Registered Nurses of Alberta, the Alberta Public Health Association, the Canadian Public Health Association, the Community Health Nurses of Alberta, and the International Union for Health Promotion and Education.

Sylvia Loewen is a senior instructor in the Faculty of Nursing at the University of Calgary. Sylvia is an RN who completed her Master of Nursing degree at the Faculty of Nursing, University of Calgary, in 1980. She teaches community health theory and practice, pediatrics, nursing inquiry, and nursing issue courses. She was the project lead for the Redesign of Community Health Courses and was responsible for course revisions for Community Practice. Sylvia's career has focused on the growing family, primarily in Canadian community settings. She has been a public health nurse for the City of Winnipeg; the Pediatric Clinical Nurse Specialist for Home Care, Calgary Health Region, where she developed and managed pediatric home care services and was the consultant for southern Alberta; and a manager in Health Promotion and Disease Prevention, where her responsibilities included developing, implementing, and evaluating population-wide initiatives to reduce the rate of low-birth-weight infants, reduce the percentage of the population that uses tobacco, and focus on creating workplace environments supportive of health. She has also worked in neonatal intensive care units and postpartum in both Canada and in New Zealand, and has been on the board of International Child Care, an organization that provides healthcare to children in Haiti and the Dominican Republic. Sylvia is a member of the College & Association of Registered Nursing of Alberta, the Alberta Public Health Association, the Canadian Public Health Association, the Canadian Association of Teachers of Community Health, the Canadian Association of International Community Health, and the National League of Nurses.

Aliyah Mawji is an instructor in the Faculty of Nursing at the University of Calgary. Aliyah is an RN who is currently in the process of completing her doctoral studies in the Department of Community Health Science, Faculty of Medicine, at the University of Calgary. She teaches community health theory and practice. Aliyah's career began as a pediatric acute care nurse. She quickly realized that she could have more impact on the health status of people if she worked at the community and population level. She worked briefly as a public health nurse, where her desire to increase her skill level in this area was cultivated. She completed an MPH from the University of Alberta in 2004, after which her career path led her to work on community health projects in developing countries. Her current doctoral work is in the area of epidemiology and population health of infants. This research will inform public health nursing practice and policy development. Other research interests include the health of immigrant women and multicultural populations. Aliyah is a member of the College & Association of Registered Nurses of Alberta, the Alberta Public Health Association, the Canadian Public Health Association, and the Canadian Association of Teachers of Community Health.

Canadian Contributors

Deborah Fraser Askin, MN, RNC-NIC
University of Manitoba
Chapter 25: Assessment of Infants, Children, and Adolescents

Margaret Dykeman, NP, PhD
University of Manitoba
Chapter 9: Nutritional Assessment

Phyllis Murray, RN dip, BN, Bed, Med, MScN (GNP/CNS)
University of New Brunswick
Chapter 9: Nutritional Assessment

Victoria Smye, RN, PhD
University of British Columbia
Chapter 4: Social and Ethnocultural Considerations and the *Social and Ethnocultural Considerations boxes*

U.S. Contributors

Lily Fountain, MS, RN
University of Maryland
Chapter 26: The Pregnant Female

Dawn Lee Garzon, PhD, APRN, BC, CPNP
University of Missouri-St. Louis
Chapter 25: Assessment of Infants, Children, and Adolescents

Dorothy G. Herron, PhD, APRN, BC
University of North Carolina
Chapter 27: Assessing the Older Adult

Sheila Tucker, MA, RD, LDN
Boston College
Chapter 9: Nutritional Assessment

PREFACE

Health & Physical Assessment in Nursing and its rich media package was written to help instructors mentor students in the art and skills of completing a comprehensive health history and physical examination, as well as to help students develop and refine the assessment skills they need to care for a diverse population of clients in a variety of settings. The focus of this book is client assessment, recognizing that each individual presents a variety of physical, social, ethnocultural, and spiritual experiences to nurses today. Our approach is holistic, advocating the principles of health promotion and client education. We introduce concepts related to health, wellness, communication, culture, and education.

The first Canadian edition of this textbook was created for undergraduate nursing students to allow them to perform a physical examination while keeping the whole person in mind. We did this by strengthening three key areas of the physical examination. The first is the *Health History* section of the examination. We begin each health history section by introducing common concerns or injuries of the body system being discussed, with follow-up questions for each concern. In organizing the health history in this manner, we are asking students to think about why the client has presented him or herself and to ask the appropriate questions, rather than simply ask a list of general questions that are related to the body system. This is followed by questions related to past health history, behaviours, the environment, and finally questions related to age.

We have also integrated concepts related to *Social and Ethnocultural Considerations* that keep the student focused on the understanding that people are more than physical body systems. The Social and Ethnocultural Considerations sections begin in Chapter 4 and are threaded throughout the chapters in Unit III. These topics go beyond the biogenetic differences between groups and include differences in gender, age, environment, and ethnicity. As the student assesses the physical being, these considerations are important to keep in mind because they can assist the examiner with planning holistic care for all clients.

Health Promotion in the Canadian healthcare system is heavily influenced by the determinants of health. We believe that health promotion begins at the first encounter with a client, which is why we have included it throughout the Unit III chapters. We have provided case studies to help students apply health promotion while conducting a physical examination, and have included action strategies at the level of the individual, family, and/or community. By including a strong health promotion thread, we integrate a clinical reasoning approach and ensure that students begin learning about health assessment with a holistic viewpoint.

ORGANIZATION OF THIS TEXTBOOK

Health & Physical Assessment in Nursing is composed of four units.

Unit I, Introduction to Health Assessment (Chapters 1–5) introduces health assessment concepts. The chapters within this unit establish a focus for comprehensive health assessment to promote health and well-being across the life span. Nursing assessment includes all of the factors that impact the client and health. Chapter 1 describes the knowledge, skills, and processes professional nurses use in holistic health assessment and health promotion. The nurse functions within the healthcare delivery system and has a responsibility to partner with other professionals and clients to maximize health. In Chapter 2 the major concepts related to health promotion in Canada are introduced. These concepts include health promotion, primary healthcare, social justice, population health promotion, levels of prevention, and the social determinants of health. The Population Health Promotion model has been used to develop the Health Promotion Assessment Tool for the case studies presented in each chapter. Chapter 3 discusses the importance of growth, development, and aging as factors that impact physical and psychosocial well-being. The client's heritage and spirituality have significant influences on the individual's health-related activities. In Chapter 4 a demographic overview of the Canadian landscape and concepts central to understanding and assessing the social and ethnocultural aspects of health and healthcare are provided in addition to guidelines for engaging in effective clinical practice with respect to ethnicity, culture, and health. Some of the topics covered include cultural sensitivity, cultural competence, and cultural safety; culture, othering, and culturalism; ethnicity, race, and racialization; and health, social, and gender inequities. Chapter 5 describes psychological and social phenomena that the nurse must consider during a comprehensive assessment.

Unit II, Introduction to Physical Assessment (Chapters 6–10), introduces physical assessment concepts. We describe techniques and equipment required for physical assessment in Chapter 6. Chapter 7 provides an in-depth explanation of the initial step of physical assessment—the general survey and measurement of vital signs. Chapters 8 and 9 discuss two important aspects of health assessment—pain and nutrition. Each chapter describes concepts related to these areas and includes measurements, methods, and tools to guide data gathering and interpretation of findings for clients across the life span. The health history interview is the mechanism through which the nurse gathers subjective data. Subjective data refer to the client's own perceptions and recollections about health, illness, values, beliefs, and practices. Chapter 10 introduces an overview of how to conduct the health history interview. The nurse's ability to communicate effectively is essential to the interview process. We include descriptions and examples of communication techniques in this chapter.

Unit III, Physical Assessment (Chapters 11–24), introduces the methods and techniques that nurses use to obtain objective data. Objective data refer to measurable and observable behaviours. The chapters in Unit III are organized by body system, and each chapter begins with a review of anatomy and physiology. These highly structured chapters use a consistent format to walk students through the steps of assessment and build their skills step-by-step:

- In **Social and Ethnocultural Considerations,** content related to social and ethnocultural factors are examined to enhance clinical practice across all of the domains of health assessment. These boxes expand on the content first introduced in Chapter 4. In addition, guidelines are provided for assessing culturally based understandings and the social, political, economic, and historical contexts that shape peoples' lives to support effective and culturally safe clinical practice.

- In **Gathering the Data,** students learn how to gather subjective data while conducting a client interview. We provide *Health History Questions* that ask the client about the most common concerns or injuries associated with the specific physiological system, as well questions related to past health history, client behaviours, environmental concerns, and those that are specific to clients according to age, including the pregnant female. We also provide follow-up questions to help the student gather more data from the interview, as well as *Rationales* so the student understands why the nurse needs to ask these questions. We provide reminders about specific communication techniques to increase student confidence and competence while performing the health assessment.

- In **Physical Assessment** we show the student how to collect objective data and conduct a physical assessment—from preparing the room and gathering the equipment, greeting the client, performing the examination, to documenting the findings in a logical and organized manner. The left column demonstrates step-by-step instructions for client preparation, position, details for each technique in assessment, and the expected findings. The right column includes corresponding abnormal findings and special considerations, such as an alternate method, technique, or finding in relation to age, development, culture, or specific client condition. This format helps the student differentiate normal from abnormal findings while interpreting and analyzing data to plan nursing care. Hundreds of photos and illustrations help the student envision how to perform the techniques precisely and thoroughly. Documentation samples for each Physical Assessment section are found at the end of each chapter. This allows the student to review and practice charting for each body system.

- In **Application Through Critical Thinking** we challenge students to apply critical thinking and diagnostic reasoning by working through a *Case Study*. After a detailed client scenario, students will answer critical thinking questions, identify possible nursing diagnoses and health promotion issues, prepare documentation, and create a sample teaching plan. Example answers are provided.

- Each Application Through Critical Thinking section in Unit III ends with a **Health Promotion Assessment Tool.** Health promotion concepts such as social justice, root causes of health issues, and levels of prevention are key to having a well-rounded understanding of the context within which nursing health promotion practice occurs with individuals, families, communities, and populations. The Health Promotion Assessment Tool highlights how nurses incorporate health promotion theory into their practice.

- In **Abnormal Findings** we provide a vivid atlas of illustrations and photographs that feature examples of abnormal findings, diseases, and conditions. This section helps the student recognize these conditions and distinguish them from normal findings before they see them in the clinical setting.

Unit IV, Physical Assessment Across the Life Span (Chapters 25–27), contains three chapters that provide information about physical assessment of specialized client groups. These chapters describe how to conduct comprehensive head-to-toe assessments of infants and children, pregnant females, and older adults. While we focus on these special groups in Unit IV, we also integrate life span considerations throughout the book and especially in the health history questions and physical assessments for each body system in Unit III. This provides instructors with the flexibility of using this book in an integrated curriculum—where assessment techniques may be integrated into courses that cover maternity, pediatrics, and aging throughout the curriculum.

MORE FEATURES THAT HELP YOU USE THIS BOOK SUCCESSFULLY

On the preceding pages we have shown you how to use the major sections and features of the textbook and media to be successful in this course. In addition, we offer the following features to further enhance the learning process and help you use this book successfully:

- **Key Terms** at the beginning of the chapter identify the terminology the student encounters in conducting assessment and the pages where the student can find the definitions. We bold key terms and define them in the text, but the student may also refer to the comprehensive Glossary at the back of the textbook.
- **Equipment boxes** at the beginning of the Physical Assessment section help you prepare for the assessment by identifying the equipment you will need to conduct the examination.
- **Clinical Tips** provide suggestions and reminders about conducting the physical assessment. We offer clinical pearls to prepare the student for the complete examination and promote client comfort.

Packaged with this book and new to this text are **Physical Assessment Prompter Cards** that students can use during their laboratory sessions and their clinical courses. The information on the cards can be used for quick recall of key health history questions and assessment techniques. The cards are based on Chapters 11 to 24. For each chapter the cards are divided into **Health History** and **Assessment**. These cards will assist the students throughout their studies and beyond.

SUPPLEMENTS

We designed teaching and learning resources to expand and extend the textbook material and to mentor students in the art and skills of health assessment. For students, MyNursingLab will help you gain a further understanding of what you have read and discussed in the text. You will find tests, activities, videos, animations, and more. For instructors, the full complement of supplemental resources is available from your Pearson Education Canada sales representative. Ask your sales representative about the comprehensive teaching and learning package that accompanies *Health & Physical Assessment in Nursing*.

MyNursingLab, (www.pearsoned.ca/mynursinglab), **Barbara Thompson,** Sault College   MyNursingLab is a user-friendly site that gives you the opportunity to test yourself on key concepts and skills in nursing. By using MyNursingLab, students can track their own progress through the course and use customized, media-rich study plan activities to help achieve success in the classroom, in clinical practice, and ultimately on the CRNE. You take a diagnostic pre-test for each chapter, receive a customized study plan to work through based on the results, and conclude with a post-test to assess competency. MyNursingLab can also help instructors monitor class progress.

CourseSmart for Instructors

CourseSmart goes beyond traditional expectations—providing instant online access to the textbooks and course materials you need at a lower cost for students. And even as students save money, you can save time and hassle with a digital eTextbook that allows you to search for the most relevant content at the very moment you need it. Whether it's evaluating textbooks or creating lecture notes to help students with difficult concepts, CourseSmart can make life a little easier. See how when you visit www.coursesmart.com/instructors.

CourseSmart for Students

CourseSmart goes beyond traditional expectations—providing instant online access to the textbooks and course materials you need at an average savings of 50%. With instant access from any computer and the ability to search your text, you'll find the content you need quickly, no matter where you are. And with online tools like highlighting and note-taking, you can save time and study efficiently. See all the benefits at www.coursesmart.com/students.

Additional Instructor Supplements

Instructor's Resource CD-ROM (ISBN 0135039746) includes the following teaching tools:

- **PowerPoint® Slides** and **Instructor's Manual,** Marianne Schneider   We offer a comprehensive set of slides specifically designed for the textbook, as well as an Instructor's Manual, which includes the learning objectives, main concepts for lecture, and suggestions for classroom activities.

Marianne Schneider has over 20 years of nursing experience that includes nursing education, clinical nursing, and nursing management, and is currently enrolled in an EdD program.

- **Test Generator,** Joanne Jones and Jeannette Murray, Thompson Rivers University   A testbank containing multiple-choice and short answer questions is provided for instructors. Each question is accompanied by rationales as to why each answer option is correct or incorrect and the page number where the correct answer can be found in the chapter material. The multiple-choice questions are similar in design to the questions found on the Canadian Registered Nurses Examination (CRNE).

Joanne Jones is a senior lecturer at Thompson Rivers University. She has over 20 years teaching experience in undergraduate nursing education with an emphasis on pathophysiology, surgical nursing, exam construction, and item writing. **Jeanette Murray** is a senior lecturer and chairperson of the School of Nursing at Thompson Rivers University. She has over 35 years of teaching experience in diploma and baccalaureate programs. Exam construction and item writing have been an interest throughout her career.

Additional Student Supplements

Clinical Handbook for Health and Physical Assessment, Shirlene Hudyma, Emily Donato, and Robyn Gorham, Laurentian University   This pocket-sized resource, which can likewise be used by both students and professional nurses, is designed to function as a practical reference for those performing health and physical assessments in the clinical setting. All essential information from *Health and Physical Assessment in Nursing* is compressed into each chapter of the *Clinical Handbook,* providing users with invaluable finger-tip information with respect to (a) the health and physical assessment process, (b) the anatomy and physiology of each major body system, (c) the special considerations that are necessary for assessing children, pregnant women, and older adults, (d) the collection of subjective and objective data as it relates to each major body system, and (e) normal and abnormal assessment findings. The handbook also includes numerous colour photographs, diagrams, charts, and figures, all of which further enhance its usefulness as a quick clinical reference. The content in this handbook is consistent with Canadian nursing and healthcare considerations in Canada.

Assessment Skills Laboratory Manual for Health & Physical Assessment in Nursing, Shirlene Hudyma, Emily Donato, and Robyn Gorham, Laurentian University   The *Laboratory Manual* is intended to reinforce the content from the main text, as well as prepare the student for the skills laboratory and clinical practice experience. Each chapter begins with a reading assignment and a list of key vocabulary terms to prepare the student for the review exercises. These exercises include anatomy and physiology labelling activities, study focus questions, multiple-choice questions, case studies, and nursing diagnosis identification activities. Each chapter also suggests various learning activities that can be carried out in both the skills laboratory and the clinical practice setting. Comprehensive assessment templates, designed to guide the student while performing focused health assessments and physical examinations of each major body system, are provided at the end of each chapter. This manual emphasizes the uniqueness of Canadian nursing and is an accurate presentation of clients and cases commonly found in Canada.

Shirlene Hudyma is a lecturer at the Laurentian University School of Nursing, where she currently teaches health and physical assessment to undergraduate nursing students. She has over 20 years of acute care nursing experience with a strong background in medical-surgical, emergency, and critical care nursing. **Emily Donato** is an assistant professor at the Laurentian University School of Nursing. She has taught in several capacities as a clinical educator, faculty advisor, course professor, and has also been the Undergraduate Program Coordinator and Coordinator for the North Eastern Ontario Collaborative Nursing Program. **Robyn Gorham** is a lecturer at the Laurentian University School of Nursing, where she currently teaches in the Nurse Practitioner program. She has a variety of nursing experience, including

acute medical, emergency nursing, and primary care. Currently, she is enrolled in the Doctorate of Education (EdD) at Athabasca University.

ACKNOWLEDGEMENTS

Pearson Education Canada and the authors would like to thank the following reviewers who provided feedback on chapters during the development of the Canadian edition manuscript:

Lynne Esson, The University of British Columbia

Sandra Longman, Seneca College

Jason Powell, Humber College

Lynn Skillen, University of Alberta

Audrey Steenbeck, Dalhousie University

Tracey Stephen, University of Alberta

Deb Wood, York University

Audrey Steenbeck, Dalhousie University

Crystal O'Connell, Algonquin College

Judy Bailey, Cape Breton University

Lynne Thibeault, Confederation College

Margaret Dykeman, University of New Brunswick

Bev William, University of Alberta

Lucia Yiu, University of Windsor

Joanne Louis, University of Toronto

Nancy Carter, McMaster University

Roberta Heale, Laurentian University

Elsie Tan, University of British Columbia

Caroline Marchionni, McGill University

Barbara E. Wendlandt, Ryerson University

Deborah Styles, Grant MacEwan University

We would also like to thank the contributors of the individual chapters of this book:

- Deborah Askin, University of Manitoba
- Margaret Dykeman, University of New Brunswick
- Candace Lind, University of Calgary
- Sylvia Loewen, University of Calgary
- Aliyah Mawji, University of Calgary
- Phyllis Murray, University of New Brunswick
- Eva Peisachovich, York University
- Victoria Smye, University of British Columbia
- Christina Rajsic, University of Toronto

No textbook is the work of one person and the influence and insights of many have contributed to the final product. Both of the authors would like to extend a warm thank you to Pearson Education Canada, especially Madhu Ranadive, Michelle Sartor, Dawn Hunter, and Leanne Rancourt, for their tireless work on this project. Your support is greatly appreciated. We would also like to personally thank the contributors who worked with us on this project. Your commitment and quality of work are both admired and respected. A special thank you to our families and friends for all their support during this project.

—Creina Twomey & Nicole Harder

It is impossible to name and acknowledge everyone who has contributed in some way to my completing this work. First and foremost I would like to thank my family and friends for their ongoing support. My thanks also go to Nicole Harder, my co-author, who has been a great source of both theoretical and practical knowledge and shares my vision of nursing education and the role of health assessment in the development of competent, caring future nurses. For those not acknowledged individually, please know that my appreciation and gratitude for your support is not diminished in any way by the omission of your name.

—Creina Twomey

A huge thank you to my past, present, and future students who have taught me more about teaching than they realize. You are the reason I wanted to work on this project. To my husband, Doug, and boys, Chaizz, Justin, and Tyler: you are the perfect balance in my life. Most importantly, to Creina Twomey: I have sincerely enjoyed our professional and personal relationship and could not imagine a better nurse to work with.

—Nicole Harder

DEDICATION

We dedicate this book to our nursing students. May you never lose

your passion for learning

CONTENTS

UNIT 2   INTRODUCTION TO PHYSICAL ASSESSMENT   86

CHAPTER 8
Pain Assessment   112

CHAPTER 9
Nutritional Assessment   124

CHAPTER 10
The Health History   145

CHAPTER 14
Ears, Nose, Mouth, and Throat   276

CHAPTER 15
Respiratory System   314

CHAPTER 16
Breasts and Axillae   353

CHAPTER 17
Cardiovascular System   378

UNIT 4 PHYSICAL ASSESSMENT ACROSS THE LIFE SPAN   684

1
HEALTH ASSESSMENT

CHAPTER OBJECTIVES

On completion of the chapter, you will be able to

1. Discuss various definitions of health.
2. Discuss the importance of the determinants of health and their relevance to health assessment.
3. Define *health assessment*.
4. Identify factors to consider in health assessment.
5. Define the steps of the nursing process.
6. Describe the critical thinking process in relation to health assessment.
7. Describe the role of the nurse in health assessment.
8. Discuss the elements of a teaching plan.

CHAPTER OUTLINE

THE HEALTHCARE DELIVERY SYSTEM in Canada is changing. Historically, the focus of care has been illness and symptom centred. The individual entered the healthcare delivery system when illness was present. Today, the focus has changed. The emphasis of care now includes wellness, prevention of disease, health maintenance, and health promotion. The client is no longer a passive recipient of care. Clients take a more active role in the planning, decision making, and treatment modalities used in care. The role of the nurse is expanding. Factors that influence the change in the healthcare delivery system are described in the following sections.

Legislation, professional organizations, nurses, and consumers nationally and internationally have influenced reform of the healthcare delivery system. In 1978 the World Health Organization (WHO) prepared a primary healthcare report that emphasized health or well-being as a fundamental right and a social goal worldwide. Within the report is a stipulation that public institutions, governments, and consumers be involved in planning and delivering healthcare.

The Canadian Nurses Association's (2010) vision asks nurses to partner with other healthcare provider groups and become leaders of health for all Canadians. By working with practice partners and other stakeholders, nurses can incorporate the principles of primary healthcare and the Canada Health Act to both achieve and sustain a healthy environment for clients and healthcare providers alike.

Consumers are encouraging reform of the healthcare system to include wellness and quality of life, rather than simply treatment of disease. In addition, consumers value community health, health promotion, and disease prevention. The many changes in the delivery of healthcare affect the role of the nurse providing care. These aspects of nursing care are explained in this chapter and incorporated throughout this text. Nurses are taking on more responsibility, and health assessment has become an integral part of the expanded role of the nurse. Health assessment was always performed in a limited manner in the acute care setting. Today, nurses perform assessment in all settings and with diverse clients. A description of the assessment process is included in a later section of this chapter. The subsequent chapters address specific areas of concern in assessment of the whole individual. The chapters in Unit III provide step-by-step guides for learning how to perform physical assessment of each system. ◌◌ Nurses use the nursing process and critical thinking skills as the basis for the implementation of safe, competent client care.

For Health Canada (2009), the federal department responsible for helping Canadians maintain and improve their health, the goal is to have Canadians be among the healthiest people in the world. To meet this goal, Health Canada (2009)

- Relies on high-quality scientific research as the basis for [its] work.

- Conducts ongoing consultations with Canadians to determine how to best meet their long-term healthcare needs.

- Communicates information about disease prevention to protect Canadians from avoidable risks.

- Encourages Canadians to take an active role in their health, such as increasing their level of physical activity and eating well.

The Public Health Agency of Canada (PHAC) works closely with Health Canada and focuses on promoting good health, reducing preventable injuries, controlling infectious diseases, and being ready to respond to emergencies. Through its research, the PHAC is working to discover what determines health and how best to support the health of Canadians. This research has shown that many different factors are involved in health:

At every stage of life, health is determined by complex interactions between social and economic factors, the physical environment and individual behavior. These factors are referred to as "determinants of health". They do not exist in isolation from each other. It is the combined influence of the determinants of health that determines health status (Public Health Agency of Canada, 2001).

When interpreting the findings from a health assessment, the nurse considers many determinants of health, including developmental factors, psychological and emotional factors, family factors, ethnocultural factors, and environmental factors, all of which are discussed later in the chapter and throughout the text.

This chapter provides an overview of the aspects of nursing practice and nursing skills required for the expanding role of the nurse. These include comprehensive assessment, nursing process, critical thinking, communication, documentation, and teaching. The skills and approaches required to meet the needs of diverse clients seeking advice and care in the changing healthcare system are illustrated throughout this text. Case studies provide opportunities to apply developing critical thinking skills. Simulated client interactions with analyses illustrate communication techniques. Teaching plans, derived from case studies, provide examples of one of the most important interventions in health promotion and illness prevention. The process of health assessment is carefully explained in regard to the health history and hands-on physical assessment of the client in general and for each system of the body. Samples of documentation for each aspect of assessment provide guidelines and exemplify the requirements for documentation explained in this initial chapter.

Additionally, the succeeding chapters provide information about developmental, cultural, psychosocial, and environmental factors that affect health and influence approaches to assessment. Learning about assessment and all related factors is enhanced through the illustrations, photographs, tables, and figures in each chapter.

HEALTH

Traditionally, **health** has been thought of as the absence of disease. The terms *health* and *wellness* have been used interchangeably to describe the state of not being sick. Today, these terms have clear distinctions in definition and description of actions.

Definitions of Health

The World Health Organization (WHO) presented a definition of health that remains active and relevant today. Health is defined as a state of complete physical, mental, and social well-being (World Health Organization, 1947). Further, the WHO describes health from a holistic approach in which the individual is viewed as a total person interacting with others. The individual functions within his or her physical, psychological, and social fields. These fields interact with one another and the external environment. The individual is capable of maximizing the potential for and fostering the most positive aspects of health. Models and mechanisms related to promotion of health are described in Chapter 2. Today, many definitions and models of health and wellness have been designed using these concepts. It is evident that health is far more than the absence of illness, disease, and symptoms.

Models of Health

The following definitions of health reflect the work of nursing theorists:

- A process and a state of being and becoming whole and integrated in a way that reflects person and environment mutuality (Roy & Andrews, 1999)
- The state of a person as characterized by soundness or wholeness of developed human structures and mental and bodily functioning that requires therapeutic self-care (Orem, 1971)
- A culturally defined, valued, and practised state of well-being reflective of the ability to perform role activities (Leininger, 1991)
- A state of well-being and use of every power the person possesses to the fullest extent (Nightingale, 1860/1969)
- A continuum with wellness and illness on opposite ends and health equated with optimal system stability, that is, the best possible wellness state at any given time (Neuman & Fawcett, 2002)

The following are examples of models that explain the concept of health:

- The ecological model developed by Leavell and Clark (1965) examines the interaction of agent, host, and environment. Health is present when these three variables are in harmony. When this harmony is disrupted, health is not maintained at its highest level and illness and disease occur.
- In the clinical model, health is defined as the absence of disease or injury. The aim of the care by the health professional is to relieve signs and symptoms of disease, relieve pain, and eliminate malfunction of physiological systems.
- The eudaemonistic model views health as the actualization of a person's potential. Actualization refers to fulfillment and complete development. Illness would prevent self-actualization.
- According to Pender, Murdaugh, and Parsons (2002), the health promotion model defines health as the actualization of inherent and acquired human potential through goal-directed behaviour, competent self-care, and satisfying relationships with others while adjustments are made to maintain structural integrity and harmony with relevant environments.

Health is highly individualized and the definition a person develops for himself or herself will be influenced by many factors, including age, gender, race, family, culture, religion, socioeconomic conditions, environment, previous experiences, and self-expectations.

Nurses must recognize that each client will have a personal definition for health, illness, and wellness. The behaviours used to maintain these changing states will be individualized. Nurses must be aware of their own personal definition of health and at the same time accept and respect the client's definition of health, for this will influence practice. When health is defined in terms of physical change, the practice focus is on improvement of physical function. When health is considered to be reflective of physical, cultural, environmental, psychological, and social factors, the focus of nursing practice is more holistic and wide ranging. Any of the previously mentioned health models could be used by the nurse and other members of the health team as a paradigm for the design and delivery of healthcare.

HEALTH ASSESSMENT

Health assessment may be defined as a systematic method of collecting data about a client to help determine the client's current and ongoing health status, predict risks to health, and identify health-promoting activities. The data include physical, social, cultural, environmental, and emotional factors that affect the overall well-being of the client. The health status includes wellness behaviours, illness signs and symptoms, client strengths and weaknesses, and risk factors. The scope of focus must be more than problems presented by the client. The nurse will use a variety of sources to gather the objective and subjective data. Knowledge of the natural and social sciences is a strong foundation for the nurse. Effective communication techniques and use of critical thinking skills are essential in helping the nurse to gather the detailed, complete, relevant, objective, subjective, and measurable data needed to formulate a plan of care to meet the needs of the client. Health assessment includes the health history, physical assessment, documentation, and interpretation of findings. Each component is described in detail in Units II and III of this text. ⏩ All planning for care is directed by interpretation of findings from objective and subjective data collected throughout the assessment process.

The Interview

In the initial health assessment interview, subjective data are gathered from primary and secondary sources: the primary or direct source is the client, and the secondary or indirect sources include family members, caregivers, other members of the health team, and medical records.

Subjective data are things that the client experiences and communicates to the nurse. Perceptions of pain, nausea, dizziness, itching sensations, and feeling nervous are examples of subjective data. Only the client can describe these feelings. Subjective data are usually referred to as *covert (hidden) data* or as *symptoms* when they are perceived by the client and cannot be observed by others. Family members or caregivers can report subjective data based on perceptions the client has shared with them. This information is helpful when the client is very ill or unable to communicate, and it is required when the client is an infant or a child. However, to ensure accuracy, the nurse must validate subjective data obtained from other sources. The accuracy of subjective data depends on the nurse's ability to clarify the information through follow-up questions and to obtain supporting data from other pertinent sources.

The Health History

The purpose of the **health history** is to obtain information about the client's health in his or her own words and based on the client's own perceptions. Biographical data, perceptions about health, past and present history of illness and injury, family history, a review of systems, and health patterns and practices are the types of information included in the health history. The health history provides cues regarding the client's health and guides further data collection. The health history is a vital aspect of the assessment process. Detailed information regarding the health history is presented in Chapter 10 of this text. ⏩

The health history enables the nurse to clarify points, to obtain missing information, and to follow up on verbal and nonverbal cues identified in the interview. The nurse does not use a prepared set of questions for the health history. The nurse applies knowledge and critical thinking when asking specific and detailed questions or requesting descriptions of symptoms, feelings, or events. Therefore, the health history provides the means and opportunity to expand the subjective database regarding specific strengths, weaknesses, problems, or concerns expressed by the client or required by the nurse to begin to make reliable judgments about information and observations as part of planning care. In-depth information about the health history in health assessment is included in each chapter in Unit III of this text. ⏩

Physical Assessment

Physical assessment is hands-on examination of the client. Components of physical assessment are the survey and examination of systems. Objective data gathered during physical assessment, when combined with all other reliable sources of information, provide a sound database from which care planning can proceed. **Objective data** are observed or measured by the nurse. These are also known as *overt data* or *signs* since they are detected by the nurse. These data can be seen, felt, heard, or measured by the nurse. For example, skin colour can be seen, a pulse can be felt, a cough can be heard, and blood pressure can be measured. These objective data are used to validate subjective data and to complete the database. The accuracy of objective data depends on the nurse's ability to avoid reaching conclusions without substantive evidence. The accuracy of objective data is also increased by attention to detail and verification. Unit II of this text provides information about the general survey and techniques for physical assessment. ⏩ Unit III includes detailed descriptions for physical assessment of systems. ⏩

In addition, data from all secondary sources, including charts, reports from diagnostic and laboratory testing, family, and all healthcare professionals involved in client care, are part of the database from which decisions about care are derived. Both subjective and objective data may further be categorized as constant or variable. *Constant data* are things that do not typically change over time, such as race, sex, or blood type. *Variable data* may change within minutes, hours, or days. Blood pressure, pulse rate, blood counts, and age are examples of variable data.

Documentation

Documentation of data from health assessment creates a client record or becomes an addition to an existing health record. The **client record** is a legal document used to plan care, to communicate information among healthcare providers, and to monitor quality of care. Further, the client record provides information used for reimbursement of services, is often a source of data for research, and is reviewed by accrediting agencies to determine adherence to standards.

Documentation is used to communicate information among the health professionals involved in the care of the client. For that communication to be effective, the nurse must adhere to the following guidelines for documentation. Documentation must be accurate, confidential, appropriate, complete, and detailed. When documenting, the nurse must use standard and accepted abbreviations, symbols, and terminology, and must reflect professional and organizational standards. Many organizations are recommending limited use of abbreviations. Consult your policy manuals for a list of accepted abbreviations in your institution or jurisdiction.

Accuracy means that documentation is limited to facts or factual accounts of observations rather than opinions or interpretations of observations. When recording subjective data, it is important to use quotation marks and quote a client exactly rather than interpreting the statement. In health assessment, accuracy also requires the use of accurate measurement and location of symptoms and physical findings. For example, rather than writing that the client had severe pain and swelling in the left lower extremity, the nurse would document that a client had pain rated 8 on a scale of 1 to 10 and edema and redness on the dorsal surface of the foot over the first through third phalanges. The use of accepted language in documentation provides for consistent interpretation of data as it is reviewed and used by healthcare professionals to monitor and oversee healthcare planning and delivery.

Confidentiality means that information sharing is limited to those directly involved in client care. Information is considered appropriate for inclusion in a health record only if it has direct bearing on the client's health. Complete documentation means that all information required to develop a plan of care for the client has been included. In comprehensive health assessment, data from the health history and physical assessment are required for a complete record.

Protection of an individual's health information is regulated provincially through legislative Acts. The main purposes of these Acts are to establish rules for the collection, use, and disclosure of personal health information about individuals, and to give individuals the right to access personal health information about themselves. Healthcare providers, hospitals, nurses, and nursing students are required to follow policies to protect the privacy of health information. The Acts protect medical records and any other individually identifiable health information, whether communicated in writing, orally, or electronically. Identifiable health information includes demographic information and anything that could identify an individual.

The types and amounts of documentation are determined by the purpose of the healthcare service and often by the setting. In emergency situations, data gathering and documentation focus on the immediate problem and factors that may influence or affect care decisions related to the emergency. For example, in an unconscious client, it would be important to know if the altered level of consciousness was a result of a head injury in an otherwise healthy individual or associated with a previously diagnosed problem. In nonemergency situations in

which a comprehensive health assessment will be conducted, documentation of all findings is required.

Data recorded during visits to healthcare providers or clinics for continued management of an existing condition are generally limited to findings indicating change, progress, or problems associated with the existing condition. Documentation for health screening and health promotion is often limited to the results of the screening process and referral information.

Data collected in health assessment should be documented as soon as possible. Recollection of details becomes difficult as time elapses. The nurse should record some details and notes during the data collection process, particularly direct client quotes and when precise information is required, such as the location of a lesion, a wound, or an abnormal finding. Immediacy of recording increases the accuracy of the information. It is important to explain the purpose of the documentation and inform the client at the outset that notes and forms will be used to record information.

Methods for documentation include narrative notes; problem-oriented charting; scales, flowsheets, or check sheets; focus documentation; charting by exception; and computer documentation. Each of these will be described in the following paragraphs, and additional documentation exercises are provided throughout this text. Examples of each type of documentation appear in Figures 1.1 through 1.5 and are based on the following case study.

Janet Lewis, a 20-year-old female, came to the university health centre. Ms. Lewis told the nurse, "I feel bloated and achy in my left side, and it has increased over the past 3 or 4 days." In response to questions about appetite, Ms. Lewis responded, "I really don't feel like eating and I'm worried because I'm supposed to eat carefully. I recently had anemia and have been taking pills for it for a month." When asked about bowel elimination, she said, "My last BM was 4 days ago; it was hard pellets and dark coloured." She responded to questions about gastrointestinal symptoms with the following: "I'm not nauseated and I haven't vomited." She further reported, "I had my last period 10 days ago." She told the nurse that her voiding was normal in amount and number of voids. Ms. Lewis brought the medication with her. The label read Fe gluconate 300 mg three times a day. Her healthcare provider instructed her to take the medication and have a follow-up visit in 1 month.

The physical examination revealed the presence of bowel sounds in all quadrants, dullness to percussion in the left upper and lower quadrants, firm distension, and tenderness in the left lower quadrant. There was no tenderness at the costovertebral angle (CVA). Hard, dry stool high in the rectum was identified on the rectal examination and a sample was applied to a slide for occult blood testing. Blood was drawn for a complete blood count (CBC).

A rectal suppository was administered with a result, within 15 minutes, of a moderate amount of hard, dark stool. Ms. Lewis stated, "I feel a little better, but still achy." She was discharged to her dormitory with 30 mL of milk of magnesia (MOM) to take at bedtime. Ms. Lewis was advised to increase her fluid intake by four glasses of fluid daily, change her diet to include whole wheat bread and more fruits, and continue to take the Fe gluconate as ordered. She was instructed to call

---

Narrative Note

A 20-year-old female seen because she "feels bloated" and has an "achiness" in her left side that has "increased over the past 3 or 4 days." She states she "really doesn't feel like eating" and that she is "worried" because she was "supposed to eat carefully" because she recently "had a problem with anemia" and has been "taking pills for it for a month." Brought medication with her. Label reads Fe gluconate 300 mg three times a day. She stated the doctor told her to take the pills until she has a return visit next month. She denies nausea and vomiting, last BM of dark hard pellets—4 days ago. LMP 10 days ago. Voiding "normal" amount and number of voids (5 to 6 times daily). On exam: VS-BP 110/66—P 88—RR 20. Colour pale, skin warm and dry. Abdomen: distended, bowel sounds present x 4 quadrants, dullness to percussion LUQ and LLQ, firm, tenderness to palpation LLQ. No CVA tenderness. Rectal exam: hard stool high in rectum, dark colour. CBC drawn, stool for OB. Dulcolax suppository administered. Result—moderate hard, dark stool after 15 minutes —"feels a little better but still achy." Discharged to dorm with medication. Advised client to increase fluid intake by at least four glasses of fluid daily, continue Fe gluconate as ordered. Education: 1. Side effects Fe—re: dark stool, constipation. 2. Schedule 2 hours after meals, take with full glass water or juice. 3. Increase roughage—fruits in diet. 4. Call in AM for follow-up . 5. Call primary healthcare provider re: follow-up visit.

Figure 1.1 ● Narrative notes.

the health centre in the morning as a follow-up measure and to call her healthcare provider to schedule a visit and to discuss her laboratory results.

The nurse provided education as follows:

- Constipation and change in stool colour are side effects of the Fe gluconate.
- Fe gluconate should be scheduled 2 hours after meals, with a full glass of water or juice.
- Increasing roughage by adding fresh fruits to the diet will help to reduce the constipation.

Narrative Notes

When implementing narrative notes, the nurse uses words, phrases, sentences, and paragraphs to record information. The information may be recorded in chronological order from initial contact through conclusion of the assessment, or in categories according to the type of data collected. The narrative record includes words, sentences, phrases, or lists to indicate judgments made about the data, plans to address concerns, and actions taken to meet the health needs of the client (see Figure 1.1).

Problem-Oriented Charting

Problem-oriented records include the SOAP and APIE methods. The letters SOAP refer to recording *s*ubjective data, *o*bjective data, *a*ssessment, and *p*lanning. Subjective data are reported by the client or reliable informant. Objective data are derived from the physical examination, client records, and reports. Assessment refers to conclusions drawn from the data. Planning indicates the actions to be taken to resolve problems or address client needs (see Figure 1.2). The letters APIE refer to *a*ssessment, *p*roblem, *i*ntervention, and *e*valuation. When using this

SOAP

S "I feel bloated and achy in my left side and it has increased over the past 3 or 4 days." "I really don't feel like eating." "I'm worried because I'm supposed to eat carefully." Because "I recently had anemia and have been taking pills for it for a month." "My last BM was 4 days ago; it was hard pellets and dark coloured." "I'm not nauseated and I haven't vomited." "I had my last period 10 days ago."

O Skin pale, warm, dry. VS-BP 110/66—P 88—RR 20 Abdomen: distended, bowel sounds + × 4, dull percussion LUQ and LLQ, firm, tender LLQ Rectal: hard stool, dark

A Constipation associated with Fe gluconate treatment for anemia.

P Rectal suppository and laxative CBC, stool for occult blood Instruct: med, diet, fluid Instructed to call clinic and primary healthcare provider in a.m. for follow up

Figure 1.2 ● SOAP notes.

method, documentation of assessment combines the subjective and objective data. The nurse will draw conclusions from the data, identify and record the problem or problems, and plan to address these problems. Interventions are documented as they are carried out. Evaluation refers to documentation of the response to the plan (see Figure 1.3).

APIE

A "I feel bloated and achy in my left side and it has increased over the past 3 or 4 days." "I really don't feel like eating." "I'm worried because I'm supposed to eat carefully." "I recently had anemia and have been taking pills for it for a month." "My last BM was 4 days ago. It was hard pellets and dark coloured." "I'm not nauseated and haven't vomited." "I had my last period 10 days ago"
Skin pale, warm, dry. VS-BP 110/66—P 88—RR 20
Abdomen: distended, bowel sounds present × 4 quadrants, dull percussion LUQ and LLQ, frim, tender LLQ
Rectal: hard stool, dark
On Fe gluconate 300 mg three times a day—Anemia
No history abdominal pain, discomfort, disease
Constipation

P Rectal suppository and laxative at bedtime CBC, stool for occult blood Instruct: diet, meds, fluids Instructed to call clinic and primary healthcare provider in a.m. for follow up

I Dulcolax suppository administered Instruction

E Moderate hard, dry dark stool "I feel a little better, but still achy."

Figure 1.3 ● APIE notes.

Flowsheets

Documentation of health assessment data can be accomplished through the use of scales, check sheets, or flowsheets. These forms are usually formatted for a specific purpose or need. They may use columns or categories for recording data and may include lists of expected findings with associated qualifiers for ranges of normal or abnormal findings. Charts and check sheets often provide space for narrative descriptions or comments (see Figure 1.4).

Focus Documentation

Focus documentation does not limit documentation to problems and can include client strengths. This type of documentation is intended to address a specific purpose or focus, that is, a symptom, strength, or need. A comprehensive health assess-

ment may result in one or more foci for documentation. The format for focus documentation is a column to address subjective and objective data, nursing action, and client response (see Figure 1.5).

Charting by Exception

In charting by exception, documentation is limited to exceptions from established norms or significant findings. Flowsheets with appropriate information and parameters are completed. This type of documentation eliminates much of the repetition involved in narrative and other forms of documentation.

Computer Documentation

Computer-generated documentation may include all of the previously mentioned methods for recording data. The amount

---

Assessment of the   Abdomen

EXAM	FINDINGS
Anterior	
INSPECTION	
Contour	__x__ Round _____ Flat _____ Protuberant _____ Scaphoid
Position of umbilicus	midline
Skin	Colour _pale, consistent with all other_
	Texture _smooth_
	Lesions _none_
Symmetry	Symmetrical
Bulging	__x__ No ____ Yes
Masses	__x__ No ____ Yes
Movements	____ Waves _____
	____ Pulsations _____
AUSCULTATION	
Bowel sounds	Present __x__ Yes ____ No
	Quadrants __4__
PERCUSSION	Tympany Dull Flat Hyperresonant
LUQ	_____ __x__ _____ _____
RUQ	_____ _____ _____ _____
RLQ	_____ _____ _____ _____
LLQ	_____ __x__ _____ _____
PALPATION	
	Pain ____ Tenderness __x__ Location _LLQ_
	Ascites ____ Yes __x__ Nonpalpable
	Bladder ____ Palpable __x__ Nonpalpable
Posterior	
PERCUSSION	
CVA	Pain __x__ No ____ Yes

Figure 1.4 ● Check sheet.

Date	Focus	Progress Note
01/20/11	Bowel Elimination	Data: "I feel bloated and achy in my left side and it has increased over the past 3 or 4 days." "I really don't feel like eating." "I'm worried because I'm supposed to eat carefully." "I recently had anemia and have been taking pills for it for a month." "My last BM was 4 days ago. It was hard pellets and dark coloured." "I'm not nauseated and haven't vomited." "I had my last period 10 days ago."
		Skin pale, warm, dry. VS-BP 110/66—P 88—RR 20
		Abdomen: distended, BS + X 4, dull percussion LUQ and LLQ, firm, tender LLQ
		Rectal: hard stool, dark
		On Fe gluconate 300 mg three times a day—Anemia, No history abdominal pain, discomfort, disease
		Constipation Action: Rectal supp administered
		Instruction Response: Moderate hard, dry dark stool
		"I feel a little better, but still achy."

Figure 1.5 ● Focus notes.

and types of information to be documented vary according to the computer program and the policies and standards of the agency in which computer documentation is used. The advantage in using most computer documentation is that it allows healthcare providers to spend more time recording appropriate information and less time determining the correct terms, spelling, and descriptors.

Development of confidence and competence in documentation is an important part of nursing education. This text provides samples of recording for the client interview. Documentation of subjective and objective data collection for body systems is provided to assist in the development of these skills.

Interpretation of Findings

Interpretation of findings can be defined as the making of determinations about all the data collected in the health assessment process. The nurse must determine whether the findings fall within normal and expected ranges in relation to the client's age, gender, and race, and then determine the significance of the findings in relation to the client's health status and immediate and long-range health-related needs. Interpretation of findings is influenced by a number of factors. These factors include the ability to obtain, recall, and apply knowledge; to communicate effectively; and to use a holistic approach. Each of these factors is discussed in the following sections.

Knowledge

Nurses obtain, recall, and apply knowledge from physical and social sciences, nursing theory, and all areas of research that affect current nursing practice. For example, knowledge includes human anatomy and physiology and the differences that are associated with growth and development across the lifespan, as well as characteristics specific to gender and race. Further, knowledge includes health-related and healthcare trends in groups and populations, such as the increased incidence of risk factors or actual illnesses in certain groups or populations. In Canada, for example, trends include increased longevity and increased incidence of obesity in children and adults. The nurse must be able to access and use reliable resources in interpretation of findings. Resources include research, scientific literature, and charts, scales, and graphs that indicate ranges of norms and expectations about physical and psychological development. Examples include Ages & Stages scores, mental status examinations, weight and body composition charts, and growth charts prepared by centres for health statistics. Examples of charts and scales or information about measures are provided throughout the text. Additionally, the nurse must be able to communicate effectively, to think critically, to recognize and act on client cues, to incorporate a holistic perspective, and to determine the significance of data in meeting immediate and long-term client needs.

Expectations about interpretation of findings change as the nurse gains experience in nursing practice and with advanced practice preparation. The nurse must be able to recognize situations that require immediate attention and initiate care or seek appropriate assistance. For example, if a client presented in an ambulatory care setting with dyspnea (trouble breathing), the nurse would focus on providing measures to alleviate some symptoms, such as positioning the client and loosening constrictive clothing. The nurse would gather data that relate to the current problem and either arrange for transport to an acute care facility or seek assistance from an advanced nurse practitioner in the facility.

A nursing student is expected to recall and apply knowledge to discriminate between normal and abnormal findings and to use resources to understand the findings in relation to wellness or illness for a particular client. Consider the findings from assessment of Julie Connor, a 12-year-old: asymmetrical shoulders and elevated right scapula on inspection of the posterior thorax, right lateral curvature of thoracic spine on palpation of vertebrae. The novice student would recall that scapulae should be symmetrical and the vertebrae should be aligned. The findings are interpreted as a deviation from the normal. The student would refer to available resources and learn that the findings are associated with scoliosis. More data would be required to confirm this diagnosis and to determine the impact on Julie's current and future health.

Continued learning and actual experiences promote the ability to discriminate between normal and abnormal findings. In addition, one can recognize patterns that predispose individuals to illness or are indicative of specific illnesses, and implement and evaluate appropriate nursing care. Consider the following findings from assessment of James Long, a 46-year-old white male: height 175 cm (5'9"), weight 100 kg (220 lb.), B/P 156/94, mother died at age 62 from cerebral vascular accident (stroke, brain attack), father died at age 42 from myocardial infarction (heart attack). Based on normal ranges for vital signs, height, and weight, this client's B/P and weight would be interpreted as abnormal findings: this client has hypertension (high blood pressure) and is obese. The nurse applies knowledge of patterns associated with health problems to interpret the significance of the findings for this client. The nurse knows that hypertension occurs more frequently in groups with lifestyle concerns and that family history of coronary artery disease, hypertension, and obesity increase the risk of acquiring both hypertension and the complications associated with it. Recommendations and plans for care for Mr. Long will be developed in collaboration with other healthcare professionals to address the immediate and long-term healthcare needs of reducing blood pressure and weight.

Communication

Effective communication is essential to the data-gathering process. **Communication** refers to the exchange of information, feelings, thoughts, and ideas. Communication occurs through nonverbal means, such as facial expression, gestures, and body language. Verbal methods include spoken or written communication. A variety of verbal techniques, such as open-ended or closed questions, statements, clarification, and rephrasing, are used to gather information. The communication techniques must incorporate regard for the individual in relation to the purposes of the data gathering, the client's age, and his or her level of anxiety. In addition, the nurse must use techniques that accommodate language differences or difficulties, ethnocultural influences, spirituality, cognitive ability, affect, demeanour, and special needs. Communication in health assessment is further discussed in Chapter 10 of this text. ⬭ Sample client–nurse interactions appear in each chapter of Unit III. ⬭

Holistic Approach

A holistic approach is an essential characteristic of nursing practice. **Holism** can best be defined as considering more than the physiological health status of a client. Holism includes all factors that affect the client's physical and emotional well-being. In a holistic approach, the nurse recognizes that developmental, psychological, emotional, family, cultural, and environmental factors will affect immediate and long-term actual and potential health goals, problems, and plans.

Developmental Factors

The developmental level of a client has an impact on health assessment. The source of information may vary depending on the age and developmental level of the client, with parents or guardians being the primary sources for information about children. Findings related to intellectual ability must be interpreted according to the assessed developmental level, not the stated age, in clients with developmental disabilities. The developmental level of the client also influences the approach to assessment, including the words and terminology. For exam-

ple, assessment of a pregnant adolescent would be different from that of a 38-year-old woman pregnant for the third time.

Psychological and Emotional Factors

Psychological and emotional factors must be recognized as affecting physiological health and must be considered as predisposing or contributing factors when interpreting findings from a health assessment. The nurse needs only to recall that anxiety triggers an autonomic response resulting in increased pulse and blood pressure to understand that relationship. Conversely, physical problems can affect emotional health. For example, childhood obesity can lead to problems with self-esteem and influence socialization and development. Psychological problems, such as anxiety and depression, may interfere with the ability to fully participate in health assessment. Grief may limit a client's ability to carry out required health practices or recognize health problems.

Family Factors

Family history of illness or health problems must be considered in health assessment and the interpretation of findings. Individuals with a family history of some illnesses are considered at higher risk for contracting that disease. For example, a female with a first-degree relative (mother, sister, daughter) with breast cancer has a risk of developing breast cancer almost three times as high as other women do. The nurse must recognize that family dynamics may influence a client's approach to healthcare. In some families, health-related decisions are not made independently but rather by the family leader or by group consensus. Circumstances within families can affect both physical and emotional health and must be considered as part of health assessment. For example, children of alcoholics are at risk not only for alcoholism but also for emotional issues not encountered by other children; therefore, the nurse must view and interpret unexpected physical or emotional behaviours in relation to the alcoholism in the family.

Ethnocultural Factors

Ethnocultural factors, which affect language, expression, emotional and physical well-being, and health practices, must be considered when collecting data and interpreting findings. Findings regarding physical and emotional health must be interpreted in relation to the ethnocultural norms for the client. Care must be taken to provide clear explanations of abnormal findings, illnesses, and treatments because views of illness, causality, and treatment may have ethnocultural influences. Refer to Chapter 4 of this text for further discussion of social and ethnocultural factors in nursing care. ⬭

Environmental Factors

Internal and external environmental factors affect health assessment and interpretation of findings. The data must always be considered in relation to norms and expectations for age, race, and gender, and in relation to factors affecting the individual client. It is essential to gather and use data from the health history and physical assessment when interpreting data.

INTERNAL ENVIRONMENTAL FACTORS. Data from the comprehensive health assessment provide cues about the client's internal environment, including emotional state, response to medication and treatment, and physiological or anatomical alterations that influence findings and interpretation. For example, the finding from assessment of Mrs. Bernice Hall, 49, is that she has dark, almost black, formed stools. This would be considered an abnormal finding since the normal finding would be brown stools. However, Mrs. Hall stated during her health history that she has taken iron pills and eaten a lot of spinach and greens for years, and her stools have been that way ever since. Therefore, considering the internal environment of medication and diet, both of which darken the stool, the nurse interprets this as a normal finding for Mrs. Hall.

EXTERNAL ENVIRONMENTAL FACTORS. External environmental factors can also affect health, health assessment, and interpretation of findings. External factors include but are not limited to inhaled toxins, such as smoke, chemicals, and fumes; irritants that can be inhaled, ingested, or contacted through the skin; noise, light, and motion; and any objects or substances a person may encounter in the home, in schools, in workplaces, while shopping, or while travelling and carrying out normal activities.

Consider the assessment of Sapna Patel, a 22-year-old with back pain. The findings from the physical assessment are all within normal limits. Ms. Patel states that the pain started 2 weeks ago and has been getting worse, with only temporary relief from Aspirin. Before referring this client for diagnostic studies, the nurse considers external environmental factors that may contribute to the back pain. The nurse asks about any activities or events associated with the onset of the pain. Ms. Patel revealed that she had taken up quilting about 2 weeks ago and has been sitting and working with an embroidery hoop almost every day for an hour or so. The additional information assists the nurse in interpretation of the back pain. The nurse recommends ways to sit and perform the quilting without straining the muscles of the back and will follow up to see if this relieves the pain.

Consider the assessment of a toddler with nausea and vomiting. The nurse must gather information about the circumstances surrounding the onset of the problem. For example, was the child in a new environment in which he could have ingested medications, cleaning fluids, or other toxic substances?

Health assessment includes the interview, physical assessment, documentation, and interpretation of findings. The preceding discussion with the accompanying examples illustrates the importance of knowledge, communication, and a holistic approach in health assessment. The collection of information and interpretation of findings are important components of nursing practice. Nursing practice is concerned with health promotion, wellness, illness prevention, health restoration, and care for the dying. The nursing process in which the nurse uses comprehensive assessment to identify a client's health status and actual or potential needs guides the practice of nursing. The nursing process then directs the nurse in the development of plans and the use of nursing interventions to meet those identified needs.

NURSING PROCESS

The **nursing process** is a systematic, rational, dynamic, and cyclic process used by the nurse to plan and provide care for the client. When first developed, the nursing process had four steps or phases: assessing, planning, implementing, and evaluating. Many nursing theorists have taken the original steps and expanded and clarified the meaning and action of each step. Most experts today accept a five-step process (see Figure 1.6). These steps are assessment, diagnosis, planning, implementation, and evaluation. The nursing process can be used in any setting, with clients of all ages, and in all levels of health and illness.

Since the nursing process is client centred, the approach to nursing care is specific to the client. The client can be the individual, family, or community. The nurse uses critical thinking, therapeutic communication skills, and the knowledge of many arts and sciences when using the nursing process. Each step of the process will be defined here; however, greatest emphasis will be placed on assessment.

In the following sections, the steps of the nursing process are identified as discrete actions. However, in practice they are interrelated and overlap to some degree. The application and effective use of the nursing process is influenced by the ability of the nurse to obtain comprehensive, accurate data.

Assessment

Assessment, step 1 of the nursing process, is the collection, organization, and validation of subjective and objective data. The data collected form the database used by the nurse. As the data change, the nurse must update the database. The database will describe the physical, emotional, and spiritual health status of the client. Strengths and weaknesses are identified, as are responses to any treatment modalities.

Assessment begins at the moment the nurse meets the client and begins to gather information. Each piece of information collected about a client is a cue, because it hints at the total health status of the client. The baseline data act as a marker during future assessment. These data become a guide for the nurse as to what questions to ask and what additional information is needed.

Consider the following situation. Mrs. Martha Jacobs is a 70-year-old female who tripped at home 2 weeks ago and sprained her right ankle. Her initial treatment included an elastic bandage wrap, ice, and a nonsteroidal anti-inflammatory drug (NSAID) for discomfort. She was instructed to elevate the extremity for 3 days and to increase weight-bearing activity gradually. She is being seen in a follow-up visit and reports that her ankle is feeling much better, but she has abdominal discomfort.

When questioned about the problem, she states, "My stomach has been kind of achy and it really started a couple of days ago." She replies to further questioning, saying, "I've had only one or two little hard bowel movements in the last five days." She denied having a problem with bowel elimination in the past and states, "I usually go once a day and it's soft." In response to further questions, she states that she has been "essentially,

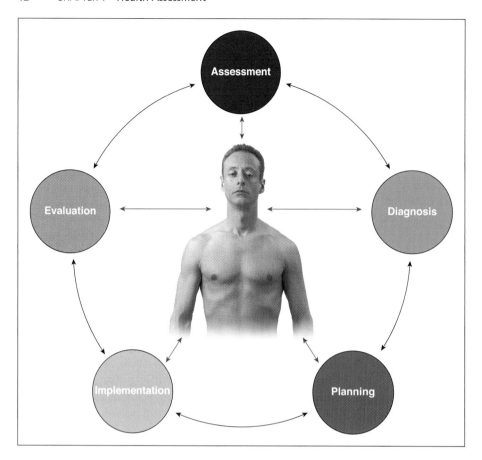

Figure 1.6 • Nursing process.

just sitting around, because I'm afraid to put too much weight on my ankle. I have been eating as usual, but I haven't been drinking so much because I hate to have to get up to use the bathroom."

A physical examination is conducted and the following results are found: bowel sounds are present in all quadrants, percussion reveals dullness in the left lower quadrant (LLQ), the abdomen is softly distended and nontender, and there are dry feces in the rectum.

Assessment refers to collecting subjective and objective data to plan and provide care for the client. Recall that subjective data are information that the client experiences and reports to the nurse. Subjective data for Mrs. Jacobs include the following: achy stomach for a couple of days; one or two hard, little bowel movements in 5 days; fear of weight bearing; limited activity; eating solid foods; and decreased fluid intake.

Objective data are observed or measured by the nurse. The objective data for Mrs. Jacobs include the following: bowel sounds in all four quadrants of the abdomen, dullness to percussion in the LLQ, no tenderness, soft distension of the abdomen, and dry feces in the rectum.

Diagnosis

Step 2 of the nursing process is diagnosis. The nurse uses critical thinking and applies knowledge from the sciences and other disciplines to analyze and synthesize the data. Client strengths, risks, and weaknesses are clearly identified. Data are compared to normative values and standards. Normative values and standards include but are not limited to charts for growth and development, laboratory values (hemoglobin, hematocrit, total cholesterol, blood glucose, etc.), the degree of flexion in the joints, the rate and characteristics of pulses, blood pressure, heart sounds, skin texture, core body temperature, language development, role performance, and interdependent functions.

Similar data are clustered or grouped together. The nurse makes a judgment after analysis and synthesis of collected data. This then becomes the **nursing diagnosis,** which is the basis for planning and implementing nursing care.

The following is an analysis of the data from the previously cited assessment of Mrs. Jacobs. The analysis will describe the comparison to normative values and standards for the subjective and objective data, respectively. The achy abdomen is a deviation from normal because the abdomen is pain free under normal conditions. One or two small, hard bowel movements in 5 days is considered an abnormal finding because stools are normally moist and because it is a deviation from the client's normal bowel pattern of soft stool, once daily. Fear of weight bearing is a normal finding. Most individuals experience anxiety after a painful injury. Older adults tend to feel anxious because they fear falling or further injury and potential loss of independence. However, "just sitting around" or immobility increases the risk, especially in older adults, for physical problems, including elimination problems, weakness, and joint discomfort. Psychologically, the older adult may lose independence or become socially isolated. Eating as usual can be considered an abnormal finding in light of the fact that this client has decreased activity, change in elimination, and abdominal discomfort. Decreased fluid intake is an abnormal finding. The client understands the relationship between the amount of intake and the frequency and amount of urination; however, her actions increase her risk for other physical problems.

The findings from the physical examination include the presence of bowel sounds in all four abdominal quadrants. This is a normal finding. Bowel sounds are indicative of peristaltic activity. Dullness to percussion in the LLQ is an abnormal but not unexpected finding. The infrequency and characteristics of this client's bowel movements indicate that feces are present in the rectum and descending colon. The abdomen is found to be nontender, which is a normal finding. Abdominal distension is an abnormal finding and indicative of stool and flatus accumulation in the bowel. Dry feces in the rectum are an abnormal but not unexpected finding because Mrs. Jacobs stated she had not been drinking much fluid. Moisture of the feces is related to fluid intake.

The analysis of assessment data includes clustering of information. The clusters consist of related pieces of information. The following clusters can be developed from the analysis of the objective and subjective data for Mrs. Jacobs:

- Achy, softly distended abdomen with dullness to percussion in the LLQ, infrequent hard stools with dry feces in rectum
- Eating regularly, decreased fluid intake
- Immobility, fear of weight bearing

After clustering the data, the nurse makes judgments and formulates diagnoses. Diagnoses are generally two-part statements. The first part identifies the problem or strength demonstrated in the data, and it is related to (R/T) the second part, that is, the likely cause of the problem. The following are three of many diagnostic statements the nurse could derive from the data for Mrs. Jacobs:

1. Constipation R/T lack of knowledge of the impact of fluid intake on bowel elimination
2. Immobility R/T fear of pain
3. Abdominal discomfort R/T constipation

A *taxonomy,* a conceptual framework for the formulation of nursing diagnoses, has been developed by NANDA International (NANDA-I). See Appendix A. ⬤⬤

Three types of nursing diagnoses are identified within the NANDA-I taxonomy: actual problems, risks for problems, and wellness issues. The following are examples of each type of diagnosis. *Ineffective breathing pattern* is a diagnostic statement, which exemplifies an actual problem. The statement *at risk for suicide* is representative of a diagnosis of a risk for a problem. An example of a diagnostic statement for wellness issues would be *readiness for enhanced family coping.*

Each NANDA-I diagnosis is composed of four components: a diagnostic label, a definition, defining characteristics, and risks or related factors. *Anxiety* is an example of a diagnostic label. Anxiety is defined as a state of mental uneasiness, apprehension, or dread in response to a perceived threat. Defining characteristics for anxiety include a verbal statement of anxiety (I feel anxious) or observed evidence, including trembling,

pallor, or a change in vital signs. Risks or related factors include physical or other factors that promote anxiety. For example, uncertainty about the outcome of a physical examination; uncertainty about the cause of a physical symptom, such as a severe and prolonged headache; a job interview; or public speaking may promote anxiety.

NANDA-I diagnoses are formulated by using a PES statement. The problem (P) is the diagnostic label, the etiology (E) includes the cause and contributing factors, and the signs and symptoms (S) are the defining characteristics. The PES statement of a diagnosis from the case study for Mrs. Jacobs would be written as follows: constipation (P) related to lack of knowledge (E) as evidenced by abdominal distension, achy abdomen, infrequent hard stool, and low fluid intake (S).

Each chapter in Unit III of this text includes a case study. ⬤⬤ The reader will be expected to analyze the data from the case studies by using critical thinking, the nursing process, and the development of nursing diagnoses.

Planning

Planning, step 3 of the nursing process, involves setting priorities, stating client goals or outcomes, and selecting nursing interventions, strategies, or orders to deal with the health status of the client. When possible, these activities need to include input from the client. Consultation or additional input may be needed from other healthcare professionals and family members. The developed nursing care plan acts as a guide for client care, helps to enhance client strengths, and helps to negate, change, or prevent a weakness or problem for the client.

Planning, as previously stated, involves setting priorities, stating client goals, and selecting strategies to address the diagnoses. The priority for Mrs. Jacobs is to decrease her abdominal discomfort. This can be accomplished by addressing the factors that contribute to the problem. The nurse uses the diagnostic statements to develop goals and interventions. The goal is stated in terms of the expected client outcome, includes a time frame, and is derived from the first part of the diagnosis. The interventions are developed by determining the strategies to address the causes of the problem and are derived from the second part of the diagnostic statement.

The first diagnosis for Mrs. Jacobs, constipation R/T lack of knowledge of the impact of fluid intake on bowel elimination, will generate the following goal: The client will resume a daily soft bowel movement within 72 hours.

The interventions are derived from the second part of the diagnosis. The intervention for Mrs. Jacobs will address her lack of knowledge about fluid intake in relation to bowel function. Therefore, the nursing intervention involves teaching Mrs. Jacobs.

Implementation

Implementation is step 4 of the nursing process. Now the care plan is put into action. Putting the nursing interventions into action, the nurse determines the client's need for assistance or the ability to function independently to achieve the stated goals. The nurse continues with the ongoing assessment of the client to update the database as behaviours change. The documentation of the implemented actions will include the client's response to nursing care. These actions will help meet the stated goals or outcomes, promote wellness, or convert illness to an improved state of health.

The intervention prescribed for Mrs. Jacobs, as previously stated, is teaching. Therefore, the nurse will teach Mrs. Jacobs by explaining the relationship of fluid intake to effective bowel function and include a discussion of the recommended amounts of fluid intake for adults. Providing information about the types of fluids that affect bowel elimination, such as fruit juices, would be part of the intervention.

Evaluation

Step 5, the final step of the nursing process, is evaluation. The nurse compares the client's present status to achievement of the stated goals or outcomes. At this time the nurse will need to modify the nursing care plan. This modification can be to continue, change, or terminate the nursing care plan based on goal achievement.

Evaluation refers to the determination that the goal has been achieved within the stated time. Recall that the goal for Mrs. Jacobs was to resume a daily soft bowel movement within 72 hours. The nurse must follow up with Mrs. Jacobs in 72 hours to determine whether she has experienced a soft bowel movement on 2 consecutive days. This would indicate a return to normal bowel function for this client. If the goal has not been reached, the plan must be modified and further assessment or action may be required.

It is important to point out that several goals and interventions are required to achieve the appropriate outcome for Mrs. Jacobs. Her bowel function is related to immobility and anxiety, as well as to decreased fluid intake. Goals would be derived for all diagnoses, and nursing interventions would be employed to address all the causative factors.

CRITICAL THINKING

Critical thinking is a cognitive skill employed in all nursing activities, and it enhances the application of the nursing process. Alfaro-LeFevre (2003) defined and explained the critical thinking process. This work provided the foundation for the following discussion. **Critical thinking** is a process of purposeful and creative thinking about resolutions to problems or the development of ways to manage situations. Critical thinking is more than problem solving; it is a way to apply logic and cognitive skills to the complexities of client care. It demands that nurses avoid bias and prejudice in their approach while using all the knowledge and resources at their disposal to assist clients in achieving health goals or maintaining well-being.

When critically thinking about the client's health status, problems, or situations, the nurse applies essential elements and skills. The five essential elements of critical thinking are collection of information, analysis of the situation, generation of alternatives, selection of alternatives, and evaluation. Figure 1.7 depicts the elements of critical thinking.

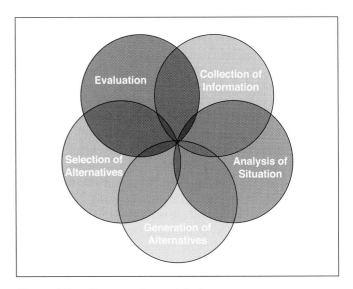

Figure 1.7 ● Elements of critical thinking.

Each element has working skills to help the nurse be complete, thorough, and competent with the cognitive processes of critical thinking. Critical thinking skills are linked with each of the essential elements. The following discussion provides information and examples of the linkage of the elements and skills of critical thinking as they are applied in health assessment. Additionally, each chapter of Unit III includes a case study and questions to provide opportunities to apply critical thinking skills. ⚭

Collection of Information

Collection of information, the first of the elements in critical thinking, involves the five skills of identifying assumptions, organizing data collection, determining the reliability of the data, identifying relevant versus irrelevant data, and identifying inconsistencies in the data (see Figure 1.8). The nurse must be able to identify assumptions that can misguide or misdirect the assessment and intervention processes. For example, when interviewing a client, the nurse must not assume that lack of eye contact indicates lack of attention, dishonesty, or apathy.

The second skill of collection of information is organizing data collection. Collection of subjective and objective data must be carried out in an organized manner. In health assessment the nurse first determines the client's current health status, level of distress, and ability to participate in the assessment process. The aim of data gathering in a client in acute distress is rapid identification of the problem and the significant predisposing and contributory factors in order to select and initiate interventions to alleviate the distress. In nonacute situations, assessment follows an accepted and organized framework of survey, health history, and physical assessment.

The third skill of collection of information is determining the reliability of the data. Client information is valuable if it is reliable and accurate, and the client is generally the best source of information, especially historical. However, physical and psychological factors may interfere with that capability. Information is then sought from a family member or caregiver who can provide reliable information. Other reliable sources

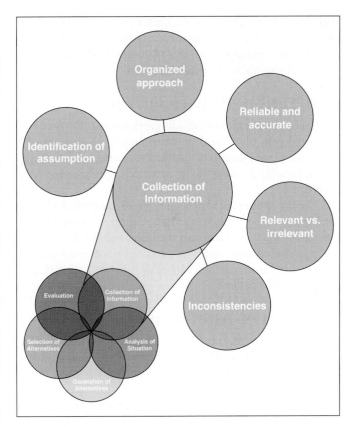

Figure 1.8 ● The five skills of the element Collection of Information.

of information include charts, medical records, and notes from other health professionals. The nurse must also be certain that objective data are accurate. Measuring devices must be standardized, calibrated, and applied correctly.

A wealth of information is obtained when carrying out a comprehensive health assessment. The nurse then applies the fourth critical thinking skill: determining the relevance of the information in relation to the client's current, evolving, or potential condition or situation. Consider the relevance of nonimmunization or contraction of German measles in a male client seeking care for a fracture versus a 26-year-old sexually active female having an annual examination.

Identifying inconsistencies is the last of the skills associated with the collection of information. The nurse must be able to recognize discrepancies in the information. Further, the nurse must determine whether the inconsistency is a result of an oversight, misunderstanding, linguistic factors, or cultural factors. Indications of confusion, memory impairment, and subtle or overt discomfort with a topic or an area of questioning must also be considered. The following is an example of an inconsistency indicating misunderstanding. During the interview a client failed to identify a surgical repair of a fracture when asked about surgical procedures, but reported it when asked about the treatment for accidents or injuries. The inconsistency may not become apparent until the physical assessment takes place. A client may say that he or she has never used street drugs, but during the assessment the nurse may see track (needle) marks on the arms. The nurse must use care in communication while dealing with the inconsistency.

Analysis of the Situation

The second element of critical thinking is analysis of the situation. Five skills are linked to this element: distinguish data as normal or abnormal, cluster related data, identify patterns in the data, identify missing information, and draw valid conclusions (see Figure 1.9).

When distinguishing normal from abnormal data, the nurse uses knowledge of human behaviour, as well as of anatomy and physiology, to compare findings with established norms in these areas. The nurse uses standards for laboratory results, diagnostic testing, charts, scales, and measures related to development and aging. The data must be analyzed in relation to expected ranges for age, gender, genetic background, and culture of the client. Consider the following situation: In a regularly scheduled checkup, John Morgan, age 31, undergoes a complete health assessment. He is found to have alopecia (hair loss) at the anterior hairline and thinning of the hair that has increased since his last visit. The nurse knows that alopecia occurs more frequently in men than in women, that in male pattern baldness the alopecia begins at the anterior hairline, and that alopecia is genetic and begins in early adulthood. When all other findings are within the normal limits for a 31-year-old male, the nurse considers the alopecia a normal finding in this client.

If the previously mentioned finding had occurred during an assessment of Su Mei Lane, a 31-year-old female, the nurse would apply the same knowledge and consider alopecia an abnormal finding. Other findings would then be carefully examined. In this situation, Ms. Lane stated in the health history, "I'm tired all the time. I must be anemic because

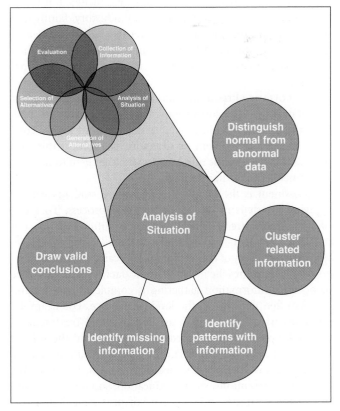

Figure 1.9 ● The five skills of the element Analysis of Situation.

I'm cold all the time, and on top of all that I'm constipated." Additionally, she said, "I think I'm becoming irregular because I'm too tired to exercise and don't eat right, and I guess that has messed up my periods too; it lasts much longer than it ever did." Findings during the physical assessment included pallor, weight gain, dry skin, and brittle nails. The nurse must now begin to apply the other skills associated with analysis of the situation.

When thinking critically, the nurse will cluster related information by sorting and categorizing information into groupings that may include but are not limited to cues, symptoms, body systems, or health practices. The following are clusters derived from the data about Ms. Lane:

- Skin dry, nails brittle, hair thinning and falling out
- Constipation, irregularity, weight gain, "not eating right"
- Lack of exercise, tired, cold, pallor, "I must be anemic"
- Prolonged menstruation

Once the clustering is complete, the nurse must apply the third skill of identifying patterns in the information. Use of this skill enables the nurse to get an idea about what is happening with the client and to determine whether more information is required. The nurse must rely on knowledge and resources in identifying patterns. The nurse might consider a pattern suggesting a nutritional or abdominal problem since information includes fatigue, changes in eating, changes in bowel elimination, and changes in the skin and hair. The data also suggest a metabolic or hormonal problem. However, the information is incomplete.

At this point the nurse would identify missing information, the fourth skill. Missing information would include but is not limited to onset of symptoms, medication history, family history of similar problems, and measures the client has taken to alleviate the problems. Additional information would include laboratory studies of hematologic, metabolic, or hormonal function.

The nurse acquires information necessary to apply the last skill of drawing valid conclusions. This skill requires the nurse to use all knowledge and reasoning skills to draw logical conclusions about a problem or situation. The critical thinking process continues as the nurse works with the client to develop a treatment plan for her problem.

Assessment is the focus of this text, and students will be applying the steps in the critical thinking process. To identify the importance of critical thinking to future practice, the remaining elements and skills are discussed. These skills are essential to delivery of competent nursing care. The nurse gathers data, determines the meaning of the data, and decides what to do once information gathering is complete. The nursing actions often depend on the level of practice. For example, autonomous decisions, such as diagnosis and treatment of disease by prescription of medication, are within the role of the advanced practice nurse. For the generalist, data are shared with physicians who prescribe medical treatment. The generalist develops interventions, such as education, support, and some modes for symptom relief, as part of professional practice.

Furthermore, the nurse brings a holistic approach to the client situation. Therefore, the nurse will collaborate with all healthcare professionals to be sure that plans are developed to meet individual physical and psychosocial needs.

Generation of Alternatives

Articulating options and establishing priorities are the two skills associated with the critical thinking element of generation of alternatives (see Figure 1.10). Articulation of options is simply stating possible paths to follow or actions to take to resolve a problem.

Once the options have been enumerated, the nurse and client work together to establish priorities. This process must reflect the acuity of the problem and the client's ability to interpret the information and weigh the advantages and disadvantages of each option in relation to health, lifestyle, cultural, and socioeconomic factors.

Selection of Alternatives

Selection of alternatives is the next element of critical thinking, and linked with it are the skills of developing outcomes and developing plans (see Figure 1.11). Outcomes are statements of what the client will do or be able to do in a specific time. The plan includes all the actions required by the client independently or in coordination with healthcare professionals and others to achieve the stated outcomes. The nurse must be sure that the client has the knowledge and skills required to follow

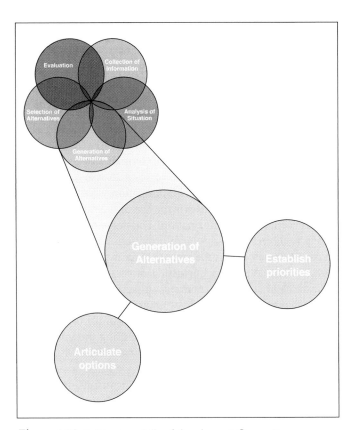

Figure 1.10 ● The two skills of the element Generating Alternatives.

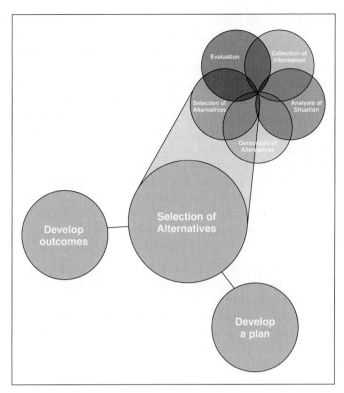

Figure 1.11 ● The two skills of the element Selection of Alternatives.

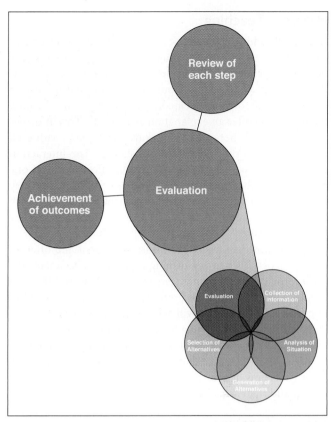

Figure 1.12 ● The two skills of the element Evaluation.

the plan. Therefore, the nurse may have to provide education, follow-up, and support for the client. A time is determined for achievement of each outcome and a plan developed to guide the client toward meeting the expectations in the stated outcome.

Evaluation

The last element in critical thinking is evaluation (see Figure 1.12). This element includes the skills of determining whether the expected outcomes have been achieved and review of the application of each critical thinking skill to be sure that omissions and misinterpretations did not occur. Ethical principles and the effects of values and biases must be considered in evaluation.

ROLE OF THE NURSE

The nurse provides care to clients needing and seeking help. Nursing care is based on a strong knowledge base and the application of critical thinking. The knowledge base of the nurse is developed over time by using information from the humanities and the biological, natural, and social sciences. By using research data, standards of care, and the nursing process, the nurse provides competent care. The client will be the individual, family, or community. The individual could be any age and at any developmental level. The actions of the nurse will be directed to promote health and wellness, treat and care for the ill, and care for the dying individual while being supportive to family members. To perform these actions, the nurse works in a variety of settings, including hospitals, clinics, nursing homes, clients' homes, schools, and workplaces.

Regardless of the setting, the role of the nurse is multifaceted. Each situation requires the nurse to use critical thinking and the nursing process. To provide care and use the nursing process, the nurse must develop strong assessment skills. The gathering of complete, accurate, and relevant data is required. While gathering the subjective and objective data from the client, the nurse must be attuned to the signs, symptoms, behaviours, and cues offered by the client. The collected data vary as the status of the client changes. The nurse functions as a teacher, caregiver, client advocate, and manager of client care.

Teacher

As a teacher, the nurse helps the client to gain knowledge required for health maintenance or improvement, to prevent illness or injury, to manage therapies, and to make decisions about health and treatment. Teaching occurs in all settings and for a variety of reasons and may be informal or formal. Teaching is an important intervention to promote wellness and prevent illness. This intervention is enacted when collection and analysis of client data reveal a knowledge deficit, a need for education about an identified risk, or the readiness to learn to enhance health. These three conditions represent the three types of diagnoses in the NANDA-I taxonomy: actual problems, risk for a problem, or a wellness issue.

Informal Teaching

Informal teaching generally occurs as a natural part of a client encounter. This type of teaching may be to provide instructions, to explain a question or procedure, or to reduce anxiety. For example, while asking about medications and the use of natural, herbal, or home remedies during the health history, the nurse may offer an explanation as follows: "This information is important because medications may interact with each other or with herbs and natural substances. The interaction can sometimes be harmful or change the effectiveness of one of your prescribed medications." The same information may be offered in response to a client statement or question, such as, "What is so important that I go over my medications every time I come here?"

Explanations are offered to inform the client and often to reduce anxiety. When performing a physical assessment, the nurse provides explanations. For example, "I would like you to take a deep breath in and out each time I place the stethoscope on your chest. This will help me to clearly hear the air as it moves in and out of your lungs." The nurse may explain a technique during assessment of the musculoskeletal system as follows: "You will notice that I've asked you to push with both arms against my hands; that is so I can compare the strength of the left and right arms."

Formal Teaching

Formal teaching occurs in response to an identified learning need of an individual, a group, or a community. Teaching plans are developed for formal teaching sessions and have six components: the identified learning need, the goal, the objectives, the content, the teaching strategies and rationales, and the evaluation, as noted in Box 1.1. Teaching plans are developed to meet distinct needs of individual clients or common needs of individuals, groups, or communities. When developing or using existing teaching plans, the nurse must consider the age, gender, developmental level, culture, linguistic ability, dexterity, physical ability or limitations, and resources of the client or group. The selection of the content and methods for teaching and evaluation of learning should be influenced by these factors. For example, use of printed materials would be inappropriate for a client with impaired vision or with limited literacy. The nurse would not include referral to internet sites for clients without computer access. It would be best to suggest walking in a park or using a public facility for exercise rather than a health club for those with limited income. The following sections address each component of the teaching plan.

BOX 1.1	Elements of a Teaching Plan

Teaching plans are developed for formal teaching sessions and have six components:

- Learning need
- Goal
- Objectives
- Content
- Teaching strategy and rationale
- Evaluation

THE LEARNING NEED. Learning needs are identified as discrete knowledge deficits for an individual or as common needs of individuals and groups. Individual learning needs can be identified through the health history or in communication with a client throughout the assessment process.

The need for learning in individuals, families, and groups arises in response to lack of knowledge about common changes or risks that occur with aging, role change and development, illness, health promotion, and disease prevention. The following provides an example of a learning need for a group. A community centre provides health promotion classes for older adults. The sessions are planned in collaboration with healthcare providers in the community. One session was developed to provide information about gastrointestinal health because the risk of developing colorectal cancer increases with age.

THE GOAL. The goal is based on an identified learning need. The goal is written as a broad statement of the expected outcome of the learning.

A goal for a group is developed in response to identification of a learning need as well. The goal for the older adults with increased risk for colorectal cancer would be as follows: The participants will follow recommended guidelines for colorectal cancer screening.

OBJECTIVES. In the teaching plan, the objectives identify specific, measurable behaviours or activities expected of the client or group. Action verbs are used to denote the behaviour or activity. Table 1.1 provides examples of action verbs. The

TABLE 1.1	Action Verbs for Development of Objectives	
DOMAIN	**ACTION VERBS**	
Cognitive	Appraises	Explains
	Changes	Generates
	Composes	Matches
	Concludes	Modifies
	Converts	Names
	Creates	Reorganizes
	Criticizes	Separates
	Defines	Solves
	Designs	States
	Diagrams	Subdivides
	Discriminates	Summarizes
Affective	Acts	Greets
	Adheres	Justifies
	Describes	Modifies
	Discusses	Presents
	Displays	Proposes
	Explains	
Psychomotor	Assembles	Fixes
	Calibrates	Makes
	Changes	Manipulates
	Demonstrates	Operates
	Dismantles	

objectives may include criteria or conditions under which the behaviour must occur. Objectives include a time for completion of the objective. An example of a time for the objectives of teaching a group about gastrointestinal health would be written as follows: At the completion of the learning session, the participants will identify three measures to promote gastrointestinal health and prevent colorectal cancer.

The type of learning or behaviour that is expected of the client also determines objectives. Objectives, therefore, are in the cognitive, psychomotor, or affective domains. Cognitive objectives include those concerning the acquisition of knowledge. Psychomotor objectives include the acquisition of skills. The affective domain refers to attitudes, feelings, values, and opinions. The example of an objective for the group learning about gastrointestinal health is in the cognitive domain because it calls for the participants to identify three measures to promote gastrointestinal health and prevent colorectal cancer.

CONTENT. The content within a teaching plan is what will actually be taught. The objective for the clients states that they will be able to identify three measures to promote gastrointes-

tinal health and prevent colorectal cancer. The clients will need to understand the risk factors for colorectal cancer. Therefore, the content must include a list of modifiable and nonmodifiable risk factors and actions that can decrease the risk. The content to address the objective of improving gastrointestinal health and preventing colorectal cancer would include information about risk factors, diets that improve gastrointestinal health, annual abdominal and rectal examinations by a healthcare provider, fecal occult blood testing, and sigmoidoscopy with biopsy.

TEACHING METHODS. Teaching methods or strategies are the channels or avenues used to present the content. They must be suited to the needs of the learner and the type of learning that is expected. Psychomotor learning requires, for example, demonstration as the nurse is teaching methodology. One-on-one discussion is a common strategy for individual client teaching. Group teaching strategies may include lecture, discussion, or role-play. Table 1.2 includes information about teaching methods.

TABLE 1.2	Teaching Methods		
TEACHING METHOD	**DOMAIN**	**ADVANTAGES**	**DISADVANTAGES**
Explanation	Cognitive	May be used for individual or group.	Passive learning.
One-on-One Discussion	Cognitive Affective	Learner participation. Clarification can be provided. Questions can be answered.	Requires time for discussion and to allow for questions.
Lecture	Cognitive	Useful for large groups. Facts presented in logical manner.	Passive learning.
Group Discussion	Cognitive Affective	Learners are more comfortable in groups. Allows participation of all members.	Can easily lose focus in a group discussion.
Case Study	Cognitive	Develops problem-solving skills. Allows learners to explore complex concepts.	Difficult to develop. Learners may have difficulty applying information to their own situation.
Role-Play	Cognitive Affective	Allows learners to appreciate different points of view. Learners actively participate.	Learners may be too anxious to participate. Effective in small groups only.
Demonstration	Cognitive Psychomotor	Can be used with individuals and groups.	Passive learning.
Practice	Cognitive Psychomotor	Learners actively involved. Hands-on experience.	Time consuming. Effective with small groups only to provide feedback.
Printed Material	Cognitive	Efficiently presents important information. Can supplement other teaching methods.	May not meet needs of low-literacy learners or those with language differences. Passive learning.
Media Audiovisual Presentation	Cognitive Affective Psychomotor	Can be used in all types of learning. Can supplement other teaching methods. Provides aural and visual stimulation.	Time consuming. Passive learning.
Computer-Assisted Instruction (CAI)	Cognitive Affective Psychomotor	Can be used with individuals and groups. Learning is active. Provides immediate feedback.	Requires equipment. Time consuming.

EVALUATION. A plan for evaluation of learning is included in the teaching plan. In evaluation, the nurse determines if the learning objectives have been achieved. The learning domain of the objective determines the methods for evaluation. Cognitive learning may be evaluated verbally through questions or in discussion with the client or by use of written measurements. Written evaluations include short answer, true-false, fill-in, multiple-choice, and other types of tests. Members of a group learning about breast cancer detection, for example, could be evaluated with a short answer quiz at the end of the session. Psychomotor learning is best evaluated by a demonstration of the skill expected in the objective. Affective objectives are difficult to evaluate. Listening to the client and observing behaviour that indicates feelings and values are effective methods. For example, the nurse could determine whether participants value prevention as part of health promotion and receive flu immunization. When evaluation reveals that learning has not taken place, the nurse may have to repeat all or part of the teaching.

Caregiver

The caregiver role has always been the traditional role of the nurse. Historically, physical care was the primary focus. Today, the nurse uses a holistic approach to nursing care. Using critical thinking and the nursing process, the nurse provides direct and indirect care to the client. Indirect care is accomplished with the delegation of activities to other members of the team. As client advocate, the nurse acts as a protector. Clients are kept informed of their rights, given information to make informed decisions, and encouraged to speak for themselves. As a case manager, the nurse helps to coordinate care, manages the multidisciplinary team, and plans client outcomes within a specific time. Providing care, maintaining cost of care, and identifying the effectiveness of the plan are all responsibilities of the case manager.

Advanced Practice Roles

The advanced formal education and expanded roles of the nurse permit the nurse to function in advanced roles. These advanced roles include but are not limited to nurse researcher, practitioner, clinical specialist, administrator, and educator.

Nurse Researcher

The nurse researcher identifies problems regarding client care, designs plans of study, and develops tools. Findings are analyzed and knowledge is disseminated. The nurse performing the research adds to the body of knowledge of the profession, gives direction for future research, and improves client care.

Nurse Practitioner

The nurse practitioner, with advanced degrees and certified by the regulatory bodies, practises independently in a variety of situations. An agency or a community-based setting may have a school nurse practitioner, family nurse practitioner, or gerontology nurse practitioner meeting the healthcare needs of clients seeking assistance.

Clinical Nurse Specialist

Clinical nurse specialists have advanced education and degrees in a specific aspect of practice. They provide direct client care, direct and teach other team members providing care, and conduct nursing research within the area of specialization.

Nurse Administrator

Today, the role of the nurse administrator varies. Professional titles include vice president of nursing services, supervisor, or nurse manager of a specific unit. The responsibilities vary and could include staffing, budgets, client care, staff performance evaluations, consulting, and ensuring that goals of the agency are being accomplished. Advanced degrees are usually required for these positions. It is common to find nurse administrators with advanced degrees in several disciplines, such as nursing and business administration.

Nurse Educator

The nurse educator, a nurse with advanced degrees, is employed to teach in a nursing program. This could be at a university, community college, or department of staff development in an agency providing nursing care. The educator is responsible for didactic and clinical teaching, curriculum development, clinical placement, and practice for students. The educator provides the student with the opportunity to practise assessment skills in a variety of settings with a diverse client population.

This chapter has presented an overview of concepts and processes important to health assessment. Aspects of nursing practice, knowledge, and skills required for the changing role of the nurse in today's healthcare arena have been introduced. These include health, comprehensive assessment, nursing process, critical thinking, communication, documentation, and teaching. An in-depth discussion of these important concepts is presented in succeeding chapters of this book. Development of knowledge, skills, and techniques is enhanced through the use of clinical examples and case studies.

APPLICATION THROUGH CRITICAL THINKING

CASE STUDY

Mary Wong is a 19-year-old university student living in the dormitory. She has come to the University Health Centre with the following complaints: nausea, vomiting, abdominal pain increasing in severity, diarrhea, a fever, and dry mouth. She tells you, the nurse, "I have had abdominal pain for about 12 hours with nausea, vomiting, and diarrhea." These symptoms, she tells you, "all started after supper in the student cafeteria on campus."

You conduct an interview and follow it with a physical examination, which reveals the following: symmetrical abdomen, bowel sounds in all quadrants, tender to palpation in the lower quadrants, guarding. Mary's skin is warm and moist, her lips and mucous membranes are dry.

▶ *Critical Thinking Questions*

1. Identify the findings as objective or subjective data.
2. Prepare a narrative nursing note from the data.
3. What factors must be considered in conducting the comprehensive health assessment of Mary Wong?
4. Before developing a nursing diagnosis, what must you do?

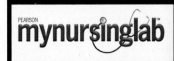

Visit the MyNursingLab website at **http://www.pearsoned.ca/mynursinglab**. This online homework and tutorial system puts you in control of your own learning with study and practice tools directly correlated to this chapter's content.

2

HEALTH PROMOTION

Canadian Authors: Candace Lind, University of Calgary; Sylvia Loewen, University of Calgary; Aliyah Mawji, University of Calgary

WHAT IS HEALTH PROMOTION?

Health promotion is the process of enabling people to increase their control over and improve their own health (World Health Organization, Health and Welfare Canada, & Canadian Public Health Association, 1986). In this definition, health promotion is described as a "process," indicating that it is a means to an end and not necessarily an outcome in its own right. Health promotion is an activity that often is focused on enabling people to take some form of action. Thus, health promotion is not something that is done *on* or *to* people; it is done *with* people, as individuals, families, communities, or population groups. Therefore, participation and partnerships are valued methods of engaging people in health promotion initiatives (Nutbeam, 1998). Empowerment is a process through which people gain greater control over the decisions and actions that affect their health (Canadian Public Health Association [CPHA], 2010). Empowerment may be a social, cultural, psychological, or political process through which people and social groups are able to express their needs; present their concerns; devise ways to become involved in decision making; and act to achieve their political, social, and cultural goals (CPHA, 2010). The purpose of health promotion activities is to strengthen the skills and capacity of individuals and their families to take action, and the capacity of communities and population groups to act collectively to exert control over the determinants of health. Thus, empowerment of individuals, families, communities, and population groups is a valued outcome of health promotion (Nutbeam, 1998).

Social Determinants of Health

Another phrase integral to the discussion of health promotion is **social determinants of health**, which are the economic and social conditions that influence the health of individuals and their communities. Extending beyond biomedical and behavioural risk factors, particular societal factors exert a large influence on health—they often determine whether individuals stay healthy or become ill (Raphael, 2004). These social determinants of health include the following (Flynn, 1999):

- Income and social status
- Social environments
- Work and working conditions
- Education
- Social support networks
- Genetic endowment
- Personal coping skills
- Health services
- Healthy child development
- Culture
- Physical environments
- Gender

These social factors make a significant contribution to an individual's health, and research has repeatedly demonstrated that people who are poor or otherwise disadvantaged experience worse health than people who live in upper socioeconomic levels of society and are more advantaged (National Institute for Health and Clinical Excellence, 2007).

Understanding determinants of health is important because they are a much stronger predictor of health status than behavioural factors, even including obesity and tobacco use (Raphael, 2006). For example, low birth weight and poor health status or child development significantly raise the probability an individual will develop type 2 diabetes or cardiovascular disease later in life. Social determinants should be considered when completing health assessments because (1) improvement in an individual's determinants of health profile will positively affect his or her health and (2) determinants have a cumulative effect. Addressing these determinants of health oftentimes requires nurses to shift the focus of their health promotion efforts away from general health improvements and toward reducing the causes of health inequities for their individual clients. Strategies that nurses use may include making referrals to social agencies and advocating for individuals to receive the services they require. Examples of nursing involvement in addressing determinants of health at a community or population level include lobbying for a living wage that enables a family to afford the basic requirements of living: affordable housing and food security (Raphael, 2006).

In tackling the social determinants of people's health, health promotion encompasses actions directed toward changing both those determinants that lie within the more immediate control of individuals (including individual health behaviours) and those factors that lie largely outside of the control of individuals (including social, economic, and environmental conditions). This kind of health promotion is exemplified in "Jason's Story" (Federal, Provincial, and Territorial Advisory Committee on Population Health, 1999, p. vii):

Jason's Story

Why is Jason in the hospital?

Because he has a bad infection in his leg.

But why does he have an infection?

Because he has a cut on his leg and it got infected.

But why does he have a cut on his leg?

Because he was playing in the junk yard next to his apartment building and there was some sharp, jagged steel there that he fell on.

But why was he playing in a junk yard?

Because his neighbourhood is kind of run down. A lot of kids play there and there is no one to supervise them.

But why does he live in that neighbourhood?

Because his parents can't afford a nicer place to live.

But why can't his parents afford a nicer place to live?

Because his dad is unemployed and his mom is sick.

But why is his dad unemployed?

Because he doesn't have much education and he can't find a job.

But why...?

From "Jason's Story," it is clear that the more powerful health promotion actions are long term and aimed at changing the root causes, the determinants of his health. The story also exemplifies the various levels at which health promotion can be implemented: the individual, the family, the community, and the population. In the past 20 years, considerable advancement has occurred in health promotion research. This rapidly expanding research base has improved nurses' knowledge and understanding of the determinants of health and how to change those determinants to improve health (Nutbeam, 1998).

Exemplary case studies are presented in the chapters throughout this textbook, along with Health Promotion Assessment Tools (including social determinants of health),

which will enable beginning nurses to see how a health assessment can identify opportunities and action strategies for health promotion. A thorough health assessment can provide information that will lead nurses to go beyond the individual and family levels, to recognize health actions nurses can take that are part of promoting the health of individuals within their communities.

HEALTH PROMOTION IN CANADA

Brief History of Health Promotion

In 1974 the importance of health promotion was recognized in Canada following the publication of a federal report called "A new perspective on the health of Canadians: A working document." This document directed the focus of health toward important factors that underlie the health of the population and was the first national health promotion strategy for Canada (Lalonde, 1974). National awareness and thinking about health began to shift toward health promotion, leading to the establishment of Canada as an initiator and international leader in health promotion. In 1985 a federal policy review led to another report: "Achieving health for all: A framework for health promotion" (Epp, 1986), which laid the foundation for Canada to host the First International Conference on Health Promotion in Ottawa. The **Ottawa Charter for Health Promotion** (WHO, Health and Welfare Canada, & CPHA, 1986) was a result of that conference, and it has led worldwide health promotion initiatives since then. The Ottawa Charter identified the components of health promotion actions: building healthy public policy, creating supportive environments, strengthening community action, developing personal skills, and reorienting health services. These are the action strategies of the population-based health promotion model used today.

Primary Healthcare

The Declaration of Alma-Ata was adopted at the International Conference on Primary Health Care, in the city of Almaty (formerly Alma-Ata), Kazakhstan, in September 1978. It expressed the need for urgent action by all governments, health and development workers, and the world community to protect and promote the health of all people in the world. It was the first international declaration underlining the importance of primary healthcare. **Primary healthcare** was developed to guide effective healthcare delivery and incorporates all levels of prevention (primary, secondary, and tertiary); it includes the concepts of accessibility, public participation, health promotion, appropriate technology, and intersectoral cooperation (WHO, 1978). The primary healthcare approach has since been accepted by member countries of the World Health Organization as the key to achieving the goal of health for all.

The Declaration of Alma-Ata emphasized the need for healthcare providers to work *with* people to assist them in making decisions about their health and help them understand how to meet health challenges in ways that are affordable, acceptable, and sustainable over the long term (Vollman, 2008). The

Declaration also identifies health system components that are necessary to achieve the goal of health for all (Vollman, 2008, p. 6):

- Education about the prevailing health problems and their prevention and control
- Safe food supply and adequate nutrition
- Adequate supply of safe water and basic sanitation
- Maternal and childcare, including family planning
- Immunization against basic infectious diseases
- Appropriate treatment of common diseases and injuries
- Essential drugs

"Primary health care is essential health care based on practical, scientifically sound, and socially acceptable methods and technology made universally accessible to individuals and families in the community through their full participation and at a cost that the community and country can afford" WHO, 1978, Article VI). It is the first level of contact between individuals, families, and communities and the national health system, and it brings healthcare as close as possible to where people live and work. But primary healthcare is more than just the first point of contact with the health system; it is the foundation that ensures public participation, social justice, and health equity at all levels of healthcare, including nursing. A system that is based on primary healthcare balances prevention and promotion with the demands of care, cure, rehabilitation, and palliation. Primary healthcare also extends beyond the health system to other societal systems, including education, politics and government, economics, and transportation, all of which have the potential to influence the determinants of health (Vollman, 2008). The principles of primary healthcare on which action on "health for all" must be based include the following (WHO, 1978):

- Equitable access to health and health services
- Public participation
- Appropriate technology
- Intersectoral collaboration
- Reorientation of the health system
- Promotion of health and prevention of disease and injury

KEY CONSIDERATIONS IN PROMOTING THE HEALTH OF INDIVIDUALS

A number of important concepts must be understood to have a well-rounded comprehension of the context in which nursing health promotion practice occurs. They also provide a foundation for understanding the Population Health Promotion model. These concepts are social justice and health equity, advocacy and activism, root causes of health issues, and upstream and downstream approaches to promoting health.

Social Justice and Health Equity

"Social justice is a matter of life and death. It affects the way people live, their consequent chance of illness, and their risk of premature death" (WHO, 2008, p. 3). Social justice and health equity are core values of health promotion (Bensaude De Castro Freire, Manoncourt, & Mukhopadhyay, 2009). **Social justice** is "the fair distribution of society's benefits, responsibilities and their consequences. It focuses on the relative position of one social group in relationship to others in society as well as on the root causes of disparities and what can be done to eliminate them" (Canadian Nurses Association [CNA], 2006, p. 7). The relationship between social justice and an individual's health is more easily understood when looked at in environments of poverty and violence. Social justice and the social context of people's lives affect their well-being, their risk of illness, and their risk of premature death (WHO, 2008). Social justice is closely linked to **health equity**, which means all persons are entitled equally to health protection, basic income levels, and opportunities to be healthy (CPHA, 2010). Inequity occurs as a result of differences in opportunity, rather than differences in personal choice. In Canada variations in health status exist depending on where an individual lives, with higher rates of illnesses, such as *tuberculosis* (TB), in remote northern communities with overcrowded homes (Canadian Broadcasting Corporation, 2010).

Social justice work includes addressing the root causes of people's health problems, not just their symptoms. Social justice and health equity are key concepts to consider in gaining a fuller understanding of individuals' health and health behaviours. These concepts help nurses understand why an individual is noncompliant with treatment or prevention messages and help nurses assess barriers that preclude participation in the activities that nurses teach and promote to improve health and well-being. For example, a nurse may suggest to her client Jim that he eat more fruits and vegetables to decrease his cardiovascular risk factors. This seemingly simple directive made by the nurse might be very challenging for him to accomplish. On exploring his life circumstances by using the social determinants of health, the nurse discovers Jim can find only part-time employment, barely has the resources to pay his monthly rent, and cannot afford the extra bus fare to travel outside his community to buy affordably priced fruits and vegetables. What appears to be noncompliance on the surface is really a larger issue of poverty and inequity for Jim: he does not have the financial resources to implement the nurse's health-promoting suggestion. The action strategies Jim's nurse needs to use must go beyond developing Jim's personal skills (i.e., his knowledge of more healthful foods) to building healthy public policy for better and more affordable access to healthful foods.

The less access people have to money, power, knowledge, and social connections, the lesser their ability to cope and gain control over those forces that affect their health—these are key considerations in health promotion activities. When people cannot gain access to resources because of their inability to pay for them, the healthcare system is inequitable. Individuals' patterns of health behaviours are strongly shaped by the social and economic environments in which they live and work. For example, high levels of stress produce behaviours aimed at decreasing tensions, such as the consumption of high-fat diets ("comfort foods"), other poor nutritional habits, and tobacco use (Raphael, 2002). Tackling health inequities therefore requires nurses to think about how individuals' social determinants of health, such as working conditions, income, education, housing, social networks, and supports, influence their health and behaviours.

Using the concepts of social justice and health equity requires nurses to better understand the causes of health issues that affect individuals in their communities, thus preventing health teaching from becoming inappropriate or unattainable for those people. The Health Promotion Assessment Tool, found in Chapters 11–27, show that many individuals' lives are complex and barriers may exist to traditional health teaching. The Chapter 19 case study involving Ms. Flett shows that she faces many inhibitors to joining a fitness facility, including affordability issues and childcare availability so she can leave home to attend an exercise class.

Nursing Role in Advocacy and Activism

Health promotion strategies are important components of nursing follow-up related to physical assessment, as they provide nurses with direction for how to proceed with issues that arise from a physical assessment of an individual. At times, nurses experience situations in which their assessment uncovers an issue that traditional health teaching or referrals may inadequately address. They are then left with the question of what else they can do to help their clients and address the root causes of the issues they are seeing in their practice. At that point, **advocacy and activism in nursing** measures may be important components of health promotion for both the individuals and the communities those individuals live in, to assist in enacting lasting health-promoting change. Nurses can engage in individual or group activities to support and garner resources for an individual, a community, or a cause. Nurses can also create awareness of a health issue, help foster social acceptance or acquire resources, and engage in policy and organizational change to achieve a health goal. Activism entails direct action (e.g., political lobbying) taken to support a health goal.

Cathy Crowe is a nurse activist in Toronto who works to end homelessness by engaging in empowering activities, such as partnering with a group of homeless people to write a book of their stories. Additionally, Cathy partnered with a filmmaker to create a series of four documentaries with the homelessness situations in Canadian cities as the subject matter. The films are being used as a community development tool to raise societal awareness and support to end homelessness.

One example of an advocacy strategy nurses can use to change risk factors and address root causes of health issues is lobbying for free transportation for older adults to attend events that help them stay active and remain involved in their communities. Many appealing and beneficial community pro-

grams for seniors fail because the seniors interested in attending have no transportation to get to the program or cannot afford to pay for transportation. As a result, low-income older adults without strong family support may become physically and socially isolated, further placing them at risk for physical mobility problems and depression.

Engaging in social action that assists individuals and the communities in which they live and work to gain mastery over their lives by changing their social and political environments (Wallerstein, 2002) is one way nurses can help address the issues they see when completing physical assessments. This action is especially important when nurses see patterns start to emerge in particular groups of people. Showing concern and interest in partnering with people to address areas that they want to see changed is an example of using empowering strategies that help raise individuals' self-esteem and improve their ability to take more control over their lives (Wallerstein, 2002). Building individuals' strengths by focusing on what they are doing well and using that to leverage what they want to do better at is another health-promoting strategy (Raeburn & Rootman, 1998) that nurses can use. Effective nursing strategies include building individuals' skills, knowledge, competencies, self-esteem, power, and social support.

To summarize, empowering individuals by valuing the strengths they bring to improving their own health is an effective tool in health promotion with individuals and communities all over the world (International Union for Health Promotion and Education & Canadian Consortium for Health Promotion Research, 2007) and is a key component of community health nursing practice (Community Health Nurses Association of Canada, 2008).

Addressing Root Causes of Health Issues

For many people, health issues keep reoccurring until the underlying root causes of those health issues are addressed. The **root cause of a health issue** is the identified reason for the presence of that health issue—the origin of the existing problem. It is the important underlying cause that is discovered when the nurse digs deep while in conversation during the physical assessments, and it is a very important starting point for creating health-promoting change for clients. When considering health-promoting activities, it is important for the nurse to step back and consider the context in which her or his client lives, works, and plays and consider from a broad viewpoint what other factors might be affecting that client's health.

The Canadian Nurses Association (CNA) recognizes that personal health practices are not the only predictors of whether individuals stay healthy or become ill. A person's life circumstances have at least as much influence on health status as do personal health behaviours (CNA, 2009). Nurses must therefore ask themselves, How are my clients' lives, personal coping skills and health behaviours, social support networks, income and social status, work and working conditions, social environments, education, physical environments, gender, or culture affecting their health? These social determinants of health affect health to a great degree; indeed, one author conducting an in-depth analysis of the literature on risk factors for cardiac disease discovered that poverty is a key cause of cardiovascular disease (Raphael, 2002).

When root causes or contributing factors of particular diseases or conditions are discovered, opportunities arise for nurses to partner more effectively with individuals to effect health-promoting change in their lives. Often, multiple strategies are required, addressing not only the individual but also her or his living conditions and public policies, even including considerations for reorienting health services to better meet the needs of that community.

"Jason's Story," discussed earlier in the chapter (Federal, Provincial, and Territorial Advisory Committee on Population Health, 1999), shows the root causes of a leg infection for a young boy. Planning health-promoting strategies for Jason and his family necessitates a larger understanding of the context of Jason's life and the reasons behind the infected cut on his leg. Many social determinants of health are exemplified in Jason's story, including healthy child development, income and social status, work and working conditions, education (parental), and physical environments. An examination of particular social determinants of health in this case leads to the understanding that the root cause of Jason's health issue is the dangerous neighbourhood that he lives in because of the family's poverty. Therefore, following his discharge from hospital, admonishing Jason to be careful of falling when playing is insufficient to promote or protect his health.

It would be important for the nurse to explore what supervision Jason's parents can provide despite the mother's illness. If in exploring the situation the nurse discovers the father is not providing supervision because he is depressed (secondary to his unemployment), the nurse could initiate tertiary prevention interventions and refer the father to the appropriate resources. Assessing the need for a referral to employment insurance or social services for Jason's family may also be important, to ensure they have adequate resources for their basic living needs. They may be struggling to pay for rent and the healthful food that is essential to assist Jason's wound healing in addition to meeting his basic needs for healthy child development.

Nursing advocacy that includes mobilizing civic and community support to address the lack of safe playgrounds for children in this neighbourhood would be a starting place for creating changes to promote and protect the health of all the neighbourhood children. Overall, a commitment to health promotion principles that include empowerment, participation of individuals and their communities, a holistic emphasis on the whole person, intersectoral action, equity, and sustainability, along with the use of multiple strategies (Raphael, 2002), should guide nurses' actions.

Population Health Promotion Model

Population health promotion is the integration of population health concepts with the principles that guide action on health promotion (Vollman, 2008). The **Population Health Promotion (PHP) model** (Figure 2.1) explains the relationship

between population health and health promotion. It shows how a population health approach can be implemented through action on the full range of health determinants by using the multiple health promotion strategies outlined in the Ottawa Charter for Health Promotion.

When undertaking health promotion at any level, the answers to three questions are critical to guiding the actions to improve health. "On WHAT should we take action?" "HOW should we take action?" and "WITH WHOM should we act?" (Public Health Agency of Canada [PHAC], 2001). Population health approaches emphasize that action must be taken on the full range of determinants of health (the WHAT). The Ottawa Charter for Health Promotion calls for a comprehensive set of action strategies to bring about the necessary change (the HOW). Both documents establish that for health promotion change to be achieved, action must be taken at various levels within society (the WHO). To explain the details of the three dimensions in the model, the evidence on the range of health determinants can be used, as well as the Ottawa Charter for a description of comprehensive action strategies.

Nurses must consider the various levels within society in which health promotion action can be taken: the individual, family, community, structural or system, or society as a whole. For example, to promote the health of young people, nurses can help them develop a positive self-image, involve families in the education of their children, and ensure that schools are healthful environments in the community (PHAC, 2001).

The following example is used to illustrate the complexity of many individuals' situations. Colleen works as a waitress and supports two young children on her own. She has been diagnosed with hypertension and placed on antihypertensive medications. Even though Colleen lives in government-subsidized housing, she does not have a drug plan through her employer—so when times are tough, she must decide between feeding her children and paying for her prescription. She places her children's needs before her own. Choosing the level for action (the WHO) to develop strategies for promoting Colleen's health therefore means going beyond teaching Colleen about the importance of taking antihypertensive medication every day (the WHO, at an individual level) to assessing what is attainable for her and determining what additional community resources can help her obtain her medication (the WHO, at a community or structural or system level).

The PHP model also exemplifies the need for evidence-based decision making to strengthen the development of population health promotion activities. Evidence-based decisions are required to ensure that policies and programs focus on the right issues, take effective action, and produce sound results. When compiling the evidence required, three sources should be consulted:

1. Research studies on health issues, their underlying factors, the interventions, and their impacts (both intended and unintended)

2. Experiential knowledge that has been gained through practice and synthesized in ways that can guide practice and policymaking

Population Health Promotion

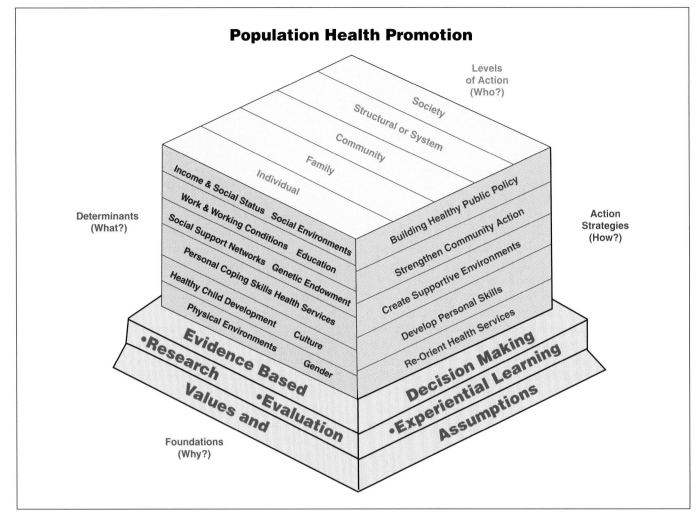

Figure 2.1 ● Population Health Promotion model.

Source: Revised by Larry Flynn, Manitoba Saskatchewan Region, HPB Health Canada, February 6, 1999. Original by Nancy Harrigan and Tarig Bhatti, Health Promotion Development Division, Health Canada, February 1996.

3. Evaluation studies (process and outcome) of policies, programs, and projects (PHAC, 2001)

When a nurse completes a comprehensive physical assessment, various determinants that affect the health of individual clients come to the forefront. By considering the WHAT, WHO, and HOW questions, the nurse can begin to formulate answers as a starting point for health promotion. Clearly, for health promotion to be long-lasting, simultaneous action must be taken at various levels, incorporating multiple determinants of health and several action strategies. By beginning with a thorough health history and comprehensive physical assessment of an individual, nurses can begin to construct a health promotion plan.

The following is an example case study and Health Promotion Assessment Tool that uses the Population Health Promotion model, identifying WHAT (in the Social Determinants of Health column), WHO (in the Levels of Action column), and HOW (in the Action Strategies column).

The Assessment Tool gives examples of multilevel health promotion actions a nurse could implement after the health assessment of an individual.

Mr. Hanslow is admitted to hospital with newly diagnosed chronic obstructive pulmonary disease (COPD). During the assessment the nurse learns he has been a two-pack-a-day smoker for 30 years, but his wife and children are nonsmokers. He is a police officer and uses smoking to cope with stress. The nurse assesses how ready and willing Mr. Hanslow is to stop smoking, whether or not he believes he can quit, the success of any past attempts to quit, and what supports he has for quitting. As Mr. Hanslow cannot smoke in the hospital, the nurse can ensure he has cessation aids, such as a nicotine patch and nicotine replacement gum, prescribed during his hospitalization. These aids will help him through the initial stages of nicotine withdrawal. The nurse will also provide information on alternative ways of dealing with stress and a referral to a community stop-smoking class or support group.

Health Promotion Assessment Tool

Social Determinants of Health	Levels of Action	Action Strategies
Personal coping skills	Individual	**Develop personal skills** • Discuss factors that increase Mr. Hanslow's stress levels • Discuss Mr. Hanslow's response to triggers • Discuss alternatives to cigarette smoking, to alleviate stress
Social support networks	Family	**Create supportive environments** • Explore factors within the family dynamic that affect (either increase or decrease) Mr. Hanslow's smoking • Discuss strategies with Mr. Hanslow's family that support a non-smoking home environment
Work and working conditions	Community	**Strengthen community action** • Discuss with Mr. Hanslow's colleagues what steps need to be put into place in order to create a non-smoking work environment **Create supportive environments** • In partnership with Mr. Hanslow and his colleagues, plan what can be done to support him in his initiative to stop smoking at work
	Structural or system	**Build healthy public policy** • Discuss opportunities to create non-smoking work environments with Mr. Hanslow's employer

Upstream and Downstream Approaches to Promoting Individual and Community Health

As seen in the Health Promotion Assessment Tool, preventing illness (and injuries) is an important nursing function that makes a measurable difference in protecting individuals' health. Although nurses know prevention and promoting health are important, it can be challenging to give prevention priority if the primary nursing focus is treating illness and injury. To help advocate for the incorporation of prevention strategies into nursing practice, a story (adapted from McKinlay, 1994) is told of a village near the edge of a fast-flowing river. People were spotted floating in the river obviously in distress and in danger of drowning. The village people were compassionate and did their best to rescue the people in the water. Over time the number of people in distress increased, and in response, villagers were hired to save the people and sophisticated equipment was purchased to enable them to do this better and faster. They

even built and staffed a first response clinic near the water's edge to ensure expert medical assistance and all the latest technology was readily available to save lives.

Several nurses in the village puzzled over why they were constantly treating so many near-drownings, and so they went upstream to assess the situation and see what was happening. When they returned, they told the other villagers about the problems they saw upstream: an unsafe bridge over a waterfall, unsupervised children playing in the water, and boaters who did not wear lifejackets. They also discovered that the river looked safe but had a strong undertow. The nurses argued it would be logical for the village to put as much, or more, effort into preventing people from going over the waterfall as they did to saving them as they floated down the river. They worked together *with* clients they had saved to begin making the upstream changes. However, most of the downstream healthcare professionals were so busy saving lives that they could not find time to engage in the prevention efforts. They would say, "If I stop helping the ones who are drowning, they will all die."

This story's usefulness in advocating for prevention has resulted in primary and secondary health prevention and promotion efforts commonly being referred to as **upstream approaches**. Interventions focused on treatment and cures are often referred to as **downstream approaches**. Upstream efforts usually focus on improving an individual's well-being and addressing the root causes of problems they are experiencing. To address upstream issues, health prevention and promotion interventions in the Population Health Promotion model often extend beyond individual care and treatment to identifying what policies, programs, environmental changes, or services are required (Stamler & Yiu, 2008). For example, adding fluoride to drinking water is an upstream policy intervention that creates an environment supportive of healthy teeth for a whole community. Planning a nonsmoking environment at Mr. Hanslow's workplace is another example of an upstream policy intervention.

Primary, Secondary, and Tertiary Prevention

Primary Prevention

Primary prevention strategies are designed to prevent or reduce the risk of disease from occurring by improving or maintaining general health, boosting the immune system, or preventing injury (Stamler & Yiu, 2008).

Improving general health includes setting goals, such as maintaining healthful weights, quitting smoking, and living actively. To achieve these requires health promotion strategies that encourage people to make positive but often difficult lifestyle changes, difficult because people's behaviours are embedded in habits, culture, and even the structural design of communities. To obtain measurable population-wide results requires complex health promotion and prevention initiatives that include all five action strategies in the Ottawa Charter. This requirement has created an increased awareness of the broader determinants of health and has shifted the focus of nursing away from solely individual care (Edgington, Pimlott, & Cobban, 2009). Observable change at the population level may take one to two generations to complete. More immediate benefits, such as increased energy and vitality and improved mental health, are available to individuals who implement strategies to improve their own health and well-being. Nurses completing health assessments in either acute care or community settings are ideally situated to reinforce positive lifestyle habits and to develop plans with individuals to address risk factors. These health-promoting interventions are labelled opportunistic because they attempt to modify behaviour for a problem that may not be related to the initial reason for the health assessment (Hyman, 2006). Below are examples of a broad spectrum of primary prevention opportunities.

Well-balanced nutritional intake maintains body functions and provides energy for the activities of daily living. A healthful diet and a healthful weight are important to remaining in good physical shape and decreasing the probability of chronic disease. Intake of a less-than-optimal diet (especially one high

in saturated fat) has been established as a contributing factor in the development of atherosclerosis and cardiovascular disease risk (Emrich & Mazier, 2009). For infants and children a nutritious, balanced diet creates a foundation from which they can grow, develop, and learn. Canada's Food Guide (Health Canada, 2007) is an excellent tool to guide nurses when educating clients on how to achieve a well-balanced, healthful diet.

It is important to encourage Canadians to be physically active at all stages of life: 63% of adult Canadians and 50% of children and youth are not active enough to achieve the health benefits derived from physical activity (PHAC, 2003). One barrier to active living is the amount of time spent in front of a computer or television (Statistics Canada, 2007).

Cultivating mental health or wellness enhances individuals' quality of life. Stress, anxiety, depression, and other mental health problems can not only affect quality of life and alter sleep, eating, and physical activity patterns, but also affect relationships, employment, studies, and social activities. Suicide is the second-leading cause of death in Canadian youth ages 10 to 24, and seniors are at even greater risk for suicide because of isolation, loneliness, and illness (Halton Suicide Prevention Coalition, 2009). To achieve mental well-being it is important to get sufficient sleep, learn effective coping skills for stress and anxiety, develop a strong social support network, engage in regular physical activity, eat a well-balanced diet, and seek professional help if signs of depression or any other mental health problem becomes evident (PHAC, 2003).

Unsafe sexual practices can have lifelong health consequences, and receiving messages about practising safer sex is important at any age. Media and social marketing have increased the public's awareness of the risks of contracting human immunodeficiency virus (HIV). However, other sexually transmitted infections, such as gonorrhea, syphilis, and chlamydia, also create significant health concerns, which include pelvic inflammatory disease, cervicitis (inflammation of the cervix), female infertility, urinary tract infections, epididymitis (inflammation of the epididymis, a common infection in males), and orchitis (painful testicular inflammation). Primary prevention strategies include providing education, providing free condoms to vulnerable populations, such as sex trade workers, and ensuring condoms are accessible in public restrooms (Canadian Federation for Sexual Health, 2007).

Seasonal influenza viruses cause illness and deaths in vulnerable populations. The Public Health Agency of Canada (2009a) has publicized the potential risk of a global influenza pandemic that would create severe illness or cause death in populations outside of those typically affected by seasonal influenza (these would include young adults and otherwise healthy populations). Nurses should be role models and teach their clients best practices for preventing influenza, which include frequent handwashing, coughing and sneezing into a sleeve (not the hands), recognizing the signs and symptoms of influenza, and receiving an annual flu vaccine (PHAC, 2009a).

Preventing injury and reducing injury severity are other significant primary prevention activities. Injury prevention requires lifelong vigilance, though the risk factors and nature of injuries differ depending on age and developmental stage.

Prevention activities focus on safety and the quality of home, school, work, and play environments; safe transportation; quality supervision of children; and falls prevention for seniors (PHAC, 2009b).

The examples given of primary prevention opportunities for general health and well-being are not exhaustive. Other areas to consider are the following:

- Food safety
- Limited exposure of unprotected skin to the sun
- Air quality
- Safe driving practices
- Prevention of hearing loss
- Folic acid supplementation in pregnancy to prevent birth defects
- Preparation of families for an emergency
- Adverse effects of ingesting, inhaling, or injecting harmful substances, such as alcohol, tobacco, and illegal drugs

Immunization in Primary Prevention

Immunization is the process of protecting people from communicable diseases through injected or oral vaccines (PHAC, 2008). Vaccines contain a minute quantity of the disease that is either very weak or dead and cannot cause illness. Common vaccine-preventable diseases include diphtheria, measles, mumps, hepatitis B, and influenza. Vaccines act by boosting a person's immune system, and they create immunity by stimulating the production of antibodies specific to the disease. Immunization is an important, safe, and successful primary prevention strategy that prevents communicable disease, controls the spread of disease, and improves health. In Canada immunizations have been so effective that some common illnesses have been almost eradicated (PHAC, 2009c). Because of high vaccination rates, many other communicable diseases are now uncommon in Canada. When a high percentage of the population is immunized, it provides protection for others who are not immunized—this protection is called herd immunity. Some children are not immunized, for various reasons: a small number of children are immunosuppressed and cannot receive some live vaccines or may experience reduced efficacy from other vaccines; parents may perceive the risk of contracting the disease to be small and so do not think vaccination is necessary; some parents refuse based on religious reasons or an inaccurate belief that disease complications are a lower risk for their child than potential vaccination complications. These unimmunized children will benefit from herd immunity.

Nurses should encourage vaccinations and discourage dangerous practices, such as "chickenpox parties" (informally arranged with the intent to expose unvaccinated children to the varicella or chickenpox virus). Parents need to be aware that such diseases as chickenpox can carry secondary complications for children, such as acute cerebellar ataxia, encephalitis, pneumonia, septic shock, and in a small percentage of cases, death.

In 2007 Health Canada started funding human papilloma virus (HPV) immunization, which, combined with cervical screening, will reduce the risk of cervical cancer by 70% (PHAC, 2009d). HPV is contracted through sexual intercourse, and the HPV vaccination is currently recommended for girls before the onset of sexual activity.

Secondary Prevention

Secondary prevention focuses on early detection of disease or conditions in a particular population, with the goal of either achieving a cure or minimizing the severity of the disease. Early detection of disease is most commonly done through screening tests, which alert the healthcare provider of abnormalities that require further testing or early treatment (Stamler & Yiu, 2008). Examples of screening tests include colonoscopies, mammograms, Pap tests, testicular examinations, and examination of skin for melanoma.

Not all diseases are caught early enough to achieve a cure or prevent disability. Secondary prevention may also include early treatment to limit disability. This treatment occurs when a person already has a disease, and the secondary prevention goal is to minimize complications or halt progression of the disease. For example, foot injuries or infections related to poor circulation can become serious health issues for people with diabetes. Education regarding foot care, thorough examinations of the feet by a healthcare provider to detect early signs of poor circulation, and early treatment can provide many disability-free years for the person with diabetes (PHAC, 2008).

Prophylaxis is the use of chemoprophylaxic or immunoprophylaxis agents to prevent illness after exposure to a communicable disease. In the case of exposure to TB, children under 6 and people who are immunosuppressed are given prophylactic medication to treat TB even though they have no symptoms of the disease. When a new case of TB is diagnosed, the nursing role includes identifying vulnerable people in close contact with the infected person and ensuring they receive prophylaxis treatment (PHAC, 2010).

Passive disease-protection agents, such as immune serum globulin, contain antibodies needed to eliminate a pathogen. Rabies is a deadly virus usually transmitted to people through a bite from an infected animal. To prevent death, immunoglobulin with the required antibodies must be given before the infected person begins to show signs and symptoms of the disease. The person is usually given an immediate injection in the area where the bite occurred and another six injections over the following 28 days (PHAC, 2010).

Tertiary Prevention

Tertiary prevention occurs later in a disease process and focuses on reducing loss of function, maximizing health, and minimizing disability (Stamler & Yiu, 2008). The nurse's role in tertiary prevention includes identifying potential complications and implementing strategies that help the person adapt while considering the person's strengths, vulnerabilities, and preferences. Strategies include providing education, monitoring treatment effectiveness, and addressing adverse side effects.

Direct observation and treatment (DOTS) is a tertiary prevention method that involves monitoring medication compliance to treat diseases, such as TB. The tertiary prevention goal for TB is to achieve a cure as quickly as possible (WHO, 2010a). DOTS is necessary because a person with TB may stop taking the medications because he or she feels well and the medications have side effects, such as nausea, vomiting, loss of appetite, jaundice, and blurred vision. However, the person has not yet been cured and remains contagious (PHAC, 2010).

APPLICATIONS OF HEALTH PROMOTION TO INDIVIDUAL HEALTH

Health Promotion Opportunities Across the Lifespan

Preconception

Women in childbearing years should be aware that if they are fit and healthy before conception, it increases the probability of healthy deliveries and healthy babies. As well, to reduce the risk of a baby developing neural tube defects, women should take a folic acid supplement daily for a minimum of three months before conception. In Canada approximately 40% of pregnancies are unplanned; therefore, all sexually active women in their childbearing years should take folic acid in case an unplanned pregnancy occurs (Darroch, Singh, & Frost, 2001).

Over the past 30 years in Canada a woman's average age at the birth of her first child has been increasing, and this trend is predicted to continue. Women and men who are planning to have a child should be provided with information on the advantages of reproduction before women are 35 and the increased genetic risks as they age (Best Start, 2007).

Pregnancy and Postpartum

During pregnancy babies experience numerous critical growth and developmental milestones, which are affected by maternal health and lifestyle. Many pregnant women are motivated to protect their infants from conception until delivery; therefore, this is an opportune time to deliver health promotion messages that benefit the baby. Maternal education is optimally received when the message communicates value for both mother and baby, which increases the likelihood that the pregnant woman will continue the healthy behaviour after delivery.

Smoking during pregnancy doubles the risk of having a low-birth-weight infant, and smoking during pregnancy is also linked to ectopic pregnancy and placental complications (Martin, Hamilton, Sutton, Ventura, Menacker, & Munson, 2003; U.S. Department of Health and Human Services, Centers for Disease Control and Prevention, & National Center for Chronic Disease Prevention and Health Promotion, 2004). Babies born to women who smoke during pregnancy are three times more likely to die from sudden infant death syndrome (DiFranza & Lew, 1995). Fetal exposure to tobacco places the baby at risk for learning difficulties, ear infections, upper respiratory tract infections, and breathing problems (Health Canada, 2008a). The less a pregnant woman smokes, the greater the likelihood of her successfully delivering a healthy full-term newborn. Pregnant women who smoke may lack the self-efficacy to quit on their own or may not fully comprehend the health risks associated with smoking. The most successful smoking cessation interventions focus on the benefits of eliminating or significantly reducing tobacco use rather than on the harmful effects of continuation.

Infants

Breast milk is the best source of nutrients for babies and for the first six months of life is recommended as the sole source of food and drink. Breastfeeding provides the infant with antibodies and immune factors that help protect against respiratory tract and gastrointestinal infections, decreases the likelihood of developing allergies, and assists with mother-baby bonding. Nurses should inform mothers of the advantages of breastfeeding but should communicate this message in a nonjudgmental way that allows a new mother to feel comfortable sharing an intention to bottle feed instead. When the mother is resolute in her desire to bottle feed, it is more advantageous to provide information related to safe and nutritious bottle feeding and how to facilitate bonding by holding the baby while bottle feeding than it is to use the small amount of teaching time available to try to convince the mother to breastfeed (College of Family Physicians of Canada, 2004).

New parents should be given coping strategies to use when their baby is not easily comforted. This knowledge may help prevent injuries, such as shaken baby syndrome. Parents should also be taught prevention strategies, such as getting adequate rest by sleeping when their baby sleeps and requesting support from family and neighbours to give the parents occasional breaks. Parents should also be provided with information on resources and supports they can access if their stress levels are high and they are concerned they might hurt their infant. Parents need to understand that although feeling frustrated with their baby is normal, intentionally harming an infant or a young child is not and is considered a criminal offence (PHAC, 2002).

Other important health promotion messages for infants' parents include the following:

- Injury risk information, including transportation safety issues and the use of approved five-point harness car seats
- The importance of creating stimulating environments and adult-infant interaction through play
- The message that babies cannot be spoiled
- The dangers of bed-sharing with a newborn
- Pet safety and babies
- The introduction of solid foods

Children

In May 2002 Canada participated in the United Nations General Assembly on Children. The results of this assembly are published in a declaration and plan of action entitled "A world fit for children" (United Nations General Assembly, 2002). Agreed-on international goals to improve the lives of children include promoting healthy lives; combating HIV/AIDS; providing quality education; protecting against abuse, exploitation, violence, and neglect; enabling social engagement and collaboration; and listening to and including children's perspectives.

For physical health, well-balanced diets and physical activity are fundamental to healthy growth and development, and to providing children with energy and vitality. The risk of childhood malnutrition and obesity increases with inactivity and diets that are low in fruits and vegetables. The Public Health Agency of Canada (2010) website reports that 20% of Canadian children are overweight, and children as young as eight or nine are being diagnosed with type 2 diabetes. Obese children have a high probability of becoming obese adults, and obese adults have an 80% greater risk of developing premature cardiac disease and type 2 diabetes, and a 40% greater risk of being diagnosed with cancer (WHO, 2010b).

Canada's Food Guide (Health Canada, 2007) is a good reference for health professionals and families. Depending on their age, children require two or three cups of milk per day and beyond that should satisfy thirst with water rather than with juice or soft drinks. Children have smaller stomachs and function better with healthful snacks between smaller meals, rather than ingesting three large meals per day.

Adolescents

Adolescents are gaining independence and making more of their own decisions; therefore, health promotion messages are primarily targeted at them rather than at their parents. Key messages must appeal to adolescents' interests to be effective. Effective strategies limit the number of messages, deliver them in clear affirmative statements, and avoid focusing on risks or what not to do (Health Canada, 2006a). An example is a message that promotes a well-balanced diet as the key to optimal performance in sport or academic achievement.

The Search Institute has completed research with more than 2.2 million young people to develop a list of 40 development assets that, if present or cultivated in a young person, will increase the probability of positive development for that person. Positive development is measured through such factors as school attendance and the avoidance of alcohol, tobacco, and drugs. Half of the assets the Search Institute has developed are internal, within the person (such as believing that he or she can make a difference for his or her own future), and half of the assets are external to the person (such as having a supportive nonparent adult to talk to). Research has confirmed that students attending schools that focus on promoting developmental assets rather than on reducing risk factors are more likely to thrive and less likely to engage in high-risk behaviour; they also have less absenteeism and lower rates of substance use, and engage in less violence (Search Institute, 2010).

Adolescent development includes a growing awareness and curiosity about their changing bodies and their sexual identity. Health promotion related to body image involves an awareness of warning signs in adolescents who are struggling with their body image and who may be eating unhealthful diets, over-exercising, or purging to remain slim. Education about safe sexual practices should include the concepts of valuing their own body and the bodies of others, mutually satisfying interpersonal relationships, and the prevention of unplanned pregnancy and sexually transmitted infections (Sex Information and Education Council of Canada, 2009). Saskatchewan researchers found that peer-led sexual education programs are effective, although teens also need the opportunity to explore their thoughts and ideas with a safe adult (Hampton, Fahlman, Goetzen, & Jeffery, 2005).

Nurses have many more opportunities to promote health with and for adolescents. Other examples of what a nurse might do include the following:

- Advocating for safe environments in which to socialize and engage in physical activity
- Advocating for affordable driver education programs available to adolescents from families of all income levels
- Encouraging adolescents to critically evaluate experimentation and participation in such activities as smoking or using drugs and alcohol, and deciding for themselves which activities will make them look smart and which will make them look stupid
- Partnering with a group of adolescents to look at the health needs of their school, and developing plans with them to address issues they are most concerned about
- Helping a group of adolescents develop and deliver an HPV vaccination promotional campaign
- Working with a school or community to establish a mentorship program in which older adolescents buddy with younger adolescents to help them feel a sense of belonging within their school or community
- Promoting a nonjudgmental environment and role-modelling acceptance of all adolescents—regardless of race, religion, gender, sexual orientation, choice of clothing, hair colour, body piercings, tattoos, and so on.

Adults

Research on the Canadian workforce indicates many employed adults are at high risk of injury and stress (Health Canada, 2004). Every year work-related injury and disease kills nearly 1000 workers in Canada (Human Resources and Skills Development Canada, 2010). Even though Canada has laws, policies, and guidelines to protect workers from hazards and dangerous substances and uses processes to ensure compliance, nurses should incorporate "safety first" messages when interacting with workers. This message may be most important with workers who are self-employed, including farmers whose workplaces may not be monitored for safety risks.

Stress is common for adults who may be simultaneously engaged in working (or seeking work), parenting, caring for their aging parents, and volunteering in the community. Stress has been linked to cardiac disease, some bowel diseases, individual herpes outbreaks, and mental health problems (Health Canada, 2008b). Methods to reduce or manage stress include identifying the root cause of the stress, making a plan to address the cause, and learning stress management techniques. Stress prevention includes such strategies as making decisions (avoiding procrastination), eating a nutritious diet, and exercising. In a descriptive pilot study of long-haul truck drivers, Layne, Rogers, and Randolf (2009) found that many had common health concerns, such as back pain, hypertension, headaches, and arthritis, but most drivers waited until they were home to seek treatment. The research results indicate that any prevention actions nurses decide to implement must be accessible and convenient to those workers. This result is equally applicable for other working adult populations.

Obesity rates have increased dramatically over the past 25 years and have contributed to increased numbers of adults with hypertension, cardiovascular disease, type 2 diabetes, stroke, gallbladder disease, sleep apnea, cancer (colon, breast, endometrial), and depression (Chen, Jiang, & Mao, 2009; Health Canada, 2006b). When deciding WHAT to take action on and with WHOM to act, nurses must consider the root causes of the health issues they see. For example, one root cause includes the evolution toward an information-based society, which has resulted in more sedentary work environments and changes to eating patterns and leisure-time activities.

Diabetes is a serious health concern for adult Canadians. Hardest hit are Aboriginal Canadians, who may be three to five times as likely to develop diabetes as non-Aboriginals; consequently, Health Canada (2010) has developed an Aboriginal Diabetes Initiative. This initiative has included training more than 300 diabetes-prevention workers, who are responsible for developing culturally relevant prevention programs. Implemented primary prevention initiatives include setting up walking clubs, fitness classes, and collective kitchens and gardens. Other prevention initiatives include screening for early signs of diabetes, as well as education and support for those already diagnosed with diabetes.

Other prevention messages for adults include the following:

- Annual physical examinations, which include Pap tests for women (although some provincial guidelines are changing to less frequent Pap tests) and testicular exams for men
- Date rape, dating violence, and spousal abuse or intimate partner violence information and resources
- Responsible and moderate consumption of alcohol

Older Adults

Older adults are often portrayed in the media as avid gardeners or frail elderly, but these stereotypes do not capture the diversity of this age group or the health risks associated with aging. Increasing numbers of young older adults are living vibrant and productive lives with only minimal use of healthcare services. Elderly older adults are much more likely to require assistance and medical intervention to maintain their health and independence.

Staying active and remaining involved in the community are protective factors for older adults. However, the biggest barriers to staying active are often inadequate income and lack of transportation to events dedicated to helping older adults stay healthy. As a result older adults with limited incomes and who lack strong social support may become isolated. Isolation is also more common in the winter months when additional

barriers to participation related to cold weather, snow, and ice are present. Isolation may contribute to depression, which is common in this population and should be screened for. Community health nurses should include an assessment of mobility and transportation options to assist in making the best health promotion recommendations. Older adults who have mobility issues may be referred to meals-on-wheels to improve their diets and provide regular, brief social contact. Meals-on-wheels volunteers are also taught to call authorities if an older adult does not answer the door.

Many aging people require an increased number of medications to help maintain their health. Nurses should ask whether a family physician or pharmacist has reviewed all the medications an older adult is taking (including self-administered over-the-counter medications, such as Tylenol, herbs, vitamins, minerals, and laxatives) to ensure that they are compatible and used appropriately. Prescription medications can be bubble-packed for home administration to avoid confusion about which medications to take at certain times of the day. If an older adult is receiving home care services, the home care worker or nurse may put prescribed medications in weekly dispensers, with separate containers marked AM and PM.

Settings for Health Promotion and Prevention

Health promotion and prevention are core nursing values that are incorporated into nurses' roles and responsibilities in acute and long-term care, as well as in the community. It is anticipated that by the year 2020, the health system will recognize the impact that social determinants of health make to the health of individuals and populations and will involve registered nurses in important roles, providing primary healthcare services (CNA, 2007). What follows are examples of how nurses are incorporating **health promotion across nursing settings**.

Acute Care Nursing

Hospitalization is an opportune time to conduct a health promotion assessment and develop a plan to improve a client's long-term health outcome. The majority of admissions are related to a health issue or injury; therefore, much of the health promotion work is downstream or tertiary. However, all clients should be asked about their tobacco use and offered health promotion strategies to quit, whether or not it directly relates to their reason for admission. Health promotion in acute care begins with the assessment of the patient's situation, including protective factors and risk factors. Nurses contribute knowledge of behavioural change theories, ideas, and strategies that support the development of a person's resiliency and an understanding of available community resources the patient may access after discharge. The patient and nurse can develop a health promotion plan together. Health promotion interventions are more likely to succeed if the nurse introduces several strategies and does not expect that education alone will change behaviour. In some situations education without strategies and resources to achieve a more healthful lifestyle may induce a sense of guilt in the patient, which subsequently increases the patient's anxiety level.

Emergency Nursing

Many clients receiving care in the emergency room (ER) have very few interactions with healthcare professionals other than the occasional visit to emergency. Therefore, the ER nurse is in an ideal position to screen for factors that place the person's health and well-being at risk and to promote healthful lifestyles.

ER nurses also compare injuries to the explanation provided for how the injury occurred, and suspected abuse is reported for further investigation. It is important that the nurse has privacy with the patient when asking questions about abuse. The reactions to questions about the possibility an adult's injury may have resulted from abuse range from gratefulness that their situation has been recognized and documented to denial and anger. Regardless of the patient's reaction, before the person leaves the ER, the nurse should offer information on prevention and community supports.

Telehealth Nursing

Telehealth nurses usually use logarithm programs to guide their responses. Some logarithm programs provide cues or a flow chart of appropriate health promotion or prevention interventions. If the problem-based logarithm does not provide preventive strategies, the telehealth nurse can begin a second intervention logarithm by using a prevention term appropriate to the situation. An example is that if a toddler has a hematoma secondary to a fall from an open window, the nurse will initially address the injury and subsequently address the safety issues related to active toddlers.

Public Health and Community Health Nursing

Public health nurses (PHN) and community health nurses have health promotion and prevention as the core areas of their practice. They use their competencies in practice areas that include prenatal classes, postpartum and new baby assessments, communicable disease control, childhood immunizations, school health, community development, older adult surveillance, and influenza immunization clinics. PHNs are integral members of the communities they work in; therefore, they are often informed of community health issues or needs by community members. PHNs may be involved in health prevention and promotion partnering with populations found in diverse settings, such as schools, seniors' homes, and community centres. They may work with small groups when teaching prenatal classes or work with individuals through new baby home visits and immunization clinics. Their work ideally positions PHNs to mobilize community resources to address current and relevant concerns of individuals.

Home Care Nursing

Home care nurses primarily provide care in ill clients' homes, which gives the nurses additional situational health assessment information, with resulting additional health promotion possibilities. A common health promotion opportunity arises with the recognition of early signs of caregiver (often a family member) burnout, and nurses can provide supports to assist caregivers to look after themselves as well as their ill family member.

Population Health Nursing

Population health nurses work in health promotion and prevention departments and look for healthcare trends and needs in population groups defined by age, gender, or location. Areas of focus can include decreasing the percentage of low-birth-weight infants in a city or province, increasing bike helmet use, increasing political awareness regarding the impact of the rising cost of living on the health of low-income older adults, or improving dental health in new immigrants. Population-based health promotion interventions include developing social marketing campaigns, such as bus or television ads, lobbying for by-law changes on smoking in public places, and advocating for increases in affordable housing—an important strategy to improve the health of low-income people.

APPLICATION THROUGH CRITICAL THINKING

CASE STUDY

Gina Clark is a 22-year-old woman who is overweight, does not exercise, and has unhealthful eating habits. She has come to see the nurse because she feels that her weight is interfering with her social life and harming her self-esteem. Gina wants to develop more healthful eating and exercising habits, but she explains that she has experienced difficulty because of her lack of coping skills and her low self-esteem, which together perpetuate the "vicious cycle" she describes herself as being in. Previous unsuccessful attempts to become healthier have led her to feel hopeless about making the changes she wants. However, the nurse knows that patterns of health behaviours are strongly shaped by the social and economic environments in which people live (Raphael, 2002).

Solutions to Gina's eating habits and health therefore will be as complex as the underlying root causes of her obesity. For example, in addition to her personal food choices, several other factors are equally important in determining her eating behaviour (Raine, 2005) and are essential for the nurse to consider when planning teaching strategies:

- Ease of access to healthful food
- Food advertising and marketing strategies that promote lower-cost junk food
- Family and peer eating habits and Gina's socialization

- A physical environment that normalizes junk food consumption (i.e., junk food is often more visible and widely available than healthful food choices)

In addition, to promote and develop strategies that encourage more healthful eating for Gina, the nurse knows that it is important for Gina to understand the connections between food and mental health, as a person's psychological state affects what and how much that person eats (Polivy & Herman, 2005). Consider this statement: "Food and eating also have social, cultural and symbolic functions; food and feeding can signify a sense of belonging, caring and community" (Raine, 2005, p. S11). This statement shows the significance of food and that eating habits are highly contextual, extending well beyond individual food choices. Therefore, to help Gina, the nurse will explore the role food plays in Gina's life (i.e., providing comfort or stress relief) and, together with Gina, brainstorm alternative ways of meeting these needs.

▶ Critical Thinking Questions

1. Describe the importance of assessing the social determinants of health in comprehensive health assessment.
2. Which social determinants of health would be relevant to consider when developing strategies to promote Gina's health?
3. Which level of prevention would a nurse be working toward in addressing healthy weight loss for Gina?
4. Describe three actions a nurse might take to address Gina's issues at an individual or community level, using the Population Health Promotion model action strategies.

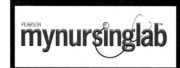

Visit the MyNursingLab website at **http://www.pearsoned.ca/mynursinglab**. This online homework and tutorial system puts you in control of your own learning with study and practice tools directly correlated to this chapter's content.

3

HEALTH ASSESSMENT ACROSS THE LIFESPAN

CHAPTER OBJECTIVES

On completion of this chapter, you will be able to

1. Identify the principles of growth and development.
2. Discuss theories of development.
3. Describe stages of development.
4. Identify a variety of measurements of growth and development across the lifespan.
5. Discuss growth and development in relation to health assessment.
6. Discuss factors that influence growth and development.

CHAPTER OUTLINE

KNOWLEDGE OF GROWTH AND DEVELOPMENT PROVIDES a framework for completing nursing assessment and planning effective nursing interventions. The focus of assessment is not on a specific aspect of an individual's health. Rather, nursing assessment requires the ability to interpret how the complex interactions of heredity, environment, and physiological, cognitive, and psychological development affect an individual at a particular time. By developing an image of what is usual or expected of people of various ages, the nurse has a basis for a comparison. This knowledge and an understanding of individual variations provide a foundation for assessment and appropriate nursing interventions that help individuals attain their maximum level of wellness.

Growth and development are dynamic processes that describe how people change over time. The two processes are interdependent and interrelated. **Growth** involves measurable physical change and increase in size. Indicators of growth include height, weight, bone size, and dentition. Growth is rapid during the prenatal, neonatal, infancy, and adolescent stages of life; slows during childhood; and is minimal during adulthood. **Development** is an orderly, progressive increase in the complexity of the total person. It involves the continual, irreversible, complex evolution of intelligence, personality, creativity, sociability, and morality. Development is continual throughout the life cycle as the individual progresses through stages in physiological maturation, cognitive development, and personality development.

The pattern of growth and development is consistent in all individuals; however, the rate of growth and development varies as a result of heredity and environmental factors. Heredity is a determinant of physical characteristics, such as stature, gender, and race. It may also play an important role in personality development as the determinant of temperament. Environmental factors affecting growth and development include nutrition, family, religion, climate, culture, school, community, and socioeconomic status.

PRINCIPLES OF GROWTH AND DEVELOPMENT

Four commonly accepted principles define the orderly, sequential progression of growth and development in all individuals:

1. Growth and development proceed in a **cephalocaudal**, or head to toe, direction. An infant's head grows and becomes functional before the trunk or limbs. A baby's hands are able to grasp before the legs and feet are used purposefully.

2. Growth and development occur in a proximodistal (proximal to distal) direction, or from the centre of the body outward. A child gains the ability to use the hand as a whole before being able to control individual fingers.

3. Development proceeds from simple to complex or from the general to specific. To accomplish an integrated act, such as putting something in the mouth, the infant must first learn to reach out to the object, grasp it, move it to the open mouth, and insert it.

4. Differentiated development begins with a generalized response and progresses to a skilled specific response. An infant responds to stimuli with the entire body. An older child responds to specific stimuli with happiness, anger, or fear.

Although the classic theories of human development provide the foundation for nursing assessment, researchers are continually evolving developmental theories that further define and explain human behaviour. Additionally, interpretation of the classic theories broadens as societal changes and advances in technology redefine individuals' relationships, expectations, and goals. Behaviour that is widely accepted or even the norm today was often considered unusual or abnormal a generation ago. For instance, the family unit is no longer assumed to be two parents with children but may now consist of a single parent, stepsiblings, half-siblings, a surrogate mother, same-sex parents, or other configurations. What are the implications for development? Researchers also study innovations in technology. Children are bombarded with stimuli through television and digital media, and they interact extensively with video games and computers. How do these affect the development of interpersonal skills? Advances in healthcare knowledge and technology have increased life expectancy, thus prolonging the span of productive years. This increase profoundly affects development, which continues until the individual dies.

THEORIES OF DEVELOPMENT

Three of the most influential classic theories of development are discussed here to provide a basic framework for nursing assessment. Although no one theory encompasses all aspects of human development, each is valuable as a framework for understanding, predicting, or guiding behaviour.

Cognitive Theory

Cognitive theory explores how people learn to think, reason, and use language. Jean Piaget theorized that cognitive development is an orderly, sequential process that occurs in four stages in the growing child. Each stage demonstrates a new way of thinking and behaving. Piaget believed that a child's thinking develops progressively from simple reflex behaviour into complex, logical, and abstract thought. All children move through the same stages, in the same order, with each stage providing the foundation for the next. At each stage, the child views the world in increasingly complex terms. Piaget's stages of cognitive development are summarized below and discussed in more detail with each specific developmental stage later in this chapter.

Stage 1, sensorimotor (birth to 2 years): The infant progresses from responding primarily through reflexes to purposeful movement and organized activity. *Object permanence* (the knowledge that objects continue to exist when not seen) and object recognition are attained.

Stage 2, preoperational skills (2 to 7 years): Highly egocentric, the child is able to view the world only from an individual perspective. The new ability to use mental symbols develops. The child's thinking now incorporates past events and anticipations of the future.

Stage 3, concrete operations (7 to 11 years): During this period, the child develops symbolic functioning. Symbolic functioning is the ability to make one thing represent a different thing that is not present. The child is able to consider another point of view. Thinking is more logical and systematic.

Stage 4, formal operations (11 to adulthood): The child uses rational thinking and deductive reasoning. Thinking in abstract terms is possible. The child is able to deal with hypothetical situations and make logical conclusions after reviewing evidence.

Psychoanalytic Theory

Sigmund Freud was an early theorist whose concepts of personality development provided the foundation for the development of many other theories. Freud believed that people are constantly adjusting to environmental changes and that this adjustment creates conflict between outside forces (environment) and inner forces (instincts). The type of conflict varies with an individual's developmental stage, and personality develops through conflict resolution.

Psychoanalytic theory defines the structure of personality as consisting of three parts: the id, the ego, and the superego. The personality at birth consists primarily of the *id*, which is the source of instinctive and unconscious urges. The *ego* is the seat of consciousness and mediates between the inner instinctual desires of the id and the outer world. The ego, a minor factor at birth, expands and gains mastery over the id. In addition, the ego is the receiving centre for the senses and forms the mechanisms of defence. The *superego* is the conscience of the personality, acting as a censor of thoughts, feelings, and behaviour. The superego begins to form after age 3 or 4 years.

According to Freud's theory, children pass through five stages of psychosexual development, with each phase blending into the next without clear separation. Individuals may become fixated at a particular stage if their needs are not met or if they are overindulged. Fixation implies a neurotic attachment and interferes with normal development.

1. The *oral phase* occurs during the first year of life when the mouth is the centre of pleasure. Sucking and swallowing give pleasure by relieving hunger and reducing tension.

2. The *anal phase* follows the oral phase and continues through about 3 years of age. The anus becomes the focus of gratification, and the functions of elimination take on new importance. Conflict occurs during the toilet-training process as the child is required to conform to societal expectations.

3. The *phallic phase* occurs during years 4 to 5 or 6, when the focus of pleasure shifts to the genital area. Conflict occurs as the child feels possessive toward the parent of the opposite sex and rivalry toward the parent of the same sex. These conflicts are referred to as the Oedipus and Electra complexes.

4. The *latency phase* occurs from 5 or 6 years of age to puberty. This is a time of relative quiet as previous conflicts are resolved and aggressiveness becomes latent. The child focuses energy on intellectual and physical pursuits and derives pleasure from peer and adult relationships and school.

5. The *genital stage* covers the period from puberty through adulthood. Sexual urges reawaken as hormonal influences stimulate sexual development. The individual focuses on finding mature love relationships outside the family.

Psychosocial Theory

Erik Erikson's psychosocial theory describes eight stages of ego development, but, unlike Freud, Erikson believed the ego is the conscious core of the personality. Erikson's **psychosocial theory** states that culture and society influence development across the entire lifespan. Erikson viewed life as a sequence of tasks that must be achieved, with each stage presenting a crisis that must be resolved. Each crisis may have a positive or negative outcome depending on environmental influences and the choices that the individual makes. Crisis resolution may be positive, incomplete, or negative. Task achievement and positive conflict resolution are supportive to the person's ego. Negative resolution adversely influences the individual's ability to achieve the next task.

Stage 1 (birth to 1 year) presents the crisis of trust versus mistrust. The child who develops trust develops hope and drive. Mistrust results in fear, withdrawal, and estrangement.

Stage 2 (1 to 2 years) is the crisis of autonomy versus shame and doubt. The child who achieves autonomy develops self-control and willpower. A negative resolution of the crisis results in self-doubt.

Stage 3 (2 to 6 years) challenges the child to develop initiative versus guilt. Initiative leads to purpose and direction, whereas guilt results in pessimism, lack of self-confidence, and feelings of unworthiness.

Stage 4 (6 to 12 years) is the crisis of industry versus inferiority. Industry results in the development of competency, creativity, and perseverance. Inferiority creates feelings of hopelessness and a sense of being mediocre or incompetent. Withdrawal from school and peers may result.

Stage 5 (12 to 18 years) presents the challenge of identity versus role diffusion. Achieving ego identity results in the ability to make a career choice and plan for the future. Role diffusion creates confusion, uncertainty, indecisiveness, and an inability to make a career choice.

Stage 6 (19 to 40 years) is the time of intimacy versus isolation. Successful resolution allows the individual to form an intimate relationship with another person. Isolation results in the development of impersonal relationships and the avoidance of career and lifestyle commitments.

Stage 7 (40 to 65 years) is the time of generativity versus stagnation. Positive crisis resolution results in creativity, productivity, and concern for others. Stagnation results in selfishness and lack of interests and commitments.

Stage 8 (65 years to death) is the time of integrity versus despair. Individuals conclude life, either appreciating the uniqueness of their lives and accepting death or feeling a sense of loss, despair, and contempt for others.

STAGES OF DEVELOPMENT

The most common and traditional approach used by developmental theorists to describe and classify human behaviour is according to chronological age. Theorists attempt to identify meaningful relationships in complex behaviours by reducing them to core problems, tasks, or accomplishments that occur during a defined age range or stage of life. Because theorists vary in their definitions of life stages, the following stages have been delineated to best illustrate the concepts of sequential development. It is important to remember that the ages are somewhat arbitrary. It is the sequence of growth, development, and observed behaviours that is meaningful during nursing assessment. For further information about infants and children, consult the Public Health Agency of Canada.

Infants

An **infant** is a baby from birth to 1 year. During infancy, change is dramatic and occurs rapidly. The totally dependent newborn is transformed into an active child with a unique personality, all within the first year of life. The infant rapidly becomes mobile, often displaying a new skill each day. The developmental tasks of infancy are (1) forming close relationships with primary caregivers and (2) interacting with and relating to the environment.

Physiological Growth and Development

Height, weight, and head circumference are the measurements used to monitor infant growth. At birth, most term infants weigh 2.5 to 4 kg (6.0 to 8.5 lb.). During the first few days of life, many infants lose up to 10% of their birth weight but usually regain it by 14 days of age. Infants gain weight at a rate of 140 to 200 g (5 to 7 oz.) weekly during the first 6 months. Weight gain occurs in spurts rather than in a steady, predictable manner, with birth weight usually doubled in 4 to 6 months and tripled by 1 year of age.

The average height of a normal term infant is 50 cm (20 in.) at birth. Height increases at a rate of about 2.5 cm (1 in.) a month during the first 6 months. An infant's height increases 50% during the first year of life.

Head circumference reflects growth of the skull and brain. At birth, the average term infant's head measures 35 cm (14 in.). Growth occurs at a monthly rate of 1.5 cm (0.5 in.) during the first 6 months, decreasing to 1 cm (0.4 in.) in the second 6 months. Ninety percent of head growth occurs during the first 2 years of life.

Dramatic changes occur within the organ systems of infants during the first year. The brain stem, which controls such functions as respiration, digestion, and heartbeat, is relatively well developed but lacks maturity at birth. As a result, these vital functions tend to be irregular during the early months of infancy, becoming regular with brain stem maturation by 1 year. The infant's nervous system is extremely immature at birth. Tremors of the extremities or chin are normal, reflecting immature myelinization. Much of the infant's physical behaviour is reflexive (see Chapter 25 ⬭). These reflexes, or infant automatisms, disappear as myelinization of the efferent pathways (nerves that carry impulses away from the brain or spinal cord) matures. Myelinization of the efferent nerve fibres follows the cephalocaudal and proximodistal principles discussed earlier.

At birth, the infant's heart lies in an almost horizontal position and is large in relation to body size. With growth, the heart gradually shifts to a more vertical position. Although the ventricles are of equal size at birth, by 2 months of age the left ventricle develops better muscularity than the right. As the heart grows larger and the left ventricle becomes stronger, the low systolic blood pressure seen in the newborn rises, and the rapid heart rate of infants becomes slower.

At birth, the lungs are filled with fluid, which is quickly eliminated and absorbed as the lungs fill with air. The full complement of conducting airways is present, and the airway branching pattern is complete. The airways increase in size and length as the infant grows. Alveoli and respiratory bronchioles continue to grow after birth. The infant's thoracic cage is relatively soft, allowing it to pull in during laboured breathing. Less tissue and cartilage in the trachea and bronchi also allow these structures to collapse more easily. Infants are obligatory nose breathers until 6 months of age. They gradually learn to breathe through their mouths by 3 or 4 months of age. Children use abdominal muscles more than thoracic muscles in respiration until 6 years of age.

Development of the eyes and visual acuity occurs rapidly during infancy. The inability of the infant to fixate consistently on an object, or not always being able to fixate the eyes together, is a result of immature eye muscles, which usually develop by 4 to 6 months of age. Infants see best at a distance of about 20 cm (7.5 in.) and have a visual acuity of about 20/150. Visual acuity rapidly develops to 20/40 by 2 years of age.

The ears and hearing are well developed at birth. The eustachian (auditory) tube, which connects the middle ear to the back of the throat in the nasopharynx, is shorter, wider, and more horizontal during infancy than during adult years. The size and position of the auditory tube gradually change with head growth.

Taste buds are present but immature at birth. Refined taste discrimination does not appear to develop until the infant is about 3 months old. Although the sense of smell is not refined in infancy, newborns are able to discriminate among distinctive odours and to recognize the smell of their mother's milk. The sense of touch is well developed at birth. Newborn infants show discriminating response to varied tactile stimuli.

Bone development, which begins before birth, continues during infancy. Ossification, the formation of bone, gradually occurs in the bony structures. Ossification is not complete until 14 years of age. While ossification is occurring, bones grow in length and width. Muscular growth occurs about twice as fast as that of bone from 5 months through 3 years. As muscle size increases, strength increases in response to appropriate stimulation.

Motor Development

Gross and fine motor skills develop in a predictable sequence, following the direction of maturation in the nervous system. Motor skill attainment in infancy provides milestones that mark normal development. Delay of early milestones may be an early indication of a developmental or neurological abnormality. Table 3.1 shows how gross and fine motor skills develop during infancy. The age of skill attainment is an average, with some infants acquiring the skill somewhat earlier, some later. The Denver II or Ages & Stages Questionnaire (ASQ) is often used to assess the development of infants and children up to 6 years of age (see Chapter 25 ∞).

TABLE 3.1	Motor Skill Development in Infancy	
AGE	**GROSS MOTOR SKILLS**	**FINE MOTOR SKILLS**
1 month	Lifts head unsteadily when prone. Turns head from side to side. "Stepping" reflex when held upright. Symmetrical Moro reflex (see Chapter 25).	Hands held in fists. Tight hand grasp. Head and eyes move together. Positive Babinski reflex (see Chapter 25).
2 months	Holds head erect in midposition. Turns from side to back. Can raise head and chest when prone.	Holds a toy placed in hand. Follows objects with eyes. Smiles.
3 months	Holds head erect and steady. Holds head at 45- to 90-degree angle when prone. Stepping reflex absent. Sits with rounded back with support. May turn from front to back.	Plays with fingers and hands. Able to place objects in mouth.
4 months	When prone, uses arms to support self at a 90-degree angle. Can turn from back to side and abdomen to back. Sits with support.	Spreads fingers to grasp. Hands held predominantly open. Brings hands to midline.
5 months	Head does not lag and back is straight when pulled to sitting position. Reaches for objects. Moro reflex disappearing. Rolls from back to abdomen.	Grasps objects with whole hand. Transfers object from hand to hand.
6 months	Sits briefly without support. May crawl on abdomen.	Bangs object held in hand. Can release an object from hand. Reaches, grasps, and carries object to mouth. Uses all fingers in apposition to thumb for grasping.
7 months	Sits briefly with arms forward for support. Bears weight when held in a standing position.	Uses tips of all fingers against the thumb. May grasp feet and suck on toes.
8 months	Sits well alone.	Uses index and middle fingers against the thumb to grasp.
9 months	Creeps and crawls. Pulls to standing position.	Uses pincer grasp (thumb and forefinger). Sucks, chews, and bites objects. Holds bottle and places it in mouth.
10 months	Stands, cruises (walks sideways holding onto something).	Can clap, wave, and bring hands together to play peekaboo.
11 months	Tries to walk alone.	Puts objects into container. Very precise pincer grasp.
12 months	Walks alone.	Positive Babinski reflex beginning to fade. Can hold a cup.

Language Development

Undifferentiated crying in early infancy communicates infants' needs. By 1 month of age, crying becomes differentiated as the pitch and intensity of the cry communicates various needs, such as hunger, discomfort, anger, or pain. Infants are cooing with pleasure by about 6 weeks and babbling by 4 months. They begin to imitate the sounds of others by 9 to 10 months, although infants do not necessarily understand the meaning of their sounds. By 1 year, most infants say two to five words with meaning.

Cognitive Development

According to Piaget, infants are in the sensorimotor phase of cognitive development, during which the infant changes from a primarily reflexive response to being able to organize sensorimotor activities in relation to the environment. At birth, the infant responds to the environment with automatic reflexes. From 1 to 4 months, the infant perceives events as centred on the body and objects as an extension of self. By 4 to 8 months, infants gradually acknowledge the external environment (see Figure 3.1). They begin to develop the notion of *object permanence,* the concept that objects and people continue to exist even though they are no longer in sight. The infant first learns to search for a partially hidden object but does not search for one completely out of sight. By 9 to 10 months, the infant learns to search behind a screen for an object if the infant saw it placed there.

Psychosocial Development

According to Freud's psychoanalytic theory of personality, the id is present at birth. The unconscious source of motive and desires, the id operates on the pleasure principle and strives for immediate gratification. Infants are egocentric and do not differentiate themselves from the outside world. The id motivates infants, and infants view the world as existing solely for their gratification. When gratification is delayed, the ego develops as infants begin to differentiate themselves from the environment.

Infants are in what Freud called the oral stage of psychosexual development until 12 months of age. Most of their

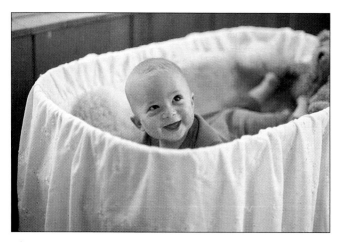

Figure 3.1 ● An infant begins to notice the external environment by the age of 4 to 8 months.

gratification is obtained from sucking nipples, hands, and objects, which satisfies the id's need for immediate gratification. Nonnutrient sucking on a pacifier, fingers, or a thumb helps satisfy infants' need for oral gratification.

Erikson believed that the quality of care infants receive during the early months determines the degree to which they learn to trust themselves, other people, and the world in general. Erikson defined the primary task of infancy as developing a sense of trust or a sense of mistrust. Trust develops as the infant's basic needs are met through sucking, feeding, warmth, comfort, sensory stimulation, and other activities that convey the sense of love and security. Basic trust versus mistrust is not resolved only during infancy but is also a component of each successive stage of development. A basically trusting child may later develop a sense of mistrust when lied to by someone the child respects. However, the foundation for all later psychosocial development is laid in infancy because, according to Erikson, the consistency and quality of the parent-infant interaction directly affect the infant's development of ego identity or self-concept.

All theorists of infant psychosocial development acknowledge the significance of the manner in which infants' needs are met. Although the concept of infant needs and the best way to meet them varies from theorist to theorist, it is clear that infants' needs extend beyond the physiological domain. Infants who lack sufficient social and cognitive stimulation exhibit signs of physical and affective imbalance. Children who receive adequate social and cognitive stimuli progress through sequentially more complex affective and social behaviours.

According to *attachment theory,* a focused, enduring relationship between the infant and the primary caregiver is imperative for the healthy attainment of infant goals and is a precursor for relating appropriately to others in the future. Occurring over months, attachment requires consistent, intimate interaction between the infant and primary caregiver. Many factors affect attachment. The infant and the primary caregiver each bring a unique temperament, personality, and style to the relationship. In addition, the primary caregiver's previous life experiences, preconceived expectations of the infant, and parenting experience influence the attachment process.

The quality of attachment depends on what is often referred to as the *goodness of fit* between the infant and primary caregiver: both the infant and the primary caregiver must receive positive feedback and evoke a positive response in the relationship for attachment to develop. The crying infant who quiets in response to being held by the primary caregiver makes the primary caregiver feel successful. The infant who is difficult to console gives negative feedback with continued crying, making the primary caregiver feel unsuccessful and perhaps unloved. The primary caregiver transmits anxiety about parenting abilities to the infant, increasing the crying. By smiling and cooing in response to the primary caregiver's vocalizations, the infant encourages the caregiver to continue vocalizations, providing the infant with environmental stimulation.

By 3 months, the infant and primary caregiver achieve social synchrony, which is apparent in reciprocal vocal and affective exchanges. This mutually satisfying synchrony signals the end of the early adjustment period. The next step in attachment occurs at 3 to 5 months when the infant develops a clear preference for primary caregivers. As memory for absent objects emerges between 7 and 9 months, the infant's preference for primary caregivers creates the reaction of stranger anxiety.

Throughout the first year of life, the infant's crying serves as the signal of the need for comfort. Research has shown that infants whose mothers respond promptly to their cries in the first months of life cry less at 1 year. It is now well accepted that responding promptly to infants' cries helps establish a sense of internal security that fosters later independence. Concern over spoiling infants by promptly responding to their cries is no longer an accepted concept. Chronically inconsistent nurturing of infants may result in infants and toddlers uninterested in exploring, even in the presence of the caregiver. Some such children appear unusually clingy; others appear actively angry and distrustful, ignoring or resisting caregivers' efforts to comfort them.

Assessment of Infants

Frequent assessments during the first year provide opportunities to monitor the infant's rate of growth and development, and to compare the infant with the norm for age. Height, weight, and head circumference measurements are plotted on an appropriate growth chart at each assessment. The three measurements should fall within two standard deviations of one another. More important, each measurement should follow the expected rate of growth, following the same percentile throughout infancy.

Accurate assessment combining information obtained by history, physical assessment, and knowledgeable observation allows early identification of common problems that may easily be resolved with early intervention. Often, basic parent education and support remedy problems that, left untreated, could result in significant health problems or disturbed parent-child interactions later.

Overnutrition and undernutrition are identified by weight that crosses percentiles. In *overnutrition,* the rate of weight gain is accelerated, and the rate of weight gain diminishes in *undernutrition.* Overnutrition may occur when caregivers do not learn to read infants' cues but instead assume that every cry signals hunger. Cultural beliefs that a fat baby is a healthy baby may also lead caregivers to overfeed infants.

Undernutrition may be caused by inadequate caloric intake resulting from lack of knowledge of normal infant feeding, a lack of financial resources to obtain formula, or inappropriate mixing of formula. Some quiet or passive infants do not demand feedings, and caregivers may misinterpret this passivity as lack of hunger.

Head growth that crosses percentiles requires evaluation as it may indicate *hydrocephalus* (enlargement of the head caused by inadequate drainage of cerebrospinal fluid). Early diagnosis and intervention for rapid head growth prevents or diminishes serious neurological sequelae (disorders caused by preceding disorders).

Parents and caregivers generally enjoy relaying infants' new developmental milestones and can accurately describe infants' abilities. An infant who seems to be lagging behind on milestones may not be receiving appropriate stimulation. Assessing caregivers' expectations and knowledge of infant development may reveal a knowledge deficit. Suggesting specific activities for caregivers to do with their infants may be the only intervention required. Infants who continue to lag behind and are not achieving normal milestones require evaluation.

Healthy attachment is observed when a caregiver holds the infant closely in a manner that encourages eye contact. The caregiver looks at the infant, smiles, talks, and interacts with the infant. The infant responds by fixing on the caregiver's face, smiling, and cooing. The caregiver stays close to the infant, providing support and reassurance during examinations or procedures.

Failure to engage the infant through eye contact, to talk, or to smile limits available opportunities for the caregiver to receive positive feedback from the infant. The infant, in turn, finds efforts to engage the parent frustrating, resulting in decreased attempts to interact. A negative pattern is quickly established, requiring more extensive intervention the longer it persists. The assessment of infants is thoroughly discussed in Chapter 25. ⚭

Toddlers

The **toddler** (1 to 3 years of age) is a busy, active explorer who recognizes no boundaries. Maturing muscles and developing language skills increase the toddler's ability to interact with the environment, allowing the child to gather information and learn with every experience. The major developmental tasks of being a toddler include the following:

- Differentiating the self from others
- Tolerating separation from primary caregivers
- Controlling body functions
- Acquiring verbal communication

Physiological Growth and Development

The rate of growth decreases during the second year. The expected weight gain is about 2.5 kg (5.5 lb.) between 1 and 2 years, and about 1 to 2 kg (2.5 to 4.5 lb.) between 2 and 3 years. The average 3-year-old child weighs about 15 kg (30 lb.).

Height growth is about 10 to 12 cm (4 to 5 in.) between 1 and 2 years, slowing to 6 to 8 cm (2.5 to 3.5 in.) between 2 and 3 years. Two-year-olds are approximately half of their adult size.

The head circumference of the toddler increases about 3 cm (1.25 in.) between the ages of 1 and 3 years. By 2 years the head is four fifths of the average adult size and the brain is 70% of the average adult size.

Alterations in the toddler's body proportions create striking changes in appearance as the child develops. Young toddlers appear chubby, with relatively short legs and large heads. After the second year, the toddler's head becomes better proportioned, and the extremities grow faster than the trunk. Young toddlers have pronounced *lordosis* (an inward curving of the back) and protruding abdomens. With growth and walking, the abdominal muscles gradually develop, and the abdomen flattens.

Neurological advances during the toddler years enable the toddler to progress developmentally. The increasing maturation of the brain contributes greatly to the child's emerging cognitive abilities. Myelinization in the spinal cord is almost complete by 2 years, corresponding to the increase in gross motor skills.

The toddler's cardiovascular system continues gradual growth. The gradual decrease in heart rate is related to the increasing size of the heart. The larger heart can pump blood more forcefully and efficiently. In addition, the toddler's capillaries constrict more efficiently to conserve body heat.

As the lungs grow, their volume and capacity for oxygenation also increase. This increased productivity of the lungs results in a decreased respiratory rate.

Visual acuity is close to 20/40 at 2 years and close to 20/30 by 3 years. Accommodation to near and far objects becomes fairly well developed in toddlers and continues with age. Taste and smell are well developed; taste and odour preferences and aversions are clearly communicated.

The toddler's changing body proportions are the direct result of musculoskeletal growth. Muscle grows faster than bone during the toddler years as muscle fibres increase in size and strength in response to increased use. Ossification slows after infancy but continues until maturation is complete. Long-shafted bones contain red marrow, which produces blood cells. The legs and feet of toddlers grow more rapidly than their trunks. The bowlegged appearance of young toddlers diminishes between 18 months and 2 years as the small-shafted bones rotate and gradually straighten the legs.

Motor Development

Gross and fine motor development continues at a rapid pace during the toddler years. The major accomplishments are listed below.

- *Fifteen months:* Walks independently, creeps upstairs, and is able to build a tower of two to three blocks.

- *Eighteen months:* Runs, climbs, pulls toys, and throws. Puts a block in large holes, scribbles, and builds a tower of four to five blocks.

- *Two years:* Tries to jump, and can walk up and down stairs. Can turn doorknobs, imitates a vertical stroke with crayon, uses a spoon without spilling, turns pages of a book, unbuttons a large button, and builds a tower of six to seven blocks.

- *Two and a half years:* Can stand on one foot for at least 1 second, can walk on tiptoe, jumps in place, goes up and down stairs by using alternating feet, and catches a ball with arms and body. Is able to make a tower of nine large blocks, likes to fill containers with objects, will take things apart, can take off some clothing, buttons a large button, twists caps off bottles, and places simple shapes in correct holes.

- *Three years:* Pedals a tricycle, jumps from a low step, is toilet trained, can undress, puts on own coat, and catches an object with both arms. Begins to use blunt scissors, strings large beads, can copy a circle, can help with simple household tasks, can wash and dry hands, and can pull pants up and down for toileting.

Language Development

Language skills develop rapidly, progressing from a few single words at 1 year to hundreds of words used in sentences by 3 years. At 1 year, children express entire thoughts by one word, saying, for instance, "out" to express "I want to go out." Simple phrases are characteristic of the speech of 2-year-olds, such as "go car." Although their speech is simple, these children understand most of what is said to them. By 3 years, sentences are more complex and include more parts of speech.

Cognitive Development

The toddler continues in Piaget's sensorimotor stage until the age of 2 years, when the preoperational stage begins. Object permanence is fully developed by 18 to 24 months. The toddler is then able to conduct a search in many places for objects hidden from sight. As object permanence develops, toddlers develop the understanding that they are separate from the environment.

By age 2 the toddler acquires mental representation: the ability to think of an external event without actually experiencing it. As a result, the toddler is now able to think through plans to reach a goal, rather than proceeding by trial and error.

With the preoperational stage, the child enters into the use of symbolic function. Instead of tying thoughts to the actual, the present, or the concrete, the child is able to think back to past events, think forward to anticipate the future, and think about what might be happening elsewhere in the present. Symbolic function enables the child to demonstrate delayed imitation: the child witnesses an event, forms a mental image of it, and later imitates it. In symbolic play, the child makes one object stand for something else, such as pretending that a laundry basket is a hat (see Figure 3.2).

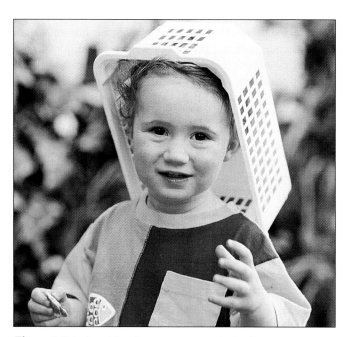

Figure 3.2 ● A toddler demonstrates symbolic play.

Psychosocial Development

According to Freud, the ego, which represents reason or common sense, continues to develop as the toddler experiences increased delays in gratification. The toddler years correspond to Freud's anal stage, during which the child takes great pleasure from expelling urine and, especially, feces. Toddlers may hold their stool, not wanting to give it up, or they may consider it a gift and object to its disposal. Toilet training takes on great significance as parents urge socially acceptable toileting while the child learns self-control and delayed gratification. Freud believed that the approach to toilet training and the child's reaction to it greatly influence the adult personality.

Toddlers' sense of trust developed during infancy leads them to a realization of their own sense of self. Realizing they have a will, they assert themselves in a quest for autonomy during Erikson's stage of autonomy versus shame and doubt. Parents are challenged to provide an environment in which toddlers may explore, while protecting them from danger and frustration above their level of tolerance. Parents provide a safe haven, with safe limits, from which the child can set out and discover the world and keep coming back to them for support.

Erikson believed that toddlers who are not provided with safe limits by adults develop a sense of shame or rage turned against themselves. Children who fail to develop a sense of autonomy, as a result of an overly controlling or permissive environment, may become compulsive about controlling themselves. Fear of losing self-control may inhibit their self-expression, make them doubt themselves, and make them feel ashamed.

Toddlers who have developed a firm attachment during infancy continue attachment behaviours during the toddler stage. Their repertoire of attachment behaviours becomes increasingly elaborate as they no longer seek prolonged body-to-body contact. Toddlers are sustained by only brief visual or physical contact with caregivers and can happily investigate new people and places. A secure attachment relationship in the first 2 years is characterized by the child's ability to seek and obtain comfort from familiar caregivers and by the child's willingness to explore and master the environment when supported by a caregiver's presence.

Assessment of Toddlers

Although the rate of growth of toddlers decreases, it proceeds in an expected manner. Height and weight continue to follow a percentile, although slight variations are often seen. Assessing caloric intake by obtaining a 24-hour recall gives clues to inappropriate feeding patterns. Toddlers generally feed themselves and begin to interact with the family at meals. A favourite food one week may be refused the next, causing frustration and confusion in caregivers. Concern for the toddler's health may precipitate a power struggle as parents try to force the toddler to eat. Poor weight gain may result as the toddler exerts a new-found independence by refusing to eat. Excessive weight gain occurs when caregivers use food to quiet or bribe their toddlers. Discussing appropriate eating expectations and weight gain helps parents resolve eating problems.

Since cooperation of the young toddler is unlikely, a health history is often the best way to assess development. Older toddlers are more willing to play with developmental testing materials or explore the environment while in proximity to a caregiver, enabling direct observations of development. Toddlers may not speak in a strange or threatening environment, making language assessment difficult. Listening to the child talk in a playroom or waiting room increases the probability of assessing the toddler's language.

The toddler wanders a short distance from a caregiver to explore, returning periodically to touch base. After receiving reassurance and encouragement, the child is ready for further exploration. Exploration provides learning opportunities but also places the toddler at risk for accidental injury or poisoning.

Tantrums are a frequent occurrence. They are the result of unwanted limits or frustration. An attitude of calm understanding limits the duration of tantrums and keeps tantrums from becoming power struggles or attention-getting behaviour.

Toddlers quickly turn to caregivers for comfort or when confronted with a stranger. Observing the adult-child interaction and listening to how the adult speaks to the child provides information on the quality of the relationship.

Continuous clinging of a toddler to a caregiver in a non-threatening situation is unusual. Failure of the child to look to a caregiver for comfort and support may indicate that trust did not develop during infancy. Inappropriate caregiver expectations, such as expecting a toddler to sit quietly in a chair, may interfere with the normal progression of the toddler's development. Caregiver inattention to the activities of the child and failure to set limits result in the child's inability to develop self-control.

Preschool Children

The busy, curious **preschooler** (3 to 5 years of age) has an appearance and proportions closer to those of adults. The preschooler's world expands as relationships include other children and adults in settings outside the home. Developmental tasks during the preschool period include the following:

- Identifying sex role
- Developing a conscience
- Developing a sense of initiative
- Interacting with others in socially acceptable ways
- Learning to use language for social interaction

Physiological Growth and Development

Preschoolers tend to grow more in height than weight and appear taller and thinner than toddlers. Weight gain is generally slow at a rate of about 2 kg (4.5 lb.) per year. The rate of height growth is about 7 cm (3 in.) per year.

The preschooler's brain reaches almost its adult size by 5 years. Myelinization of the central nervous system continues, resulting in refinement of movement. Most physiological systems continue to grow and are nearing maturity. Visual acuity remains approximately 20/30 throughout the preschool years. The musculoskeletal system continues to develop. Muscles are growing, and cartilage is changing to bone at a faster rate than previously. From 4 to 7 years, the active red bone marrow of earlier ages is gradually replaced by fatty tissue.

Motor Development

Gross and fine motor skills continue to be refined during the preschool years:

- *Three and a half years:* Skips on one foot, hops forward on both feet, kicks a large ball, and catches an object with hands. Cuts straight lines with scissors, manipulates large puzzle pieces into position, places small pegs in a pegboard, copies a circle, and unbuttons small buttons.
- *Four years:* Jumps well, hops forward on one foot, walks backward, and catches an object with one hand. Cuts around pictures with scissors, can copy a square, and can button small buttons.
- *Five years:* Can jump rope, and alternates feet to skip. May be able to print own name, copies a triangle, dresses without assistance, threads small beads on a string, and eats with a fork.

Language Development

Language becomes a tool for social interaction. As the preschooler's vocabulary increases, sentence structure becomes more complex, and the child becomes better able to understand another's point of view and share ideas. Speech should be 80% to 90% understandable by age 4. Sentences evolve from three or four words between 3 and 4 years, to six to eight words in grammatically correct sentences by 5 to 6 years.

Cognitive Development

Preschoolers are in the middle of Piaget's preoperational stage. Although symbolic thought is an immense milestone begun as a toddler, the preschooler's thinking continues to be rudimentary. Preschoolers continue to be egocentric and unable to see another's point of view. In addition, they feel no need to defend their point of view, because they assume that everyone else sees things as they do. Preschoolers demonstrate centration: they focus on one aspect of a situation and ignore others, leading to illogical reasoning. In addition, preschoolers believe that their wishes, thoughts, and gestures command the universe. The child believes that these "magical" powers of thought are the cause of all events.

Preschoolers enter Piaget's stage of intuitive thought at about 4 years. While egocentricity continues, older preschoolers are developing the ability to give reasons for their beliefs and actions and to form some concepts. They are limited by their inability to consider more than one idea at a time, making it impossible for them to make comparisons. Fantasy play begins to give way to play that imitates reality (see Figure 3.3).

Psychosocial Development

The superego, or conscience, develops as the preschooler becomes more aware of other people's interests, needs, and values. The child learns right from wrong, developing an understanding of the consequences of actions. At this stage, the child's conscience is rigid and often unrealistic. With maturity, the conscience becomes more realistic and flexible.

As preschoolers become further aware of their separateness, gender awareness develops. They learn what makes girls differ-

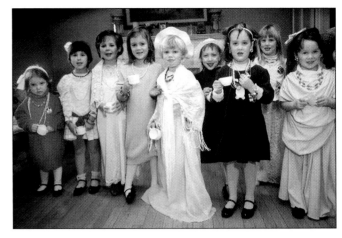

Figure 3.3 ● Preschoolers imitate reality in their play.

ent from boys during what Freud called the phallic phase. At this time, Freud believed that children have a romantic attraction to the parent of the opposite sex, making them rivals with their same-sex parent. The resulting fear and guilt are resolved as children identify with the same-sex parent, realizing they are unable to compete with the bigger, powerful parent. According to Freud, sexual urges are repressed, and the sex-related behaviours, attitudes, and beliefs of the same-sex parent are imitated.

Erikson believed that children's primary conflict at this stage is between initiative, which enables them to plan and carry out activities, and guilt over what they want to do. Their high level of energy, eagerness to try new things, and ability to work cooperatively characterize preschoolers. Children who are encouraged, reassured, and cheered on in their pursuits learn self-assertion, self-sufficiency, direction, and purpose. They develop initiative. Children who are ridiculed, punished, or prevented from accomplishing initiative develop guilt.

Preschoolers turn from a total attachment to their caregivers and begin to identify with them. A firm attachment during the early years allows preschoolers to detach from caregivers at this stage. This ability to detach enables children to explore new territory, learn new games, and form new relationships with peers.

Assessment of Preschool Children

Preschoolers' slowed rate of growth is often of concern to caregivers. The nurse can allay anxiety by showing the preschooler's growth chart and discussing eating expectations.

Preschoolers are generally pleasant, cooperative, and talkative. They continue to need the reassurance of a caregiver in view but do not need to return to the caregiver for comfort except in threatening situations. Talking with preschoolers about favourite activities allows the nurse to assess language ability, cognitive ability, and development. The nurse evaluates the child's use of language to express thoughts, sentence structure, and vocabulary. It may be possible to identify centration, magical thinking, and reality imitation as the child relays play activities. Lack of appropriate environmental stimulation may become evident, and the nurse may need to educate caregivers about age-appropriate activities for their children.

A clinging, frightened preschooler in a nonthreatening situation may be a child who lacks trust. Lack of communication between caregiver and child limits the child's ability to learn appropriate social interaction. In addition, the child does not have the opportunity to practise language skills or to obtain information by having questions answered. A thorough discussion of the assessment of children is found in Chapter 25 of this text. ∞

School-Age Children

School age begins about the age of 6 years, when deciduous teeth are shed, and ends with the onset of puberty at about 12 years. Tasks of the school-age child include the following:

- Mastering physical skills
- Building self-esteem and a positive self-concept
- Fitting in with a peer group
- Developing logical reasoning

Physiological Growth and Development

Most children during the years from 6 to 10 reach a relative plateau, with growth occurring in a slow but steady manner. The average child gains about 3 kg (6.5 lb.) and grows about 5 cm (2 in.) per year. Growth accelerates again at the onset of puberty, which occurs about age 10 for girls and age 12 for boys. During preadolescence (10 to 12 or 13 years), the growth of boys and girls differs. Growth in boys is generally slow and steady, and growth in girls is rapid. Growth is variable, especially among girls at this age. Some girls of 11 years look like children, while others are starting to look like adolescents. By 12 years, some boys are beginning their growth spurt and demonstrating the onset of secondary sexual characteristics.

The body proportions of the school-age child are different from those of the preschooler. Children often appear gangly and awkward because of their proportionately longer legs, diminishing body fat, and a lower centre of gravity. As increases in organ maturity and size occur, the child responds physiologically to illness in a more adult manner. The continuing maturation of the central nervous system (CNS) allows the child to perform increasingly complex gross and fine motor skills. Brain growth is slowed, with 95% of growth achieved by 9 years of age. Myelinization continues and is partly responsible for the transformation of the clumsy 6-year-old into the coordinated 12-year-old.

As cardiac growth continues, the diaphragm descends, allowing more room for cardiac action and respiratory expansion. The respiratory tissues achieve adult maturity, with lung capacity proportional to body size.

Most children achieve 20/20 vision by age 5 or 6 years. Visual maturity, including fully developed peripheral vision, is usually achieved by 6 or 7 years.

The most rapid growth during the school-age years occurs in the skeletal system. Ossification continues at a steady pace. Muscle mass gradually increases in size and strength, and the body appears leaner as baby fat decreases. As muscle tone increases, the loose movements, knock knees, and lordosis of early childhood disappear.

Motor Development

The gross motor skills of the 6- to 7-year-old are far better developed than fine motor coordination. Children of this age greatly enjoy gross motor activity, such as hopping, roller-skating, bike riding, running, and climbing. The child seems to be in perpetual motion. Balance and eye-hand coordination gradually improve. The 6-year-old is able to hammer, paste, tie shoes, and fasten clothes. Right- or left-hand dominance is firmly established by age 6. By age 7, the child's hands become steadier. Printing becomes smaller, and reversal of letters during writing is less common. Many children have sufficient finger coordination to begin music lessons.

Less restlessness is seen in 7- and 8-year-old children, although they retain their high energy level. Increased attention span and cognitive skills enhance their enjoyment of board games. Improved reaction time increases sports ability.

Children between 8 and 10 years of age gradually develop greater rhythm, smoothness, and gracefulness of movements. They are able to participate in physical activities that require more concentrated attention and effort. They have sufficient coordination to write rather than print words, and they may begin sewing, building models, and playing musical instruments.

Energy levels remain high in children between 10 and 12 years of age, but activity is well directed and controlled. Physical skills are almost equal to those of the adult. Manipulative skills are also comparable to the precision exhibited by adults. Complex, intricate, and rapid movements are mastered with practice.

Language Development

The school-age child uses appropriate sentence structure and continues to develop the ability to express thoughts in words. Comprehension of language continues to exceed the school-age child's ability of expression. Vocabulary increases as the child is exposed to a wider range of reading materials and ideas in school and through association with peers.

Cognitive Development

Sometime around 6 or 7 years of age, children become what Piaget called operational. They are now able to use symbols to carry out operations, or mental activities, enabling them to perform such activities as reading and using numbers. The child becomes able to serialize, that is, order objects according to size or weight. In addition, the child begins to understand how to classify objects by something they have in common. Children commonly practise this new skill by collecting and frequently sorting collections of rocks, sports cards, shells, or dolls (see Figure 3.4).

The school-age child develops an understanding of the principle of conservation, the ability to tell the difference between how things seem and how they really are. The child is able to see that transformation of shape or position does not change the mass or quantity of a substance. For instance, the child understands that two equal balls of clay remain equal when one ball is rolled into a cylindrical shape. In contrast, a younger child who has not mastered the principle of conservation believes the cylindrical shape is bigger because it is longer.

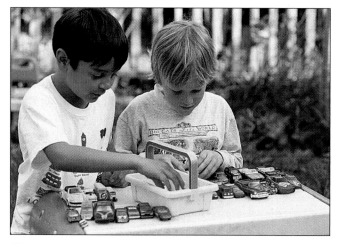

Figure 3.4 • School-age children enjoy classifying objects.

School-age children develop logical reasoning and understand cause-and-effect relationships. They can consider various sides of a situation and form a conclusion. Egocentrism decreases as the child becomes able to consider another's point of view. Although able to reason, the child is still somewhat limited by the inability to deal with abstract ideas.

Psychosocial Development

School-age children have accepted their sex roles and are now able to turn their energies to acquiring new facts, mastering skills, and learning cultural attitudes. Freud termed this the latency stage, considering it a time of relative sexual quiet. Curiosity about sex, and sexual and bathroom jokes demonstrate the ongoing sexual awareness of school-age children; however, the sexual turbulence of earlier and later stages is absent.

Erikson described the crises of this stage as industry versus inferiority. If children are motivated by activities that provide a sense of worth, they focus their attention on mastering skills in school, sports, the arts, and social interaction. Approval and recognition for their achievements result in feelings of confidence, competence, and industry. When children feel that they cannot meet the expectations of family or of society, they lose confidence, lack the drive to achieve, and develop feelings of inferiority and incompetence. The challenge of caregivers and teachers is to praise accomplishments and encourage skill development while avoiding criticism in areas in which children fail to excel. Providing successful experiences and positive reinforcement for children increases their opportunities to achieve.

Belonging to groups and being accepted by peers take on a new significance for school-age children. Children form clubs and gather in groups, often implementing strict rules or secret codes. They gradually become less self-centred and selfish as they learn to cooperate as part of a group. With this increased social exposure, children begin to question parental values and ideas. The family, however, remains the major influence on behaviour and decisions.

As children enter the late school-age or preadolescent years (10 to 12 or 13 years), the caregiver-child relationship becomes strained as children begin to drift away from the family. Preadolescent children increasingly challenge parental authority and reject family standards as they discover that the family is "not perfect and does not know everything." Identification with a peer group increases, and children form a close relationship with a best friend. Some children begin to show an interest in others of the opposite sex. Preadolescents continue to want and need some restrictions, because their immaturity makes determining their own rules too frightening.

Assessment of School-Age Children

The slow, steady growth and changing body proportions of school-age children make them appear thin and gangly. Assessing children's intake of nutrients and calories and reviewing their growth charts reassures parents that their children are not too thin. The nurse can relieve family stress resulting from parents pushing their children to eat by educating parents to evaluate objectively their children's diets during the early school-age years. Older school-age children have an increase in appetite as they enter the prepubertal growth spurt. During the growth spurt, height and weight increase and may normally cross percentiles.

School-age children are eager to talk about their hobbies, friends, school, and accomplishments. Increasing neurological maturity allows them to master activities requiring gross and fine motor control, such as playing sports, dancing, playing a musical instrument, following artistic pursuits, or building things. School-age children enjoy showing off newly acquired skills, and the family displays pride in their children's accomplishments.

School-age children frequently sort and classify collections of rocks, sports cards, dolls, coins, stamps, or almost anything. They are industrious in school, feeling pride in their accomplishments as they master difficult concepts and skills. The family provides positive feedback and encouragement to their children and speaks of their children's successes with pride.

Adult family members and school-age children communicate openly, with adults setting needed limits. Although peer relationships are becoming more important, the family remains the major influence during most of the school-age years. As children approach adolescence, the relationship with family may become strained as the children are drawn closer to peer groups and seek greater independence.

Children who lack hobbies or cannot think of any accomplishments may be environmentally deprived. Caregivers who are unable to think of anything positive to say about their children or who speak of them as a burden likely have a disturbed parent-child relationship. Children who lack encouragement and positive reinforcement at home for their achievements are at risk for gang recruitment. Gangs provide the "family" support children lack at home, increasing children's risk for violence, drug use, and illegal activity.

Problems in school may evolve at this time, with conflicts over grades and study time. The nurse can encourage the caregiver to help the child set a consistent place and time for homework. Caregivers should also be encouraged to communicate actively with the child's teacher. Teachers, adults, family members, and healthcare providers may identify learning disabilities at this time by careful observation.

Adolescents

Adolescence marks the transition from childhood to adulthood (12 to 19 or 20 years). Although all children undergo this transformation, passing through the stages of growth and development in a predictable sequence, the age and rate at which it occurs are highly variable. In a group of children of the same age, some look and act like children and some look and act like young adults. Adolescence is divided into three phases: early (12 to 14 years), middle (14 to 17 years), and late (17 to 21 years). The search for a unique self or identity is the foundation of the tasks of this stage. Tasks of this period include the following:

- Searching for identity
- Increasing independence from parents
- Forming close relationships with peers
- Developing analytic thinking
- Forming a value system
- Developing a sexual identity
- Choosing a career

Physiological Growth and Development

An increase in physical size is a universal event during puberty, with maximum growth occurring before the onset of discernible sexual development. Pubertal weight gain accounts for about 50% of an individual's ideal adult body weight. While the percentage of body fat increases in females during puberty, it decreases in adolescent males. Pubertal height growth accounts for 20% to 25% of final adult height. The growth spurt generally begins between the ages of 12 and 14 in girls, and between 12 and 16 in boys, and lasts 24 to 30 months. Girls experience their fastest rate of growth at about 12 years, gaining 4.5 kg (10 lb.) to 10.5 kg (23.5 lb.) and growing 5 cm (2 in.) to 11 cm (4.5 in.). Boys experience their fastest rate of growth at about 14 years, gaining 5.5 kg (12.5 lb.) to 13 kg (29 lb.) and growing 5.5 cm (2.25 in.) to 13 cm (5.25 in.).

During puberty, the period of maturation of the reproductive system, primary and secondary sexual characteristics develop in response to endocrine changes. Primary sexual development includes the changes that occur in the organs directly related to reproduction, such as the ovaries, uterus, breasts, penis, and testes. Secondary sexual development includes the changes that occur in other parts of the body in response to hormonal changes, such as development of facial and pubic hair, voice changes, and fat deposits. Some changes, such as increased activity in sebaceous and sweat glands, occur as early as 9.5 years of age in girls and at 10.5 years of age in boys. Further information about changes in secondary sex characteristics is included in Chapters 21 and 22 of this text. ⚭

Brain tissue appears to reach maturity with puberty, and myelinization continues until the middle adult years. Because growth of the cerebrum, cerebellum, and brain stem is essentially complete by the end of the 10th year, the central nervous system (CNS) does not experience substantial growth during the pubertal period.

A cardiac growth spurt occurs during the prepubertal growth period, increasing cardiac strength, elevating the blood pressure, and stabilizing the pulse at a lower rate. Cardiac output becomes more dependent on stroke volume than heart rate.

During the growth spurt, rapid growth of the hands and feet occurs first, then growth of the long bones of the arms and legs, followed by trunk growth. Skull and facial bones change proportions as the forehead becomes more prominent and the jawbones develop. The growth rate slows after the onset of the external signs of puberty as ossification slows, and the epiphyseal maturation (the fusing of the end of a long bone with the shaft, which halts bone growth) of the long bones occurs in response to hormonal influences. Since androgen influences bone density, the bones of males become more dense than those of females. Androgen also appears to be directly related to the significant increase in male muscle mass.

Cognitive Development

Adolescence corresponds to Piaget's stage of formal operations in which abstract thinking develops. Adolescents develop the ability to integrate past learning and present problems to plan for the future. They learn to use logic and solve problems by methodically analyzing each possibility. They use this new ability in scientific reasoning, and they create hypotheses and test them by setting up experiments. Analytic thinking extends to the adolescent's development of values. No longer content to accept what others say in an unquestioning manner, the adolescent can reason through inconsistencies and consider value options.

Psychosocial Development

According to Freud, sexual urges repressed during latency reawaken as adolescents enter the genital stage. Sexual gratification comes with finding a partner outside the family.

Erikson described the conflict of adolescence as ego identity versus role diffusion. Homogeneous cliques support adolescents through the difficult search for their identity. They become very concerned with their bodies, their appearances, and their abilities, avoiding anything that would make them appear different. According to Erikson, the intolerance of others outside the clique displayed by adolescents is a temporary defence against identity confusion.

Adolescents' search for identity is stressful for adolescents and their families. The peer group becomes even more important than during the school-age years, providing a sense of belonging. Peer group participation allows adolescents to develop comfort in social participation (see Figure 3.5). Peer group influence on clothing and hairstyles, beliefs, values, and actions may create tension between adolescents and their families. As personal identity evolves, adolescents begin to plan for a future career and prepare to enter adulthood.

Assessment of Adolescents

Caregivers rarely express concern that their adolescents are not eating. The pubertal growth spurt requires adolescents to increase their caloric intake dramatically, causing parents

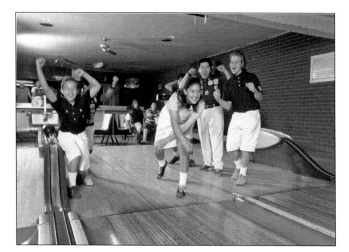

Figure 3.5 ● Peer group activity of adolescents.

concern that they eat constantly but never seem full. Adolescents (particularly women) are at risk for developing eating disorders; feelings surrounding changes in the body should be explored.

Adolescents often communicate better with peers and adults outside of the family than with family members. Assessing adolescents with their parents and then one-on-one affords a more complete picture of their relationship and provides adolescents with an opportunity to freely express themselves and discuss concerns.

Adolescents are able to hold an adult conversation and are often happy to discuss school, friends, activities, and plans for the future. They tend to be anxious about their bodies and the rapid changes occurring. Often adolescents are unsure if what is happening to them is normal, and they frequently express somatic complaints.

As adolescents become more independent, adult family members become anxious over their evolving lack of control. Parents may be uncomfortable with adolescents' sexuality, rebellious dress and hairstyles, and developing values, which may differ from those of the parents. Communication between parents and adolescents is often challenging at this stage.

Severely restricting the activities and freedom of adolescents inhibits their ability to progress toward independence. Adolescents who lack social contacts and tend to spend much time alone may be depressed and at high risk for suicide. Acting out and risk-taking behaviours place adolescents at risk for serious injury from accidents or drug or alcohol use. Alliance with gangs places adolescents at risk for violence and participation in illegal activities.

Young Adults

The **young adult** (21 to 40 years) establishes a new life on a chosen career path and in a lifestyle independent of parents. Tasks of this period include the following:

- Leaving the family home
- Establishing a career or vocation
- Choosing a mate and forming an intimate relationship
- Managing a household
- Establishing a social group
- Beginning a parenting role
- Developing a meaningful philosophy of life

Physiological Development

During young adulthood, the body reaches its maximum potential for growth and development, and all systems function at peak efficiency. Skeletal system growth is completed around 25 years of age, with the final fusion of the epiphyses of the long bones. The vertebral column continues to grow until about 30 years, adding perhaps 3 to 5 mm to an individual's height. Adult distribution of red bone marrow is achieved at about 25 years of age. Muscular efficiency reaches its peak performance between 20 and 30 years and declines at a variable rate thereafter.

Cognitive Development

According to Piaget, by young adulthood, cognitive structures have been completed. During the formal operations stage in adolescence, abstract thinking has been achieved. Formal operations characterize thinking throughout adulthood. Young adults continue to develop, however, as egocentrism diminishes and thinking evolves in a more realistic and objective manner.

Psychosocial Development

According to Erikson, the central task of young adults in their early 20s is intimacy versus isolation. During this stage, the young adult forms one or more intimate relationships. A secure self-identity must be established before a mutually satisfying and mature relationship can be formed with another person. The mature relationship requires the ability to establish mutual trust, cooperate with another, share feelings and goals, and completely accept the other person.

Other theorists believe that young adulthood consists of several stages. The 20s are generally accepted as the time of establishing oneself in adult society by choosing a mate, friends, an occupation, values, and a lifestyle. Around the age of 30, life is reassessed and the person either reaffirms past choices or deliberates changes. During the 30s, life again settles down, with the adult striving to build a better life in all aspects. It is a time of financial and emotional investment, and career advancement (see Figure 3.6).

The decision whether to have children usually is made sometime during the young adult years. The addition of children requires major role adjustment and causes readjustment in a couple's relationship.

Assessment of Young Adults

Young adults are busy, productive, and healthy. At their maximum physical potential, young adults actively pursue sports and physical fitness activities. They refine their creative talents and enjoy activities with peers.

Young adults form an intimate partnership with another in a mature, cooperative relationship. Traditionally, this intimate relationship involved marriage. Increasingly, the relationship is formed and maintained without a formal marriage between

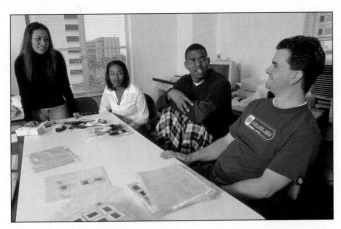

Figure 3.6 ● Young adults strive to advance their careers.

two people of the same or opposite sex. Developmentally, the important concept is the formation of the mature, intimate relationship.

People deciding to have children have many more choices than previously: surrogate motherhood, artificial insemination, in vitro fertilization, and other technological innovations. Deciding not to have children or delaying having children is increasingly accepted, as is the decision of single women to have children.

Young adults have chosen an occupation, established their values, and adopted a lifestyle. Career advancement, financial stability, and emotional investment characterize the young adult years.

The young adult without a steady job may lack direction and self-confidence. Marital discord can trigger feelings of failure and insecurity. Failing to achieve intimacy may place the young adult at risk for depression, alcoholism, or problematic drug use.

Middle-Aged Adults

Middle adulthood (40 to 65 years) signals a halfway point, with as many years behind an individual as potentially ahead. This is a time of evaluation and adjustment, and its tasks include the following:

- Accepting and adjusting to physical changes
- Reviewing and redirecting career goals
- Developing hobbies and leisure activities
- Adjusting to aging parents
- Coping with children leaving home

Physiological Development

Functioning of the CNS during the early years of middle adulthood is normally maintained at the same high level achieved in young adulthood. Some individuals may experience a gradual decline in mental or reflex functioning after age 50 because of changes in enzyme function, hormones, and motor and sensory functions. Decreased CNS integration may result in a slower, more prolonged, and more pronounced response to stressors.

Both men and women experience decreasing hormonal production during middle adulthood. During menopause, which usually occurs between ages 40 and 55, the ovaries decrease in size, and the uterus becomes smaller and firmer. Progesterone is not produced, and estrogen levels fall, resulting in the atrophy of the reproductive organs, vasomotor disturbances, and mood swings. Men experience a gradual decrease in testosterone, causing decreased sperm and semen production and less intense orgasms.

In individuals who become more sedentary over time, the heart begins to lose tone, and rate and rhythm changes become evident. Blood vessels lose elasticity and become thicker. Degeneration of cardiovascular tissues becomes a leading cause of death in individuals over age 45.

Lung tissues become thicker, stiffer, and less elastic with age, resulting in gradually decreased breathing capacity by age 55 or 60. Respiratory rates increase in response to decreasing pulmonary function.

Visual acuity declines, especially for near vision, and auditory acuity for high-frequency sounds decreases. Skin turgor, elasticity, and moisture decrease, resulting in wrinkles. Hair thins, and grey hair appears. Fatty tissue is redistributed in the abdominal area.

Bone mass decreases from age 40 until the end of middle adulthood. Calcium loss from bone tissues becomes pronounced in females. Muscle mass and strength are maintained in individuals who continue active muscle use. In those who lead a sedentary lifestyle, muscles decline in mass, structure, and strength. Muscle loss may also result from changes in collagen fibre, which becomes thicker and less elastic.

Cognitive Development

The middle adult's cognitive and intellectual abilities remain constant, continuing the abilities characteristic in Piaget's stage of formal operations. Memory and problem solving are maintained, and learning continues, often enhanced by increased motivation at this time of life. Life experiences tend to enhance cognitive abilities as the middle adult builds on past experiences.

Psychosocial Development

Erikson defined the developmental task of middle adulthood as generativity versus stagnation. He defined generativity as the concern for establishing and guiding the next generation. People turn from the self- and family-centred focus of young adulthood toward more altruistic activities, such as community involvement, charitable work, and political, social, and cultural endeavours. Erikson believed that stagnation results if the need for sharing, giving, and contributing to the growth of others is not met. Stagnation refers to feelings of boredom and emptiness, which lead individuals to become inactive, self-absorbed, self-indulgent, and chronic complainers.

Some theorists believe the middle adult years begin with a transition during which a major reassessment of life accomplishments occurs. Typically the middle adult asks the question, "What have I done with my life?" People confront reality, accept that they cannot meet some goals, and emerge with redirected goals. Reassessment involves areas of career, personal identity, and family. The middle adult may reorder career goals or choose a new career path. Adjusting in a positive manner to children leaving home helps parents to focus attention on other relationships, find satisfying leisure activities, or pursue intellectual activities (see Figure 3.7). Successful coping with the death of a parent helps people in middle adulthood come to terms with their own aging and death. Making financial plans and preparing for productive use of leisure time in retirement strengthen effective adaptation to retirement.

Assessment of Middle-Aged Adults

The adult in the middle years of life is satisfied with past accomplishments and involved in activities outside the family. Adjusting to the physical changes of aging, individuals develop appropriate leisure activities in preparation for an active retirement. Good financial planning during the middle adult years ensures financial security during retirement.

The middle adult years signal the end of childbearing and, most often, the end of child rearing. Individuals adjust to never having had children or to children leaving home. Couples renew their relationships or sometimes find they have little in common and separate. Some women choose to delay childbearing until their late 30s or early 40s, after establishing their careers. They begin their child-rearing years as many of their peers are completing this phase of life. Older mothers must make the transition from having careers to being mothers, even if they continue working.

The dissatisfied middle adult is unhappy with the past and expresses no hope for the future. Sedentary and isolated, the individual complains about life, avoids involvement, and fails to plan appropriately for retirement.

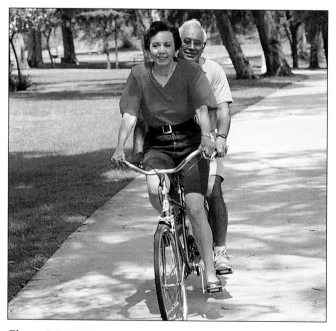

Figure 3.7 • Middle adults usually have more time to focus attention on their relationships.

Older Adults

Individuals in **older adulthood** (65 years and older) vary greatly in their physical and psychosocial adaptation to aging. Developmental tasks of older adults include the following:

- Adjusting to declining physical strength and health
- Forming relationships within a peer group
- Adjusting to retirement
- Developing postretirement activities that maintain self-worth and usefulness
- Adjusting to the death of spouse, family members, and friends
- Conducting a life review
- Preparing for death

Physiological Development

During the later years, people experience an inevitable decline in body functions. The body becomes less efficient in receiving, processing, and responding to stimuli. The CNS experiences a decrease in electrical activity, resulting in slowed or altered sensory reception and decreases in reaction time and movement.

The cardiovascular system demonstrates degenerative effects in old age. Fatty plaques are deposited in the lining of blood vessels, decreasing their ability to supply blood to tissues. Systolic blood pressure increases as a result of the inelasticity of the arteries and an increase in peripheral resistance. Endocardial thickening and hardening throughout the heart decrease the efficiency of its pumping action. The valves become more rigid and less pliable, leading to reduced filling and emptying abilities. Cardiac output and reserve diminish, resulting in an inability to react to sudden stress efficiently.

The efficiency of the lungs decreases with age, increasing the respiratory effort required to obtain adequate oxygen. Vital capacity decreases, and residual air increases with age. The bronchopulmonary tree becomes more rigid, reducing bronchopulmonary movements. Ciliary activity decreases, allowing mucus secretions to collect more readily in the respiratory tree. As a result of diminished muscle tone and decreased sensitivity to stimuli, the ability to cough decreases.

Visual changes include loss of visual acuity, decreased adaptation to darkness and dim light, loss of peripheral vision, and difficulty in discriminating similar colours. Gradual loss of hearing is the result of changes in nerve tissues in the inner ear and a thickening of the eardrum. The senses of taste and smell decrease, and older adults are less stimulated by food than before. The gradual loss of skin receptors increases the threshold for sensations of pain and touch in older adults.

Renal function is slowed by structural and functional changes associated with aging. Arteriosclerotic changes can reduce blood flow, impairing renal function. The kidney's filtering abilities become impaired as the number of functioning nephrons decreases with age. An enlarged prostate gland causes urinary urgency and frequency in men, and in women the same complaints are often due to weakened muscles supporting the bladder or weakness of the urethral sphincter. The capacity of the bladder and its ability to empty completely diminish with age in both men and women.

All bones are affected by a decrease in skeletal mass. Decreased density causes bones to become brittle and fracture more easily. Range of motion decreases as the tissues of the joints and bones stiffen.

Cognitive Development

Research continues into the effects of aging on cognitive abilities. Different kinds of cognitive functions seem to undergo different types, amounts, and rates of change in individual older adults. Functions dependent on perception rely on the acuity of the senses. When senses become impaired with aging, the ability to perceive the environment and react appropriately is diminished. Changes in the aging nervous system may also affect perceptual ability. Impaired perceptual ability diminishes the aging adult's cognitive capability.

Studies suggest that people who live in a varied environment that provides for continued use of intellectual function are often the ones who maintain or even strengthen these skills throughout life. Conversely, those who live in a static environment that lacks intellectual challenge may be the ones who most likely show some decline in intellectual ability with aging. Although learning and problem solving may not be as efficient in old age as in youth, both processes still occur to a greater extent than is often portrayed in stereotypes of older adults (see Figure 3.8).

Psychosocial Development

The developmental task of late adulthood, according to Erikson, is ego integrity versus self-despair. When a review of life events, experiences, and relationships makes the adult content with life, the person attains ego integrity. Failure to resolve this last developmental crisis results in a sense of despair, resentment, futility, hopelessness, and fear of death.

Late adulthood requires lifestyle changes and a review of life. The adult adjusting to retirement must develop new activities to replace work and the role of worker. New friendships are established with peers of similar interests, abilities, and means. The person may pursue projects or recreational activities deferred

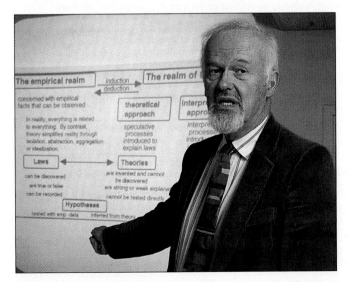

Figure 3.8 ● The ability to solve problems may be highly efficient in the older adult.

during the working years, but activities are limited to those compatible with the physical limitations of old age. Lack of adequate income limits the activities and lifestyle of many older adults; financial resources enable them to be independent and look after themselves.

The lifestyle of later years is, to a large degree, formulated in youth. The person who was once gregarious and spent time with people continues to do so, and the person who avoided involvement with others continues toward isolation. Those who learned early in life to live well-balanced and fulfilling lives are generally more successful in retirement. The later years can foster a sense of integrity and continuity, or they can be years of despair.

Through the late adult years, the deaths of friends, siblings, and partners occur with increasing frequency. Reminded of the limited time left, the older adult comes to terms with the past and views death as an acceptable completion of life.

Assessment of Older Adults

Well-adjusted older adults maintain an active lifestyle and involvement with others and often do not appear their age. Lifestyle changes occur in response to declining physical abilities and retirement. Participation in activities that promote the older adult's sense of self-worth and usefulness also provides opportunities for developing new friendships with others of similar abilities and interests. Intellectual function is maintained through continued intellectual pursuits. Content with their life review, older adults enjoy their retirement years and accept death as the inevitable end of a productive life.

The older adult who has not successfully resolved developmental crises may feel that life has been unfair. Despair and hopelessness may be evident in the individual's lack of activity and bitter complaining. A thorough discussion of the assessment of middle adults and older adults is found in Chapter 27 of this text. ◯◯

GROWTH AND DEVELOPMENT IN HEALTH ASSESSMENT
●●●

Health assessment includes gathering objective and subjective data, which are used to develop plans to maintain health or address health needs in clients of all ages. A comprehensive assessment includes data about physical, cognitive, and emotional growth and development. When conducting health assessments, the nurse must be able to obtain accurate data and interpret findings in relation to expectations and predicted norms and ranges for clients at various stages of physical and emotional development. Knowledge of anatomical and physiological changes and of theoretical information about cognitive, psychoanalytic, and psychosocial events and expectations at each stage of human development is invaluable for the nurse.

Physical growth and development change across the age span. Stages from infancy through adolescence are marked by spurts of rapid growth and development. Health assessment includes the use of clinical growth charts to index individual client measurements of height and weight (and head circumference in infants) as expected normal values for age and gender (see Chapter 25 ⬤). Additional indicators for normal growth and development throughout these stages are eating, sleeping, elimination, and activity patterns. Neurological and sensory functions are assessed by monitoring development of speech and language, muscular growth, strength and coordination, and tactile sensibility.

Puberty is a period of rapid physiological growth and development. It occurs between the ages of 10 and 14 years in females and is marked by menarche (the first menstruation), breast development, presence of pubic hair, and a spurt in height. In males, puberty occurs between the ages of 12 and 16 years and is characterized by a spurt in height, development of the penis and testicles, and presence of pubic hair. Young adulthood is the stage marked by completed growth in physical and mental structures. Physical development continues to be assessed by comparing individual findings with clinical growth charts and by assessing eating, sleeping, and activity patterns.

Middle age, occurring between the ages of 45 and 60 years, is another period in which dramatic changes in physical development occur. Primary changes are related to hormonal changes of the male and female climacteric (menopause). In addition, changes occur in all systems and include decreases in basal metabolic rate, muscle size, nerve conduction, lung capacity, glomerular filtration, and cardiac output. Adipose tissue deposit increases, skeletal changes lead to decreases in height, and changes in tactile sensibility, vision, and hearing occur. The physical changes continue into the stage of older adulthood. The middle and older adult is at risk for obesity and the health problems associated with it. Therefore, health assessment will include use of the body mass index (BMI) to assess weight and risk for disease. Information about calculation of BMI is included in Chapter 9 of this text. ⬤ In addition, assessment will include checking the ability to carry out activities of daily living (ADLs) and regular testing of vision and hearing.

In addition to expectations about physical growth and development, there are also expectations about cognitive, psychosocial, and emotional development across the age span. For example, attachment is an essential element in infant development. Attachment refers to the tie between the infant and caregivers that promotes physical and psychosocial well-being.

TABLE 3.2	**Instruments to Measure Growth and Development**
Ages & Stages Questionnaire (ASQ)	This parent-completed questionnaire covers developmental areas of communication, gross motor, fine motor, problem solving, and personal-social.
Battelle Developmental Inventory	It tests developmental domains of cognition, motor, self-help, language, and social skills in children from birth through 8 years of age.
Brigance Screens	The screens assess speech-language, motor, readiness, and general knowledge at younger ages and reading and math. Used from 21 to 90 months of age.
Eyberg Child Behavior Inventory (ECBI)	The ECBI is a parent report scale of conduct problem behaviours in children ages 2 to 16 years.
Family Psychosocial Screening	A clinic intake form identifies psychosocial risk factors associated with developmental problems, including parental history of physical abuse as a child, parental substance abuse, and maternal depression.
Hassles and Uplifts Scale	This measures adult attitudes about daily situations defined as "hassles" and "uplifts." It focuses on evaluation of positive and negative events in daily life rather than on life events.
Life Experiences Survey	This self-administered questionnaire reviews life-changing events of a given year. Ratings are used to evaluate the level of stress a person is experiencing.
McCarthy Scale of Children's Abilities	The McCarthy evaluates the general intelligence level of children ages 2.5 to 8.5 years. The scale identifies strengths and weaknesses in verbal, perceptual-performance, quantitative, memory, motor, and general cognitive skills.
Neonatal Behavioural Assessment Scale	The scale is used to assess newborns and infants up to 2 months of age. It measures 28 behavioural and 18 reflex items. It provides information about the baby's strengths, adaptive responses, and potential vulnerabilities.
Pediatric Symptom Checklist	This checklist of short statements identifies conduct behaviours and behaviours associated with depression, anxiety, and adjustment in children from 4 to 16 years of age. Item patterns determine the need for behavioural or mental health referrals.
Stanford-Binet Intelligence Scale: Fourth Edition	This test measures general intelligence. The areas of verbal reasoning, quantitative reasoning, abstract/visual reasoning, and short-term memory can be tested from age 2 to 23 years.
The Child Development Inventory	The scales measure social, self-help, gross motor, fine motor, expressive language, language comprehension, letters, numbers, and general development in children from 15 months to 6 years of age.
The Denver II	This test is administered to well children between birth and 6 years of age. The Denver II is designed to test 20 simple tasks and items in four sectors: personal-social, fine motor adaptive, language, gross motor.
The Mini-Mental Status Examination	This brief quantitative measure of cognitive status in adults can be used to screen for cognitive impairment, to estimate the severity of cognitive impairment at a given point in time, to follow the course of cognitive changes in an individual over time, and to document an individual's response to treatment.
Wechsler Preschool and Primary Scale of Intelligence—Revised (WPPSI-R)	This is a standardized test of language and perception for children ages 4.5 to 6 years.

Assessment of attachment includes observation of interactions between the infant and caregivers for eye contact, apparent interest in the child, talking or cooing to the child, response to infant needs, and communication. Children are expected to develop language and cognitive abilities that enable them to learn and, over time, become independent beings. Young adults are expected to develop relationships with others and to become productive members of society. Maturity and aging lead individuals to contribute to the well-being of communities and their families and often to adapt to change and loss. Developmental milestones and crises occur in all stages of development and must be assessed. A variety of instruments and scales can be used to identify developmental delays, behavioural patterns, and responses that indicate potential or actual problems with emotional, cognitive, and psychosocial development and adaptation in children and adults of all ages. Table 3.2 includes a list and description of some of the instruments available to measure aspects of growth and development.

Health assessment also includes reviewing the immunization history and ensuring that children are up-to-date. Be aware that not all parents consent to the immunization of their children. Routine schedules are included in Box 3.1.

FACTORS THAT INFLUENCE GROWTH AND DEVELOPMENT

Factors that influence growth and development include nutrition, family, culture, and socioeconomic status. The following discussion provides examples of ways in which these factors affect growth and development.

Nutrition

Nutrition is essential to physical and mental development. Growth patterns, in large part, are genetically determined. However, malnutrition can delay or prevent growth and development. Healthcare professionals routinely use measures of height and weight in comparison to clinical growth charts to identify slowed growth in children. Slowed growth is an early indicator of inadequate nutrition. The body is made up of

---

BOX 3.1   Routine Immunization Schedules

Table 1. Routine Immunization Schedule for Infants and Children

Age at vaccination	DTaP-IPV	Hib	MMR	Var	HB	Pneu-C-7	Men-C	Tdap	Inf
Birth					Infancy 3 doses ★				
2 months	⊙	✦				⊠	⊙		
4 months	⊙	✦				⊠	(⊙)		
6 months	⊙	✦				⊠	⊙ or ⊙		6-23 months ⊗ 1-2 doses
12 months			■	●	or	⊠ 12-15 months	if not yet given		
18 months	⊙	✦	■						
4-6 years	⊙		or ■						
14-16 years					Pre-teen/teen 2-3 doses		⊙ if not yet given	▲	

Table 2. Routine Immunization Schedule for Children < 7 Years of Age Not Immunized in Early Infancy

Timing	DTaP-IPV	Hib	MMR	Var	HB	Pneu-C-7	Men-C	Tdap
First visit	⊙	✦	■	●	★	⊠	⊙	
2 months later	⊙	(✦)	■		★	(⊠)	(⊙)	
2 months later	⊙					(⊠)		
6-12 months later	⊙	(✦)			★			
4-6 years of age	(⊙)							
14-16 years of age								▲

BOX 3.1 | Routine Immunization Schedules *(continued)*

Table 3. Routine Immunization Schedule for Children ≥ 7 Years of Age up to 17 Years of Age Not Immunized in Early Infancy

Timing	Tdap	IPV	MMR	Var	HB	Men-C
First visit	▲	♠	■	●	★	◉
2 months later	▲	♠	■	(●)	(★)	
6-12 months later	▲	♠			★	
10 years later	▲					

Table 4. Routine Immunization Schedule for Adults (≥ 18 Years of Age) Not Immunized in Childhood

Timing	Tdap	Td	MMR	Var	Men-C	Pneu-C-23	Inf
First visit	▲		■	●	(◉)		
2 months later		▯	(■)	●		(▣)	(✇)
6-12 months later		▯					
10 years later		▯					

Notes

( ) Symbols with brackets around them imply that these doses may not be required, depending upon the age of the child or adult. Refer to the relevant chapter [of the *Canadian Immunization Guide*] for that vaccine for further details.

◎ **Diphtheria, tetanus, acellular pertussis and inactivated polio virus vaccine (DTaP-IPV):** DTaP-IPV(± Hib) vaccine is the preferred vaccine for all doses in the vaccination series, including completion of the series in children who have received one or more doses of DPT (whole cell) vaccine (e.g., recent immigrants). In Tables 1 and 2, the 4–6 year dose can be omitted if the fourth dose was given after the fourth birthday.

✦ **Haemophilus influenzae type b conjugate vaccine (Hib):** the Hib schedule shown is for the *Haemophilus* b capsular polysaccharide–polyribosylribitol phosphate (PRP) conjugated to tetanus toxoid (PRP-T). For catch up, the number of doses depends on the age at which the schedule is begun (see *Haemophilus Vaccine* chapter [of the *Canadian Immunization Guide*]). Not usually required past age 5 years.

■ **Measles, mumps, and rubella vaccine (MMR):** a second dose of MMR is recommended for children at least 1 month after the first dose for the purpose of better measles protection. For convenience, options include giving it with the next scheduled vaccination at 18 months of age or at school entry (4–6 years) (depending on the provincial/territorial policy) or at any intervening age that is practical. In the catch-up schedule (Table 2), the first dose should not be given until the child is ≥12 months old. MMR should be given to all susceptible adolescents and adults.

● **Varicella vaccine (Var):** children aged 12 months to 12 years should receive one dose of varicella vaccine. Susceptible individuals ≥13 years of age should receive two doses at least 28 days apart.

★ **Hepatitis B vaccine (HB):** hepatitis B vaccine can be routinely given to infants or pre-adolescents, depending on the provincial/territorial policy. For infants born to chronic carrier mothers, the first dose should be given at birth (with hepatitis B immunoglobulin), otherwise the first dose can be given at 2 months of age to fit more conveniently with other routine infant immunization visits. The second dose should be administered at least 1 month after the first dose, and the third at least 2 months after the second dose, but these may fit more conveniently into the 4 and 6 month immunization visits. A two-dose schedule for adolescents is an option (see *Hepatitis B Vaccine* chapter [of the *Canadian Immunization Guide*]).

✉ **Pneumococcal conjugate vaccine—7-valent (Pneu-C-7):** recommended for all children under 2 years of age. The recommended schedule depends on the age of the child when vaccination is begun (see *Pneumococcal Vaccine* chapter [of the *Canadian Immunization Guide*]).

▣ **Pneumococcal polysaccharide—23-valent (Pneu-P-23):** recommended for all adults ≥65 years of age (see *Pneumococcal Vaccine* chapter [of the *Canadian Immunization Guide*]).

◉ **Meningococcal C conjugate vaccine (Men-C):** recommended for children under 5 years of age, adolescents and young adults. The recommended schedule depends on the age of the individual (see *Meningococcal Vaccine* chapter [of the *Canadian Immunization Guide*]) and the conjugate vaccine used. At least one dose in the primary infant series should be given after 5 months of age. If the provincial/territorial policy is to give Men-C to persons ≥12 months of age, one dose is sufficient.

▲ **Diphtheria, tetanus, acellular pertussis vaccine–adult/adolescent formulation (Tdap):** a combined adsorbed "adult type" preparation for use in people ≥7 years of age, contains less diphtheria toxoid and pertussis antigens than preparations given to younger children and is less likely to cause reactions in older people.

▯ **Diphtheria, tetanus vaccine (Td):** a combined adsorbed "adult type" preparation for use in people ≥7 years of age, contains less diphtheria toxoid antigen than preparations given to younger children and is less likely to cause reactions in older people. It is given to adults not immunized in childhood as the second and third doses of their primary series and subsequent booster doses; Tdap is given only once under these circumstances as it is assumed that previously unimmunized adults will have encountered *Bordetella pertussis* and have some pre-existing immunity.

✇ **Influenza vaccine (Inf):** recommended for all children 6–23 months of age and all persons ≥65 years of age. Previously unvaccinated children <9 years of age require two doses of the current season's vaccine with an interval of at least 4 weeks. The second dose within the same season is not required if the child received one or more doses of influenza vaccine during the previous influenza season (see *Influenza Vaccine* chapter [of the *Canadian Immunization Guide*]).

♠ **IPV Inactivated polio virus**

water, fat, ash, and protein, and nutritional intake determines the amounts of each of these essential components. Alteration in one or more of the components affects development and health. Balanced nutrition promotes brain development in children and has been reported to prevent some forms of dementia in older adults. Further discussion of these concepts is included in Chapter 9 of this text.

Family

Family refers to a social system made up of two or more individuals living together, who are related by blood, marriage, or agreement. Families today may be identified as nuclear families, extended families, same-sex families, single-parent families, stepfamilies, or single-state families. Families share bonds of affection or love, loyalty, commitment of an emotional or financial nature, continuity, and common shared values and rituals. Families help members to develop physically and emotionally by providing for the economic and safety needs of one another. Included in safety needs is provision of appropriate nutrition to foster physical growth and development, as well as objects, interactions, and activities that promote cognitive and emotional well-being. Family members provide support for one another during physical and emotional crises, and serve as models for social interaction, all of which affect individual members as they move through the stages of development from infancy to old age.

Culture

Growth and development are influenced by cultural factors, that is, by beliefs, attitudes, and values. They are also affected by the aspects of people's lives that influence how they are in relationship with others, such as spirituality, religion, ethnicity, nationality, age, class, sexual orientation, gender, and so on. For example, parenting roles and practices are influenced by the beliefs and values parents have regarding children.

Different experiences associated with culture, such as the immigrant and refugee experience, influence growth and development. For example, language differences influence the ability to communicate and to form social bonds outside the cultural community and to identify and use resources that foster development and support for individuals and families experiencing developmental situational crises.

Socioeconomic Status

Socioeconomic status is a major influence on growth and development. Overall, school-age children of low socioeconomic status have been found to have lower height and weight than those in other economic groups. Poverty affects the ability to meet nutritional needs at all stages of development and increases exposure to environmental elements that influence health status and physical well-being. Socioeconomic status influences values and role expectations and behaviours regarding marriage, family, and gender responsibilities in parenting, education, and occupation. Income, values, and role expectations affect physical and psychosocial development across the age span. Further information about culture and psychosocial development is included in Chapters 4 and 5 of this text.

Planning care for individuals is dependent on comprehensive health assessment of health status and all the factors that affect health. Accurate interpretation of data requires the nurse to use knowledge and resources in formulating judgments about findings. The previous discussion provided information about measures that assist in health assessment of physical and psychosocial growth and development across the lifespan.

APPLICATION THROUGH CRITICAL THINKING

CASE STUDY

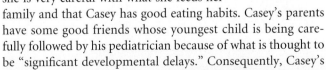

Casey is a 2-year-old girl whose mother brought her in for a checkup. Her mother states that Casey does not have any problems that she has identified; she has no history of medical problems or diseases and her immunizations are up-to-date. The mother states she is very careful with what she feeds her family and that Casey has good eating habits. Casey's parents have some good friends whose youngest child is being carefully followed by his pediatrician because of what is thought to be "significant developmental delays." Consequently, Casey's mother is very concerned about developmental milestones and wants her daughter "checked to make sure everything is all right." The mother states she has "read a lot of books" on child development but asks many questions regarding care and needs of her child.

▶ Critical Thinking Questions

1. What are the expectations regarding physical development for a 2-year-old child, such as Casey?
2. What level of language development is expected for a toddler?
3. Identify at least two standardized tools that are used to assess physical and psychosocial development across the age span.

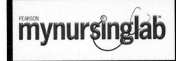

4

SOCIAL AND ETHNOCULTURAL CONSIDERATIONS

CHAPTER OBJECTIVES

On completion of this chapter, you will be able to

1. Describe concepts that are central to understanding social and ethnocultural aspects of health assessment.
2. Distinguish among cultural sensitivity, cultural competence, and cultural safety.
3. Provide examples of ethnocultural diversity within the Canadian population.
4. Provide examples of health, social, and gender inequities in Canada.
5. Identify guidelines for assessing culturally based understandings and the social and economic contexts shaping people's lives.

CHAPTER OUTLINE

Canadian Contributor: Victoria Smye, University of British Columbia

CANADIAN DEMOGRAPHICS

Canada is a diverse nation across many dimensions, including languages spoken, urban-rural population distribution, age, ethnocultural identities, religion, and so on. For example, in the 2006 census by Statistics Canada, 200 different ethnic origins were declared by Canadians (Statistics Canada, 2008a), and although European countries were once the main source of immigrants to Canada, newcomers from Asia and the Middle East far surpassed them in 2006 (see Table 4.1).

On July 1, 2008, Canada's population was estimated at 33 311 400, an increase of 1.2% over the previous year. This growth was the strongest since 1991–1992 (Statistics Canada, 2008b). The rise in Canada's population in 2007–2008 was mainly attributed to a strong increase in international net migration, which in turn was a result of a rise in both the number of immigrants and the number of nonpermanent residents. In 2007–2008, 249 600 people immigrated to Canada, up 11 478 over the previous year.

Seventy percent of people who immigrated to Canada in 2006 reported a first language (mother tongue) other than English or French (Statistics Canada, 2007c), Canada's two official languages. Fifty-eight percent of Canadians reported English and 22% reported French as their first language. The Chinese languages are the third-largest first-language group, at 3%.

According to the 2006 census, **Aboriginal peoples** in Canada—First Nations, Metis, and Inuit—numbered more than 1 million for the first time. Between 1996 and 2006, the Aboriginal population grew by 45%, compared with 8% for the non-Aboriginal population. The census counted 698 025 First Nations, 389 785 Metis, and 50 485 Inuit people in 2006 (Statistics Canada, 2008c). Several factors accounted for the growth of the Aboriginal population, including demographic factors, such as high birth rates. In addition, more individuals identified themselves as Aboriginal, and the number of incompletely enumerated Indian reserves decreased after 1996 (Statistics Canada, 2008c). Nearly 60 different languages were spoken by First Nations people in 2006, with Cree being spoken by the largest number (Statistics Canada, 2008c). The Inuktitut language was strongest in the region of Nunavik and in Nunavut.

In 2006, about 6 million people lived in rural areas, and more than four fifths of Canadians lived in urban areas (Statistics Canada, 2009; see Figure 4.1). Of those urban areas, six cities (census Metropolitan Areas, with populations greater than 1 million people) are home to 45% of Canada's population. Toronto, Vancouver, and Montreal remained the top choices for immigrants to Canada, who make up between one fifth and almost half of the populations of those cities (see Table 4.2).

Immigration to these cities was related to job prospects and connections to support networks of family and friends. Recently, immigrants to Canada have been attracted to other large cities, such as Calgary, Ottawa-Gatineau, Edmonton, Winnipeg, Hamilton, and London. Overall, the young-working-age population (ages 20 to 44) was much larger in urban areas than in rural ones. The differences are due primarily to internal migration of young adults, who often leave the rural areas to pursue their education or find work in

TABLE 4.1	Top Countries of Origin for Newcomers to Canada, 2006
COUNTRY	**PERCENTAGE OF IMMIGRANTS**
Asia and Middle East	58.3
Europe	16.1
Central and South America and the Caribbean	10.8
Africa	10.6

Source: Statistics Canada, 2007a.

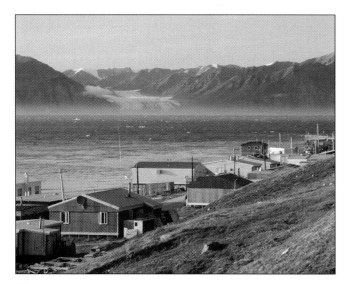

Figure 4.1 • How does living in a rural and remote area shape health?

urban areas, and to international immigration, which is heavily concentrated in large urban centres (Statistics Canada, 2008b).

According to Statistics Canada (2008c), in 2006, fewer First Nations people lived on reserve (40%) than off reserve (60%). Some 98% of the First Nations people living on reserve were Status Indians (those registered under the Indian Act). In 2006, about 76% of the off-reserve First Nations population lived in urban areas, along with 69% of Metis. Seventy-eight percent of Inuit live in four regions: 49% in Nunavut, 19% in Nunavik in northern Quebec, 6% in the Inuvialuit region in the Northwest Territories, and 4% in Nunatsiavut in Labrador. An estimated 17% lived in urban centres and 5% in rural areas outside Inuit Nunaat (Statistics Canada, 2008c).

The 2006 census reports that the 65-and-over population made up a record 13.7% of the total population of Canada in 2006 (Statistics Canada, 2007b). The proportion of the under-15 population fell to 17.7%, its lowest level ever. The number of people aged 55 to 64, many of whom are workers approaching retirement, had never been so high in Canada, at close to 3.7 million in 2006; similarly, since the first national census in 1871, the 80-years-and-older group also had never been so large (1.2 million people in 2006). The median age for the general population was 39.6 years. However, in all parts of the country, the Metis were younger than non-Aboriginal people, with 25% of the Metis population ages 14 and under, well above the 17% in the non-Aboriginal population. The proportion was highest in Saskatchewan, where children made up 29% of the Metis

TABLE 4.2	Foreign-Born People as a Percentage of City Population, 2006
CITY	PERCENTAGE
Toronto	45.7
Vancouver	39.6
Montreal	20.6

Source: Statistics Canada, 2007a.

population. In 2006, the median age of the Inuit population was 22 years. Inuit were also younger than First Nations people, whose median age was 25 years, and Metis, whose median age was 30 years (Statistics Canada, 2008c).

Life expectancy for women in the general population is 82.5 years, compared with 77.5 years for men; however, nearly two out of three people over 80 years are women (see Figure 4.2). Comparatively, in 2000, life expectancy for the registered Indian population was 76.6 years for women and 68.9 years for men, 5 and 8.6 years less than other Canadians, respectively (Statistics Canada, 2007b). In addition, infant mortality rates, one of the most powerful indicators of the social determinants of health, are almost twice as high for Status Indian infants than for other Canadians, and the poverty rate for First Nations children is at least double the national average (Assembly of First Nations, 2005)—health inequities related to social and structural issues that will be discussed later in the chapter.

The rich ethnocultural, linguistic, and social diversity within Canada requires that health policies and practices support health professionals to work across difference. Box 4.1 outlines guidelines adapted from standards developed in the United States to support services for culturally and linguistically diverse populations (U.S. Department of Health and Human Services, 2001). According to Doane and Varcoe (2005), attending to cultural differences is central to nurses' ability to provide high quality care to increasingly diverse client groups—a perspective shared by the Canadian Nurses Association (CNA) (2004) and the Aboriginal Nurses Association of Canada (ANAC) (2009).

According to the CNA (2004), cultural competency needs to be achieved to ensure best possible outcomes. The three main reasons provided by the CNA are (1) nurses have a duty to provide ethical care to their patients as per clear guidelines provided by the CNA Code of Ethics with respect to professional responsibilities and culture; (2) there is greater diversity in the Canadian population associated with ethnicity, language, religion, notions of family, and so on; (3) in Canada, culture is one of the 12 key determinants of health (Health Canada, 2001)—understanding and providing culturally competent care will

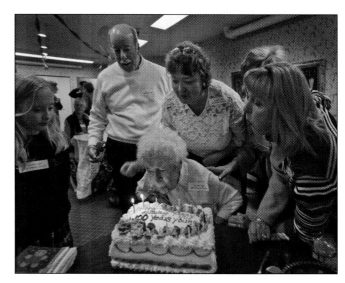

Figure 4.2 • What does this 100th birthday party in a long-term care facility mean for this family?

BOX 4.1	Standards for Culturally, Linguistically, and Socially Appropriate Services in Healthcare

1. Promote and support the attitudes, openness, behaviours, knowledge, and skills necessary for staff to work respectfully and effectively with patients and one another in a culturally, linguistically, and socially diverse work environment.
2. Have a comprehensive management strategy to address culturally, linguistically, and socially safe and appropriate services, including strategic goals, plans, policies, procedures, and designated staff responsible for implementation.
3. Use formal mechanisms for community and consumer involvement in the design and execution of service delivery, including planning, policymaking, operations, evaluation, training, and, as appropriate, treatment planning.
4. Develop and implement a strategy to recruit, retain, and promote diverse administrative, clinical, and support staff that are trained and qualified to address the needs of the various communities being served.
5. Require and arrange for ongoing education and training for administrative, clinical, and support staff to foster safe, responsive, and appropriate services for culturally, linguistically, and socially diverse people.
6. Provide all clients who have limited English or French proficiency with access to interpretation services.
7. Provide oral and written notices, including translated signage at key points of contact, to clients in their primary languages to inform them of their right to receive free interpreter services.
8. Translate and make available signage and commonly used written client educational material and other materials for members of the predominant language groups in the local service areas.
9. Ensure that interpreters and bilingual staff can demonstrate bilingual proficiency and receive training that includes the skills and ethics of interpreting and knowledge in both languages of the terms and concepts relevant to clinical or nonclinical encounters. Family or friends are not considered adequate substitutes because they usually lack these abilities.
10. Ensure that the client's primary spoken language is included in the healthcare organization's information system and in any patient records used by staff or healthcare professionals.
11. Use a variety of methods to collect and use accurate demographic, cultural, epidemiological, and clinical outcome data for groups and populations in the service area, and become informed about the cultural, linguistic, and social needs, resources, and assets of the surrounding community.
12. Undertake ongoing organizational self-assessments, internal audits, and performance improvement programs, and integrate measures of access, satisfaction, quality, and outcomes of services with attention to culturally, linguistically, and socially diverse people.
13. Develop structures and procedures to address ethical and legal conflicts in healthcare delivery and complaints or grievances by patients or staff about unfair, unsafe, or discriminatory treatment, perceived inequities in accessing services or denial of services.
14. Prepare an annual progress report documenting the organization's progress with implementing services that are culturally, linguistically, and socially safe, appropriate, and responsive, including information on programs, staffing, and resources.

Source: Adapted from the U.S. Department of Health and Human Services. (2001). *National Standards for Culturally and Linguistically Appropriate Services in Health Care, Final Report.* Washington, DC: Author, pp. 7–20.

make a difference to the health outcomes of Canadians. It is the responsibility of nurses to acquire, maintain, and continually enhance cultural competence in all phases of the nursing process and across all domains of nursing practice: clinical practice (direct practice), education, research, and administration (CNA, 2004). In addition to cultural competence, nursing organizations (e.g., the Aboriginal Nurses Association of Canada, 2009; and the College of Registered Nurses of Nova Scotia [CRNNS], 2006) and other institutions and agencies (e.g., the Mental Health Commission of Canada, 2009; the National Aboriginal Health Organization, 2008; and the Native Mental Health Association of Canada, 2009) have taken up the notion of cultural safety. *Cultural competence* and *cultural safety* are gradually replacing the notion of *cultural sensitivity* as the standard of care for healthcare professionals.

CULTURAL SENSITIVITY, CULTURAL COMPETENCE, AND CULTURAL SAFETY

In response to cultural diversity and multiculturalism in Canada, there has been a call for healthcare professionals to provide culturally sensitive healthcare. **Cultural sensitivity** is the practice of being sensitive to the values, beliefs, and practices of all people—a sensitivity that requires a recognition of

difference and active engagement to provide care in keeping with that recognition. However, because cultural sensitivity is tied to a notion of culture as individual or group values, beliefs, and practices, it does not address context and the structural determinants of health (Doane & Varcoe, 2005, p. 310). In addition, culturally sensitive approaches run the risk of generating a cookbook response to cultural differences, which can do more harm than good; for example, nurses learn about the values, beliefs, and practices of "others," such as "Muslim values," "Aboriginal beliefs," or "Chinese practices." As Doane and Varcoe note, this places the dominant white Eurocentric norm at the centre and leaves the healthcare professional open to generalizations and stereotypes about the "cultural other" that are often based on race, class, gender, sexual orientation, ability, religion, age, and so on (p. 310).

Cultural competence is the "application of knowledge, skills, attitudes and personal attributes required by nurses to provide appropriate care and services in relation to the cultural characteristics of their clients" (CNA, 2004, p. 1). Similar to cultural sensitivity, cultural competence includes valuing diversity, knowing about the cultural mores and traditions of the populations being served, and being sensitive to these while caring for a client. However, it also has been used to consider the broader context of health and healthcare (Spector, 2004) and, in Canada, to draw attention to power relations and dynamics and to consider culture in ways that directly address issues of racism and inequity (Srivastava, 2007). Currently, many health professional organizations and health institutions and agencies are incorporating the notion of cultural competence into Canadian healthcare settings (e.g., British Columbia Provincial Health Services Authority, 2009; CNA, 2004; CRNNS, 2006). Nurses need to be aware of the limitations of brief diversity or cross-cultural training programs that fail to address the structural and power inequities that affect healthcare and health (Browne & Varcoe, 2009). In this chapter, the concept of cultural safety is used as a lens for nurses to address cultural competence.

Moving Beyond Cultural Sensitivity: Cultural Safety

Cultural safety was developed in the early 1990s in New Zealand by Maori nurse educators and leaders, in collaboration with other Maori, to address persistent health disparities related to inequities in Maori access to healthcare—inequities often associated with discriminatory health policies and practices (Ramsden, 2000; Wepa, 2005). Over the past decade in Canada, the concept of cultural safety has been used increasingly across many health disciplines, including nursing. The notion of **cultural safety** encourages nurses to be aware of the assumptions and stereotypes they hold about particular groups of people that may influence how the nurses provide care; to consider the uniqueness of each client within the context of the social, political, historical, and cultural realities of the client's life that shape or influence health and healthcare (e.g., immigration laws, class, age, geographic location, stigma, racism, and discrimination); and to consider and address power (the nurses' power and the power of the institutions in which nurses work) and social and structural inequities that influence health and well-being, such as poverty, social isolation, lack of access to education, and so on (Anderson et al., 2003; Browne, 2005, 2007; Browne & Fiske, 2001; Browne & Smye, 2002; Browne & Varcoe, 2006; Browne, Varcoe, Smye, Reimer Kirkham, Lynam, & Wong, 2009; Reimer Kirkham et al., 2002; Smye & Browne, 2002).

Cultural safety requires actions that recognize and nurture the unique cultural identity of clients to safely meet their needs, expectations, and rights (Ramsden, 2000); that is, care needs to be provided in a way that is respectful and preserving of human dignity—it reflects ethical standards (Polaschek, 1998) and relational practice. Cultural safety requires nurses to shift attention from the *culture* of their clients to the culture of the healthcare system and the culture of nursing and other health professions, and to how health practices, education, research, and policies can themselves perpetuate marginalizing conditions and inequities (Browne & Varcoe, 2006, 2009; Browne, Smye, & Varcoe, 2005; Smye & Browne, 2002). Cultural safety begins with the nurse—nurses are required to reflect on their own cultural reality in the process of practice, such as direct patient care. As bearers of culture, that is, as "powerful bearers of their own life experiences and realities and the impact this may have on others" (Ramsden, 2000, p. 117), nurses need be aware of cultural and power differences between the nurse and client—differences that need to be recognized and addressed so

they do not negatively influence healthcare and client health. In relation to culture and power, nurses need to consider the historical, social, political, and economic realities of people's lives and other factors that influence health status, such as age, gender, class, ability, sexual orientation, religion, spirituality, ethnicity, race, and so on.

Nurses have a social mandate to support the health of all people. To achieve this, they need to be willing to address power inequities within healthcare—inequities that exist at the bedside, in the classroom, in research partnerships, and in policy. This includes a willingness to challenge structural inequities and everyday stereotyping and discrimination. Cultural safety is strongly connected with a relational approach to nursing that understands relationships among health professionals and clients as located within particular historical, social, political, economic, and cultural contexts. To understand cultural safety and relational approaches, the nurse first needs to critically reflect on the notion of culture both personally and as a theoretical construct (see Box 4.2).

BOX 4.2   Health Assessment Guidelines: Cultural Competence and Cultural Safety

Nursing practice reflects acceptance of, respect for, and honouring of difference in relational experience and processes, beliefs, values, practices, and traditions across people, by, for example, age or generation, gender, language, sexual orientation, occupation and socioeconomic status, education, ethnic origin or migrant experience, religious or spiritual belief, ability, and so on.

1. The nurse understands the notion of difference within his or her own cultural reality and the impact that may have on a person who differs from the nurse, and recognizes that both the nurse and the client are influenced by their own cultures in relationship.

2. The nurse understands and accepts that the attitudes and beliefs, policies, and practices of health providers and healthcare agencies, organizations, and institutions can act as barriers to service access, and works to shift the status quo, as appropriate.

3. The nurse recognizes inequalities within healthcare interactions and their fit with inequalities in health from a sociocultural, political, and historical perspective and as lived out in the everyday world.

4. The nurse understands the importance of the power relationship between the service provider and people using the service, is able to reflect critically on personal factors and institutional processes that affect power dynamics, and works to equalize power in practice.

5. The nurse understands that power imbalances can be examined, negotiated, and changed to provide equitable, effective, efficient, and safe delivery of services, minimizing risk for people who might otherwise be alienated.

6. The nurse demonstrates flexibility in relationships with people who are different from the nurse.

7. The nurse demonstrates an ability to build trusting relationships such that, for example, clients and families will ask health questions relevant to them.

Source: Adapted from the Nursing Council of New Zealand. (2002). *Guidelines for Cultural Safety, the Treaty of Waitangi and Maori Health in Nursing and Midwifery Education and Practice.* Wellington, New Zealand: Author; and Smye, V. (2007, July). *Integrating Culture into Practice: Developing a Peer Review Framework for Nurses.* Victoria, BC: Intertribal Health, University of Victoria & Vancouver Island Health Authority, Aboriginal Programs, pp. 10–11.

CULTURE, "OTHERING," AND CULTURALISM

Culture

Culture remains difficult to define. As Culley (1996) notes, in nursing and other healthcare literature, **culture** is commonly presented as comprising the beliefs, practices, and values of particular ethnic or religious groups, and as Reimer Kirkham and Anderson (2002, p. 4) observe, it is also commonly used as a framework for human behaviour. With its roots in cultural pluralism, multiculturalism—the official state policy in Canada since 1983—embraces the liberal notion of respect for diversity. However, according to Lock (1990) one of the difficulties is

> that in establishing boundaries as to what exactly is a culture or an ethnic group... a 19th century style of thinking is usually drawn upon in which nation states, or large regional areas, language, religion, and even skin colour or other physical features are taken as immutable markers. (p. 240)

Although acknowledging and celebrating cultural diversity in this way has resulted in increased public awareness and appreciation for the diversity of people in Canada, critically oriented scholars are concerned with a primary attachment of culture with differences (and identity) and the lack of analysis of culture as mediated by historical, economic, and political conditions (Gilroy, 2000, 2001; McConaghy, 2000; Narayan, 2000; Reimer Kirkham & Anderson, 2002). Descriptions of cultural values, beliefs, and practices have been useful to healthcare professionals and researchers, but when they are seen as unchallengeable markers of culture, these descriptions can reinforce stereotypes and simplistic views of particular groups as outsiders, as different, and as "other," a process known as *culturalism*. Of particular concern, from this perspective, is that all facets of social experience can be attributed to culture and can exclude those societal influences, such as colonialism and neocolonialism, consumerism, multiculturalism, medicalization, globalization, nationalism, self-governance, and health policy—factors that also shape health and healthcare.

"Othering"

Despite growing concerns about images of the other being reproduced through a variety of discourses, static notions of culture continue to predominate in healthcare textbooks and healthcare settings. As Narayan (2000) writes, groups of people are presented as homogeneous without recognition of the diversity across and within people in the group—people with diverse values, interests, ways of life, moral political commitments, and so on. This process of "othering" confers cultural characteristics, differences, or identities onto members of diverse groups, based not on real or actual identities but rather on stereotyped identities and as such erases the complexity of human identity and experience in favour of essentialized accounts. For example, it is not uncommon to hear people attribute particular child-rearing practices, family relations, dietary restrictions, body postures, and so on, to particular groups of people without considering the myriad factors that influence people's identities, preferences, and behaviours.

Culturalism

Most insidiously, culturalism masks the way in which culture is transformed through the historical, social, and political contexts in which it is used. In this way, it obscures the dynamic, ever-changing quality of culture (Anderson & Reimer Kirkham, 1998). From a culturalist perspective, issues of access, compliance, and poor health status are often viewed as stemming from cultural characteristics that conflict with mainstream, routine healthcare practices rather than as being shaped by larger social and political structures. Research has shown that healthcare professionals frequently attribute people's social problems to their cultural characteristics (Anderson et al., 2003; Browne, 2005, 2007; Varcoe, 2001, 2008). For example, the high rates of type 2 diabetes in First Nations populations are sometimes attributed to culture rather than to the historical, social, political, and economic processes that have profoundly influenced health and well-being for this group: forced loss of land, place, traditional foods, and geographic location, and consequent limited access to fresh fruits and vegetables. Intimate partner violence, experienced for the first time after immigration by some families, could mistakenly be attributed to their culture rather than to the immigration experience and the loss of traditional gender roles and meaningful employment (Guruge & Gastaldo, 2008; Hyman, Guruge, & Mason, 2008). Oversimplistic representations of culture as transparent, ahistorical, or apolitical are problematic because of the way they divert attention away from the underlying structural inequities that influence healthcare and health (Anderson & Reimer Kirkham, 1999).

To address the issue of culturalism, it can be useful to use a critical cultural perspective. From this perspective, culture is viewed as dynamic, lived, and evolving within multiple contexts—as something through which meanings are produced and exchanged. Culture is a relational process that is influenced by history, past experiences, and social, professional, and gendered location, and people's perception of how they are viewed by others in society (Anderson & Reimer Kirkham, 1999, p. 63; Browne & Varcoe, 2006, 2009). To view culture in this way *does not* exclude considering people's values, beliefs, and practices, for example, in health assessment; rather it draws attention to those aspects of the client and how they intersect with historical, social, political, economic, and cultural contexts.

Many cultures exist within healthcare: nursing culture, medical culture, and so on. Western-educated health professionals tend to embrace the values of dominant healthcare culture, including beliefs about health, illness, and healing (see Figure 4.3). For example, in the dominant culture, disease is often attributed to the individual: exposure to bacteria and viruses, lack of sleep or exercise, lifestyle choices, and so on. Cure is highly valued and "getting well usually means cooperation with technical procedures applied to the body such as medicines and surgery" (Waxler-Morrison & Anderson, 2005, p. 3). Because healthcare professionals often do not think of their interactions as reflecting a particular culture, history taking and interventions tend to reflect a dominant-culture stance without consideration of client *difference*.

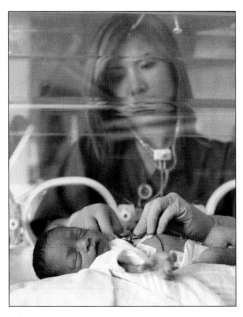

Figure 4.3 ● What does Western medical technology mean for this baby's family?

ETHNICITY, RACE, AND RACIALIZATION

As social constructs that categorize and ascribe *difference*, the terms *culture*, *ethnicity*, and *race* are often used interchangeably and with little consistency (McConaghy, 2000; Reimer Kirkham & Anderson, 2002, p. 3). According to Henry, Tator, Mattis, and Rees (2005) **ethnicity** involves notions of blood, kinship, a common sense of belonging, and often a common geographic or national origin, and an **ethnic group** is a group or "community maintained by a shared heritage, culture, language or religion" (p. 350). In healthcare contexts (including research), ethnicity is often used interchangeably with *race,* contributing to the reduction of ethnicity to such categories as white, Black, and so on—categories that often are associated with how people look rather than with individual characteristics that have real meaning or connection to health and well-being (Browne & Varcoe, 2009). For purposes of health assessment, it is important to understand that people's ethnic identities are dependent on how they see themselves. For example, in research examining the hospitalization experiences of Canadians of South Asian and Chinese ancestry who immigrated to Canada and Canadians of European ancestry who were born in Canada, Anderson et al. (2003) found that many people being recruited to the study resisted the categories that had been constructed (South Asian, Chinese Canadian, and Anglo Canadian), noting emphatically that they saw themselves as Canadian. In addition, in some health contexts people may choose to report that they are Aboriginal, Ethiopian, Serbian, or Jewish, for example, and in others, they may be reluctant to identify themselves in these ways because of concerns that they might be treated differently (Browne & Varcoe, 2009, p. 37).

Although genes do contribute to some traits, such as skin colour and other physical characteristics, it is society that con-stitutes these traits as **race** and marks racial difference among people (Drevdahl, Philips, & Taylor, 2006, p. 53). Race does not refer to physical or phenotypical categorizations; race is understood as a socially constructed category that orders the world and provides differential access to resources (e.g., resources for health and well-being) for members of various groups (Gustafson, 2007; Tang & Browne, 2008). However, although continuing scientific evidence dispels the existence of such categories as "race" (Dei, 1996) in the United States, *race* and *ethnicity* continue to be used interchangeably to cat-egorize people, for example, as Black, Latina, Asian, or white— categories that signal social categories rather than genetically linked groups of people.

Although the notion of race as socially constructed takes us beyond the understanding of race as biologically determined, controversies about its significance and the dilemmas of racial injustice and conflict that accompany it are transferred to politics (Omi & Winant, 2002, p. 128). In this way, race has been manipulated "to define, structure, and organize relations between dominant and subordinate groups" (Reimer Kirkham & Anderson, 2002, p. 4).

Racialization is a process that "assumes that 'race' is the primary, natural, and neutral means of categorization, and that the groups also are distinct in behavioral characteristics, which result from their 'race'" (Ahmad, 1993, p. 18). Race cannot be neatly sifted apart from processes of racialization, issues of gender, class relations, and other social relations that struc-ture people's lives, such as their education level, employment status, health, and well-being. Issues of race and racialization are inherent in the construction of the Canadian nation and entrenched in the fabric of Canadian society: they are not insig-nificant processes that people simply move beyond (Anderson & Reimer Kirkham, 1998; Henry et al., 2005; Reimer Kirkham & Anderson, 2002). For example, in a study funded by the Canadian Institutes of Health Research (2006–2009), called *Aboriginal Peoples' Experiences of Mental Health and Addictions Care,* many Aboriginal participants described experiences of racialization and discrimination within the healthcare system; assumptions were made about them based on being "read" as Aboriginal, with consequent iniquitous treatment (Smye, Browne, & Varcoe, under review).

HEALTH, SOCIAL, AND GENDER INEQUITIES

It is important to note the difference between health inequality and health equity to understand how inequities affect health. According to Kawachi, Subramanian, and Almeida-Filho (2002) **health inequality** is a term used to designate differ-ences, variations, and disparities in the health status of individ-uals and groups. An example of a health inequality is the larger death burden due to sex-specific causes of death for women (e.g., breast cancer) than men (e.g., prostate cancer and testicu-lar cancer) (Varcoe, Hankivsky, & Morrow, 2007, p. 5). *Health inequity* refers to those inequalities or disparities in health that are deemed to be unfair or unjust differences because they stem from some form of injustice related to social, political, or historical inequities: "an unfair distribution of the underlying social determinants of health (for example, access to educational opportunities, safe jobs, health care, and the social bases of self respect)" (Kawachi et al., 2002, p. 647). People are differentially likely to experience ill health and inadequate healthcare related, for example, to where they live, their social class, and the income group they find themselves in, whether they are of European or non-European descent, Aboriginal or not, male or female (Raphael, 2006). However, people are also more likely to experience barriers to healthcare access because of discrimination, racism, and stigma associated with other factors, such as mental health problems, ability, addictions, language, and so on (Henry et al., 2005). Racism has long been associated with health disparity (e.g., Kendall & Hatton, 2002). In the assessment of risk and promotion of health, the nurse needs to be aware of the way in which behavioural and biological risk factors (e.g., smoking, risky drug-sharing practices, high blood pressure) intersect with historical, social, economic, and political factors.

According to Raphael (2007) the evidence is now conclusive that poverty is a primary cause of poor health among Canadians. In 2002, 15.6% of Canadians were living in poverty. Women and children are particularly vulnerable. For example, as noted by Browne and Varcoe (2009), the poverty rate for lone-mother families was 51% in 2004, which is exceptionally high in comparison with other wealthy industrialized nations and is another figure that is likely to grow. Poverty among women is related to such factors as family breakdown and lone parenting, labour market inequities, clawbacks to welfare payments for women with small children, and wage disparities with men (Reid, 2007) and is particularly problematic because of its immediate and long-term effects on children.

Aboriginal Peoples in Canada

The provision of healthcare to Aboriginal people has been shaped by more than a century of internal colonial practices, policies, and politics that have profoundly disrupted the lives of many Aboriginal people (Kelm, 1998; Waldram, Herring, & Young, 2006). As a consequence, the current health system is plagued by the same problems, and the health inequities experienced by many Aboriginal peoples are alarming. Despite a number of important events over the past two decades which have drawn attention to the health concerns of Aboriginal people and the attendant systems of healthcare, Aboriginal health is largely glossed over by the health authorities.

Nurses need to understand the significance of previous colonial relations to understand the current social, political, and economic conditions influencing Aboriginal health, such as lack of employment opportunities, limited access to educational programs, inadequate and often crowded housing, and high levels of poverty (Waldram et al., 2006). In particular, colonizing attitudes continue to influence the way in which healthcare is provided to Aboriginal peoples.

The systematic subjugation of Aboriginal peoples has its origins in the colonial laws and policies enacted on Aboriginal peoples in 1876 in the Indian Act—an Act that continues to direct the lives of First Nations people, shaping life opportunities, economic conditions, and the overall health and social status of individuals, families, and communities. For example, although the Act has been amended many times, it continues to pose restrictions on self-governance, land claims, matrimonial rights, and economic development in Aboriginal communities. Although the Act was premised on the pretext of assisting "Indians" (now often referred to as First Nations), the underlying intent of assimilation was pursued at many levels: Aboriginal lands were taken and reserves established; residential schools and boarding homes were instituted with the goal of indoctrinating children into the dominant culture—a collaborative effort between church and state (the last residential school closed in Saskatchewan in 1996)—and cultural spiritual practices were outlawed, with profound health and social consequences for Aboriginal people. In fact, the Act gradually took control of most aspects of Aboriginal life. Notably, Aboriginal people were not able to vote in federal elections until 1960. In 2006, the federal government announced the approval of the Indian Residential School Agreement and the new Truth and Reconciliation Commission (Indian Residential Schools Adjudication Secretariat, 2008) in response to the devastating effects of residential schools on the health and well-being of Aboriginal peoples: disruption to family, abuses experienced by many, and consequent intergenerational trauma.

In accordance with the Indian Act, health services are provided to people living on reserves and deemed "Indian," and the services are explicitly related to disease control and, more ambiguously, to the broader provision of healthcare. Thus, additional uncertainty is created concerning which level of government has responsibility for what population of Aboriginal peoples. Limited health benefits, called non-insured health benefits, paid by the federal government both on- and off-reserve are provided to First Nations and Inuit and include selected prescription drugs, limited medical supplies and equipment, short-term counselling, limited coverage for glasses and vision care, medical transportation (limited by allocation and need), and dental care (however, many dentists do not accept "status" people because the dentists must wait for reimbursement from the federal government) (Health Canada, 2009).

Off-reserve, the provinces provide many services to First Nations people through the mainstream service delivery system. The provinces continue to be the chief legislative body for First Nations services, a perpetuation of earlier notions of integrating First Nations services with regular provincial services. Metis peoples and non-status Indians are caught in the jurisdictional struggle because the provinces generally disclaim any responsibility for them, given the provinces' position that the federal government is responsible for all matters not related to the Canada Health Act (Cairns, 2000). In addition, First Nations and Inuit Health, the branch of Health Canada that oversees the delivery of health services on-reserve and in Inuit communities, does not provide services to non-status Indians and Metis, whether living in urban or rural settings. However, the federal government provides some resources for "targeted programming" to the Metis and non-status Indians (O'Neil, Lemchuk-Favel, Allard, & Postl, 1999, p. 147).

In summary, tremendous heterogeneity exists across Aboriginal people in Canada, even those people from the same tribal group, band, family, and so on. Aboriginal health and well-being cannot be understood without understanding the historical, social, political, cultural, and economic context of Aboriginal peoples' lives. Colonialism continues today (referred to as neocolonialism), and the social suffering of many Aboriginal people in Canada continues because of inequities in access to health and social services, racism and discrimination, and social inequities related to the legacy of colonization. Despite these disparities, it is important to note that many Aboriginal people are doing very well—it is for the more marginalized Aboriginal people that attention is drawn to health inequities.

Newcomers to Canada

Nurses and other healthcare professionals need to be aware of the potential challenges of migration and resettlement and how those may affect health and well-being (see Figure 4.4). Research shows that for non-Europeans who were healthy when they immigrated to Canada, health often deteriorates over time compared with Canadian-born residents and those immigrants born in Europe (Pederson & Raphael, 2006). Many immigrants face downward job mobility, and consequently lower socioeconomic status, and lack fluency in English or French. Of course, there is variability in this regard, however; as an example, research in immigrant health shows that non-European immigrants are more likely to have lower-paying jobs that require little education than European immigrants. Even for those people with higher levels of education, finding good jobs can be very difficult. In addition, many immigrants are disconnected from social support networks, leading to extreme stress and sometimes distress. Some people did not choose to migrate; instead, they fled or were forced to leave. Others chose to come in search of a better life. The nurse needs to remember that people who chose to migrate bring different sets of experiences and expectations than do refugees (Anderson, Reimer Kirkham, Waxler-Morrison, Herbert, Murphy, & Richardson, 2005, p. 329). For example, many refugees have endured extreme hardships and may have lost their

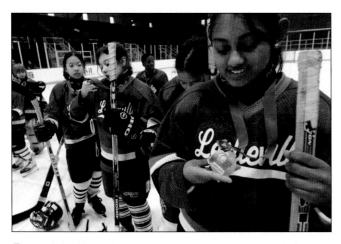

Figure 4.4 ●; What does the immigration experience mean for this family?

life belongings. Some have also endured torture, witnessed murder, and lost family and friends.

Both men and women go through a process of readjustment in Canada; however, Vissandjee, Thurston, Apale, and Nahar (2007) found that women were particularly vulnerable to the stress created by the immigration experience—they often were socially isolated because they had left friends and families behind in their country of origin, were trying to learn a new language, and at the same time were trying to meet the basic needs of the family. Some older adults are also vulnerable to social isolation because of the loss of role definition and position within the family, and because they may not speak English and may be afraid to venture out on their own.

Negotiating the healthcare system can also be challenging (Anderson et al., 2005). One of the most trying times for immigrants and refugees occurs when a family member needs healthcare. Language differences, the lack of available interpreters, and the unfamiliarity with the practices within the Canadian healthcare system can be confusing and anxiety provoking. For example, women may not be used to having male physicians examine them, and wearing hospital gowns may be untried. Long, detailed histories and examinations may be unsettling and generate a lack of confidence in the healthcare professional because these do not fit with previous experience. Also, when using hospitals, many families find the idea of leaving their loved one alone incomprehensible, and tensions sometimes arise when large numbers of family want to stay with their family member. The nurse needs to be willing to negotiate these differences to ensure the well-being of individuals and families, to understand that for some families, illness and assessment, care planning, and treatment is a family affair. Discharge planning and home care also create challenges for families. For example, responsibility is increasingly being placed on families to provide care at home, care that some new immigrant families may not completely understand or may feel overwhelmed about providing. The nurse needs to be careful not to assume that families can carry out this care—for some, it may mean lost wages and an added burden.

Although most immigrants and refugees perceive Canadian healthcare to be excellent and are eager to receive the best that Western medicine has to offer, the organization of the healthcare system may be a barrier to care (Anderson et al., 2005). As Anderson and colleagues note, "the restructuring of hospitals has meant increased workloads for staff, and a cutback in the in-service education needed for professionals to respond to an increasingly complex patient population" (p. 350). However, this is not a sufficient rationale for poor communication and inadequate care. For example, Tang (1999) notes that it is important for nurses and other healthcare professionals to use and advocate for interpreter services in healthcare settings—unfortunately, interpreters are not always used, even when they are available. In addition, research (e.g., Anderson & Reimer Kirkham, 1998; Browne & Fiske, 2001; Browne, Fiske, & Thomas, 2000; Browne & Smye, 2002; Smye, Browne, & Varcoe, under review; Tang & Browne, 2008) with people marginalized by social and structural inequity, such as immigrants, refugees, Aboriginal people, mental health clients, and people who use illegal substances, shows that discrimination continues to be problematic, both within and outside healthcare—an experience that undermines trust and strong provider-client alliances, as well as outside social attachments.

In summary, tremendous variability exists across the people who immigrate to Canada—even among those persons coming from the same country, there are cultural, linguistic, and social differences. Further, previous experiences (e.g., histories), education, socioeconomic status, proficiency in English or French, and familiarity with the healthcare system mitigate people's experiences.

Culturally safe care means that the nurse responds to the linguistic, cultural, and social differences across people and understands that those differences intersect with the context of people's lives to shape health—the nurse responds relationally. Applying a relational approach in assessment will help the nurse to assess the unique contexts, histories, and experiences that shape a client's health and well-being.

HEALTHCARE PRACTICE

Canadians draw from a range of health and healing approaches based on their historical, social, and economic location. For example, today, more people want to know about complementary and alternative healthcare and natural health products. People's exposure to Western medicine, their life experiences, and their experiences with the healthcare system shape their perspective on health, well-being, and healing. Some people engage primarily with allopathic (Western) medicine; some with a mixture of approaches, for example, allopathic and Chinese medicine or Aboriginal traditional herbs and remedies; and others with primarily traditional methods. Perspectives on acceptable healthcare practices have changed over time, that is, they are socially mediated. For example, acupuncture, Chinese medicine, and other therapies have become more commonly accepted in Canada over the past decade.

Conventional therapies are the treatments that are currently accepted and widely used in the Canadian healthcare system—for example, surgery, pharmacotherapy, and chemotherapy and radiation, among others—those treatments supported with scientific evidence. Complementary therapies are used *together with* conventional treatments to assist in managing the illness experience and/or to promote health, healing, and well-being. Alternative therapies are used *instead of* conventional treatments. An example of an alternative therapy is using a special diet to treat cancer instead of undergoing chemotherapy or another conventional treatment. Research in the area of "complementary and alternative therapies" has increased over the past several years.

When completing a health assessment, it is important for the nurse to remember that people often use a combination of therapies and approaches, many of which are not accessible to everyone by virtue of their economic, social, and geographic location (e.g., most of these therapies and approaches are not covered by provincial or territorial healthcare plans). In addition, when used with conventional therapies, some complementary therapies may create a toxic or negative effect, such as the potential for some nutritional supplements to increase the effects of certain anticoagulants (blood thinners). This means that an accurate and nonjudgmental assessment of all therapies is essential so that a positive dialogue can be initiated.

Religion, Spirituality, and Health

Spirituality has long been recognized as central to human experience and health and healing. Often confused with religion, **spirituality** is that dimension of the self that is most often associated with the search for meaning (Browne & Varcoe, 2009). Religions have most often been established through the formalizing of institutional structures, rituals, and beliefs. However, both religion and spirituality can play a significant role in the human response to illness, health, well-being, and healing (see Figure 4.5). In response to the increasing social diversity of healthcare recipients, nurse scholars (e.g., Pesut, Fowler, Johnston Taylor, Reimer Kirkham & Sawatzky, 2008; Reimer Kirkham, Pesut, Meyerhoff, & Sawatzky, 2004) have turned their attention to developing theoretical foundations for culturally responsive and spiritually sensitive nursing practice. However, despite the potential overlap between culture and spirituality, there has been little exploration of these. According to Reimer Kirkham et al. (2004), nurses and other healthcare professionals need to cultivate a space in which to provide spiritual care and to seek spiritual points of connection amid diverse faith and cultural traditions. The contexts of current practice environments, as well as the social setting of a diverse and secular state, shape the dynamics of spiritual caregiving.

In relation to health assessment, it is important for the nurse to remain open to a discussion of religion and spirituality. The nurse needs to be respectful of differences—there is no need to know the specifics of particular religions and spiritual practices, but there is a need to convey an openness, interest, and acceptance of religious and spiritual traditions. It is important that the nurse does not make assumptions about people based on their affiliations in this realm (e.g., the client may be part of a particular ethnocultural group but not part of a religious group). In addition, it is important for the nurse to note that his or her own affiliations may get in the way of asking pertinent

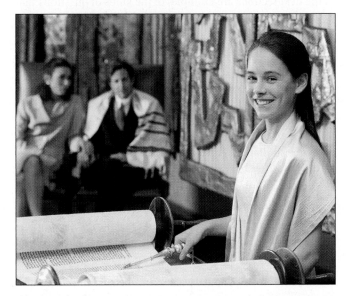

Figure 4.5 ● How might religion and spirituality shape health?

questions and lead to making assumptions and using language that is not appropriate, such as referring to a mosque or temple as a church. The nurse should invite clients to discuss what is important to them, such as asking "Do you have any religious beliefs or practices that you think it is important for me to know about in relation to your health and healthcare?"

GUIDELINES FOR CLINICAL NURSING PRACTICE

"Assessment is a clinical art that combines sensitivity, judgment, and scientific knowledge" (Anderson et al., 2005). It can occur in one short encounter or over an extended period, in an acute care or a community setting. In the context of the Canadian healthcare system, assessment may seem very strange or anxiety producing for some, even those who have been born and raised in Canada. For example, questions about education, employment, health and illness beliefs, violence, and so on may be extremely intrusive to some people and as such, some questions require particular care in timing and phrasing—noticing verbal and nonverbal cues is important to ensure the nurse is "in sync" with the client. Importantly, the nurse needs to assess the ability of the client to speak and write the local language and to assess the need for an interpreter; mistakenly, some health professionals use families as translators, including children, instead of using an interpreter.

As nurses tend to be task-oriented, they sometimes forget about how their behaviour might be interpreted by the client. It is good practice for the nurse to stop for a moment before doing an assessment to reflect on what is happening. Regardless of when an assessment is conducted, several key components ensure a culturally safe encounter: critical reflective practice, the building of trust, authentic inquiry, active listening, respectful engagement, and attention to the context of people's lives. Of importance, in this kind of assessment, questions arise out of what is meaningful and significant to the client—the nurse follows the lead of the client. The questions in the next sections are examples of the kinds of questions that might be asked of anyone, regardless of their *culture*.

Critical Reflective Practice

When working with people with backgrounds different from their own it is important for nurses to examine how their own social location and how their values, beliefs, and assumptions might influence the interaction. To develop trust and connection, it is particularly important to recognize points of difference and similarity. The nurse might begin with reflection by asking herself or himself the following questions:

- Who are the people I learn from and who are the people I *could* learn from?
- What kinds of knowledge, judgment, and/or skill would be expected to provide culturally safe care? What does cultural competence look like in my practice?

In addition to personal values and beliefs, the nurse also needs to reflect on the values and beliefs of the healthcare environment that shape her or his practice, such as the restructuring of the healthcare environment founded on ensuring efficiency and its impact on healthcare (Anderson et al., 2005).

The nurse might continue with self-reflection by using other kinds of questions that Anderson et al. (2005) suggest, such as the following:

- What are my own beliefs about newcomers to Canada and how might I interact with this person?
- What assumptions do I hold about this person and about this particular ethnocultural group?
- Why do I think this way?
- Where did I get my information?
- What might I learn if I talk to the person?
- What may we have in common?

Critical reflection often results in addressing the assumptions and biases every nurse brings to the healthcare encounter—it is a continual process of moving back and forth between the nurse-client encounter and self-reflection. Critical reflection is an approach "to aid in the production of knowledge from experience by examining the impact of one's position and action" (Lipp, 2007, p. 19). Critical reflection has the goal of social transformation, that is, nurses are expected to take this new knowledge and use it for change (Lipp, 2007; Timmins, 2006).

Building Trust

Anderson et al. (2005) caution the nurse not to ask clients to share sensitive information until trust has been established—some people may be reluctant to share health information, such as their health beliefs, because of a fear of being "ridiculed" (p. 339). For example, questions should be framed in a nonjudgmental way; asking "Have you found anything else that has helped you?" may be more appropriate than asking "Are you taking medicines other than those prescribed by a doctor?" (Anderson et al., 2005, p. 339). Establishing trust often takes time.

Authentic Inquiry: Getting a Sense of the Person

Authentic inquiry presumes that the nurse wants to get to know the client. As noted above, people affiliated with various ethnocultural groups may or may not hold to the beliefs about health and illness of that group—there is tremendous variability. To avoid stereotyping, the pattern of questioning might be directed at locating the patient's social position before asking those questions to get a sense of the person. As Anderson et al. (2005) note, questions should put the patient at ease. For example, some clients may not be comfortable discussing their country of origin, particularly if they are refugees and have entered Canada for safety reasons. However, if the nurse feels that the client *is* comfortable, such questions or comments as those suggested by Doane and Varcoe (2005) might be asked to get a sense of who the client is:

I am interested in how you have been.

Could you tell me a bit about what has been happening for you?

What stands out as you think about things in your day-to-day life?

What stands out to you as really important for me to know about your situation?

What is OK and what has been challenging?

What has changed as a result of (your situation or health challenge)? (p. 233)

The following represent a series of questions based on examples of "crucial things" Anderson et al. (2005, p. 341) suggest healthcare professionals attend to:

- Tell me about what it was like where you were born.
- Do you live in a rural or urban setting?

If the client was born outside of Canada, consider asking the following:

- How long have you been in Canada and do you have family and/or friends in Canada?
- What did you do in your country of origin and what do you do now?
- What were the health services like in your country of origin? When did you access healthcare and what was that like?
- What do you expect from your healthcare here in Canada?

Active Listening

Nurses, other health professionals, and clients often bring different ideas and key priorities to the clinical encounter. The identification of a key priority governing and explaining a whole perspective is referred to as an *explanatory model* or the way a person understands the world and health, illness, and approaches to healing (Anderson et al., 2005; Kleinman, 1980; Kleinman & Benson, 2006). A clash in perspectives can have devastating consequences if these differences are not acknowledged and worked through. The following are adaptations by Browne and Varcoe (2009, p. 46) of sample questions from Kleinman (1980, p. 106) and Anderson et al. (2005, p. 343) who suggest them as either direct or "listening for cues" questions—that is, the nurse does not necessarily ask them but listens for them, notices them, and perhaps follows up on them with a question:

- What do you call this problem? What term or name do you give to it?
- What do you think has caused this problem?
- Why do you think it started when it did?
- What concerns you most?
- What do you usually do to stay healthy? Have you been able to continue with these approaches (activities, food, medications)?

These questions are not posed in isolation from the rest of the interview; rather, they are woven throughout—timing and phrasing should be adapted to the client (Anderson et al., 2005, p. 344).

Respectful Engagement

The ability to convey respect for difference is one of the hallmarks of cultural safety and excellent relational practice. This skill will help to build trust and allow the nurse to engage in collaborative practice with clients. Research shows that people know when they are being negatively evaluated. For some, there is an acute awareness of and sensitivity to a lack of respect given their group history and personal and collective experiences of racialization. Asking questions about what people have done to address their health and illness concerns can convey respect while at the same time exploring people's various health practices. The following are adapted from sample questions posed by Anderson et al. (2005, p. 346):

- Have you found any treatments or medications that have worked for you in the past?
- How did they help you?
- Are you using them now? If so, are they helping?
- (For those people who have come from another country): did you use any special treatments or medicines in your home country that seemed to work for you?

Questions that convey an interest in hearing about traditional or complementary healing practices may include those suggested by Browne and Varcoe (2009): "Have you used any traditional medicines or healing methods that you have found helpful? Are you able to access those medicines or healing methods?" (p. 47).

Relational Practice: Connecting Across Differences

From a relational perspective, it is important to identify "differences" that are operating and to be aware that those differences arise from multiple simultaneous sources—self, other, and context. Similarities and differences illustrate issues of meaning, experience, history, culture, health, and sociopolitical systems. Relational practice requires that nurses connect across difference by engaging in respectful relationships fostered by "unconditional positive regard and openness" (Doane & Varcoe, 2005, p. 295). A relational approach in nursing practice recognizes that health, illness, health promotion, and the meanings they hold are shaped by people's economic, social, cultural, family, community, historical, and geographical contexts and intersect with gender, age, ability, and other personal factors. Although the quality of relationships is central to nursing, relational practice goes beyond a sole focus on interpersonal relationships and communication to the ways in which people's lives, their health, and their healthcare are shaped in relation to their social contexts. By using a relational practice approach in health assessment, the nurse's attention is focused on the importance of understanding what is significant to people in the context of their everyday lives and how capacities and socioenvironmental influences shape opportunities, possibilities, and choice, as well as people's health and agency.

These factors also influence how nurses view, relate, and work with clients and families. Nursing as a relational practice is also focused on action; that is, nurses will be able to respond to the complex ways in which the health experiences and the wider contexts of clients' lives are shaped, and to participate in change (UBC School of Nursing Undergraduate Curriculum, 2009).

Culturally safe relational approaches provide nurses with the tools necessary to make connections across difference, that is, "joining people as they are and where they are" (Doane & Varcoe, 2005, p. 295). Finding "the join" begins with critical self-reflection relative to health, illness, and health promotion—to become aware of, and in some cases challenge, the assumptions, biases, prejudices, and judgments that become evident. In addition, the nurse needs to become aware of those aspects of the healthcare system, such as policies and practices, that act as barriers to access. The nurse also needs to be aware of the societal factors that influence people's health and healthcare, including stigma and discrimination, social welfare policies and practices, the availability of transportation, and so on. Finally, good practice begins with cultivating the skills of relational practice to work effectively with people from a wide range of backgrounds, including people whose primary language is different from the nurse's.

Cultivating the Skills of Relational Practice

Verbal communication includes spoken and written language and is essential to the provision of healthcare. The tone of voice and the words chosen are important to good communication. Language difference is one of the most problematic issues in the provision of appropriate, culturally and physically safe healthcare (Anderson et al., 2005). For example, assuming that a client understands a prescription label, or that someone else in the family understands it, is dangerous. Access to timely healthcare can be difficult when a client does not speak or write the local language. Nonverbal communication is also important because it can relay emotions and feelings. However, it is essential that the nurse does not make assumptions about nonverbal language, such as silence. For example, silence and a lack of eye contact have been attached to some ethnocultural groups, that is, to the "culture" rather than to the nature of the healthcare encounter. For some people simply being in an institution is intimidating, given historical factors and personal experiences—they may experience discomfort in response to power differentials or worry that questions and concerns may be trivialized. The nurse needs to be sure her or his perceptions of the client are appropriate to the level of trust and comfort of the client.

Doane and Varcoe (2005) provide a list of particular skills to enhance the relational capacities that the nurse already brings to practice: the skills of letting be, listening, self-observation, questioning to look beyond the surface, intentionality, interrupting contextual constraints, and reimagining—all are important in the process of health assessment. The following provides a snapshot of each.

"Letting be" is both a skill and a process. It is the skill of "joining into the flow" of health that individuals and families are living instead of seeking to change people. It is helpful for the nurse to be open to the possibilities that the client offers, that is, to be with the client where they are and learn from the individual or family—to take the time to see the person and be with them (Doane & Varcoe, 2005, pp. 200–202).

Listening is an essential ingredient to good communication. Many people listen to others with one ear while they are busy preparing a response or do not listen to the answer and continue with questions. As Doane and Varcoe (2005) note, there is a vast difference between "listening" and "wanting to speak." Listening involves multiple senses. The nurse comes to know what people mean not just from what they are saying "but from what they communicate energetically, bodily, contextually and so forth" (p. 202). The practice of clarifying and repeating an answer is helpful in ensuring good listening.

Self-observation is part of critical reflection. By attending to and reflecting on his or her thoughts, emotions, and bodily responses in the moment, the nurse enhances the opportunity to respond with intention, that is, the nurse is more likely to choose to act in a way that is supportive of the individual or family (Doane & Varcoe, 2005, p. 204).

Questioning and looking beyond the surface begins with the strategy of seeing what may have contributed to the difficulty being experienced by an individual or family, such as the structural issues and the actual lived experience of the individual or family (Doane & Varcoe, 2005, pp. 204–206). Noticing discrepancies and asking related questions to clarify what the nurse is hearing and seeing and what might lie beyond is an important aspect of looking beyond the surface. The nurse should look for patterns that arise in communication, such as ways in which an individual or a family is treated in healthcare that undermine their well-being. For example, when someone is reported as "noncompliant" by health professionals, the nurse may find that noncompliance is actually an inability to do something rather than a refusal. This finding is common in diabetes management where historical, social, and economic factors may intrude on a person's ability to adhere to his or her diet and exercise regime.

The skill of intentionality involves a clear and expressed congruence between what the nurse values and believes and her or his practice—the nurse becomes increasingly able to question and see beyond his or her own concerns to enhance the ability to be with individuals and families as they are and engage in intentional action to support them (Doane & Varcoe, 2005, p. 207).

The skill of interrupting contextual constraints by intentionally interrupting involves voicing questions and concerns, refusing to participate in oppressive practices, and countering with questions and countering alternative views. For example, a lone nurse can refuse to use such labels as "bed blockers" but will need the collaboration of other health professionals and families to scrutinize the practice of co-ed rooms in hospitals in Canada or the lack of access to interpreters (Doane & Varcoe, 2005, p. 208).

The skill of reimagining refers to addressing the problem of "what is" by imagining "what might be." In this way, the nurse can create opportunities for clients to tap into their capacity and transform their health and healing experiences (Doane & Varcoe, 2005, p. 208).

In the process of assessment, the nurse has an opportunity to support individuals and families as they enter healthcare and to ensure appropriate, culturally safe care. By supporting an understanding of their health and healing experiences in context, clarifying the meaning those experiences have for them, and supporting their choices and power within their experiences and ability to act on their choices, the nurse creates a climate in which the health-promoting quality of relationships is understood and supported (Doane & Varcoe, 2005, p. 210).

In summary, excellence in relational practice requires an acquisition of the skills described by Doane and Varcoe (2005) and a curiosity about the everyday lives of the clients, families, and communities the nurse meets. It is important to be interested in the work people do (whether or not they are employed), their housing, financial resources, children and how they are managed, extended family and responsibilities related to elders and others, transportation and access to healthcare, and so on (Anderson et al., 2005). This curiosity is essential to the provision of care—to health-promoting practice. For example, the nurse could begin by simply asking the client how things are going— this question will often end up providing an incredible amount of information related to how people are managing health and illness in the context of their everyday lives. Further information about the social circumstances of people's lives can be sought by asking such questions as the following, which are based on example questions posed by Anderson et al. (2005, p. 345):

- What is particularly challenging or difficult? *or* What is needed to manage your health or illness?
- Are you working currently? Can you tell me a little about the job you have? *or* What would you like to be doing?

- What do you need help with at home? Do you live alone?
- Do you have family or friends nearby who can help if needed?
- What kinds of things do you need help with?
- Are you able to get the things you need, such as medications, glasses, dental work, and assistive devices, such as a cane or wheelchair? (This is a delicate question that needs to be asked carefully.)
- Are you able to travel where necessary to access services or support?

These kinds of questions provide the contextual information necessary to assess the kinds of things people need to consider when they are challenged by a health issue. For example, healthcare professionals are often unaware of the challenges people face when they are discharged home from hospital, assuming that they have the resources necessary to manage (Anderson et al., 2005). This lack of resources could mean that there is nobody to care for an older adult who is immobile because it will mean lost wages or even loss of a job for the caregiver, or it could mean that a homeless person will be discharged to the street or that an Aboriginal person living on-reserve will need to find accommodation off-reserve while seeking healthcare there, with profound implications for others, such as her or his children.

The social context of people's lives has an incredible influence on health and healthcare—an important consideration in the process of health assessment.

APPLICATION THROUGH CRITICAL THINKING

CASE STUDY

Jeannette is a 21-year-old nursing student who is conducting health assessments in a core city health clinic. The people using this clinic are from a wide range of backgrounds and include a significant South Asian population, many with a long history living in this area, many different First Nations, a large gay community, and a growing population of young families with children. There is a small group of older adults in this area. Many people in the community are actively engaged in advocacy related to health and social inequities. Jeanette will be engaged in home visits in addition to her work in the clinic.

▶ *Critical Thinking Questions*

1. What should Jeannette do to prepare for this experience?
2. How might Jeanette begin her time in this community?
3. What can she expect from this experience?

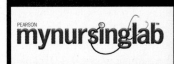

Visit the MyNursingLab website at **http://www.pearsoned.ca/mynursinglab**. This online homework and tutorial system puts you in control of your own learning with study and practice tools directly correlated to this chapter's content.

5

PSYCHOSOCIAL ASSESSMENT

PSYCHOSOCIAL FUNCTIONING INCLUDES THE WAY a person thinks, feels, acts, and relates to self and others. It is the ability to cope and tolerate stress, and the capacity for developing a value and belief system. Psychosocial functioning is part of an intricate set of subsystems making up the human organism. These subsystems are interrelated components that make up an individual who is greater than the sum of the parts. Assessment of the client must consider the interaction of body, mind, and spirit in their entirety rather than as separate body systems. When one part is missing or dysfunctional, all other parts of the individual are affected. Illness, developmental changes, or life crises may bring about changes in psychosocial functioning. The client may become stressed, may lose self-esteem, or may experience positive changes, such as greater closeness with family. Changes in psychosocial functioning may, in turn, affect the client's physical health or response to treatment. For example, a client who is extremely stressed may not be able to understand or remember instructions for self-care, and a client who is socially isolated may not be able to get needed help at home. Increasing evidence supports the theory that mind-body interactions play a key role in both health and illness. No matter what the source of the client's concern, a psychosocial assessment can provide significant insights that help to individualize client care.

PSYCHOSOCIAL HEALTH

Psychosocial health can be defined as being mentally, emotionally, socially, and spiritually well (see Figure 5.1). Psychosocial health includes mental, emotional, social, and spiritual dimensions. The mental dimension refers to an individual's ability to reason, to find meaning in and make judgments from information, to demonstrate rational thinking, and to perceive realistically. The emotional dimension is subjective and includes feelings. Social functioning refers to the individual's ability to form relationships with others. Included in the spiritual dimension are beliefs and values that give meaning to life.

FACTORS THAT INFLUENCE PSYCHOSOCIAL HEALTH

Psychosocial health is influenced by internal and external factors. Internal factors consist of a person's genetic makeup, physical health, and physical fitness. External factors include the influence of those responsible for a person's upbringing, and experiences in the social environment in which culture, geography, and economic status are contributory aspects.

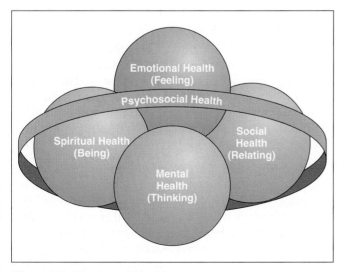

Figure 5.1 ● Psychosocial health.

Additional factors to consider when addressing psychosocial health are self-concept, role development, interdependent relationships, and the abilities to manage stress, to cope with and adapt to change, and to develop a belief and values system.

Internal Factors

Internal factors that influence psychosocial health include hereditary characteristics or those related to genetic makeup. In addition, the individual's physical health and level of fitness contribute to psychosocial health.

Genetics

As stated by the International Council of Nurses (2005), every health problem (with the exception of trauma) has a basis in genetics. With the completion of the Human Genome Project, gene-based testing and treatment are expected to dominate healthcare.

An individual's genetic makeup may influence physical and psychosocial health throughout life. Research indicates that 60% to 65% of hypertension is inherited, children whose parents have bipolar disorder have a slightly higher risk of experiencing that illness, and shyness is reportedly an inherited personality trait (International Council of Nurses, 2005). Parents with attention deficit hyperactivity disorder have an increased likelihood of having offspring with the disorder, and such conditions as alcoholism and hypoglycemia appear to have a genetic link. Some studies of identical twins reveal that they often have the same habits, mannerisms, and perceptions of anxiety, even when raised separately.

Hereditary differences affect a person's development in two ways. First, experiences affect hereditary predisposition for certain health problems. For example, whether an individual with a genetic predisposition to develop schizophrenia will develop the disease can depend, in part, on the environment in which the person lives. Second, genetic characteristics result in reactions from others that can influence the developing personality. Consider the fact that body structure, appearance, and overall physical attractiveness are inherited. Most people respond more positively to children who are physically attractive than to those who are not. Repeated responses of a positive or negative nature can affect a child's developing self-concept and self-esteem, as well as overall behaviour and interaction with others. Positive responses result in feelings of self-worth and confidence. Negative responses lead to low self-concept and may result in unmanageable levels of stress causing unacceptable behaviour or mental health problems. Furthermore, cognitive processes, including the abilities to think, perceive, remember, and make judgments, are dependent on an innate or inherited capacity and are enhanced or diminished in response to environmental and educational factors.

Physical Health

Physical health may be associated with satisfaction of basic needs, quality of life, and psychosocial well-being. Physical health enables an individual to respond to stressors and, therefore, to adapt, cope with change, and grow as a functioning individual capable of personal and social interaction.

Conversely, problems with health, particularly chronic illness, can negatively affect coping, adaptation, and personal and emotional fulfillment.

The mind-body-spirit connection is further explained as the body's response to thoughts and feelings. Positive and negative stress and anxiety can result in physical symptoms. Situations of positive and negative stress include marriage, childbirth, success in school or job performance, financial difficulties, the death of a friend or family member, or the loss of a job. Physical symptoms that may indicate a problem related to emotional stress or distress include the following:

- Back pain
- Chest pain
- Breathlessness
- Constipation
- Fatigue
- Hypertension
- Palpitations
- Dry mouth
- Nausea
- Weight loss or gain

Emotional **stress** affects health in several ways. First, stress affects the immune system, resulting in increased susceptibility to infection. Second, during periods of stress or change, individuals are less likely to attend to habits that promote health, such as eating nutritious meals or following an exercise routine. Last, some individuals use alcohol, tobacco, or drugs to feel better.

Measures to deal with stress and reduce the negative impact on physical and emotional health include talking openly about feelings; thinking about positive aspects of life; using relaxation techniques, such as meditation, yoga, prayer, or positive imagery; and following a regimen to promote health that includes healthy eating, exercise, and sleep.

Physical Fitness

Physical fitness is to the human body what fine-tuning is to an engine. It enables the body to perform up to its potential. Fitness can be described as a condition that helps individuals look, feel, and do their best. More specifically, physical fitness is

a set of attributes that are either health related or performance (or skill) related. Health related fitness comprises those components of fitness that exhibit a relationship with health status. Performance/skill related fitness involves those components of fitness that enable optimal work or sport performance. (Public Health Agency of Canada, 2003)

Physical fitness involves the performance of the heart, lungs, and muscles. Fitness, to some degree, influences such qualities as mental alertness and emotional stability, because what humans do with their bodies affects what they can do with their minds. To maintain fitness, a person must meet the needs for exercise, nutrition, rest, and relaxation, and follow practices to promote and preserve health. Recommendations related to physical activity were described in Chapter 2 of this text. ∞

External Factors

An individual's personality, sense of self, and role as a member of a larger society are influenced by a number of external factors. The manner and conditions in which a child is raised are an important influence. Additionally, the experiences during childhood and throughout life that are framed by family, culture, geography, and economic status contribute in great part to psychosocial well-being.

Family

Research indicates that children who receive consistent love, attention, and security grow into adults who are able to adapt to change and stress. Child rearing or caregiving generally occurs within a family unit. Families are social units of individuals who are related or live together. Individual members in families have ongoing contact with one another; share goals, values, and concerns; and develop practices common to that specific group. Today, families involved in child rearing can be two-parent, single-parent, heterosexual or same-sex marriages or common-law partnerships, blended or stepfamilies, adoptive families, or those in which grandparents, members of the extended family, or others provide childcare in the absence of parents.

Families influence psychosocial health because they are expected to provide for physical safety and economic needs; to help members develop physically, emotionally, and spiritually; and to help each individual develop an identity as self and a member of the family. Families foster development of social skills, spiritual beliefs, and a value system. Families promote adaptive and coping skills and assist members to become part of the greater society. The ability to provide these basic needs is dependent on the maturity of the caregivers and the support system available to them from family, community, and society.

Culture

Culture is a relational concept and therefore is highly complex. It is a process that exists between and within groups of people; it is created and lived; it is dynamic (Anderson & Reimer Kirkham, 1999, p. 63). Although culture includes shared beliefs, attitudes, values, and so on, it is important to consider culture more broadly as including those aspects of people's lives that contribute to their life experiences, the way they respond to those experiences, and the way they are in relationship with others, such as their identity as it relates to spirituality, religion, ethnicity, nationality, age, class, sexual orientation, gender, and so on. Healthcare, health, and well-being are strongly influenced and shaped by culture and associated sociopolitical, historical, and economic factors, such as globalization. Recall the details about the relationship between culture and health described in Chapter 4. ⬭

Geography

Geography refers to the country, region, section, community, or neighbourhood in which a person was born and raised or in which that person currently resides. The geography of an area affects family life and the development of individuals within families. Psychosocial health is influenced by the climate, terrain, resources, and aesthetics of a location. Community resources, including schools, places of worship, healthcare facilities, transportation systems, support services, and safety systems affect the social development and emotional well-being of individuals within the community. Individuals in urban areas are subjected to stressors associated with crowded conditions, congestion, and crime rates higher than in other areas. Residents of rural areas may experience the stressors of limited resources and isolation.

In addition, the nurse must consider the geographic impacts on psychosocial health that accompany regional characteristics, immigration, and the increased mobility of individuals and families. These characteristics shape the individual's self-concept and the ways that person appraises, is appraised, and interacts with others from within and without the regional or ethnic norm. Immigrants face the stress of adapting to new geographical characteristics and cultural norms. Communities into which immigrants settle and the individuals within them must adapt to the differences in language, customs, morals, values, and roles of the immigrant population. Children of immigrants may face the difficulty of being raised in a family with "old world" values and norms while growing and developing as members of their adopted community and culture. Because of economic demand or opportunity, families tend to move more frequently today than in the past. Adults and children then must adjust to the culture of the new location, the loss of the familiar, and the stress of separation from family and friends.

Economic Status

Economic status affects the formation of values and attitudes. Values and role expectations related to marriage, gender roles, family roles, sex, parenting, education, housing, leisure activities, clothing, occupation, and religious practice are influenced by an individual's or a family's economic status. The higher the income, the more likely it is that individuals and families will have achieved higher levels of education or provide for higher levels of education for their children. Better education leads to greater occupational opportunity, better housing, and the ability to participate in a variety of leisure activities. These advantages contribute to the development of high self-worth and self-esteem and result in individuals and families who are better equipped to manage and adapt to life changes. Those in lower economic groups or in poverty are focused on the present, that is, the immediate needs of self or family, including the basic needs of food, clothing, and shelter. Self-esteem and self-image are often lower in poor individuals and families. Continual confrontation with the results of the disparities in income may result in anger, frustration, difficulty in coping, family disturbances, abnormal behaviours, and mental health problems. Many times these individuals do not know how to access the healthcare delivery system.

Additional Factors in Psychosocial Health

Additional factors to consider in psychosocial health are self-concept, role development, interdependent relationships, and the abilities to manage stress, to cope and adapt to change, and to develop a belief and value system.

Self-Concept

Self-concept refers to the beliefs and feelings a person holds about himself or herself. A positive self-concept is essential to a person's mental and physical health. Individuals with a positive self-concept are better able to develop and maintain interpersonal relationships and cope with psychological and physical illness.

Self-concept develops over time as a person reacts to and learns from interactions with others. As an individual develops across the lifespan, the interactions move from the immediacy of contact with caregivers as children to contact with individuals in the greater environment.

Body image and self-esteem are components of self-concept. Body image is the way people think about their own physical appearance, size, and body functioning. Self-esteem refers to the sense of worth or self-respect of an individual. All aspects of self-concept affect psychosocial health. Psychosocially healthy people have a realistic sense of self, adapt to change, develop ways to cope with problems, and form relationships that promote growth and development. In contrast, psychosocially unhealthy individuals often have problems with self-concept, which manifest as pessimism, social isolation, feelings of worthlessness, neglect of physical health, depression, anxiety, problematic drug or alcohol use, or suicidal thoughts (see Figure 5.2).

Role Development

Role development refers to the individual's capacity to identify and fulfill the social expectations related to the variety of roles assumed in a lifetime. Roles are reciprocal relationships in which expectations exist for each participant. Examples of reciprocal roles are child-parent, student-teacher, employee-employer, as well as the reciprocal roles of spouse, sibling, friend, and neighbour. Roles are learned through socialization. The earliest learning generally occurs within the family when children observe and model adult behaviour. When role development is healthy and occurs in a supportive environment, self-concept and psychosocial well-being are enhanced as the individual gains confidence in the ability to interact with others according to societal norms. However, unsupportive, violent, or abusive family relationships are stressful and can

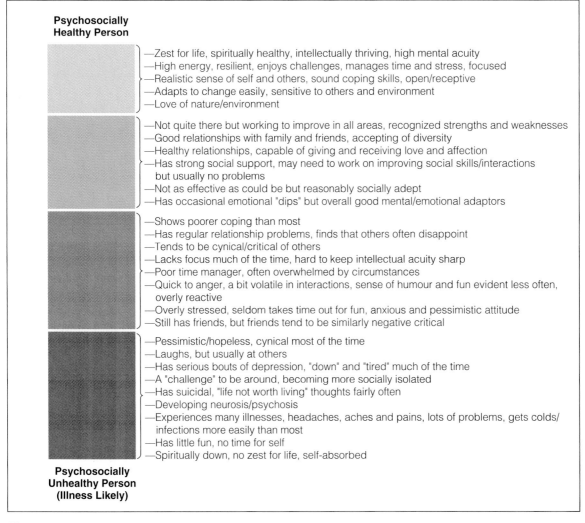

Psychosocially Healthy Person

—Zest for life, spiritually healthy, intellectually thriving, high mental acuity
—High energy, resilient, enjoys challenges, manages time and stress, focused
—Realistic sense of self and others, sound coping skills, open/receptive
—Adapts to change easily, sensitive to others and environment
—Love of nature/environment

—Not quite there but working to improve in all areas, recognized strengths and weaknesses
—Good relationships with family and friends, accepting of diversity
—Healthy relationships, capable of giving and receiving love and affection
—Has strong social support, may need to work on improving social skills/interactions but usually no problems
—Not as effective as could be but reasonably socially adept
—Has occasional emotional "dips" but overall good mental/emotional adaptors

—Shows poorer coping than most
—Has regular relationship problems, finds that others often disappoint
—Tends to be cynical/critical of others
—Lacks focus much of the time, hard to keep intellectual acuity sharp
—Poor time manager, often overwhelmed by circumstances
—Quick to anger, a bit volatile in interactions, sense of humour and fun evident less often, overly reactive
—Overly stressed, seldom takes time out for fun, anxious and pessimistic attitude
—Still has friends, but friends tend to be similarly negative critical

—Pessimistic/hopeless, cynical most of the time
—Laughs, but usually at others
—Has serious bouts of depression, "down" and "tired" much of the time
—A "challenge" to be around, becoming more socially isolated
—Has suicidal, "life not worth living" thoughts fairly often
—Developing neurosis/psychosis
—Experiences many illnesses, headaches, aches and pains, lots of problems, gets colds/infections more easily than most
—Has little fun, no time for self
—Spiritually down, no zest for life, self-absorbed

Psychosocially Unhealthy Person (Illness Likely)

Figure 5.2 ● A psychosocially healthy person versus a psychosocially unhealthy person.

lead to unsuccessful role relationships. Individuals who receive support and understand role expectations are able to meet the challenges of changing roles as they develop and mature. Individuals who have experienced family stress have conflicting views of role expectations or are unclear about social norms. They often experience frustration or a sense of inadequacy associated with fear or negative judgment from others if their performance is not in accordance with expectations for new or changing roles.

Interdependent Relationships

Interdependent relationships are those in which the individual establishes bonds with others based on trust. Interdependent relationships are characterized by mutual reliance and support. According to Roy and Andrews (1999), these relationships are based on the human needs of love, respect, and value for another. These important relationships include the individuals that a person identifies as the significant other and as a support system. The ability to form, maintain, and adapt to changes in interdependent relationships is affected by the individual's self-esteem. Individuals generally choose loving and close relationships with those who have similar levels of self-esteem. For example, when two people with high self-esteem form a loving and caring relationship, the high self-esteem is reinforced. Conversely, individuals with low self-esteem typically choose relationships with others with low self-esteem. As a result, feelings of negative self-worth are reinforced. Positive self-esteem enhances psychosocial health and enables the individual to grow and develop, adapt to change, solve problems, make decisions, maintain physical well-being, and seek help when needed for physical or emotional difficulties. Further, quality of life and length of life, which are measures of psychosocial health, have been linked to positive interdependent relationships.

Stress and Coping

Stress and coping are the individual's physical and emotional response to psychosocial or physical threats called stressors. An automobile accident, a failing grade, an illness, and loss of a job are examples of stressors. However, stress is not the event itself but the individual's response to it. Events that are highly stressful for one individual may not be stressful for another. The stress response may include familiar physical symptoms, such as sweaty palms or a pounding heart. The immediate physical reaction to stress is also referred to as the fight-or-flight response. Physical response to long-term stress may include such symptoms as habitually cold hands or suppression of immune function. The emotional reactions to stress may include difficulty sleeping, inability to concentrate, or anxiety. Positive and negative events can produce stress. The physical signs of stress include the following:

- Increased heart rate
- Decreased blood clotting time
- Increased rate and depth of respirations
- Dilated pupils
- Elevated glucose levels
- Dilated skeletal blood vessels
- Elevated blood pressure
- Dilated bronchi
- Increased blood volume
- Contraction of the spleen
- Increased blood supply to vital organs
- Release of T lymphocytes

Stress, in itself, is not bad. In fact, stress can sometimes motivate or enhance performance. Coping mechanisms are what an individual uses to deal with threats to physical and mental well-being. Like other patterns of behaviour, patterns of coping with stress stem from early development, when the child models the ways significant people in his or her life have coped with and dealt with stress.

Spiritual and Belief Patterns

Spiritual and belief patterns reflect an individual's relationship with a higher power or with something, such as an ideal, a group, or humanity itself, that gives meaning to life and that the person sees as larger than the self. The outward demonstration of spirituality may be reflected in religious practice, lifestyle, or relationships with others. A moral code is often included in a person's belief patterns. A moral code is the internalized values, virtues, and rules learned from significant others. It is developed by the individual to distinguish right from wrong. An individual's spiritual beliefs and moral code are affected by culture and ethnic background.

According to McSherry and Ross (2001), methods to assess spirituality and spiritual needs include direct questioning, indicator tools, and values clarification tools. Stoll (1979) introduced direct questioning as a method to assess spirituality. Stoll incorporated four basic areas for questioning: the client's concept of God (or a higher power), sources of hope and strength, religious practices, and the relationship between spiritual beliefs and health.

When using indicator tools, the nurse will observe verbal or nonverbal behaviours that indicate a spiritual need. Expressions of anger and crying are behaviours indicative of distress. Verbal cues would include such statements as "Why do I deserve this?"

Additional measures for spiritual assessment include the spiritual well-being scale (SWBS; Ellison & Paloutzian, 1982). This scale is a 20-item instrument that examines religious and existential well-being. The SWBS is a paper-pencil instrument currently available in English and Spanish. The standard method is for the scale to be self-administered, and it takes 10 to 15 minutes to complete. The SWBS is available for purchase online.

Anandarajah and Hight (2001) developed the use of HOPE questions to use as a formal spiritual assessment in the client interview. In the mnemonic HOPE, **H** refers to questions about the client's spiritual resources, including sources of hope, meaning, love, and comfort. **O** refers to participation in or association with organized religion. **P** includes personal spiritual practices. **E** refers to the effects of healthcare and end-of-life issues. Table 5.1 includes questions for the HOPE approach to spiritual assessment.

TABLE 5.1	HOPE Approach to Spiritual Assessment
H Spiritual resources	What are your sources of **hope** or comfort? What helps you during difficult times?
O Organized religion	Are you a member of an **organized religion?** What religious practices are important to you?
P Personal spirituality	Do you have **spiritual beliefs,** separate from organized religion? What **spiritual practices** are most helpful to you?
E Effects on care	Is there any conflict between your beliefs and the **care** you will be receiving? Do you hold beliefs or follow practices that you believe may affect your **care?** Do you wish to consult with a religious or spiritual leader when you are ill or making decisions about your **healthcare?**

Source: Adapted from Anandarajah, G., & Hight, E. (2001). Spiritutality and medical practice: Using the HOPE questions as a practical tool for spiritual assessment. *American Family Physician, 63,* 81–89. Retrieved from http://www.aafp.org/afp/2001/0101/p81.html

Hodge (2001) described a narrative framework for spiritual assessment. This qualitative instrument incorporates a spiritual history and a framework to identify spiritual strengths as shown in Table 5.2.

PSYCHOSOCIAL ASSESSMENT

The nurse uses knowledge, effective communication skills, and critical thinking while completing a psychosocial assessment. In conducting a psychosocial assessment, the nurse uses a holistic approach in assessing the client's responses to life experiences and the environment. The information is used to formulate nursing diagnoses and to plan care for the client.

Assessment

When assessing psychosocial health, the nurse gathers data related to several important areas, including psychosocial concern, self-concept and beliefs, stress and coping mechanisms, and reasoning ability.

Psychosocial assessment begins before the health history, when the nurse gathers information from the medical record relating to past emotional or psychiatric problems and physiological illnesses that may have affected the client's psychological or social functioning. For example, psychosocial problems may be related to brain tumours, multiple sclerosis, or bipolar disorder.

During the health history the nurse gathers more information about the client's social history (e.g., marital status and occupation), history of growth and development, past psychological problems, response to crises and illnesses, and family history of psychological or psychiatric illness. If an area of heightened concern is discovered, the nurse may focus on that area during the health history and may also conduct a health history later in the client's care. During the health history, the nurse uses information obtained from the medical history, the

TABLE 5.2	Narrative Spiritual Assessment

Part I. Narrative Framework—Spiritual History Sample Interview

1. Describe your personal and family religious traditions. (Include the importance of religion and religious practices.)
2. What practices were important to you in youth? How have those experiences influenced your life?
3. How would you describe your religiosity or spirituality today? Do you believe your spirituality provides strength? How?

Part II. Interpretive Framework—Evokes Spiritual Strengths

1. Affect: How does spirituality affect joy, sorrow, coping? What part does spirituality play in providing hope?
2. Behaviour: What rites or rituals do you use or follow? Do you have a relationship with a religious community or leader?
3. Cognition: Describe your current beliefs. Do your beliefs affect the ways you deal with difficulties or affect healthcare decisions?
4. Communion: What is your relationship with God? How do you communicate? Does your relationship help you in difficult times?
5. Conscience: Describe your values. How do you determine right and wrong?
6. Intuition: Have you experienced spiritual hunches, premonitions, or insights?

Source: Adapted from Hodge, D. R. (2001). Spiritual assessment: A review of major qualitative methods and a new framework for assessing spirituality. *Social Work, 46*(3), 8037–8046.

health history, and subsequent client interactions to help the client do a careful inventory of past and current psychosocial health status.

Psychosocial Well-Being

The nurse conducts a health history focused on psychosocial well-being in these cases:

- The information collected during the health history indicates psychosocial dysfunction.
- The client's behaviour during the health history is anxious, depressed, erratic, or bizarre.
- More information is needed to determine if any relationships exist between past disease processes and potential psychological or psychiatric concerns.

In some situations a psychosocial concern is not apparent during the health history but becomes apparent later, such as when a client learns of a negative prognosis or undergoes disfiguring surgical procedures. In these cases, the nurse should conduct a focused psychosocial health history when the psychological problem becomes apparent.

In some situations, the client's primary health concern is psychosocial in nature. Clients who experience problematic drug or alcohol use, depression, neurosis, or psychosis fall into this category. In these situations, the nurse should integrate the questions outlined here as part of the health history into the initial interview during the first contact with the client, family, or friends.

The health history should be structured to obtain the most information with the fewest questions. Clients may feel uncomfortable answering questions about themselves, making it difficult for the nurse to gather accurate and detailed data regarding the psychosocial aspects of the client's life. The following sections include a variety of questions to use as a guide for collecting information about the client's past history of psychosocial and physiological problems, as well as the five areas of psychosocial functioning.

History of Psychosocial Concerns

Some psychosocial concerns begin early in life and reappear whenever a client faces a major stressor or life crisis. The way the client coped with problems and treatment modalities in the past can be useful information for planning care for the client's current problems. The following questions are helpful in eliciting this information:

1. Describe any emotions you frequently experience or have frequently experienced in the past. *When the nurse assesses a client, a complete psychosocial history is helpful in determining whether the current health problem is related to previous psychosocial dysfunction.*

2. If you have had a psychological problem in the past, were you treated for it? What kind of treatment did you have? Was the treatment successful? Who gave you the treatment? When? Do you still have the problem? *This information is helpful in developing the current nursing care plan if previous methods of treatment were successful.*

3. Do you use alcohol or drugs? If so, what do you use, how much, and how often? Have you had any treatment for substance abuse? What kind of treatment? Where? *Substance abuse may be the underlying cause of physiological or psychosocial health problems or may be the result of some other underlying problem.*

4. Have you had any eating disorders, such as anorexia, bulimia, or binge eating? Were you treated? How? By whom? When? *A client who has an eating disorder may be in denial and unable to give accurate information on this question. If an eating disorder is suspected, the nurse should look for the diagnostic cues during the physical assessment.*

History of Diseases or Physical Alterations

When being treated for medical-surgical conditions, clients and their families may be unaware that the physical problems may be related to or caused by an underlying psychosocial problem. An understanding of the body-mind interaction, both positive and negative, can help nurses and clients realize when covert cognitive, perceptual, or affective problems are related to the overt signs and symptoms. Sometimes the underlying problem does not surface immediately but becomes apparent only after several days of nursing care.

The following questions are helpful for uncovering additional information:

1. Describe any chronic illnesses you have had. *Clients with recent onset of chronic illnesses often have problems complying with treatment or adjusting to living with the condition.*

2. How has your illness changed your mood or feelings? When you are nervous or anxious, how does your body feel? *A physiological condition may be an underlying cause of anxiety, nervousness, or other abnormal behaviour. Conversely, abnormal psychosocial behaviour may aggravate or cause a physiological condition.*

3. Have you had any of the following health problems: arthritis? asthma? bowel disorders? heart problems? glandular problems? headaches? stomach ulcer? skin disorders? If so, describe how the condition has affected your life. *These conditions sometimes have both a psychological and a physiological component.*

Self-Concept

It is difficult to gather significant data about self-concept, because most clients find it embarrassing to answer questions about themselves. Clients feel more comfortable divulging this information after a positive nurse-client relationship has been established and when the nurse integrates questions into general conversation.

The following questions are helpful in obtaining additional information about self-concept:

1. How would you describe yourself to others? *Asking clients to describe themselves is an excellent technique for determining how they perceive themselves.*

2. What are your best characteristics? What do you like about yourself?

3. What would you change about yourself if you could? *This is a positive way of asking a client to talk about negative self-perceptions.*

4. Would you describe yourself as shy or outgoing?

5. Do you consider yourself attractive? Sexually appealing? If no, why not? *The client's self-perception of attractiveness and sex appeal may reveal problems with self-image.*

6. Have your feelings about your appearance changed with this illness? If so, how? *Self-image may change if the illness or treatment has caused a change in appearance.*

7. Who comes first in your life: your spouse, children, friends, parents, or yourself?

8. Do you have difficulty saying no to others? *Clients who are depressed, feel hopeless, or feel powerless have difficulty with assertiveness.*

9. Do you like to be alone? *Clients with positive self-concept enjoy spending time by themselves, but those who indicate that they'd rather be alone most of the time may be experiencing psychological problems.*

10. Describe your social life. What do you do for fun? *Clients who are unable to answer this question may be depressed or out of touch with reality.*

11. What are your hobbies or interests? Do you spend much time pursuing them?

12. For heterosexuals only. Are you comfortable relating to the opposite sex? If no, why not? *Persons with self-concept or self-image problems may experience difficulty relating to the opposite sex.*

13. Are you comfortable with your sexual orientation? If no, why not? *Clients who are gay or lesbian and have not learned to accept their sexuality may experience a self-image problem.*

14. Do you have any concerns about your sexual function? If so, what?

15. Do you have problems with intimacy?

Family History

The nurse should explore this area more fully if the health history indicates a family history of psychosocial dysfunction. Although no member of the family may have been diagnosed as being mentally ill, the nurse should explore individual as well as family dysfunction.

The nurse should ask the following questions in relation to the client's parents, siblings, and extended family in the case of a child, and in relation to the client's current family, if an adult:

1. Describe any problems your family may have had with mental disorders. *Some mental disorders, such as schizophrenia, are familial, that is, the illness recurs in the same family over several generations.*

2. What were your major responsibilities in your family?

3. Describe your relationships with your parents and extended family. *The nurse should look for family dysfunction problems, such as schisms (families in chronic controversy), disengagement (detached relationships), or enmeshment (family interactions that are intense and focus on power conflicts rather than affections) as the client describes his or her family life.*

4. What is your birth order in your family? How many brothers and sisters? Are your sisters and brothers older or younger? *Age and gender birth order influence how an individual relates to other men and women throughout life.*

5. Describe your relationship with your siblings growing up at home. Did you and your siblings have problems getting along? If so, how did you solve them? *The way a client learned to handle stress and conflict with siblings as a child influences the way the client handles these issues throughout life.*

6. What members of your extended family (grandparents, aunts, uncles, cousins) were important to you as you grew up? How did they influence you? *Significant others shape an individual's self-concept and self-esteem. Descriptions of significant others help the nurse understand why clients feel and act as they do.*

7. Did you have death or losses in your family as you grew up? How did your parents teach you to cope with the loss? How did they cope with the loss? *Clients who are depressed may not have learned how to deal with loss as a child and may have difficulty dealing with the loss of a loved one or with their own or a significant other's declining health status.*

8. Were your parents divorced or remarried during your childhood? If so, whom did you live with? Describe your life growing up with a single parent or stepparent. *Children who are products of a divorce may carry scars into adulthood, affecting their psychosocial health and indirectly affecting their physical health status.*

9. Describe how your parents raised you. How did it affect you? *Clients who were raised by parents who had serious psychological problems, or who were abused by their parents, are more likely to have psychological problems as adults.*

10. How did your family deal with adversity and conflict? *Clients learn their approach to problem solving from their family. Knowing how the client learned to deal with problems as a child helps the nurse understand how the client might deal with the present health problem.*

11. When disagreement arose in your family, how was it solved? Who sided with whom? *In dysfunctional families, schisms result causing family members to align themselves into coalitions against other family members, such as parents against children, father and sons against mother and daughters, and sisters against brothers.*

12. Did you experience or observe physical or psychological abuse as a child?

Other Roles and Relationships

It is also important for the nurse to ask questions about other roles and relationships in the client's life:

1. Describe your relationships with your friends, neighbours, and co-workers.

2. Do you belong to any social groups? community groups?

3. Who is your closest friend? How do you maintain your friendship? *An individual's ability to form close relationships indicates a healthy self-concept. An individual who consistently fails to form close relationships may have a self-concept problem.*

4. Is your closest friend the most important person in your life? If not, who is the most important person in your life? Explain why.

Stress and Coping

A person learns coping mechanisms from significant others during early childhood and throughout life. The ability to cope is also greatly affected by the number and severity of stressors that have occurred in a person's life. One method for assessing stress in a client's life is to administer the Holmes social readjustment rating scale (see Table 5.3). The items on this scale represent stressors that may occur in a person's life. Since stress is a response to events, not the events themselves, not all people are equally stressed by these events. However, on average, the higher the client's score, the more likely it is that the individual has responded with stress. As a result, the individual is more likely to experience stress-related disorders (e.g., headaches, skin rashes, back pain, frequent colds, anxiety). The scale demonstrates that positive life events should also be part of a psychosocial assessment, because these positive events can be just as stressful as negative events in a person's life.

The following questions are helpful to gather additional information about the client's stress and coping mechanisms:

1. What do you do for relaxation? for recreation?

2. What is your greatest source of comfort when you are feeling upset? *This question identifies the client's coping mechanisms.*

TABLE 5.3	Holmes Social Readjustment Scale	

EVENT	EVENT VALUE
1. Death of a spouse	100
2. Divorce	73
3. Marital separation	65
4. Jail term	63
5. Death of a close family member	63
6. Personal injury or illness	53
7. Marriage	50
8. Fired at work	47
9. Marital reconciliation	45
10. Retirement	45
11. Change in health of family member	44
12. Pregnancy	40
13. Sex difficulties	39
14. Gain of a new family member	39
15. Business readjustment	39
16. Change in financial state	38
17. Death of a close friend	37
18. Change to different line of work	36
19. Change in number of arguments	35
20. Mortgage or loan over $10 000	31
21. Foreclosure of mortgage or loan	30
22. Change in responsibilities at work	29
23. Son or daughter leaving home	29
24. Trouble with in-laws	29
25. Outstanding personal achievement	28
26. Spouse begins or stops work	26
27. Begin or end school	26
28. Change in living conditions	25
29. Revision of personal habits	24
30. Trouble with boss	23
31. Change in work hours or conditions	20
32. Change in residence	20
33. Change in schools	20
34. Change in recreation	19
35. Change in church activities	19
36. Change in social activities	19
37. Change in sleeping habits	16
38. Change in number of family get-togethers	15
39. Vacation	13
40. Christmas	12
41. Minor violations of the law	11
Total Points	

Directions for completion: Add up the point values for each of the events that you have experienced during the past 12 months.

Scoring

Below 150 points:

The amount of stress you are experiencing as a result of changes in your life is normal and manageable. There is only a 1 in 3 chance that you might develop a serious illness over the next 2 years based on stress alone. Consider practising a daily relaxation technique to reduce your chance of illness even more.

150 to 300 points:

The amount of stress you are experiencing as a result of changes in your life is moderate. Based on stress alone, you have a 50/50 chance of developing a serious illness over the next 2 years. You can reduce these odds by practising stress management and relaxation techniques on a daily basis.

(continued)

Over 300 points:

The amount of stress you are experiencing as a result of changes in your life is high. Based on stress alone, your chances of developing a serious illness during the next 2 years approaches 90%, unless you are already practising good coping skills and regular relaxation techniques. You can reduce the chance of illness by practising coping strategies and relaxation techniques daily.

Source: From Holmes, T., & Rahe, R. J. (1967). Social readjustment rating scale. *Journal of Psychosomatic Research, 11,* 213–218. Elsevier Science Ltd., Pergamon Imprint, Oxford, England.

3. Who do you call when you need help? *This question identifies important persons in the client's support system.*

4. What is the greatest source of stress in your life? How have you coped with similar situations in the past? *A person who has successfully coped with stress in the past may be able to call on these coping skills to deal with current problems.*

5. Describe how you are dealing with your illness. Have you had difficulty adjusting to changes in your appearance? ability to carry out activities of daily living? relationships? If so, describe how you feel. *Clients who have undergone severe, sudden changes that are apparent to others frequently have difficulty adjusting to these changes.*

6. Do you take any drugs, medications, or alcohol to cope with your stress? If so, describe what you are taking. *Clients who are experiencing stress are at risk for becoming addicted to these substances, especially if there is a family history of problematic drug or alcohol use.*

7. Are you experiencing any of the following: sadness? crying spells? insomnia? lack of appetite? weight loss? weight gain? loss of sex drive? constipation? fatigue? hopelessness? irritability? indecisiveness? confusion? pounding heart or pulse? trouble concentrating? *These may indicate a high level of stress or major depression.*

8. Have you ever considered taking your life? If so, describe what you would do. *Clients who are suicidal often admit their intentions if questioned directly. Clients are at high risk for suicide if they can describe a method for committing the suicide and have the necessary means at their disposal. (See Box 5.1 for characteristics of the suicidal client.)*

The Senses and Cognition

Clients who are out of contact with reality may display illusional, delusional, and hallucinatory speech and behaviours, such as talking to themselves (auditory hallucinations); reacting to objects, noises, or other people in strange ways (illusions); or discussing false beliefs (delusions). Direct questioning may increase the client's anxiety and escalate the abnormal behaviour or cause confusion. The nurse should use direct questioning only when the client appears to be in control and in touch with reality.

The following questions are helpful to gather additional information. The nurse should preface these questions by first explaining to the client that some of the questions may seem

BOX 5.1	Characteristics of the Client Who Is at the Highest Risk for Suicide

The following characteristics may indicate that a client is at increased risk for suicide. While one of the following items alone may not indicate a client is contemplating suicide, the more factors present, the more likely that the client is at increased risk:

- Single, divorced, or widowed
- Socially isolated or little or no support system
- History of suicide attempts
- Family history of suicide
- Recent loss, such as divorce, threat of or loss of a loved one; loss of a job, money, or social status
- History of problematic drug use or alcoholism
- History of mental illness
- Depression or recovering from depression
- Severe anxiety or fear
- Serious or physical illness, with impaired lifestyle or altered body image
- Sleep dysfunction
- Expression of feelings of hopelessness, powerlessness, rejection, or punishment
- Arrangement of personal affairs, such as taking out an insurance policy, planning a funeral, cancelling social engagements, preparing a will, or giving possessions away
- Verbalization of suicidal thoughts, such as "Sometimes I think I'd be better off dead" or "I give up"
- Sudden or unexplained behaviour change
- Feelings of ineffective communication or family members rejecting attempts at communication
- Feelings of increased life responsibilities
- Crying for no obvious reason
- Certain demographic variables, such as gender (suicide rates are higher for men), race (suicide rates are higher for white people and Aboriginal Canadians), age (suicide rates are higher between 15 and 24 years), both ends of the socioeconomic scale

silly or unimportant but that they are helpful in assessing memory. Questions 1 through 5 determine whether the client is oriented to person, place, and time.

CLINICAL TIP!

Don't ask a question you don't know the answer to.

1. What is your name?

2. How old are you?

3. Where were you born?

4. Where are you right now?

5. What day of the week is it? What is the date?

6. What would you take with you if a fire broke out? *The client's ability to make a judgment is tested here.*

7. Count backward from 10 to 1. *This task tests cognitive function.*

8. What did you have for breakfast? *This question tests recent memory.*

9. Who was the last premier? *This question tests remote memory.*

10. Describe what the following statement means: People who live in glass houses shouldn't throw stones. *This task tests the client's ability to do abstract or symbolic thinking.*

11. Are you having any problems thinking? If so, describe what happens. *The client may not be able to answer this question if a thought disorder is present. Clients with bipolar disorder and who experience mania describe their thoughts as "racing."*

12. Do you have trouble making decisions? Describe what happens when you have to make a decision. *The inability to make decisions may indicate depression or low self-esteem.*

13. Do you ever hear voices, see objects, or experience other sensations that don't make sense? If so, describe your experiences. *The client who is out of touch with reality may experience auditory, visual, gustatory, somatic, and olfactory hallucinations (hearing, seeing, tasting, feeling, and smelling stimuli that are not real). Discussing hallucinatory experiences in detail may reinforce them for the client; therefore, it is important not to dwell on these symptoms.*

14. If you hear voices, do they tell you what you must do? *The nurse asks this question to determine if the client is experiencing command hallucinations. These are dangerous hallucinations that may lead the client to self-destructive behaviour or to harm others.*

15. Do you ever misinterpret objects, sounds, or smells? If so, please describe. *Clients who are very anxious or out of contact with reality may experience illusions (misinterpretation of environmental stimuli).*

It is important to assess the content of a client's hallucinations and delusions to provide for the client's safety and the safety of others. Command hallucinations tell clients to carry out acts that are usually harmful against themselves or others. The command hallucinations may be part of an elaborate delusional system in which clients feel persecuted or in danger. In some cases, clients are disturbed by these thoughts and share them with others. In other situations, however, clients keep their thoughts to themselves, and these thoughts do not become apparent until clients commit some violent act. A client who demonstrates these symptoms should be referred to a psychiatric or mental health nurse or clinical specialist who has the skill and expertise needed to uncover hallucinatory and delusional thinking without exacerbating the symptoms.

Spiritual and Belief Systems

The questions in this section determine how clients' ethical, moral, and religious values affect their health status. Often the client's statements about values play an important role in how the nurse should implement care. It is important to be sensitive to the client's reaction to these questions when assessing this area, because the client's spiritual life and belief systems may be very personal.

The nurse should also be careful about querying a client who is having hallucinations or has a delusional disorder, because the questions can exacerbate delusional or hallucinatory behaviour.

The spiritual and belief systems of clients usually derive from their culture and ethnic background. A client may have beliefs about health and illness, God, or the supernatural that are culturally derived. The nurse needs to understand that these issues play an important role in the client's ability to cope with a psychosocial health concern or illness.

The following questions are used to assess the client's spiritual and belief systems and the cultural and ethnic considerations surrounding them. While collecting this information, the nurse should observe the client's verbal and nonverbal behaviour, interpersonal relationships, and immediate environment.

1. Describe your ethnic and cultural background. *Clients from some ethnic and cultural groups are more likely to have health-related beliefs and practices that have an impact on nursing care (see Chapter 4 ⬭).*

2. To whom do you go for help regarding your health (doctor, nurse practitioner, folk healer, medicine man, or other healer)? *The nurse is more likely to gain the client's compliance if the client's folk healer is included in the planning stage.*

3. What are your beliefs about life, health, illness, and death? *The nurse needs this knowledge about the client's health-related beliefs to develop an individualized plan of care.*

4. Does religion or God or a higher power play a part in your life? If so, what is it? *The nurse should incorporate the client's religion and faith in God or a higher power in the plan of care if they are important to the client.*

5. What part do hope and faith play in your life? Is your faith helpful to you during times of stress? If so, describe how.

6. Has your present health concern affected your spiritual life? If so, describe how.

7. Do your spiritual beliefs help you cope with illness or stress? If so, describe how.

8. Have you experienced any anger with God or a higher power because of things that have happened to you? If so, describe how you feel. *Clients who feel anger toward God or a higher power may project this anger toward family, friends, and healthcare providers.*

9. Do you believe your illness is a punishment for past sins or wrongdoing? *Clients who feel they are being punished may feel guilty and lose the ability to cope with the illness.*

10. If you use prayer, describe how you use it to cope with life or stress. *The nurse should incorporate the client's use of prayer in the plan of care if it is meaningful to the client.*

11. Are you affiliated with any religion?

12. Describe any religion-related nutrition or health practices that you must follow.

13. Are you concerned about the morality or ethical implications of any of the treatments planned for you?

Physical Observation

During the health history, the nurse should also observe the client's general appearance, posture, gait, body language, and speech patterns. The client's general appearance includes the manner of dress, personal hygiene, and grooming.

- The client should be clean and well groomed. The clothes should be clean, worn properly, and appropriate for the client's age and the time and place. The nurse must be careful not to impose his or her own standards when judging a client's clothing.

- Abnormal speech patterns may indicate anxiety, fear, or altered thought processes (see Box 5.2). The nurse should observe the coherence and organization of the client's speech. The client's speech should be logical and sequential.

- Clients may demonstrate the following: talking to themselves (auditory hallucinations); reacting to objects, noises, or other people in strange ways (illusions); or manifesting erratic beliefs (delusions). The client may appear to be aphasic or incoherent. These clients may be experiencing altered communication, altered thought processes, and ineffective coping.

- The client who is dirty, dishevelled, or unshaven or who has a body odour may have an altered body image caused by a low self-esteem. The nurse should further assess the client for changes in skin integrity caused by unclean conditions and look for signs of ringworm, pediculosis (lice infestation), or other skin problems (see Chapter 11 ⬭).

The nurse should next observe the client's posture, gait, and general body language.

- The client's posture should be erect and relaxed. The body language should be open with direct eye contact unless inappropriate for the client's ethnic group. Movements should be fluid, relaxed, and spontaneous. A closed, guarded posture with poor eye contact may indicate fear, anxiety, or defence mechanisms. The client who paces, wrings hands, appears restless, or exhibits tics (involuntary movements) may also be experiencing anxiety. A slow, shuffling gait may indicate depression or poor contact with reality.

The nurse must also observe the client's facial expression and affect. The expression and affect should be appropriate for the conversation and circumstances.

- An unusually sad (depressed) or extremely happy (euphoric) demeanour that is inappropriate for the circumstances, labile (rapid) mood swings, or flat affect (absence of emotional expression) may indicate difficulty coping.

BOX 5.2	Abnormal Speech Patterns Associated with Altered Thought Processes

Certain speech patterns can point to a client's altered thought process:
- Loud, rapid, pressured, and high-pitched
- Circumlocution (inability to communicate an idea because of numerous digressions)
- Flight of ideas (jumping from one subject to another)
- Word salad (a conglomeration of multiple words without apparent meaning)
- Neologisms (coining new words that have symbolic meaning to the client)
- Clanging (rhyming conversation)
- Echolalia (constant repetition of words or phrases that the client hears others say)

Finally, the nurse should notice the content and manner of speech. The content, tone, pace, and volume of the speech should be appropriate for the situation.

Measures, scales, and instruments are available to assess particular aspects of psychosocial health including quality of life, social support, stress, and psychosocial well-being. For example, in the United States the Centers for Disease Control and Prevention (CDC) uses "healthy day measures" to assess quality of life in populations. Box 5.3 includes questions used in healthy day measures. This tool is widely used in Canada as well.

Other measures to assess particular aspects of psychosocial health include the Multidimensional Health Profile–Psychosocial Functioning (MHP–P). An instrument designed to screen for psychosocial problems, the MHP–P assesses life stress, coping, social supports, and mental health.

The nurse may also use the Duke Social Support and Stress Scale (DUSOCS). This is a 24-item self- and interviewer-administered instrument to measure family and nonfamily support and stress. Psychological well-being can be assessed with a variety of scales, including the delighted-terrible scale, the faces scale, the ladder scale, and the life satisfaction index. Each of these provides a system to rank the client's perceptions of well-being. More information is available on the website of the Department of Community and Family Medicine at Duke University.

In 2008, the Canadian Institute of Wellbeing was established and headed by the Honourable Roy J. Romanow. Its mission is to report on the quality of life of Canadians and promote a dialogue on how to improve it through evidence-based policies that are responsive to the needs and values of Canadians. All aspects of health, including psychosocial health, are assessed by using the Canadian Index of Wellbeing. In June 2009, the Canadian Institute of Wellbeing released its first report titled "How Are Canadians *Really* Doing?" The report and index are available through the Institute's website.

BOX 5.3	HEALTHY DAY MEASURES

The CDC uses a set of questions called the "healthy day measures." These questions include the following:

1. Would you say that in general your health is
   a. Excellent
   b. Very good
   c. Good
   d. Fair
   e. Poor

2. Now thinking about your physical health, which includes physical illness and injury, for how many days during the past 30 days was your physical health not good?

3. Now thinking about your mental health, which includes stress, depression, and problems with emotions, for how many days during the past 30 days was your mental health not good?

4. During the past 30 days, for about how many days did poor physical or mental health keep you from doing your usual activities, such as self-care, work, or recreation?

Source: United States Department of Health and Human Services, Centers for Disease Control and Prevention, National Center for Chronic Disease Prevention and Health Promotion. Retrieved from http://www.cdc.gov/hrqo/hrqo/14_measures.htm

Organizing the Data

Once the nurse has collected the data from all of the various sources, the information is sorted, grouped, and categorized. Each diagnostic cue falls under one of the psychosocial functioning groups mentioned earlier in this chapter: self-concept, roles and relationships, stress and coping, the senses and cognition, and spiritual and belief systems. After the diagnostic cues have been grouped and clustered under one of the psychosocial groups, the nurse determines the final nursing diagnoses.

The following case study demonstrates how diagnostic cues obtained during the assessment lead to nursing diagnoses related to psychosocial well-being and function.

Mr. Abe Johnson, a transient passing through town, was admitted to the local hospital emergency room after being arrested for disturbing the peace and possession of heroin. The guards at the jail had brought him to the hospital after they were unable to control his violent behaviour. When approached by the admitting nurse, Ms. Quan, Mr. Johnson shouted, "Don't come near me with that gas machine! The High Lord has told me that I control the secret of life and death, and if you touch me you must die!" The nurse recognized that Mr. Johnson had seen the stethoscope she carried as a "gas machine." After observing Mr. Johnson's manner and tone for a few minutes, she also noted that he was hearing voices. Ms. Quan knew that Mr. Johnson's behaviour could become violent if he continued to experience command hallucinations. She removed the stethoscope from around her neck and showed it to Mr. Johnson. She said, speaking in a quiet calm voice, "This is the stethoscope that I use to listen to a client's heart. Sometimes I use it to take blood pressures. Would you like to look at it?" As Mr. Johnson doubtfully held the stethoscope and rapidly and repeatedly turned it over, she said, "Most stethoscopes are black and silver but mine is white and gold. I think it's a pretty colour, don't you?" Mr. Johnson threw the stethoscope back at Ms. Quan, mumbling, "Okay." After a few minutes she said, "You've been brought to the hospital, Mr. Johnson. I'm Ms. Quan, your nurse, and I'm here to take care of you. Have you noticed that even though I've been helping you remove your clothes, nothing has happened to me?"

In this clinical situation, the nurse showed Mr. Johnson respect and concern for his feelings and well-being. She did not, however, validate his perceptions about the stethoscope or acknowledge the voices he heard. Instead, she reinforced reality for him by describing the white and gold stethoscope and pointing out that he had no special power to harm her.

The nurse then clustered the information gained from the assessment and identified the significant cues demonstrated by Mr. Johnson:

- Hallucinations
- Delusions
- Illusions
- Fearful thoughts
- Irritability
- Inaccurate interpretation of environment

Ms. Quan reviewed all the data and saw the following factors as contributing to Mr. Johnson's problems:

- Problematic drug use
- Transient lifestyle

Then, after reviewing the assessment data, identifying contributing factors, and clustering the information, Ms. Quan formulated diagnoses and a plan of care.

The holistic approach to nursing holds that the individual must be viewed as a total being in which body, mind, and spirit continuously interact with the self and with the environment. The psychosocial assessment is a key component that must be integrated into the nurse's holistic approach to data collection. This assessment guides the nurse toward a true and accurate picture of the client as a total human being.

APPLICATION THROUGH CRITICAL THINKING

CASE STUDY

Luke Van Hoff, a 44-year-old engineer, has recently been transferred from a suburban town office to a larger firm in an urban area. His wife and three school-age children will join him at the completion of the school year.

Luke is currently residing in company housing while house hunting on the weekends. He was eager to take the new position because it meant a significant increase in income.

You are the nurse in the corporate health office who will conduct a comprehensive health assessment of this new employee.

▶ *Critical Thinking Questions*

1. What psychosocial issues will be addressed in the interview?
2. Analyze the data in the case study and describe how the psychosocial health of Mr. Van Hoff will be impacted.
3. Select which psychosocial functioning groups would be included in an assessment of Mr. Van Hoff.

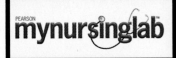

6

TECHNIQUES AND EQUIPMENT

CHAPTER OBJECTIVES

On completion of the chapter, you will be able to

1. Describe the four basic techniques used by the nurse when performing physical assessment.
2. Explain the purpose of equipment required to perform a complete physical assessment.
3. Describe client safety and comfort measures to be considered when performing physical assessment.
4. Apply critical thinking when using the four basic techniques of physical assessment.
5. Apply the principles of routine practices.

CHAPTER OUTLINE

Unit I of this book identified and discussed many concepts to be considered when assessing the overall health status of the client. These concepts include but are not limited to health, wellness, growth and development, culture, and psychosocial considerations. Much of the data gathered in relation to these concepts is subjective and is obtained through client interviews during the health history sessions. For example, when a client reports feeling "pins and needles" in his left foot, or feelings of "nausea" after drinking cold water, subjective data are being reported and collected.

Objective data must be gathered as part of the **database**. This task is accomplished through the physical assessment of the client. The objective data are obtained by using the four basic or cardinal techniques of physical assessment: inspection, palpation, percussion, and auscultation. Special equipment and the nurse's senses are used to measure, observe, touch, and listen to sounds of the body. A safe, comfortable environment conducive to client comfort, dignity, and privacy is essential. Individual clients will react differently to each situation. The nurse must obtain client permission to proceed, make the client feel comfortable, and communicate with the client throughout the physical assessment.

BASIC TECHNIQUES OF PHYSICAL ASSESSMENT

When performing physical assessment, the nurse will use four basic techniques to obtain objective and measurable data. These techniques are inspection, palpation, percussion, and auscultation and are performed in an organized manner. This pattern changes when assessing the abdomen. The sequence for abdominal assessment is inspection, auscultation, percussion, and palpation. Percussion and palpation could alter the natural sounds of the abdomen; therefore, it is important to auscultate and listen to the unaltered sounds. This sequence is further discussed in Chapter 19 of this text. ◎

Inspection

Inspection is the skill of observing the client in a deliberate, systematic manner. It begins the moment the nurse meets the client and continues until the end of the client-nurse interaction (see Figure 6.1). Inspection always precedes the other assessment skills and is never rushed. Most novice nurses feel uncomfortable staring at the client; nevertheless, careful scrutiny provides critical assessment data. The nurse should talk to the client, help

KEY TERMS

auscultation, 91
cues, 95
database, 87
dullness, 91
flatness, 91
fremitus, 88
hyperresonance, 91
inspection, 87
palpation, 88
percussion, 89
pleximeter, 90
plexor, 90
resonance, 91
tympany, 91

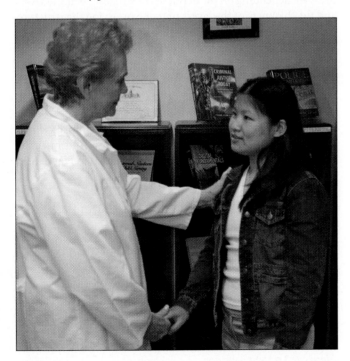

Figure 6.1 ● Inspection of client.

the client relax before proceeding with inspection. It is important to complete inspection of the client before using any of the other techniques. However, if the client is a child, the nurse may need to vary the approach to secure the child's attention and cooperation.

Inspection begins with a survey of the client's appearance and a comparison of the right and left sides of the client's body, which should be nearly symmetrical. As the nurse assesses each body system or region, he or she inspects for colour, size, shape, contour, symmetry, movement, and drainage. When inspecting a large body region, the nurse should proceed from general overview to specific detail. For example, when inspecting the leg, the nurse surveys the entire leg and then focuses on each part, including the thigh, knee, calf, ankle, foot, and toes in succession. The nurse should remember to look at the client, listen for natural sounds, and use the sense of smell to detect odours. Use of each of the senses enhances the findings.

Throughout inspection, the nurse applies the skills of critical thinking to analyze the observations and determine the significance of the findings to the general health of the client. The nurse must know the anticipated findings regarding inspection of a body part. The nurse thinks about the following questions: Are the findings considered to be within normal parameters, or are they unexpected findings? Are the findings consistent with other diagnostic cues? What other information is needed to support this finding?

Although the nurse will perform most of the inspection without the help of instruments, some special tools for visualizing certain body organs or regions are important. For example, the ophthalmoscope is used to inspect the inner aspect of the eye. This instrument and others used to enhance inspection are discussed later in this chapter.

Palpation

Palpation is the skill of assessing the client through the sense of touch to determine specific characteristics of the body. These characteristics include size, shape, location, mobility of a part, position, vibrations, temperature, texture, moisture, tenderness, and edema. The approach used by the nurse to obtain these data is important. The nurse must be gentle and obtain the client's confidence. The nurse's hand must move slowly and intentionally. The nurse must learn how much pressure to use during palpation with the examination hand. Too much pressure may produce pain for the client. Too little pressure may not permit the nurse to perceive the data accurately. This skill requires practice and is developed over time.

The hand has several sensitive areas; therefore, it is important to use the part of the hand most responsive to body structures and functions. The nurse will use the fingertips, fingerpads, base of the fingers, palmar surface of the fingers, and the dorsal and ulnar surfaces of the hand (see Figure 6.2).

The fingerpads are used for discrimination of underlying structures and functions, such as pulses, superficial lymph nodes, or crepitus. Vibratory tremors felt through the chest wall are known as **fremitus**. Fremitus can be vocal, when the client speaks, or tussive, during coughing. Vibrations are perceived by the examiner when using the metacarpophalangeal

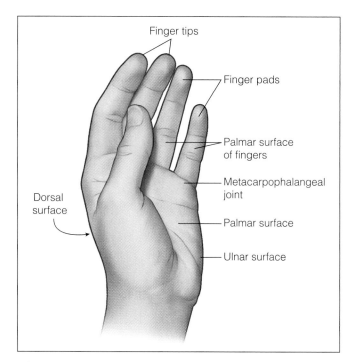

Figure 6.2 ● Sensitive areas of the hand.

joints (base of the fingers). The palmar aspect of the fingers is used to determine position, consistency, texture, size of structures, pain, and tenderness. The ulnar surface of the hand, including the finger, is sensitive to vibrations, such as fremitus. Remember, the dominant hand is always more sensitive than the nondominant hand. The fingertips are used in percussion and will be discussed later in this chapter.

Light Palpation

During palpation, the nurse should use light, moderate, or deep pressure depending on the depth of the structure being assessed and the thickness of the layers of tissue overlying the structure. One must always begin with light palpation. This is the safest, least uncomfortable method and allows the client to become accustomed to the nurse's touch. Light palpation is used to assess surface characteristics, such as skin texture, pulse, or a tender, inflamed area near the surface of the skin. For light palpation, the fingerpads of the dominant hand are placed on the surface of the area to be examined. The hand is moved slowly and the fingerpads, at a depth of 1 cm (0.25 in.), form circles on the skin during assessment, as demonstrated in Figure 6.3.

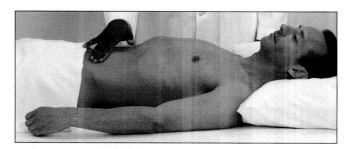

Figure 6.3 ● Light palpation.

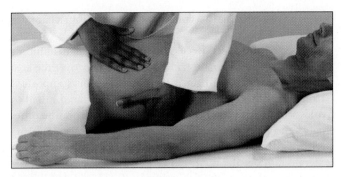

Figure 6.4 ● Moderate palpation.

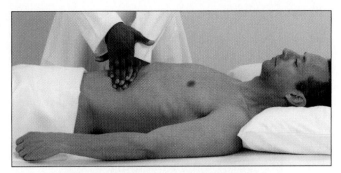

Figure 6.5 ● Deep palpation.

Moderate Palpation

Moderate palpation is used to assess many of the other structures of the body. For moderate palpation, the nurse uses moderate pressure, places the palmar surface of the fingers of the dominant hand over the structure to be assessed, and presses downward approximately 1 to 2 cm (0.25 to 0.5 in.), rotating the fingers in a circular motion. Now the nurse can determine the depth, size, shape, consistency, and mobility of organs, as well as any pain, tenderness, or pulsations that might be present (see Figure 6.4).

Deep Palpation

Deep palpation is used to palpate an organ that lies deep within a body cavity, such as the kidney or spleen, or when overlying musculature is thick, tense, or rigid, such as in obesity or with abdominal guarding. The nurse should use more than moderate pressure by placing the palmar surface of the fingers of the dominant hand on the skin surface. The extended fingers of the nondominant hand are placed over the fingers of the dominant hand, pressing and guiding the fingers downward. This technique provides extra support and pressure and allows the nurse to palpate at a deeper level, from 2 to 4 cm (1 to 1.5 in.), but as much as 5 to 8 cm (2 to 3 in.). All palpation must be used with caution; however, greatest caution must be used with deep palpation. Deep palpation can cause pain and disrupt underlying pathology (see Figure 6.5).

Before beginning the technique of palpation, the nurse should explain to the client what is about to happen. It is difficult to feel underlying structures if the client is tense or frightened. Therefore, it is important to help the client relax and become comfortable before proceeding. To help prevent discomfort, the nurse should warm the hands; keep fingernails short, smooth, and trimmed; and not wear jewellery. Nonsterile gloves should be used if open skin areas or drainage were noted during inspection. Gloves should be nonlatex material as many individuals have latex allergies.

The nurse should proceed slowly, using smooth, deliberate movements, and avoid abrupt changes. Most clients will be more relaxed if the nurse talks to them during the examination, explaining each movement in advance. For example, during an abdominal assessment, the nurse might say, "I'm going to place my hand on your abdomen next. Tell me if you feel any discomfort and I will stop right away. How does it feel when I press down in this area?" It is a good idea to touch each area before palpating it. This touch informs the client that the examination of the area is about to begin and may prevent a startled reaction. Known painful areas of the body are usually the last area to be palpated.

Through palpation the nurse perceives data from the assessment and applies critical thinking. The nurse must be able to anticipate the findings regarding palpation of a body structure. Examples of critical thinking questions include the following: Should light, moderate, or deep pressure be used? If so, why? Are the findings consistent with normative parameters, or are they unexpected findings? Does the client report any discomfort or pain during the process of palpation? Are the findings consistent with other diagnostic cues? What other information is needed to support this finding?

Percussion

Percussion is the third technique used by the nurse to obtain data when performing physical assessment. **Percussion** comes from the Latin word *percutire,* meaning "to strike through." Therefore, the nurse strikes through a body part with an object, fingers, or a reflex hammer, ultimately producing a measurable sound. The striking or tapping of the body produces sound waves. As these waves travel toward underlying structures, they are heard as characteristic tones. The procedure is similar to a musician striking a drum, creating a vibration heard as a musical tone. Percussion is used to determine the size and shape of organs and masses, and whether underlying tissue is solid or filled with fluid or air.

Three methods of percussion can be used: direct percussion, blunt percussion, and indirect percussion. The part of the body to be percussed indicates the method to be used.

Direct Percussion

Direct percussion is the technique of tapping the body with the fingertips of the dominant hand. It is used to examine the thorax of an infant and to assess the sinuses of an adult, as illustrated in Figure 6.6.

Blunt Percussion

Blunt percussion involves placing the palm of the nondominant hand flat against the body surface and striking the nondominant hand with the dominant hand. A closed fist of the dominant hand is used to deliver the blow. This method is used for assessing pain and tenderness in the gallbladder, liver, and kidneys, as shown in Figure 6.7.

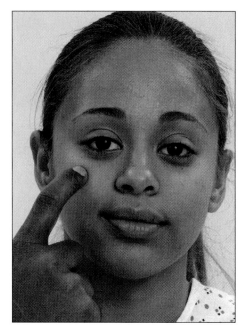

Figure 6.6 ● Direct percussion.

Indirect Percussion

Indirect percussion is the technique most commonly used because it produces sounds that are clearer and more easily interpreted. A hammer or tapping finger used to strike an object is called a **plexor**, derived from the Greek word *plexis*. **Pleximeter,** from the Greek word *metron*, meaning "measure," refers to the device that accepts the tap or blow from a hammer (see Figure 6.8).

To perform indirect percussion, the hyperextended middle finger of the nondominant hand is placed firmly over the area being examined. This finger is the pleximeter. It is important to keep the other fingers and the palm of this hand raised to avoid contact with the body surface. Pressure from the other fingers and palm on the adjacent surface muffles tones being produced. By using only wrist action of the dominant hand to generate motion, the nurse delivers two sharp blows with the plexor. The plexor is the fingertip of a flexed middle finger of the dominant hand. The plexor makes contact with the distal phalanx of the pleximeter and is immediately removed. When the plexor maintains contact with the distal phalanx, the sound waves are muffled. Enough force should be used to generate vibrations and ultimately a sound without causing injury to the client or self. Some helpful percussion hints follow:

- Ensure that motion is from the wrist, not the forearm or plexor finger.
- Release the plexor finger immediately after the delivery of two sharp strikes.
- Ensure that only the pleximeter makes contact with the body.
- Use the tip of the plexor finger, *not* the fingerpad, to deliver the blow.
- Use two strikes and then reposition the pleximeter. Delivery of more than two rapid consecutive strikes creates "woodpecker syndrome" and sounds are muffled.

Sounds

Interpreting a percussion tone is an art that takes time and experience to develop. The amount of air in the underlying structure being percussed is responsible for the tone being produced. The more dense the tissue is, the softer and shorter the

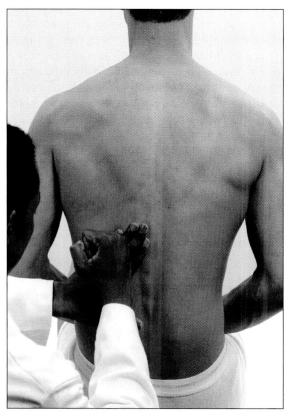

Figure 6.7 ● Blunt percussion.

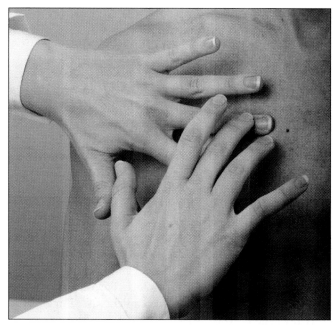

Figure 6.8 ● Indirect percussion.

tone. The less dense the tissue is, the louder and longer the tone. The five percussion sounds are classified as follows:

1. **Tympany** is a loud, high-pitched, drumlike tone of long duration characteristic of an organ that is filled with air. It is heard commonly over the gastric bubble in the stomach or over air-filled intestines.

2. **Resonance** is a loud, low-pitched, hollow tone of moderate-long duration. It is the normal finding over the lungs.

3. **Hyperresonance** is an abnormally loud, low tone of longer duration than resonance. It is heard when air is trapped in the lungs.

4. **Dullness** is a high-pitched tone that is soft and of short duration. It is usually heard over solid body organs, such as the liver.

5. **Flatness** is a high-pitched tone, very soft, and of very short duration. It occurs over solid tissue, such as muscle or bone.

Percussion sounds have characteristic features the nurse learns to interpret. These features include intensity, pitch, duration, and quality.

Intensity or *amplitude* of a sound refers to the softness or loudness of the sound. The louder the sound is, the greater the intensity or amplitude of the sound. This characteristic is influenced by the amount of air in the structure and the ability of the structure to vibrate.

Pitch or *frequency* of the sound refers to the number of vibrations of sound per second. Slow vibrations produce a low-pitched sound while a high-pitched sound comes from more rapid vibrations.

Duration refers to the length of time of the produced sound. This time ranges from very short to very long with variation in between.

Quality refers to the recognizable overtones produced by the vibration. This characteristic will be described as clear, hollow, muffled, or dull.

As with other assessment skills, the nurse perceives data from the assessment of the client and applies critical thinking. The nurse must be able to anticipate and identify the produced sound. Is this sound the expected sound? Is this sound considered to be within the normative range for this body part? Does the client report any discomfort or pain during percussion? Are the findings consistent with other diagnostic cues? What other information is needed to support this finding?

Auscultation

Auscultation is the skill of listening to the sounds produced by the body. When auscultating, the nurse uses both the unassisted sense of hearing and special instruments, such as a stethoscope. Body sounds that can be heard with the ears alone include speech, coughing, respirations, and percussion tones. Many body sounds are extremely soft, and a stethoscope is needed to hear them. Stethoscopes work not by amplifying sounds but by blocking out other noises in the environment. Use of the stethoscope is described later in this chapter.

Auscultating body sounds requires a quiet environment in which the nurse can listen not just for the presence or absence of sounds but also for the characteristics of each sound. External distractions, such as radios, televisions, and loud equipment, should be eliminated whenever possible. The nurse should avoid rubbing against client's clothes or drapes, or touching the stethoscope tubing since these actions produce sounds that will obscure the sounds of the body. It is important to keep the client warm, because shivering is uncomfortable and also obscures body sounds.

Sounds are described in terms of intensity, pitch, duration, and quality. For example, the nurse might note that a client's respirations are loud, high-pitched, long, and raspy. Many times the nurse will hear more than one sound at a time. It is important to focus on each sound and identify the characteristics of each sound. Closing the eyes and concentrating on each sound might help the nurse focus on the sound.

The nurse uses critical thinking with the technique of auscultation. The nurse must know the expected sound in the body region being auscultated. Is this sound considered to be within the normative range for this body region? Are unusual sounds heard? Are these findings consistent with other diagnostic cues? What other information is needed to support this finding?

EQUIPMENT

Throughout physical assessment the nurse will use various instruments and pieces of equipment that help in visualizing, hearing, and measuring data. It is the responsibility of the nurse to know how to operate and when to use all equipment for client safety. Before beginning the physical assessment, the nurse should gather all the equipment, organize it, and place it within easy reach. Table 6.1 gives a complete list of the equipment needed for a typical screening exam. Some of the more complex items on the list are discussed in greater detail below or in later chapters.

Stethoscope

The stethoscope is used to auscultate body sounds, such as blood pressure, heart sounds, respirations, and bowel sounds. The stethoscope has three parts: the binaurals (earpieces), the flexible tubing, and the end piece. The end piece contains the diaphragm and the bell (see Figure 6.9). To be effective in blocking out environmental noise, the stethoscope must fit. The binaurals should fit snugly but comfortably, sloping forward, toward the nose, to match the natural slope of the ear canals. (Most manufacturers supply several different binaurals from which to choose.)

The tubing that joins the binaurals to the diaphragm and bell is thick, flexible, and as short as possible (approximately 30 to 36 cm, or 12 to 18 in.). Longer tubing may distort the sound.

The flat end piece, called the diaphragm, screens out low-pitched sounds and, therefore, is best for transmitting high-pitched sounds, such as lung sounds and normal heart sounds. The nurse should place the diaphragm evenly and firmly over the client's exposed skin. The deep, hollow end piece, called the bell, detects low-frequency sounds, such as heart murmurs. It is placed lightly against the client's skin so that it forms a seal but does not flatten to a diaphragm. Either end piece may be held

TABLE 6.1	Equipment Used During the Physical Assessment

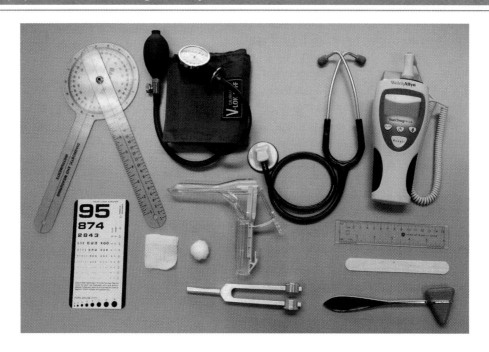

EQUIPMENT	USE
Cotton balls or wisps	Test the sense of touch
Cotton-tipped applicators	Obtain specimens
Culture media	Obtain cultures of body fluids and drainage
Dental mirror	Visualize mouth and throat structures
Doppler, hand-held	Obtain readings of blood pressure, pulse, and fetal heart rate
Flashlight	Provide a direct source of light to view parts of the body
Gauze squares	Obtain specimens; collect drainage
Gloves	Protect the nurse and client from contamination
Goggles	Protect the nurse's eyes from contamination by body fluids
Lubricant	Provide lubrication for vaginal or rectal examinations
Nasal speculum	Dilate nares for inspection of the nose
Ophthalmoscope	Inspect the interior structures of the eye
Otoscope	Inspect the tympanic membrane and external ear canal
Penlight	Provide a direct light source and test pupillary reaction
Reflex hammer	Test deep tendon reflexes
Ruler, marked in centimetres	Measure organs, masses, growths, and lesions
Skin-marking pen	Outline masses or enlarged organs
Slides	Make smears of body fluids or drainage
Specimen containers	Collect specimens of body fluids, drainage, or tissue
Sphygmomanometer	Measure systolic and diastolic blood pressure
Sterile safety pin	Test for sensory stimulation
Stethoscope	Auscultate body sounds
Tape measure, flexible, marked in centimetres	Measure the circumference of the head, abdomen, and extremities
Test tubes	Collect specimens
Thermometer	Measure body temperature
Tongue blade	Depress tongue during assessment of the mouth and throat
Tuning fork	Test auditory function and vibratory sensation
Vaginal speculum	Dilate the vaginal canal for inspection of the cervix
Vision chart	Test near and far vision
Watch with second hand	Time heart rates, fetal pulse, or bowel sounds when counting

TABLE 6.1	Equipment Used During the Physical Assessment *(continued)*
SPECIAL EQUIPMENT	**USE OR DESCRIPTION**
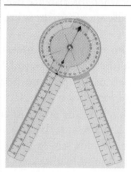 Goniometer	Measures the degree of joint flexion and extension. Consists of two straight arms of clear plastic usually marked in both inches and centimetres. The arms intersect and can be angled and rotated around a protractor marked with degrees. The nurse places the centre of the protractor over a joint and aligns the straight arms with the extremity. The degree of flexion or extension is indicated on the protractor.
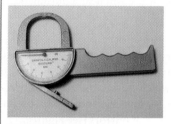 Skinfold calipers	Measures the thickness of subcutaneous tissue. The nurse grasps a fold of skin, usually on the upper arm, waist, or thigh, keeping the sides of the skin parallel. The edges of the caliper are placed at the base of the fold and the calipers tightened until they grasp the fold without compressing it.
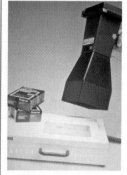 Transilluminator	Detects blood, fluid, or masses in body cavities. Instruments manufactured for transillumination are available, or a flashlight with a rubber adapter can be used. In either case, the light beam produced is strong but narrow. When directed through a body cavity, the beam produces a red glow that reveals the presence of air or fluid.
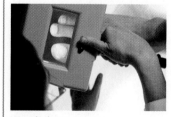 Wood's lamp	Detects fungal infections of the skin. The Wood's lamp produces a black light, which the nurse shines on the skin in a darkened room. If a fungal infection is present, a characteristic yellow-green fluorescence appears on the skin surface.

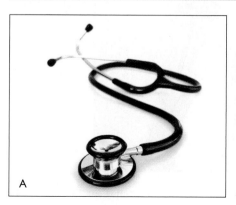

A

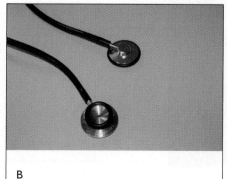

B

Figure 6.9 ● A. Stethoscope with both a bell-shaped and flat-disc amplifier.
B. Close-up of a flat-disc amplifier (left) and a bell amplifier (right).

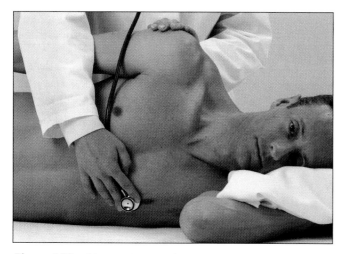

Figure 6.10 ● Nurse using a stethoscope.

between the index and middle fingers of the examiner against the client's skin (see Figure 6.10).

Friction on the diaphragm or bell from coarse body hair may cause a crackling sound easily confused with abnormal breath sounds. This problem can be avoided by wetting the hair before auscultating the area. Stethoscopes usually include an assortment of interchangeable diaphragms and bells in different sizes for different purposes; for example, smaller diaphragm pieces are used for examining children.

Hand-Held Doppler

A hand-held Doppler or a Doppler ultrasound stethoscope uses ultrasonic waves to detect sounds that are difficult to hear with a regular stethoscope, such as fetal heart sounds and peripheral pulses (see Figure 6.11). It operates on a principle discovered in the nineteenth century by Christian Johann Doppler, the Austrian physicist who found that the pitch of a sound varies in relation to the distance between the source and the listener. To the listener, the pitch sounds higher when the distance from the source is small and lower when the distance from the source is great.

The way to eliminate interference is to apply a small amount of gel to the end of the Doppler probe (the transducer), which may resemble a wand or a disc. When using the hand-held Doppler to assess the pulse, the nurse turns it on and places the probe gently against the client's skin over the artery to be auscultated. It is important to avoid heavy pressure, because it may impede blood flow. The probe sends a low-energy, high-pitched sound wave toward the underlying blood vessel. As the blood ebbs and flows, the probe picks up and amplifies the subtle changes in pitch, and the nurse will hear a pulsing beat.

Ophthalmoscope

An ophthalmoscope is used to inspect internal eye structures. Its main components are the handle, which holds the battery or power source, and the head, which houses the aperture selector, viewing aperture, lens selector disc, lens indicator, lenses of varying powers of magnification, and mirrors (see Figure 6.12).

The light source shines light through the viewing aperture, which is adjusted to select one of five apertures (see Figure 6.13):

1. The large aperture is used most often. It emits a large, full spot for viewing dilated pupils.

2. The small aperture is used for undilated pupils.

3. The red-free filter shines a green beam used to examine the optic disc for pallor or hemorrhaging, which appears black with this filter. In conjunction with fluorescein dye, the red-

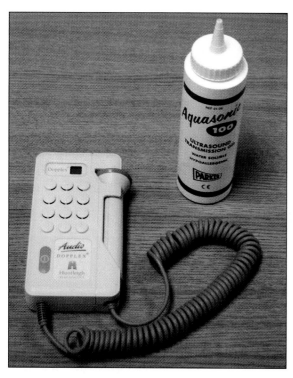

Figure 6.11 ● Doppler ultrasound stethoscope.

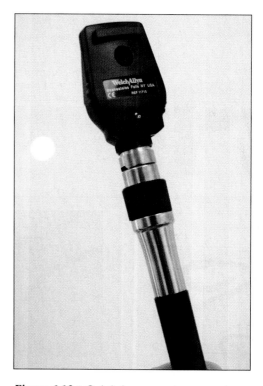

Figure 6.12 ● Ophthalmoscope demonstrating aperture.

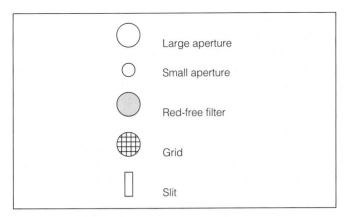

○ Large aperture

○ Small aperture

● Red-free filter

⊞ Grid

▯ Slit

Figure 6.13 ● Apertures of ophthalmoscope.

free filter can be used to detect corneal abrasions and other lesions.

4. The grid allows the examiner to assess the size, location, and pattern of any lesions.

5. The slit allows for examination of the anterior eye and aids in assessing the elevation or depression of lesions.

The lens selector dial must be rotated to bring the inner eye structures into focus. While looking through the viewing aperture, the nurse rotates the lens selection dial to adjust the convergence or divergence of the light. At the zero setting, the lens neither converges nor diverges the light. The lens dial is moved clockwise to access the numbers in black, which range from +1 to +40. These lenses improve visualization in a client who is farsighted. The lens dial is moved counterclockwise to access the red numbers, which range from 1 to 20. These lenses improve visualization if the client is nearsighted. See Chapter 13 for a more detailed discussion of assessment of the eye. ⬯

Otoscope

The otoscope is used to inspect internal ear structures. The main components of the otoscope are the handle, which is similar to that of the ophthalmoscope, the light, the lens, and specula of various sizes (see Figure 6.14). The specula are used to narrow the beam of light. The nurse should select the largest one that will fit into the client's ear canal. If a nasal speculum is not available, the otoscope can be used to inspect the nose. In this case, the nurse should use the shortest, broadest speculum and insert it gently into the client's naris. See Chapter 14 for a more detailed discussion of assessment of the ears and nose. ⬯

Special equipment is required for assessment of several body systems. For example, the reflex hammer is used in the neurological assessment and the vaginal speculum in assessment of the female reproductive system. Each chapter in Unit III of this text provides a discussion of specialized equipment and uses in physical assessment of a particular system. ⬯

PROFESSIONAL RESPONSIBILITIES

Throughout all aspects of the assessment process, the nurse must apply critical thinking while providing a safe and com-

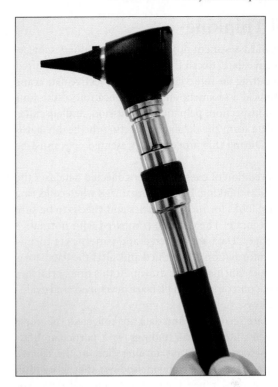

Figure 6.14 ● Otoscope.

fortable environment for the client. The nurse must identify cues presented by the client and apply critical thinking to determine the relevance of these data. The safe external environment created by the nurse includes comfort, warmth, privacy, and the use of routine practices.

Cues

In addition to developing the skills of inspection, palpation, percussion, and auscultation, the nurse must be able to recognize the relative significance of the many visual, palpable, or auditory cues that may be present during an assessment. **Cues** are bits of information that hint at the possibility of a health problem. In other words, the nurse needs to know what to look for. To become skilled at cue recognition, nurses should cultivate their senses until they readily perceive even slight cues. For example, some things that are noticed during an initial survey or inspection of the client may hint at an underlying health problem. Edema (swelling) of the legs provides a cue to assess for heart problems. Ecchymosis (bruising) of the skin is a cue to ask the client about recent falls, trauma, injury, anticoagulant medication, or a bleeding problem. Grimacing, guarding (protective posture), or wincing when a client moves or a body part is moved during assessment are cues to examine for underlying joint and muscle problems or masses. Cues that suggest hearing loss include not following directions, looking at the examiner's lips during conversation, or speaking in a loud voice. Asymmetry of facial expression is a cue to assess function of the cranial nerves. Odours are cues to suggest a problem with hygiene or drainage from an orifice or a wound. Cue recognition develops with practice, but beginners can acquire the skill by observing an experienced nurse, by practising on partners, and by studying the visual aids in this text.

Critical Thinking

Throughout the assessment process, the nurse gathers subjective and objective data. Recall that subjective data are reported by the client during the interviews, and the objective data come from the physical assessment and the application of the four techniques of inspection, palpation, percussion, and auscultation. These data form the database reflecting the health status of the client. During this process the presented cues must be interpreted.

The interpretation of cues and other collected data uses the process of critical thinking. By being organized when collecting data, the nurse looks for inconsistencies and checks to be sure the data are accurate. The data are compared with normative values and ranges. Data are clustered and patterns are identified. Missing information is identified and, after the database is completed, valid conclusions are drawn. At this time, priorities are established, outcomes and a plan are developed, and evaluation then follows.

Once cues are recognized and data are collected, the nurse must be able to interpret the findings. Is a particular finding normal, or does it indicate an alteration in the client's health? Normal data are assessment findings that fall within an accepted standard range for a specific type of data. For example, the normal range for the adult pulse rate is 60 to 100 beats per minute. A pulse of 76 is therefore considered normal. Some healthy individuals exhibit characteristics that are outside the standard range for a specific type of data. Such findings are considered variations from the norm. For example, a long-distance runner with a pulse of 48 resulting from regular cardiovascular conditioning exhibits a variation from the norm for pulse rate. Findings that are outside the range for a specific type of data and that may indicate a threat to the client's health are considered unexpected findings or deviations from the norm. For example, an irregular, thready pulse rate of 120 is an unexpected finding that could indicate the presence of a harmful condition. It is important to note that not all unexpected findings indicate the presence of a disease or disorder. For example, fatigue in a 20-year-old student may indicate anemia or infection, or it may be caused simply by a lack of sleep.

Providing a Safe and Comfortable Environment

The physical assessment can be performed in any one of a variety of settings, including a clinic, a hospital room, or a client's home. No matter where the location, the nurse is responsible for preparing a setting that is conducive to the client's comfort and privacy. The examination room should be warm, private, and free from distractions and interruptions. Overhead lighting must ensure good visibility and be free of distortion. A portable lamp to highlight body surfaces and contours may be needed.

The client should be positioned on a sturdy examination table with a firm surface that is covered with a clean sheet or paper cover. Though not as efficient, a firm bed will suffice if an examination table is not available. The table must be placed to allow the nurse easy access to both sides of the client's body.

The table's height should allow the nurse to perform the examination without stooping. The nurse should also have a stool to sit on during certain parts of the examination and a small table or stand to hold the examination equipment.

The examination should be individualized according to the client's personal values and beliefs. Some clients, for example, may request that a family member be present during the examination. Some may ask for a nurse of the same sex. Some female clients may object to breast and vaginal examinations, regardless of the gender of the examiner, and some male clients may refuse penile, scrotal, and rectal examinations. A thorough assessment of the client's culture, religious beliefs, and environment, as described in previous chapters, can help the nurse to anticipate these needs. Although explaining the reason for a certain procedure may help the client understand its benefit, a nurse must never attempt to influence or coerce the client to agree to any procedure. In all cases, the nurse must document which procedures took place and any that were refused.

Many clients experience anxiety before and during a physical examination. These feelings may stem from fear of pain, embarrassment at being looked at and touched by a stranger, or worry about the outcome of the examination. The nurse can alleviate the client's anxiety by approaching the examination gradually, first by communicating with the client, then by performing simple measurements, such as height, weight, temperature, and pulse, which most clients find familiar and nonthreatening. As these measurements are taken, the client will have the opportunity to ask additional questions and to become accustomed to the nurse's presence.

In most cases, clients should urinate before the examination. Voiding helps clients feel more comfortable and relaxed and facilitates palpation of the abdomen and pubic area. If urinalysis is to be done, the client should be instructed in obtaining a clean-catch specimen and given a container for the urine sample.

After ensuring that the examination room is warm, the nurse shows the client how to put on the examination gown and leaves the client to undress in privacy. It may be helpful to assure the client that it is all right to leave underpants on until just before the genital examination. Before reentering the examination room, the nurse should knock to alert the client.

Drapes are used to preserve the client's privacy and to provide warmth. When invasive procedures, such as vaginal or rectal examinations, are performed, drapes provide an aseptic field. When used properly, a drape exposes only the part of the body being examined and covers the surrounding area. Drapes are available in a variety of shapes and materials, from simple rectangular sheets made of linen to disposable drapes made of paper lined with waterproof plastic (see Chapter 22 ⬭).

The physical examination may be an exhausting experience for a client who is older, debilitated, frail, or suffering from a chronic illness, since the nurse must examine every part of the body, and the client must make frequent changes in position. Consequently, the nurse should consider the client's age, health status, level of functioning, and severity of illness at all times and adapt the examination accordingly. In addition, the nurse can conserve the client's energy by moving around the client during the examination, rather than asking the client to move, and by carrying out the examination as quickly and efficiently as possible. The techniques and approaches for physical assessment vary for children, pregnant females, and older adults. Special considerations for assessment of these groups are included in each assessment chapter in Unit III. ◯ Further, Chapters 25 through 27 provide in-depth information about assessment of infants, children, adolescents, pregnant females, and older adults. ◯

Before beginning the physical examination, the nurse should perform hand hygiene in the presence of the client. Hand hygiene not only protects the nurse and the client but also signals that the nurse is providing for the client's safety. Nonsterile exam gloves should be available and used appropriately during the examination. The bell and diaphragm of the stethoscope should be cleaned after the assessment of each client to prevent the spread of infection.

Some situations that arise during a physical examination pose a potential hazard for the client. For example, a client might become light-headed and dizzy from taking deep breaths during a respiratory assessment, or fall when asked to touch the toes during a musculoskeletal assessment. A client who is frail, weak, debilitated, or suffering from a chronic illness is at greatest risk. Throughout the procedure, it is necessary to anticipate potential hazards and modify the examination to prevent them. In addition, some examination techniques may injure the client if used indiscriminately. For example, vigorous, deep palpation of a throbbing mass might lead to a ruptured abdominal aneurysm.

Before beginning the examination, the nurse should thoroughly explain to the client what is to follow and encourage the client to ask questions. If the client does not speak the nurse's language, it is important to secure the assistance of a translator. If the client's hearing is impaired, the nurse must find someone who knows sign language.

During the examination, the nurse should explain each step in advance so that the client can anticipate the nurse's movements. Clients are more relaxed and cooperative during the procedure when they understand what is about to happen. This is also an opportunity to provide client teaching. For example, while inspecting the client's skin, the nurse may want to discuss the long-term effects of sun exposure. Sharing information with clients during the examination may alleviate their anxiety, enhance their understanding, and give them a sense of partnership in their healthcare.

At times, the nurse may note an unexpected finding and want to call in another examiner to check the finding. In such instances, it is best simply to inform the client that another examiner is being asked to check the assessment. Because the finding may be normal, it is best to avoid alarming the client.

Routine Practices

Throughout the physical assessment, the nurse is required to apply the principles of asepsis. Hand hygiene, the use of gloves, the use of protective barriers, the disposal of sharps, the handling of specimens, and the proper disposal of body wastes are included in the guidelines. Each healthcare agency has created agency policies based on these guidelines. A nurse working at an agency is responsible for knowing the policies and following the guidelines. Refer to Appendices B, C, and D to review routine practices.

APPLICATION THROUGH CRITICAL THINKING

CASE STUDY

As part of a comprehensive health assessment course, Ian Martens, a student nurse, must conduct a physical assessment of a child between the ages of 2 and 5 years and an adult over the age of 65. Ian contacts the parents of a 3-year-old white female for consent to carry out the assessment. The parents have asked Ian to meet with them and explain in detail what he will be doing before giving consent.

In addition, a 73-year-old Asian male residing in an assisted living facility has consented to the physical assessment.

▶ *Critical Thinking Questions*

1. What should be included in the explanation of the assessment procedures to the parents and the older adult?
2. What factors will influence application of physical assessment techniques for each of the clients?
3. Identify the equipment Ian must prepare for the physical assessment.
4. What safety and comfort issues must be addressed when conducting the assessment for the child and the adult?

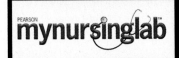

7

GENERAL SURVEY

The **general survey** begins during the interview phase of a comprehensive health assessment (see Figure 7.1). While collecting subjective data, the nurse observes the client, develops initial impressions about the individual's health, and formulates strategies for the physical assessment. The observation includes what is seen, heard, or smelled during the initial phase of assessment. Clues that are uncovered during the general survey will guide the nurse during later assessment of body regions and systems. These clues will help to determine the client's ability to participate in all aspects of the assessment process. For example, the client having pain will need to have pain relief. The client with dyspnea (trouble breathing) will need assistance before proceeding. Remember, pain and dyspnea are two of the many factors that will influence the client's ability to participate in the assessment. These concepts are discussed in detail in Chapters 8 and 15 of this text. ⊂⊃ On completion of the general survey, the nurse will assess height, weight, and vital signs. Information about each of these important phases of comprehensive health assessment is discussed in the sections that follow. The data obtained in the general survey form a guide for all physical assessment.

COMPONENTS OF THE GENERAL SURVEY

The general survey is composed of four major categories of observation: physical appearance, mental status, mobility, and behaviour of the client. Specific observations are required in the general survey. The following sections identify these required observations. During the general survey the nurse will determine if the observed behaviours fall within an expected range for the gender, age, genetic background, and culture of the client. The nurse must also determine the ability of the client to participate in all aspects of the process before proceeding.

Physical Appearance

The client's physical appearance provides immediate and important cues to the level of individual wellness. Thus, beginning with the initial meeting, the nurse notes any factors about the client's physical appearance that are in any way unexpected. For example, the nurse might note that a client appears undernourished, seems older than his or her stated age, has a frown, is smiling, or has skin that is pale, flushed, ruddy, or cyanotic.

Body shape and build may indicate the client's general level of wellness. The body should be symmetrical and the proportions regular: the client's arm span should approximate the

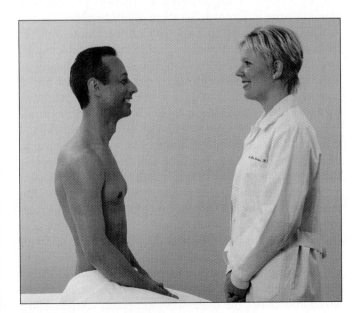

Figure 7.1 ● The nurse begins the general survey.

height, and the distance from the pubis to the crown of the head should roughly equal the distance from the pubis to the sole of the foot. The client's height and weight should be within normal ranges for age and body build. Extreme thinness or obesity may indicate an eating disorder. The nurse must consider the client's lifestyle, socioeconomic level, and environment.

Mental Status

The nurse assesses the client's mental status while the client is responding to questions and giving information about the health history. The nurse notes the client's affect and mood, level of anxiety, orientation, and speech. Findings in these areas may be evaluated further during the assessment of the client's psychosocial status and neurological system.

The nurse assesses the client for orientation to person, place, and time. A client should typically be able to state his or her name, the name of the location, and the date, month, season, and time of day. In most cases, the nurse will be able to sense a client's orientation during the initial interview. If the client appears confused, the nurse should ask him or her to respond to the following: "Tell me your name." "Where you are now?" "What is today's date?" and "What time is it?" If the client cannot respond or responds incorrectly, a more detailed assessment of mental status must be performed. See Chapter 25 for details on how to perform this assessment in children. ⚭

Mobility

The nurse observes the client's gait, posture, and range of motion (the complete movement possible for a joint). Normally, the client walks in a rhythmic, straight, upright position with arms swinging at each side of the body. The shoulders are level and straight. Difficulty with gait and posture, such as stumbling, shuffling, limping, or the inability to stand erect, calls for further evaluation. Range of motion should be fluid and appropriate to the age of the client. The nurse will observe deviations from the normal that include weakness, stiffness, or involuntary motor activity. See Chapter 23 for information on assessing the musculoskeletal system and range of motion. ⚭

Behaviour of the Client

An assessment of the client's behaviour includes information about the following factors: dress and grooming, body odours, facial expression, mood and affect, ability to make eye contact, and level of anxiety. The way in which clients dress may provide clues to their sense of self-esteem and body image. However, the nurse must consider many factors before drawing conclusions based on a client's appearance. For example, a client who wears clothing that is inappropriate for the situation or weather may be blind, have a mental illness, be experiencing situational grief or anxiety, or be mentally fit but unable to buy other clothes because of financial constraints.

The nurse observes the client for cleanliness and personal hygiene. The client who is dirty or has a strong body odour or poor dental hygiene may be depressed, have poor self-concept, or lack knowledge about personal hygiene practices. However, the nurse must consider the client's environment before drawing conclusions. For example, a client who is dirty may have just come from working on a construction site.

The nurse assesses the client's emotional state by noting what the client says, the client's body language and facial expression, and the appropriateness of the client's behaviour in relation to the situation and circumstances. The client should exhibit comfort in talking with the examiner. Giggling when answering questions about bowel movements may simply indicate embarrassment, whereas giggling when describing the death of a loved one may be an example of inappropriate affect.

The nurse also assesses the client for apprehension, fear, and nervousness. Like affect and mood, the client's level of anxiety is revealed through speech, body language, and facial expression. During the health assessment, the client may exhibit anxiety because of embarrassment, fear of pain, or worry about the outcome of the examination. If the client's anxiety seems to have no cause, the client must be evaluated further. To obtain a relative impression of the level of anxiety, clients may be asked to rate their feelings of anxiety on a scale of 0 to 10. The nurse uses the client's response as an indicator of the need for further assessment and as a baseline for future assessment of anxiety levels.

The nurse assesses the client's speech for quantity, volume, content, articulation, and rhythm. The client should speak easily and fluently to the nurse or to an interpreter. Disorganized speech patterns, silence, or constant talking may indicate normal nervousness or shyness, or may signal a speech defect, a neurological deficit, depression, or another disorder.

Age-Related Considerations

It is important to consider the developmental stage of the child or adolescent when assessing for each of the previous factors. The appearance of the younger child reveals a great deal of information about the child's parents or caretakers, and the appearance of an older child gives clues about self-care. For instance, a child 3 years of age whose skin and clothes are dirty may be a victim of neglect, while a 13-year-old in the same condition may lack knowledge about proper hygiene.

The nurse should note the child's interaction with the parents or caretakers. Their relationship should exhibit mutual warmth and caring. Signs of child abuse include clinging to a parent or strong attachment to a parent because of fear of parental anger; absence of separation anxiety in a child who, because of developmental stage, would ordinarily demonstrate it; avoidance of eye contact between caretaker and child; a caretaker's demonstration of disgust with a child's behaviour, illness, odour, or stool; flinching by the child when people move toward her or him; and regression to infantile behaviour.

The dress, grooming, and personal hygiene of an older adult may be affected by limitations in mobility from arthritis, cardiovascular disease, and other disorders, or by a lack of funds.

The gait of an older adult is often slower and the steps shorter. To maintain balance, older adults may hold their arms away from the body or use a cane. The posture of an older adult may look slightly stooped because of a generalized flexion, which also causes the older adult to appear shorter. A loss in height may also be due to thinning or compression of the intervertebral disks.

The behaviour of the older adult may be affected by various disorders common to this age group, such as vascular insufficiency and diabetes. In addition, medications may affect the client's behaviour. Some medications may cause the client to feel anxious, and others may affect the client's alertness, orientation, or speech. Older adults are more likely to have one or more chronic conditions associated with age, such as arthritis, hypertension, or diabetes. As a result, many older adults take several prescription medications. Overmedication may occur when older adults seek care from multiple healthcare providers without collaboration regarding treatment. Multiple medications may combine to produce dangerous side effects. Additionally, the schedules for multiple medications may be confusing and result in overmedication, forgotten doses, negative side effects, or ineffectiveness of medication. Therefore, the nurse must conduct a thorough assessment of the client's medication schedule and history.

MEASURING HEIGHT AND WEIGHT

The nurse measures the client's height and weight to establish baseline data and to help determine health status. The client should be asked about height and weight before taking any measurements. Large discrepancies between the stated height and weight and the actual measurements may provide clues to the client's self-image. Alternatively, discrepancies in weight may indicate the client's lack of awareness of a sudden loss or gain in weight that may be due to illness.

Height

The nurse uses a measuring stick attached to a platform scale or to a wall to measure height. The client should look straight ahead while standing as straight as possible with heels together and shoulders back. When using a platform scale, the nurse raises the height attachment rod above the client's head, then extends and lowers the right-angled arm until it rests on the crown of the head. The measurement is read from the height attachment rod (see Figure 7.2). When using a measuring stick, the nurse should place an L-shaped level on the crown of the client's head at a right angle to the measuring stick (see Figure 7.3).

Weight

A standard platform scale (see Figure 7.4) is used to measure the weight of older children and adults. It is best to use the same scale at each visit and weigh the client at the same time of day in the same kind of clothing (e.g., the examination gown) and without shoes. If using a digital scale, the nurse simply reads the weight from the lighted display panel. Otherwise, the scale is calibrated by moving both weights to 0 and turning the knob until the balance beam is level. The nurse moves the large and small weights to the right and takes the reading when the balance beam returns to level. Special bed and chair scales are available for clients who cannot stand.

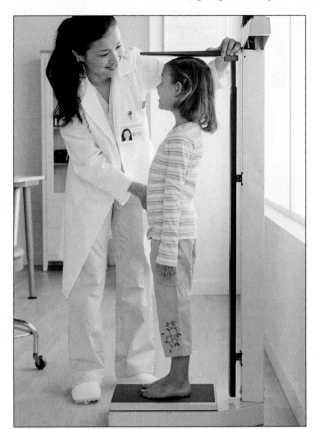

Figure 7.2 ● Measuring the client's height with a platform scale.

Average height and weight for adult men and women are available in charts prepared by governmental agencies and insurers. The body mass index (BMI) is considered a reliable indicator of healthy weight. The BMI and other measures in relation to weight are discussed in Chapter 9 of this text.

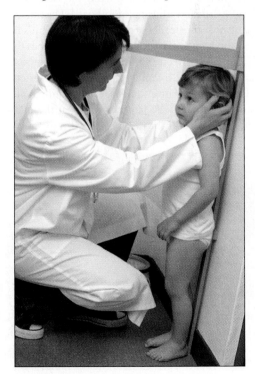

Figure 7.3 ● Measuring a child's height with a measuring stick.

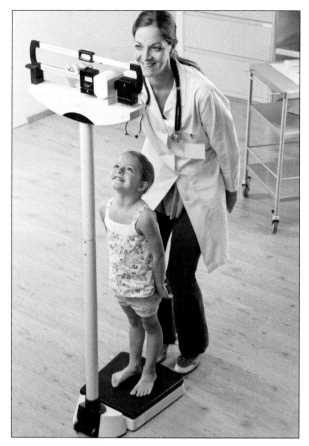

Figure 7.4 • Measuring the client's weight with a standard platform scale.

Age-Related Considerations

To measure an infant's length, the nurse places the child in a supine position on an examining table that is equipped with a ruler, headboard, and adjustable footboard. The nurse positions the head against the headboard, extends the infant's leg nearest the ruler, and adjusts the footboard until it touches the infant's foot. The space between the headboard and footboard represents the length of the infant (see Figure 7.5). Alternatively, the nurse places the infant on a standard examination table, extends the infant's leg, marks the paper covering at the infant's head and foot, and measures the distance between the markings.

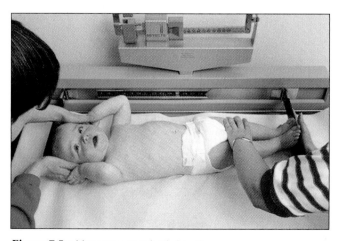

Figure 7.5 • Measuring an infant's length.

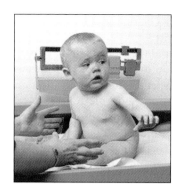

Figure 7.6 • Weighing an infant.

Infants are weighed on a modified platform scale with curved sides to prevent injury. The scale measures weight in grams and in ounces. The nurse places the unclothed baby on the scale on a paper drape and watches the baby to prevent a fall (see Figure 7.6). Measurements are taken to the nearest 10 g (0.5 oz.).

Children over the age of 2 or 3 years may be weighed on the upright scale or seated on the infant scale. The child's underpants should be left on. To measure height, the nurse uses the platform scale or a measuring stick attached to the wall, as for an adult. By the age of 4, most children enjoy being weighed and measured and finding out how much they have grown. Growth and development are discussed in Chapter 3 of this text. ⬭

The height of older adults may decline somewhat as a result of thinning or compression of the intervertebral disks and a general flexion of the hips and knees. Body weight may decrease because of muscle shrinkage. The older client may appear thinner, even when properly nourished, because of loss of subcutaneous fat deposits from the face, forearms, and lower legs. At the same time, fat deposits on the abdomen and hips may increase.

MEASURING VITAL SIGNS

Vital signs include body *temperature, pulse, respiratory rate, blood pressure,* and *pain.* Measurement of oxygen saturation may be included when taking vital signs. The nurse measures vital signs to obtain baseline data, to detect or monitor a change in the client's health status, and to monitor clients at risk for alterations in health.

Measuring Body Temperature

The body's surface **temperature**—the temperature of the skin, subcutaneous tissues, and fat—fluctuates in response to environmental factors and is therefore unreliable for monitoring a client's health status. Instead, the nurse should measure the client's core temperature: the temperature of the deep tissues of the body (e.g., the thorax and abdominal cavity). This temperature remains relatively constant at about 37°C (98.6°F).

Sensors in the hypothalamus regulate the body's core temperature. When these hypothalamic sensors detect heat, they signal the body to decrease heat production and increase heat loss (e.g., by vasodilation and sweating). When sensors in the hypothalamus detect cold, they signal the body to increase heat production and decrease heat loss (e.g., by shivering, vasoconstriction, and inhibition of sweating).

Factors That Influence Body Temperature

A variety of factors may influence normal core body temperature:

- *Age.* The core temperature of infants is highly responsive to changes in the external environment; therefore, infants need extra protection from even mild variations in temperature. The core body temperature of children is more stable than that of infants but less so than that of adolescents or adults. However, older adults are more sensitive than middle adults to variations in external environmental temperature. This increased sensitivity may be due to the decreased thermo-regulatory control and loss of subcutaneous fat common in older adults, or it may be due to environmental factors, such as lack of activity, inadequate diet, or lack of central heating.

- *Diurnal variations.* Core body temperature is usually highest between 8:00 p.m. and midnight, and lowest between 4:00 and 6:00 a.m. Normal body temperature may vary by as much as 1°C (2°F) between these times. Some individuals have more than one complete cycle in a day.

- *Exercise.* Strenuous exercise can increase core body temperature by as much as 2°C (5°F).

- *Hormones.* A variety of hormones affect core body temperature. For example, in women, progesterone secretion at the time of ovulation raises core body temperature by about 0.35°C (0.5°F).

- *Stress.* The temperature of a highly stressed client may be elevated as a result of increased production of epinephrine and norepinephrine, which increase metabolic activity and heat production.

- *Illness.* Illness or a central nervous system disorder may impair the thermostatic function of the hypothalamus. **Hyperthermia**, also called fever, may occur in response to viral or bacterial infections, or from tissue breakdown following myocardial infarction, malignancy, surgery, or trauma. **Hypothermia** is usually a response to prolonged exposure to cold.

Routes for Measuring Body Temperature

Core body temperature was once typically measured with a mercury-in-glass thermometer. Mercury, a toxic liquid metal, can pose a health threat to the individual and community. Although the amount of mercury in each thermometer is small, the adverse effects are high and multidimensional when the instrument breaks and the liquid escapes from the container. Agencies are banning the sale and use of mercury-filled glass thermometers. Alcohol and galinstan are two products replacing mercury in glass thermometers. Today, nurses are more likely to use an electronic thermometer (see Figure 7.7), which gives a highly accurate reading in 2 to 60 seconds. These portable, battery-operated devices consist of an electronic display unit, a probe, and disposable probe sheaths. The nurse attaches the appropriate probe to the unit, covers it with a sterile sheath, and inserts it into the body orifice. The probe is left in place until the temperature appears on the liquid crystal display (LCD) screen. Five routes are used for measuring core body temperature: oral, rectal, axillary, tympanic, or temporal.

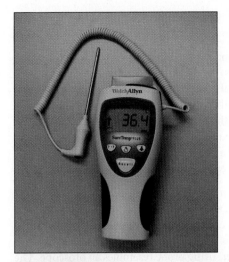

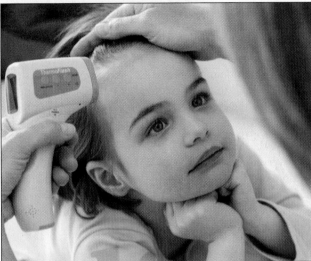

Figure 7.7 ● Electronic thermometers.

ORAL. The oral temperature is the most accessible, accurate, and convenient method. While glass thermometers may be used in the home setting, because of the possibility of breakage and mercury exposure, they are no longer used in the clinical setting. Oral temperatures may be evaluated by using an electronic or a digital probe device. Place the covered probe at the base of the tongue in either of the sublingual pockets to the right or left of the frenulum, and instruct the client to keep the lips tightly closed around the thermometer. The thermometer is left in place until the device beeps or shows indication that the measurement is completed. After removing the thermometer, the nurse either discards the disposable sheath or cleans the device. The temperature reading will be in the display window.

RECTAL. A rectal temperature is taken if the client is comatose, confused, having seizures, or unable to close the mouth. It is important to use lubricated thermometer covers and put on disposable examination gloves. The client should be in a side-lying position. The nurse asks the client to take a deep breath and then inserts the thermometer from 1.5 to 4 cm (0.75 to 1.5 in.) into the anus, being careful not to force insertion of the thermometer. The probe is left in place until there is a beep or the device indicates that the reading is completed. Remove the probe, dispose of the disposable sheath, and obtain the reading in the display window.

AXILLARY. Occasionally, the nurse needs to take an axillary temperature. This is the safest method and is less invasive than the oral or rectal routes, especially for infants and young children. Because of the variability of probe positioning, many authorities consider the axillary route to be least accurate. For an axillary temperature, the nurse places the thermometer in the client's axilla and assists the client in placing the arm tightly across the chest to keep the thermometer in place.

TYMPANIC. The tympanic temperature can be taken only with an electronic thermometer. By using infrared technology, it measures a client's core body temperature quickly and accurately. This method is the most comfortable and least invasive for the client. The measuring probe resembles an otoscope. The nurse gently places the covered tip of the probe at the opening of the ear canal, being careful not to force the probe into the ear canal or occlude the canal opening. After about 2 seconds, the client's temperature reading will appear on the LCD screen. Tympanic thermometers are no longer commonly used as they have been found to be inaccurate. This inaccuracy is due, in large part, to the inconsistent placement of the thermometer in the ear canal.

TEMPORAL. The temporal thermometer is relatively new and is very useful for assessing children's temperatures. The thermometer works by scanning the area over the temporal artery across the forehead. By taking more than 1000 readings per second, the temporal thermometer measures ambient skin temperatures and displays the temperature readings on an LCD display.

Measuring the Pulse Rate

The heart is a muscular pump. The left ventricle of the heart contracts with every beat, forcing blood from the heart into the systemic arteries. The amount of blood pumped from the heart with each heartbeat is called the *stroke volume*. The force of the blood against the walls of the arteries generates a wave of pressure that is felt at various points in the body as a **pulse**. The ability of the arteries to contract and expand is called *compliance*. When compliance is reduced, the heart must exert more pressure to pump blood throughout the body.

Location of Pulse Points

The apical pulse is felt at the apex of the heart. Figure 7.8 illustrates the location of the apical pulse for a child under 4 years, a child 4 to 6 years, and an adult. The peripheral pulse is the pulse as felt in the body's periphery, for example, in the neck, wrist, or foot. Figure 7.9 shows eight sites where the peripheral pulse is most easily palpated. In a healthy client, the peripheral pulse rate is equivalent to the heartbeat. Alterations in the client's health can weaken the peripheral pulse, making it difficult to detect. Thus, assessment of the peripheral pulse is an important component of a thorough health assessment.

Factors That Influence Pulse Rate

A variety of factors may influence the normal pulse rate:

- *Age.* The average pulse rate of infants and children is higher than that of teens and adults. After age 16, the pulse stabilizes to an average of about 70 beats per minute (bpm) in males and 75 bpm in females.
- *Gender.* As previously noted, the average pulse rate of the adult male is slightly lower than that of the adult female.
- *Exercise.* The pulse rate normally increases with exercise.
- *Stress.* In response to stress, fear, and anxiety, the heart rate and the force of the heartbeat increase.
- *Fever.* The peripheral vasodilation that accompanies an elevated body temperature lowers systemic blood pressure, in turn causing an increase in pulse rate.
- *Hemorrhage.* Pulse rate increases in response to significant loss of blood from the vascular system.
- *Medications.* A variety of medications may either increase or decrease the heart rate.
- *Position changes.* When clients sit or stand for long periods, blood may pool in the veins, resulting in a temporary decrease in venous blood return to the heart and, consequently, reduced blood pressure and lowered pulse rate.

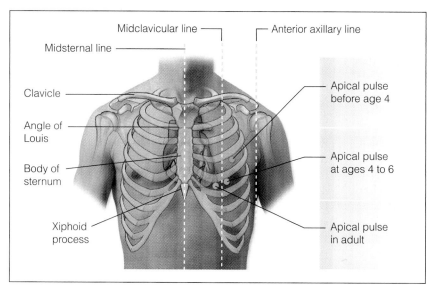

Figure 7.8 ● Location of the apical pulse in a child under age 4, a child ages 4 to 6, and an adult.

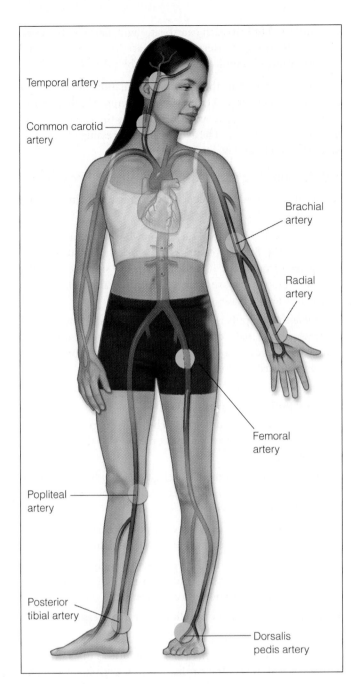

Figure 7.9 ● Body sites where the peripheral pulse is most easily palpated.

Palpation of the Radial Pulse

The peripheral pulse site most commonly used is the radial pulse. The radial pulse is palpated by placing the pads of the first two or three fingers on the anterior wrist along the radius bone (see Figure 7.10). If the pulse is regular, the nurse counts the beats for 30 seconds and multiplies by 2 to obtain the total bpm. If the pulse is irregular, the nurse counts the beats for a full minute.

Four factors are considered when assessing the pulse: rate, rhythm, force, and elasticity. A pulse rate of less than 60 bpm, called *bradycardia,* may be found in a healthy, well-trained athlete. A pulse rate over 100 bpm, called *tachycardia,* may also be found in the healthy client who is anxious or has just finished exercising.

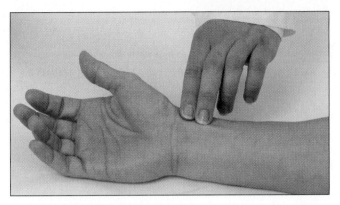

Figure 7.10 ● Palpating the radial pulse.

The pulse of a healthy adult has a relatively constant rhythm; that is, the intervals between beats are regular. Irregularities in heart rhythm are discussed fully in Chapter 17 of this text. ⚭

The nurse assesses the force of a pulse, or its stroke volume, by noting the pressure that must be exerted before the pulse is felt. A full, bounding pulse is difficult to obliterate. It may be caused by fear, anxiety, exercise, or a variety of alterations in health. A weak, thready pulse is easy to obliterate. It also may indicate alterations in health, such as hemorrhage. The nurse palpates along the radial artery in a proximal-to-distal direction to assess the elasticity of the artery. A normal artery feels smooth, straight, and resilient.

Measuring Respiratory Rate

The human body continuously exchanges oxygen and carbon dioxide through the act of respiration. Normal respiratory rates are dependent on age.

Assessment of Respiratory Rate

Counting the number of respirations per minute assesses **respiratory rate.** The nurse observes the full respiratory cycle (one inspiration and one expiration) for rate and pattern of breathing. The client's respiratory rate is assessed by counting the number of breaths for 30 seconds and then multiplying by 2. If the nurse detects irregularities or difficulty breathing, the respirations are counted for a full minute.

Factors That Influence Respiratory Rate

The respiratory rate in some clients may increase if they become aware that their breaths are being counted. For this reason, the nurse should maintain the posture of counting the radial pulse while counting breaths per minute. Other factors that may increase respiratory rate include exercise, stress, increased temperature, and increased altitude. Some medications may either increase or decrease respiratory rate. Table 7.1 lists normal respiratory rates for newborns through older adults. See Chapter 15 for a more detailed discussion of respiration. ⚭

Oxygen Saturation

Oxygen saturation of the hemoglobin is measured by using a pulse oximeter. The pulse oximeter uses a sensor and a photodetector to determine the light sent and absorbed by the hemoglobin. The reported percentage represents the light absorbed

TABLE 7.1	Normal Respiratory Rates for Newborns Through Older Adults
AGE	**RESPIRATIONS PER MINUTE**
Newborn	30–80
3–9 years	20–30
10–15 years	16–22
16–adult	15–20
Adult	12–20
Older adult	15–25

by oxygenated and deoxygenated hemoglobin. A value of 95% to 100% is considered normal, while a value of 70% is considered to be life threatening. This noninvasive procedure allows oxygen saturation values to be easily obtained and rapidly updated. Pulse oximetry can detect hypoxemia (low blood oxygen) before symptoms, such as cyanosis (blue colour) of the skin, appear.

Measuring Blood Pressure

Blood ebbs and flows within the systemic arteries in waves, causing two types of pressure. The **systolic pressure** is the pressure of the blood at the height of the wave, when the left ventricle contracts. This number is the first recorded in a **blood pressure** measurement. The **diastolic pressure** is the pressure between the ventricular contractions, when the heart is at rest. This number is the second recorded in a blood pressure measurement.

Circulatory Factors That Influence Blood Pressure

Factors that influence blood pressure include but are not limited to the following:

- *Cardiac output* is the amount of blood ejected from the heart. Cardiac output is equal to the stroke volume, or amount of blood ejected in one heartbeat (measured in millilitres per beat), multiplied by the heart rate (measured in bpm). Cardiac output averages about 5.5 L/min (litres per minute).
- *Blood volume* is the total amount of blood circulating within the entire vascular system. Blood volume averages about 5 L in adults. A sudden drop in blood pressure may signal sudden blood loss, as with internal bleeding.
- *Peripheral vascular resistance* is the resistance the blood encounters as it flows within the vessels. Peripheral resistance is in turn influenced by various factors, such as vessel length and diameter. Two of the most important factors influencing peripheral resistance are blood viscosity and vessel compliance.
- *Blood viscosity* is the ratio between the blood cells (the formed elements) and the blood plasma. When the total amount of formed elements is high, the blood is thicker, or more viscous. The molecules pass one another with greater difficulty, and more pressure is required to move the blood.
- *Vessel compliance* describes the elasticity of the smooth muscle in the arterial walls. Highly elastic arteries respond

readily and fully to each heartbeat. Rigid, hardened arteries, as are found with arteriosclerosis, are less responsive, and greater force is required to move the blood along.

Note that blood in the systemic circulation flows along a pressure gradient from central to peripheral; in other words, pressure is higher in the arterioles than in the capillaries and higher still in the aorta. The average blood pressure of a healthy adult is 120/80 mm Hg.

Additional Factors Affecting Blood Pressure

Additional factors that influence blood pressure include but are not limited to the following:

- *Age.* Systolic blood pressure in newborns averages about 78 mm Hg. Blood pressure rates tend to rise with increasing age through age 18 and then tend to stabilize. In older adults, blood pressure rates tend to rise again as elasticity of the arteries decreases.
- *Gender.* After puberty, females tend to have lower blood pressure than males of the same age. Reproductive hormones may influence this difference because blood pressure in women usually increases after menopause.
- *Race.* Black males over the age of 35 tend to have higher blood pressures than other males.
- *Obesity.* Blood pressure tends to be higher in people who are overweight and obese than in people of normal weight of the same age.
- *Physical activity.* Physical activity (including crying in infants and children) increases cardiac output and therefore increases blood pressure.
- *Stress.* Stress increases cardiac output and arterial vasoconstriction, resulting in increased blood pressure.
- *Diurnal variations.* Blood pressure is usually lowest in the early morning and rises steadily throughout the day, peaking in the late afternoon or early evening.
- *Medications.* A variety of medications can increase or decrease blood pressure.

Blood pressure is also affected by alterations in health. Any condition that affects the cardiac output, peripheral vascular resistance, blood volume, blood viscosity, or vessel compliance can affect blood pressure.

Assessment of Blood Pressure

An accurate measurement of blood pressure is an essential part of any complete health assessment.

CLIENT PREPARATION. It is important to reassure the client that the procedure for taking blood pressure is generally quick and painless. The client should be at rest for at least 5 minutes before taking a blood pressure measurement and up to 20 minutes if the client has been engaging in heavy physical activity. Client anxiety may also cause a temporary elevation of blood pressure.

EQUIPMENT. The nurse measures blood pressure with a blood pressure cuff, a **sphygmomanometer,** and a stethoscope. There are various cuff sizes, as shown in Figure 7.11. The cuff consists

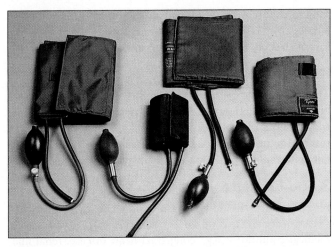

Figure 7.11 ● A variety of cuff sizes: a small cuff for an infant, small child, or frail adult; a normal adult-size cuff; and a large cuff for measuring the blood pressure on the leg or on the arm of an obese adult.

of an inflatable bladder, which is covered by cloth and has two tubes attached to it. One of these tubes ends in a rubber bulb with which to inflate the bladder. A small valve on the side of the bulb regulates air in the bladder. When the valve is loosened, air in the bladder is released. After the valve is tightened, pumped air remains in the bladder. The second tube attached to the bladder ends in a sphygmomanometer, a device that measures the air pressure in the bladder. There are two types of sphygmomanometers: aneroid and mercury. The aneroid sphygmomanometer has a small, calibrated dial with a needle. It is more portable but less reliable than the mercury type. The mercury sphygmomanometer has a calibrated cylinder filled with mercury. To determine the blood pressure, the nurse reads the measurement corresponding to the crescent-shaped top of the column of mercury. (*Note:* The use of mercury sphygmomanometers is being discontinued in healthcare settings.)

The bladder of the blood pressure cuff must fit the length and width of the client's limb. If the bladder is too narrow, the blood pressure reading will be falsely high. The width of the bladder should equal 40% of the circumference of the limb. The length of the bladder should equal 80% of the circumference of the limb. Note that the circumference of the client's limb, and not the age of the client, determines the cuff used. Automatic monitors can be used to measure blood pressure. These devices include a cuff attached to an electronic monitor. Application of the cuff is the same as in the manual method. The monitor provides a reading on an LCD screen of the systolic, diastolic, and mean blood pressures.

THE PROCEDURE. Blood pressure measurements are usually taken by placing the cuff on the client's arm and auscultating the pulse in the brachial artery. The nurse must use common sense when choosing which arm to use for the measurement. For example, blood pressure should not be measured in an arm on the same side as a mastectomy or an arm with a shunt. If blood pressure cannot be measured in either arm because of disease or trauma, a thigh blood pressure may be taken, using the popliteal artery, or a leg blood pressure may be taken, using the posterior tibial or dorsalis pedis arteries.

To measure the blood pressure in the client's arm, the nurse follows these steps:

1. Place the client in a comfortable position in a quiet room.
2. Confirm that the blood pressure cuff is the appropriate size for the client's arm.
3. Remove any clothing from the client's arm.
4. Slightly flex the arm and hold it at the level of the heart with the palm upward.
5. Palpate the brachial pulse.
6. Place the cuff on the arm with the lower border 3 cm (1.25 in.) above the antecubital area, making sure that the cuff is smooth and snug. One finger should fit between the cuff and the client's arm. Be sure that the centre of the bladder is over the brachial artery. Many cuffs have an arrow to indicate the centre of the bladder and thus the part of the cuff to be over the artery.
7. Palpate the radial pulse.
8. Close the release valve on the pump.
9. Inflate the cuff until the radial pulse is no longer palpable and note the reading on the sphygmomanometer. This is the palpatory systolic blood pressure. Deflate the cuff.
10. Wait 30 seconds before reinflating the cuff.
11. Place the diaphragm of the stethoscope over the brachial pulse (see Figure 7.12).
12. Pump up the cuff until the sphygmomanometer registers 30 mm Hg above the palpatory systolic blood pressure (the point at which the radial pulse disappeared).
13. Release the valve on the cuff carefully so that the pressure decreases at the rate of 2 to 3 mm Hg per second.
14. Note the manometer reading at each of the five Korotkoff phases (see Box 7.1). The first sound is recorded as the systolic blood pressure and the last sound is recorded as the diastolic blood pressure.
15. Deflate the cuff rapidly and completely.
16. Remove the cuff from the client's arm.

Age-Related Considerations

The client's age can affect the methods and equipment used to assess vital signs. The following sections address age-related considerations.

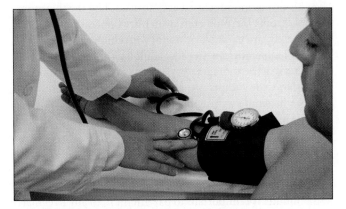

Figure 7.12 ● Measuring the client's blood pressure.

BOX 7.1	Korotkoff's Sounds
Phase I	The pressure level at which the first faint, clear tapping or thumping sounds are heard. These sounds gradually become more intense. To ensure that they are not extraneous sounds, the nurse should identify at least two consecutive tapping sounds. The first tapping sound heard during deflation of the cuff is called the systolic blood pressure.
Phase II	The period during deflation when the sounds have a muffled, whooshing, or swishing quality.
Phase III	The period during which the blood flows freely through an increasingly open artery and the sounds become crisper and more intense and again assume a thumping quality but softer than in phase I.
Phase IV	The time when the sounds become muffled and have a soft blowing quality.
Phase V	The pressure level when the last sound is heard. This is followed by a period of silence. The pressure at which the last sound is heard is known as the diastolic blood pressure in adults.*

*In agencies in which the fourth phase is considered the diastolic pressure, three measures are recommended (systolic pressure, diastolic pressure, and phase V). These may be referred to as systolic, first diastolic, and second diastolic pressures. The phase V (second diastolic pressure) reading may be zero; that is, the muffled sounds are heard even when there is no air pressure in the blood pressure cuff. In some instances, muffled sounds are never heard, in which case a dash is inserted where the reading would normally be recorded (e.g., /–/110).

Source: Kozier, B., Erb, G., Berman, A., Snyder, S., Bouchal, S., Hirst, S., Yiu, L., Stamler, L., & Buck, M. (2009). *Fundamentals of Canadian nursing* (2nd ed.). Toronto, ON: Pearson Education Canada, p. 692.

Temperature

Respirations and pulse rate are assessed before measuring rectal temperature in infants because taking a rectal temperature may cause an infant to cry. Holding the infant in a lateral position with the knees flexed onto the abdomen, or prone on the nurse's lap, the nurse separates the infant's buttocks with the nondominant hand and inserts the thermometer with the dominant gloved hand. The nurse should use a blunt-tipped thermometer, insert it no more than 2.5 cm (1 in.), and hold on to the exposed end. To avoid the risk of rectal perforation, an axillary temperature may be taken rather than a rectal temperature in newborns. The nurse should take the axillary temperature also in toddlers and older children whenever possible to eliminate their anxiety over the invasive rectal procedure. An oral route may be used as early as age 5 if the child is able to keep his or her mouth closed and does not bite the thermometer. Electronic thermometers, which are unbreakable and register quickly, are particularly useful with children.

Body temperature in the older adult may be reduced because of decreased thermoregulatory control and loss of subcutaneous fat. Older adults are more sensitive to environmental changes in temperature, possibly because of lack of physical activity, inadequate diet, or inability to afford adequate heating.

Pulse

The apical site is used for children younger than age 2. In older children, the nurse uses the radial site and counts the pulse for a full minute. It is important to pay attention to any irregularities in rhythm, such as sinus arrhythmia, which is not uncom-

mon in children. The pulse rate of the healthy older adult is in a range from 60 to 100 bpm. The radial artery may feel rigid if loss of elasticity in the arterial walls has occurred.

Respirations

The nurse should count respirations for a full minute in infants, because the breathing pattern may show considerable variation, from a series of rapid breaths to brief episodes of apnea. The respiratory rate in older adults may be increased to accommodate a decrease in vital capacity and inspiratory reserve volume.

Blood Pressure

Blood pressure should be measured in all children more than 3 years of age and in children less than 3 years of age with certain medical conditions (e.g., congenital heart disease, renal malformation, medications that affect blood pressure). The nurse uses a pediatric stethoscope with a small diaphragm. As with adults, the width of the cuff bladder should be 40% of the arm circumference, but the length should be 80% to 100% of the arm circumference. The lower edge of the blood pressure cuff can be closer to the antecubital space of an infant. The nurse uses the palpation method if auscultation with a stethoscope or Doppler ultrasound stethoscope is unsuccessful, or if the child is under 3 years of age. In children, the diastolic pressure is considered to be the onset of phase IV, where the sounds become muffled. Arm and thigh pressures are equivalent in children less than 1 year of age, and in children over 3, the thigh pressure is about 10 mm Hg higher. One quick way to determine the normal systolic blood pressure of a child is to use the following formula: normal systolic B/P $= 80 + (2 \times$ child age in years).

PAIN: THE FIFTH VITAL SIGN

Assessment of **pain** is essential in comprehensive health assessment. Pain is an entirely subjective and personal experience. When pain is present, it affects every aspect of an individual's health and well-being. Pain can be acute and chronic, severe or mild, but overall it is an experience unique to the individual. The perception of pain and the ways in which the individual responds to pain vary according to age, gender, culture, and developmental level. When conducting a pain assessment, the nurse must consider all factors influencing the individual's experience with pain. Refer to Chapter 8 of this text for a thorough discussion of pain. ⚭

Pain Assessment

The nurse typically initiates pain assessment because many individuals do not discuss their pain until asked about it. Pain assessment consists of two phases. The first phase is a pain history, and the second phase is observation of behaviours and responses to pain.

Pain History

A pain history includes collection of data about the location, intensity, quality, pattern, precipitating factors, actions aimed at relief of pain, impact on activities of daily living (ADLs), coping strategies, and emotional responses.

LOCATION. The nurse should ask the client to point to the specific location of pain. Charts in which body outlines are depicted are a useful method for children and adults to accurately identify the site of pain. When recording the location, the body outline charts may be used. The nurse is also expected to record locations using appropriate terminology in relation to the proximity or distance from known landmarks (e.g., pain in substernal area 3 cm (1.25 in.) below the xiphoid process).

INTENSITY. The intensity of pain is most accurately assessed through the use of **pain rating scales** (see Figure 7.13). Most scales use a numerical rating of 0 to 5 or 0 to 10, with 0 indicating the absence of pain. Descriptors accompany the number ratings in many scales. The descriptors assist the client to "quantify" the intensity of the pain. For children and adults who cannot read or are unable to numerically rate their pain, faces rating scales are available (see Figure 7.14). Numbers accompany each facial expression so that pain intensity can be identified.

QUALITY. Quality of pain is assessed by asking the client to apply an adjective to the pain. For example, pain may be experienced as burning, stabbing, piercing, or throbbing. Children may have difficulty describing pain; therefore, it is important to use familiar terminology, such as "boo-boo," "feel funny," or "hurt." The nurse must use quotation marks to record the description of the pain in the exact words spoken by the client.

PATTERN. The pattern of pain refers to the onset and duration of the pain experience. In addition, the nurse assesses whether the pain is constant or intermittent. If the pain is intermittent, the nurse must assess the length of time without pain or between episodes of pain.

PRECIPITATING FACTORS. A variety of factors can precipitate pain, including activity, exercise, and temperature or other climatic changes. Fear, anxiety, and stress can also precipitate pain.

ACTIONS TO ACHIEVE PAIN RELIEF. Assessment of pain includes gathering data about the measures taken by the client

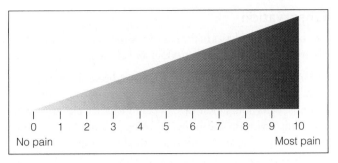

Figure 7.13 ● Pain rating intensity scale.

to relieve or alleviate the pain. The nurse will inquire about the use of medications, home and folk remedies, and alternative or complementary therapies, such as acupuncture, massage, and imagery. The nurse must also gather data about the effectiveness of the measures.

IMPACT ON ACTIVITIES OF DAILY LIVING. Assessment of the impact of pain on ADLs enables the nurse to understand the severity of the pain and the impact of the pain on the client's quality of life. ADLs include work, school, household and family management, mobility and transportation, leisure activities, and marital and family relationships. The nurse may ask the client to rate the impact of the pain on each of the ADLs.

COPING STRATEGIES. Individuals cope with pain in a variety of ways. Various coping strategies include but are not limited to prayer, yoga, Tai Chi, chi quong, support groups, distraction, relaxation techniques, or withdrawal. The strategies are often unique to the individual or reflect cultural values and beliefs. The nurse attempts to identify coping strategies employed by the client and to determine if they are effective in pain management.

EMOTIONAL RESPONSES. An assessment of the client's emotional response to pain is important. Pain, especially chronic or debilitating pain, can result in depression, anxiety, and physical and emotional exhaustion. The emotional response to pain is often related to the type, intensity, and duration of pain.

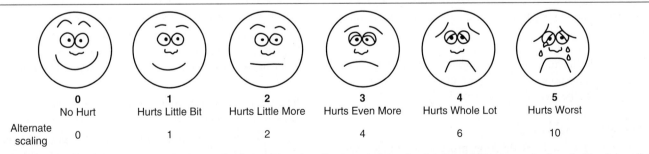

Brief word instructions: Point to each face using the words to describe the pain intensity. Ask the child to choose the face that best describes their own pain and record the appropriate number.

Original instructions: Explain to the person that each face is for a person who feels happy because he has no pain (hurt) or sad because he has some or a lot of pain. Face 0 is very happy because he doesn't hurt at all. Face 1 hurts just a little bit. Face 2 hurts a little more. Face 3 hurts even more. Face 4 hurts a whole lot. Face 5 hurts as much as you can imagine, although you don't have to be crying to feel this bad. Ask the person to choose the face that best describes how he is feeling.

Rating scale is recommended for persons age 3 years and older.

Figure 7.14 ● The Wong-Baker "Faces" pain rating scale.

Source: From Hockenberry, M. J., Wilson D., Winkelstein, M. L. *Wong's Essentials of Pediatric Nursing*, ed. 7, St. Louis, 2005, p. 1259. Used with permission. Copyright Mosby.

Observation

The observation phases of the pain assessment includes the direct observation of the client's behaviour and physiological responses.

BEHAVIOUR. A variety of behaviours indicate the presence of pain. Many of these behaviours are nonverbal or consist of vocalizations. Behaviours indicative of pain include facial grimacing, moaning, crying or screaming, guarding or immobilization of a body part, tossing and turning, and rhythmic movements.

PHYSIOLOGICAL RESPONSES. The site of the pain and the duration of the pain influence physiological responses to pain. The sympathetic nervous system is stimulated in the early stage of acute pain. The response is demonstrated in elevation of blood pressure, pulse and respiratory rates, pallor, and diaphoresis. Parasympathetic stimulation often accompanies visceral pain. This results in lowered blood pressure and pulse rate, and warm, dry skin.

THE FUNCTIONAL ASSESSMENT AS PART OF THE GENERAL SURVEY

Nurses use their observational skills in many situations. When making observations, nurses are continually thinking about the data and using their knowledge of the physical, behavioural, and social sciences to interpret the findings. The findings are interpreted according to the expected norms for clients in relation to age, gender, race, development, and culture.

Functional Assessment Defined

The **functional assessment** is an observation to gather data while the client is performing common or routine activities.

Functional Assessment During the General Survey

During the general survey of a healthy client, the nurse will observe the client while performing the following common activities: walking into the examination room, taking a seat for the interview, and moving the arms and hands to arrange clothing or to shake hands as an introduction. The nurse will also observe the facial expression while these acts occur. From this brief encounter, the nurse applies knowledge to begin to gather and interpret data about the client's mobility and strength, and the symmetry of the face and parts of the body.

Critical Thinking

When applying the critical thinking process, the nurse uses a variety of skills that culminate in assisting clients to make healthcare decisions.

The following case study and analysis are presented to demonstrate the application of critical thinking in the functional assessment of a client as part of the general survey.

The nurse conducted a comprehensive health assessment of a 70-year-old Aboriginal female who was new to the clinic. The interaction began when the nurse went to the waiting area to bring the client to the interview area. The following occurred: As the nurse entered the waiting area, all the clients looked up.

The nurse called out "Jane Carter" and looked about the room. An Aboriginal female with grey hair seen under a brightly coloured scarf said, "Here I am. I'll be right there." The woman rose slowly, pushing herself up with her hands placed on the arms of the chair. The nurse heard a soft "mmm, oh my." The client gathered her purse and reached for a cane resting next to the chair. As the client approached, the nurse noted that she had smooth skin on her face and hands. She was approximately 1.5 m (5′4″) and obese. She walked slowly toward the nurse, with the c ane in her right hand. She moved her left leg stiffly. As she moved through the door, she asked, "Will I have to sit down again now? I'm very stiff."

As stated early in this chapter, the general survey begins with the initial encounter with the client and provides cues about the client. The observations from the brief case study include the following:

- All the clients looked up when the nurse entered the waiting area.
- When a name was called, an Aboriginal female with grey hair responded.
- The woman rose slowly.
- The woman used her arms to push herself out of the chair.
- The woman uttered "oh my" while rising.
- The woman gathered her purse and reached for a cane.
- The woman had smooth skin on her face and hands.
- The woman was approximately 1.5 m (5′4″) tall and was obese.
- She walked slowly.
- She held the cane in her right hand.
- The movement of the left leg was stiff.
- As she entered the exam area, she asked, "Will I have to sit down again now? I'm very stiff."

In applying critical thinking the nurse will begin to sort information and determine an approach to continue data gathering. The nurse considers each of the observations in terms of normal and abnormal findings in relation to the age, gender, race, and culture of the client. Interpretations of the nurse's observations in the preceding case study are as follows:

- All the clients looked up when the nurse entered the room. *The client was aware that someone entered the room; this indicates that her vision and hearing are intact. This is considered a normal finding.*
- The client responded when her name was called. *This is further indication that hearing is intact. This is a normal finding.*
- The client had grey hair. *This is an expected finding in a 70-year-old female.*
- The client rose slowly. *This is an expected finding in an older adult because of decreased muscle tone and strength.*
- The client used her arms to push herself out of the chair. *This is an indication of diminished strength in the lower extremities. This is an expected finding in an older adult because of decreased muscle tone and strength. This requires follow-up to determine the actual muscle strength of the client.*
- The client uttered "oh my" while rising. *This indicates discomfort or surprise. This is initially interpreted as an abnormal*

finding. *Discomfort is indicative of an underlying problem. In this case, the problem may be musculoskeletal.*

- The client gathered her purse and reached for a cane. *This indicates that the client is alert and cognizant of her surroundings and the need to gather her personal items. This is a normal finding. The reaching for the cane suggests she has a musculoskeletal problem requiring its use. This is an abnormal finding and requires follow-up to ascertain the underlying problem.*

- The client had smooth skin on her face and hands. *This finding suggests that the client is in a state of fluid and nutritional balance and that she follows hygiene practices. This has the suggestion of being a normal finding. However, the nurse will consider other factors during the assessment.*

- The client was approximately 1.5 m (5′4″) tall and was obese. *Obesity is an abnormal finding. However, the nurse knows that weight gain occurs with aging.*

- She walked slowly. *This is expected in older adults who have lost muscle and skeletal mass and strength. This requires further evaluation in relation to the client's need to push herself up from the chair while uttering "oh my."*

- She held the cane in her right hand. *The ability to hold the cane indicates coordination in the right extremity. The nurse must follow up to determine the reason for the use of the cane and whether the client has been using the cane appropriately in relation to the underlying problem.*

- The movement of the left leg was stiff. *This is an abnormal finding. The nurse must determine the underlying cause. This is suggestive of a musculoskeletal problem. However, there may be a neurological problem.*

- As she entered the exam area, she asked, "Will I have to sit down again now? I'm very stiff." *This response indicates the client's concern with movement. The statements are not unexpected in relation to observations about the movements and gait of the client. This statement forces the nurse to make a rapid decision about the process of the health assessment. The nurse must quickly gather more data to determine the client's ability to participate in all aspects of the assessment.*

The preceding analyses demonstrate that a great deal of information can be obtained through observation. In this situation, much information is missing. As this information is gathered, the nurse will determine the relevance of each piece of data to the overall situation. The nurse applies critical thinking throughout the comprehensive health assessment while working with the client to meet health-related needs.

APPLICATION THROUGH CRITICAL THINKING

CASE STUDY

It was a Friday morning. You were the nurse who conducted a physical examination of Joseph Miller, a 73-year-old white male. You began with a client interview during which the following occurred.

The client entered the room, looked right at you, smiled, and stated, "How do you do?" in a clear voice. When you introduced yourself, he gave a firm handshake, then held both of your hands in his and commented, "Boy, you sure have cold hands." He walked steadily to the chair you indicated, but held onto the desk while sitting down. You informed the client of the purpose of the interview. He stated "no" when asked if he had any specific complaints or problems. He then shrugged his shoulders and commented, "I don't think I have anything special going on. I'm here for my three-month check and I expect to get a clean bill of health." You asked him to sign an admission form. He put on reading glasses, perused the form, and signed.

When asked about current medications, the client stated, "I have them with me, let me show you." He then took out three medicine bottles. He read each label and commented as follows about each. "This is captopril, and it's for my blood pressure; this one is ferrous sulphate, that's iron, I have some anemia; this last one is digoxin, I take it every other day for my heart." He frowned and said, "This bottle is nearly empty." After opening the bottle and looking at the contents he said, "Yup, just as I thought, I only have three pills left so I'll have to fill it. I'll be out of pills by Thursday and the drug store is always packed just before the weekend."

You continued the interview and concluded it by telling the patient you were going to check his blood pressure, pulse, temperature, and weight before escorting him to the examination room.

▶ Critical Thinking Questions

1. What are the findings from the case study for Mr. Miller?
2. How would you interpret the findings in relation to the categories for observation in the general survey?
3. Which findings indicate the need for follow-up in the interview or physical assessment?
4. What factors must be considered when evaluating the vital signs assessment for Mr. Miller?

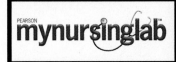

8

PAIN ASSESSMENT

PAIN IS A HIGHLY UNPLEASANT SENSATION that affects a person's physical health, emotional health, and well-being. Healthcare professionals include pain as the fifth vital sign and as a component of vital signs assessment.

Assessment of pain requires a strong knowledge base regarding the concept of pain and methods to collect information about the pain experience. Accurate assessment of pain is essential to develop, monitor, and evaluate the effectiveness of pain relief interventions.

Pain assessment, treatment, and relief present one of the greatest challenges to the nurse and other members of the healthcare team. The nurse has a primary role regarding the collection and analysis of data, the implementation of treatment modalities, and the evaluation of the client regarding pain experiences.

DEFINITION OF PAIN

Pain comes from the Greek word *poin[[emacron]]* meaning penalty, implying the person is paying for something. An individual's perception of pain is influenced by age, gender, culture, and previous experience with pain.

Pain has been defined as "whatever the experiencing person says it is, existing whenever he or she says it does" (McCaffery & Pasero, 1999, p. 5). Pain is a universal experience. Everyone experiences pain at some time and to some degree. It is a highly subjective, unpleasant, and personal sensation that cannot be shared with others. This sensation can be associated with actual or potential tissue damage. Pain can be the primary problem or associated with a specific diagnosis, treatment, or procedure.

No two people experience pain in the same manner. It can occupy all of a person's thinking, force changes in the ability to function on a daily basis, and produce changes in the individual's life. For the client, it is a difficult concept to describe, thus making pain treatment and relief most difficult.

The nurse cannot see or feel the pain being experienced by the client; however, the effects produced by the pain can be assessed. These changes can be physiological, psychological, and behavioural in nature.

PHYSIOLOGY OF PAIN

Pain is a complex, subjective, multidimensional phenomenon that is not clearly understood. Theories that have been developed to explain the conceptual and physiological aspects of pain include specific theory, pattern theory, and gate control theory.

Theories of Pain

The concept of specific theory explains the complexity of pain. This theory demonstrates that pain neurons are as specific and unique as other specific neurons (taste, smell) in the body. The special pain neurons transport the sensation to the brain for interpretation. The transport occurs in a straight line to the brain, making the pain equal to the injury. This theory does not include a consideration of any psychological component to pain.

The pattern theory indicates that individuals will respond in a different manner to a similar stimulus. This theory implies the pattern of the stimulus is more important than the specific stimulus. It does not take into consideration the psychosocial component to pain.

According to Melzack and Wall's gate control theory (1965), peripheral nerve fibres carrying pain impulses to the spinal cord can have their input modified at the spinal cord level before transmission to the brain. Synapses in the dorsal horns act as gates that close to keep impulses from reaching the brain or open to permit impulses to ascend to the brain.

Small-diameter nerve fibres carry pain stimuli through a gate, but large-diameter nerve fibres going through the same gate can inhibit the transmission of those pain impulses—

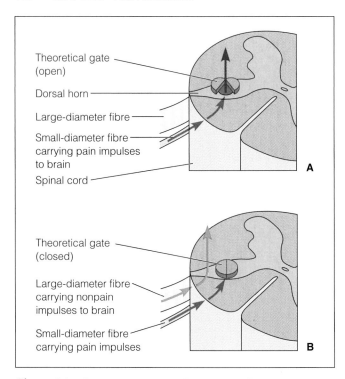

Figure 8.1 ● Gate control theory. A. open gate, B. closed gate.

that is, close the gate (see Figure 8.1). The gate mechanism is thought to be situated in the substantia gelatinosa cells in the dorsal horn of the spinal cord. Because a limited amount of sensory information can reach the brain at any given time, certain cells can interrupt the pain impulses. The brain also appears to influence whether the gate is open or closed. For example, previous experiences with pain affect the way an individual responds to pain.

The involvement of the brain helps explain why painful stimuli are interpreted differently by different people. Although the gate control theory is not unanimously accepted, it does help explain why electrical and mechanical interventions, as well as heat and pressure, can relieve pain. For example, a back massage may stimulate impulses in large nerves, which in turn close the gate to back pain.

Nervous System

The nervous system must receive and interpret a stimulus to allow the individual to recognize the pain process. How pain is transmitted and perceived is not completely understood. Whether pain is perceived and to what degree depends on the interaction between the body's analgesia system and the nervous system's transmission and interpretation of stimuli.

Nociception

The peripheral nervous system includes primary sensory neurons specialized to detect tissue damage and to evoke the sensations of touch, heat, cold, pain, and pressure. The receptors that transmit pain sensation are called **nociceptors**. These pain receptors or nociceptors can be excited by mechanical, thermal, or chemical stimuli (see Table 8.1). The physiological processes related to pain perception are described as **nociception**. Four processes are involved in nociception: transduction, transmission, perception, and modulation (Paice, 2002).

TRANSDUCTION. During the transduction phase, noxious stimuli (tissue injury) trigger the release of biochemical mediators (e.g., prostaglandins, bradykinin, serotonin, histamine, substance P) that sensitize nociceptors. Noxious or painful stimulation also causes movement of ions across cell membranes, which excites nociceptors. Analgesics (pain medications) can work during this phase by blocking the production of prostaglandin (e.g., ibuprofen) or by decreasing the movement of ions across the cell membrane (e.g., local anaesthetic).

TRANSMISSION. The second process of nociception, transmission of pain, includes three segments (McCaffery & Pasero, 1999). During the first segment, the pain impulse travels from the peripheral nerve fibres to the spinal cord. Substance P serves as a neurotransmitter, enhancing the movement of impulses across the nerve synapse from the primary afferent neuron to the second-order neuron in the dorsal horn of the spinal cord (see Figure 8.2). Two types of nociceptor fibres cause this transmission to the dorsal horn of the spinal cord: C fibres, which transmit dull, aching pain; and A-delta fibres, which transmit sharp, localized pain. The second segment is transmission from

TABLE 8.1	Types of Pain Stimuli
STIMULUS TYPE	**PHYSIOLOGICAL BASIS OF PAIN**
Mechanical	
1. Trauma to body tissues (e.g., surgery)	Tissue damage; direct irritation of the pain receptors; inflammation
2. Alterations in body tissues (e.g., edema)	Pressure on pain receptors
3. Blockage of a body duct	Distension of the lumen of the duct
4. Tumour	Pressure on pain receptors; irritation of nerve endings
5. Muscle spasm	Stimulation of pain receptors (also see chemical stimuli)
Thermal	
Extreme heat or cold (e.g., burns)	Tissue destruction; stimulation of thermosensitive pain receptors
Chemical	
1. Tissue ischemia (e.g., blocked coronary artery)	Stimulation of pain receptors because of accumulated lactic acid (and other chemicals, such as bradykinin and enzymes) in tissues
2. Muscle spasm	Tissue ischemia secondary to mechanical stimulation (see above)

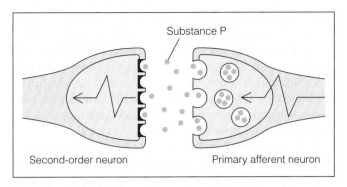

Figure 8.2 • Substance P assists the transmission of impulses across the synapse from the primary afferent neuron to a second-order neuron in the spinothalamic tract.

the spinal cord, and ascension, via spinothalamic tracts, to the brain stem and thalamus (see Figure 8.3). The third segment involves transmission of signals between the thalamus and the somatic sensory cortex where pain perception occurs.

Pain control can take place during this second process of transmission. For example, opioids (narcotics) block the release of neurotransmitters, particularly substance P, which stops the pain at the spinal level.

PERCEPTION. The third process, perception, occurs when the client becomes conscious of the pain. It is believed that pain perception occurs in the cortical structures, which allows

for different cognitive-behavioural strategies to be applied to reduce the sensory and affective components of pain (McCaffery & Pasero, 1999). For example, nonpharmacological interventions, such as distraction, guided imagery, and music, can help direct the client's attention away from the pain.

MODULATION. Often described as the descending system, this fourth process occurs when neurons in the brain stem send signals back down to the dorsal horn of the spinal cord (Paice, 2002, p. 75). These descending fibres release substances, such as endogenous opioids, serotonin, and norepinephrine, which can inhibit the ascending noxious (painful) impulses in the dorsal horn. These neurotransmitters are taken back by the body, which limits their analgesic usefulness (McCaffery & Pasero, 1999). Clients with chronic pain may be prescribed tricyclic antidepressants, which inhibit the reuptake of norepinephrine and serotonin. This action increases the modulation phase that helps inhibit painful ascending stimuli.

RESPONSES TO PAIN. The body's response to pain is a complex process that has both physiological and psychosocial aspects. Initially the sympathetic nervous system responds, resulting in the fight-or-flight response. The body adapts to the pain as the parasympathetic nervous system takes over, reversing many of the initial physiological responses. This adaptation to pain occurs after several hours or days of pain. The actual pain receptors adapt very little and continue to transmit the

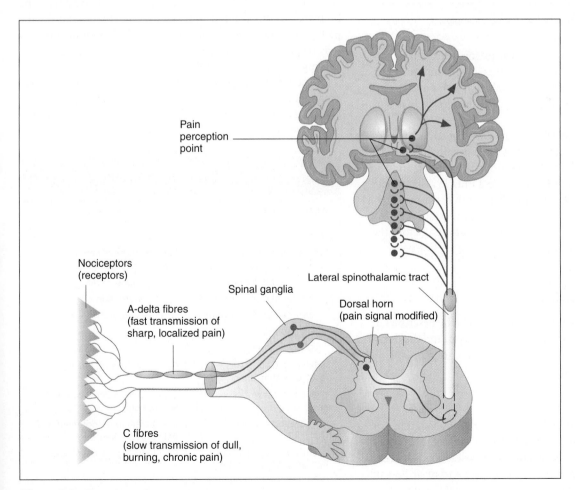

Figure 8.3 • Physiology of pain perception.

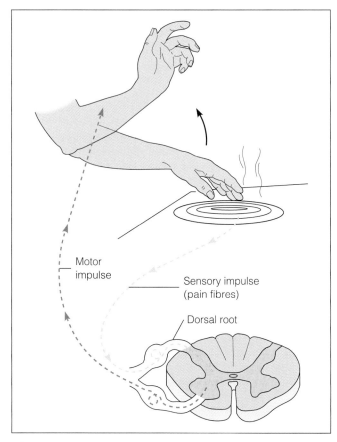

Figure 8.4 ● Proprioceptive reflex to a pain stimulus.

pain message. The person may learn to cope through cognitive and behavioural activities, such as diversions, imagery, and excessive sleeping. The individual may seek out physical interventions to manage the pain, such as analgesics, massage, and exercise.

A proprioceptive reflex also occurs with the stimulation of pain receptors. Impulses travel along sensory pain fibres to the spinal cord. There they synapse with motor neurons, and the impulses travel back via motor fibres to a muscle near the site of the pain (Figure 8.4). The muscle then contracts in a protective action. For example, when a person touches a hot stove, the hand reflexively draws back from the heat even before the person is aware of the pain.

NATURE OF PAIN

Pain, a subjective and personal experience, can be described in many ways. The type of pain, the point of origin, and the duration of pain are several ways that the nurse and other members of the healthcare team may describe pain.

Types of Pain

Pain may be described in terms of duration, location, or etiology. When pain lasts only through the expected recovery period from illness, injury, or surgery, it is described as **acute pain**, whether it has a sudden or slow onset and regardless of the intensity. **Chronic pain** is prolonged, usually recurring or

persisting over 6 months or longer, and interferes with functioning. Chronic pain can be further classified as chronic malignant pain when associated with cancer or other life-threatening conditions or as chronic nonmalignant pain when the etiology is a nonprogressive disorder. Such disorders include cluster headaches, low back pain, and myofascial pain dysfunction. Acute pain and chronic pain result in different physiological and behavioural responses, as shown in Table 8.2.

Pain can be categorized according to its origin as cutaneous, deep somatic, or visceral. **Cutaneous pain** originates in the skin or subcutaneous tissue. A paper cut causing a sharp pain with some burning is an example of cutaneous pain. **Deep somatic pain** arises from ligaments, tendons, bones, blood vessels, and nerves. It is diffuse and tends to last longer than cutaneous pain. An ankle sprain is an example of deep somatic pain. **Visceral pain** results from stimulation of pain receptors in the abdominal cavity, cranium, and thorax. It tends to appear diffuse and often feels like deep somatic pain, that is, burning, aching, or a feeling of pressure. Visceral pain is frequently caused by stretching of the tissues, ischemia, or muscle spasms. For example, an obstructed bowel will result in visceral pain.

Pain can also be described according to where it is experienced in the body. **Radiating pain** is perceived at the source of the pain and extends to nearby tissues. For example, cardiac pain may be felt not only in the chest but also along the left shoulder and down the arm. **Referred pain** is felt in a part of the body that is considerably removed from the tissues causing the pain. For example, pain from one part of the abdominal viscera may be perceived in an area of the skin remote from the organ causing the pain (see Figure 8.5).

Intractable pain is highly resistant to relief. One example is the pain from an advanced malignancy. When caring for a client experiencing intractable pain, nurses are challenged to

TABLE 8.2	Comparison of Acute and Chronic Pain

ACUTE PAIN	CHRONIC PAIN
Mild to severe	Mild to severe
Sympathetic nervous system responses:	Parasympathetic nervous system responses:
Increased pulse rate	Vital signs normal
Increased respiratory rate	Dry, warm skin
Elevated blood pressure	Pupils normal or dilated
Diaphoresis	
Dilated pupils	
Related to tissue injury; resolves with healing	Continues beyond healing
Client appears restless and anxious	Client appears depressed and withdrawn
Client reports pain	Client often does not mention pain unless asked
Client exhibits behaviour indicative of pain: crying, rubbing area, holding area	Pain behaviour often absent

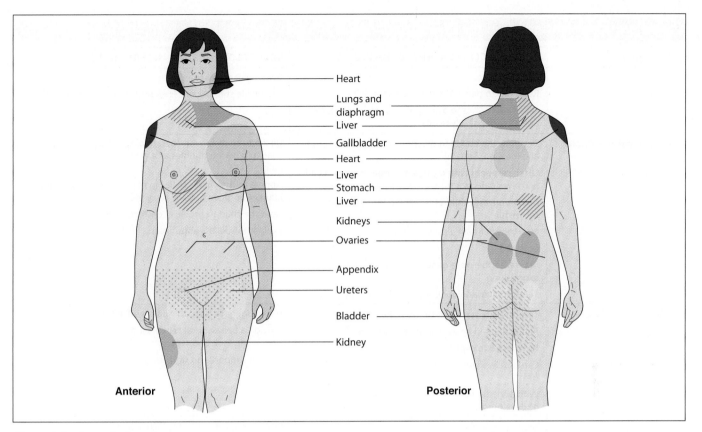

Figure 8.5 ● Sites of referred pain.

use a number of methods, pharmacological and nonpharmacological, to provide pain relief.

Neuropathic pain is the result of current or past damage to the peripheral or central nervous system and may not have a stimulus, such as tissue or nerve damage, for the pain. Neuropathic pain is long lasting, is unpleasant, and can be described as burning, dull, and aching. The health history is the most important component of the diagnosis of neuropathic pain. The physical examination and other specific tests are also used and should support this diagnosis (Gilron, Watson, Cahill, & Moulin, 2006). Examples of this pain include trigeminal neuralgia and peripheral neuropathy.

Phantom pain, which is perceived in a body part that is missing (e.g., an amputated leg) or paralyzed by a spinal cord injury, is an example of neuropathic pain. This pain can be distinguished from *phantom sensation*, that is, the feeling that the missing body part is still present. The incidence of phantom pain can be reduced when analgesics are administered via epidural catheter before the amputation.

Concepts Associated with Pain

When a person perceives pain from injured tissue, the pain threshold is reached. An individual's **pain threshold** is the amount of pain stimulation the person requires to feel pain. A person's pain threshold is fairly uniform; however, it can change. For example, the same stimuli that once produced mild pain can at another time produce intense pain. Excessive sensitivity to pain is called **hyperalgesia.**

Two additional terms used in the context of pain are *pain sensation* and *pain reaction*. **Pain sensation** can be considered the same as pain threshold; **pain reaction** includes the autonomic nervous system and behavioural responses to pain. The autonomic nervous system response is the automatic reaction that often protects the individual from further harm, such as the automatic withdrawal of the hand from a hot stove. The behavioural response is a learned response used as a method of coping with pain.

Pain tolerance is the maximum amount and duration of pain that an individual is willing to endure. Some clients are unable to tolerate even the slightest pain, whereas others are willing to endure severe pain rather than be treated for it. Pain tolerance is widely influenced by psychological and sociocultural factors.

FACTORS INFLUENCING PAIN

Factors that influence the individual's perception of and reaction to pain include developmental stage, psychosocial development, and the environment.

Developmental Considerations

The age and developmental stage of a client will influence both the reaction to and the expression of pain. Age variations and related nursing interventions are presented in Table 8.3.

The field of pain management for infants and children has grown significantly. It is now accepted that anatomical,

TABLE 8.3	Age Variations in the Pain Experience	
AGE GROUP	**PAIN PERCEPTION AND BEHAVIOUR**	**SELECTED NURSING INTERVENTIONS**
Infant	Perceives pain. Responds to pain with increased sensitivity. Older infant tries to avoid pain; for example, turns away and physically resists.	Give a glucose pacifier. Use tactile stimulation. Play music or tapes of a heartbeat.
Toddler and Preschooler	Develops the ability to describe pain and its intensity and location. Often responds with crying and anger because child perceives pain as a threat to security. Reasoning with child at this stage is not always successful. May consider pain a punishment. Feels sad. May learn there are gender differences in pain expression. Tends to hold someone accountable for the pain.	Distract the child with toys, books, pictures. Involve the child in blowing bubbles as a way of "blowing away the pain." Appeal to the child's belief in magic by using a "magic" blanket or glove to take away pain. Hold the child to provide comfort. Explore misbeliefs about pain.
School-Age Child	Tries to be brave when facing pain. Rationalizes in an attempt to explain the pain. Responsive to explanations. Can usually identify the location and describe the pain. With persistent pain may regress to an earlier stage of development.	Use imagery to turn off "pain switches." Provide a behavioural rehearsal of what to expect and how it will look and feel. Provide support and nurturing.
Adolescent	May be slow to acknowledge pain. Recognizing pain or "giving in" may be considered weakness. Wants to appear brave in front of peers and not report pain.	Provide opportunities to discuss pain. Provide privacy. Present choices for dealing with pain. Encourage music or TV for distraction.
Adult	Behaviours exhibited when experiencing pain may be gender-based behaviours learned as a child. May ignore pain because to admit it is perceived as a sign of weakness or failure. Fear of what pain means may prevent some adults from taking action.	Deal with any misbeliefs about pain. Focus on the client's control in dealing with the pain. Allay fears and anxiety when possible.
Older Adult	May have multiple conditions presenting with vague symptoms. May perceive pain as part of the aging process. May have decreased sensations or perceptions of the pain. Lethargy, anorexia, and fatigue may be indicators of pain. May withhold complaints of pain because of fear of the treatment, of any lifestyle changes that may be involved, or of becoming dependent. May describe pain differently, that is, as "ache," "hurt," or "discomfort." May consider it unacceptable to admit or show pain.	Taking a thorough history and conducting assessment are essential. Spend time with the client and listen carefully. Clarify misbeliefs. Encourage independence whenever possible.

physiological, and biochemical elements necessary for pain transmission are present in newborns, regardless of their gestational age. The Canadian Paediatric Society and the American Academy of Pediatrics (2007) recommended that nonpharmacological and pharmacological interventions be used to prevent, reduce, or eliminate pain in neonates. Physiological indicators may vary in infants, so behavioural observation

is recommended for pain assessment (Ball & Bindler, 2008). Children may be less able than adults to articulate their experience or needs related to pain, which may result in their pain being undertreated.

Older adults constitute a major portion of the individuals within the healthcare system. The prevalence of pain in the older population is generally higher because of both acute and chronic disease conditions. Pain threshold does not appear to change with aging, although the effect of analgesics may increase because of physiological changes related to drug metabolism and excretion (Eliopoulos, 2005).

Psychosocial Considerations

Family, culture, religion, and other factors influence the individual's ability to express and accept treatment modalities regarding pain.

Ethnic background and cultural heritage have long been recognized as influencing both a person's reaction to pain and the expression of that pain. Behaviour related to pain is part of the socialization process. For example, individuals in one culture may learn to be expressive about pain, whereas individuals from another culture may learn to keep those feelings to themselves and not bother others.

People's culture, including their religion and other social factors, can influence their ability to express and accept treatment modalities regarding pain. Ethnocultural background may influence both a person's reaction to pain, the expression of that pain, and the level of pain the person is willing to tolerate. For some people, self-infliction of pain is a sign of mourning or grief; for others, pain may be anticipated as part of ritualistic practices, and tolerance of pain may signify strength and endurance. Significant variations exist in the expression of pain, depending on a person's acculturation history and experiences.

Nurses have their own attitudes and expectations about pain and must identify their own personal attitudes about pain to provide culturally competent care. According to the Canadian Nurses Association (2004), cultural competence is essential in nursing practice and includes valuing diversity and being sensitive to those receiving nursing care. The provision of culturally competent care is necessary to ensure the best possible patient outcomes for clients in pain.

Environmental Considerations

Environmental factors will influence a person's ability to identify and seek relief for pain. The external environment includes a variety of stimuli for pain. Objects that may contribute to pain include restrictive clothing, ill-fitting shoes, or furniture and other objects in the work and home environments that cause pressure, strain, discomfort, or pain in healthy or already painful areas of the body. The ability to move freely influences the person's ability to avoid or control painful stimuli.

Family members and support systems, including members of the health team, are factors in the external environment that must be considered. A strange environment, such as a hospital, with its noises, lights, and activity, can compound pain. The lonely person who is without a support network may perceive pain as severe, whereas the person who has supportive people around may perceive less pain. Some people prefer to withdraw when they are in pain; others prefer the distraction of people and activity around them. Family caregivers can be a significant support for a person in pain. With the increase in outpatient and home care, families are assuming an increased responsibil-

ity for pain management. Education related to the assessment and management of pain can positively affect the perceived quality of life for both clients and their caregivers (McCaffery & Pasero, 1999).

Expectations of significant others can affect a person's perceptions of and responses to pain. In some situations, girls may be permitted to express pain more openly than boys. Family role can also affect how a person perceives or responds to pain. For instance, a single mother supporting three children may ignore pain because of her need to stay on the job. The presence of support people often changes a client's reaction to pain. For example, toddlers often tolerate pain more readily when supportive parents or nurses are nearby.

The internal environment includes individual perceptions and experiences related to pain. Previous pain experiences alter a client's sensitivity to pain. People who have experienced pain or who have been exposed to the suffering of someone close are often more threatened by anticipated pain than people without a pain experience. The success or lack of success of pain relief measures influences a person's expectations for relief. For example, a person who has tried several pain relief measures without success may have little hope about the helpfulness of nursing interventions.

Some clients may accept pain more readily than others, depending on the circumstances. A client who associates the pain with a positive outcome may withstand the pain amazingly well. For example, a woman giving birth to a child or an athlete undergoing knee surgery to prolong his career may tolerate pain better because of the benefit associated with it. These clients may view the pain as a temporary inconvenience rather than a potential threat or disruption to daily life.

By contrast, clients with unrelenting chronic pain may suffer more intensely. They may respond with despair, anxiety, and depression because they cannot attach a positive significance or purpose to the pain. In this situation, the pain may be looked on as a threat to body image or lifestyle and as a sign of possible impending death.

Anxiety often accompanies pain. The threat of the unknown and the inability to control the pain or the events surrounding it often augment the pain perception. Fatigue also reduces a person's ability to cope, thereby increasing pain perception. When pain interferes with sleep, fatigue and muscle tension often result and increase the pain; thus a cycle of pain–fatigue–pain develops. People who believe that they have control of their pain have decreased fear and anxiety, which decreases their pain perception. A perception of lacking control or a sense of helplessness tends to increase pain perception. Clients who are able to express pain to an attentive listener and participate in pain management decisions can increase a sense of control and decrease pain perception.

ASSESSMENT

Accurate and timely client assessment is imperative for effective pain management. Poorly managed or untreated pain will influence every aspect of an individual's health and well-being.

Pain assessment is considered the fifth vital sign. The strategy of linking pain assessment to routine vital sign assessment and documentation ensures pain assessment for all clients. Because pain is subjective and experienced uniquely by each person, nurses need to assess all factors affecting the pain experience: physiological, psychological, behavioural, emotional, and sociocultural.

The extent and frequency of the pain assessment varies according to the situation. For clients experiencing acute or severe pain, the nurse may focus only on location, quality, severity, and early intervention. Clients with less severe or chronic pain can usually provide a more detailed description of the experience. Frequency of pain assessment usually depends on the pain control measures being used and the clinical circumstances. For example, in the initial postoperative period, pain is often assessed whenever vital signs are taken, which may be as often as every 15 minutes and then extended to every 2 to 4 hours. Following pain management interventions, pain intensity should be reassessed at an interval appropriate for the intervention. For example, following the intravenous administration of morphine, the severity of pain should be reassessed in 20 to 30 minutes.

Because many people will not voice their pain unless asked about it, pain assessments must be initiated by the nurse. It is also essential that nurses listen to and rely on the client's perceptions of pain. Believing the person experiencing and conveying the perceptions is crucial in establishing a sense of trust.

Pain assessments consist of two major components: (1) a pain history to obtain facts from the client and (2) direct observation of behavioural and physiological responses of the client. The goal of assessment is to gain an objective understanding of a subjective experience.

Pain History

A detailed history to obtain subjective data from the client is essential for successful treatment and relief from pain. During the health history, the nurse provides clients an opportunity to express in their own words how they view pain. It also gives the nurse an opportunity to observe the body language or nonverbal communication of the client. The responses made by the client will help the nurse understand the meaning of pain to the client and the coping strategies being used. Each person's pain experience is unique, and the client is the best interpreter of the pain experience.

Health History

During the health history, qualitative and quantitative information regarding pain will be collected. The qualitative data will include location, duration, and characteristics of the pain. The quantitative data will provide information regarding the severity of the pain. The subjective data will be obtained by using closed and open-ended questions. Follow-up questions may be needed for greater clarification regarding the pain experience. Sample questions are provided for the nurse to use to obtain the subjective data. This list of questions is not all-inclusive but represents the types of questions required in a comprehensive health history. The mnemonic O-P-Q-R-S-T-U, which stands for onset (chronology), precipitating (or palliating), quality, region (or radiation), severity, timing, and understanding will help the learner remember the dimension of pain assessment. Additional questions specific to pain relief, the activities of daily living, coping strategies, and emotional responses are also included.

Questions Regarding Onset (Chronology)

1. When did you first notice the pain?
2. How long does it last?

Questions Regarding Precipitating/ Palliating Factors

1. What makes the pain worse?
2. What makes the pain better?

Questions Regarding Quality

1. Can you describe the pain?
2. An alternative method would be to list the possible descriptive terms and ask the client to respond yes or no to each descriptor. The terms include *deep, superficial, burning, aching, dull, sharp, shooting, stabbing, crushing, or tingling.*

Questions Regarding Region (Radiation)

1. Where is the pain located?
2. Does the pain radiate?
3. Are you able to point to or put your finger on the painful area?
4. An alternative method to assess the location or radiation of the pain would be to give the client a picture of the body and ask him or her to colour or point to the areas of the body affected by the pain.

Questions Regarding Severity

1. How bad is the pain now?
2. How would you rate the pain on a scale of 0 to 10, with 0 being no pain and 10 being the worst pain?
3. An alternative method would be to give the client a pain rating intensity scale (see Figure 7.13) and ask the client to place a mark to correspond to the pain being experienced. The nurse should be sure to use an appropriate tool for the client. Rating scales include the use of numbers and pictures, and they are language specific.

Questions Regarding Timing

1. Is the pain constant or intermittent?
2. How long does it last?
3. What were you doing just before the pain started?
4. Is the pain associated with a time of day or other symptoms?

Question Regarding Understanding

1. What do you think is causing the pain?

   This question attempts to understand the client's perception of the cause of pain and may yield information not previously elicited.

Questions Regarding Pain Relief

1. What have you done to relieve the pain? Ask the client about pharmacological and nonpharmacological approaches to pain relief.

2. Did it work?

3. Have you used this before? When?

4. Why do you think it worked (or didn't work) this time?

   Questions 1 to 4 provide the client the opportunity to discuss what actions have been taken to help decrease or eliminate the pain.

5. An alternative method to questions 1 to 4 would be to list the possible strategies and ask the client to respond yes or no to each strategy:

   Do you take a prescribed pain pill?

   Do you take an over-the-counter medicine for the pain?

   Do you change your diet in any way when you have pain?

   Do you use an ice pack or heating pad on the pain?

   Do you use prayer?

   Do you or a family member perform some ritual?

   Do you rest when you have the pain?

   Do you do anything that has not been mentioned?

   When the client responds yes, the nurse must then determine the effectiveness of the strategy.

Questions Regarding Impact on Activities of Daily Living

1. Describe your daily activities.

2. How well are you able to perform these activities?

3. Does the pain in any way hinder your ability to function?

4. An alternative method would be to list possible daily activities and ask the client to respond with a yes or no if the pain hinders the ability to perform the actions:

   Do you have difficulty sleeping?

   Has your appetite changed?

   Are you able to get out of bed without help?

   Do you have difficulty walking, standing, sitting, or climbing stairs?

   Are you able to perform your work activities?

   Are you able to concentrate at school, work, or home?

   Are you able to drive? to ride in a car?

   Do you have mood swings?

   Do you find yourself being short with family members and friends?

Questions Related to Coping Strategies

1. Describe how you deal or cope with the pain.

2. Are you in a support group for pain?

3. What do you do to decrease the pain so you can function and feel better?

   Questions 1 to 3 enable the client to share his or her coping strategies. These may be unique to the individual and may reflect family values and cultural beliefs.

Questions Related to Emotional Responses

1. Emotionally, how does the pain make you feel?

2. Does your pain make you feel depressed?

3. Does your pain ever make you feel anxious, tired, or exhausted?

4. Have you been under a great deal of stress lately?

   These questions attempt to determine a link to psychosocial factors or psychogenic sources of pain.

Physiological Responses

Assessment of client behaviours will include the collection of objective data. Nonverbal responses to pain vary widely. For clients who are very young, aphasic, confused, or disoriented, nonverbal expressions may be the only means of communicating pain. Facial expression is often the first indication of pain, and it may be the only one. Clenched teeth, tightly shut eyes, open sombre eyes, biting of the lower lip, and other facial grimaces may be indicative of pain. Vocalizations like moaning and groaning or crying and screaming are sometimes associated with pain.

Immobilization of the body or a part of the body may also indicate pain. The client with chest pain often holds the left arm across the chest. A person with abdominal pain may assume the position of greatest comfort, often with the knees and hips flexed, and move reluctantly.

Purposeless body movements can also indicate pain—for example, tossing and turning in bed or flinging the arms about. Involuntary movements, such as a reflexive jerking away from a needle inserted through the skin, indicate pain. An adult may be able to control this reflex; however, a child may be unable or unwilling to do so.

Rhythmic body movements or rubbing may indicate pain. An adult or a child may assume a fetal position and rock back and forth when experiencing abdominal pain. During labour a woman may massage her abdomen rhythmically with her hands. Because behavioural responses can be controlled, they may not be very revealing. When pain is chronic, overt behavioural responses are rarely seen because the individual develops personal coping styles for dealing with pain, discomfort, or suffering.

Physiological responses vary with the origin and duration of the pain. Early in the onset of acute pain the sympathetic nervous system is stimulated, resulting in increased blood pressure, pulse rate, respiratory rate, pallor, diaphoresis, and pupil dilation. The body does not sustain the increased sympathetic function over a prolonged period. Therefore, the sympathetic nervous system adapts, making the physiological responses less evident or even absent. Physiological responses are most likely to be absent in people with chronic pain because of central nervous system adaptation. Thus, it is important that the nurse assess more than the physiological responses, because they may be poor indicators of pain.

ASSESSMENT TOOLS

Assessment tools have been developed to help the client use measurable terms to describe the pain being experienced. The same tool will help the nurse obtain precise data needed to implement treatment modalities and evaluate pain relief.

The tool should be easy to use, tabulate, and score. It should be in the language of the client, and it should be used consistently. The nurse must teach the client, family members, and other members of the healthcare team correct use of the tool. All tools have advantages and disadvantages. It is the nurse's responsibility to identify these factors before implementation of the appropriate tool.

Tools used for pain assessment are designed and classified as unidimensional or multidimensional tools. A unidimensional tool will seek data regarding one aspect of pain. Many times this single element relates to the intensity of pain. Numerical rating scales, visual analog scales, the Oucher Scale, and the Poker Chip Scale are examples of unidimensional tools.

A multidimensional tool will seek data regarding more than one factor of pain. These tools look at intensity and other elements, including affective and sensory elements. The McGill Pain Questionnaire, short and long form, is an example of a multidimensional tool.

Unidimensional Tools

Assessment tools employed by the nurse help clients describe their pain. Unidimensional tools are used to help determine the client's level of acute pain. The tool is called unidimensional since it assesses one aspect of pain. These tools can be used in any clinical setting across the age span. It is important for the nurse to use the tool consistently throughout the assessment, treatment, and reassessment of the client. Because they measure just one element of the pain experience, unidimensional tools can lead to inadequate use of treatment modalities.

The Numeric Rating Scale asks the client to describe pain intensity with a number. The selected number then equates to pain severity. The Simple Verbal Descriptive Scale is another unidimensional tool. The individual is presented with six descriptive words and is asked to select one that corresponds to the present level of intensity.

The Body Diagram tool presents an outline of the body. The individual is asked to mark the picture showing the location of the pain. Shading of the body parts by the client will describe the intensity of the pain. The Oucher Scale has been designed for children. Pictures of faces ranging from neutral to distressed are presented, and the child selects the one representing his or her level of pain.

Multidimensional Tools

The multidimensional assessment tools assess two or more elements of pain. These tools go beyond pain intensity. They assess the nature, location, mood, and impact of pain regarding activities of daily living. The McGill Pain Questionnaire is available in a long and short form, and it is used when pain is prolonged. The long form measures intensity, location, pattern, sensory dimensions, and affective dimensions of pain. The short form measures intensity, sensory dimensions, and affective dimensions of pain.

The Brief Pain Inventory is another multidimensional scale used for assessment of pain. This tool provides information on pain and how pain interferes with the person's ability to function. Questions on this tool address medications, relief, individual beliefs, and quality of life.

Many tools are available to assist the client and nurse to assess, treat, and evaluate pain, and to measure the effectiveness of the treatment modalities. Tools must be appropriate for the age, culture, language, and cognitive abilities of the individual.

This chapter emphasizes pain as both physiological and emotional. Pain perception may be increased when a client also experiences anxiety, fatigue, or depression. The psychological aspect of pain is a subjective and personal experience influenced by age, culture, religion, and past experience with pain.

Pain assessment requires respect for the client's beliefs and attitudes about pain. Establishing a caring relationship, listening to the client, and using comprehensive interview techniques are essential in the assessment of pain. Numeric scales and surveys assist the nurse in quantifying pain.

Successful management of pain is dependent on an accurate assessment of the type and degree of pain the client is experiencing as well as the identification of underlying causes.

The assessment data are used by the nurse in interaction with the client and other health professionals to develop a plan for pain management. The holistic approach to nursing assessment of pain permits the plan to reflect the individual beliefs, needs, and wants of the client.

APPLICATION THROUGH CRITICAL THINKING

CASE STUDY

John Taylor, age 12, was hit by a car while riding his bicycle. He has several injuries and is brought to the emergency department at the local community hospital. The paramedic informs the staff John's right leg was splinted at the scene, right pedal pulse was 56, and left pedal pulse was 76. John has had no loss of consciousness; however, his respirations are 32 and shallow. He is crying and tells the nurse he has a lot of pain in his right leg and cannot seem to catch his breath.

The emergency department physician asks for a chest X-ray immediately, starts supportive oxygen therapy, and gives direction for administration of analgesic.

▶ *Critical Thinking Questions*

1. How and when should the nurse assess the pain in this patient?
2. What pain scale tool, if any, would be appropriate to use?
3. What additional information regarding pain is needed?
4. What role will the parents have at this time?

▶ *Applying Nursing Diagnoses*

1. What diagnostic statement from NANDA-I is appropriate for the client experiencing pain?
2. Identify the subjective and objective data for John Taylor that support the NANDA-I nursing diagnosis of *pain, acute*.

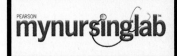

Visit the MyNursingLab website at **http://www.pearsoned.ca/mynursinglab**. This online homework and tutorial system puts you in control of your own learning with study and practice tools directly correlated to this chapter's content.

9

NUTRITIONAL ASSESSMENT

Canadian Contributors: Margaret Dykeman, University of New Brunswick, and Phyllis Murray, University of New Brunswick

Nᴜᴛʀɪᴛɪᴏɴᴀʟ ʜᴇᴀʟᴛʜ is a crucial component of overall health across the lifespan. The nutritional health of a pregnant female will influence pregnancy outcome. Nutritional health in growing children plays a central role in growth and development. In adults and older adults, nutritional health can be associated with prevention or development of chronic disease in conditions involving both undernutrition and overnutrition. **Undernutrition,** also called **malnutrition,** describes health effects of insufficient nutrient intake or stores. Undernutrition can be a deficit of either calories or specific nutrients. **Overnutrition** results from excess nutrient intake or stores and can manifest itself in conditions such as obesity, hypertension, hypercholesterolemia, or toxic levels of stored vitamins or minerals.

The determination of an individual's nutritional status is based on the foundation of a thorough nutritional assessment. The assessment portion of the nursing care process incorporates the gathering and interpretation of data often used as part of a nutritional assessment. These data then create the base for later development of appropriate nursing and nutritional interventions aimed at preserving or improving nutritional health.

DEFINING NUTRITIONAL HEALTH

Nutritional health can be defined as the physical result of the balance between nutrient intake and nutritional requirements. For example, an individual who consumes excess saturated fat may be at risk for elevated blood cholesterol and cardiovascular disease. This person may therefore be considered to have poor nutritional health because of overnutrition. A pregnant female who consumes less than required amounts of folic acid may place her unborn child at risk for certain birth defects, such as neural tube defects, and could be considered in poor nutritional health because of undernutrition. The incidence of gestational diabetes is dramatically increasing and producing more high-risk pregnancies and neonates. A client who consumes adequate nutrition to meet individual needs and avoids habitual excesses and insufficiencies would be considered in good nutritional health.

Many factors influence nutritional health, which in turn influences weight-related problems. The Provincial Working Group on the Problems of Weight in Quebec (2004) adapted a diagram developed by Ritenbaugh, Kamunvika, Morabia, Jeffery, and Antipatis to depict the "web of factors influencing weight-related problems." This causal web, shown in Figure 9.1, clearly shows the many factors that have an influence on nutritional health, both at the microlevel (individual) and at the macrolevels (environmental, social, cultural). Therefore, an assessment of nutritional health needs to include not only an assessment of the individual but also an assessment of the circumstances in which the individual lives.

When gathering data for a nutritional assessment, it is important to consider all the risk factors for a poor nutritional status, those that cause overnutrition and those that cause undernutrition. Overnutrition in the form of excess dietary intake of fat, especially saturated fat, has been associated with an increased risk of atherosclerosis. Overweight and obesity are linked with increased risk of hypertension, cardiovascular disease, type 2 diabetes, some cancers, degenerative joint disease, and other conditions. Overnutrition can occur when caloric input exceeds demands to sustain life and exercise level. Overnutrition also can be secondary to overeating specific elements, such as salt, simple sugar, and supplements, or to unique eating habits.

In the 2004 Canadian Community Health Survey (Health Canada, 2006), 58.8% of adults (65.2% of men and 52.4% of women) were either overweight or obese. These numbers are likely low since they are self-reported and not clinical measurements. The most striking increases since 1978–1979 were in the age groups 25 to 34 and 75+. The 2004 Canadian Community Health Survey also indicated that, based on measured heights and weights, 18.1% of children ages 2 to 17 were overweight and another 8.2% were obese, for a total of 26.3%. Comparing 2004 data with 1978–1979 data from a representative Canadian population sample shows that the problem of overweight and obesity has

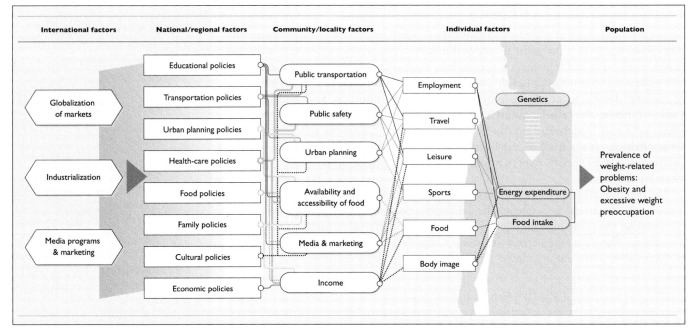

Figure 9.1 ● Causal web of factors influencing weight-related problems.

Source: Provincial Working Group on the Problems of Weight in Quebec. (2004). *Weight problems in Quebec: Getting mobilized*. Montreal, PC: ASPQ. p. 12. Retrieved from http://www.aspq.org/DL/gettingmob.pdf

tripled. When obesity was considered separately from overweight, approximately 23% of Canadians were obese (Health Canada, 2006), considerably below that in United States (30%). Health Canada (2006) reports indicate that cardiovascular disease, for which obesity is a risk factor, accounted for 37% of male deaths and 41% of female deaths in 2004. In comparison, cancer accounted for 28% of male and 27% of female deaths in 2004.

Undernutrition is less common than caloric excess, but it can have devastating physical health consequences when **protein-calorie malnutrition** or other specific nutrient deficiencies develop. Undernutrition can lead to growth faltering, compromised immune status, poor wound healing, muscle loss, physical and functional decline, and lack of proper development. Generally, individuals at risk for undernutrition include those who have a chronic illness, experience severe prolonged stress, or are older adults, poor, hospitalized, restrictive eaters (from chronic dieting, anorexia, or disordered eating), or alcoholics. An individual can have both caloric overnutrition and nutrient-specific undernutrition, such as when an older adult eats a diet of tea and toast, or a child overeats bread but consumes no fruits or vegetables.

Overall in Canada, 5.7% of newborns have low birth weight, but in some populations (inner-city dwellers, First Nations, smokers), the percentage rises as high as 10%, which is comparable to that in developing countries (Health Canada, 2002). Breastfeeding is strongly associated with the health of both mothers and children. Breastfeeding rates vary greatly in Canada, but only 30% of the 75% of mothers who initially begin breastfeeding continue until the child is 4 to 6 months old (Health Canada, 2002).

Box 9.1 outlines additional risk factors for overnutrition and undernutrition to consider when conducting a nutrition assessment.

Health Canada's document *Nutrition for Health: An Agenda for Action* (2002) builds on the Canadian Framework for Population Health initiated in the Ottawa Charter. Various provincial governments have developed health strategies to guide the provincial departments administering the healthcare system. For example, in Manitoba the document *Quality Health*

BOX 9.1	Risk Factors for Poor Nutritional Health

The nurse must consider all risk factors for poor nutritional health when conducting a nutrition assessment:

Undernutrition

- Chronic disease, acute illness, extreme stressors or injury
- Multiple medications
- Food insecurity—lack of access to adequate food or of ability to acquire and prepare
- Restrictive eating caused by chronic dieting, disordered eating, faddism, or food beliefs
- Alcohol abuse
- Depression, bereavement, loneliness, social isolation (some may overeat and others undereat)
- Poor dental health
- Decreased knowledge or skills about food preparation and recommendations (health literacy)
- Extreme age—premature infants or adults over 80 years of age

Overnutrition

- Excess intake of fat, sugar, calories, salt, or specific nutrients (energy, soft drinks)
- Alcohol abuse
- Sedentary lifestyle or altered mobility
- Decreased knowledge about or skills for food preparation and recommendations
- Depression, loneliness, or isolation

Care for Manitobans: The Action Plan (Manitoba Health, 1992) outlined a health policy framework. In New Brunswick, *Health 2000: Toward a Comprehensive Health Strategy*(New Brunswick Government, 1990) set goals and encouraged government, healthcare providers, consumers, and community groups to translate the goals into action plans. Concurrently in New Brunswick the Department of Public Health was charged to measure, assess, and track progress toward the goals, according to the plan identified in *Public Health Service: Vision, Mission, Goals and Objectives* (New Brunswick Government, 1993).

In Canada nutritional and weight concerns vary across jurisdictions because of regional differences that affect food choices and activity. For example, in the eastern and northern areas of Canada, which are colder and more isolated, the availability of fresh vegetables and fruit is reduced throughout the year. Low population densities reduce the availability of public transit, forcing people to drive more and walk less, which contribute to higher obesity rates. Awareness of the determinants of health guides all comprehensive health assessments in Canada; therefore, assessment of nutritional health also must take the determinants into consideration.

The increasing prevalence of overweight and obesity in North America, as well as the statistics on nutritional health disparities, illustrate the importance of nutritional screening and assessment as the first step toward reaching the goals for a healthy population. Box 9.2 outlines the cultural and socioeconomic influences that may affect nutritional health.

BOX 9.2	Cultural and Socioeconomic Influences on Nutritional Health

Several cultural and socioeconomic factors can affect nutritional health.

Overweight and Obesity

- In 1972, 40% of Canadian adults ages 20 to 74 were overweight or obese; in 1998, 50.7% were (Starky, 2005). In addition, one third of the adults who were of normal weight in the 1994–1995 census had become overweight by 2002–2003, and nearly 25% of the people who were previously overweight were reported as obese (Starky, 2005).
- The incidence of gestational diabetes is a national health problem that produces very large neonates at risk of premature delivery.
- In Canada the prevalence of overweight and obesity in children ages 7 to 13 is unclear. In 1996, 32.6% of boys and 26.6% of girls were reported to be overweight or obese. By 2001 the numbers dropped to 29% and 27%, respectively, but this information was given by parents in census data and as such isn't reliable.

Undernutrition

- Undernutrition can contribute to growth retardation.
- Up to 60% of older adults in dependent care facilities or hospitals experience both nutrient and calorie deficits.
- Adequate folic acid and iron are important for healthy outcomes during pregnancy. Planning pregnancies and boosting folate intake before pregnancy can prevent serious deficits in the neonate. Females of lower economic status and those with less education are more likely to have both unplanned pregnancies and inadequate folic acid or iron intake.
- Calcium and vitamin D needs vary throughout the lifespan, and many girls and women have significant lifelong deficits.

NUTRITIONAL ASSESSMENT

A nutritional assessment is the foundation on which related nursing diagnoses are developed and the goals and objectives for nutritional health are implemented. The prevention or treatment of malnutrition and overnutrition first requires a nutritional assessment. Determination of an individual's nutritional status should be accomplished while gathering data for an inclusive nursing assessment.

Nutritional assessment techniques and tools vary in their level of sophistication and depth. No one piece of data can give a complete nutritional assessment. Many parameters used to assess nutritional status can be affected by nonnutritional influences, such as disease, medication, culture, or environment. This fact illustrates the need to gather data from several resources. Generally, an assessment done by using multiple variables will be more valuable than an assessment made with limited data. In some healthcare situations, not all parameters or data are available. The nurse must rely on available information and sharp clinical judgment when making an assessment.

Various medical diagnoses or issues specific to the lifespan also influence pertinent parameters and techniques used in assessing a client's nutritional status. For example, measuring **waist circumference (WC)** may be of use when assessing overnutrition and cardiovascular risk status in adults, or protein malnutrition, but would be of little nutritional use when assessing a client with ascites or a pregnant female. WC also is not reliable if the client has a large abdominal pannus that will not be reflected in a simple measure of waist size.

A registered dietitian (RD) is generally responsible for completing a comprehensive nutritional assessment in most acute or long-term-care settings. However, as a frontline clinician, a nurse is ideally situated to identify nutritionally at-risk clients and initiate screening for those requiring further intervention targeting nutritional health. To perform age-appropriate screening, nurses require an awareness of age-related risk factors and body composition changes, for example, to differentiate normal versus abnormal height loss and subsequent health-related issues. In community and home care, the nurse is often both an assessor and an interventionist in relation to nutrition issues.

A nutritional assessment consists of a physical assessment, anthropometric measurements, and laboratory values, as well as a health history that includes nutrition. Several validated assessment tools exist to streamline the nutritional assessment process for use in a variety of healthcare settings or with specific populations. Most common standardized tools used to screen for nutritional status are specific to individual risk factors or populations. General tools for assessing nutrition in a general population are scarce. A Mini Nutritional Assessment is included in Appendix E.

Cultural factors influence both perception of nutritional status and assessment. Assessment tools need to be culturally specific for a population. In cases where tools are not already in existence, nurses must develop their own to ensure that assessments are relevant to the specific individual and situation.

Nutritional History

A careful nutritional history is part of a comprehensive nutritional assessment and is best accomplished by using more than one tool. A diet recall, a food frequency questionnaire, and a food record are components of a nutritional history that may be complemented with a health history for more specific information.

Diet Recall

A **diet recall,** also called a 24-hour recall, can be done quickly in most settings to obtain a snapshot assessment of dietary intake. A client is asked to verbally recall all food, beverages, and nutritional supplements or products consumed in a 24-hour period. Obtaining a recall for both a weekday and one weekend day will strengthen the data obtained. The nurse should ask primarily open-ended questions to appear nonjudgmental and not hint at "correct" answers to questions. The nurse should begin the diet recall by asking, "Tell me what you ate yesterday [or on a specific day]. When was the first time you had something to eat or drink in the day?" This type of questioning avoids the assumption of asking, "What did you have for breakfast?" Clients may feel judged if they admit they skip breakfast or too embarrassed to admit missing a meal. The result may be an inaccurate recall in which clients contrive answers they feel the nurse is seeking. Gentle prompting to obtain complete information is often needed. The nurse should ask about all food from meals and snacks; all liquids, including alcohol; and any use of nutritional supplements, such as herbs, vitamins and minerals, or diet and sports nutritional products. The nurse must determine whether fortified versions of common foods are consumed to assess nutrient intake accurately. Many foods are now fortified and should not be overlooked as significant sources of vitamins and minerals. Cereals and juices are examples of fortified foods to which nutrients not normally found in the product, such as calcium, have been added. A family member may participate in the interview with the permission of the client or if the client is unable to give a recall. Accuracy of a second-hand recall, even from a family member, has been found to be variable.

A best estimate of portion sizes will improve the accuracy of a recall. It is easy to over- and underestimate portion sizes of foods and liquids without a visual comparison. Life-size culturally appropriate food models are available. Digital photographs are less cumbersome and easily available as well. It is not always convenient to carry facsimiles to different settings where the nurse may be interviewing a client. In such cases, use of the food analogies in Figure 9.2 can be helpful.

Exclusive use of a diet recall for a nutritional history has drawbacks. A 24-hour recall is simply a 1-day example of intake and may not be indicative of normal habits. Other types and amounts of intake may occur on different days that were not assessed. Clients may have significant food habits that occur occasionally but not on the day recalled. The use of dietary supplements or alcohol often does not occur in the same fashion each day, yet it is crucial information to assess. Many other important data related to diet could be overlooked by relying on the recall alone. The accuracy of the recall relies heavily on the memory of the client and good interviewing skills of the

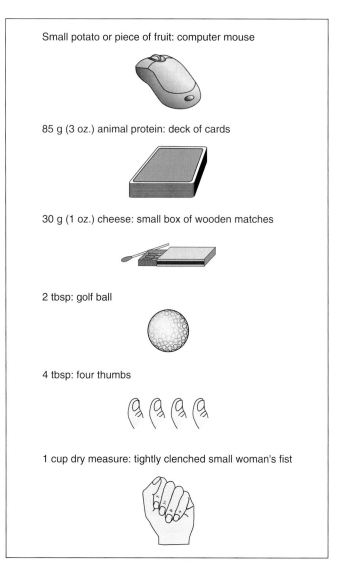

Figure 9.2 ● Analogies for estimating portion size.

nurse. Repeated diet recalls taken during subsequent healthcare visits can be used for comparison purposes and validation of intake. If the client is visited at home, an examination of the types of food in the cupboards and refrigerator may be informative, also.

Underreporting bias can occur with all parts of a nutritional history and may become apparent during the recall. Clients seeking the social approval of the nurse or wanting to avoid disapproval for their habits may underreport. Underreporting occurs for all ages and is seen more often in people who smoke, those who are obese, and individuals with lower educational and socioeconomic levels. Additionally, alcohol and drug use are frequently underreported. A nonjudgmental approach during the nutritional history will provide an environment conducive to the client giving full answers. Combining the recall with a food frequency assessment and an interview will yield the best information on which to base an assessment.

Food Frequency Questionnaire

A **food frequency questionnaire** assesses intake of a variety of food groups on a daily, weekly, or longer basis. This questionnaire helps to fill in some of the missing data not captured by a 24-hour recall to provide a more balanced assessment of intake.

For example, a 24-hour recall may indicate no fruit intake while a food frequency assessment finds two servings of fruit and one serving of juice daily. Food frequency questionnaires can be formal instruments composed of a checklist of food groups and foods or shorter questionnaires aimed at gathering general information. All food, beverage, and supplement groups should be included. Clients can fill out longer checklists before or after an interview but may find such tools cumbersome. Shorter questionnaires can be administered verbally and are more practical. Table 9.1 is an example of a completed basic food frequency questionnaire.

Food Record

Keeping a food record or diary for up to 3 days can provide supplemental information for a nutritional history. Recording intake for two sequential weekdays and a weekend day works well. Food diaries longer than 3 days in length tend to be recorded retrospectively with a loss of accuracy. Underreporting bias should also be considered when evaluating a food diary.

Health Literacy: The New Factor in Nutritional Assessment

Those unable to use information from various sources of media, print or electronic, have a serious disadvantage and may be noncompliant because of low health literacy skills. They may fail to follow instructions, miss appointments, and not get the help available for health resources because of inabilities related to either the language of material or the reading level of the clients. Health history forms may be incomplete and lead to the assumption that the clients have no problems rather than a revelation of illiteracy. Unfortunately, illiteracy often coexists in clients with chronic health conditions and multiple comorbidities and is misinterpreted by healthcare professionals. Health and progress through the healthcare system are negatively affected by low literacy skills. Behaviours suggestive of inadequate health literacy include (1) asking for help, (2) bringing someone who does the reading, (3) making excuses, (4) not complying with medication regimes, (5) adhering poorly to other prescribed interventions, (6) postponing a decision until others are consulted, and (7) mimicking or copying others (Safer & Keenan, 2005). One quick and easy health literacy assessment strategy is based on asking the client to read and explain the label on an ice cream container (Weiss et al., 2005). This strategy incorporates the issue of literacy being more than reading; the client needs the ability to see, read, interpret, and act on printed information. The six questions take only 3 minutes to administer.

Nutritional History Interview

A diet recall, food frequency questionnaire, or food record can be used alone or in combination as parameters in a quick

TABLE 9.1	Food Frequency Questionnaire				
FOOD	**VARIETY**	**TYPE**	**AMOUNT PER DAY**	**AMOUNT PER WEEK**	**LESS THAN ONCE PER WEEK (LIST)**
Fruit	Juice	Apple	350 mL (12 fl.oz.)		
	Fresh	Melon		1 cup	
	Canned/frozen	None			
Vegetables	Green	Varied		1–2×	
	Other	Squash		1×	
Dairy	Milk	Low Fat	2 cups		
	Cheese				1× month
	Yogurt	Never			
Protein	Animal	Poultry or Fish	Each night		
	Plant	Soyburger or Tofu		1–2×	
Fats	Saturated	Butter	1–2 pats		
	Unsaturated	Olive oil		tbsp	
Fluids	General	Water	120 mL (4 fl.oz.) 4× with meds		
	Caffeine	Tea	Each a.m.		
	Alcohol	Wine		3×	
Sweets and sugars		Cookies		2×	
Supplements	Vitamin/mineral	Multivitamin	One		
	Herbal	Echinacea			4–5× year for cold
	Other: Over-the-counter weight-loss product	Cannot recall ingredients			Tried once and stopped, complained of feeling dizzy

nutritional assessment. Conducting a nutritional history interview along with these tools, either as part of a nursing assessment or just concerning nutrition, will give the clearest picture of nutritional status.

A nutritional interview often incorporates a diet recall to glean specific details. It can be unreliable, as it is affected by memory, but it often gives information that leads to further questions regarding dietary choices. For example, a client may report drinking cranberry juice at breakfast because of intolerance to citrus fruits. The nurse could then use that cue to ask if the client has other intolerances or food allergies, before returning to the recall. The remainder of the needed nutritional history data can be gathered from the client and the medical chart after the recall portion of the interview. This more extensive form of a nutritional history assesses current habits but also can assess former habits. Past chronic dieting, supplement use, and therapeutic diets are examples of important historical data to gather.

BOX 9.3	Nutritional History Data

The nurse should address these topics when conducting a nutritional history interview:

Food
- All meals and snacks
- All liquids, including water, alcohol, and caffeinated beverages
- Use of fortified foods
- Preparation methods
- Portion sizes
- Grocery habits

Beliefs and Practices
- Adherence to a therapeutic diet for medical reasons or because of food allergy or food intolerance
- Cultural or religious influences on food choices and practices
- Faddism—trendy food and nutrition beliefs
- Lifestyle diet choices—vegetarianism, vegan diet, avoidance of certain foods or food groups
- **Pica** (abnormal craving for or eating of nonfood items)—if present: types of substances eaten, source, and amounts
- Meal patterns—number and frequency of meals and snacks, missed meals, location of meals

Supplement and Medication Use
- Vitamin and mineral use—dose, frequency, and constituents
- Herbal use—dose, frequency, and constituents
- Over-the-counter weight-loss or sports supplements—dose, frequency, and ingredients
- Over-the-counter and prescription medications to assess for drug-nutrient interactions or drug-herb interactions

Socioeconomic and Educational Influences
- Education and literacy level
- Knowledge and skills related to food and nutrition
- Social environment—assess for isolation and social support system
- General economic status and access to adequate food (food security)
- Independent activities of daily living, such as shopping, meal preparation, and self-feeding
- Activity level
- Functional capacity related to activities of daily living
- Presence of problematic substance use—drugs, alcohol, which can interfere with adequate diet

Box 9.3 outlines data topics to gather during the nutritional history interview, in addition to diet recall data. Table 9.2 is an example of a nutritional history form combining diet recall, food frequency, and nutritional history data. Health literacy must be considered before giving any client a form to complete.

Physical Assessment

The physical assessment portion of a nutritional assessment consists of two parts: **anthropometric** measurements and a head-to-toe physical assessment of a client. Anthropometric measurements include any scientific measurement of the body. Pertinent data from the medical history and examination should be considered during this portion of a nutritional assessment. The healthcare setting and the client's needs dictate the depth of data gathered. At times, estimated measurements and alternative techniques for obtaining anthropometric data may be necessary because of specific circumstances that make standard measurement difficult or impossible.

Anthropometric Measurements

Specific assessment of body fat and lean muscle mass may be better than weight or height alone as a measure of nutrition. Body fat can be measured by using skinfold measurements or technological instruments. Muscle mass is also referred to as **somatic protein** stores or skeletal muscle. Body mass index (BMI) is a widely used index relating weight and height. The first-tier assessments of weight and height used to be pillars of nutritional assessment but these are less dominant today as primary indicators. A second tier of anthropometric measurements assess body composition of various components, fat and fat-free mass, or of multiple components, which can include more precise analysis of fat-free mass: muscle, bone, and fluid components, for example. Racial differences have been observed in body composition that may warrant specific BMI classifications for various population groups. Asian adults have been reported to have a higher proportion of body fat mass at a given BMI than white adults. Black adults have greater muscle mass and bone mineral density at a given BMI than white adults. Additionally, ethnic differences within race categories have been observed. For example, Chinese adults have been observed to have proportionately higher body fat mass at a given BMI than Polynesians. Increasing levels of technology and updating of older reference values to include multicomponent factor analysis will allow more valid assessment of body composition in the future. The height-weight comparisons (tables) commonly used in the United States are not used in the Health Canada literature but are seen in practice because of the influence of American literature.

HEIGHT. Measurement of height is needed in adults as well as children to make an accurate assessment of nutritional status. In children and older adults, height is monitored on a continuum to assess skeletal growth and, indirectly, nutritional status. See Chapter 7 for accurate height assessment methods ∞.

When no means of obtaining measured height is feasible, self-reported height can be used. Every effort should be made to obtain a current measured height in centimetres, but this is not always possible. The accuracy of self-reported heights

TABLE 9.2	Nutrition Assessment Form

NUTRITION EVALUATION

Name: _____ DOB/age: _____

Address: _____ Date: _____

_____

Phone: _____ Referral source: _____

Date consent signed: _____

Ht: _____ Wt: _____ Wt change in last 3/6 M: _____ Ht & Wt at 20: _____

Client goal wt: _____ Body fat %: _____ Exercise pattern: Freq & duration: _____ Other activities: _____

Concurrent medical conditions _____ List Rx & OTC meds: _____ Allergies: _____

Food intolerances: _____ Food prep/storage concerns (who shops): _____

Hx: Food restriction, binging, purging, laxatives, other: _____

List supplements—Vit, Minerals, Herbals: _____ Diet history: _____

M–F _____ Weekends: Sa/Su _____

Dental Status: _____ natural teeth _____ dentures _____ caries _____

Eating Well with Canada's Food Guide (Indicate frequency: Qd, Qw, & other) _____

Vegetables & fruit (4-10)	**Grain products (3-8)**	**Milk and alternatives (2-4)**	**Meat and alternates (1-3)**
Vit C	White flour	Milk	Animal protein
Other	Whole grain	Cheese	Plant protein
Veg Yel/Green		Yogurt	
Other		Other	

Sugars/Sweets	**Fats (type)**	**Fluids**	
Substitute type & amount	Saturated	Water	
	Monounsaturated	Caffeinated soft drinks	
	Polyunsaturated	Alcohol	
		Other	

Source: Adapted, based on recommended number of food servings per day, from Health Canada. (2007). *Eating well with Canada's food guide.* Retrieved from http://www.hc-sc.gc.ca/fn-an/food-guide-aliment/index-eng.php

can be questionable. Men, women, and adolescents have been reported to overstate self-reported height by up to 2 cm (1 in.). Aging adults normally experience height loss, particularly in the trunk, which worsens with time, and older adults may consistently (unintentionally) overstate height by approximately 2.5 cm (1 in.) or more, just by stating their normal adult height. Self-estimates of height given in feet and inches are problematic since they must be converted to metres or centimetres and can become a source of error. When self-reported heights are used, documentation should note this. However, the nurse should ask what the client's height was at 20 years of age to test whether the potential for height loss is known by the individual.

WEIGHT. Current body weight and weight history are essential components of a nutritional assessment. Measured weight in kilograms should be obtained if physically possible since both men and women consistently underreport actual weight. Self-estimates of weight given in pounds are problematic since they must be converted to kilograms and can become a source of error. See Chapter 7 for accurate methods to determine the client's weight. ∞

Weight history is crucial to determining the presence of any intentional or unplanned weight losses. Unintentional weight loss could delay proper nutritional intervention or recognition of significant risk. Planned weight loss may lead to a readiness to initiate or adjust efforts to improve health. Weight history is also followed in children and pregnant females to monitor growth and development. Biochemical and weight assessment parameters for children and pregnant females are outlined in the section Nutritional Assessment Across the Lifespan. When obtaining a weight history, the nurse should look for prior documentation of actual weight if available. Otherwise, open-ended questions can be asked, such as "When was the last time you were weighed?" "What did you weigh then?" The nurse may also ask for weights at specific points in time as a cross-check: "What did you weigh this past summer before coming to college?" The nurse should not simply ask, "Has your weight changed recently?" Loose or tight clothing may be personal preference or an indicator of weight change, so the nurse can ask whether the fit of clothing has changed. The nurse can discern whether weight change has occurred by asking for specific weight information and calculating any noted differences.

Unintentional weight loss of 5% of body weight or more over a month or 10% or more over 6 months is considered clinically significant and warrants attention. These parameters are a required national standard for nutritional assessment of older adults in assisted living centres. Weight change is calculated by using the following formula:

$$[(\text{Prior weight} - \text{Current weight}) / \text{Prior weight}] \times 100 = \% \text{ weight change}$$

Box 9.4 provides an example of the calculations used to determine the percentage of weight change.

BODY MASS INDEX. The **body mass index (BMI)** is widely used to assess appropriate weight for height using the following formula: BMI = weight (kg)/height^2 (metres) (Starky, 2005). Parameters have been established to delineate underweight, healthy weight, and overweight standards in adults based on current scientific findings of morbidity and mortality prevalence associated with various BMI values. The World Health Organization (2000) established internationally used classifications for BMI, which were adapted by Health Canada and are outlined in Table 9.3. Health Canada (2003a) also uses BMI to indicate the severity of the health risk for each group as shown in Table 9.3. Adults with a BMI of less than 18.5 or between 25 and 29 have an increased risk of health problems. Those with a BMI in the Class II and III obesity ranges, respectively, have very high and extremely high risk of developing health problems. Health Canada (2003b) has a graphic chart that can be used to make rapid clinical comparisons regarding height and weight available on its website.

Exclusive use of BMI as an indicator of weight status makes the assumption that all individuals have equal body composition at each given weight. It also assumes that every person of the same weight has the same amount of muscle mass, body fat, and bone mineral content. This generalization has not been found to be true and therefore represents a clinical limitation to the use of BMI alone when assessing weight. Athletic people with little body fat and ample muscle mass can be classified as overweight by using BMI, despite a visual assessment that reveals a high level of fitness. Likewise, an individual's BMI may fall within the classification of healthy, yet the person may have little muscle mass and excess body fat.

BMI classifications exist as generic standards of height-weight comparisons for the general population. Racial differences have been observed in body composition that may warrant more specific BMI classifications for various population groups, as noted earlier in the chapter. Further study is warranted to establish valid BMI health classifications for various population groups. These drawbacks show the problem of using BMI as a sole indicator of weight status or nutritional health and are an excellent example of the need to use multiple parameters when conducting an assessment.

WAIST CIRCUMFERENCE (WC). Excess, centrally located abdominal fat deposition is considered to be an independent risk factor for cardiovascular disease in adults 18 years and older. Measurement of adults' WC in specific BMI categories should be included in a comprehensive nutritional assessment. WC validity can be limited when large amounts of abdominal fat become pendulous because of the effects of gravity and are no longer situated along the waistline. Increases in abdominal subcutaneous fat and increases in body weight may not always be reflected by increases in WC, such as in people with weight distribution that creates a pear shape versus an apple shape. Additionally, waist circumference is not a valid nutritional assessment tool for pregnant (or lactating) females or for those with other medical conditions associated with increases in abdominal girth, such as polycystic kidney disease or ascites (fluid in the abdomen).

The cutoff point for women is a WC of 88 cm (35 in.) and for men is a WC of 102 cm (40 in.) (Health Canada, 2003a). For adults with a BMI greater than 35, a high WC does not contribute additional health risk. An adult with a BMI of 18.5 to 34.9 and a WC above the appropriate cutoff has an additional risk of developing type 2 diabetes, coronary artery disease, and hypertension. Use of the bony landmark on the lateral border of the ilium is recommended when marking a site guide for the measurement. Figure 9.3 depicts the location of this landmark. By standing behind the client and palpating the right hip, the nurse can locate the lateral ilium. A line should be drawn at the uppermost lateral line of the ilium at the midaxillary point. WC should be measured with a spring-loaded measuring tape to ensure reliable tension is applied with each measurement.

Other references suggest measuring WC just below the umbilicus, but this can be unreliable since obesity can change the position of the umbilicus. WC should be measured at the

TABLE 9.3	Classification of Body Mass Index (BMI) in Adults	
BMI	CLASSIFICATION	RISK OF DEVELOPING HEALTH PROBLEMS
<18.5	Underweight	Increased
18.5–24.9	Normal weight	Least
25.0–29.9	Overweight	Increased
30–34.9	Obese class I	High
35–39.9	Obese class II	Very high
40+	Obese class III	Extremely high

Source: Health Canada. (2003). *Canadian guidelines for body weight classification in adults, Table 3: Health risk classification according to body mass index (BMI)*. Retrieved from http://www.hc-sc.gc.ca/fn-an/nutrition/weights-poids/guide-ld-adult/weight_book-livres_des_poids-03-table1-eng.php

BOX 9.4	Calculating Weight Loss Percentage

A community health nurse is visiting the assisted living centre for a seasonal flu shot clinic. Miss M., an 80-year-old female, complains that she needs to sew new elastic into her skirt as the old elastic is not working to keep the skirt on her waistline. The nurse wonders if Miss M. has lost some weight since the last visit and weighs her. Miss M. weighs 49.5 kg, down from 55 kg 6 months ago.

(55 kg prior weight − 49.5 kg current weight)/55 kg prior weight = 5.5/55 = 0.10.1 × 100 = 10% weight loss in 6 months

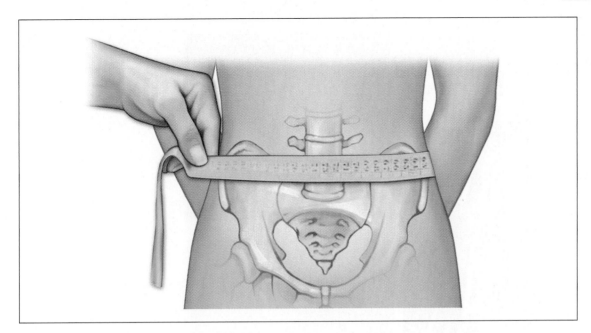

Figure 9.3 ● Landmarks for waist circumference.

marked midaxillary line while keeping the measuring tape parallel to the floor. Measurement should be done directly on the surface of the skin and not over clothing. It has been suggested that taking measurements with the client in front of a mirror is helpful to ensure a true horizontal extension of the measuring tape, especially in those who are obese or have wider hips than waist. The spring-loaded measuring tape should be pulled taut but should not compress the skin. Uneven tension on the measure between sequential measurements will alter reliability of WC measurements. Statistical evidence exists of the superiority of central body obesity measures, such as the waist to height ratio, for detecting the risk for cardiovascular disease in men and women (Lee, Huxley, Wildman, & Woodard, 2008).

SKINFOLD MEASUREMENTS. Skinfold thickness measurements can estimate subcutaneous body fat stores. People who perform these measurements need training, experience, and frequent use to maintain competence. Kinesiologists or dietitians rather than nurses may perform this aspect of the nutritional assessment, but it can be done by a nurse specialist.

Measurements taken at up to eight sites on the body are believed to be indicative of overall body fat composition. Skinfold measurements are made by using professional-grade metal (not plastic) calipers and a flexible measuring tape. The technique for properly grasping the skinfold layers and subcutaneous fat takes practice before reliable measurements can be made. Both skinfold layers and subcutaneous fat are pinched and then held gently between the thumb and forefinger, with care taken not to grasp underlying muscle. The fold is then measured with the caliper for each marked site on the body. If a distinct separation of subcutaneous fat and muscle cannot be accomplished when grasping the skinfold, body composition results will not be representative. The caliper jaws should be placed perpendicular to the fold and left in place for several seconds after tension is released to allow for even compression before the reading is taken. Three measurements should be

taken at each site and then averaged. The right side of the body is used for taking skinfold measurements to ensure consistency. Repeat tests should be done by the same tester at the same time of day, after rest and not after exercise.

The tricep skinfold (TSF) is the site most often used to estimate subcutaneous fat because of easy access to this measurement in most situations. Tricep measurements are done at the midpoint of the arm equidistant from the uppermost posterior edge of the acromion process of the scapula and the olecranon process of the elbow. A measuring tape should be used to determine this midpoint on the back of the upper arm, and the site should be marked for reference. It is helpful to have the client flex the arm at a 90-degree angle while the nurse locates the bony landmarks and measures the midpoint. However, the arm should hang freely during the skinfold measurement itself. Figure 9.4 illustrates the location of the TSF measurement. Other sites that can be used for skinfold measurements include the chest, subscapular, midaxillary, suprailiac, abdomen, and upper thigh.

Measurement values for each skinfold site can be evaluated in two ways. First, they may be compared with reference values that are specific for gender, age, race, and fitness level. Reference values are simply descriptions of body composition compiled from subjects in population studies and should not be considered the same as a standard. Reference values allow the clinician to assess an individual's measurements compared with others in a similar, well-defined population group. Standards, however, are values that are known to be desirable targets for health regardless of population norms.

Commonly used reference values to assess skinfold measurements in some populations are more than 20 years old. Older references were not obtained from diverse population groups, making them difficult to apply to the wider population that exists today. Newer reference standards are constantly being published and are becoming more population specific, but no widely used single reference exists. Therefore, even

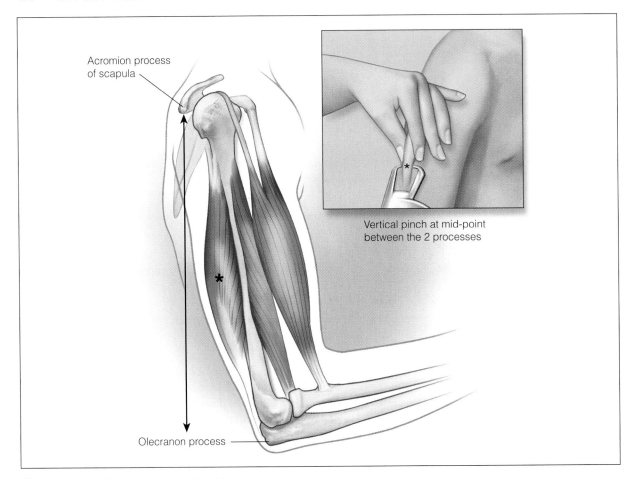

Acromion process
of scapula

Vertical pinch at mid-point
between the 2 processes

*

Olecranon process

Figure 9.4 • Landmarks for tricep skinfold measurement.

more research needs to be done in this area to produce the variety of reference values needed for racial, ethnic, age, fitness, and gender categories. Age-related differences in body fat distribution necessitate specific skinfold references for older adults as the relationship between specific-site subcutaneous fat measurements and total body fat is different from that in younger adults. Changes in skin elasticity and connective tissue also affect skinfold accuracy with age.

MIDARM MUSCLE CIRCUMFERENCE AND CALF CIRCUMFERENCE. Circumference measurements of limbs can be used alone or in conjunction with skinfold measurements to provide additional or confirmational body composition information. Midarm muscle circumference is obtained by measuring midarm circumference at the same site as the tricep skinfold. A spring-loaded flexible measure is used to provide tension without compressing the skin. Calf circumference is measured at the site of maximum calf width, which can be determined by placing the measure around the calf and sliding it along the calf until a maximum value is noted. Limb circumferences are measured in centimetres in adults.

BIOELECTRICAL IMPEDANCE ANALYSIS. Bioelectrical impedance analysis (BIA) is a noninvasive tool for assessing body composition by employing the principles of electroconduction through water, muscle, and fat. In traditional BIA, electrodes are placed on the dorsal surfaces of the right foot and hand with the client in the supine position on a nonconductive surface. Calculations are based on the knowledge that muscle and fluids have a higher electrolyte and water content than does fat and thus conduct electrical current differently. Altered hydration and altered skin temperature will cause measurement error by altering electrical current flow. Clients should be well hydrated when employing BIA technology, or dehydration will slow conductivity and give a falsely high body fat measurement. Equations used to predict body fat composition with BIA need to be population specific. Standard error for BIA measurements approximates skinfold measurements at 3% to 4%, provided correct equations are used and the client is hydrated. In comparison with the difficult and sometimes unreliable measuring of skinfold thickness in older adult clients and those who are obese, BIA technology may provide more accurate results in these two groups. Newer BIA devices are being manufactured for easier clinical use (see Figure 9.5). Hand-held body fat analyzer devices measure segmental electrical impedance from arm to arm rather than the traditional whole-body method.

NEAR-INFRARED INTERACTANCE. Infrared interactance devices measure body fat at specific sites by passing infrared light through tissue and measuring the reflected light. Predictive equations estimate body fat composition at the site. Gender, body weight, height, frame size, and fitness level are included in the calculation to determine total body fat percentage. Generally

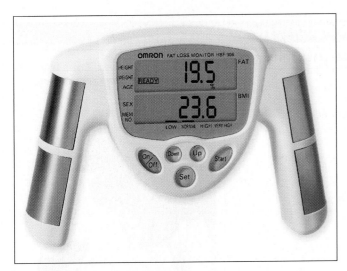

Figure 9.5 ● Hand-held BIA device.

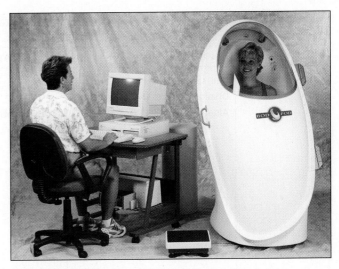

Figure 9.6 ● Bod Pod Body Composition Tracking System.

this measurement is performed on the bicep. Small, hand-held near-infrared devices are available for clinical use. Standard error for near-infrared measurement exceeds 3.5% and can be as high as 5.5%; error is greater with increased body fat.

LABORATORY BODY COMPOSITION. Several other more sophisticated and expensive tools exist for measuring body composition. These are primarily used in laboratory research and not in clinical situations. Underwater weighing, dual X-ray absorptiometry (DEXA), and body plethysmography are examples of research tools. Underwater weighing requires the client to be completely submersed underwater to measure water displacement by the body. Regression equations calculate body fat based on known density of fat-free and fat tissue. Underwater weighing has long been called the gold standard for body composition although it uses only a two-component model and does not measure bone mineral content or total body water. DEXA takes advantage of X-ray technology to measure a multicomponent model of body composition and is quickly becoming the research tool of choice. Plethysmography measures air volume displacement by the body by using similar methodology to underwater weighing. Clients are measured in a small chamber called a Bod Pod Body Composition Tracking System (see Figure 9.6).

Body Fat References or Standards

Standards of body fat percentage that are associated with health or morbidity and mortality have not been established. Many sources agree that a minimum essential body fat percentage exists. A minimum of 3% body fat in men and 12% in women is considered essential. These minimums are the lowest value compatible with health, but optimal body fat is higher and should be determined on an individual basis. It is recommended that a range of body fat be given rather than a specific target because of the errors associated with predicting specific values. A range of 12% to 20% body fat in men and 20% to 30% in women has been suggested for health, but more research is necessary to develop population-specific recommendations. Research aimed at the development of standards and references

for body fat percentage must address the relationship between BMI and body fat percentage and allow the nurse to make a clearer assessment of body composition traits associated with health risks. Age-specific recommendations are also needed.

Head-to-Toe Examination

A visual head-to-toe physical assessment can yield findings that may be indicative of normal or abnormal nutritional status. Like all other components of a nutritional assessment, the physical assessment is most useful when used in conjunction with other nutritional assessment parameters. Table 9.4 outlines physical findings associated with poor nutritional health.

Data that are gathered as part of the physical assessment are also pertinent to the nutritional assessment. Existing medical diagnoses and treatment, such as medication or surgical plans, are important when evaluating nutritional status. Physical findings, such as poor dental health, problems with chewing or swallowing, gastrointestinal complaints, functional decline in physical or mental status, and declining vision, taste, or smell, all have negative effects on nutritional health.

Biochemical Assessment: Laboratory Measurements

Several biochemical parameters are commonly used in a nutritional assessment. No one laboratory value is unique in its sensitivity to predict nutritional status as each has confounding reasons for abnormal values. As in the case of physical findings of malnutrition, laboratory values may not reflect current known nutrition status as half-lives and body pools of plasma components vary. The biochemical assessment and laboratory measurements along with their significance, values, and findings are summarized in Table 9.5 on page 139.

Cultural Considerations for the Nutritional Assessment

Religious and cultural influences on health, nutrition beliefs, and food habits vary among and within ethnic groups. It is

TABLE 9.4	Clinical Findings Associated with Poor Nutritional Health		
BODY PART	**FINDING**	**POTENTIAL DEFICIENT NUTRIENT**	**EXAMPLE**
Hair	Dull, spaces, brittle hair Dyspigmentation (flag sign) Alopecia	Protein Protein, biotin, or zinc	 Alopecia
Face	Moon face Pallor	Protein Iron	
Eyes	Dry mucosa (xerophthalmia), blindness and night blindness, Bitot's spot Pale conjunctiva Yellow subdermal fat deposits around lids (xanthelasma)	Vitamin A Iron High cholesterol	 Night blindness Bitot's spot
Mouth Lips	Cracks at corners (angular stomatitis), inflammation (cheilosis)	Riboflavin	 Angular stomatitis

(continued)

TABLE 9.4	Clinical Findings Associated with Poor Nutritional Health *(continued)*		
BODY PART	**FINDING**	**POTENTIAL DEFICIENT NUTRIENT**	**EXAMPLE**
Tongue	Smooth, beefy red or magenta (glossitis)	Niacin, pyridoxine (B_6), riboflavin	
	Atrophic papillae	Iron	
	Diminished tasten (hypogeusia)	Zinc	
Teeth	Delayed eruption	Vitamin D	
	Caries in baby	May indicate baby-bottle tooth decay	
	Mottled enamel	Excess fluoride	 Glossitis Atrophic papillae
Gums	Spongy, bleeding	Vitamin C	 Spongy, bleeding
Glands	Increased thyroid (goitre)	Iodine	
	Increased parotid size	Protein-calorie or bulimia	 Goitre

(continued)

TABLE 9.4	Clinical Findings Associated with Poor Nutritional Health *(continued)*		
BODY PART	**FINDING**	**POTENTIAL DEFICIENT NUTRIENT**	**EXAMPLE**
Skin	Poor wound healing/decubitus ulcer	Protein, calories, vitamin C, zinc	 Pellagra
	Follicular hyperkeratois (goosebump flesh**)**	Vitamin A	
	Dry, scaly	Vitamin A, essential fatty acids, zinc	
	Photosensitive symmetrical rash (pellagra)	Niacin	
	Bruising (purpura)	Vitamin C and K	
	Pinpoint hemorrhages (petechiae)	Vitamin C	
Skeleton/Trunk	Stunted growth	Protein-calorie, zinc	 Rickets
	Ascites	Protein	
	Beading on ribs (rachitic rosary), bowed legs (rickets), widened epiphysis, narrow chest (pigeon breast)	Vitamin D	
	Loss of fat, muscle wasting	Protein, calories	
Genitalia	Hypogonadism	Zinc	
Limbs	Pitting edema Loss of fat, muscle wasting	Protein Protein, calories	 Depression of pitting edema lower leg

(continued)

TABLE 9.4	Clinical Findings Associated with Poor Nutritional Health *(continued)*		
BODY PART	**FINDING**	**POTENTIAL DEFICIENT NUTRIENT**	**EXAMPLE**
Nails	Spoon-shaped (koilonychia) ridges	Iron	
Nervous System	Hyporeflexia, confabulation	Thiamine	
	Dementia, confusion, ataxia, neuropathy	Vitamin B_{12}	
	Neuropathy	Excess vitamin B_6	
	Tetany	Calcium, magnesium	
Cardiac	Arrhythmia	Potassium, magnesium	

TABLE 9.5	Laboratory Measurements to Assess Biochemical Nutrition Status		
LABORATORY TEST	**VALUES**	**PHYSICAL SIGNIFICANCE**	**INDICATOR OF DEFICIT OR EXCESS**
Protein malnutrition			
Albumin	N:3.8–5.0 g/dL Critical value: <3.5 g/L	Dehydration or overhydration will falsely raise or lower the results. Low albumin can indicate depleted visceral stores or malnutrition of chronic disease. Twenty day half-life.	Low: Edema, poor healing, thin dry hair.
Prealbumin (thyroid-binding prealbumin)	15.0–35.0 mg/dL (150 to 350 mg/L) <10 mg/dL: significant risk <5 mg/dL: severe risk	Best indicator of nutrition in last 2 to 3 weeks. Two day half-life, can be restored after 48 hours of supplement. Not altered by hydration status. Decreased if zinc is low.	Drops after 48 hours of less than 60% of optimal nutritional intake.
Transferrin	M:10%–50% F:15%–50% Normal: >0.2 g/dL	Binds to iron to transport it in the body. Increased in iron deficiency, pregnancy, or estrogen therapy. Decreased in micro-cytic anemia, low protein states, liver and renal disease. Ten day half-life.	Decreased hormone functions. Moderate malnutrition : >160 g/d L <180 g/d L Severe malnutrition: <160 g/d L
Nitrogen balance			
Urea nitrogen (BUN)	Adult: 7–18 mg/dL (2.5–6.4 mmol/L)	Indicator of dietary intake and hydration, metabolic deficits and/or indicator of renal failure, diuretic overdose. Better indicator of uremia than creatinine.	Signs of muscle wasting (catabolism). Low in protein malnutrition; high in salt and water depletion.
Creatinine	0.6–1.5 mg/dL (62–125 mmol/L)	Indicator of ability of body to save or excrete water and selected nutrients. Falsely up in high meat diet or vitamin C supplementation.	Retained metabolic wastes. B/P increased with muscle breakdown.
Hydration status		Water is a nutrient essential for cellular function. Potential losses from GI, exudating wounds.	Dry mucous membranes, tenting skin.
Electrolytes			
Sodium	135–145 mmol/L	Kidney functions to actively save or excrete; indicator of water balance.	Dehydration, weakness, heart failure.
Chloride	98–106 mmol/L	Influences acid-base, water, and osmotic pressure balance.	Excess dilute urine or GI losses.
Potassium	3.5–5.3 mmol/L	Metabolic acidosis drives K+ out of cells. Diabetic ketoacidosis: decreased insulin alters K+ pump.	Nausea, vomiting, and/or diarrhea. Hypo: weakness, increased pulse, decreased respirations, tetany. Hyper: Tremors, cardiac arrest/block.
Anemia assessment: CBC			
Lymphocytes (WBC)	Lymphocytes: 25%–40% of leukocytes. Relative value: <1500 cells indicates malnutrition or immunoincompetence.	White blood cells require adequate protein for differentiation. Production of immunoglobins and antibodies is a function of lymphocytes.	Fatigue, frequent infections. Malignancies. Leukemias.

(continued)

TABLE 9.5	Laboratory Measurements to Assess Biochemical Nutrition Status *(continued)*		
LABORATORY TEST	**VALUES**	**PHYSICAL SIGNIFICANCE**	**INDICATOR OF DEFICIT OR EXCESS**
Hemoglobin	F: 115–150 g/L M: 140–174 g/L	Oxygen-carrying capacity of the red blood cell is based on the Hgb, which is also an acid-base pH buffer playing a role in elimination of both kidneys and lungs.	Pallor, fatigue if low. Increased in CHF, COPD, polycythemia vera. Decreased in liver and renal disease, blood loss, and other chronic disease.
Hematocrit (Hct)	F: 36%–48% M: 42%–52%	Hct is an indicator of RBC mass.	Drops in anemia due to iron deficiency but not for all causes of anemia.
B_{12}	Traditionally considered 100–700 pg/mL, but new research suggests neuro deficits can appear below 200–300; Japan recommends a value above 500.	Necessary for neurological and emotional health, should be tested at same time as supplementing one can mask deficits of the other. Can be from dietary restriction or malabsorption. No toxic effects known. Can take 2 to 5 years to deplete stores.	Symptoms develop insidiously. Neuropsychiatric, cognitive deficits, balance, gait disorders, and peripheral neuropathy. Macrocytic anemic. Vegetarians or those who self-limit nutrients (e.g., tea and toast in seniors) are at risk.
Folate	2.7–17.0 mg/mL	Dietary deficits, restriction, or malabsorption are common causes. All women should supplement as soon as planning to get pregnant.	Neural tube deficits in fetuses. Angular cheilosis, macrocytic anemia, anxiety states.

Source: "Assessing the nutritional status of wound-care patients" (2008); Dawson and Favaloro (2009); Fischbach and Dunning (2009); Hess (2009).

important to ask specific questions about these influences to understand how they affect or are interpreted by the individual client. Assumptions and generalizations based on the client's association with a cultural or an ethnic population will not provide the nurse with accurate personal information about the client.

During the physical assessment and anthropometric portion of the assessment, careful and sensitive questioning of the client or a translator is needed to determine whether issues exist that may interfere with the gathering of data. Removal of certain garments may be prohibited; this can interfere with obtaining accurate weight, determining body measurements, or assessing clinical signs and symptoms. Examination or touching by a member of the opposite sex may be taboo. The nurse should engage in decision making with the client on how best to proceed when such issues are present. Box 9.5 outlines cultural nutritional considerations.

Nutritional Assessment Across the Lifespan

From infancy to older adulthood, specific consideration needs to be given to each population's unique, nutritional health parameters. Normal growth and development during childhood, the nutritional needs for a healthy pregnancy, and health maintenance and disease prevention in adulthood all provide additional parameters to consider when conducting a nutritional assessment.

The Pregnant Female

Nutritional health plays a primary role in a successful pregnancy. A mother's nutritional status before conception, and appropriate weight gain and adequate nutrition during pregnancy are important contributing factors to the health of a newborn. A comprehensive nutritional assessment of a pregnant female includes all the parameters of a general assessment, with some additional pregnancy-specific data assessed. See Chapter 26 for further details. ⬤

Infants, Children, and Adolescents

Nutrition plays a crucial role in the growth, physical development, and cognitive development of infants and children. Undernutrition can lead to growth faltering and developmental delays or stunting, the effects of which can be permanent. Overnutrition can set the stage for chronic disease. Overweight and obese children, especially those with one or more overweight or obese parents, are more likely to become overweight adults. Accurate assessment of nutritional health can help ensure positive health outcomes or serve as the necessary foundation for needed nutritional interventions. It is essential for a nurse to have the knowledge and skills to identify nutritionally at-risk children. In many community settings, such as schools, early intervention clinics, or well-child clinics, the nurse is often the only healthcare professional conducting an assessment that includes nutritional parameters. See Chapter 25 for a discussion of nutritional assessment of infants, children, and adolescents. ⬤

Adults

Nutritional assessment of the adult focuses on evaluating the issues of both overnutrition and undernutrition. Overnutrition and undernutrition are not mutually exclusive conditions. For example, an obese individual can have nutrient deficiencies from poor quality intake that contains excess calories. Food habits developed early in life and maintained may help to promote good health well into adulthood and older adulthood.

The general components of a nutritional assessment are all pertinent when assessing an adult. The presence of a chronic disease or condition may become a significant factor affecting nutritional health. Medications can have nutritional health

BOX 9.5 | Cultural Diet Influences

Some cultural nutritional considerations can affect health:

- Cultural and religious beliefs and traditions can affect food choices, beliefs, and practices in many ways, from the number of meals eaten in a day to choices of foods, preparation methods, and overall food beliefs.
- Diversity exists within cultural and religious groups. It is important to avoid applying general knowledge about cultural and religious food practices to all people within a group; instead explore individual interpretation and influences.
- Assess common dietary staples, as well as foods believed to be associated with health or symbolic benefits. Some food is thought to promote health or cure conditions. Other beliefs may be related to lifespan issues, such as the proper diet during pregnancy for easy delivery or to make the "hot" condition "colder."
- Many religious groups have dietary laws that are observed differently by subgroups within the population. Consumption of kosher meats, fasting, and avoidance of certain foods, such as pork, crustaceans, birds of prey, beef, or other animal products, are examples.
- Ask about food practices and special meals for special occasions and holidays. Some religious groups fast during parts of some religious holy days.
- Discuss food preparation methods. A variety of cultures make similar dishes but prepare them differently—for example, by using different fats, such as bacon drippings, lard, oils, or ghee (clarified butter).
- Ask about medicinal herb use as this varies among cultures and is often an important aspect of health beliefs.
- Explore to what extent any acculturation has taken place and traditional practices changed once living in a new dominant culture. Ask whether new foods have been added along with traditional foods, whether foods have been substituted for different newer versions, and whether any traditional foods have been omitted. In some cases, traditional diets are more healthful than the diet in the new culture, and encouragement to maintain healthful traditions may be helpful.

implications, such as anorexia or weight gain. Drugs that reduce gastric acid production may lead to malabsorption syndromes, such as of B_{12}, in a person who otherwise does not have risk factors. Patients with wounds may have specific multivitamin, mineral, or protein needs that are difficult to meet without supplementation or parenteral nutrition. Lifestyle choices, socioeconomic status, education, and cultural influences can affect nutrition status in addition to dietary habits. Box 9.3 outlines pertinent nutritional history data to obtain when assessing the adult.

The Older Adult

Regular nutritional assessment of the older adult is essential. Good nutritional health is an important component of ensuring autonomy into older adulthood. Undernutrition can affect quality of life, morbidity, and mortality. Protein-energy malnutrition is considered an independent risk factor for mortality in older adults recently discharged from the hospital. Skeletal muscle loss, functional decline, altered pharmacokinetics, depressed immune status, and increased risk of institutionalization may all result from malnutrition in the older adult. The prevalence of malnutrition in the older adult population unfortunately is significant, affecting up to 60% of institutionalized or hospitalized older adults and up to 13% of those in the community.

Quality of life issues related to overnutrition are also important in the older population. Overweight and obesity are risk factors for degenerative joint disease and functional and mobility problems. Comorbid conditions associated with overweight, such as diabetes and cardiovascular disease, may require treatment intervention, therapeutic diets, and medications that affect nutritional health. Poor nutrition occurs along a continuum. In the older adult, changes in nutrition health can go undetected if strict cutoff values are observed to diagnose nutrition issues. Most general nutritional assessment parameters are applicable to the older adult population, but the nurse should be mindful of any change in nutrition status in the older adult, even when measured values and parameters remain within normal limits. See Chapter 27 for a discussion of nutritional assessment in the older adult.

NUTRITIONAL SCREENING AND ASSESSMENT TOOLS

Nutritional assessment data can be gathered and evaluated in a comprehensive fashion, or a more formal validated tool can be used to streamline the process. Numerous nutritional screening and assessment tools exist, but none is considered the gold standard for use in most populations. Until a consensus is reached defining malnutrition, a variety of nutritional screening and assessment tools will continue to be published.

Nutritional screening tools are used for quick assessment of risk factors for poor nutritional health. Screening tools are not meant for diagnostic purposes but are instead used to triage clients who may require further assessment or intervention. Screening tools give a rough estimate of nutrition risk or status. Nutritional assessment tools are generally more comprehensive than screening tools for the goal of identifying or diagnosing malnutrition. Not all assessment or screening tools are validated for use in the populations where they are being used. Lack of validation may lead to frequent missed diagnoses or incorrect diagnoses of poor nutritional health. Sharp clinical judgment by the nurse is a necessary adjunct to any tool.

Eating Well with Canada's Food Guide

Eating Well with Canada's Food Guide is published by Health Canada (2007). The Food Guide provides authoritative advice for people 2 years and older about how good dietary habits can promote health and reduce risk for major chronic diseases. The most recent Food Guide, released in 2007 (see Figure 9.7), provides a *new*, comprehensive food guide and an interactive website that can be used for individual food guide planning and diet analysis. The nurse can compare the diet recall or nutritional history data with the distribution of food groups recommended and make a general assessment of diet adequacy. The number and size of food servings included in the Food Guide are generic and should be adjusted for more active or less active individuals. An interactive section of the website allows

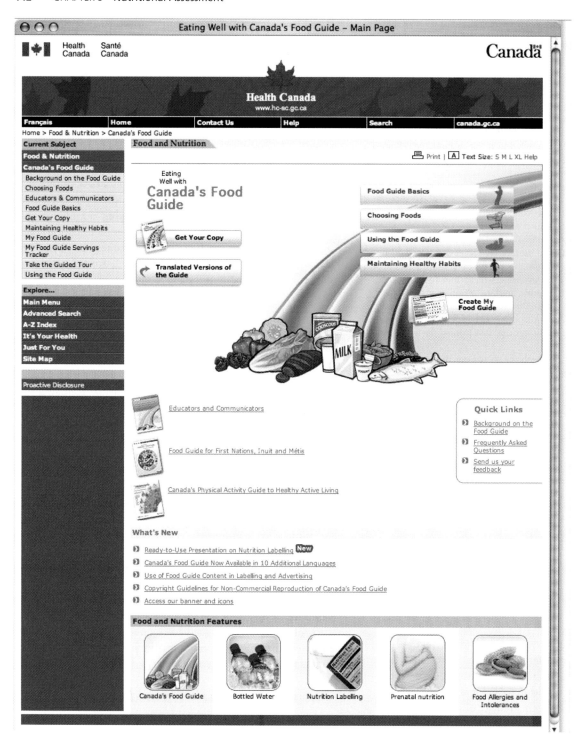

Figure 9.7 ● Eating Well with Canada's Food Guide.

Source: Health Canada. (2007). *Eating well with Canada's food guide.* Retrieved from http://www.hc-sc.gc.ca/fn-an/food-guide-aliment/index-eng.php

the user to develop and personalize a food guide. The benefit of the new Food Guide is that it is flexible and adaptable to the individual. It includes a Food Guide servings tracker and food intake record. Instead of needing special food guides for various ages or cultural groups, the new website has the richness of choice to meet the needs of people from a number of cultures as it is has been translated into 10 languages. However, a specific edition of the Food Guide is available for First Nations, Inuit, and Metis.

Other Assessment Tools

In addition to comprehensive resources, such as *Eating Well with Canada's Food Guide* (Health Canada, 2007), there are specialized screening tools that many clinicians have found helpful.

The REAP Tool

The REAP (Rapid Eating and Activity Assessment for Patients/Clients) tool is a food and eating questionnaire for clients to complete before a clinic or an office visit. The questions, which range from diet and food choices to activity and exercise, are intended to provide a nutritional interview during a comprehensive assessment.

The WAVE Tool

WAVE is an acronym for **w**eight, **a**ctivity, **v**ariety in diet, and **e**xcess related to overnutrition, calories, foods, and alcohol. This handy pocket card reminds the healthcare professional of the important components to assess during the examination.

The DETERMINE Checklist

DETERMINE is an acronym for **d**isease, **e**ating poorly, **t**ooth loss/mouth pain, **e**conomic hardship, **r**educed social contact, **m**ultiple medicines, **i**nvoluntary weight loss/gain, **n**eeds assistance in self-care, and **e**lder above 80 years.

The DETERMINE checklist can be used to assess the nutritional status of the older adult. The mnemonic scores the nine warning signs of poor nutrition in the older adult. The scoring of the tool provides a stratified nutritional risk score. This tool has been validated for use with community-based older adults.

Mini Nutritional Assessment and Subjective Global Assessment

The Mini Nutritional Assessment (MNA) and Subjective Global Assessment (SGA) have both been validated for use in the nutritional assessment of older adults. The SGA has also been used in assessment of other populations since its development more than 20 years ago. The MNA is a newer tool with extensive data validating its use with older adults. The MNA can be included as a routine component of a physical examination or as a quick bedside tool. The Mini Nutritional Assessment is also located in Appendix E.

APPLICATION THROUGH CRITICAL THINKING

CASE STUDY

Harry Brown is an 89-year-old widower brought to the clinic by his niece, who is concerned about his diminished dietary intake. His past medical history is significant for mild hypertension, which is treated with a diuretic and a 2000 mg sodium therapeutic diet. Physical examination reveals blood pressure of 110/75 and pulse of 72. Height is 173 cm (5′8″), and weight is 71 kg (156 lb.). Weight 6 months prior was 79 kg (175 lb.). Significant laboratory measures: albumin 3.0 mg/dL. Urinalysis sent: sample dark and scant volume. His skin appears dry with dry axillae and petechiae on trunk and arms. His eyes are sunken. Temporal wasting is noted, as are diminished subcutaneous fat stores on limbs. The exam of the oral cavity reveals poorly fitting dentures, spongy gums, and deep tongue furrows.

On talking to Mr. Brown, the nurse learns that food does not taste the same to him anymore. He blames this on his low-sodium diet. His niece reports that she takes her uncle grocery shopping each week and has noticed that his pantry at home still has many of the items from the previous week. She tells the nurse that her uncle is a retired professional chef and loved to cook until a few months ago. He has resorted to heating food in the microwave and often overcooks it. Mr. Brown states he overheats the food because the microwave is unpredictable. His niece is reading her concerns from a list she has made and passes the list to her uncle for further comment. The nurse notices he squints at the list and then says he has nothing to add.

The nurse conducts a diet recall that reveals the following:

Breakfast:	Large mug black coffee
	Either cold cereal (flake type, not fortified) and whole milk, or 2 pieces of toast or 1 English muffin with butter and jelly
	180 mL (6 fl.oz.) apple juice or cider, unfortified
Midday meal:	Sandwich on white bread—either tuna salad, peanut butter and jelly, or sliced turkey, mayonnaise, and iceberg lettuce. Used to add tomato to sandwich but "can't be bothered cutting up one."
	Occasionally heats leftovers from restaurant meal with niece; usually has enough for two or three reheated meals during week. Pasta or meat-and-potato or rice-type meals. No vegetables.
	Overheats and discards often.
	Cookie
	Cup of tea with whole milk and 2 tsp sugar
Evening:	180 mL (6 fl.oz.) ready-to-eat pudding
	120 mL (4 fl.oz.) milk with comment "no liquids after 7 p.m. or I have to get up all night"

Mr. Brown takes no nutritional supplements of any kind. The nurse asks further questions about the lack of fruit and vegetables and learns that it has been almost 6 months since Mr. Brown had fruit other than applesauce or apple juice. He has stopped eating vegetables in the same time frame. He stated that he cannot be bothered preparing either type of food, but on further questioning, he admits that he is having difficulty chewing some foods and that some vision problems make food preparation difficult or unsafe.

► Complete Documentation

The following is sample documentation from the nutrition assessment of Harry Brown.

SUBJECTIVE DATA: Brought by niece who notes diminished intake. c/o low NaCl rx causing hypogeusia with secondary anorexia. Also c/o difficulty chewing, vision changes. Diet recall 2 meal/day pattern with no liquids after 7 p.m. Liquid intake, 910 mL (32 fl.oz.)/day (only 285 mL [10 fl.oz.] noncaffeinated). No fruit/vegetable 3–6 mos.

OBJECTIVE DATA: VS: B/P 110/75—Pulse 72. Height 173 cm (5′8″), weight 71 kg (156 lb.) BMI 23.5. Weight 6 months ago 79 kg (175 lb.). Albumin 3.0 mg/dL, UA pdg: sample dark and scant. Skin and axillae dry/petechiae present. Temp/limb wasting noted. Eyes sunken. Oral cavity: spongy gums, poorly fitting dentures, tongue furrows. Medications: Hydrochlorothiazide.

► Critical Thinking Questions

1. How would the data from the case study be clustered to identify the problem areas?
2. How should the nurse interpret the data related to Mr. Brown's fruit and vegetable intake?
3. What additional data would the nurse require to develop a plan of care for Mr. Brown?

► Applying Nursing Diagnoses

The NANDA-I taxonomy (see Appendix A ⬯) includes the following nursing diagnoses: *dentition, impaired; skin integrity, impaired;* and *oral mucous membrane, impaired.*

1. Do the data from the case study support these nursing diagnoses? If so, identify the data.
2. Identify nursing diagnoses from the NANDA-I taxonomy that address the self-care and dependency issues for Mr. Brown and identify the data that support your conclusions.
3. Develop additional nursing diagnoses from Mr. Brown and provide PES (problem, etiology, and signs and symptoms) statements.

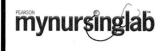

10

THE HEALTH HISTORY

CHAPTER OBJECTIVES

On completion of this chapter, you will be able to

1. Discuss the purpose of the nursing health history.
2. Describe communication skills used by the nurse when conducting a health history.
3. Identify barriers to effective nurse-client communication.
4. Describe the influence of culture on nurse-client interactions.
5. Discuss the professional characteristics used in establishing a nurse-client relationship.
6. Discuss the phases of the client interview.
7. Describe the components of the nursing health history.
8. Obtain a health history.
9. Develop a genogram.

CHAPTER OUTLINE

THE HEALTH ASSESSMENT INTERVIEW PROVIDES an opportunity to gather detailed information about events and experiences that have contributed to a client's current state of health. The **health history** is a comprehensive record of the client's past and current health. The health history is gathered during the initial health assessment interview, which usually occurs at the client's first visit to a healthcare facility. This database is updated with each visit. The purpose of the health history is to document the responses of the client to actual and potential health concerns. Thus, the health history includes a wellness assessment covering questions on how the client optimizes health and well-being in such areas as nutrition, stress management, and social interaction.

The health history performed by the nurse has a different focus from the medical history performed by the physician. Although both consist of subjective data, the focus of the medical history is to gather data about the cause and course of disease. Thus, the medical history focuses on the disease rather than on the client and the client's lifestyle practices. For example, the physician may ask a client to relate the details of the range of motion in the left hip to determine the cause of abnormal movement and to prescribe a specific treatment. The nurse obtains the same information but uses it to determine the extent to which the client will need support and teaching regarding ambulation and performance of activities of daily living (ADLs), such as getting dressed independently at home. The nurse and the physician gather the same information for different purposes. The nursing health history may produce information about a medical diagnosis, but the focus is on the client's response to the health concern as a whole person, not just on one or two body parts or systems.

COMMUNICATION SKILLS

Effective communication skills play an important role in developing a nurse-client relationship, conducting the health assessment interview, and collecting data for the health history. Communication is also important in educating, guiding, facilitating, directing, and counselling the client. The nurse cannot develop trust, establish rapport, or carry out nursing interventions for clients without knowledge of communication techniques. For example, nurses may need to modify their communication skills when dealing with younger or older clients. The younger nurse teaching the older adult client about ways to add fibre to the diet may need to use a serious and respectful communication technique. Conversely, an older nurse counselling a teenage client regarding safe and responsible sexual practices may need to make special efforts to create an informal atmosphere that allows the teenager to open up and speak freely.

Communication is the exchange of information between individuals. During the communication process, an individual, sometimes called the sender, develops an idea and transmits it in the form of a message to another person, or receiver. The receiver perceives the message (the sender's transmitted idea) and interprets it. Once the receiver interprets the meaning, the receiver formulates a response and transmits it back to the sender as feedback. **Encoding** is the process of formulating a message for transmission to another person. To encode an idea, the sender has to choose the words, body language, signs, or symbols that will be used to convey the message. Decoding is the process of searching through memory, experience, and knowledge to determine the meaning of the intended message (see Figure 10.1).

To communicate successfully, the client must be able to accurately decode the messages the nurse sends. For example, communication may break down if the nurse uses words the client does not understand or behaves in a manner that is frightening to the client. Communication may also break down if the nurse fails to decode the client's messages accurately by not listening actively and attentively.

Interactional Skills

Interactional skills are actions that are used during the encoding and decoding process to obtain and disseminate information, develop relationships, and promote understanding

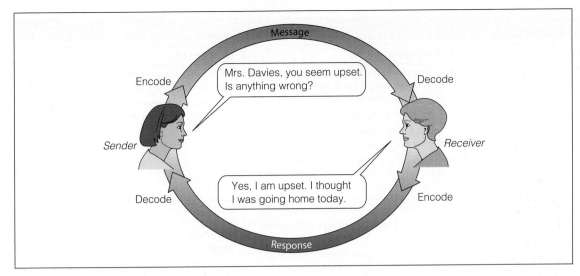

Figure 10.1 • The communication process.

of the self and others. Nurses use a variety of interactional skills during the communication process to gather assessment data from the client, family, significant others, and healthcare personnel. The interactional skills that are helpful during an interview include listening, attending, paraphrasing, leading, questioning, reflecting, and summarizing (see Table 10.1). The nurse uses these interactional techniques to help the client communicate information thoroughly and to confirm that the nurse has understood the client's communication correctly.

Listening

Listening is paying undivided attention to what the client says and does. It involves interpretation of what has been said. Listening is a basic part of the communication process and is the most important interactional skill. People who have not developed listening skills have problems relating to others and difficulty attaining their goals. Successful listening involves taking in the client's whole message by hearing the words and interpreting body language. Successful listening is an active process that requires effort and attention by the nurse (see Figure 10.2). It is important for the nurse to push thoughts about the day's schedule or the next client from her or his mind while listening to a client and to give full attention to the client so as not to miss some of the message. The nurse should note not only the words the client speaks but also the tone of voice and even what the client does not say. The woman who states, "My mother died last week," and immediately moves on to another topic of discussion has told the nurse a lot about how she is dealing with a death in her family.

Attending

Giving full attention to verbal and nonverbal messages is called **attending.** Body language can convey as much as 93% of the message a client sends. Body language, or nonverbal messages, also provides significant information that the nurse might otherwise overlook, and it can signal information that the client may have omitted intentionally or unintentionally. For example, a male client who feels that expressing pain is a weakness may deny that he is in pain. However, his facial expression, guarded reaction to abdominal palpation, and drawn position in bed send a message of severe pain. Because body language can send such messages as hostility, defensiveness, or confusion, the nurse must tune in to the client's nonverbal and verbal messages. Nonverbal cues, such as posture, eye contact, makeup, dress, accessories, and items in the client's environment (books, a rosary, or photographs), tell a story and add more depth to the intended message. Attentive listening skills also include the nurse encouraging the client to speak by making such comments as "I see" and "Go on."

Paraphrasing

Communication skills include the nurse checking to make sure that she or he has understood the client accurately by paraphrasing. **Paraphrasing** means that the nurse restates the client's basic message. For example, the client may say, "I don't really know if I should have this test." The nurse would paraphrase by saying, "You haven't received enough information yet to make a decision."

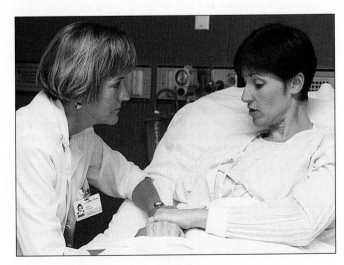

Figure 10.2 • The nurse conveys attentive listening through a posture of involvement.

TABLE 10.1 | Interactional Skills

SKILL/DEFINITION	TECHNIQUE	EXAMPLES
Attending: Giving the client undivided attention.	• Use direct eye contact if appropriate for the client's culture. Look at the client during the conversation. • Lean toward the client slightly. • Select a quiet area with no distractions for the interview. • Convey an unhurried manner; avoid fidgeting and looking at your watch or a clock.	The nurse arranges with peers for no interruptions during the interview. The nurse sits facing the client, remains alert, and focuses on what the client is saying.
Paraphrasing: Restating the client's basic message to test whether you have understood.	• Listen for the client's basic message. • Restate the client's message in your own words. • Ask the client if your words are an accurate restatement of the message.	*Client:* "I toss and turn all night. Sometimes I can't get to sleep at all. I don't know why this is happening. I've always been a deep sleeper." *Nurse:* "It sounds like you're not getting enough sleep. Is that right?"
Direct leading: Directing the client to obtain specific information or to begin an interaction.	• Decide what area you want to explore. • Tell the client what you want to discuss. • Encourage the client to follow your lead.	"Describe how you feel when you can't sleep." "Did you say you were angry and frustrated before you went to bed? Go over that again."
Focusing: Helping the client zero in on a subject or get in touch with feelings.	• Use focusing when the client strays from the topic or uses tangential speech. • Listen for themes, issues, or feelings in the client's rambling conversation. • Ask the client to give more information about a specific theme, issue, or feeling. • Encourage the client to emphasize feelings when giving this information.	"Let's discuss the pain in your back." "When did your symptoms begin?"
Questioning: Gathering specific information on a topic through the process of inquiry.	• Use open-ended questions whenever possible. Avoid using questions that can be answered with "yes," "no," "maybe," or "sometimes." • Ask the client to express feelings about what is being discussed. • Ask questions that help the client gain insight.	"What did you mean when you said your back was breaking?" "How did you feel after you talked to your boss?"
Reflecting: Letting the client know that you empathize with the thoughts, feelings, or experiences expressed.	• Take in the client's feelings from verbal and nonverbal body language. • Determine which combination of cues you should reflect back to the client. • Reflect the cues back to the client. • Observe the client's response to the reflected feelings, experience, or content.	*Feelings:* "It sounds as if you're feeling lonely." "It must really be frustrating not to be able to get enough sleep." *Experience:* "You're yawning. You must be tired." "You act as if you're in pain." *Content:* "You think you're going to die." "You believe the medication is helping."
Summarizing: Tying together the various messages that the client has communicated throughout the interview.	• Listen to verbal and nonverbal content during the interview. • Summarize feelings, issues, and themes in broad statements. • Repeat them to the client, or ask the client to repeat them to you.	"Let's review the health problems you've identified today."

Leading

Nurses use leading skills to encourage open communication. These skills are most effective when starting an interaction or when trying to get the client to discuss specific health concerns.

Leading skills are especially helpful in getting clients to explore their feelings and to elaborate on areas already introduced in the discussion. The leading techniques nurses commonly use when interviewing a client include direct leading, focusing, and questioning.

Questioning

Questioning is a very direct way of speaking with clients to obtain subjective data for decision making and planning care. Questioning techniques include closed and open-ended questions. *Closed questions* limit the client's response to yes, no, or one-word answers ("Were you feeling angry when your mother said that?"). *Open-ended questions* are purposely general and encourage the client to provide additional information. Examples of open-ended questions include "Tell me what brought you here today" or "You said that your ankle hurts. Tell me more about that."

Reflecting

Reflecting is repeating the client's verbal or nonverbal message for the client's benefit. It is a way for the nurse to show the client that she or he empathizes or is in tune with the client's thoughts, feelings, and experiences. For example, Mr. Bates, a 60-year-old with diabetes, is admitted to an outpatient clinic to be evaluated for a possible amputation of his right lower leg because of gangrene. During the clinic visit, Mr. Bates sits in a chair in the examination room with his head in his hands. When the nurse begins to question him, he looks up and says, "Leave me alone. Nothing you can do will help. I might as well be dead." The nurse's response might be, "Mr. Bates, may I sit here for a while? I can see that you are upset" (reflecting feeling). "You must feel angry that this is happening to you" (reflecting content). This example demonstrates that thoughts, feelings, and experiences are reflected at the same time.

Summarizing

Summarizing is the process of gathering the ideas, feelings, and themes that a client has discussed throughout the interview and restating them in several general statements. Summarizing is a useful tool because it shows clients that the nurse has listened and understood their concerns. It also allows clients to know that progress is being made in resolving their health concerns and signals closure of the interview. One strategy is to read back to the client what has been documented and then ask, "Is that correct?"

BARRIERS TO EFFECTIVE CLIENT INTERACTION

In some situations the nurse may unknowingly hinder the flow of information by using nontherapeutic interactions (interactions that are harmful rather than helpful). Nontherapeutic interactions interfere with the communication process by making the client uncomfortable, anxious, or insecure. Some interactions that can be most harmful if used during the health assessment interview are giving false reassurance, interrupting or changing the subject, passing judgment, cross-examining, using technical terms, and being insensitive.

False Reassurance

False reassurance occurs when the nurse assures the client of a positive outcome with no basis for believing in it. False reassurance deprives clients of the right to communicate their feelings. Examples include "Everything will be all right" or "Don't worry about not being able to sleep at night. You'll be fine." False reassurance can be implied by the nurse's tone of voice.

Interrupting or Changing the Subject

Interrupting the client or changing the subject shows insensitivity to the client's thoughts and feelings. In most cases this happens when the nurse is ill at ease with the client's comments and is unable to deal with their content. Clients who show extreme emotion (e.g., anger, weeping) during the interview, who ask intimate questions about the nurse's personal life, or who are sexually aggressive in the presence of the nurse may make the nurse uncomfortable during the interview. In these instances, the nurse must recognize what it is about the client's behaviour that is making him or her uncomfortable and deal with the situation in a professional manner rather than by changing the subject. For example, "Your questions about my personal life are making me feel uncomfortable. We need to talk about what is concerning you today instead."

Passing Judgment

Judgmental statements convey a strong message that the client must live up to the nurse's value system to be accepted. These statements imply nonacceptance and discourage further interaction. Examples include "Abortion is the same as murder" or "You must stay strong for your family."

Cross-Examination

Asking question after question during an assessment interview may cause the client to feel threatened, and the client may seek refuge by revealing less information. Because all interviews include many questions, the nurse should be careful not to make clients feel that they are being cross-examined. It is helpful to pause between questions and ask how the client is tolerating the interview. Encouraging clients to express their feelings about the pace and nature of the interview makes them feel more at ease.

Technical Terms

Whenever possible, the nurse should use lay rather than technical terms and avoid jargon, slang, or clichés. Such terms as *anterior* and *posterior* are useful for nursing and medical personnel but are more confusing to the client than the terms *front* and *back*. It is best to avoid the use of initials and acronyms unless they are commonly accepted as everyday language. For instance, most clients will understand the term AIDS but not prn (as necessary).

Sensitive Issues

Nurses often need to ask clients questions that are sensitive and personal. The client may feel uncomfortable providing information about such concerns as abuse, homelessness, emotional and psychological problems, use of drugs and alcohol, self-image, sexuality, or religion. Discomfort with these issues may cause the client to lapse into silence. It is important to be sensitive to the client's need for silence. The client may need to reflect on what was said or to come to grips with emotions the question has evoked before proceeding. The nurse also watches for nonverbal signs, such as tear-filled eyes or wringing of the hands, which indicate the client's need to pause for a moment. After a period of silence, if the client does not resume the conversation, the nurse may need to prompt the client by saying, "After that, what happened?" or "You were saying..." Certain questions may cause a client to cry. The nurse should offer tissues, let the client cry, and wait until the client is ready to proceed before asking additional questions. Some clients may feel that they need permission to cry. A nurse who sees that the client is holding back tears can give the client permission to cry by saying, "I know that you are upset. It is all right to cry." If the client reacts to questions about sensitive issues with anger, the nurse should acknowledge what the client is feeling: "I can see that you are angry. Please tell me why." If the client becomes angry, the nurse should acknowledge the anger, empathize with the client's situation, apologize (as appropriate), and wait to resume the interview until the client's anger dissipates.

Asking the client sensitive questions may make the nurse uncomfortable. A nurse who anticipates being uncomfortable with certain questions should take time to reflect on and come to terms with these feelings before beginning the interview. Role-playing the situation with another nurse as the client or mentally visualizing how to react in the anticipated situation will help avoid uncomfortable feelings during the interview. When asking sensitive questions, it is best to be direct and honest with the client: "I feel uncomfortable asking you such personal questions, but I need the information to complete your plan of care." Communication strategies like these will help the nurse conduct a thorough and effective interview in these sensitive situations.

INFLUENCE OF CULTURE ON NURSE-CLIENT INTERACTIONS

Differences in culture and the ways in which they are demonstrated have a significant impact on the interactions that occur in the nurse-client relationship. The nurse must be prepared to recognize and adapt the interactional processes to cultural differences. Further, nurses must not allow their own cultural values and practices to bias the impressions of the client or to impair the interaction.

Diversity

How a sender encodes a message and a receiver decodes it depends on a combination of factors, such as culture, ethnicity, religion, nationality, education, health status, and level of intelligence. When two people differ in any of these ways, each must be more open to the other person's way of thinking and foster mutual understanding.

The nurse should be careful not to bring cultural stereotypes to the communication process. Each individual, whether client

or nurse, has some degree of ethnocentrism; that is, the individual sees a culturally specific way of life as being the "normal" way. Nurses must not impose their own culturally specific values on clients. Avoiding cultural bias requires effort because these values may be so ingrained that they may surface unconsciously during communication. All people have a right to have their cultural heritage recognized as valuable. No one culture is better than another. The nurse who works in a community with clients from many cultures and nationalities should learn as much as possible about the culture, values, and belief systems of the clients who present for healthcare. The best way to learn is by asking and observing the cultural experts: clients and clients' families.

Body Language

Body language is extremely important when developing the nurse-client relationship. If the nurse and the client are from different cultures, body language is an even more critical part of the communication process. Simple body movements, such as eye contact, handshakes, or posture, may carry different messages in different cultures.

Although nurses should attempt to individualize communication styles to ethnic groups, they must not make assumptions about the ethnicity of clients. The differences among individuals in a group are often greater than the differences between the groups themselves. Nurses must never stereotype clients because they are of a different culture, are from a different country, or practise a different religion. Rather, it is the nurse's responsibility to learn about a client's culture and use this knowledge as a basis for developing a meaningful nurse-client relationship.

Communicating with Language Differences

Communication is challenged if the client does not speak the same language as the nurse or uses the language of the dominant culture, such as English, as a second language. If the client does not speak the same language, the nurse should bring in a translator to assist with the interview. It is helpful to meet with the translator before approaching the client to discuss the purpose of the interview, the terms the nurse needs to use, the kinds of information the nurse needs to collect, and the confidentiality of the subject matter. Learning a few key health-related terms in the client's language contributes to developing trust and establishing an effective nurse-client relationship.

During the interview, the seating should be arranged so that the client can see the nurse and the translator at the same time without turning the head from side to side. The nurse looks at the client, not at the translator, as the interview progresses. It is important to avoid discussing the client with the translator and leaving the client out of the conversation. Throughout the interview, the nurse asks questions one at a time and uses clear, concise terms. Even clients who are not bilingual may understand some of the words. Although some clients speak English extremely well as a second language, they may have some difficulty communicating their thoughts when under

BOX 10.1 | Guidelines for Interviewing Clients Who Do Not Speak English

The following guidelines are helpful when interviewing clients who do not speak English:

- Be open to ways you can communicate effectively. Imagine yourself entering a care setting in which few people speak your language. Your sensitivity to this fear and unease will be your greatest strength in providing quality care for your client.
- Determine what language your client speaks. Your first assumption may not be correct.
- Make sure the client can read and write, as well as speak, in his or her language. Do not assume. Be alert for any confusion.
- Learn key foreign phrases that will help you communicate with the client.
- Find out if your healthcare facility has access to translators. It is best to have an official translator when you give instructions or obtain consent.
- Look at your *client* while telling the translator what to say. This approach helps your client feel connected to you and conveys meaning through body language and facial expression.
- Use clear, simple language. For example, don't tell the translator to ask for a clean-catch specimen; instead, explain what you mean step by step.
- Pause frequently for the translator.
- Ask the translator to provide the proper context for any colloquial expressions your client may use.

If You Can't Find a Translator

- Develop cards with phrases or illustrations to aid communication. Have several translators review the cards before using them.
- Use written handouts for client teaching. These can be developed or purchased. Look for handouts with plenty of diagrams.

stress. It is not uncommon for clients who speak fluent English to revert back to their first language during times of stress. If this is the case, the nurse should follow the recommendations for clients who do not speak English. A translator is usually not needed unless the client is extremely stressed or in severe pain. Some clients communicate better in writing or understand the written word better than the spoken word, so it is a good idea to have a pencil and paper available. Box 10.1 provides guidelines for interviewing clients who do not speak English.

PROFESSIONAL CHARACTERISTICS THAT ENHANCE THE NURSE-CLIENT INTERACTION

Clients are more willing to discuss their health issues if they perceive that they are in a trusting, helping relationship and have developed a sense of rapport or mutual trust and understanding with the interviewing nurse. Carl Rogers, founder of the humanities psychology movement, developed client-centred therapy. Rogers defined the helping relationship as one "in which at least one of the parties has the intent of promoting the growth, development, maturity, improved functioning, and improved coping with life of the other" (1957, pp. 27–32). Nurses who establish helping relationships with their clients

believe that the positive aspects are shared by the nurse as well as by the client.

The nurse interviewer's attitude plays an important role in the success of the interview. The client is more likely to cooperate if the nurse conveys a willingness to help and assist the client. According to Rogers (1951), Brammer, Abrego, and Shostrum (1993), Carkhuff (2000), and other social psychologists, a helping person possesses the characteristics of positive regard, empathy, genuineness, and concreteness.

Positive Regard

Positive regard is the ability to appreciate and respect another person's worth and dignity with a nonjudgmental attitude. Nurses who respect their clients value their individuality and accept them regardless of race, religion, culture, ethnic background, country of origin, or any other characteristic. Clients sense positive regard in nurses by their demeanour, attitudes, and verbal and nonverbal communication.

Empathy

Empathy is "the capacity to respond to another's feelings and experiences as if they were your own" (Cormier, Cormier, & Weiser, 1984, p. 22). Nurses demonstrate empathy by showing their understanding and support of the client's experience or feelings through actions and words. Empathy allows the nurse to see the issues through the client's eyes, fostering understanding of the client's health concerns.

Genuineness

Genuineness is the ability to present oneself honestly and spontaneously. People who are genuine present themselves as down-to-earth and real. To be genuine, nurses must convey interest in, and focus on, the situation at hand, giving the client their full attention. They use direct eye contact, facial expressions appropriate to the situation, and open body language. Facing the client, leaning forward during conversation, and sitting with arms and legs uncrossed are examples of open body language. A genuine person communicates in a congruent manner, making sure that verbal and nonverbal messages are consistent. The nurse who tells a client to "take your time" during the interview but constantly looks at the clock gives a mixed or incongruent message. Genuineness and congruent communication promote rapport and trust with the client.

Concreteness

For the nurse, **concreteness** means speaking to the client in specific terms rather than in vague generalities. For instance, saying, "I need this information to help you to plan a diet to lower your cholesterol level," is more specific than saying, "I need this information to plan your nursing care." The more specific statement promotes understanding and a sense of security in the client. Speaking to the client in concrete terms implies that the nurse respects the client's ability to understand and recognizes the client's right to know the details of the plan of care.

HEALTH HISTORY INTERVIEW

The health history interview is the exchange of information between the nurse and the client. This information, along with the data from the physical assessment, is used to develop nursing diagnoses and design the nursing care plan. Unlike other types of interviews nurses conduct, the health history interview is a formal, planned interaction to inquire about the client's health patterns, ADLs, past health history, current health issues, self-care activities, wellness concerns, and other aspects of the client's health status. In most situations, nurses use a special health history tool to collect assessment data. The health history is a critical component of the comprehensive health interview.

Sources of Information

A variety of sources of information are included in a comprehensive health assessment. In the health history portion, subjective data are gathered. Therefore, the nurse will seek to obtain information from the most reliable source.

The Primary Source

The best and **primary source** of information for the health assessment interview is the client. The client is the only one who can describe personal symptoms, experiences, and factors leading to the current health concern. In some situations, the client may be unable or unwilling to provide information. For example, a client who has had a cerebral vascular accident (brain attack) may not be able to understand what is being said or verbalize a response. The nurse carefully evaluates the client who is unable to give accurate and reliable information and uses another source of information if indicated. The following clients may be unable to provide accurate and reliable information:

- Infants or children
- Clients who are seriously ill, comatose, sedated, or in substantial pain
- Clients who have a developmental disability
- Clients disoriented to person, place, or time
- Clients with mental health problems
- Clients who cannot speak the common language
- Aphasic clients

In some situations an adult client is able but unwilling to provide certain types of information because of fear, anxiety, embarrassment, or distrust. Some reasons why clients may be hesitant to share information include the following:

- *Fear of a terminal diagnosis.* A client may not be ready to cope with the stress of a terminal illness and deny its possibility.
- *Fear of undergoing further physical examination.* A claustrophobic client may deny problems because of fear of a magnetic resonance imaging (MRI) scan.
- *Embarrassment.* A male client may refuse to discuss urinary problems because he fears catheterization or rectal examination.

- *Fear of legal implications.* An alcoholic client involved in a car accident may fear revealing the addiction to alcohol.
- *Fear of losing a job.* An airline pilot may be reluctant to admit vision problems or hearing loss.
- *Lack of trust.* A client with AIDS who wants the diagnosis to remain private may fear a breach in confidentiality.

Secondary Sources

A **secondary source** is a person or record that provides additional information about the client. The nurse uses secondary sources when the client is unable or unwilling to communicate. For example, the parent or caregiver is the source of information for a child who cannot communicate. Secondary sources are used to augment and validate previously obtained data. The most commonly used secondary sources are significant others to whom the client has expressed thoughts and feelings about lifestyle or health status, and medical and other records containing descriptions of the client's subjective experience. The interviewing nurse should not overlook the attending physician and other healthcare personnel who have cared for the client as excellent secondary sources of information.

Clients often share their personal experiences, feelings, and emotions with significant others. A significant other is a person who has the client's respect and who holds a position of importance in the client's life. A significant other may be a family member, lover, cohabitant, legal guardian (if the client is a minor or legally incompetent), close friend, co-worker, pastor, teacher, or health professional. These individuals often provide a different viewpoint or perspective about the client's stresses and thoughts, attitudes, and concerns about daily life and illness. The significant other who has the closest relationship with the client is usually the source of the most accurate information when the client is unable or unwilling to speak.

Whenever possible, the nurse should obtain the client's consent before requesting information from another person. This simple act of courtesy demonstrates respect for the client's privacy and goes a long way in establishing a mutual sense of trust. Obtaining the client's verbal and written permission also prevents potential accusations concerning invasion of privacy.

The nurse must be cautious when collecting client data from another person. This information may be prejudiced by that person's own bias, life experience, and values, and may not be a true reflection of the client's own thinking. Every attempt must be made to validate secondary information by verifying it with the client, by observing, or by confirming the information with at least one other source. The nurse does not seek secondary information if the client is competent but unwilling to provide personal information and has not granted the nurse permission to explore information with secondary sources. The nurse should respect the wishes and confidentiality of the client and attempt to obtain the information at a later time.

The medical record is an excellent source of accurate subjective and objective data about the client. The subjective statements made by the client and recorded in the nursing progress notes provide insight about the client's symptoms and feelings. Nursing progress notes, descriptions of client responses to treatment, physicians' progress notes, treatment plans, medical histories, laboratory results, and vital signs are examples of excellent secondary resources the nurse can use to develop the nursing care plan. The nurse also investigates medical records from previous hospitalizations or clinic visits. If the medical record is available, it should be reviewed before the health assessment interview because it provides cues to actual and potential health problems to explore. During the interview, the nurse should always validate any information from a secondary source, especially if it conflicts with the client's statements during the interview.

Phases of the Health Assessment Interview

The health assessment interview is divided into three phases: preinteraction, the initial or formal interview, and the health history. The first two phases provide information the nurse uses along with information from the physical assessment to develop the total client database, formulate nursing diagnoses, and initiate the nursing care plan. The third phase, the health history, occurs throughout all stages of the nursing process. Its purpose is to gather, clarify, and update additional client data as it becomes available.

The health history is used to validate probable or hypothetical nursing or collaborative diagnoses. After the initial interview, the nurse develops several hypothetical nursing diagnoses. Before making a final diagnosis, the nurse conducts a health history along with a physical assessment to gather additional data. These additional data are then compared with defining characteristics of the probable diagnoses to determine the most appropriate nursing diagnosis for the client. The chapters in Unit III contain health history questions for each body region or system. ⬭

Phase I: Preinteraction

The **preinteraction** phase is the period before meeting with the client. During this time, the nurse collects data from the medical record, previous health-risk appraisals, health screenings, therapists, dietitians, and other healthcare professionals who have cared for, taught, or counselled the client, and family members or friends. The nurse reviews the client's name, age, sex, nationality, medical and social history, and current health concern. If necessary, the nurse also reviews literature describing recent research, new treatments, medication, prevention strategies, and self-care interventions that might have a bearing on the client's care.

The nurse uses information obtained during the preinteraction phase to plan and guide the direction of the initial interview. Nurses are more likely to conduct a successful interview if they know in advance, for example, that the client has a psychological problem, is deaf, speaks a foreign language, or is a triathlete.

Information about the client is not the nurse's only consideration during the preinteraction phase. During this phase, the nurse reflects on his or her own strengths and limitations. For example, a nurse opposed to abortion may have difficulty interviewing a client who is considering an abortion. In this situation, the nurse's anxiety could interfere with the collection of data and the provision of nursing care. Nurses should be aware of their own feelings and prejudices and plan how to interact with the client.

The nurse chooses the setting and time before the initial interview takes place. A quiet, private place where few distractions or interruptions will occur is most conducive to a successful interview. The client will feel more relaxed and comfortable if the area has subdued lighting, a moderate temperature, and comfortable seating. More chairs should be provided if family members or an interpreter will be present. A glass of water and tissues should be available for the client's use. The ideal setting is one that is private because the presence of another person might hinder the client's ability to be free and open. If the client is hospitalized, the nurse should hold the interview in a private conference room, if one is available. The nurse can also hold the interview in the client's room, preferably with no roommates present. If this is not possible, the nurse should select a quiet time of day for the interview, draw the bedside curtains or place a screen for privacy, and use a subdued level of speech. In the home setting, a quiet room or even the backyard can be used as long as the client is comfortable and no distractions are present.

The nurse should sit facing the client at a comfortable distance, without using a table, a desk, or any other barrier that might make communication difficult. When possible, the nurse and the client should be on the same level. If the nurse sits in a chair that is higher than the client's or stands at the bedside, it places the client in an inferior position that might make the client uncomfortable. A distance of approximately 0.5 to 2 m (1.5 to 4 ft.) between the nurse and the client is most likely to make the client feel at ease. Moving closer than 0.5 m (1.5 ft.) may invade the client's intimate space, which some clients may consider aggressive or seductive. Although 0.5 to 2 m (1.5 to 4 ft.) is the average distance, each person's personal space differs slightly. If the client moves back in the chair, suddenly crosses arms and legs, or seems anxious, the nurse may be invading the client's intimate space. If so, the nurse should move back until the client seems more relaxed. A translator or family member who is present to assist with the interview should sit on one side of the client so that conversation flows easily (see Figure 10.3).

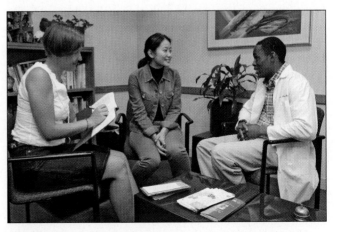

Figure 10.3 ● A translator may help facilitate interaction with a client who does not speak English.

The interview should be scheduled at a time that is convenient for the nurse and the client. The interview should not interfere with cooking dinner, picking up the children after school, or work. If the client is hospitalized, the nurse takes care not to schedule the interview during times when diagnostic tests or treatments are scheduled, during mealtimes, or during visiting hours. The interview should be postponed if the client is in pain, has been sedated recently, is upset, or is confused.

Phase II: The Initial Interview

The initial interview is a planned meeting in which the nurse gathers information from the client. The nurse gathers information about every facet of the client's health status and state of wellness at this time. These data will be used to develop hypothetical nursing diagnoses. In addition to providing data, the initial interview also helps establish a nurse-client relationship based on mutual trust and communication, and gives the nurse insight into the client's lifestyle, values, and feelings about wellness, health, and illness. The health assessment interview is an anxiety-producing situation for most clients. In few other situations is a person required to tell a stranger such intimate details about personal history, health habits, or physical and psychological problems. The nurse has a responsibility to allay these fears and anxieties so that the client can communicate as effectively as possible. One way to make clients feel at ease is to address them by their title (Dr., Mrs., Mr., Ms.) and family name (last name) rather than given name (first name). It is important to ask permission to use the client's given name, since some clients may feel that the nurse is being overly familiar or inappropriate. In this case, the client will be reluctant to divulge personal information.

The nurse begins by describing the interviewing process, explaining its importance, and telling the client what to expect. The nurse might say something like this: "Good morning, Mr. Lavoie. I'm Janet Goebel, the nurse responsible for your care today. To plan the care, I need some additional information. For about the next 45 minutes, I would like to find out as much as possible about you and why you are here. Since we will be talking about a variety of things, I'll be jotting down some notes as we speak. Please stop me at any time if you don't understand a question or need more information about something. Some questions have to do with personal and private subjects, such as your beliefs, family, income, emotions, and sexual activity. Everything we discuss will be held in strict confidence. However, you may choose not to disclose some information."

Notice several things about these introductory remarks. First, the nurse introduced herself and described the purpose of the interview in a friendly, caring tone intended to make the client feel at ease. Second, the nurse gave the client a time frame and said notes would be taken during the interview. This advance notice is important, because some clients become threatened or anxious when the nurse writes down information. Third, the nurse encouraged the client to interrupt or ask questions at any point during the interview. Finally, the nurse reinforced the privacy and confidentiality of the interview.

After making the introductory comments, the nurse will begin to seek information about the client's health status. The opening questions are purposely broad and vague to let the client adjust to the questioning nature of the interview. For instance, "Why did you request a visit by a home health nurse?" or "What led up to your seeking assistance with your health?" If the nurse begins the interview with a series of very specific personal questions, the client may begin to shut down, giving less and less information until no exchange takes place. The nurse continually assesses the client's anxiety level as the interview continues. Restlessness, distraction, and anger are signs that the client perceives the interview as threatening. The nurse will elicit the best information from clients by asking carefully thought-out and clearly stated, open-ended questions throughout the interview.

After gathering sufficient information, the nurse proceeds with closure of the interview. The nurse indicates that the interview is almost at an end and gives the client an opportunity to express any final questions or concerns. For example, "Is there anything else you would like to discuss or ask about, since our time is just about at an end?" It is important to take a few minutes to summarize the information gathered in the interview and to identify key health strengths and concerns. The nurse should review what the client can expect next with regard to nursing care. A final step is to thank the client: "I've appreciated your time and cooperation during the interview."

Phase III: The Health History

The nurse uses the health history throughout the physical assessment, during treatment, and while caring for the client. The purpose of the health history is to clarify previously obtained assessment data, gather missing information about a specific health concern, update and identify new diagnostic cues as they occur, guide the direction of a physical assessment as it is being conducted, and identify or validate probable nursing diagnoses.

Consider the following situation: Mr. Joseph Lavoie is a 36-year-old stockbroker who is a new client at the outpatient clinic. He told the nurse during the initial interview that he experiences severe abdominal pain, nausea, and bloating after eating spicy foods and that this is why he has decided to seek help. Later that day when Mr. Lavoie was admitted to the hospital, the same nurse used the health history interview to elicit the following information from the client: He drinks at least 10 cups of coffee and smokes two packages of cigarettes a day, tends to forget to eat when feeling stressed, uses over-the-counter medication to treat his heartburn, and recently lost a large amount of money in the stock market. When questioned further, Mr. Lavoie confirmed that his pain sometimes occurs at times when he has not eaten spicy foods. By using a health history interview, the nurse clarified information that had been previously obtained (the client's abdominal pain is not associated with spicy foods), included additional needed information, and identified several new cues not observed before (caffeine and nicotine intake, stress, and anxiety). It is not unusual for clients like Mr. Lavoie to fail to give complete information during the initial interview because of anxiety, distrust, discomfort, or confusion.

Nurses use the health history continually to update diagnostic cues because signs, symptoms, and client health concerns often change from moment to moment or day to day. Nurses perform most health history interviews during routine nursing care. For example, while bathing a man who recently had surgery, the nurse focuses on the client's discomfort by asking pertinent questions about his pain. Examples of focusing questions or statements a nurse might use in this situation to update information include "Is the pain as severe as it was yesterday?" "Describe the pain you are experiencing now."

In some cases, the information that the nurse learns during the healthy history plays an important part in how physical assessment is performed. For example, if the client states that he is experiencing severe pain in the upper right quadrant of the abdomen, the nurse would examine this area last. Beginning the assessment with the nontender areas permits the nurse to establish the borders of the affected area. Examination of a painful area can exacerbate symptoms, increase the pain, and force termination of the assessment process.

In Mr. Lavoie's situation, the nurse's initial hypothetical nursing diagnosis was pain related to consumption of spicy foods, as evidenced by abdominal discomfort, nausea, and abdominal distension. However, with the additional information obtained during the health history, the nurse changed the nursing diagnosis to *Pain related to nicotine and caffeine intake, stress, and missed meals, as evidenced by abdominal discomfort, nausea, and abdominal distension.* In view of the new information, the nurse added the following nursing diagnosis: *Anxiety related to financial losses, as evidenced by chain smoking, forgetting meals, increased intake of coffee, and agitation.*

GOAL OF THE HEALTH HISTORY

The goal of the interview process is to obtain a health history containing information about the client's health status. In many healthcare settings, both inpatient and outpatient settings, the nurse and physician complete separate health histories regarding the client. The nursing health history focuses on the client's physical status, patterns of daily living, wellness practices, and self-care activities, as well as psychosocial, cultural, environmental, and other factors that influence health status. As nurses gather information during the nursing history, they allow clients an opportunity to express their expectations of the healthcare staff and the agency or institution. The information in a nursing health history is used along with the subsequent data from the physical assessment to develop a set of nursing diagnoses that reflect the client's health concerns.

A medical history, by contrast, focuses on the client's past and present illnesses, medical problems, hospitalizations, and family history. The major aim of the medical history is to determine a medical diagnosis that accounts for the client's physiological alteration.

Although nursing and medical histories tend to overlap in some areas, neither format alone presents a true picture of the client's total health status and health needs. Combining the nursing and medical history into one format, the complete health history, provides the most comprehensive source of information for assessing the client's total health needs. Integrating the salient features from the nursing and medi-

cal history has distinct advantages for both the client and the caregivers. The information in the health history directs coordinated or collaborative medical and nursing treatment plans that complement one another. The health history saves both the staff and the client time and energy, because the client has to provide significant information only once. Using a health history fosters communication among members of the healthcare team, because they all share its contents. The health history, therefore, fosters effective communication and collaboration among the nurse, physician, and other healthcare providers.

Components of the Health History

Most healthcare settings have developed nursing and medical health history forms for collecting the data, organizing it, and ensuring that the interviewer does not omit any information. The nursing health history form is organized in different ways in different institutions, agencies, or facilities. That organization often reflects a conceptual framework or nursing model used by that facility. The required information remains constant regardless of which framework or nursing model is used, how the information is labelled, or how the data are categorized. For instance, Orem's model is organized according to self-care deficits (Orem, 1991); Gordon's, according to 11 functional health patterns (Gordon, 1990); and Doenges's, according to 13 diagnostic divisions (Doenges & Moorhouse, 1990). Nonetheless, all models focus on the current health concerns, along with an additional broad focus on all aspects of the client's lifestyle and response to the environment.

In general, health histories include the following groups of information (see Table 10.2):

- Biographical data
- Present health or illness
- Past history
- Family history
- Psychosocial history
- Review of body systems

The information gathered for each of the components of the health history serves a purpose in health assessment and in application of the nursing process for each client. Responses to the questions asked in the health history provide specific information about the individual. The nurse will use professional judgment in determining the significance of the responses, the need for follow-up questioning, and the relevance of information to meeting the health needs of the client.

Biographical Data

The biographical data include the client's name and address, age and date of birth, birthplace, gender, marital status, race, religion, occupation, information about health insurance, and the reliability of the source of information. When possible, the client completes a form that elicits these data. Otherwise, the interviewing nurse documents it.

Gathering biographical data is an important initial step in understanding the client. The biographical data provide a data set from which the nurse can begin to make judgments. The

TABLE 10.2	Health History Format	

I. Biographical Data	III. Past History	VI. Review of Body Systems
Name	Medical	Skin, Hair, and Nails
Address	Surgical	Head, Neck, and Lymphatics
Age	Hospitalization	Eyes
Date of Birth	Outpatient Care	Ears, Nose, Mouth, and Throat
Birthplace	Childhood Illnesses	Respiratory
Gender	Immunizations	Breasts and Axillae
Marital Status	Mental and Emotional Health	Cardiovascular
Race	Allergies	Peripheral Vascular
Ethnic Identity/Culture	Substance Use	Abdomen
Religion and Spirituality	IV. Family History	Urinary
Occupation	Immediate Family	Male Reproductive
Source of Information/Reliability	Extended Family	Female Reproductive
II. Present Health or Illness	Genogram	Musculoskeletal
Reason for Seeking Care	V. Psychosocial History	Neurological
Health Beliefs and Practices	Occupational History	
Health Patterns	Education	
Medications, Prescription and Over the Counter	Financial Background	
	Roles and Relationships	
	Family	
	Social Structure/Emotional Concerns	
	Self-Concept	

biographical data will be used to relate individual characteristics to and compare them with established expectations and norms for physical and emotional health. Furthermore, the biographical data provide information about social and environmental characteristics that affect physical and emotional health.

A thorough discussion of each piece of information in the biographical data section of the health history is presented in the following sections. This information is presented to assist the reader in developing and refining the skills required in meeting the healthcare needs of clients.

NAME AND ADDRESS. The client's name and address are generally the first pieces of biographical data to be collected. Listening to the client state his or her name and address provides the first opportunity to assess the client's ability to hear and speak. The client's address reveals information about the client's environment. The nurse will associate the environment with known health benefits and risks. For example, individuals living in crowded urban environments are at risk for problems associated with heavy vehicular traffic including respiratory problems from the exhaust. Conversely, access to a variety of healthcare facilities and services is usually greater in urban areas than in rural areas.

AGE AND DATE OF BIRTH. The client's age and date of birth are requested in the biographical data. Establishing the age of the client permits the nurse to begin evaluation of individual characteristics in relation to norms and expectations of physical and social characteristics across the age span. For example, the skin of a 20-year-old is expected to be smooth and elastic,

while the skin of a 70-year-old would be expected to have wrinkles and decreased elasticity. The client's age also influences behaviour, communication, and dress. For example, the nurse would expect that the vocabulary of an 18-year-old would be greater than that of a 6-year-old.

GENDER. The client's gender is an element of the biographical data. Differences according to gender exist in terms of physical development, secondary sex characteristics, and reproduction. For example, males have greater muscle mass than do females. Fat distribution in the thighs, hips, and buttocks is seen in females in greater amounts than in males. Males develop coarse facial hair as a beard while females do not. Moreover, health risks are associated with sexual differences. For example, although breast cancer can occur in males, it occurs more frequently in females. Osteoporosis occurs in both sexes; however, postmenopausal females are at greater risk.

BIRTHPLACE. The biographical data include identification of the client's birthplace. Identification of the birthplace allows the nurse to determine the environmental and cultural factors that affected or contributed to the client's current state of health and well-being.

It is important to determine the length of time the client spent in and near the place of birth and the places in which the client lived before locating to the current residence. Cultural, environmental, and geographic characteristics of regions and nations influence the health and well-being of the inhabitants. Further, geographic moves force the individuals to adapt and adjust to new cultural norms. Problems in development may result when frequent moves prohibit individuals from forming and maintaining attachments to family and friends. It is important to understand the characteristics of the areas in which clients were born and where they resided throughout their lives. Knowledge of the characteristics of cities, communities, and regions beyond the nurse's own experience is difficult. Persons who immigrated to Canada may have knowledge about their location of origin and the region in which they now reside. However, they may not be able to describe the physical environment of regions beyond their experience. All nurses encounter clients who were born or lived in cities, regions, or countries with which the nurses have little specific knowledge. Therefore, nurses must ask clients to describe the locations in which they were born or resided over time, using such questions or statements as the following:

- Is the place you were born in a city?

- Is the region in which you lived close to a large city?

- Tell me about the place where you were born.

To find out about the physical and environmental characteristics of each location, the nurse will include such questions as these:

- Was the area you grew up in an industrial area?

- Was the place where you were born a farming area?

- How far did you have to travel to shop or go to school or get to a healthcare facility?

- How many people reside in that city?

MARITAL STATUS. Marital status is another element of the biographical data. Marital status indicates if the client is single, married, widowed, or divorced, both for heterosexual and gay or lesbian clients. It is helpful to determine the length of marriage, relationship, widowhood, and divorced status.

The client's marital or relationship status provides initial information about the presence of significant others who may provide physical or emotional support for the client. In addition, when a client relates the loss of a significant other through death or divorce, the nurse begins to evaluate emotional responses and coping ability expected in relation to the event and length of time from the event. The nurse also considers the information in relation to expectations for development. Developmental theorists, such as Erikson, discussed in Chapter 3 of this text, ⬭ have described stages across the lifespan, which include the establishment of intimate relationships. Marriage and establishing intimate relationships is a hallmark of young adulthood. Intimacy and sharing in relationships outside of marriage is an essential developmental process when a person is single and during middle and older adulthood when a person is widowed.

RACE. Race refers to classification of people according to shared biological and genetic characteristics. The nurse can begin to identify characteristics of the client in relation to expectations, norms, and risk factors associated with race.

It is important to note that racial blurring is occurring in Canada. Many individuals identify themselves as having mixed racial origins. Therefore, expectations, norms, and risks are not as clearly delineated as they have been in the past. Assessment requires careful history taking.

RELIGION. Religion generally refers to an organizing framework for beliefs and practices and is associated with rites, rituals, and ceremonies that mark specific life passages, such as birth, adulthood, marriage, and death. Religious beliefs often influence perceptions about health and illness. Religions can impose certain restrictions that affect health, such as not eating pork in the Jewish and Muslim religions.

The nurse will ask the client the following questions or use the following statements to elicit information:

- What is your religion or religious preference?

- Have you ever belonged to a religious group?

- How long have you followed the religion?

- Do you adhere to all the rules of the religion?

- Tell me how your religion influences your health.

- Are there beliefs that govern your life?

- Tell me how your beliefs affect your relationships with others.

Additional information about the role of religion in the client's life is obtained when asking about health practices, when asking about family history, and when obtaining psychosocial information.

OCCUPATION. The client's occupation is part of the biographical data. Information about the client's occupation is important in determining if physical, psychological, or environmental factors associated with work affect the client's health.

SOURCE OF INFORMATION. The biographical data must identify the source of the information for the health history. The usual source of information is the client, who is the primary source. Secondary sources of information include family members, friends, healthcare professionals, and others who can provide information about the client's health status. The use of translators or interpreters must be indicated when recording the source of information.

RELIABILITY OF THE SOURCE. Reliability of the source means that the person providing information for the health history is able to provide a clear and accurate account of present health, past health, family history, psychosocial information, and information related to each body system. The client is considered to be the most reliable source. Determining the reliability of the client includes assessing the client's ability to hear and speak and the ability to accurately recall health-related past events. However, parents or guardians must serve as the source of information for children. Secondary sources are used when the client cannot participate in the interview because of physical or psychological problems. Secondary sources are selected when their knowledge of the client is sufficient to provide thorough and accurate information. A complete health history may be impossible, for example, when a person has no living relatives or friends who can provide information, when the client is unable to provide information because of a language barrier and no translator is available, and in an emergency when the client is unable to respond and sources of information cannot be identified.

Present Health or Illness

The history of present health or illness includes information about all the client's current health-related issues, concerns, and problems. The history includes determination of the reason for seeking care and identification of health beliefs and practices, health patterns, health goals, and information about medication and therapies.

REASON FOR SEEKING CARE. The client usually gives the reason for seeking care when the nurse asks, "Why are you seeking help today?" or "What is bothering you?" The reason for seeking care, sometimes written as the chief complaint, is an important part of the health history picture. The nurse explores the reason for seeking care because it provides the first indicators for possible nursing diagnoses and sets the direction of the rest of the health history interview. It is not appropriate, however, to attempt to develop nursing diagnoses at this point. The client has given minimal information, and no physical assessment or diagnostic testing has been performed. Instead, the nurse develops a list of statements that reflect the client's major reasons for seeking care. Each statement is a brief, concise, and time-oriented description of the client's concern. Here are some examples of statements describing reason for seeking care:

- Substernal chest pain since 9:00 a.m.
- Swelling in lower legs and feet for the past 2 weeks
- Physical examination needed for football team by next Tuesday
- Weight gain of 5 kg (11 lb.) since discontinuing daily walking regimen

The client's own words should be used to document the reason for contact whenever possible: "I've lost 7 kg [15 lb.] in the last 3 weeks" or "I've lost the feeling in my right arm and hand." The nurse explores the onset and progression of each behaviour, symptom, or concern the client relates. Also, the nurse asks clients how their concern has affected their lives and what expectations they have for recovery and subsequent self-care. The answers to these questions provide valuable information about clients' ability to tolerate and cope with the stress brought on by their health concern and healthcare.

HEALTH BELIEFS AND PRACTICES. A person's beliefs about health and illness are influenced by heritage, exposure to information, and experiences. Culture and heritage influence an individual's perceptions about internal and external factors that contribute to health and cause illness and the practices the individual follows to prevent and treat health problems.

In Canada and in many Westernized countries, beliefs about health and illness are derived from a scientific approach. The scientific approach includes *germ theory* as applied in infectious diseases; knowledge of changes in body structures and functions associated with aging, including arthritis, menopause, and vision changes; and the understanding that diet and lifestyle choices influence health and illness. Health practices include seeking healthcare from healthcare providers who use scientific methods to diagnose and treat illness. Healthcare practices include following recommendations for disease prevention, including screening for risks, screening for early detection of problems, and immunization.

Two factors have influenced perceptions of health and healthcare practices in Canada. The first factor is that people of all nations have immigrated and continue to immigrate to Canada. As a result, the beliefs and practices of these individuals, families, and groups influence the ways in which individual healthcare is managed. Many of the immigrant populations have adapted to and use the healthcare system in Canada but retain cultural practices. The adoption of Westernized or scientific beliefs and practices is influenced by the length of time from immigration and often by the age of the client. Conversely, the exposure to and knowledge of a variety of cultural beliefs and healthcare practices has promoted the adoption of many treatments, remedies, and therapies from those cultures by healthcare practitioners in Canada. For example, acupuncture, which is part of traditional Chinese medicine, has become a widely accepted therapy.

The second factor to influence health beliefs and practices is the availability of information. Healthcare information is widely available in all forms of media, through educational programs, and in literature provided by healthcare and community organizations. The internet is responsible for dissemination of healthcare information to a growing number of computer users. The increased amount of information about preventive and treatment services has promoted a different approach to healthcare. Clients who use a variety of information sources are more likely to be informed about recommendations for screening and preventive measures for themselves or family members. Informed clients are more likely to seek therapies they have read or heard about, to question recommended therapies, or to seek many opinions about therapy. The use of the internet for healthcare information has its risks, such as clients not being able to judge the reliability of the source. In addition, healthcare products are available for purchase online. Clients may purchase and use products that interfere with current therapies or are harmful.

The following are questions or statements used to obtain information about the client's health beliefs and practices:

- What do you think it means to be healthy?
- What are the reasons people become sick?
- Do the members of your family think about health and illness the same way that you do?
- Tell me about your own health.
- What do you do to take care of your health?
- Where do you go for healthcare?
- Does a doctor provide your healthcare?
- Does a nurse provide your healthcare?
- Does a healer associated with your culture or religion provide your healthcare?
- Do you have concerns about the people who will provide your healthcare?

- Are there special practices that need to be carried out by you or your family while you are receiving healthcare?

- Do you use cultural remedies for illness?

- Do you use any home remedies for illness?

- Where do you get information about healthcare?

- Have your healthcare practices changed over time?

The preceding questions and statements are used to elicit information about a client's health beliefs and practices. Many of them are closed questions and require follow-up if a client responds positively. For example, if a client responds that a faith healer is used or a cultural remedy is used, the nurse must follow up. Such statements as "Tell me about the healing" or "Tell me about the kinds of remedies you use" are nonjudgmental and allow clients to describe the treatments or healing in their own words.

HEALTH PATTERNS. A **health pattern** is a set of related traits, habits, or acts that affect a client's health. The client's health patterns play a key role in the client's total health history because they are the lifestyle threads that, woven throughout the fabric of the health history, give it depth, detail, and definition. For example, the number of hours a client sleeps, the time a client awakens and falls asleep, the number of times a client awakens during the night, and any dream activity are the behaviours that define a client's sleep patterns. Inadequate sleep can contribute to stress, which in turn can be related to gastrointestinal symptoms, such as nausea.

The nurse compares a client's health behaviour with predetermined standard health patterns. For example, most people sleep 8 to 10 hours per night, seldom awaken once asleep, and can recall some dream activity. When assessing a client's rest and sleep patterns, the nurse compares the client's behaviour with the health pattern standard. Health pattern assessment includes information about diet and nutrition. Chapter 9 of this text provides details about nutritional assessment. ∞ The nurse usually collects information about a client's health patterns when assessing the system or section of the body with which the health pattern is associated. For example, the nurse might collect information on patterns related to rest and sleep as the neurological system is assessed, on activity and exercise as the musculoskeletal system is assessed, and on sexuality as the reproductive system is assessed.

Health patterns also refer to the types and frequency of healthcare in which a client participates. The nurse will ask questions related to the frequency of healthcare visits, preventive and screening measures used by the client, including laboratory and other diagnostic testing, and the results if known. For example, the nurse will ask the client to give the dates of the last physical and dental, hearing, and eye examinations. In addition, the nurse will inquire about preventive measures, such as flu or hepatitis immunization, and ask the client about screening for health problems (e.g., mammography for breast cancer, stool examination for bleeding as a sign of rectal cancer, and laboratory screening of cholesterol and glucose levels because of the links with heart disease and diabetes, respectively).

MEDICATIONS. Information about the use of medications is obtained during this part of the health history. The information should include the use of prescription and over-the-counter (OTC) medications. The nurse should determine the name, dose, purpose, duration, frequency, and desired or undesired effects of each of the medications. When the client provides information about medications, the nurse is able to determine the level of knowledge about the medication regimen, whether the client has an understanding of the problem for which the medication has been prescribed, and if the client has noted or received information about the therapeutic effects of the medication.

The medication history includes the use of home remedies, folk remedies, herbs, teas, vitamins, dietary supplements, or other substances. The use of traditional medicines and herbs is common among many groups in Canada. The use of herbal remedies, teas, vitamins, and traditional remedies can interfere with the action of some prescribed medications and can in some instances be harmful. For example, exceeding the recommended daily allowance of vitamins can result in side effects and toxicity. Large doses of vitamin E can increase levels of cholesterol, produce headaches or blurred vision, and increase the risk of bleeding in clients who are taking Coumadin. The nurse uses the medication history to identify any potential drug interactions and to determine if the client requires education about medications, dosing, side effects, and interactions.

When gathering information about medications, it is helpful to ask if the client has the container. Reading the name and dosage provides the specific information the nurse needs to make judgments about client data. It is also helpful to ask clients about categories of OTC medications. Categories include laxatives; vitamins; herbs; pain relievers, including Aspirin and nonsteroidal anti-inflammatory drugs (NSAIDs); dietary supplements; cold remedies; drops for the eyes, nose, or ears; enemas; allergy preparations; appetite stimulants or suppressants; sleeping aids; and medicated lotions, creams, or unguents. Asking about each category is an efficient method to obtain a comprehensive assessment of medication use.

Past History

The past history includes information about childhood diseases; immunizations; allergies; blood transfusions; major illnesses; injuries; hospitalizations; labour and deliveries; surgical procedures; mental, psychological, or psychiatric health problems; and the use of alcohol, tobacco, and other substances. Many health history forms include a checklist of the most commonly occurring illnesses or surgical procedures to help the client recall information. The nurse asks the client to recall all childhood diseases. A history of German measles, polio, chickenpox, streptococcal throat infections, or rheumatic fever is especially significant because these diseases have sequelae (diseases caused by previous diseases) that may affect the client's health status and health concerns in adulthood. The nurse also ascertains a history of the client's immunizations. If the client is a child, the nurse checks whether the immunizations are up to date. If possible, the immunization data should be verified through immunization records. The nurse questions adult clients concerning the administration of recent tetanus immunizations or boosters, flu shots, or immunizations required for foreign travel. The complete immunization history includes the name of the immunization, the number of doses, and the date of each dose. Chapter 3 provides information about recommended immunization schedules across the age span.

The nurse elicits information about any history of major illnesses, injuries, surgical procedures, hospitalizations, major outpatient care, or therapies. The client should describe each incident, including the date, treatment, healthcare provider, and any other pertinent information. If the client has had a surgical procedure, the nurse elicits specific information concerning the type of surgery and postoperative course. Complicated labour and deliveries are recorded here, as well as in the reproductive section of the review of the systems.

It is important to obtain a thorough history of any chronic illness and major health concerns. Such disease processes as diabetes, heart disease, or asthma are examples of chronic illnesses. The nurse records the onset, frequency, precipitating factors, signs and symptoms, method of treatment, and long-term effects so that this information can be used to meet the learning needs of the client and develop appropriate nursing interventions in the nursing care plan.

Information about the client's psychological, mental, or psychiatric health should include the description of the problem. The nurse asks the client to identify whether care was received through a healthcare provider, through a support group, from a religious leader, or within the family or community. The information should include a description of the therapy or remedy and the outcome of treatment. The nurse's questioning must reflect sensitivity to individual and cultural reluctance to describe problems of a psychological or psychiatric dimension.

The following questions or statements are used to obtain information about psychological and mental health:

- Have you ever had an emotionally upsetting experience?
- Tell me about any emotional upsets you have experienced.
- Have you ever sought assistance for a psychological problem?
- Where did you go to get assistance?
- Did the assistance help you with the problem?
- Have you ever been told that you have a mental illness or psychiatric disorder?
- What were the circumstances that led to the mental or psychiatric problem?
- What care did you receive for the mental or psychiatric problem?
- Has the care helped the problem?
- Do you take any medication for a mental or psychiatric problem?
- Are you experiencing problems now?
- What kind of help would you like to receive for the psychological, mental, or psychiatric problem?

Information about allergies and the use of illicit drugs, caffeine, alcohol, and tobacco is included in the health history.

Information about allergies should include determination of the allergy as food, drug, or environmentally occurring, and the symptoms, treatment, and personal adaptation. It is important to determine the extent of the client's knowledge about allergens, especially when exposure to allergens can result in anaphylactic reactions. The nurse should ask the client to describe the ways allergies are managed. The information should indicate if a client's allergies have been identified through testing, through confirmation of a cause by a healthcare professional, or by informal means. Eliciting information about adaptation includes identification of client practices, such as avoidance of allergens, the use of environmental controls (e.g., filters, air conditioners, or other devices) in the home or work environment, and the use of ingested remedies or medications. The information enables the nurse to begin to identify educational needs about allergies. The learning needs may include general or specific details about avoidance of allergens, methods to manage allergy symptoms, and measures to employ in severe allergic reactions. For example, the nurse may suggest that a client obtain and wear a MedicAlert bracelet when an allergy to medications is identified.

When gathering information about the use of alcohol, tobacco, caffeine, and illicit drugs, the nurse will want to know the type, amount, duration, and frequency of use of each substance. The information is elicited whether the client is currently using any substances or reports that he or she has stopped using the products. Tobacco use includes cigarettes, cigars, and products that are chewed or inhaled as snuff. Use of any of these products has an impact on the physical and emotional health of the client and family. Smoking is a causative factor in lung cancer and emphysema. Family members of smokers are at risk for asthma, emphysema, and cancer from second-hand smoke. Alcohol abuse can lead to liver disease, increases risk of injury or death in accidents, and is associated with disruptions in families.

Family History

The family history is a review of the client's family to determine if any genetic or familial patterns of health or illness might shed light on the client's current health status. For example, if the client has a family history of type 1 diabetes, the nurse will question the client closely about signs of the disease. These signs include increased appetite, frequent urination, and weight loss. The family history begins with a review of the immediate family: parents, siblings, children, grandparents, aunts, uncles, and cousins. The nurse should encourage the client to recall as many generations as possible to develop a complete picture. If the client provides data about a genetic or familial disease, it is helpful to interview older members of the family for additional information. Adopted children, spouses, and other individuals living with the client may not be related by blood; however, their health history should be reviewed because the client's concern may have an environmental basis. For example, illnesses may be associated with second-hand smoke in the spouse or child of a smoker, or illness may be associated with exposure to toxins or fumes carried into the home on the clothing of a spouse or family member. The nurse documents information collected from the client and the family in a family genogram. A **genogram** is a pictorial representation of family relationships and medical history. The family genogram, also known as a pedigree or family tree, is the most effective method of recording the large amount of data gathered from a family's health history (see Figure 10.4).

Psychosocial History

The psychosocial history includes information about the client's occupational history, educational level, financial background, roles and relationships, ethnicity and culture, family, spirituality, and self-concept. The information about occupation, education, and finances provides the nurse with cues about previous experiences that may affect current or future health. A client's occupational history can reveal risk factors for a variety of problems. For example, coal mining increases the risk for respiratory diseases, and exposure to asbestos in the shipbuilding and construction industries is associated with lung cancer. Determining the client's level of education establishes expectations related to the ability to comprehend verbal and written language. These abilities are significant during the assessment process, in discussion of health problems or needs, and in education of the client. The types of words that will be used and the choice of educational approaches and materials are influenced by the client's abilities to read, write, and in some cases perform calculations. The client's financial situation has an impact on health, health practices, and health-seeking behaviours. Low income is associated with a lowered health status and predisposition to illness. A client may report that he now enjoys a secure financial situation. However, he may have been born and raised in poverty. Poverty in youth is associated with physical and mental health problems, poor nutrition, and lack of dental care (Human Resources and Social Development Canada, the Public Health Agency of Canada, & Indian and Northern Affairs Canada, 2007). These deficiencies can have long-term consequences for the client.

The nurse will also gather information about the client's roles and relationships, family, ethnicity and culture, spirituality, and self-concept. The nurse will ask the client to identify a significant other and support systems. Support systems include family members, friends, neighbours, club members, clergy and church members, and members of the healthcare team. The information provides an initial impression of the family dynamics and informs the nurse of the religious and spiritual needs of the client. Remember that culture influences roles and relationships within families and society. Determination of roles and relationships is important when planning healthcare and assisting the client to make healthcare decisions. The nurse must respect the practices of the client and prepare to include recognized decision makers in the planning process.

The following are questions and statements to elicit information about roles and relationships, family, and self-concept:

- Tell me about your family.
- How many people are in your family?
- Who is the head of the family?
- What is your role in the family?

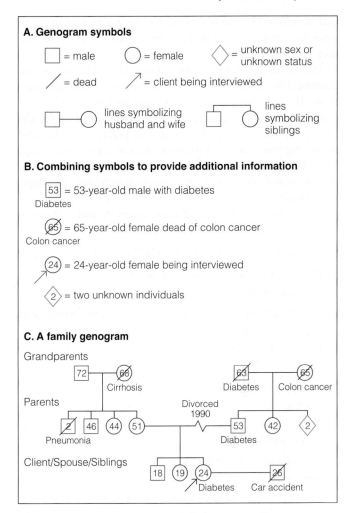

Figure 10.4 • Genogram. A. Standard symbols used in constructing the family genogram. B. Combining symbols to provide additional information. C. A family genogram.

- Who makes decisions about healthcare in your family?
- Who is involved in discussing health or psychological problems in your family?
- Are there certain roles for children in the family?
- Who is your significant other?
- Tell me about your support system.
- Tell me how you feel about yourself.
- How would you describe yourself to someone else?
- Tell me about your body image.

When conducting the assessment of culture, the nurse must be careful to avoid stereotyping. That is, the nurse must not assume because a client looks a certain way or has a certain name that he or she belongs to or identifies with a certain cultural or religious group. In addition, even if the nurse is of the same cultural or ethnic background as the client, the nurse cannot assume they share the same beliefs and practices. The nurse should ask clients to describe what identification with a specific culture means to them. The use of open-ended questions helps to obtain information about the meaning of the client's statements about ethnic or cultural identity. Often, the follow-up question about the family's cultural or ethnic identity can reveal areas to explore in relation to beliefs about illness or disease, diet, and relationships.

Information about ethnicity and culture is gathered because it enables the nurse to determine the physical and social characteristics that influence healthcare decisions. Ethnicity or culture influences a number of health-related factors for the client, including health beliefs, health practices, verbal and nonverbal methods of communication, roles and relationships in the family and society, perceptions of healthcare professionals, diet, dress and rituals, and rites associated with birth, marriage, child rearing, and death.

Information about the client's ethnicity and culture is obtained by asking the following questions:

- Do you identify with a specific ethnic group?
- How strong would you say that identity is?
- What language do you speak at home?
- Do you or members of your family speak a second language?
- Are you comfortable receiving information about your health in English?
- Would you like an interpreter during this interview?
- Would you like to have an interpreter during the physical examination?
- Are there rules in your culture about the ways an examination must be carried out?
- Are there rules about the gender of the person who is examining you?
- Do you need to have someone in your family participate in the interview or examination?

Information about health beliefs and practices, family, roles and relationships, cultural influences on diet, activity, emotional health, and other topics are included in other components of the health history including the review of systems. For example, when asking about the client's health patterns, the nurse will gather information about cultural healing or rituals associated with health and health maintenance. Further, when asking about nutrition, the nurse will gather information about cultural influences on food selection, preparation, and consumption.

Spirituality refers to the individual's sense of self in relation to others and a higher being, and what the person believes gives meaning to life. Assessment of spirituality can be evaluated by asking the following questions:

- Tell me how you meet your spiritual needs.
- Do you have special objects of a religious or spiritual nature that you carry with you or are in your home?
- Are there any religious or spiritual objects that you would want with you if you were ill or hospitalized?
- Is there a member of your place of worship you would want to contact if you were ill or hospitalized?
- Is there a person who you would want to contact to help you with prayer or spiritual practices if you were ill or hospitalized?
- Do you use spiritual healers?

- Are there rituals that are important to you when you are ill or have a health problem?
- Tell me about the rituals you use when you are ill or need healthcare.

Chapter 5 of this text provides information about spirituality and spiritual assessment. ⬤⬤

Review of Body Systems

The focus of this portion of the health history is to uncover current and past information about each body system and its organs. The nurse asks the client about system function and any abnormal signs or symptoms, paying special attention to gathering information about the functional patterns of each system. For example, when assessing the gastrointestinal system, the nurse should ask the client to describe digestive and elimination patterns ("How many bowel movements do you have each day?") as well as function ("Are your bowel movements usually hard or soft?"). Open-ended questions or statements are best for eliciting information about abnormal signs or symptoms: "Describe the abdominal pain you've been experiencing. What other symptoms are associated with the pain?" The nurse carefully explores the characteristics and quality of each subjective symptom the client identifies to obtain a total picture of each system.

Some health history formats use a cephalocaudal or head-to-toe approach for collecting data. In this approach, the nurse considers regions of the body rather than systems. Other formats use an approach related to a nursing theory. Regardless of the method, each area of the body must be reviewed until all systems are covered in each region.

Unit III of this text provides information related to the systems of the body. ⬤⬤ Each chapter provides suggestions for questions to gather data about a particular system. Health history questions are included and follow-up information is provided to elicit details when symptoms are reported. Examples of the types of information required for comprehensive system review are included in the sample documentation of the health history. Box 10.2 lists the systems included in this part of the health history.

BOX 10.2	Review of Body Systems

The following systems are included in health history:

- Skin, hair, and nails
- Head, neck, and related lymphatics
- Eye
- Ear, nose, mouth, and throat
- Respiratory system
- Breasts and axillae
- Cardiovascular system
- Peripheral vascular system
- Abdomen
- Urinary system
- Reproductive system
- Musculoskeletal system
- Neurological system

DOCUMENTATION

The data collected during the interview is recorded as the nurse's health history. The type of recording is often influenced by the agency or facility in which the interview is carried out. Forms for documentation are varied and include checklists, fill-in forms, and narrative records. The nurse's health history becomes part of the client record and is a legal document. Principles of documentation must be applied.

The subjective data are recorded by using quotes. The nurse uses communication skills to elicit as much detail as possible about each area and topic within the health history. The nurse should ask the client to explain his or her meaning of such words as *good, average, okay, normal,* and *adequate.* The nurse must be sure to record what the client intended by use of such terms.

When recording data, the information must be presented in a clear and concise manner. For example, the nurse uses dates and writes them in descending order from present to past when providing details about events. Sample documentation of the health history is included in Boxes 10.3 and 10.4. Box 10.3 is a case study presented in narrative form. Box 10.4 represents a fill-in form for documentation of the health history. The fill-in form does not use quotation marks because all entries are as stated by the client.

BOX 10.3	Narrative Recording of the Health History

Biographical Data　Mrs. Amparo Bellisimo, age 31, comes to the health centre for a health assessment. She is employed as an account representative for a large clothing retail establishment. She lives in a single-family residence at 22 Highland Avenue, Regina, Saskatchewan. Mrs. Bellisimo lives with her husband, who she names as her emergency contact. Mrs. Bellisimo was born on July 20, 1980, in Santa Clara, Cuba. She immigrated to Canada 9 years ago. She speaks English with an accent. Mrs. Bellisimo can read and write in English and Spanish. Mrs. Bellisimo has no immediate family in Canada. She completed 12 years of schooling in Cuba and took several accounting courses in a community college in Regina. She has no formal religious affiliations, because religious practice was not permitted in Cuba when she was there. Some of her family were "hidden" Catholics. She states, "I am happy with my life. I have made adjustments to being in Canada. I have many friends and have a close relationship with my husband's family. I like my job, except when it gets crazy."

Present Health Status: Reason for Seeking Healthcare　Mrs. Bellisimo has no complaints except "weight gain and occasional headaches relieved with Aspirin." The weight gain has occurred "over 3 years since I started dating my husband and more since we got married last year." The headaches occur "when I'm tired, stressed, or reading too much."

Health Beliefs and Practices　Mrs. Bellisimo has no current health problem, except as stated above. She believes "health is important and you need to take care of yourself, but sometimes it's out of your control." When she was a child her mother used to tell her things like "no bathing when you have your period, no water at all" and she "prepared certain foods for certain illnesses and sometimes got medicines from a botanica for ailments." She has had regular physical, gynecological, dental, and eye examinations, all of which have been completed annually for 3 years.

Mrs. Bellisimo states she "sleeps well most nights about 8 hours, unless I stay up and read." She "feels rested most mornings." She tries to exercise but finds it hard "after work and when it's cold out."

Mrs. Bellisimo would like to lose weight. She would "feel healthier, my clothes would fit, and I'd feel good about myself." People in Cuba would not have a problem with this weight, but "I don't like it." Eating patterns include "fast foods at dinner, bread at every meal, and dessert or snacks at night."

Medications　Mrs. Bellisimo has used oral contraceptives "for 4 years," without problems, and takes a multivitamin every day. She is not undergoing any therapy and "really have never needed any specific care."

Past History, Surgeries, and Illnesses　Mrs. Bellisimo had measles as a child. She received smallpox, polio, mumps, tetanus, and other "vaccines" as a child. She has had no major illnesses. She has never been hospitalized, received a blood transfusion, been pregnant, or had allergies. Mrs. Bellisimo cut her lower left leg on glass as a child and had sutures, and a scar remains. She had four wisdom teeth extracted 2 years ago with no complications, "no other surgery."

Psychological History　Mrs. Bellisimo states, "I miss my family and get sad when I can't see them. I get frustrated when I don't understand some Canadian ways. I'm pretty emotional. I cry over books and movies, but I haven't had a mental health problem." She doesn't smoke, but her whole family smoked when she was in Cuba. "I drink some beer, wine, and tequila on weekends or at dinner with my in-laws. I have never used drugs or anything like that."

Family History　Mrs. Bellisimo's father died at age 56 from "some cancer." "He didn't live with us, so I don't know for sure and my mother doesn't say." Her mother is 49 and well. She has a brother, 33, and a sister, 27. Both are "well." Her grandparents were not really known to her but were "old when they died."

Psychosocial History: Occupation　Mrs. Bellisimo held jobs in hotels as a teenager in Cuba. "Since coming to Canada, I have worked in a factory making clothes, been a receptionist in a hair salon, and in some form of accounting for the past 5 years." She states, "I have not been poor but just okay almost all my life until the last 4 or 5 years. Things are really bad in Cuba, no proper food or medicine. They were better when I was there, but not like here."

(continued)

BOX 10.3	Narrative Recording of the Health History *(continued)*

Roles and Relationships She states, "I love my family, but I can't see them. I have friends here that are like my family. My friends were a big part of my wedding. One walked me down the aisle. I call home to Cuba, but it's hard to be far away. My husband is Canadian and we dated for 2 years before we got engaged. He helped me a lot and we love each other very much. His family are like my new family. We see them a lot, they help us, and they treat me like a daughter, so it's very good."

Ethnicity and Culture Mrs. Bellisimo says she will always consider herself Cuban, but "I am a Canadian citizen now. I have come to like Canadian food, especially pasta, but still make my beans and rice and other Cuban foods. My husband likes it too but not every day. I laugh sometimes when I call my mother in Cuba and speak English sometimes."

Spirituality Mrs. Bellisimo states, "I have no real religion; family and honesty are important to me. I believe in God and sometimes pray but really believe your family helps you when you are in need."

Self-Concept Mrs. Bellisimo says of herself, "I am a good person. I worry about others. I want to have a family, with children who understand about being Cuban. I take care of myself and other than some extra weight, I think I look pretty good."

Review of Systems

Skin, Hair, and Nails No reported problems. "I use sunscreen, shower daily, use conditioner on my hair and lotion to prevent dry skin. I would like to have a professional manicure more often but keep my nails looking nice."

Head and Neck No reported problems except "occasional headache relieved by Aspirin."

Eyes Annual eye exam for 3 years. Glasses for "driving."

Ear, Nose, Mouth, and Throat No problems with hearing, has "never had an official exam." Regular dental exams. Wisdom teeth extracted with no problems. No trouble eating or swallowing.

Respiratory No reported problems. "A cold once a year." No exposure to pollutants. No history of tobacco use. Exposure to second-hand smoke from birth to 22 years of age at home. Denies cough, difficulty breathing.

Breasts and Axillae "I have had large breasts since I was 12. I don't like to examine my breasts; I get scared I might find something. I do get them checked every year by the doctor." No changes, discharge, discomfort.

Cardiac No reported problems. No history of heart disease. Never has palpitations.

Peripheral Vascular No reported problems. "The doctor says my blood pressure is fine. I have two veiny spots on my legs, but they don't hurt. They are flat and stringy."

Gastrointestinal No reported problems. "My bowels move every day with no problem. I get diarrhea when I'm nervous sometimes."

Urinary No reported problems. "I pass urine five or six times a day and more if I drink more."

Reproductive Onset of menses age 11. "Regular every 28 days for 3 or 4 days. I take birth control pills." Denies pregnancy, abortion. "Relations are good with my husband."

Musculoskeletal No reported problems. "I don't get enough exercise."

Neurological No history of head injury, seizure, tremor, loss of consciousness. "Other than headache, I'm okay."

BOX 10.4	Documentation of a Health History

Health History

Date: June 30

Name:	Amparo Bellisimo
Address:	22 Highland Avenue, Regina, SK S4S 6X6
Telephone:	306-555-0000
Age:	31
Date of birth:	July 20, 1980
Birthplace:	Santa Clara, Cuba. Came to Canada 9 years ago.
Gender:	Female
Marital status:	Married (Chris, age 33, emergency contact)
Race:	Cuban
Religion:	None really, religious practice was forbidden in Cuba. Some family are hidden Catholics.
Occupation:	Account representative. Retail clothing establishment.
Source:	Client
Reliability:	Reliable, alert, oriented, recall of information intact (nursing assessment).

Present Health or Illness

Reason for seeking care

Scheduled health assessment. No complaints except weight gain and occasional headaches, relieved with Aspirin. Weight gain of 10 kg (22 lb.) more than 3 years since I started dating my husband, most since we got married last year. I get headaches when I'm stressed, tired, or read too much.

Health beliefs and practices

Health is important and you need to take care of yourself, but sometimes it's out of your control. When I was younger my mother would tell me no bathing when you have your period, no water at all. My mother prepared certain foods for certain illnesses and sometimes got medicine from a botanica for ailments. All medical care was done well because it was all free.

(continued)

BOX 10.4	Documentation of a Health History *(continued)*

Health patterns

At first in Canada I didn't see doctors. My husband reminds me to make appointments. I have medical, dentist, gynecologist, and eye doctor exams. I have had them all every year for the last 3 years. I don't examine my breasts but the doctor does it each year. I haven't had any vaccines since I came here and I think my blood tests are okay. I sleep well most nights for about 8 hours, unless I stay up and read. I try to exercise but it is so hard after work and when it's cold out. Diet is crazy sometimes. I have coffee and toast in the morning. Lunch depends on my schedule, sometimes a sandwich, sometimes a salad. Dinner is probably pizza or fast food three or four times a week. I have a sweet at night. I like all kinds of foods and I still like Cuban foods like beans, pork, and rice. I eat all kinds of Canadian foods. I especially like pasta and I like bread, I have it at almost all meals.

Medications

I take birth control pills.
I have been on them for 4 years.
I have not had a problem.
I take a vitamin "one-a-day" every day, my doctor told me to.
I take Aspirin for headaches but that's all.
I don't use stuff like my mother did in Cuba and that some of my friends do.

Health goals

To lose weight so my clothes fit and I feel better about myself. In Cuba people would not have a problem with this weight, but I don't like it.

Past History

Childhood illnesses

Measles when I was little. I don't remember other illnesses.

Immunizations

Smallpox, polio, and other vaccines like tetanus as a child.
I don't remember other specifically.

Medical illnesses

A cold every year—but really no serious illnesses.

Hospitalization

I've never been in the hospital.

Surgery

Never had any except wisdom teeth. All four out 2 years ago because the dentist said they were packed in. I did okay.

Injury

Cut my leg on glass, had stitches and have a scar by my knee.

Blood transfusion

Never had one.

Psychological or psychiatric problems

I miss my family and get sad when I can't see them. I get frustrated when I don't understand some Canadian ways, and I'm pretty emotional. I cry over books and movies, but I haven't had a mental health problem.

Allergies

Food: None I know of.
Medication: I don't know of any.
Environment: No, I don't have a problem.

Use of tobacco

I don't smoke, never have, but my family smoked when I was in Cuba.

Use of alcohol

I have a glass of beer or wine or tequila on weekends or at dinner with my in-laws. One or two glasses maybe two times a week.

Use of illicit drugs

I have never used drugs or anything like that.

Family History

Father

He died at age 56 from "some cancer." He didn't live with us, so I don't know for sure and my mother doesn't say.

Mother

Her mother is 49 and well.

Siblings

She has a brother, 33, and a sister, 27. Both are "well."

Grandparents

Her grandparents were not really known to her but were "old" when they died.

Psychosocial History

Occupational history

Jobs in hotels as teenager in Cuba.
In Canada—a factory making clothes, a receptionist in a hair salon, and in some form of accounting for 5 years.

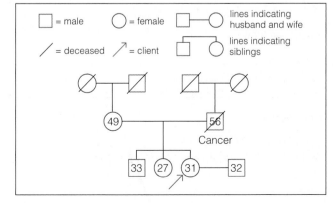

BOX 10.4	Documentation of a Health History *(continued)*

Educational level

Completed 12 years in Cuba.

A few courses in accounting in community college in Canada 6 years ago.

Reads: English, Spanish

Financial background

I have not been poor but just okay for all my life until the last 4 or 5 years. Things are really bad in Cuba. No food or medicine. They were better when I was there but not like here.

Roles and relationships

I love my family but I can't see them. I have friends here that are like my family. My friends were a big part of my wedding. One walked me down the aisle. I call home to Cuba but it's hard to be far away.

Ethnicity and culture

I will always consider myself Cuban but I am a Canadian citizen now and am so much more gringo than my friends. I like all Canadian things, especially food. I still make beans and rice and other Cuban foods. My husband likes it too but not every day.

Family

My family is in Cuba. Oh, I miss them bad. Would like them to come here someday. My husband is Canadian. We dated for 2 years before we got married. He helped me a lot and we love each other very much. His family is my new family. We see them a lot, they help us out, they treat me like a daughter so it's very good.

Spirituality

I have no real religion. Family and honesty are important to me. I believe in God and sometimes pray but I really believe your family helps you when you are in need.

Self-concept

I am a good person. I worry about others. I want to have a family with children who understand being Cuban. I take care of myself and other than some extra weight, I think I look pretty good.

Review of Systems

Skin, hair, nails

No changes, rashes, lesions, colour changes, sweating.

No birthmarks.

Scar left knee. Shower daily, hair shampoo every other day.

No use of hair dyes for 2 years. Would like professional manicure more often but keeps nails nice.

Head, neck, related lymphatics

Occasional headaches relieved by Aspirin. No history of injury, seizure, tremor, dizziness. No neck swelling.

Eye

Annual exam; no change in 2 years.

Glasses for distance.

Next exam 3 months.

Ears, nose, mouth, and throat

No hearing problems, never had specific exam.

Nose patent, no injury, sense of smell intact, clear drainage with cold.

No trouble eating or swallowing.

Dental exam annually, last exam 1 month ago. Brushes and flosses twice daily.

Respiratory

No respiratory problems. A cold once a year. No exposure to pollutants.

No history of tobacco use. Exposure to second-hand smoke birth to 22 years. Denies cough, difficult breathing.

No history of respiratory problems.

Unsure of TB screening.

Breasts and axillae

Annual exam by physician.

No SBE.

Large breasts with no masses, lumps, or discharge.

Cardiovascular

No history of heart disease. Never has palpitations. No edema or cyanosis.

Peripheral vascular

The doctor says my blood pressure is fine. I have two veiny spots on my legs, but they don't hurt.

Abdomen

No reported problems. My bowels move every day with no problem. I get diarrhea when I'm nervous sometimes.

Urinary

No reported problems. No history of UTI. I pass urine five or six times a day and more if I drink more.

Reproductive

On oral contraceptives. Onset menses age 11. Regular every 28 days for 3 to 4 days.

Para 0

Gravida 0

Relations are good with my husband.

Musculoskeletal

No problems.

I don't get enough exercise.

Range of motion normal. No problems with strength.

Neurological

Other than headache, I'm okay.

Denies falls, balance problems, memory problems.

Right-handed. Can sense touch and temperature.

NURSING CONSIDERATIONS

The nurse must consider the ability of the client to participate in the interview process. As stated previously, culture and language are important considerations in establishing a positive relationship. Additional factors that can affect the interview process are alterations in the senses, such as blindness or hearing deficits, developmental level, and pain. The nurse may have to develop written questions for use with clients with hearing deficits.

It is important to consider the client's developmental level when conducting an interview. Word usage and overall communication will differ when interviewing children and adolescents. In addition, the nurse may find that the developmental level of a client differs from that expected for a stated age. Clients who have experienced neurological problems congenitally or as a result of injury or aging may not be able to participate effectively in an interview. Last, when a client is experiencing unrelieved acute or chronic pain, the ability to participate in a lengthy interview is diminished. The nurse must then focus on the immediacy of the problem and gather in-depth information at another time.

The nurse uses the health history and interview in various healthcare settings to create a comprehensive account of the client's past and present health. The completed health history is a compilation of all the client data collected by the nurse, and it is combined with information obtained during the nursing physical assessment to form the total health database for the client. The nurse can use this database, which provides a total picture of the client's past and present physical, psychological, social, cultural, and spiritual health, to formulate nursing diagnoses and plan the client's care.

The process of interviewing to obtain a complete picture of the client can be uncomfortable. To obtain the required information the nurse will be asking clients to provide information about their physical and psychosocial well-being, family, personal habits, body functions, and lifestyle. The nurse may believe that clients will perceive questions about religion, culture, economic status, body functions, and sexuality as intrusive. The nurse may feel that he or she is prying or being nosy by asking certain questions. Remember that the nurse-client interaction is different from social interaction. When taking on the role of the nurse, the questions are intended to guide healthcare decisions. It is helpful to practise the communication techniques that were discussed earlier in the chapter. The nurse will also find it helpful to prepare a list of questions or statements for each category of the health history before conducting the interview. For example, when asking about the financial status of the client, the nurse may state, "Tell me about your financial situation," or "How would you classify your economic situation?" The nurse may want to use a list of categories in the following way: "Of the following economic levels—low, middle, or high income—how would you rate your current situation?"

The nurse should be prepared to address areas concerned with the client's self-esteem and emotional state. For example, clients may be asked to describe their image in a mirror. The nurse could ask each client to describe the following in a few sentences: self-perception of strengths and weaknesses, personality, or how a friend or loved one would describe him or her. Often, when addressing sensitive areas, such as mental health, a straightforward question is the best approach. For example, "Have you ever experienced an emotional upset?" If the response is yes, the nurse should ask the client to describe it. The nurse might ask the client, "Have you ever had a strong emotional response to a person or situation?" If the response is yes, the nurse would ask the client to describe it. The nurse may also list a number of emotional behaviours and ask the client to respond yes or no to each item on the list. Examples of emotional behaviours include anxiety, depression, fear, grief, loneliness, or joy.

Questions about body functions, habits, adaptation, and lifestyle may be difficult for a novice nurse. It is helpful to use the words and terms associated with parts of the body, body functions, and habits regularly when speaking and writing. The health history questions provided in each chapter of Unit III of this text are intended to guide the nurse in eliciting information about functions, practices, and behaviours associated with each body system. ⏳ The nurse should refer to these frequently and use them in preparation for client interviews.

APPLICATION THROUGH CRITICAL THINKING

CASE STUDY

The nurse conducted a health history interview with Mrs. Martha Cruzat, a 77-year-old Filipino woman. The following are excerpts from the health history.

Mrs. Cruzat, I am going to ask you a lot of questions before your physical. I need to have correct responses, and I have to tell you, there will be a lot of them if we are to get to the root of your problem. I will use the information to develop a plan of care.

What are you here for? Did someone come with you? I see on your chart that you have some problems with urination; are you incontinent? How long have you had the problem?

The nurse included the following questions: What is your economic status? Do you go to church? What do you do when you are ill?

We need information about your family, so let's start out with your parents. Are they alive? Do you have siblings?

The nurse completed a review of symptoms and prepared the client for the physical examination by showing her into a room and telling her to get undressed.

▶ Critical Thinking Questions

1. Critique the nurse's actions in the initial interview phase of the case study.
2. Identify the types of information sought in the questions in the case study.
3. Create alternative approaches to the interview and questioning techniques in the case study.
4. Describe your preparation for an interview of Mrs. Cruzat.

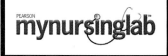

11

SKIN, HAIR, AND NAILS

CHAPTER OBJECTIVES

On completion of this chapter, you will be able to

1. Relate knowledge of anatomy and physiology to the physical examination of a client.
2. Identify landmarks that guide assessment of the skin, hair, and nails.
3. Relate knowledge of the principles of communication to the health history interview.
4. Conduct a health history interview that represents a comprehensive account of the client's physical and psychosocial health status in relation to the skin, hair, and nails.
5. Explain client preparation for assessment of the skin, hair, and nails.
6. Describe the different assessment techniques required for examination of the skin, hair, and nails.
7. Perform a physical examination of a client's skin, hair, and nails by using appropriate equipment and assessment techniques.
8. Differentiate between normal and abnormal findings in assessment of the skin, hair, and nails.
9. Describe developmental, psychosocial, ethnocultural, and environmental variations in assessment techniques and findings in relation to the skin, hair, and nails.
10. Apply critical thinking in selected situations related to assessment of the skin, hair, and nails.
11. Document findings of the skin, hair, and nail examination by using appropriate terminology.

CHAPTER OUTLINE

THE SKIN, HAIR, AND NAILS ARE THE MAJOR COMPONENTS of the integumentary system. The integumentary system consists of the skin and the accessory structures, the sweat and oil glands, the hair, and the nails. The largest organ of the body, the skin weighs approximately 4 kg (9 lb.) and has a surface area of about 4.5 to 6 m (15 to 20 ft.) in adults. Every 6.5 cm^2 (1 in.^{2}) of the skin contains 3 to 4.5 m (10 to 15 ft.) of blood vessels and nerves, hundreds of sweat and oil glands, and more than 3 million cells that are constantly dying and being replaced. This complex shield protects the body against heat, ultraviolet rays, trauma, and invasion by bacteria. In addition, the skin works with other body systems to regulate body temperature, synthesize vitamin D, store blood and fats, excrete body wastes, and help humans sense the world around them.

A thorough assessment of the skin, hair, and nails provides valuable clues to a client's general health. The skin, hair, and nails can suggest the status of a client's nutrition, airway clearance, thermoregulation, and tissue perfusion. The skin, hair, and nails can also reveal alterations in activity, sleep and rest, level of stress, and self-care ability. A client's ancestry, cultural practices, and physical environment, both at home and at work, can greatly influence integumentary health and are an integral part of the assessment data. Assessing for risk factors related to skin cancer and occupational skin disorders will also assist the nurse in reducing the client's exposure.

A client's developmental stage has a tremendous influence on the appearance and functioning of these structures. Skin is very thin at birth and thickens throughout childhood. Sweat and oil glands are activated during adolescence. The function of these glands diminishes in the older adult. The appearance of the skin, hair, and nails affects the self-concept of the individual. Skin disorders may interfere with social relationships, roles, and sexuality. Stress may also trigger or exacerbate skin disorders. The type of soap or agents used as part of the cleansing routine may contribute to dry, oily, itchy skin, or rashes. Hairstyling methods, use of hair products, and chemical curling or bleaching may be factors in damage, breakage, or loss of hair.

ANATOMY AND PHYSIOLOGY REVIEW

The skin is composed of the epidermal, dermal, and subcutaneous layers. The cutaneous glands, which are located in the dermal layer, release secretions to lubricate the skin and to assist in temperature regulation. The hair and nails are composed of keratinized (hardened) cells and serve to protect the skin and the ends of the fingers and toes. Each of these anatomical structures is described in the following paragraphs.

Skin and Glands

The skin has two distinct layers. The outer layer, called the **epidermis**, is firmly attached to an underlying layer called the **dermis**. Deep in the dermis is a layer of subcutaneous tissue that anchors the skin to the underlying body structures.

Epidermis

The epidermis is a layer of epithelial tissue that forms the outermost portion of the skin. Where exposure to friction is greatest, such as on the fingertips, palms, and soles of the feet, the epidermis consists of five layers (or strata), as shown in Figure 11.1. These five layers are, from deep to superficial, the stratum basale, stratum spinosum, stratum granulosum, stratum lucidum, and stratum corneum.

New skin cells are formed in the stratum basale, or basal layer, which is also known as the stratum germinativum (germinating layer). These new skin cells consist mostly of a fibrous protein called **keratin**, which gives the epidermis its tough, protective qualities. About 25% of the cells in the stratum basale are *melanocytes*, which produce the skin pigment called **melanin**. All humans have the same relative number of melanocytes, but the amount of melanin they produce varies according to genetic, hormonal, and environmental factors.

Cells produced in the stratum basale gradually move through the layers of the epidermis toward the stratum corneum, where they are sloughed off. The abundance of keratin in

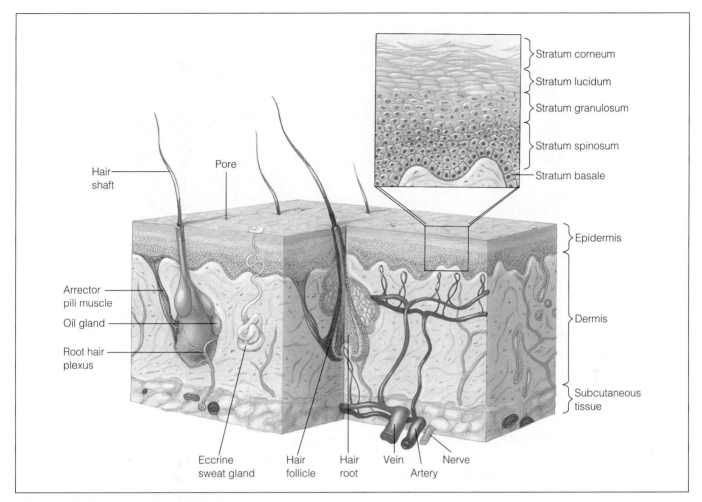

Figure 11.1 • Skin structure. Three-dimensional view of the skin, subcutaneous tissue, glands, and hairs.

this tough "horny layer" protects against abrasion and trauma, repels water, resists water loss, and renders the body insensitive to a variety of environmental toxins.

Dermis

The dermis is a layer of connective tissue that lies just below the epidermis. The dermis consists mainly of two types of fibres: collagen, which gives the skin its toughness and enables it to resist tearing, and the elastic fibres, which give the skin its elasticity. The dermis is richly supplied with nerves, blood vessels, and lymphatic vessels, and it is embedded with hair follicles, sweat glands, oil glands, and sensory receptors.

Subcutaneous Tissue

The subcutaneous tissue (or **hypodermis**) is a loose connective tissue that stores approximately half of the body's fat cells. Thus, it cushions the body against trauma, insulates the body from heat loss, and stores fat for energy.

Cutaneous Glands

The cutaneous glands are formed in the stratum basale and push deep into the dermis. They release their secretions through ducts onto the skin surface.

Sudoriferous (sweat) glands come in two types: eccrine and apocrine. **Eccrine glands** are more numerous and more widely distributed. They produce a clear perspiration made up mostly of water and salts, which they release into funnel-shaped pores at the skin surface. **Apocrine glands** are found primarily in the axillary and anogenital regions. They are dormant until the onset of puberty. Apocrine glands produce a secretion made up of water, salts, fatty acids, and proteins, which is released into hair follicles. When apocrine sweat mixes with bacteria on the skin surface, it assumes a musky odour.

Oil Glands

Oil glands, or **sebaceous glands**, are distributed over most of the body except the palms of the hands and soles of the feet. They produce *sebum,* an oily secretion composed of fat and keratin that is usually released into hair follicles.

The major functions of the skin are the following:

- Perceiving touch, pressure, temperature, and pain via the nerve endings
- Protecting against mechanical, chemical, thermal, and solar damage
- Protecting against loss of water and electrolytes
- Regulating body temperature

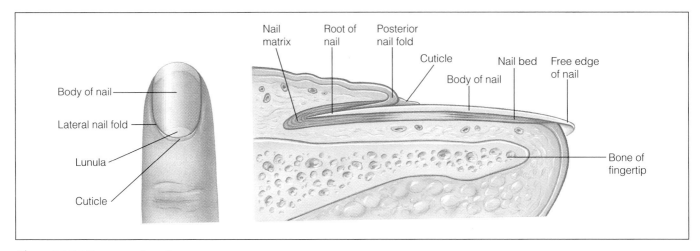

Figure 11.2 ● Structure of a nail.

- Repairing surface wounds through cellular replacement
- Synthesizing vitamin D
- Allowing identification through uniqueness of facial contours, skin and hair colour, and fingerprints

The major functions of the cutaneous glands are the following:

- Excreting uric acid, urea, ammonia, sodium, potassium, and other metabolic wastes
- Regulating temperature through evaporation of perspiration on the skin surface
- Protecting against bacterial growth on the skin surface
- Softening, lubricating, and waterproofing skin and hair
- Resisting water loss from the skin surface in low-humidity environments
- Protecting deeper skin regions from bacteria on the skin surface

Hair

A **hair** is a thin, flexible, elongated fibre composed of dead, keratinized cells that grow out in a columnar fashion (Figure 11.1). Each hair shaft arises from a follicle. Nerve endings in the follicle are sensitive to the slightest movement of the hair. Each hair follicle also has an arrector pili muscle that causes the hair to contract and stand upright when a person is under stress or exposed to cold.

The deep end of each follicle expands to form a hair bulb. New cells are produced at the hair bulb. Hair growth is cyclic; scalp hair typically has an active phase of about 4 years and a resting phase of a few months. Because these phases are not synchronous, only a small percentage of a person's hair follicles shed their hair at any given time.

Hair colour is determined by the amount of melanin produced in the hair follicle. Black or brown hair contains the greatest amount of melanin.

The type and distribution of hair vary in different parts of the body. **Vellus hair**, a pale, fine, short strand, grows over the entire body except for the lips, the nipples, the palms of the hands, the soles of the feet, and parts of the external genitals.

The **terminal hair** of the eyebrows and scalp is usually darker, coarser, and longer. At puberty, hormones signal the growth of terminal hair in the axillae, pubic region, and legs of both sexes, and on the face and chest of most males.

The major functions of the hair are to insulate against heat and cold, protect against ultraviolet and infrared rays, perceive movement or touch, protect the eyes from sweat, and protect the nasal passages from foreign particles.

Nails

Nails are thin plates of keratinized epidermal cells that shield the distal ends of the fingers and toes (see Figure 11.2). Nail growth occurs at the nail matrix as new cells arise from the basal layer of the epidermis. As the nail cells grow out from the matrix, they form a transparent layer, called the body of the nail, which extends over the nail bed. The nail body appears pink because of the blood supply in the underlying dermis. A moon-shaped crescent called a **lunula** appears on the nail body over the thickened nail matrix. A fold of epidermal skin called a **cuticle** protects the root and sides of each nail. The major functions of the nails are to protect the tips of the fingers and toes and aid in picking up small objects, grasping, and scratching.

SPECIAL CONSIDERATIONS

Throughout the assessment process, the nurse gathers subjective and objective data regarding the client's state of health. By using critical thinking and the nursing process, the nurse identifies many factors to be considered when collecting the data, including age, developmental level, race, ethnicity, work history, living conditions, social economics, and emotional well-being.

Developmental Considerations

Growth and development are dynamic processes that describe change over time. Data collection and interpretation of these findings in relation to normative values is important. The following discussion presents specific variations for different age groups.

Infants and Children

At birth, the newborn's skin typically is covered with **vernix caseosa**, a white, cheeselike mixture of sebum and epidermal cells. The skin colour of newborns is often bright red for the first 24 hours of life and then fades. Some newborns develop physiological jaundice 3 to 4 days after birth, resulting in a yellowing of the skin, sclera, and mucous membranes. Jaundice can occur within the first 24 hours after birth or as late as 7 days postnatally. Physiological jaundice is a temporary condition treated with fluids and phototherapy. The skin of dark-skinned newborns normally is not fully pigmented until 2 to 3 months after birth. An infant's skin is very thin, soft, and free of terminal hair.

Many harmless skin markings are common in newborns. For example, they may have areas of tiny white facial papules. These are called **milia** and are due to sebum that collects in the openings of hair follicles (see Figure 11.3). Milia usually disappear spontaneously within a few weeks of birth. Vascular markings are also common. These may include stork bites, which are irregular red or pink patches found most commonly on the back of the neck. Vascular markings disappear spontaneously within a year of birth. The newborn may also have transient mottling or other transient colour changes, such as harlequin colour change, in which a side-lying infant becomes markedly pink on the lower side and pale on the higher side. **Mongolian spots** are grey, blue, or purple spots in the sacral and buttocks areas of newborns (see Figure 11.4). Mongolian spots occur in about 90% of Black newborns and in about 80% of Asian or Aboriginal newborns. Mongolian spots fade during the first year of life. Because the subcutaneous fat layer is poorly developed in infants and the eccrine sweat glands do not secrete until the first few months of life, their temperature regulation is inefficient and absorption of topical medications is increased. The fine, downy hair of the newborn, called **lanugo**, is replaced within a few months by vellus hair. Hair growth accelerates throughout childhood.

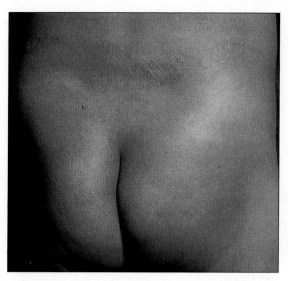

Figure 11.4 Mongolian spots.

Throughout childhood, the epidermis thickens, pigmentation increases, and more subcutaneous fat is deposited, especially in females during puberty. During adolescence, both the sweat glands and the oil glands increase their production. Increased production of sebum by the oil glands predisposes adolescents to develop acne (see Figure 11.5). Increased axillary perspiration occurs as the apocrine glands mature, and body odour may develop for the first time. Pubic and axillary hair appears during adolescence, and males may develop facial and chest hair.

The Pregnant Female

Pigmentation of the skin commonly increases during pregnancy, especially in the areolae, nipples, vulva, and perianal area. Approximately 70% of pregnant women develop hyperpigmented patches on the face referred to as **chloasma**, melasma, gravidum, or "the mask of pregnancy" (see Figure 11.6). This

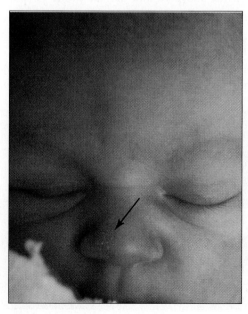

Figure 11.3 ● Milia.

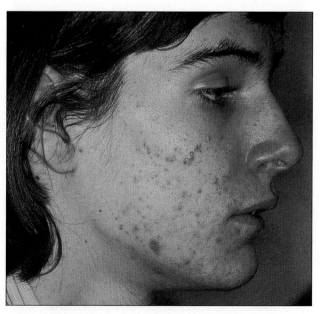

Figure 11.5 Acne.

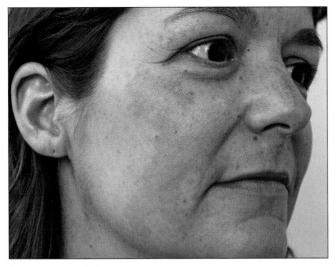

Figure 11.6 • Melasma.

normal condition disappears after pregnancy in some women but may be permanent in others. Some pregnant clients may also have a dark line called a **linea nigra** running from the umbilicus to the pubic area (see Figure 11.7), increased pigmentation of the areolae and nipples, and darkened moles and scars. These are all normal findings.

Many pregnant females develop striae gravidarum (stretch marks) across the abdomen. These usually fade after pregnancy but do not disappear entirely. Cutaneous tags are not uncommon, especially on the neck and upper chest.

Hormonal changes may cause the oil and sweat glands to become hyperactive during pregnancy. This increased secretion may in turn lead to a worsening of acne in the first trimester of pregnancy and an improvement in the third trimester. As more hairs enter the growth phase under hormonal influences in pregnancy, more than the usual number of hairs reach maturity and fall out in the postpartum period during months 1 to 5. Usually all hair grows back by 6 to 15 months postpartum.

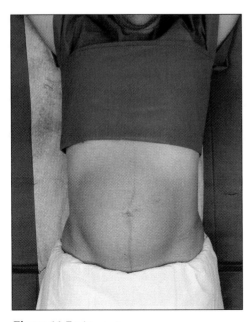

Figure 11.7 • Linea nigra.

The Older Adult

As the skin ages, the epidermis thins and stretches out, and collagen and elastin fibres decrease, causing decreased skin elasticity and increased skin wrinkling. The skin becomes slack and may hang loosely on the frame. It may sag, especially beneath the chin and eyes, in the breasts of females, and in the scrotum of males.

The older client's skin is also more delicate and more susceptible to injury. Decreased production of sebum leads to dryness of both the skin and the hair. The skin may appear especially thin on the dorsal surfaces of the hands and feet and over the bony prominences. Tenting of the skin is common (see Figure 11.8). The sweat glands also decrease their activity, and the older adult perspires less. Decreased melanin production leads to a heightened sensitivity to sunlight, and skin cancer rates increase with age.

Some light-skinned older clients may appear pale because of decreased vascularity in the dermis, even though they may be healthy and well oxygenated. The colour of a dark-skinned elderly person may appear dull, grey, or darker for the same reason.

A variety of lesions are common in older adults. For example, the skin of many older clients may develop senile *lentigines* (liver spots), which look like hyperpigmented freckles, most commonly on the backs of the hands and the arms (see Figure 11.9). Cherry angiomas are small, bright-red spots common in older adults (see Figure 11.10). They increase in number with age. Cutaneous tags may appear on the neck and upper chest (see Figure 11.11), and cutaneous horns may occur on any part of the face (see Figure 11.12).

The hair becomes increasingly grey as melanin production decreases. Hair thins as the number of active hair follicles decreases. Facial hair may become coarser.

The nails may show little change, or they may show the effects of decreased circulation in the body extremities, appearing thicker, harder, yellowed, oddly shaped, or opaque. They may be brittle and peel, and may be prone to splitting and breaking.

Psychosocial Considerations

Stress may exacerbate certain such skin conditions as rashes or acne. Stress may also be a factor in compulsive behaviours, such

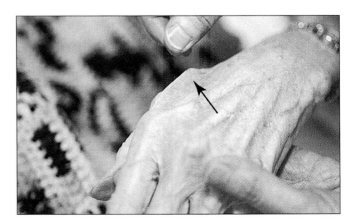

Figure 11.8 • Tenting.

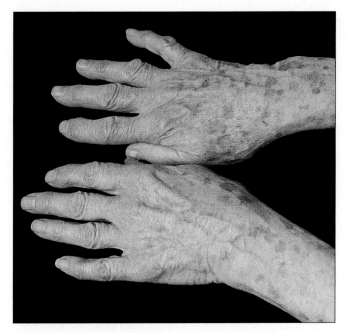

Figure 11.9 ● Senile lentigines.

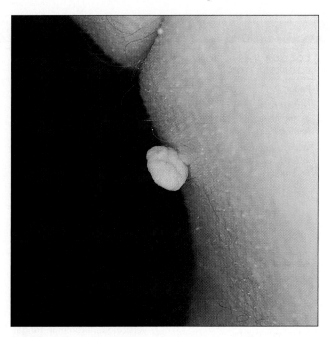

Figure 11.11 ● Cutaneous tag.

as trichotillomania (hair twisting or plucking) and nail biting, signalled by nails that have no visible free edge or that have short, jagged edges. A lack of cleanliness of the skin, hair, or nails also may result from emotional distress, poor self-esteem, or a disturbed body image. If appropriate, the nurse should refer the client to social services or a mental health professional for assistance.

A visible skin disorder may trigger psychosocial health problems leading to social isolation, a body image disturbance, or a self-esteem disturbance. If appropriate, the client should be assessed further for the presence of emotional distress or anxiety related to a skin disorder.

Social and Ethnocultural Considerations

A client's culture, socioeconomic status, home environment, and means of employment may affect the health of the skin, hair, and nails. If the client's skin, hair, and nails appear unclean, the nurse should consider the client's job, socioeconomic status,

and living situation. A client who seems unkempt may have just come from a physically demanding job or may be ill, have a disability, or be depressed.

Changes in skin colour may be difficult to evaluate in clients with dark skin. It is helpful to inspect areas of the body with less pigmentation, such as the lips, oral mucosa, sclerae, palms of the hands, and conjunctivae of the inner eyelids. The nurse must be careful not to mistake the normal deposition of melanin in the lips of some olive to dark-skinned people for cyanosis. Some individuals with dark skin have increased pigmentation in the creases of the palms and soles, and yellow or brown-tinged sclerae. These are normal findings (see Table 11.1 for evaluating colour variations in light and dark skin).

Dry skin does not necessarily indicate dehydration and in fact may be normal for the dark-skinned client. Additionally, since many clients use petroleum-based products to lubricate their skin, the nurse should ask about self-care before concluding that the client has oily skin.

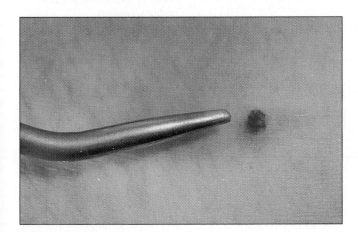

Figure 11.10 Cherry angioma.

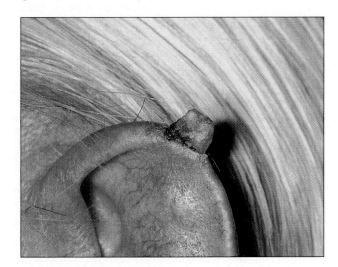

Figure 11.12 Cutaneous horn.

TABLE 11.1 | Colour Variations in Light and Dark Skin

COLOUR VARIATION/ LOCALIZATION	POSSIBLE CAUSES	APPEARANCE IN LIGHT SKIN	APPEARANCE IN DARK SKIN
Pallor *Loss of colour in skin caused by the absence of oxygenated hemoglobin.* Widespread, but most apparent in face, mouth, conjunctivae, and nails.	May be caused by sympathetic nervous stimulation resulting in peripheral vasoconstriction caused by smoking, a cold environment, or stress. May also be caused by decreased tissue perfusion caused by cardiopulmonary disease, shock and hypotension, lack of oxygen, or prolonged elevation of a body part. May also be caused by anemia.	White skin loses its rosy tones. Skin with natural yellow tones appears more yellow; may be mistaken for mild jaundice.	Black skin loses its red undertones and appears ash-grey. Brown skin becomes yellow-tinged. Skin looks dull.
Absence of Colour *Congenital or acquired loss of melanin pigment.* Congenital loss is typically generalized, and acquired loss is typically patchy.	Generalized depigmentation may be caused by albinism. Localized depigmentation may be due to vitiligo or tinea versicolour, a common fungal infection.	Albinism appears as white skin, white or pale blond hair, and pink irises. Vitiligo appears as patchy milk-white areas, especially around the mouth. Tinea versicolour appears as patchy areas paler than the surrounding skin.	Albinism appears as white skin, white or pale blond hair, and pink irises. Vitiligo is very noticeable as patchy milk-white areas. Tinea versicolour appears as patchy areas paler than the surrounding skin.
Cyanosis *Mottled blue colour in skin caused by inadequate tissue perfusion with oxygenated blood.* Most apparent in the nails, lips, oral mucosa, and tongue.	Systemic or central cyanosis is due to cardiac disease, pulmonary disease, heart malformations, and low hemoglobin levels. Localized or peripheral cyanosis is due to vasoconstriction, exposure to cold, and emotional stress.	The skin, lips, and mucous membranes look blue-tinged. The conjunctivae and nail beds are blue.	The skin may appear a shade darker. Cyanosis may be undetectable except for the lips, tongue, and oral mucous membranes, nail beds, and conjunctivae, which appear pale or blue-tinged.
Reddish Blue Tone *Ruddy tone caused by an increased hemoglobin and stasis of blood in capillaries.* Most apparent in the face, mouth, hands, feet, and conjunctivae.	Polycythemia vera, an overproduction of red blood cells, granulocytes, and platelets.	Reddish purple hue.	Difficult to detect. The normal skin colour may appear darker in some clients. Check lips for redness.
Erythema *Redness of the skin caused by increased visibility of normal oxyhemoglobin.* Generalized or on face and upper chest or localized to area of inflammation or exposure.	Hyperemia, a dilatation and congestion of blood in superficial arteries. Caused by fever, a warm environment, local inflammation, allergy, emotions (blushing or embarrassment), exposure to extreme cold, consumption of alcohol, dependent position of body extremity.	Readily identifiable over entire body or in localized areas. Local inflammation and redness are accompanied by higher temperature at the site.	Generalized redness may be difficult to detect. Localized areas of inflammation appear purple or darker than surrounding skin. May be accompanied by higher temperature, hardness, swelling.
Jaundice *Yellow undertone caused by increased bilirubin in the blood.* Generalized but most apparent in the conjunctivae and mucous membranes.	Increased bilirubin may be due to liver disease, biliary obstruction, or hemolytic disease following infections, severe burns, or resulting from sickle-cell anemia or pernicious anemia.	Generalized. Also visible in sclerae, oral mucosa, hard palate, fingernails, palms of the hands, and soles of the feet.	Visible in the sclerae, oral mucosa, junction of hard and soft palate, palms of the hands, and soles of the feet.

(continued)

The skin's response to stressors, such as ultraviolet radiation, is similar in all races. Dark-skinned clients tan, and their skin suffers the same damaging effects from the sun, although skin damage may take longer to occur. Therefore, assessment of colour, texture, moles, and other lesions should be as thorough as for light-skinned clients.

Calluses (circumscribed, painless thickenings of the epidermis) tend to form on parts of the body that are regularly

TABLE 11.1	Colour Variations in Light and Dark Skin *(continued)*			
Carotenemia *Yellow-orange tinge caused by increased levels of carotene in the blood and skin.* Most apparent in face, palms of the hands, and soles of the feet.	Excess carotene from ingestion of foods high in carotene, such as carrots, egg yolks, sweet potatoes, milk, and fats. Also may be seen in clients with anorexia nervosa or endocrine disorders, such as diabetes mellitus, myxedema (skin changes and swelling usually caused by hypothyroidism), and hypopituitarism (decreased production of pituitary hormones).	Yellow-orange seen in forehead, palms, soles. No yellowing of sclerae or mucous membranes.	Yellow-orange tinge most visible in palms of the hands and soles of the feet. No yellowing of sclerae or mucous membranes.
Uremia *Pale yellow tone caused by retention of urinary chromogens in the blood.* Generalized if perceptible.	Chronic renal disease, in which blood levels of nitrogenous wastes increase. Increased melanin may also contribute, and anemia is usually present as well.	Generalized pallor and yellow tinge but does not affect conjunctivae or mucous membranes. Skin may show bruising.	Very difficult to discern because the yellow tinge is very pale and does not affect conjunctivae or mucous membranes. Rely on laboratory and other data.
Brown *An increase in the production and deposition of melanin.* Generalized or localized.	May be due to Addison's disease or a pituitary tumour. Localized increase in facial pigmentation may be caused by hormonal changes during pregnancy or the use of birth control pills. More commonly caused by exposure to ultraviolet radiation from the sun or from tanning beds.	With endocrine disorders, general bronzed skin. Hyperpigmentation in nipples, palmar creases, genitals, and pressure points. Sun exposure causes red tinge in pale skin, and olive-toned skin tans with little or no reddening.	With endocrine disorders, general deepening of skin tone. Hyperpigmentation in nipples, genitals, and pressure points. Sun exposure leads to tanning in various degrees from brown to black.

exposed to pressure, weight bearing, or friction. Common sites of calluses include the fingers, palms, toes, and soles of the feet.

Differences in hair colour and texture are widely variable among cultural groups. Individuals of Asian origins tend to have straight, dark hair. Scandinavians typically have very light, blond hair. Black people may have straight, kinky, or braided hair, and it can often be dry.

The client's occupation (e.g., gardener, mechanic) may make it difficult to keep the fingers and nails unstained. Chemicals used in certain occupations and tobacco may stain the nails. The client's occupation may require frequent or prolonged immersion of the hands in water, which may lead to paronychia (an infection that occurs at the sides or base of a nail). The nail plates of dark-skinned clients may show dark pigmented streaks, which are normal findings.

Many clients use therapies that are not part of standard Western treatment. Among some cultures, coining and cupping are used in treatment for a variety of illnesses. These alternative therapies include using coins, cups, or pinching on areas of the body. The use of this therapy results in lesions, welts, or bruises. These lesions can suggest abuse. Therefore, the nurse must inquire about cultural healing practices.

Social and Ethnocultural Considerations

- Skin colour variations exist across all ethnic groups. Assessment for oxygenation, jaundice, and petechiae in dark-skinned clients requires examination of nail bed refill, sclera, and mucous membranes, respectively.
- Light-skinned clients are at higher risk for skin cancer than dark-skinned clients.
- Black clients have an increased incidence of inflammatory skin diseases.
- Clients who are Black or of Chinese or Aboriginal ancestry have an increased incidence of Mongolian spots on the sacral area.
- Melasma (mask of pregnancy) occurs more frequently in dark-skinned women.
- Dark-skinned individuals may have pigmented streaks in their nails.

- Clients may have religious or spiritual beliefs regarding the cutting of hair.
- Covering the head and hair are common for some groups of people.
- Touching the head is discouraged in some ethnocultural groups.
- Tattoos and body piercing are common and, for some, are part of religious or spiritual practices.
- Some clients will be sensitive about disrobing for the assessment of the skin.
- Linguistic and ethnocultural factors need to be considered to avoid miscommunication and misinterpretation of information about assessment and diagnosis, such as when caring for new immigrants and refugees.
- Females may require the presence of another female during physical assessment of the skin, especially when the examiner is male.

GATHERING THE DATA

Assessment of the integumentary system includes gathering subjective and objective data about the skin, hair, and nails. Subjective data collection occurs during the health history, before the actual physical assessment. The nurse will use a variety of communication techniques to elicit general and specific information about the condition of the client's skin, hair, and nails. Health records and the results of laboratory tests are important secondary sources to be reviewed and included in the data-gathering process. In physical assessment of the integumentary system, the techniques of inspection and palpation will be used. The questions in the health history form part of the subjective data and provide valuable information to meet the objectives related to integumentary health.

HEALTH HISTORY

The health history for the integumentary system concerns data related to the structures and functions of that system. Subjective data related to the condition of the skin, hair, and nails are gathered during the health history. The nurse must be prepared to observe the client and listen for cues related to the integumentary system. The nurse may use closed or open-ended questions to obtain information. A number of follow-up questions or requests for descriptions may be required to clarify data or gather missing information. Follow-up questions are used to identify the source of problems, determine the duration of difficulties, identify measures to alleviate problems, and provide clues about the client's knowledge of his or her own health.

The health history guides the physical assessment of the integumentary system. The information is always considered in relation to norms and expectations about the function of the integument. Therefore, the nurse must consider age, gender, race, culture, environment, health practices, and past and concurrent problems and therapies when forming questions and using techniques to elicit information. To address all the factors when conducting a health history, specific questions related to the skin, hair, and nail status and function have been developed. These questions focus on the most common concerns or injuries associated with the skin, hair, and nails; questions related to past health history; questions related to behaviours; questions that address environmental concerns; and those that are specific to clients according to age, including the pregnant female.

The nurse must consider the client's ability to participate in the health history and physical assessment. Further, the nurse must consider that the appearance of the skin has an impact on self-image. A client with clear, healthy skin may have a heightened self-esteem. Clients with changes in the skin caused by the normal aging process or from skin disorders may be anxious about the way they appear to others. Clients with visible skin disorders are often sensitive about the condition and their appearance. The nurse must select communication techniques that demonstrate caring and preserve the dignity of the client.

As the nurse gathers the data, she or he will shift the type of questions to direct questions that give the client room to explain or qualify. The mnemonic O-P-Q-R-S-T-U, which stands for onset (chronology), precipitating (or palliative), quality, region (or radiation), severity, timing, and understanding, will help the learner remember the dimensions of the symptoms. The nurse will keep in mind that not all these qualifiers will apply to each symptom.

GATHERING THE DATA

HEALTH HISTORY QUESTIONS

RATIONALES

The following sections provide sample questions and follow-up questions. Rationales for some questions are provided. The list of questions is not all-inclusive but rather represents the more common concern or injury questions required in a health history related to the skin, hair, and nails. An example of using O-P-Q-R-S-T-U with pain is provided.

Questions Related to Common Concerns or Injuries

The most common concerns related to illness or injury of the skin, hair, and nails are as follows:

Skin
- Pain
- Rash or lesions
- Pruritus (itching)
- Changes in skin colour

HEALTH HISTORY QUESTIONS	RATIONALES

1. Pain
- Are you having any pain to your skin at this time? *If yes:*
- When did you first notice the pain? How long does it last? *Onset (chronology)*
- What makes the pain worse? What makes the pain better? *Precipitating (palliative)*
- Can you describe the pain? Is it sharp? dull? burning? *Quality*
- Does the pain radiate or spread to other locations? *Radiation*

▶ Pain in particular areas, such as in body folds (between the toes, under the breast, etc.), may signal bacterial and fungal infections.

- How often do you experience the pain? How would you rate the pain on a scale of 1 to 10, with 10 being the worst pain? *Severity*
- Is the pain associated with anything that you have noticed? *Timing*
- What do you think is causing the pain? *Understanding*

2. Rashes or lesions
- Have you ever had a skin problem?

▶ The client has an opportunity to provide information about specific skin problems or illnesses.

- Do you have any sores or ulcers on your body that are slow in healing?

▶ Delayed healing or frequent skin infections may be a sign of diabetes mellitus or inadequate nutrition.

- Have you noticed any rashes on your body? Where did it start? Did it spread? When did you first notice it?

▶ These factors may help in determining the cause.

- Does the rash occur more after wearing certain clothes or jewellery?

▶ Rashes related to clothing, jewellery, or cosmetics may be due to contact dermatitis, a type of allergy.

- Does the rash occur after taking medication?

▶ Many medications, such as Aspirin, antibiotics, and barbiturates, cause allergic skin reactions. A drug reaction can occur even if the client has been taking the drug for a long time.

- Have you noticed any other lesions, lumps, bumps, tender spots, or painful areas on your body?

▶ The time of onset and pattern of development may help determine the sources of the problem. For instance, certain patterns of bruises may signal frequent falls or physical abuse.

3. Pruritis
- Does your skin itch? If so, where? How severe is it? When does it occur?

▶ These questions may help in determining if the itching is due to an allergic reaction or eczema.

- Has your skin become either oilier or drier recently?

▶ Metabolic disorders or simple age-related changes in the production of sebum may produce changes in the texture of the skin. Pruritis associated with dryness needs to be examined and may indicate other disorders.

4. Changes in skin colour
- Have you noticed any changes in the colour of your skin? If so, has the change occurred over your entire body or only in one area?

▶ Widespread or localized colour changes may indicate the presence of a disorder.

- Have you noticed a change in the size, colour, shape, or appearance of any moles or birthmarks? Are they painful? Do they itch? bleed?

▶ Any changes in a mole or birthmark may signal a skin cancer.

GATHERING THE DATA

Health History Questions

Rationales

- Do you perform a self-examination of your skin on a routine basis?

▶ The nurse should provide teaching on how to perform a skin self-examination. (see Box 11.1).

BOX 11.1	Self-Examination of the Skin

The nurse should teach all clients the steps for examining their own skin:

1. Use a room that is well lit and has a full-length mirror. Have a hand-held mirror and chair available. Remove all your clothes.

2. Examine all your skin surface, front and back. Begin with your hands, including the spaces between your fingers. Continue with your arms, chest, abdomen, pubic area, thighs, lower legs, and toes. Next examine your face and neck. Make sure you inspect your underarms, the sides of your trunk, the back of your neck, the buttocks, and the soles of your feet.

3. Next, sit down with one leg elevated. Use the hand-held mirror to examine the inside of the elevated leg, from the groin area to the foot. Repeat on the other leg.

4. Use the hand-held mirror to inspect your scalp.

5. Consult your physician promptly if you see any newly pigmented area or if any existing mole has changed in colour, size, shape, or elevation. Also report sores that do not heal; redness or swelling around a growth or lesion; a change in sensation, such as itching, pain, tenderness, or numbness, in a lesion or the skin around it; and a change in the texture or consistency of the skin.

Hair

1. **Changes in hair patterns, distribution, or texture**
   - Have you noticed an increase in hair loss recently?

▶ Progressive diffuse hair loss is natural in some men. Hair loss in women that follows a male pattern may be due to an imbalance of adrenal hormones. When patches of hair fall out, the nurse should suspect trauma to the scalp caused by chemicals, infections, or blows to the head. Some people with psychological disorders pull or twist their hair, causing it to fall out. If hair loss is distributed over the entire head, it may be caused by a systemic disease or fungal infection. Abnormal hair loss sometimes follows an illness with fever.

   - Are you taking any prescription or over-the-counter medication?

▶ Certain medications can change the texture of the hair or lead to hair loss. For instance, oral contraceptives may change the hair texture or rate of hair growth in some women, and drugs used in the treatment of circulatory disorders and cancer may result in a temporary generalized hair loss over the entire body.

HEALTH HISTORY QUESTIONS	RATIONALES

Nails

1. **Changes in nail colour, consistency, or shape**
   - Describe your nails now.

▶ Ridged, brittle, split, or peeling fingernails may be caused by protein or vitamin B deficiencies. Changes in circulation may affect the nails. Newly acquired longitudinal lines may signal a nevus or melanoma in the nail root. Dark lines may be normal, especially in dark-skinned clients, or associated with some medications, including antiretrovirals.

   - Have you noticed any pain, swelling, or drainage around your cuticles?

▶ Infection of the cuticles could be due to an ingrown nail or the use of contaminated instruments during a manicure or pedicure.

   - Are you taking any prescription or over-the-counter medication?

▶ Some medications may cause nail changes in some clients. For example, clients who have been treated with the antiretroviral drug zidovudine (Retrovir, AZT) can develop dark, longitudinal lines on all of their fingernails.

Questions Related to Past Health History

1. **Have you ever been diagnosed with an illness of the skin, hair, or nails?**

2. **History of skin disorders**
   - Is there a history of allergies, rashes, or other skin problems in your family?

▶ Some allergies and skin disorders are familial; thus, the client may be predisposed. Follow-up is required to obtain details about specific problems and their occurrence, treatments, and outcomes.

   - Do you have or have you had a skin infection?

▶ If an infection is identified, follow-up about the date of infection, treatments, and outcomes is required. Data about each infection identified by the client are essential to an accurate health assessment. Infections can be classified as acute or chronic, and follow-up regarding each classification will differ.

Questions Related to Behaviours

Healthcare behaviours include both health practices and health patterns. Health practices consist of following recommendations for disease prevention, including screening for risks, screening for early detection of problems, and immunization. Health patterns are habits or acts that affect the client's health. Health behaviours may also include seeking healthcare from healthcare providers who use alternative methods to diagnose and treat illness. Clients should be questioned in a nonjudgmental way and areas for health teaching should be identified.

1. **Do you sunbathe? Have you ever sunbathed or used tanning beds?**

▶ Excessive exposure to ultraviolet radiation thickens and damages the skin, depresses the immune system, and alters the DNA in skin cells, predisposing an individual to cancer.

2. **Do you spend time in the sun exercising or playing sports? Do you work outdoors?**

3. **How does your skin react to sun exposure?**
   - Do you use a sunscreen with sun protection factor (SPF) when spending time in the sun?

HEALTH HISTORY QUESTIONS	RATIONALES
• What SPF sunscreen do you use? Do you reapply the lotion after several hours or after swimming?	► The ultraviolet radiation that causes a sunburn is capable of disabling cells that initiate the normal immune response. Individuals who burn easily or have a history of serious sunburns may have a greater risk for developing skin cancer.
4. Do you remember having a sunburn that left blisters?	► A history of blistering sunburn increases the risk for skin cancer, especially if the sunburn occurred in childhood.
5. How do you care for your skin? • What kind of soap, cleansers, toners, or other treatments do you use? • How do you clean your clothes? • What kind of detergent do you use? • How often do you bathe or shower?	► Some skin products and laundry detergents may affect the skin of some clients. Infrequent cleansing of the skin increases the likelihood of skin infections, whereas excessive bathing decreases protective skin oils.
6. Do you now have or have you ever had a tattoo? • How long have you had the tattoo? Have you had any problems with that area of the skin? • Further follow-up would include questions related to treatment and outcomes if skin problems accompanied tattoos.	► Tattoos can cause skin irritation, and the process of tattooing puts an individual at risk for infection, hepatitis C, and HIV.
7. Do you now have or have you ever had a piercing of any part of your body? • Where are the sites of the piercing? • How long have you had the piercing? • Have you ever had a problem at the piercing site? What was the problem? Was it treated? • What is the current condition of piercing sites?	► Piercing of any body part puts an individual at risk for infection and hepatitis C and can result in the development of scar tissue at the site.

Questions Related to the Environment

Environment refers to both internal and external environments. Questions related to the internal environment include all the previous questions and those associated with internal or physiological responses. Questions regarding the external environment include those related to home, work, or social environments.

Internal Environment

1. How would you describe your level of stress? Has it changed in the past few weeks? few months? Please describe how.	► Emotional stress may aggravate skin disorders.
2. Are you taking any prescription or over-the-counter medications?	► Clients may experience rashes or other skin eruptions in response to various drugs. Some drugs, such as antibiotics, antihistamines, antipsychotics, oral hypoglycemic agents, and oral contraceptives, can cause an adverse effect if the client is exposed to the sun.
3. Have you changed your diet recently? Have you recently tried any unfamiliar types of food? Please describe.	► Changes in diet or eating new foods may cause rashes and other skin reactions.
4. Has the condition of your skin affected your social relationships in any way? Has it limited you in any way? If so, how?	► Skin problems may affect a person's self-concept and body image and interfere with social relationships, roles, and sexuality, especially in adolescents and young adults. Serious skin problems may also affect a person's ability to maintain a job.

HEALTH HISTORY QUESTIONS	RATIONALES

5. Female clients: Are you pregnant? If not, are you menstruating regularly? Describe your menstrual periods.

▶ The skin may be affected by changes in hormonal balance.

External Environment

The following questions deal with substances and irritants found in the physical environment of the client. The physical environment includes the indoor and outdoor environments of the home and the workplace, those encountered for social engagements, and any encountered during travel.

1. Have you been exposed recently to extremes in temperature?
- If so, when? How long was the exposure? Where did this occur?

▶ Extremes in environmental temperature may exacerbate skin disorders.

2. Do you work in an environment where radioisotopes or X-rays are used?
- If so, are you vigilant about following precautions and using protective gear?

▶ Excessive exposure to X-rays or radioisotopes may predispose a client to skin cancer.

3. Do you wear gloves for work? If so, what types of gloves?

▶ Certain types of gloves, especially latex, can cause mild to severe skin allergic reactions.

4. How often do you travel?
- Have you travelled recently?
- If so, where?
- Have you come into contact with anyone who has a similar rash?

▶ The nurse should suspect unfamiliar foods, water, plants, or insects as potential causes of rashes and other skin problems if the client has travelled recently. In addition, some rashes, such as measles and impetigo, are contagious.

5. Does your job or hobby require you to perform repetitive tasks? to work with any chemicals?
- Does your job or hobby require you to wear a specific type of helmet, hat, goggles, gloves, or shoes?

▶ Regular work with certain tools or regular wearing of ill-fitting helmets, hats, goggles, or shoes may cause skin abrasions. Additionally, the skin absorbs some organic solvents used in industry, such as acetone, dry-cleaning fluid, dyes, formaldehyde, and paint thinner. Excessive exposure to these and other types of irritants may contribute to rashes, skin cancers, or other skin reactions.

Questions Related to Age

The health history must reflect the anatomical and physiological differences that exist along the age span.

Questions Regarding Infants and Children

1. Does the child have any birthmarks? If so, where are they?

2. Has the infant developed an orange hue in the skin?

▶ Ingestion of large amounts of carotene in such vegetables as carrots, sweet potatoes, and squash can cause an orange hue.

3. Does the child have a rash? If so, what seems to cause it?
- Have you introduced any new foods into your child's diet?
- How do you clean the child's diaper area?

▶ Many children may have allergic reactions to certain foods, especially milk, chocolate, and eggs. Infrequent changing of diapers may lead to diaper rash. Harsh detergents may cause skin reactions in some children.

Questions for the Pregnant Female

1. What changes have you noticed in your skin since you became pregnant?

▶ The hormonal changes of pregnancy may cause various benign changes in skin pigmentation, moisture, texture, and vascularity that are entirely normal.

GATHERING THE DATA

Health History Questions

Rationales

2. Do you use any topical medications for problems with the skin, hair, or nails?

▶ Topical medications that can result in birth defects include Retin-A for acne, antifungal agents, and minoxidil for hair growth.

3. Do you use topical medications for other problems? If so, identify the medications.

▶ Many medications that are absorbed through the skin can reach the baby through the bloodstream. Some of these medications, such as antibiotics, steroids, and medications for muscle pain, may harm the developing fetus.

Questions for the Older Adult

1. What changes have you noticed in your skin in the past few years?

▶ The normal changes of aging, such as increased dryness and wrinkling of the skin, may cause distress for some clients.

2. Does your skin itch?

▶ **Pruritus** (itching) increases in incidence with age. It is usually due to dry skin, which may in turn be caused by excessive bathing or use of harsh skin cleansers.

3. Do you experience frequent falls?

▶ Older adults bruise easily. Multiple bruises may result from frequent falls.

Physical Assessment

ASSESSMENT TECHNIQUES AND FINDINGS

Physical assessment of the skin, hair, and nails requires the use of inspection and palpation. Inspection includes looking at the skin, hair, and nails to determine colour, consistency, shape, and hygiene-related factors. Knowledge of norms or expected findings is essential in determining the meaning of the data as the nurse performs the physical assessment.

The skin of the adult should be clean, free from odour, and consistent in colour. It should feel warm and moist and should have a smooth texture. The skin should be mobile with blood vessels visible beneath the surfaces of the abdomen and eyelids. It should be free of lesions except for findings of freckles and birthmarks. The skin is sensitive to touch and temperature.

The scalp and hair in the adult should be clean. Hair colour is determined by the amount of melanin. Grey hair can occur as a result of decreased melanin, genetics, or aging. Hair texture may be coarse or thin. Hair distribution is expected to be even over the scalp. Male pattern baldness is a normal finding. Fine hair is distributed over the body with coarser, darker, longer hair in the axillae and pubic regions in adults. The nails should have a pink undertone and lie flat or form a convex curve on the nail bed.

Physical assessment of the skin, hair, and nails follows an organized pattern. It begins with a survey and inspection of the skin, followed by palpation of the skin. Inspection and palpation of the hair and nails is then carried out. When lesions are present, measurements are used to identify the size of the lesions and the location in relation to accepted landmarks.

> **EQUIPMENT**
> examination gown and drape
> magnifying glass
> examination light
> penlight
> examination gloves, clean and nonsterile
> Wood's lamp (filtered ultraviolet light) for special procedures
> centimetre ruler

PHYSICAL ASSESSMENT

HELPFUL HINTS

- A warm, private environment will reduce client anxiety.
- Provide special instructions and explain the purpose for removal of clothing, jewellery, hairpieces, nail enamel.
- Maintain the client's dignity by using draping techniques.
- Monitor verbal responses to skin conditions that already threaten the client's self-image.
- Be sensitive to cultural issues. In some cultures touching or examination by members of the opposite sex is prohibited.
- Covering the head, hair, face, or skin may be part of religious or cultural beliefs. Provide careful explanations regarding the need to expose these areas for assessment.
- Direct sunlight is best for assessment of the skin; if it is not available, lighting must be strong and direct. Tangential lighting may be helpful in assessment of dark-skinned clients.
- Use routine practices throughout the assessment.

TECHNIQUES AND NORMAL FINDINGS

ABNORMAL FINDINGS AND SPECIAL CONSIDERATIONS

SURVEY

A quick survey enables the nurse to identify any immediate problem and the client's ability to participate in the assessment. The nurse inspects the overall appearance of the client, notes hygiene and odour, and observes for signs of anxiety.

CLINICAL TIP!

The nurse must be alert for the possibility of impending shock if the client has pallor accompanied with a drop in blood pressure, increased pulse and respirations, and marked anxiety. If these cues are present, a physician should be consulted immediately.

▶ Clients experiencing pain or discomfort may not be able to participate in the assessment. Severe pain or distress may require referral to an emergency care facility.

Clients experiencing anxiety may demonstrate pallor and **diaphoresis** (profuse sweating). Acknowledgment of the problem and discussion of the procedures often provide relief.

INSPECTION OF THE SKIN

1. Position the client.
   - The client should be in a sitting position with all clothing removed except the examination gown (see Figure 11.13).

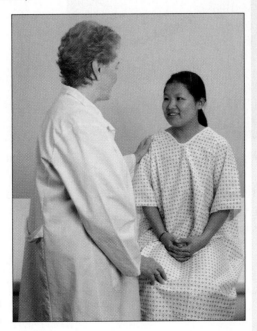

Figure 11.13 ●
Positioning of client.

TECHNIQUES AND NORMAL FINDINGS

ABNORMAL FINDINGS AND SPECIAL CONSIDERATIONS

2. Instruct the client.

- Explain that you will be looking carefully at the client's skin.

3. Observe for cleanliness and use the sense of smell to determine body odour.

- Body odour is produced when bacterial waste products mix with perspiration on the skin surface. During heavy physical activity, body odour increases. Amounts of urea and ammonia are excreted in perspiration.

▶ Urea and ammonia salts are found on the skin of clients with kidney disorders.

4. Observe the client's skin tone.

- Evaluate any widespread colour changes, such as cyanosis, pallor, erythema, or jaundice. For example, always assess cyanotic clients for vital signs and level of consciousness. Use Table 11.1 to evaluate colour variations in light and dark skin.

- The amount of melanin and carotene pigments, the oxygen content of the blood, and the level of exposure to the sun influence skin colour. Dark skin contains large amounts of melanin, while fair skin has small amounts. The skin of most Asians contains a large amount of carotene, which causes a yellow cast.

▶ Cyanosis or pallor indicates abnormally low plasma oxygen, placing the client at risk for altered tissue perfusion. Pallor is seen in anemia.

5. Inspect the skin for even pigmentation over the body.

- In most cases, increased or decreased pigmentation is caused by differences in the distribution of melanin throughout the body. These are normal variations. For example, the margins of the lips, areolae, nipples, and external genitalia are more darkly pigmented. Freckles (see Figure 11.14) and certain *nevi* (congenital marks; see Figure 11.15) occur in people of all skin colours in varying degrees.

▶ For unknown reasons, some people develop patchy depigmented areas over the face, neck, hands, feet, and body folds. This condition is called **vitiligo** (see Figure 11.16). Skin is otherwise normal. Vitiligo occurs in all races in all parts of the world but seems to affect dark-skinned people more severely. Clients with vitiligo may suffer a severe disturbance in body image.

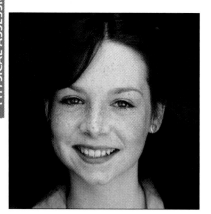

Figure 11.14 ● Freckles.

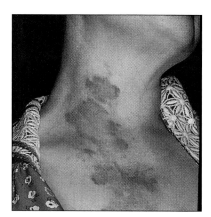

Figure 11.15 ● Nevus.

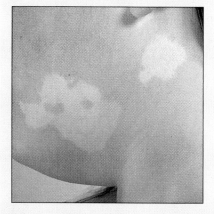

Figure 11.16 ● Vitiligo.

6. Inspect the skin for superficial arteries and veins.

- A fine network of veins or a few dilated blood vessels visible just beneath the surface of the skin are normal findings in areas of the body where skin is thin (e.g., the abdomen and eyelids).

TECHNIQUES AND NORMAL FINDINGS	ABNORMAL FINDINGS AND SPECIAL CONSIDERATIONS

PALPATION OF THE SKIN

1. **Instruct the client.**
   - Explain that you will be touching the client in various areas with different parts of your hand.

2. **Determine the client's skin temperature.**
   - Use the dorsal surface of your hand, which is most sensitive to temperature. Palpate the forehead or face first. Continue to palpate inferiorly, including the hands and feet, comparing the temperature on the right and left side of the body (see Figure 11.17).

   ▶ The temperature of the skin is higher than normal in the presence of a systemic infection or such metabolic disorders as hyperthyroidism, after vigorous activity, and when the external environment is warm.

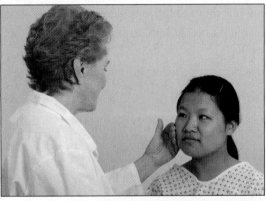

Figure 11.17 ●
Palpating skin temperature.

   - Local skin temperature is controlled by the amount and rate of blood circulating through a body region. Normal temperatures range from mildly cool to slightly warm.

   ▶ The temperature of the skin is lower than normal in the presence of such metabolic disorders as hypothyroidism, or when the external environment is cool. Localized coolness results from decreased circulation caused by vasoconstriction or occlusion, which may occur from peripheral arterial insufficiency.

   - The skin on both sides of the body is warm when tissue is perfused. Sometimes the hands and feet are cooler than the rest of the body, but the temperature is normally similar on both sides.

   ▶ A difference in temperature *bilaterally* may indicate an interruption in or lack of circulation on the cool side caused by compression, immobilization, or elevation. If one side is warmer than normal, inflammation may be present on that side.

3. **Assess the amount of moisture on the skin surface.**
   - Inspect and palpate the face, skin folds, axillae, and palms, where perspiration is most easily detected.

   ▶ Diaphoresis occurs during exertion, fever, pain, and emotional stress and in the presence of some metabolic disorders, such as hyperthyroidism. It may also indicate an impending medical crisis, such as a myocardial infarction.

   - A fine sheen of perspiration or oil is not an abnormal finding, nor is moderately dry skin, especially in cold or dry climates.

   ▶ Severely dry skin typically is dark, weathered, and fissured. Pruritus frequently accompanies dry skin and may lead to abrasion and thickening if prolonged. Generalized dryness may occur in an individual who is dehydrated or has a systemic disorder, such as hypothyroidism.

   ▶ Dry, parched lips and mucous membranes of the mouth are clear indicators of systemic dehydration. These areas should be checked if dehydration is suspected. Dry skin over the lower legs may be due to vascular insufficiency. Localized itching may indicate a skin allergy.

PHYSICAL ASSESSMENT

Techniques and Normal Findings

ABNORMAL FINDINGS AND SPECIAL CONSIDERATIONS

4. Palpate the skin for texture.

- Use the palmar surface of fingers and fingerpads when palpating for texture. Normal skin feels smooth, firm, and even.

▶ The skin may become excessively smooth and velvety in clients with hyperthyroidism, whereas clients with hypothyroidism may have rough, scaly skin.

5. Palpate the skin to determine its thickness.

- The outer layer of the skin is thin and firm over most parts of the body, except the palms, soles of the feet, elbows, and knees, where it is thicker. Normally, the skin over the eyelids and lips is thinner.

▶ Very thin, shiny skin may signal impaired circulation.

6. Palpate the skin for elasticity.

- Elasticity is a combination of turgor (resiliency, or the skin's ability to return to its normal position and shape) and mobility (the skin's ability to be lifted).

- Using the forefinger and thumb, grasp a fold of skin beneath the clavicle or on the medial aspect of the wrist (see Figure 11.18).

▶ When skin turgor is decreased, the skinfold "tents" (holds its pinched formation) and slowly returns to the former position. See Figure 11.8. Decreased turgor occurs when the client is dehydrated or has lost large amounts of weight.

Increased skin turgor may be caused by scleroderma, literally "hard skin," a condition in which the underlying connective tissue becomes scarred and immobile.

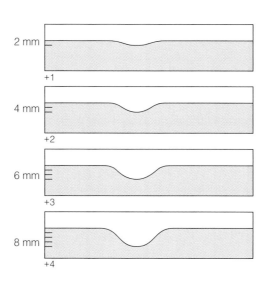

Figure 11.18 ●
Palpating for skin elasticity.

- Notice the reaction of the skin both as you grasp and as you release. Healthy skin is mobile and returns rapidly to its previous shape and position.

- Finally palpate the feet, ankles, and sacrum. Edema is present if your palpation leaves a dent in the skin.

- Grade any edema on a four-point scale: 1 indicates mild edema, and 4 indicates deep edema (see Figure 11.19).

▶ **Edema** is a decrease in skin mobility caused by an accumulation of fluid in the intercellular spaces. Edema makes the skin look puffy, pitted, and tight. It may be most noticeable in the skin of the hands, feet, ankles, and sacral area (see Figure 11.20).

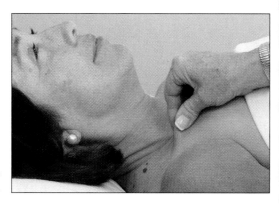

Figure 11.19 ●
Four-point scale for grading edema.

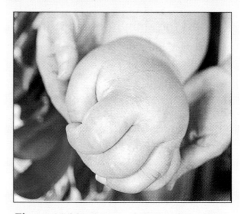

Figure 11.20 ● Edema of the hand.

TECHNIQUES AND NORMAL FINDINGS	ABNORMAL FINDINGS AND SPECIAL CONSIDERATIONS

- Note that because the fluid of edema lies above the pigmented and vascular layers of the skin, skin tone in the client with edema is obscured.

7. **Inspect and palpate the skin for lesions.**

- Lesions of the skin are changes in normal skin structure. **Primary lesions** develop on previously unaltered skin. Lesions that change over time or because of scratching, abrasion, or infection are called **secondary lesions**.

- Carefully inspect the client's body, including skin folds and crevices, by using a good source of light.

- Wear gloves if there are body fluids present. When lesions are observed, palpate lesions between the thumb and index finger. Measure all lesion dimensions (including height, if possible) with a small, clear, flexible ruler.

- Document lesion size in centimetres. If necessary, use a magnifying glass or a penlight for closer inspection (see Figure 11.21).

▶ The periumbilical and flank areas of the body should be observed for the presence of **ecchymosis** (bruising). Ecchymoses in the periumbilical area may signal bleeding somewhere in the abdomen (Cullen's sign). Ecchymoses in the flank area are associated with pancreatitis or bleeding in the peritoneum (Grey Turner's sign). Certain systemic disorders may produce characteristic patterns of lesions on particular body regions. Widespread lesions may indicate systemic or genetic disorders, or allergic reactions. Localized lesions may indicate physical trauma, chemical irritants, or allergic dermatitis. The nurse may want to photograph the client's skin to document the presence, pattern, or spread of certain lesions.

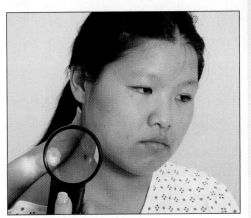

Figure 11.21 •
Using a magnifying glass.

- Shine a Wood's lamp on the skin to distinguish fluorescing lesions.
- Assess any drainage for colour, odour, consistency, amount, and location. If indicated, obtain specimen of the drainage for culture and sensitivity.
- Some fungal infections, including tinea capitis, do not fluoresce.
- Healthy skin is typically smooth and free of lesions; however, some lesions, such as freckles, insect bites, healed scars, and certain birthmarks, are expected findings.

8. **Palpate the skin for sensitivity.**

- Palpate the skin in various regions of the body and ask the client to describe the sensations.
- Give special attention to any pain or discomfort that the client reports, especially when palpating skin lesions.
- Ask the client to describe the sensation as closely as possible. Document the findings.
- The client should not feel any discomfort from your touch.

▶ Physical abuse should be suspected if the client has any of the following: bruises or welts that appear in a pattern suggesting the use of a belt or stick; burns with sharply demarcated edges suggesting injury from cigarettes, irons, or immersion of a hand in boiling water; additional injuries, such as fractures or dislocations; or multiple injuries in various stages of healing. A nurse must be especially sensitive if the client is fearful of family members, is reluctant to return home, and has a history of previous injuries. When any of these diagnostic cues are evident, it is important to obtain medical assistance and follow the legal requirements to notify the police or local protective agency.

The injection of drugs into the veins of the arms or other parts of the body results in a series of small scars called *track marks* along the blood vessel. A nurse who sees track marks and suspects substance abuse should refer the client to a mental health or substance abuse professional.

CLINICAL TIP!

Localized hot, red, swollen painful areas indicate the presence of inflammation and possible infection. These areas should not be palpated, because the slightest disturbance may spread an infection deeper into skin layers.

PHYSICAL ASSESSMENT

TECHNIQUES AND NORMAL FINDINGS	ABNORMAL FINDINGS AND SPECIAL CONSIDERATIONS

INSPECTION OF THE SCALP AND HAIR

1. **Instruct the client.**
   - Explain that you will be looking at the client's scalp and hair. Tell the client you will be parting the hair to observe the scalp.

2. **Observe for cleanliness.**
   - Ask the client to remove any hairpins, hair ties, barrettes, wigs, or hairpieces and to undo braids. If the client is unwilling to do this, examine any strands of hair that are loose or undone.
   - Part and divide the hair at 2.5 cm (1 in.) intervals and observe (see Figure 11.22).
   - A small amount of **dandruff** (dead, scaly flakes of epidermal cells) may be present.

   ▶ Excessive dandruff occurs on the scalps of clients with certain skin disorders, such as psoriasis or seborrheic dermatitis, in which large amounts of the epidermis slough away. Dandruff should be distinguished from head lice.

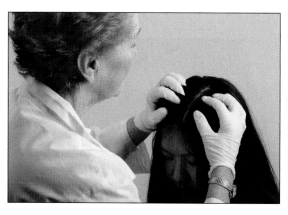

Figure 11.22 ●
Inspecting the hair and scalp.

3. **Observe the client's hair colour.**
   - Like skin colour, hair colour varies according to the level of melanin production. Greying is influenced by genetics and may begin as early as the late teens in some clients.

   ▶ Greying of the hair in patches may indicate a nutritional deficiency, commonly of protein or copper.

4. **Assess the texture of the hair.**
   - Roll a few strands of hair between your thumb and forefinger.

   ▶ Hypothyroidism and other metabolic disorders, as well as nutritional deficiencies, may cause the hair to be dull, dry, brittle, and coarse.

   - Hold a few strands of hair taut with one hand while you slide the thumb and forefinger of your other hand along the length of the strand.
   - Hair may be thick or fine and may appear straight, wavy, or curly.

5. **Observe the amount and distribution of the hair throughout the scalp.**
   - The amount of hair varies with age, gender, and overall health. Healthy hair is evenly distributed throughout the scalp.

   ▶ When hair loss occurs in women, it is thought to be caused by an imbalance in adrenal hormones.

   - In most men and women, atrophy of the hair follicles causes hair growth to decline by the age of 50. Male pattern baldness (see Figure 11.23), a genetically determined progressive loss of hair beginning at the anterior hairline, has no clinical significance. It is the most frequent reason for hair loss in men.

   ▶ Widespread hair loss may also be caused by illness, infections, metabolic disorders, nutritional deficiencies, and chemotherapy. **Alopecia areata** (patchy hair loss) may be due to infection.

PHYSICAL ASSESSMENT

TECHNIQUES AND NORMAL FINDINGS	ABNORMAL FINDINGS AND SPECIAL CONSIDERATIONS

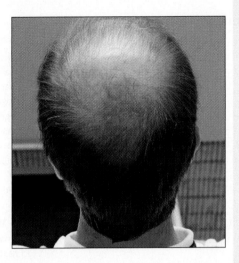

Figure 11.23 ●
Male pattern baldness.

- Remember to assess the amount, texture, and distribution of body hair. Some practitioners prefer to perform this assessment with the regions of the body.

6. **Inspect the scalp for lesions.**
   - Dim the room light and shine a Wood's lamp on the client's scalp as you part the hair (see Figure 11.24).

▶ Grey, scaly patches with broken hair may indicate the presence of a fungal infection, such as ringworm. Regions of infection will fluoresce when exposed to the ultraviolet light of a Wood's lamp.

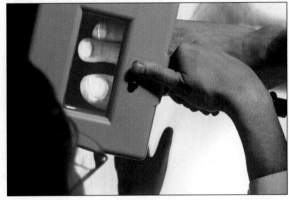

Figure 11.24 ●
Using a Wood's lamp on a client's foot.

- The healthy scalp is free from lesions and areas of fluorescent glow.

▶ Infestation by **pediculosis capitis** (head lice) is signalled by tiny, white, oval eggs (nits) that adhere to the hair shaft. Head lice usually cause intense itching. The scalp should be checked for excoriation (abrasion) from scratching.

ASSESSMENT OF THE NAILS

1. **Instruct the client.**
   - Explain that you will be looking at and touching the client's nails and that you will ask the client to hold the hands and fingers in certain positions while you are inspecting the fingernails.

2. **Assess for hygiene.**
   - Confirm that the nails are clean and well groomed.

▶ Dirty fingernails may indicate a self-care deficit but could also be related to a person's occupation.

TECHNIQUES AND NORMAL FINDINGS

ABNORMAL FINDINGS AND SPECIAL CONSIDERATIONS

3. Inspect the nails for an even, pink undertone.
   - Small, white markings in the nail are normal findings and indicate minor trauma.

▶ The nails appear pale and colourless in clients with peripheral arteriosclerosis or anemia. The nails appear yellow in clients with jaundice, and dark red in clients with *polycythemia*, a pathological increase in production of red blood cells. Fungal infections may cause the nails to discolour. Horizontal white bands may occur in chronic hepatic or renal disease. A darkly pigmented band in a single nail may be a sign of a melanoma in the nail matrix and should be referred to a physician for further evaluation.

4. Assess capillary refill.
   - Depress the nail edge briefly to blanch, and then release. Colour returns to healthy nails instantly on release.

▶ The nail beds appear blue, and colour return is sluggish in clients with cardiovascular or respiratory disorders.

5. Inspect and palpate the nails for shape and contour.
   - Perform the Schamroth test to assess for clubbing. Ask the client to bring the dorsal aspect of corresponding fingers together, creating a mirror image.

   - Look at the distal phalanx and observe the diamond-shaped opening created by nails. When clubbing is present, the diamond is not formed and the distance increases at the fingertip (see Figure 11.25). The angle between the skin and the nail base is greater than 160 degrees.

▶ Clubbing of the fingernails occurs when there is hypoxia or impaired peripheral tissue perfusion over a long time. It may also occur with cirrhosis, colitis, thyroid disease, or long-term tobacco smoking. The ends of the fingers become enlarged, soft, and spongy, and the angle between the skin and the nail base is greater than 160 degrees (see Figure 11.26).

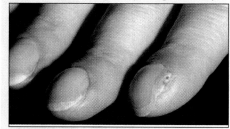

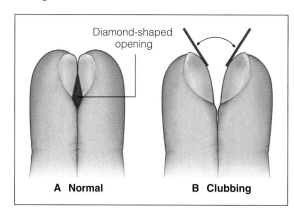

Figure 11.25 ●
Schamroth test.
A. Healthy nail.
B. Clubbing.

Figure 11.26 ● Clubbing of fingernails.

   - The nails normally form a slight convex curve or lie flat on the nail bed. When viewed laterally, the angle between the skin and the nail base should be 160 degrees or less (see Figure 11.27). Curved nails are also considered normal.

▶ Spoon nails form a concave curve and are thought to be associated with iron deficiency (see Figure 11.28).

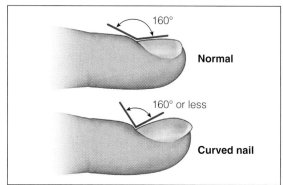

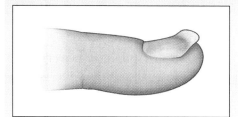

Figure 11.27 ●
Angle of fingernail.

Figure 11.28 ● Spoon nail.

TECHNIQUES AND NORMAL FINDINGS	ABNORMAL FINDINGS AND SPECIAL CONSIDERATIONS

6. Palpate the nails to determine their thickness, regularity, and attachment to the nail bed.

   - Healthy nails are smooth, strong, and regular and are firmly attached to the nail bed, with only a slight degree of mobility.

   ▶ Nails may be thickened in clients with circulatory disorders. **Onycholysis**, separation of the nail plate from the nail bed, occurs with trauma, infection, or skin lesions.

7. Inspect and palpate the cuticles.

   - The cuticles are smooth and flat in healthy nails.

   ▶ Hangnails are jagged tears in the lateral skin folds around the nail. An untreated hangnail may become inflamed and lead to a **paronychia**, an infection of the cuticle.

SAMPLE DOCUMENTATION

Subjective: No past history of skin disease, no changes in colour or texture. Denies rashes, lesions, or pruritus. Washes hands frequently with mild soap. Denies changes to texture or patterns of hair growth. Patient colours hair with chemical, no problems reported. Reports no problems with nail growth or contour.

Objective: Skin uniform in colour, no redness, lesions, or ulcerations noted. Warm and dry to touch, no tenting. Hair long with coarse texture. Evenly distributed. Scalp free of redness or lesions. Nails pink, no clubbing, cuticles smooth, capillary refill 1 second.

APPLICATION THROUGH CRITICAL THINKING

CASE STUDY

Mr. Shelley is a 54-year-old groundskeeper for a large corporation. Today, he visited the company's health and wellness office saying, "My wife told me to have someone check my leathery skin."

Julieta Caredenas, RN, asked Mr. Shelley how much time he spends outdoors. He revealed that he is outside from about 8:00 a.m. until 4:00 p.m. each day, except for his lunch break, which he usually takes in the cafeteria. He reported that he does not use sunscreen. In the summertime, he works in a short-sleeved shirt, shorts, and a hat. He doesn't recall ever having had a bad sunburn. He stated that he has a mole on his left thigh that has been present since birth, but to his knowledge it has not changed. He is not aware of any other birthmarks or skin lesions. He has never performed a skin self-assessment. He reported no family history of skin cancer. He stated that he never sunbathes or swims and that he plays outdoor sports only at the annual family picnic. He showers each day before going home and uses deodorant soap. He admitted that his skin is often quite dry but said he feels that sunscreens and lotions "are for women."

The nursing assessment of Mr. Shelley's skin revealed the following data: His skin was clean. It was a ruddy brown colour where frequently exposed to the sun and a pinkish tan elsewhere. His temperature was warm bilaterally, and he had a mild sheen of perspiration on his face, neck, and upper trunk. Where exposed to the sun, his skin was thick, with decreased elasticity. There were no unexpected visible blood vessels or vascular lesions. There was a mole approximately 2 cm by 2 cm (1 in. by 1 in.) on the anterior surface of his left thigh. No drainage was noted. Mr. Shelley's scalp and hair appeared dry but clean and free of lesions. Soil was embedded beneath the free edge of his nails. He stated that he had been transplanting cuttings.

▶ Complete Documentation

The following information is summarized from the case study.

SUBJECTIVE DATA: Seeks checkup for "leathery skin." Works as groundskeeper. Outdoors 7 hours a day. No sunscreen, protective clothing. No recall of sunburn. Mole left thigh since birth, reports unchanged. No other lesions. No self-skin assessment. No family history of skin cancer. Denies sunbathing or swimming. Occasional outdoor baseball. Showers daily with deodorant soap. Feels skin is "dry." "Sunscreens and lotions are for women."

OBJECTIVE DATA: Skin clean, ruddy brown where exposed, pinkish tan in unexposed areas. Temperature warm, bilaterally, mild perspiration face, neck, upper trunk. Exposed skin thick, decreased elasticity. No unexpected vessels, vascular lesions. Mole 2 cm × 2 cm (1 in. × 1 in.) anterior (L) thigh, no drainage. Scalp and hair, no lesions. Nails, soil embedded beneath free edge.

A sample assessment form appears below.

ASSESSMENT FORM

HISTORY

Problems

Skin: *No family history, mole left thigh (unchanged) skin*
   dry

Hair: *N/A*

Nails: *N/A*

Hygiene: *Shower daily—deodorant soap*

Environment: *Works outdoors 7 hrs./day. No sunscreen or*
   protective clothing

PHYSICAL FINDINGS

Skin

Color: *Ruddy brown where exposed, pinkish tan in unexposed areas*

Turgor: *Decreased in exposed areas*

Moisture: *Perspiration face, neck, and upper trunk*

Temperature: *Warm*

Odours: *None*

Lesions: *2 cm X 2 cm mole anterior (L) thigh, no drainage*

Hair

Distribution:

Texture:

Hygiene: *Dry scalp, no lesions*

Nails

Contour:

Nail bed:

Hygiene: *Soil under free edge*

▶ *Critical Thinking Questions*

1. Describe the findings from the case study.
2. Identify the findings as normal or abnormal.
3. Determine the categories that emerge from clustering of the data.
4. Analyze the categories to identify the physical and psychosocial nursing care priorities for Mr. Shelley.

▶ *Applying Nursing Diagnoses*

1. The NANDA-I taxonomy includes the nursing diagnosis *risk for impaired skin integrity*. Do the data support this diagnosis? If so, identify the data.
2. Use the NANDA-I taxonomy (see Appendix A ⬯) to formulate additional diagnoses for Mr. Shelley. For each diagnosis identify the following:
   a. Type of diagnosis
   b. Defining characteristics
   c. Risks or related factors

▶ *Prepare Teaching Plan*

LEARNING NEED: The data from the case study reveal that Mr. Shelley is concerned about his "leathery skin." His skin condition is associated with unprotected skin exposure to the sun for long periods of the daytime. Mr. Shelley is at risk for skin cancer.

The case study provides data that are representative of risks, symptoms, and behaviours of many individuals. Therefore, the following teaching plan is based on the need to provide information to members of any community about skin cancer.

GOAL: The participants in this learning program will have increased awareness of risk factors and strategies to prevent skin cancer.

OBJECTIVES: At the completion of this learning session, the learner will be able to

1. Identify risk factors associated with skin cancer.
2. List the symptoms of skin cancer.
3. Describe the types of skin cancer.
4. Discuss strategies to prevent skin cancer.

Following is an example of the teaching plan for Objective 1. After reviewing this sample teaching plan for Objective 1, go to the MyNursingLab website for this text to complete the teaching plan for the other objectives.

APPLICATION OF OBJECTIVE 1: Identify risk factors associated with skin cancer.

Content	Teaching Strategy	Evaluation
• *Moles.* Usually harmless pigmented growth. Multiple moles or large moles indicate risk. • *Fair complexion.* Skin cancer risk is higher in those with fair skin, freckles, blue eyes, and blond hair. • *Family history of skin cancer.* • *Past exposure.* Too much time in the sun or tanning booth. Severe sunburn as child or teen. • *Age.* Half of skin cancer occurs after age 50.	• Lecture • Discussion • Audiovisual materials • Printed materials Lecture is appropriate when disseminating information to large groups. Discussion allows participants to bring up concerns and to raise questions. Audiovisual materials, such as illustrations of the moles, reinforce verbal presentation. Printed material, especially to be taken away with learners, allows review, reinforcement, and reading at the learner's pace.	• Written examination May use short answer, fill-in, or multiple-choice items, or a combination of items. If these are short and easy to evaluate, the learner receives immediate feedback.

HEALTH PROMOTION ASSESSMENT TOOL

Social Determinants of Health	Level of Action	Action Strategies
Personal coping skills	Individual	**Develop personal skills** • Teach Mr. Shelley about the risks of prolonged sun exposure. • Encourage use of daily sunscreen when outside. • Teach Mr. Shelley how to conduct a skin self-assessment. • Explore Mr. Shelley's beliefs about lotion use. Discuss the importance of skin care for both men and women and the appropriateness of lotions to combat dry skin. • Discuss the importance of using gardening gloves to protect his hands from abrasions and toxins.
	Family	**Create supportive environments** • Discuss with Mr. Shelley the opportunities to have sunscreen available for all family members, for example at annual family picnics. • Encourage Mr. Shelley to support all family members wearing protective clothing such as hats when outdoors in the sun at family functions.
Work and working conditions	Community: All groundskeepers that work for the same large corporation as Mr. Shelley	**Building healthy public policy** • Provide gardening gloves and sunscreen in all groundskeepers' toolboxes. • Develop educational posters on the risks of prolonged sun exposure with tips on how to minimize risks and post them in the lunchroom and outdoor equipment storage sheds. **Creating supportive environments** • Develop health and wellness lunchtime seminars on the importance of skin care and sun protection.

ABNORMAL FINDINGS

Abnormal findings of the integumentary system include alterations in the skin, hair, or nails. Skin abnormalities include lesions, vascular lesions, and malignant lesions. Figures 11.29 through 11.75 depict these skin abnormalities. Abnormalities of the hair are depicted in Figures 11.76 through 11.81. Splinter hemorrhage, clubbing, and paronychia are among the abnormalities of the nail depicted in Figures 11.82 through 11.87.

Vascular Lesions

Hemangioma

Hemangioma is a bright red, raised lesion about 2 to 10 cm (1 to 4 in.) in diameter. It does not blanch with pressure. It is usually present at birth or within a few months of birth. Typically, it disappears by age 3. The lesion pictured in Figure 11.29 is located on the dorsal surface on the hand.

Cause: A cluster of immature capillaries.

Localization/Distribution: Can appear on any part of the body.

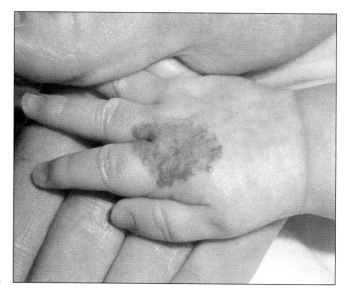

Figure 11.29 ● Hemangioma.

Port-Wine Stain

A port-wine stain is a flat, irregularly shaped lesion ranging in colour from pale red to deep purple-red. Colour deepens with exertion, emotional response, or exposure to extremes of temperature. It is present at birth and typically does not fade (see Figure 11.30).

Cause: A large, flat mass of blood vessels on the skin surface.

Localization/Distribution: Most commonly appears on the face and head but may occur in other sites.

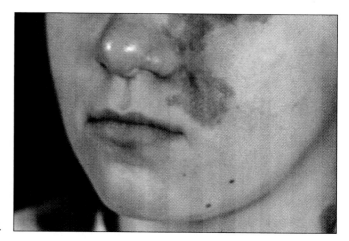

Figure 11.30 ● Port-wine stain (nevus flammeus).

Spider Angioma

Spider angioma is a flat, bright red dot with tiny radiating blood vessels ranging in size from a pinpoint to 2 cm (1 in.). It blanches with pressure (see Figure 11.31).

Cause: A type of telangiectasis (vascular dilatation) caused by elevated estrogen levels, pregnancy, estrogen therapy, vitamin B deficiency, or liver disease, or may not be pathological.

Localization/Distribution: Most commonly appears on the upper half of the body.

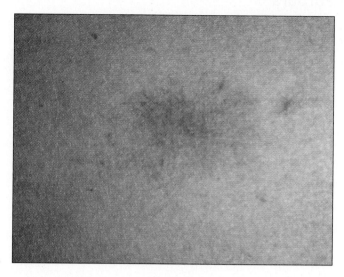

Figure 11.31 ● Spider (star) angioma.

Venous Lake

Venous lake is a flat blue lesion with radiating, cascading, or linear veins extending from the centre. It ranges in size from 3 to 25 cm (1.25 to 10 in.; see Figure 11.32).

Cause: A type of telangiectasis (vascular dilatation) caused by increased intravenous pressure in superficial veins.

Localization/Distribution: Most commonly appears on the anterior chest and the lower legs near varicose veins.

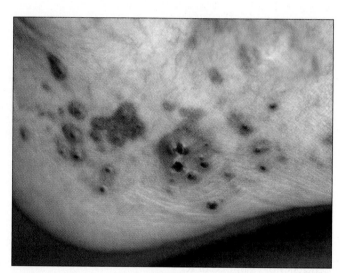

Figure 11.32 ● Venous lake.

Petechiae

Petechiae are flat red or purple rounded "freckles" approximately 1 to 3 mm (0.04 to 0.12 in.) in diameter (see Figure 11.33). They are difficult to detect in dark skin. They do not blanch.

Cause: Minute hemorrhages resulting from fragile capillaries, petechiae are caused by septicemias, liver disease, or vitamin C or K deficiency. They may also be caused by anticoagulant therapy.

Localization/Distribution: Most commonly appear on the dependent surfaces of the body (e.g., back, buttocks) but may occur elsewhere on the body. In the client with dark skin, may be seen in the oral mucosa and conjunctivae.

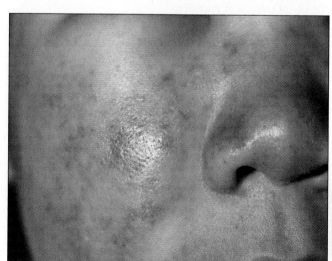

Figure 11.33 ● Petechiae.

Purpura

Purpura are flat, reddish blue, irregularly shaped extensive patches of varying size (see Figure 11.34).

Cause: Bleeding disorders, scurvy, and capillary fragility in the older adult (senile purpura).

Localization/Distribution: May appear anywhere on the body but are most noticeable on the legs, arms, and backs of hands.

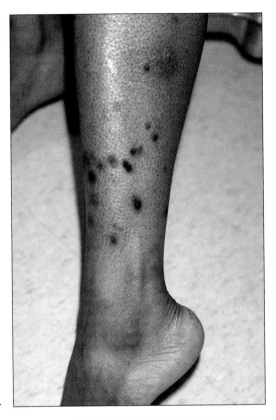

Figure 11.34 ● Purpura.

Ecchymosis

Ecchymosis is a flat, irregularly shaped lesion of varying size with no pulsation (see Figure 11.35). It does not blanch with pressure. In light skin, it begins as a bluish purple mark that changes to greenish yellow. In brown skin, it varies from blue to deep purple. In black skin, it appears as a darkened area.

Cause: Release of blood from superficial vessels into surrounding tissue caused by trauma, hemophilia, liver disease, or deficiency of vitamin C or K.

Localization/Distribution: Occurs anywhere on the body at the site of trauma or pressure.

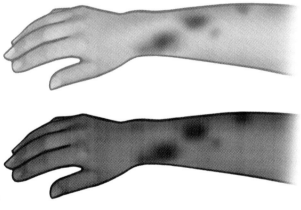

Figure 11.35 ● Ecchymosis (bruise).

Hematoma

A hematoma is a raised, irregularly shaped lesion similar to an ecchymosis except that it elevates the skin and looks like a swelling (see Figure 11.36).

Cause: A leakage of blood into the skin and subcutaneous tissue as a result of trauma or surgical incision.

Localization/Distribution: May occur anywhere on the body at the site of trauma, pressure, or surgical incision.

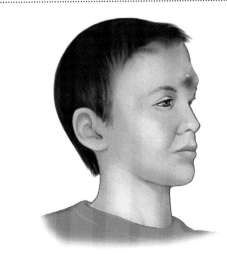

Figure 11.36 ● Hematoma.

Primary Lesions

Macule and Patch

A macule or patch is a flat, nonpalpable change in skin colour. Macules are smaller than 1 cm (0.5 in.), with a circumscribed border (see Figure 11.37), and patches are larger than 1 cm (0.5 in.) and may have an irregular border.

Examples: Macules: freckles, measles, and petechiae. Patches: Mongolian spots, port-wine stains, vitiligo, and chloasma.

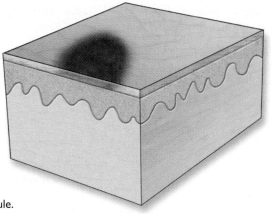

Figure 11.37 ● Macule.

Papule and Plaque

A papule or plaque is an elevated, solid, palpable mass with circumscribed border (see Figure 11.38). Papules are smaller than 0.5 cm (0.25 in.); plaques are groups of papules that form lesions larger than 0.5 cm (0.25 in.).

Examples: Papules: elevated moles, warts, and lichen planus. Plaques: psoriasis, actinic keratosis, and also lichen planus.

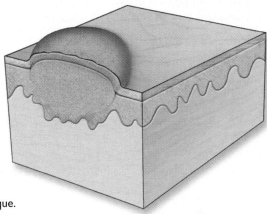

Figure 11.38 ● Papule, plaque.

Nodule and Tumour

A nodule or tumour is an elevated, solid, hard or soft, palpable mass extending deeper into the dermis than a papule (see Figure 11.39). Nodules have circumscribed borders and are 0.5 to 2 cm (0.25 to 1 in.); tumours may have irregular borders and are larger than 2 cm (1 in.).

Examples: Nodules: small lipoma, squamous cell carcinoma, fibroma, and intradermal nevi. Tumours: large lipoma, carcinoma, and hemangioma.

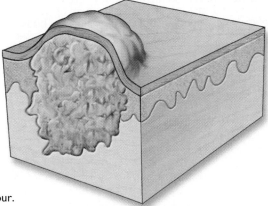

Figure 11.39 ● Nodule, tumour.

Vesicle and Bulla

A vesicle or bulla is an elevated, fluid-filled, round or oval-shaped, palpable mass with thin, translucent walls and circumscribed borders (see Figure 11.40). Vesicles are smaller than 0.5 cm (0.25 in.); bullae are larger than 0.5 cm (0.25 in.).

Examples: Vesicles: herpes simplex/zoster, early chickenpox, poison ivy, and small burn blisters. Bullae: contact dermatitis, friction blisters, and large burn blisters.

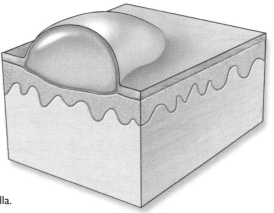

Figure 11.40 ● Vesicle, bulla.

Wheal

A wheal is an elevated, often reddish area with an irregular border caused by diffuse fluid in tissues rather than free fluid in a cavity, as in vesicles (see Figure 11.41). Size varies.

Examples: Insect bites and hives (extensive wheals).

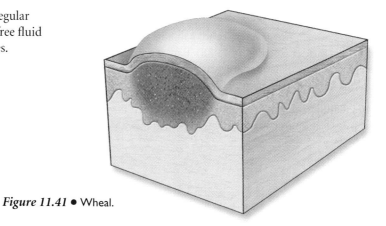

Figure 11.41 ● Wheal.

Pustule

A pustule is an elevated, pus-filled vesicle or bulla with a circumscribed border (see Figure 11.42). Size varies.

Examples: Acne, impetigo, and carbuncles (large boils).

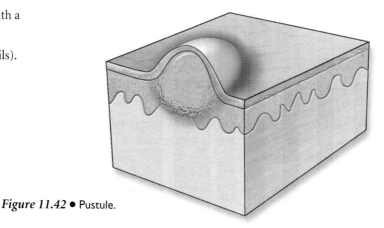

Figure 11.42 ● Pustule.

Cyst

A cyst is an elevated, encapsulated, fluid-filled or semisolid mass originating in the subcutaneous tissue or dermis, usually 1 cm (0.5 in.) or larger (see Figure 11.43).

Examples: Varieties include sebaceous cysts and epidermoid cysts.

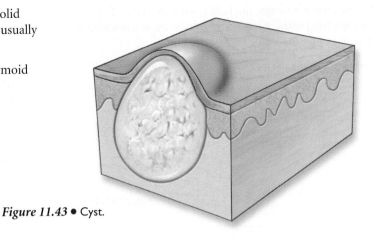

Figure 11.43 ● Cyst.

Secondary Lesions

Atrophy

Atrophy is a translucent, dry, paperlike, sometimes wrinkled skin surface resulting from thinning or wasting of the skin caused by loss of collagen and elastin (see Figure 11.44).

Examples: Striae, aged skin.

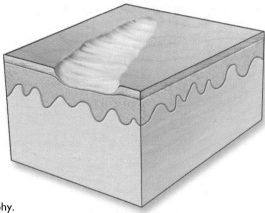

Figure 11.44 ● Atrophy.

Erosion

Erosion is wearing away of the superficial epidermis, causing a moist, shallow depression. Because erosions do not extend into the dermis, they heal without scarring (see Figure 11.45).

Examples: Scratch marks, ruptured vesicles.

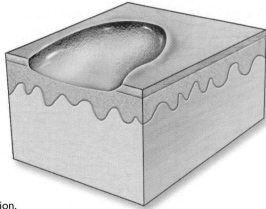

Figure 11.45 ● Erosion.

Lichenification

Lichenification is a rough, thickened, hardened area of epidermis resulting from chronic irritation, such as scratching or rubbing (see Figure 11.46).

Examples: Chronic dermatitis.

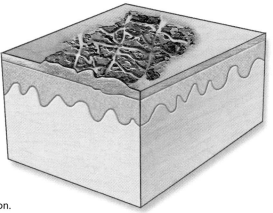

Figure 11.46 ● Lichenification.

Scales

Scales are shedding flakes of greasy, keratinized skin tissue. Colour may be white, grey, or silver. Texture may vary from fine to thick (see Figure 11.47).

Examples: Dry skin, dandruff, psoriasis, and eczema.

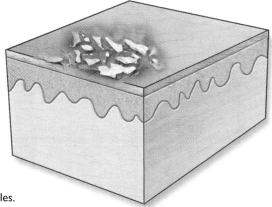

Figure 11.47 ● Scales.

Crust

Crust is dry blood, serum, or pus left on the skin surface when vesicles or pustules burst (see Figure 11.48). It can be red-brown, orange, or yellow. Large crusts that adhere to the skin surface are called scabs.

Examples: Eczema, impetigo, herpes, or scabs following abrasion.

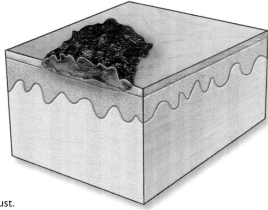

Figure 11.48 ● Crust.

Ulcer

An ulcer is a deep, irregularly shaped area of skin loss extending into the dermis or subcutaneous tissue (see Figure 11.49). It may bleed or leave a scar.

Examples: Decubitus ulcers (pressure sores), stasis ulcers, chancres.

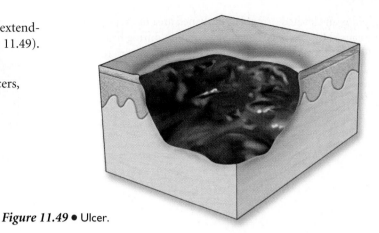

Figure 11.49 ● Ulcer.

Fissure

A fissure is a linear crack with sharp edges, extending into the dermis (see Figure 11.50).

Examples: Cracks at the corners of the mouth or in the hands, athlete's foot.

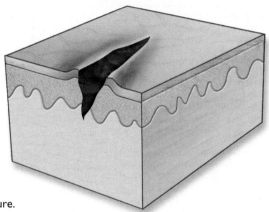

Figure 11.50 ● Fissure.

Scar

A scar is a flat, irregular area of connective tissue left after a lesion or wound has healed (see Figure 11.51). New scars may be red or purple; older scars may be silvery or white.

Examples: Healed surgical wound or injury, healed acne.

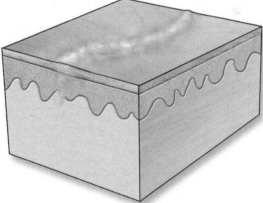

Figure 11.51 ● Scar.

Keloid

A keloid is an elevated, irregular, darkened area of excess scar tissue caused by excessive collagen formation during healing (see Figure 11.52). It extends beyond the site of the original injury. There is higher incidence in Black people.

Examples: Keloid from ear-piercing or surgery.

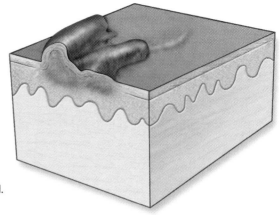

Figure 11.52 ● Keloid.

Configurations and Shapes of Lesions

Annular

Annular lesions are lesions with a circular shape (see Figure 11.53).

Examples: Tinea corporis, pityriasis rosea.

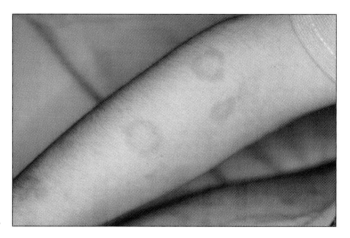

Figure 11.53 ● Annular lesions.

Confluent

Confluent lesions are lesions that run together (see Figure 11.54).

Example: Urticaria (hives).

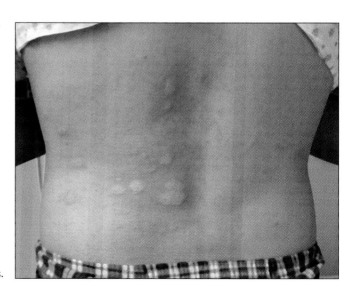

Figure 11.54 ● Confluent lesions.

Discrete

Discrete lesions are lesions that are separate and distinct (see Figure 11.55).

Example: Molluscum.

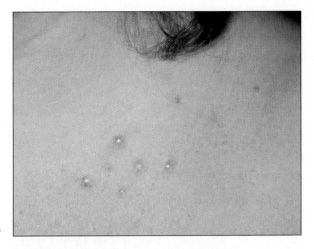

Figure 11.55 ● Discrete lesions.

Grouped

Grouped lesions are lesions that appear in clusters (see Figure 11.56).

Example: Purpural lesion.

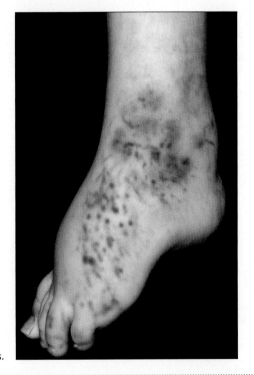

Figure 11.56 ● Grouped lesions.

Gyrate

Gyrate lesions are lesions that are coiled or twisted (see Figure 11.57).

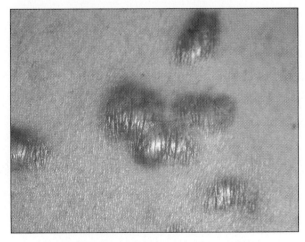

Figure 11.57 ● Gyrate lesions.

Target

Target lesions are lesions with concentric circles of colour (see Figure 11.58).

Example: Erythema multiforme.

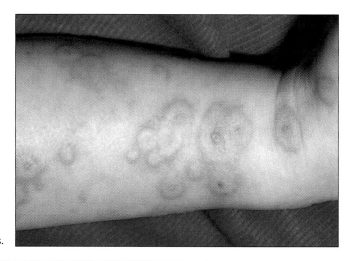

Figure 11.58 ● Target lesions.

Linear

Linear lesions are lesions that appear as a line (see Figure 11.59).

Example: Scratches.

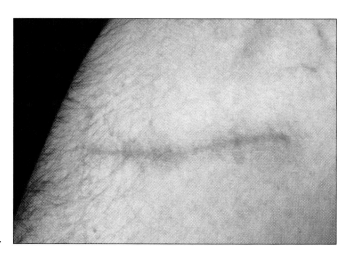

Figure 11.59 ● Linear lesions.

Polycyclic

Polycyclic lesions are lesions that are circular but united (see Figure 11.60).

Example: Psoriasis.

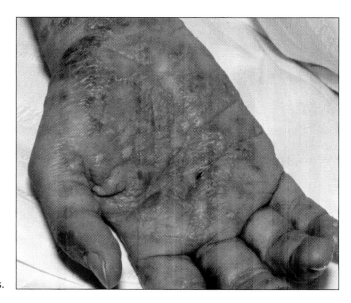

Figure 11.60 ● Polycyclic lesions.

Zosteriform

Zosteriform lesions are arranged in a linear manner along a nerve route (see Figure 11.61).

Example: Herpes zoster.

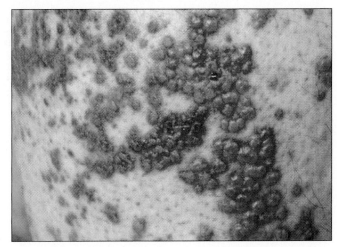

Figure 11.61 ● Zosteriform lesions.

Common Skin Lesions

Tinea

Tinea is a fungal infection affecting the body (tinea corporis), the scalp (tinea capitis), or the feet (tinea pedis, also known as athlete's foot). Secondary bacterial infection may also be present. The appearance of the lesions varies, and they may present as papules, pustules, vesicles, or scales (see Figure 11.62).

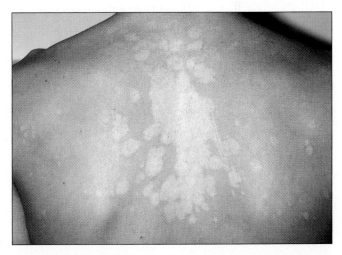

Figure 11.62 ● Tinea corporis.

Measles (Rubeola)

Measles is a highly contagious viral disease that causes a rash of red to purple macules or papules (see Figure 11.63). The rash begins on the face, then progresses over the neck, trunk, arms, and legs. It does not blanch. It may be accompanied by tiny white spots that look like grains of salt (called Koplik's spots) on the oral mucosa. It occurs mostly in children.

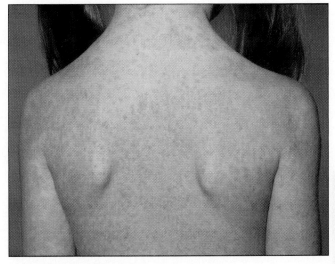

Figure 11.63 ● Measles (rubeola).

German Measles (Rubella)

German measles is a highly contagious disease caused by a virus. Typically it begins as a pink, papular rash that is similar to measles but paler (see Figure 11.64). Like measles, it begins on the face, then spreads over the body. Unlike measles, it may be accompanied by swollen glands. It is not accompanied by Koplik's spots. It occurs mostly in children.

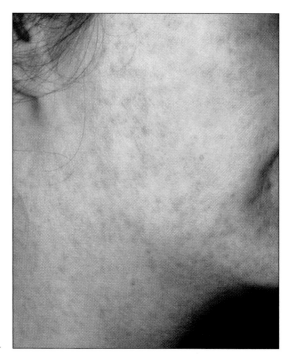

Figure 11.64 • German measles (rubella).

Chickenpox (Varicella)

Chickenpox is a mild infectious disease caused by the herpes zoster virus. It begins as groups of small, red, fluid-filled vesicles, usually on the trunk, and progresses to the face, arms, and legs (see Figure 11.65). Vesicles erupt over several days, forming pustules and then crusts. The condition may cause intense itching. It occurs mostly in children.

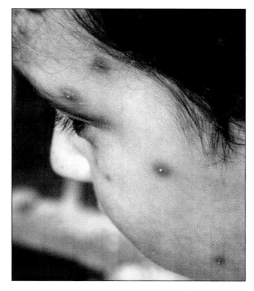

Figure 11.65 • Chickenpox (varicella).

Herpes Simplex

Herpes simplex is a viral infection that causes characteristic lesions on the lips and oral mucosa (see Figure 11.66). Lesions progress from vesicles to pustules and then crusts. Herpes simplex also occurs in the genitals.

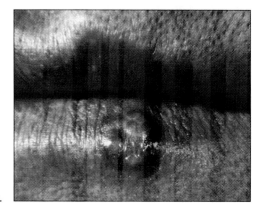

Figure 11.66 • Herpes simplex.

Herpes Zoster

Herpes zoster is an eruption of dormant herpes zoster virus, which typically has invaded the body during an attack of chickenpox. Clusters of small vesicles form on the skin along the route of sensory nerves. Vesicles progress to pustules and then crusts (see Figure 11.67). It causes intense pain and itching. The condition is more common and more severe in older adults.

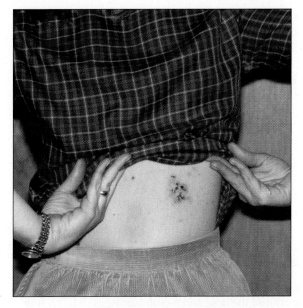

Figure 11.67 ● Herpes zoster (shingles).

Psoriasis

Psoriasis is thickening of the skin in dry, silvery, scaly patches (see Figure 11.68). It occurs with overproduction of skin cells that results in a buildup of cells faster than they can be shed. It may be aggravated by stress. It may be located on any area, including the scalp, elbows and knees, lower back, perianal area, trunk, and hands.

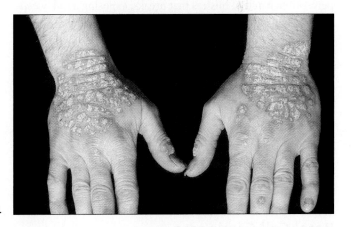

Figure 11.68 ● Psoriasis.

Contact Dermatitis

Contact dermatitis is inflammation of the skin caused by an allergy to a substance that comes into contact with the skin, such as clothing, jewellery, plants, chemicals, or cosmetics. The location of the lesions may help identify the allergen. It may progress from redness to hives, vesicles, or scales (see Figure 11.69) and is usually accompanied by intense itching.

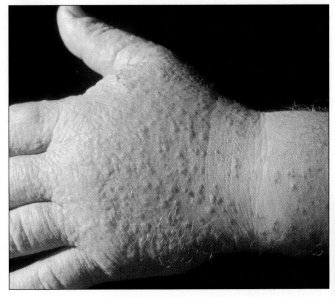

Figure 11.69 ● Contact dermatitis.

ABNORMAL FINDINGS

Eczema

Eczema is internally provoked inflammation of the skin causing reddened papules and vesicles that ooze, weep, and progress to form crusts (see Figure 11.70). The lesions are usually located on the scalp, face, elbows and knees, and forearms and wrists. Eczema usually causes intense itching.

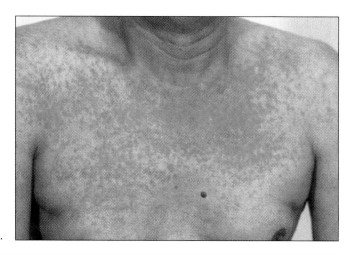

Figure 11.70 ● Eczema (atopic dermatitis).

Impetigo

Impetigo is a bacterial skin infection that usually appears on the skin around the nose and mouth (see Figure 11.71). It is contagious and common in children. It may begin as a barely perceptible patch of blisters that breaks, exposing a red, weeping area beneath. A tan crust soon forms over this area, and the infection may spread out of the edges.

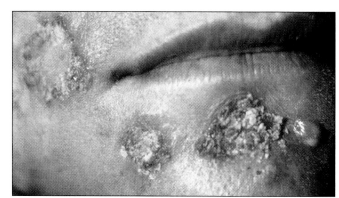

Figure 11.71 ● Impetigo.

Malignant Skin Lesions

Basal Cell Carcinoma

Basal cell carcinoma is the most common but least malignant type of skin cancer. Basal cell carcinoma is a proliferation of the cells of the stratum basale into the dermis and subcutaneous tissue. The lesions begin as shiny papules that develop central ulcers with rounded, pearly edges (see Figure 11.72). Lesions occur most often on skin regions regularly exposed to the sun.

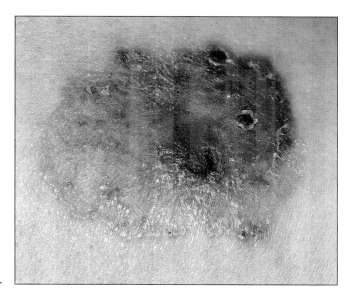

Figure 11.72 ● Basal cell carcinoma.

Squamous Cell Carcinoma

Squamous cell carcinoma arises from the cells of the stratum spinosum. It begins as a reddened, scaly papule, then forms a shallow ulcer with a clearly delineated, elevated border (see Figure 11.73). It commonly appears on the scalp, ears, backs of the hands, and lower lip, and is thought to be caused by exposure to the sun. It grows rapidly.

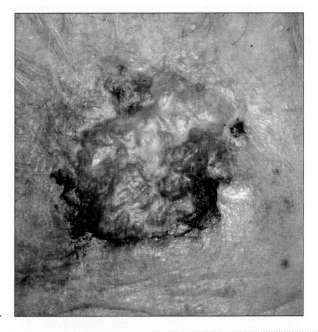

Figure 11.73 ● Squamous cell carcinoma.

Malignant Melanoma

Malignant melanoma is the least common but most serious type of skin cancer, because it spreads rapidly to lymph and blood vessels. The lesion usually contains areas of varied pigmentation, from black to brown to blue or red. The edges are often irregular, with notched borders, and the diameter is greater than 6 mm (see Figure 11.74).

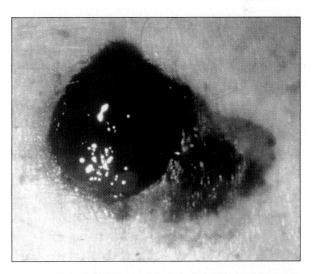

Figure 11.74 ● Malignant melanoma.

Kaposi's Sarcoma

Kaposi's sarcoma is a malignant tumour of the epidermis and internal epithelial tissues. Lesions are typically soft, blue to purple, and painless (see Figure 11.75). Other characteristics are variable: they may be macular or papular and may resemble keloids or bruises. Kaposi's sarcoma is common in people who are HIV positive.

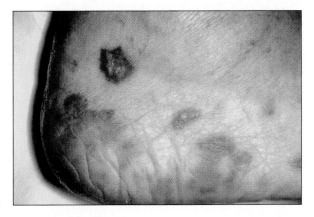

Figure 11.75 ● Kaposi's sarcoma.

ABNORMAL FINDINGS

Abnormalities of the Hair

Seborrheic Dermatitis

Seborrheic dermatitis is common in infants. It appears as eczema of yellow-white greasy scales on the scalp and forehead. It is also known as cradle cap (see Figure 11.76).

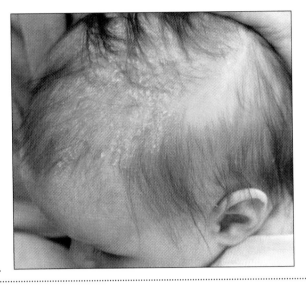

Figure 11.76 ● Seborrheic dermatitis (cradle cap).

Tinea Capitis

Tinea capitis is patchy hair loss on the head with pustules on the skin (see Figure 11.77). This highly contagious fungal disease is transmitted from the soil, from animals, or from person to person.

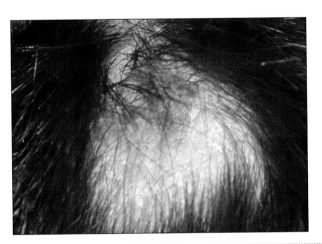

Figure 11.77 ● Tinea capitis (scalp ringworm).

Alopecia Areata

There is no known cause for the sudden loss of hair in a round balding patch on the scalp (see Figure 11.78).

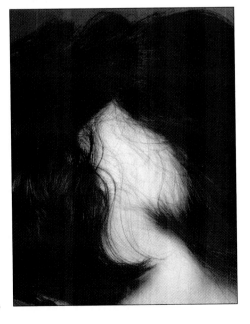

Figure 11.78 ● Alopecia areata.

Folliculitis

Folliculitis, infections of hair follicles, appears as pustules with underlying erythema (see Figure 11.79).

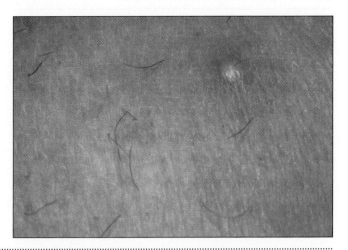

Figure 11.79 ● Folliculitis.

Furuncle and Abscess

Infected hair follicles give rise to furuncles (see Figure 11.80). These are hard, erythematous, pus-filled lesions. Abscesses are caused by bacteria entering the skin. These are larger lesions than furuncles.

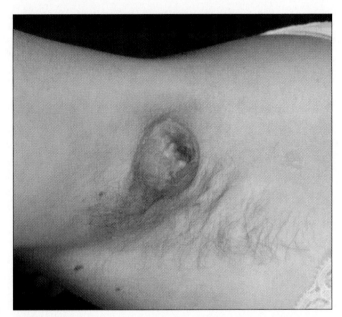

Figure 11.80 ● Furuncle or abscess.

Hirsutism

Hirsutism is excess body hair in females on the face, chest, abdomen, arms, and legs, following the male pattern. This example shows excessive hair on the female chin (see Figure 11.81). It is typically due to endocrine or metabolic dysfunction, though it may be idiopathic.

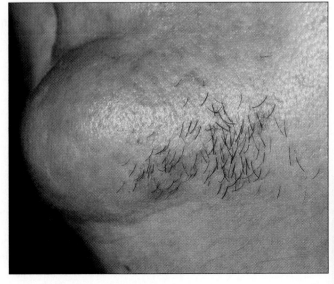

Figure 11.81 ● Hirsutism.

Abnormalities of the Nails

Spoon Nails

Concavity and thinning of the nails (see Figure 11.82), which is commonly a congenital condition.

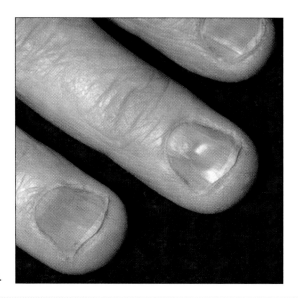

Figure 11.82 • Spoon nails (koilonychia).

Paronychia

Paronychia is an infection of the skin adjacent to the nail, usually caused by bacteria or fungi (see Figure 11.83). The affected area becomes red, swollen, and painful, and pus may ooze from it.

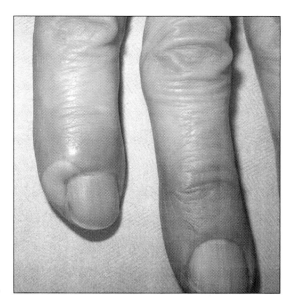

Figure 11.83 • Paronychia.

Beau's Line

Beau's line occurs from trauma or illness affecting nail formation. A linear depression develops at the base and moves distally as the nail grows (see Figure 11.84).

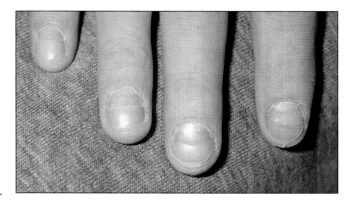

Figure 11.84 • Beau's line.

Splinter Hemorrhage

Splinter hemorrhage can occur as a result of trauma or in endocarditis. These appear as reddish-brown spots in the nail (see Figure 11.85).

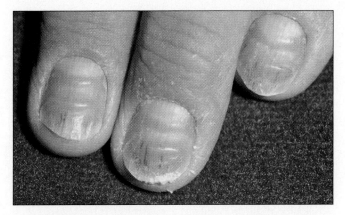

Figure 11.85 ● Splinter hemorrhages.

Clubbing

In clubbing, the nail appears more convex and wide (see Figure 11.86). The nail angle is greater than 180 degrees. It occurs in chronic respiratory and cardiac conditions in which oxygenation is compromised.

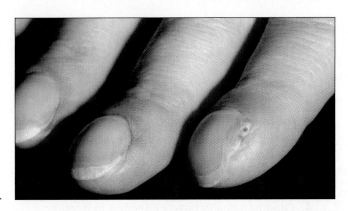

Figure 11.86 ● Nail clubbing.

Onycholysis

In onycholysis, the nail plate loosens from the distal nail and proceeds to the proximal portion (see Figure 11.87).

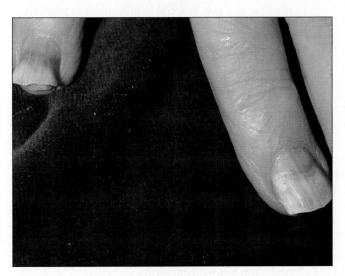

Figure 11.87 ● Onycholysis.

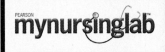

ABNORMAL FINDINGS

12

HEAD, NECK, AND RELATED LYMPHATICS

THE HEAD AND NECK REGION IS, IN MANY WAYS, the most important region in the body. Several systems are integrated in the head and neck. For example, the musculoskeletal system permits movement of the neck and face, while the bones protect the brain, spinal cord, and eyes.

Several body systems overlap in the head and neck region. The nurse will be assessing several systems at the same time. For instance, the integumentary system provides covering and protection. Food is taken in through the mouth, which is the beginning of the gastrointestinal system. Air enters the lungs through the nose, mouth, and trachea, which make up the upper respiratory system. The cardiovascular system carries oxygen and other nutrients to the region and transports wastes. The nurse must consider this close interrelationship of systems when assessing the client's head and neck, where clues to the client's nutritional status, airway clearance, tissue perfusion, metabolism, level of activity, sleep and rest, level of stress, and self-care ability may be apparent.

When performing an assessment of the head and neck, the nurse must be aware of psychosocial factors, such as stress and anxiety, that can influence the health of this body area. It is also important for the nurse to consider the client's self-care practices. Many clients spend a great deal of time caring for this area of the body, and alterations in health may affect their ability to provide this care. A client's ancestry, cultural practices, socioeconomic status, and physical environment both at home and at work can greatly influence the health of the head and neck, and they are an integral part of the assessment data. Additionally, a client's developmental stage has a tremendous influence on the appearance and functioning of the region.

ANATOMY AND PHYSIOLOGY REVIEW

The structures of the head include the skull and facial bones. The vertebrae, hyoid bone, cartilage, muscles, thyroid gland, and major blood vessels are found within the neck. A large supply of lymph nodes is located in the head and neck region. Each of these structures is described in the sections that follow.

Head

The skull is a protective shell made up of the bones of the cranium (see Figure 12.1) and face. The major bones of the cranium are the frontal, parietal, temporal, and occipital bones. These bones are connected to each other by means of **sutures,** or nonmovable joints. The solidification process of the sutures is completed by the second year of life. The primary function of the skull is to protect the brain. The bones of the skull are covered by muscles and skin, which is commonly called the scalp. The bones provide landmarks for assessment. Fourteen bones form the anterior region of the skull, commonly called the face. These bones are the frontal, maxillae, zygomatic, nasal, ethmoid, lacrimal, sphenoid, and mandible. The intricate fusion of these bones provides structure for the face and cavities for the eyes, nose, and mouth. It also allows movement of the mandible at the temporomandibular joint (TMJ). The TMJ is located anterior to the tragus of the ear and allows a person to open and close the mouth, protract and retract the chin, and slide the lower jaw from side to side. These actions are used for chewing and speaking.

The skin, muscles, and bones of the face provide landmarks for assessment, as do the bones of the skull. The eyebrows, appendages of the skin, are over the supraorbital margins of the skull. The lateral canthus of the eye forms a straight line with the pinna, and the nasolabial folds are equal (see Figure 12.2).

Figure 12.3 identifies the main muscles of the scalp, face, and neck. These muscles play a major role in expressing emotions through facial expressions. They also contribute to movement of the head and neck. Details regarding movement of the structures of the head and neck are discussed in Chapter 23 of this text. ⬭ Cranial nerve innervation of muscles, senses, and balance are discussed in detail in Chapter 24 of this text. ⬭

KEY TERMS

acromegaly, 237
anterior triangle, 219
atlas, 218
axis, 218
Bell's palsy, 237
craniosynostosis, 237
Cushing's syndrome, 238
Down syndrome, 238
goitre, 222
hydrocephalus, 236
hyoid, 219
hyperthyroidism, 230
hypothyroidism, 240
lymphadenopathy, 231
posterior triangle, 219
sutures, 217
thyroid gland, 220
torticollis, 239

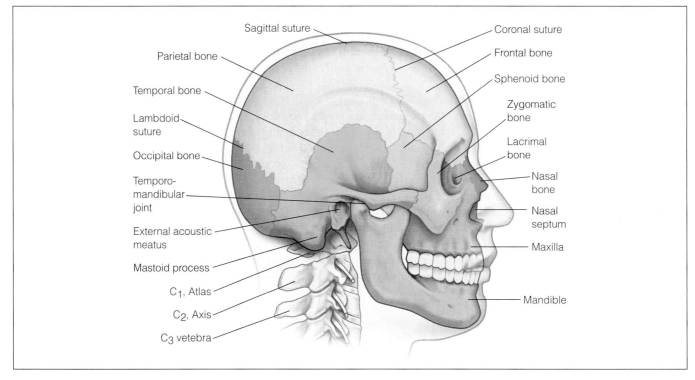

Figure 12.1 ● Bones of the head.

Neck

The neck is formed by the seven cervical vertebrae, ligaments, and muscles, which support the cranium. The first cervical vertebra (C_1), commonly called the **atlas,** carries the skull. The second cervical vertebra (C_2), commonly called the **axis,** allows for movement of the head (see Figure 12.1). The greatest mobility is at the level of C_4, C_5, and C_6. The seventh cervical vertebra (vertebra prominens) has the largest spinous process. This vertebral process is visible and easily palpated, making it a landmark during client assessment.

The sternocleidomastoid and trapezius muscles are the primary muscles of the neck. The sternocleidomastoid muscles, innervated by cranial nerve XI, originate at the manubrium of the sternum and the medial portion of the clavicles. The insertion of this muscle is at the mastoid process of the temporal bones.

Each trapezius muscle, also innervated by cranial nerve XI, originates on the occipital bone of the skull and spine of several vertebrae. The insertion of these muscles is on the scapulae and lateral third of the clavicles.

These two muscle groups form the anterior and posterior triangles of the neck. The mandible, the midline of the neck,

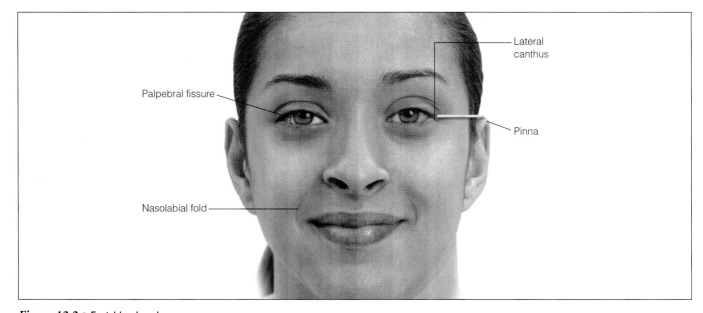

Figure 12.2 ● Facial landmarks.

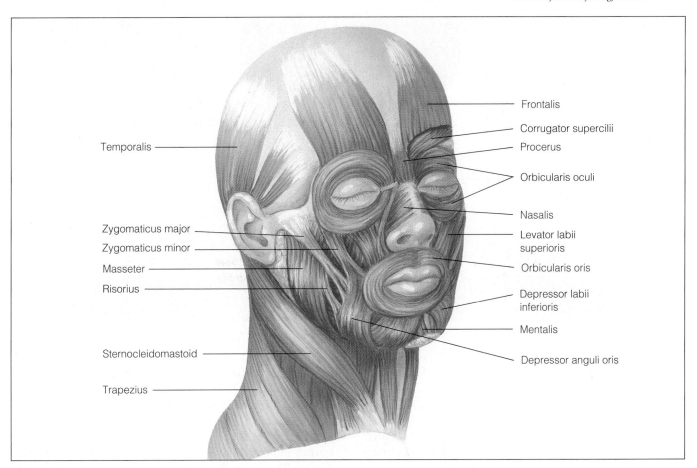

Temporalis

Frontalis

Corrugator supercilii

Procerus

Orbicularis oculi

Zygomaticus major

Zygomaticus minor

Masseter

Risorius

Nasalis

Levator labii superioris

Orbicularis oris

Depressor labii inferioris

Mentalis

Sternocleidomastoid

Trapezius

Depressor anguli oris

Figure 12.3 ● Muscles of the head and neck.

and the anterior aspect of the sternocleidomastoid muscles border the **anterior triangle.** The trapezius muscle, the sternocleidomastoid muscle, and the clavicle form the **posterior triangle** (see Figure 12.4).

The hyoid bone is suspended in the neck (see Figure 12.5) approximately 2 cm (1 in.) above the larynx. The **hyoid** is the only bone in the body that does not articulate directly with another bone. The base of the tongue rests on the curved body of this bone. The curved shape of the bone produces a horn at each end that is palpable just inferior to the angle of the jaw. This serves as a landmark for assessing structures of the neck, especially the trachea and thyroid gland.

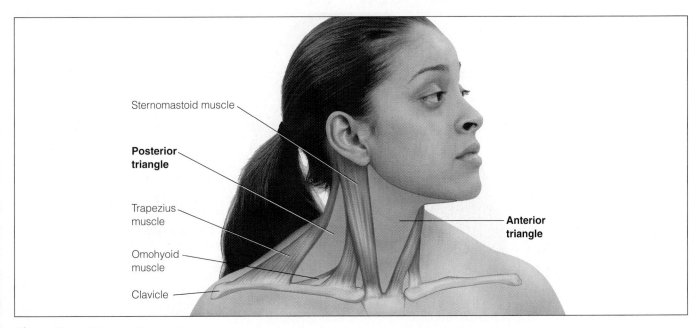

Sternomastoid muscle

Posterior triangle

Trapezius muscle

Omohyoid muscle

Clavicle

Anterior triangle

Figure 12.4 ● Triangles of the neck.

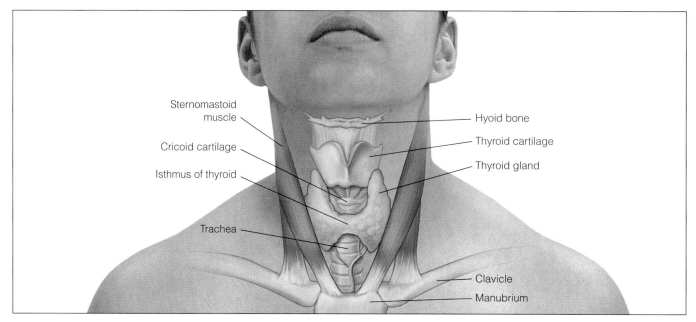

Figure 12.5 ● Structures of the neck.

The thyroid cartilage is the largest cartilage of the larynx and is formed by the joining of two pieces of cartilage. This fusion forms a ridge and forms the Adam's apple. This ridge is significantly larger in males (Figure 12.5). The cricoid cartilage, a C-shaped ring, is the first cartilage ring anchored to the trachea. The trachea, commonly called the windpipe, descends from the larynx to the bronchi of the respiratory system. The trachea has slight mobility and flexibility. The C-shaped rings help maintain the shape of the trachea and are palpable superior to the sternum at the midline of the neck (Figure 12.5).

The **thyroid gland,** the largest gland of the endocrine system, is butterfly shaped. It is located in the anterior portion of the neck. The isthmus of the thyroid connects the right and left lobes of the thyroid gland. The thyroid gland lies over the trachea, and the sternocleidomastoid muscles cover the lateral aspects of the lobes (Figure 12.5).

The carotid arteries and the jugular veins are located in the neck. The carotid artery is palpated in the groove between the trachea and the sternocleidomastoid muscle below the angle of the jaw. The external and internal jugular veins are also in the neck, in proximity to the common carotid artery. The external jugular veins are more superficial and smaller than the internal jugular veins. These vessels are lateral to the sternocleidomastoid muscle. The internal jugular vein is larger and not visible; however, a reflection of the undulation is seen (see Figure 12.6). The carotid arteries and jugular veins are discussed in detail in Chapter 17 of this text. ⚭

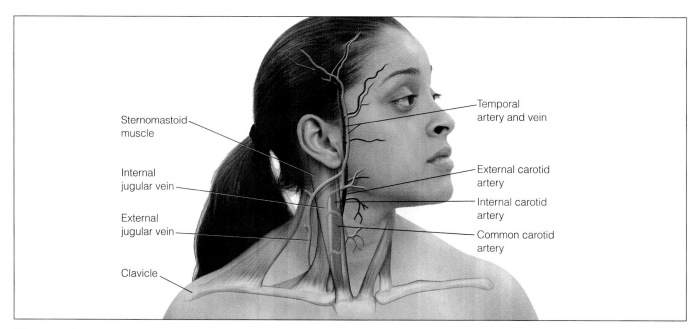

Figure 12.6 ● Vessels of the neck.

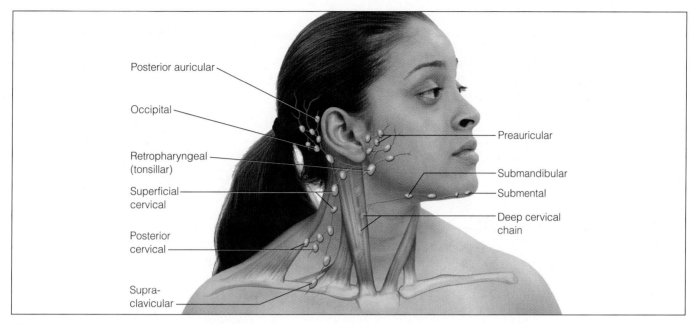

Figure 12.7 ● Lymph nodes of the head and neck.

Lymphatics

A large supply of lymph nodes is located in the head and neck region of the body. These nodes provide defence against invasion of foreign substances by producing lymphocytes and antibodies. The lymph nodes are clustered along lymphatic vessels that infiltrate tissue capillaries and pick up excess fluid called *lymph.* The nurse palpates various areas of the head and neck looking for lymph nodes. Normally, the nodes are nonpalpable. Occasionally, an isolated node is found on palpation, which is usually not considered an abnormal finding. Nodes are palpable when infected or enlarged. Finding several enlarged nodes may be significant in recognizing signs of early infection. The names of the nodes vary depending on the author or practitioner; however, they usually correspond to adjacent anatomical structures or locations (see Figure 12.7). The nodes most commonly assessed are the following:

- *Preauricular:* in front of the ear
- *Occipital:* at the base of the skull
- *Posterior auricular:* behind the ear, over the outer surface of the mastoid bone
- *Submental:* behind the tip of the mandible at the midline
- *Submandibular:* on the medial border of the mandible
- *Retropharyngeal (tonsillar):* at the junction of the posterior and lateral walls of the pharynx at the angle of the jaw
- *Superficial cervical:* anterior to and over the sternocleidomastoid muscle
- *Deep cervical:* posterior to and under the sternocleidomastoid muscle
- *Supraclavicular:* above the clavicle

A detailed description of the lymphatic system is provided in Chapter 18 of this text. ◯◯

SPECIAL CONSIDERATIONS

Throughout the assessment process, the nurse gathers subjective and objective data about the client's state of health. By using critical thinking and the nursing process, the nurse identifies many factors to be considered when collecting the data, including age, developmental level, race, ethnicity, work history, living conditions, social economics, and emotional well-being.

Developmental Considerations

Growth and development are dynamic processes that describe change over time. It is important to understand data collection and interpretation of findings regarding growth and development in relation to normative values. The following discussion presents specific variations in the head and neck for different age groups.

Infants and Children

An infant's head should be measured at each visit until 2 years of age. The newborn's head is about 34 cm (13 to 14 in.), and this is generally equal to the chest circumference. The shape of the head may indicate *moulding,* the shaping of the head by pressure on the bony structures as the head moves through the vaginal canal during delivery. The degree of moulding will be influenced by the presenting part of the head and type of delivery. Usually, it takes several days for the head to take on the more normal round shape. Suture lines should be open, as should the fontanelles. The anterior fontanelle is diamond shaped, and the posterior fontanelle is triangular in shape (see Figure 12.8). The fontanelles should be firm and even with the skull. Slight pulsations are normal. The neck of the newborn is short with many skin folds and begins to lengthen over time. By about 4 months of age the infant begins to demonstrate control of the head. In toddlers, the head is relatively large and the

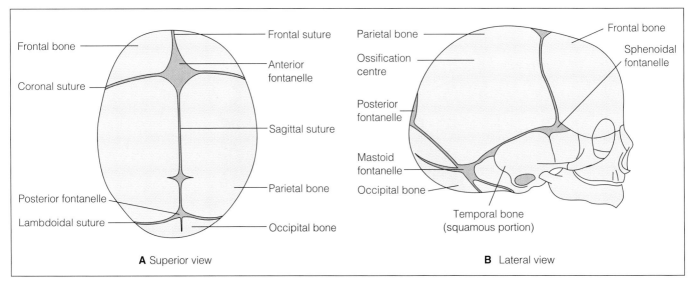

Figure 12.8 ● The newborn's skull.

muscles of the neck are underdeveloped compared with adults. The proportions change throughout the preschool years, and by school age the proportions are similar to those of adults.

The thyroid gland, located in the neck, plays an important role in growth and development. The thyroid is difficult to palpate on an infant, but it can be accomplished on a child by using two or three fingers. Abnormalities in thyroid function are generally detected by assessment of growth and development and through laboratory testing. Further information related to the structures of the head and neck in infants and children is included in Chapter 25 of this text. ⚭

The Pregnant Female

The pregnant female may develop blotchy pigmented spots (melasma) on her face (see Figure 11.6), facial edema, and enlargement of the thyroid. All these symptoms are considered normal and subside after childbirth. The pregnant female may also complain of headaches during the first trimester, which may be related to increased hormones; however, severe, persistent headaches should be evaluated. Serious headaches, especially in late pregnancy, are associated with preeclampsia. Preeclampsia is a serious pregnancy-induced syndrome of high blood pressure, fluid retention, and protein excretion in the urine. Preeclampsia can result in restricted blood flow to the placenta and harm to the developing fetus.

The Older Adult

The older adult loses subcutaneous fat in the face. This increases the wrinkles in the skin, yielding an older appearance. A decrease in reproductive hormones results in the development of coarse, long eyebrows and nasal hair in males and coarse hair, usually on the chin, in females. Loss of teeth or improperly fitting dentures may change facial expressions and symmetry. Rigidity of the cervical vertebrae is common, causing limited range of motion of the neck. The thyroid gland produces fewer hormones with age.

Psychosocial Considerations

A client who is under a great deal of stress may be prone to headaches, including tension headaches, neck pain, and mouth ulcers. Pain in the TMJ may be due to unconscious clenching of the jaw during stressful situations, such as driving in heavy traffic or taking an exam. It may also be caused by teeth grinding during sleep. Chronic TMJ syndrome may eventually result in a wearing down of the teeth, and the client may need to consult a dentist or orthodontist.

Other indications of psychosocial disturbances include tics (involuntary muscle spasms), hair twisting or pulling, lip biting, and excessive blinking. Relaxation techniques, such as meditation and guided imagery, may help relieve head and neck symptoms related to stress. If appropriate, the nurse should refer the client to a mental health professional for assistance.

Social and Ethnocultural Considerations

Within some cultures, eye contact and smiling are considered rude or aggressive. Furthermore, sharing of personal information with strangers is not permitted. These factors make obtaining a detailed health history difficult. Some cultures and religions require the individual to cover the head or face.

Facial malformations are a frequent occurrence in children with fetal alcohol syndrome (FAS). Some infants have a flat occipital prominence (plagiocephaly), which may result from putting them to sleep on their backs. Placing infants on their backs for sleep has become a common practice to reduce the incidence of sudden infant death syndrome (SIDS). Flattening of the head may also occur when infant boards are used.

Thyroid disease is common in areas where iodine is limited. Iodine deficiency disorders, including **goitre** (enlarged thyroid) and hypothyroidism, are significant health problems in India and China. Iodine deficiencies occur in areas with soil poor in iodine. These areas include eastern Europe, parts of South America, Australia, and the western United States. Use of iodized salt has generally eliminated iodine deficiencies in Canada. The World Health Organization (WHO) is overseeing global programs to increase the use of iodized salt to prevent these deficiencies.

Social and Ethnocultural Considerations

- Covering the hair or face is required in some cultures.
- Facial malformations may occur in infants with fetal alcohol syndrome (FAS).

- Immigrants from countries in which millet is a staple food are more likely to have goitre.
- Conduct a nutritional assessment with all individuals exhibiting signs of goitre or other thyroid-related problems.

GATHERING THE DATA

Health assessment of the head and neck includes gathering subjective and objective data. Recall that subjective data collection occurs during the client interview, before the physical assessment, with the collection of the objective data. During the interview, the nurse uses a variety of communication techniques to elicit general and specific information about the structures of the client's head and neck. Health records, the results of laboratory tests, and radiological and imaging reports are important secondary sources to be reviewed and included in the data-gathering process. During physical assessment of the head and neck, the techniques of inspection, palpation, and auscultation will be used to gather the objective data.

HEALTH HISTORY

The health history for the head and neck concerns data related to the head, the face, and the structures of the neck, including the thyroid, trachea, and lymph nodes. Subjective data are gathered during the health history. The nurse must be prepared to observe the client and listen for cues related to the functions of structures within the head and neck. The nurse may use open-ended or closed questions to obtain information. Follow-up questions are intended to identify the source of problems, explain the duration of problems, discuss ways to alleviate problems, and provide clues about the client's knowledge about his or her own health.

The health history guides the physical assessment of the head and neck. The information is always considered in relation to normative values and expectations regarding function of the specific structure. Therefore, the nurse must consider age, gender, race, culture, environment, health practices, past and concurrent problems, and therapies when framing questions and using techniques to elicit information. To address all the factors when conducting a health history, specific questions related to the head, neck, and related lymphatic status and function have been developed. These questions focus on the most common concerns or injuries associated with the head, neck, and lymphatic system; questions related to past health history; questions related to behaviours; questions that address environmental concerns; and those that are specific to clients according to age, including the pregnant female.

The nurse must consider the client's ability to participate in the health history and physical assessment of the head and neck. If a client is experiencing pain, stiffness, or anxiety that accompanies any of these problems, attention must focus on relief of symptoms.

As the nurse gathers the data, she or he will shift the type of questions to direct questions that give the client room to explain or qualify. The mnemonic O-P-Q-R-S-T-U, which stands for onset (chronology), precipitating (or palliative), quality, region (or radiation), severity, timing, and understanding, will help the learner remember the dimensions of the symptoms. The nurse will keep in mind that not all these qualifiers will apply to each symptom.

HEALTH HISTORY QUESTIONS	RATIONALES

The following sections provide sample questions and follow-up questions. Rationales for some questions are provided. The list of questions is not all-inclusive but rather represents the more common concern or injury questions required in a health history related to the head, neck, and related lymphatics. An example of using O-P-Q-R-S-T-U with pain is provided.

HEALTH HISTORY QUESTIONS	RATIONALES

Questions Related to Common Concerns or Injuries

The most common concerns related to illness or injury of the head, neck, and related lymphatics are as follows:

- Pain
- Mass or lumps
- Stiffness

1. **Pain**
   - Are you having any pain or headaches at this time? *If yes:*
   - How long have you been bothered with this type of headache? When does it begin? How long does it last? Where is the pain felt? *Onset (chronology)*

     ▶ Encourage the client to provide a detailed description of the headache to help determine the cause, and possible treatments.

   - What makes the pain worse? What makes it better? Is the pain triggered by any other factors? *Precipitating (palliative)*
   - Can you describe the pain? Is it throbbing? sharp? dull? *Quality*
   - Does the pain radiate or spread to other locations? *Radiation*
   - How often do you experience the pain? How would you rate the pain on a scale of 1 to 10, with 10 being the worst pain? *Severity*
   - Is the pain associated with any particular time of day or activity, such as resting, sleeping, or eating? *Timing*
   - What do you think is causing the pain? *Understanding*

2. **Mass or lumps**
   - Have you noticed any swelling, lumps, bumps, or skin sores on your head that did not heal?

     ▶ Swelling, masses, and lesions that do not heal may indicate cancer.

   - Have you noticed any lumps or swelling on your neck?

     ▶ Lateral neck masses are usually due to enlargement of the cervical lymph nodes, which can be a sign of infection or malignancy.

3. **Stiffness**
   - Do you have or have you experienced stiffness in your neck?
   - Was the stiffness sudden or did it occur gradually?
   - Do you have any other symptoms associated with the stiffness, such as fever?

     ▶ These questions may help in determining if the stiffness is related to muscle stiffness or possible meningeal irritation.

Questions Related to Past Health History

1. **Is there a history of headaches or thyroid problems in your family?**

   ▶ This question may elicit information about illnesses with a familiar or genetic predisposition. Follow-up is required to obtain details about specific problems related to occurrence, treatment, and outcomes.

2. **Do you have or have you had problems affecting your head, face, or neck, including your thyroid gland?**

   ▶ Oversecretion or undersecretion by the thyroid gland may cause rapid weight gain or loss, erratic temperature regulation, fatigue, dyspnea, mood swings, and other alterations in health.

3. **Describe any recent or past injury to your head.**

   ▶ The neurological system assessment is explained in detail in Chapter 24. ○○

   - Did you have any symptoms afterward? Describe them.
   - How did your injury occur?
   - Did you lose consciousness? For how long?
   - Have any problems recurred? *(acute)* How are you managing the problem now? *(chronic)*

     ▶ Head injury can result in acute or chronic neurological problems.

HEALTH HISTORY QUESTIONS	RATIONALES

Questions Related to Behaviours

Healthcare behaviours include both health practices and health patterns. Health practices consist of following recommendations for disease prevention, including screening for risks, screening for early detection of problems, and immunization. Health patterns are habits or acts that affect the client's health. Health behaviours may also include seeking healthcare from healthcare providers who use alternative methods to diagnose and treat illness. Clients should be questioned in a nonjudgmental way and areas for health teaching should be identified.

1. **Do you now use or have you ever used alcohol, recreational drugs, tobacco products, or caffeine?**
   - How much of the product do you use? When did you start?
   - How long have you used the product?
   - Have you had problems associated with the product?
   - What have you done to deal with the problem?

▶ Use of alcohol, tobacco, street drugs, and large amounts of caffeine can affect neurological function and increase headaches.

Questions Related to the Environment

Environment refers to both internal and external environments. Questions related to the internal environment include all the previous questions and those associated with internal or physiological responses. Questions regarding the external environment include those related to home, work, or social environments.

Internal Environment

1. **Are you now experiencing or have you ever had an experience of intermittent or prolonged anxiety or upset?**

▶ Anxiety and upset affect the sympathetic nervous system, producing hormonal responses that affect vascular function. The vasoconstriction can contribute to headache, hypertension, and risk for neurological problems. Stress and tension precipitate and increase neck pain or stiffness.

2. **Do you now use or have you used prescribed or over-the-counter (OTC) medications, home remedies, alternative treatments or therapies, or herbs for problems with your head and neck or for any other purpose?**

▶ Medications can have side effects and interactions that exacerbate or enhance symptoms. Knowledge of medication usage provides information that assists in the analysis of client situations and determination of the significance of findings in a comprehensive assessment.

External Environment

The following questions deal with substances and irritants found in the physical environment of the client. These include the indoor and outdoor environments of the home and the workplace, and those encountered during travel.

1. **Have you ever had irradiation of the head or neck?**

▶ Radiation exposure increases the risk for thyroid tumours.

2. **Are you exposed to chemicals or toxins in your home or work environment?**

▶ Environmental chemicals and toxins can be precipitating factors for headache and neurological problems.

Questions Related to Age

The health history must reflect the anatomical and physiological differences that exist along the age span. The following questions are examples of those that would be specific for infants and children, the pregnant female, and the older adult.

GATHERING THE DATA

HEALTH HISTORY QUESTIONS	RATIONALES
Questions Regarding Infants and Children	
1. Did you use alcohol or recreational drugs during your pregnancy?	▶ Fetal alcohol syndrome causes some deformities of the face. Use of cocaine during pregnancy can result in neurological problems in the infant.
2. Have you noticed any depression or bulging over the infant's soft spots (fontanelles)?	▶ A depressed fontanelle can indicate dehydration, and a bulging fontanelle can indicate an infection.
Questions for the Pregnant Female	
1. Do you have frequent headaches?	▶ Headaches are common during the first trimester, but it is important to rule out other possible complications of pregnancy, such as preeclampsia.
2. Have you noticed changes in the skin on your face? If yes, what changes have occurred?	▶ Hormonal changes can result in melasma or chloasma, pigmented areas on the face. In addition, hormonal changes cause increased secretions of oils in the skin, which may result in acne.
3. Do you have a history of thyroid disease? If yes, what is the disease and treatment?	▶ Thyroid diseases can result in problems with the developing fetus. Existing thyroid problems require careful monitoring of medications.
Questions for the Older Adult	
1. Do you carry out safety precautions in your home? when driving or away from home?	▶ Safety precautions can reduce the risk for falls and injuries to the head and neck. Older adults are at increased risk for falls.

PHYSICAL ASSESSMENT

ASSESSMENT TECHNIQUES AND FINDINGS

Physical assessment of the head and neck requires the use of inspection, palpation, and auscultation. During each procedure, the nurse is gathering objective data related to the structures of the head and neck, and the functions of the structures within them. Inspection includes looking at skin colour, the scalp, the skull, and the face for symmetry of bones and structure. The trachea is palpated for position. The thyroid is palpated for movement, texture, and identification of size or abnormalities. The lymph nodes of the head and neck are palpated. The temporal artery is auscultated. Knowledge of normal parameters and expected findings is essential to interpreting data as the nurse performs the assessment.

In adults, the skull should be normocephalic, that is, a rounded and symmetrical shape. The frontal parietal and occipital prominences are present and symmetrical. The scalp is clear and free of lesions; the hair is evenly distributed. The face is symmetrical; the eyes, ears, nose, and mouth are symmetrically placed. The facial movements are smooth, coordinated, and demonstrate a variety of expressions. The temporal artery feels smooth and firm with no tenderness to palpation and without bruits. The TMJ has nonpainful, full, and smooth range of motion. The head is held erect, without tremors. The neck is symmetrical without swelling and has full range of motion. Carotid artery pulsation is visible bilaterally. The trachea is midline, and the hyoid bone and tracheal cartilage move with swallowing. The thyroid is not enlarged and is without palpable nodules. The lymph nodes of the head and neck are nonpalpable in adults.

EQUIPMENT

examination gown
glass of water
clean, nonsterile examination gloves
stethoscope

TECHNIQUES AND NORMAL FINDINGS	ABNORMAL FINDINGS AND SPECIAL CONSIDERATIONS

THE HEAD

1. **Position the client.**
   - Ask the client to sit comfortably on the examination table (see Figure 12.9).

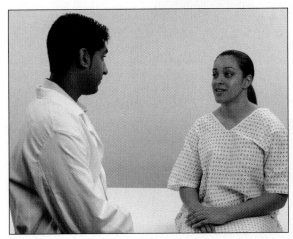

Figure 12.9 ●
Client is positioned.

2. **Instruct the client.**
   - Explain that you will be looking at the client and touching the head, hair, and face. Explain that no discomfort should occur, but if the client experiences pain or discomfort you will stop that part of the examination.

3. **Inspect the head and scalp.**
   - Note size, shape, symmetry, and integrity of the head and scalp. Identify the prominences—frontal, parietal, and occipital—that determine the shape and symmetry of the head.
   - Part the hair and look for scaliness of the scalp, lesions, or foreign bodies. (Refer to Figure 11.22.)
   - Check hair distribution and hygiene.

4. **Inspect the face.**
   - Note the facial expression and symmetry of structures. The eyes, ears, nose, and mouth should be symmetrically placed. The nasolabial folds should be equal. The palpebral fissures should be equal. The top of the ear should be equal to the canthi of the eyes (see Figure 12.2).

5. **Observe movements of the head, face, and eyes.**
   - All movements should be smooth and with purpose. Cranial nerves III, IV, and VI control movement of the eye. Cranial nerve V stimulates movement for mastication (chewing of food). Cranial nerve VII controls movement of the face. A detailed discussion of the cranial nerves is found in Chapter 24. ⚭

▶ Jerky movements or tics may be the result of neurological or psychological disorders.

PHYSICAL ASSESSMENT

TECHNIQUES AND NORMAL FINDINGS	ABNORMAL FINDINGS AND SPECIAL CONSIDERATIONS

6. Palpate the head and scalp.

- Note contour, size, and texture. Ask the client to report any tenderness as you palpate. Normally there is no tenderness with palpation.

▶ Note any tenderness, swelling, edema, or masses, which require further evaluation.

7. Confirm skin and tissue integrity.

- The skin should be intact.

▶ Note any alteration in skin or tissue integrity related to ulcerations, rashes, discolourations, or swellings.

8. Palpate the temporal artery.

- Palpate between the eye and the top of the ear (see Figure 12.10). The artery should feel smooth.

▶ Any thickening or tenderness could indicate inflammation of the artery.

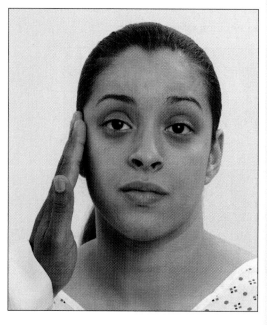

Figure 12.10 ●
Palpating the temporal artery.

9. Auscultate the temporal artery.

- Use the bell of the stethoscope to auscultate for a bruit (a soft blowing sound). Bruits are not normally present.

▶ A bruit is indicative of stenosis (narrowing) of the vessel.

10. Test the range of motion of the TMJ.

- Place your fingers in front of each ear and ask the client to open and close the mouth slowly. There should be no limitation of movement or tenderness. You should feel a slight indentation of the joint. (For more detail on assessment of the TMJ, see Chapter 23. ⟲)

  Soft clicking noises on movement are sometimes heard and are considered normal.

▶ Crepitation, a crackling sound on movement, may indicate joint problems.

▶ Any limitation of movement or tenderness on movement requires further evaluation.

THE NECK

1. Instruct the client.

- Explain that you will be looking at and touching the front and sides of the client's neck. Tell the client that you will provide specific instructions for special tests. Advise the client to inform you of any discomfort.

PHYSICAL ASSESSMENT

Techniques and Normal Findings

2. Inspect the neck for skin colour, integrity, shape, and symmetry.
   - Observe for any swelling of the lymph nodes below the angle of the jaw and along the sternocleidomastoid muscle.
   - The head should be held erect with no tremors.

▶ Excessive rigidity of the neck may indicate arthritis. Inability to hold the neck erect may be due to muscle spasms. Swelling of the lymph nodes may indicate infection and requires further assessment.

3. Test the range of motion of the neck.
   - Ask the client to slowly move the chin to the chest, turn the head right and left, then touch the left ear to left shoulder and the right ear to right shoulder (without raising the shoulders). Then ask the client to extend the head back.
     There should be no pain and no limitation of movement (for further discussion, see Chapter 23 ⬭).

▶ Any pain or limitation of movement could indicate arthritis, muscle spasm, or inflammation. Rapid movement and compression of cerebral vertebrae may cause dizziness.

4. Observe the carotid arteries and jugular veins.
   - The carotid artery runs just below the angle of the jaw, and its pulsations can frequently be seen. Assessment of the carotid arteries and jugular veins is discussed fully in Chapter 18. ⬭

▶ Any distension or prominence may indicate a vascular disorder.

5. Palpate the trachea.
   - Palpate the sternal notch. Move the finger pad of the palpating finger off the notch to the midline of the neck. Lightly palpate the area. You will feel the C rings (cricoid cartilage) of the trachea.
     Move the finger laterally, first to the right and then to the left. You have now identified the lateral borders of the trachea (see Figure 12.11).
   - The trachea should be midline, and the distance to the sternocleidomastoid muscles on each side should be equal. Place the thumb and index finger on each side of the trachea and slide them upward. As the trachea begins to widen, you have now identified the thyroid cartilage. Continue to slide your thumb and index finger high into the neck. Palpate the hyoid bone. The greater horns of the hyoid bone are most prominent. Confirm that the hyoid bone and tracheal cartilages move when the client swallows.

▶ Tracheal displacement is the result of masses in the neck, mediastinum, pneumothorax, or fibrosis.

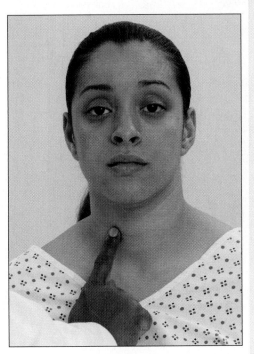

Figure 12.11 ●
Palpating the trachea.

TECHNIQUES AND NORMAL FINDINGS	ABNORMAL FINDINGS AND SPECIAL CONSIDERATIONS

6. Inspect the thyroid gland.

- The thyroid is not observable normally until the client swallows. Give the client a cup of water.
- Distinguish the thyroid from other structures in the neck by asking the client to drink a sip of water.
- The thyroid tissue is attached to the trachea, and, as the client swallows, it moves superiorly. You may want to adjust the lighting in the room, if possible, so that shadows are cast on the client's neck. This may help you to visualize the thyroid.

▶ If the client has any enlargement of the thyroid or masses near the thyroid, they appear as bulges when the client swallows.

7. Palpate the thyroid gland from behind the client.

- Normally, the thyroid gland is nonpalpable, and so you need to be patient as you learn this technique.
- Stand behind the client.
- Ask the client to sit up straight, lower the chin, and turn the head slightly to the right.
- This position causes the client's neck muscles to relax.
- Use the fingers of your left hand to gently push the trachea to the right. Use light pressure during palpation to avoid obliterating findings.
- With the fingers of the right hand, palpate the area between the trachea and the sternocleidomastoid muscle. Slowly and gently retract the sternocleidomastoid muscle, and then ask the client to drink a sip of water. Palpate as the thyroid gland moves up during swallowing (see Figure 12.12). Normally, you will not feel the thyroid gland, although in some clients with long, thin necks, you may be able to feel the isthmus. Reverse the procedure for the left side.

▶ An enlarged thyroid gland may be due to a metabolic disorder, such as **hyperthyroidism.** Palpable masses of 5 mm (0.2 in.) or larger are alterations in health. Their location, size, and shape should be documented, and the client should be evaluated further. In pregnancy, a slightly enlarged thyroid can be a normal finding. Most pathological hyperthyroidism in pregnancy is caused by Graves' disease, an autoimmune disorder that causes increased production of thyroid hormones.

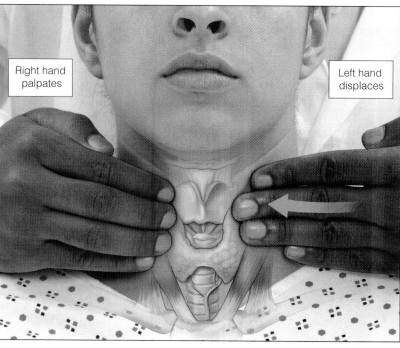

Right hand palpates

Left hand displaces

Figure 12.12 ● Palpating the thyroid by using a posterior approach.

PHYSICAL ASSESSMENT

TECHNIQUES AND NORMAL FINDINGS	ABNORMAL FINDINGS AND SPECIAL CONSIDERATIONS

8. **Palpate the thyroid gland from in front of the client.**
   - This is an alternative approach. Stand in front of the client. Ask the client to lower the head and turn slightly to the right. Using the thumb of your right hand, gently push the trachea to the left (see Figure 12.13).
   - Place your left thumb and fingers over the sternocleidomastoid muscle and feel for any enlargement of the right lobe as the client swallows. Have water available to make swallowing easier. Reverse the procedure for the left side.

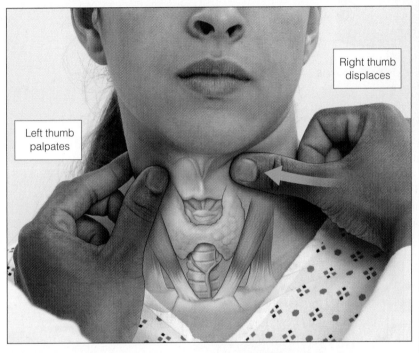

Right thumb displaces

Left thumb palpates

Figure 12.13 ● Alternative technique for palpating the thyroid.

9. **Auscultate the thyroid.**
   - If the thyroid is enlarged, the area over the thyroid is auscultated to detect any bruits. In an enlarged thyroid, blood flows through the arteries at an accelerated rate, producing a soft, rushing sound. This sound can best be detected with the bell of the stethoscope.

   ▶ The presence of a bruit is abnormal and is an indication of increased blood flow.

10. **Palpate the lymph nodes of the head and neck.**
    - Palpate the lymph nodes by exerting gentle circular pressure with the fingerpads of both hands. It is important to avoid strong pressure, which can push the nodes into the muscle and underlying structures, making them difficult to find. It is also important to establish a routine for examination; otherwise, it is possible to omit one or more of the groups of nodes. The following is one suggested order of examination (see Figure 12.14).

      1. Preauricular
      2. Postauricular
      3. Occipital
      4. Retropharyngeal (tonsillar)
      5. Submandibular
      6. Submental (with one hand)
      7. Superficial cervical chain
      8. Deep cervical chain
      9. Posterior cervical lymph node palpation
      10. Supraclavicular

    ▶ Enlargement of lymph nodes is called **lymphadenopathy** and can be due to infection, allergies, or a tumour.

PHYSICAL ASSESSMENT

TECHNIQUES AND NORMAL FINDINGS	ABNORMAL FINDINGS AND SPECIAL CONSIDERATIONS

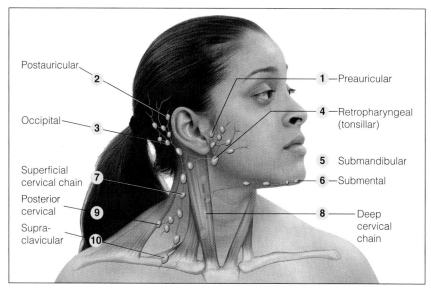

Figure 12.14 ● Suggested sequence for palpating lymph nodes.

- Ask the client to bend the head toward the side being examined to relax the muscles and make the nodes easier to palpate. If any lymph nodes are palpable, make a note of their location, size, shape, fixation or mobility, and tenderness (see Figure 12.15).

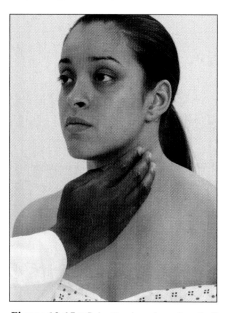 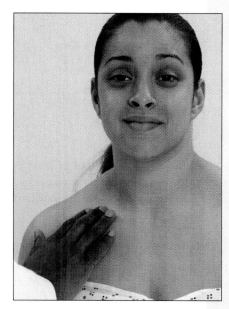

Figure 12.15 ● Palpating lymph nodes. A. Cervical. B. Supraclavicular.

SAMPLE DOCUMENTATION

Subjective: No history of head injury or surgery to the head or neck. Complains of occasional headache but attributes this to "stress." No complaints of dizziness or neck pain. Has not noticed any lumps, swelling, or lesions to the head or neck.

Objective: Head normocephalic. No rashes or lesions seen. No masses palpable. No temporal bruits heard. Full range of motion with TMJ, no clicks. Trachea midline, thyroid nonpalpable. Lymph nodes of the head and neck nontender and nonpalpable.

APPLICATION THROUGH CRITICAL THINKING

CASE STUDY

A married couple has come to the clinic for renewal of prescriptions and annual flu shots. During the encounter, the husband mentions to the nurse that he is concerned about his 69-year-old wife. He tells the nurse his wife has become very forgetful. She eats very little but seems to have gained weight. She seems "down" all the time. When questioned, the wife states she "just hasn't been herself." She admits she doesn't have much of an appetite. She explains that she has not been as active as she used to be and as a result her bowels are not as regular. She thinks those are the reasons she feels "out of sorts." She chides her husband that his memory "isn't so hot either." He insists that she is forgetting simple things while he has always forgotten birthdays and to write down phone messages and such.

A simple health history indicates that Mr. and Mrs. Currie live in a rural farming region that has, in the past, used a number of pesticides that are now banned. Mrs. Currie remains a very active individual and is the primary support for her husband, who is in his 80s.

The nurse is concerned about this client and carries out a further interview, which reveals the following findings: The client is generally cold, feels tired all of the time, and really doesn't have the energy to do much around the house. She finds the thought of going out exhausting. She tells the nurse that her tongue feels thick and she thinks her voice has changed.

The client agrees to a physical examination. The findings include a weight gain of 4.5 kg (10 lb.) from her last clinic visit, 6 months ago. Her thyroid is enlarged and palpable. Her skin is dry, she has 1+ edema of the lower extremities, and her speech is slow. Her abdomen is distended with bowel sounds in all quadrants.

The nurse recommends that this woman have laboratory testing for thyroid dysfunction and arranges for consultation with a physician. The nurse schedules a follow-up appointment and makes some recommendations for this client that include increasing fluid intake and fibre to improve bowel function. The client is advised to wear warm clothing and to rest frequently. The nurse explains the functions of the thyroid and that medication can improve all aspects of her current condition when taken regularly.

Complete Documentation

The following information is summarized from the case study.

SUBJECTIVE DATA: "Just haven't been myself." Loss of appetite, decreased activity, irregular bowel function. Generally cold, tired, lack of energy, thick tongue, and change in voice. Husband states that wife is forgetful, eats very little, has gained weight, and seems "down."

OBJECTIVE DATA: B/P 120/76—P 64—T 36.9°C (98.4°F). Alert and oriented. Unable to repeat list of five words after 5 minutes. Weight gain 4.5 kg (10 lb.) over 6 months. Thyroid enlarged and palpable. Skin cool and dry, edema lower extremities. Slow speech. Abdomen distended. Bowel sounds present all quadrants.

A sample assessment form appears below.

ASSESSMENT FORM

Vital Signs: *BP 120/76—P 64—T 36.9*

Neur: *Alert and oriented*

Speech: *Slow, slurred, unable to recall list of words at 5 minutes*

Skin: *Cool, dry, 1+ edema lower extremities*

Nutrition: *Lack of appetite, weight gain 4.5 kg in 6 months*

Neck: *Thyroid enlarged, palpable*

Abdomen: *Distended, BS present X 4*

▶ Critical Thinking Questions

1. What may be responsible for the findings about this 69-year-old female?
2. What further data should the nurse collect?
3. What aspects of physical assessment and what tests are important in arriving at a diagnosis for this client?

▶ Applying Nursing Diagnoses

1. *Activity intolerance* is a diagnostic statement in the NANDA-I taxonomy (see Appendix A 👓). Do the data in the case study support this diagnosis? If so, identify the data.
2. Use the NANDA-I taxonomy to formulate additional diagnoses for the female client in the case study. Identify the data required for the PES (problem, etiology, signs or symptoms) statements.

▶ Prepare Teaching Plan

LEARNING NEED: The case study includes subjective and objective data indicative of a thyroid dysfunction. The nurse provides for diagnostic studies and follow-up with a physician, and provides information about the thyroid gland and medication as treatment for the problem. The nurse's actions are based on the determination that the client needs suggestions to ease current symptoms, information that will reassure her and assist her in decision making about the diagnosis and treatment of her problem.

The client is representative of a population at risk for hypothyroidism, that is, female and over 50 years of age. Aging individuals could benefit from education about hypothyroidism. The following teaching plan is intended to provide information about hypothyroidism for a group of learners.

GOAL: The participants will acquire information of value in promotion of thyroid health.

OBJECTIVES: On completion of the learning session, the participants will be able to do the following:

1. Discuss thyroid function.
2. Describe hypothyroidism.
3. List symptoms of hypothyroidism.
4. Identify diagnostic tests for hypothyroidism.
5. Discuss treatment for hypothyroidism.

Following is an example of the teaching plan for Objective 2. After reviewing this sample teaching plan for Objective 2, go to the MyNursingLab website for this text to complete the teaching plan for other objectives.

APPLICATION OF OBJECTIVE 2: Describe hypothyroidism.

Content	Teaching Strategy	Evaluation
• Hypothyroidism occurs when the thyroid does not produce enough of the thyroid hormones. • Hypothyroidism can occur as a result of inflammation of the thyroid, leading to failure of parts of the gland. • Hashimoto's disease is an autoimmune disease that leads to thyroid failure. The immune system attacks the thyroid. • Other causes include surgical removal of part of the gland, irradiation of the gland, or inflammatory processes. • Hypothyroidism occurs more frequently in females and after 50 years of age. • Risk factors include obesity, X-ray exposure in the neck area, or radiation treatment of the thyroid.	• Lecture • Discussion • Printed materials Lecture is appropriate when disseminating information to large groups. Discussion allows participants to bring up concerns and to raise questions. Printed material, especially to be taken away with learners, allows review, reinforcement, and reading at the learners' pace.	• Written examination. May use short answer, fill-in, or multiple-choice items or a combination of items. If these are short and easy to evaluate, the learner receives immediate feedback.

HEALTH PROMOTION ASSESSMENT TOOL

Social Determinants of Health	Level of Action	Action Strategies
Personal coping skills	Family	**Develop personal skills** • Teach Mrs. and Mr. Currie about the importance of good hydration and nutrition, and provide tips to ensure their meals are balanced. • Encourage them to use multivitamins that are appropriate for seniors. • Discuss the importance of incorporating 30 minutes of physical activity three times per week into their routine; give examples of what this may look like for them in relation to their age and lifestyle. • Discuss the need for frequent rest periods and how to accommodate these when at home and when out. • Discuss the importance of increasing fluid intake and fibre to maintain bowel function. • Encourage various options to keep Mrs. Currie warm in the house, such as increasing the thermostat, using shawls and throws, and taking warm showers. • Teach the couple the importance of skin care, including the use of moisturizers and sunscreen.
Health services	Individual and family	**Create supportive environments** • Complete a cognitive assessment of Mrs. Currie with referrals to other healthcare professionals as necessary. • Provide memory prompt tools (e.g., a Day-Timer) the couple can use to plan their daily activities.
Social support networks	Family and community	**Create supportive environments** • Assess the couple's social supports. Are there family or friends they connect with regularly who can check in on them and help them decide whether they need further assistance at home? • Assess mobility level of this family. Are resources required to help with household tasks, including purchasing groceries or other necessities?

Abnormal Findings

Abnormal findings in the head and neck include headaches, abnormalities in the size and contour of the skull, malformations or abnormalities of the face and neck, and thyroid disorders. Examples of common abnormalities of the head and neck are presented in the following pages.

Headaches

Classic Migraine

A classic migraine is usually preceded by an aura during which the client may feel depressed, restless, or irritable; see spots or flashes of light; feel nauseated; or experience numbing or tingling in the face or extremities. The pain of the migraine itself may be mild or debilitating, requiring the client to lie down in the darkness in silence. It is usually a pulsating pain that is localized to the side, front, or back of the head, and it may be accompanied by nausea, vertigo, tremors, and other symptoms. The acute phase of a classic migraine typically lasts from 4 to 6 hours.

Cluster Headache

A cluster headache is so named because numerous episodes occur over days or even months and then are followed by a period of remission, during which no headaches occur. Cluster headaches have no aura. Their onset is sudden and may be associated with alcohol consumption, stress, or emotional distress. They often begin suddenly at night with an excruciating pain on one side of the face spreading upward behind one eye. The nose and affected eye water, and nasal congestion is common. Cluster headaches may last for only a few minutes or up to a few hours.

Tension Headache

A tension headache, also known as a muscle contraction headache, is due to sustained contraction of the muscles in the head, neck, or upper back. The onset is gradual, not sudden, and the pain is usually steady, not throbbing. The pain may be unilateral or bilateral and typically ranges from the cervical region to the top of the head. Tension headaches may be associated with stress, overwork, dental problems, premenstrual syndrome, sinus inflammation, and other health problems.

Abnormalities of the Skull and Face

Hydrocephalus

Hydrocephalus is enlargement of the head caused by inadequate drainage of cerebrospinal fluid, resulting in abnormal growth of the skull (see Figure 12.16).

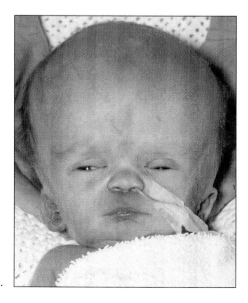

Figure 12.16 ● Hydrocephalus.

Craniosynostosis

Craniosynostosis is early closure of sutures (see Figure 12.17). With early closure of the sagittal sutures, the head elongates. With early closure of the coronal sutures, the head, face, and orbits are altered.

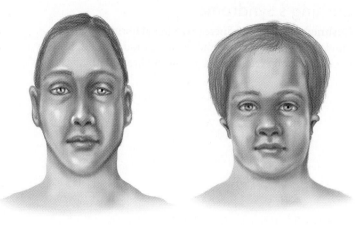

Figure 12.17 ● Craniosynostosis.

Acromegaly

Acromegaly is enlargement of the skull and cranial bones cause by increased growth hormone (see Figure 12.18).

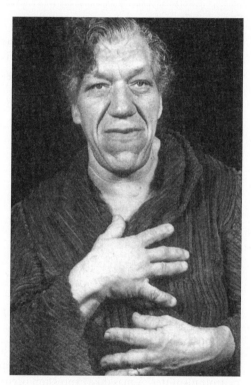

Figure 12.18 ● Acromegaly.

Bell's Palsy

Bell's palsy is a temporary disorder affecting cranial nerve VII and producing a unilateral facial paralysis (see Figure 12.19). It may be caused by a virus. Its onset is sudden, and it usually resolves spontaneously in a few weeks without residual effects.

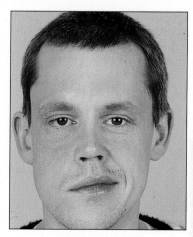

Figure 12.19 ● Bell's palsy.

Cushing's Syndrome

Cushing's syndrome is increased adrenal hormone production leading to a rounded "moon" face, ruddy cheeks, prominent jowls, and excess facial hair (see Figure 12.20).

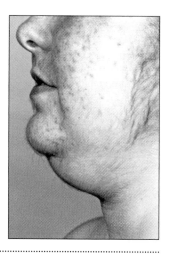

Figure 12.20 ● Cushing's syndrome.

Down Syndrome

Down syndrome is a chromosomal defect causing varying degrees of intellectual disability and characteristic facial features, such as slanted eyes, a flat nasal bridge, a flat nose, a protruding tongue, and a short, broad neck (see Figure 12.21).

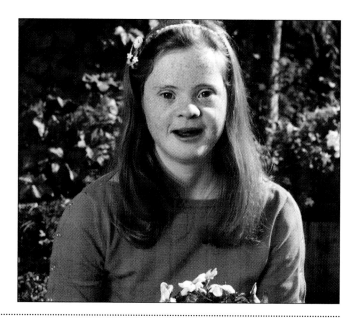

Figure 12.21 ● Down syndrome.

Parkinson's Disease

Parkinson's disease is the result of a decrease in dopamine, a neurotransmitter. A masklike expression occurs in the disease (see Figure 12.22).

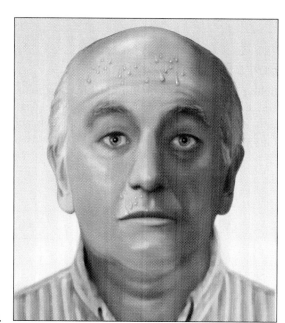

Figure 12.22 ● Parkinson's disease.

Brain Attack

A brain attack, stroke, or cerebrovascular accident (CVA) can result in neurological deficits that include facial paralysis (see Figure 12.23).

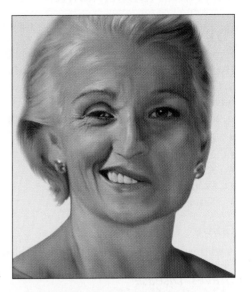

Figure 12.23 ● Brain attack.

Fetal Alcohol Syndrome

Fetal alcohol syndrome is a disorder characterized by epicanthal folds, narrow palpebral fissures, a deformed upper lip below the septum of the nose, and some degree of intellectual disability (see Figure 12.24). FAS is seen in infants of mothers whose intake of alcohol during pregnancy was significant.

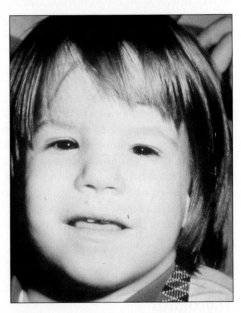

Figure 12.24 ● Fetal alcohol syndrome.

Torticollis

Torticollis is spasm of the sternocleidomastoid muscle on one side of the body, which often results from birth trauma (see Figure 12.25). If left untreated, the muscle becomes fibrotic and permanently shortened.

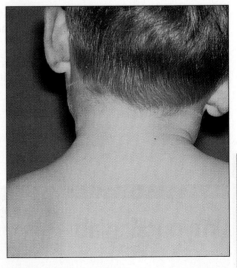

Figure 12.25 ● Torticollis.

Thyroid Abnormalities

Hyperthyroidism

Hyperthyroidism is excessive production of thyroid hormones. Hyperthyroidism results in enlargement of the gland, exophthalmos (bulging eyes), fine hair, weight loss, diarrhea, and other alterations.

Symptoms of hyperthyroidism include the following:

- Irritability or nervousness
- Muscle weakness or tremors
- Amenorrhea
- Weight loss
- Visual disturbances

Goitre

A goitre is an enlargement of the thyroid gland.

Graves' Disease

Graves' disease is the most common type of hyperthyroidism. There is no known cause. Graves' disease may be an autoimmune response or related to hereditary factors.

Thyroid Adenoma

Thyroid adenoma refers to benign thyroid nodules that occur most frequently in older adults. There is no known cause for thyroid adenomas.

Thyroid Carcinoma

Thyroid carcinoma can occur following radiation of the thyroid, chronic goitre, or as a result of hereditary factors. Thyroid carcinomas are malignant tumours in hormone-producing cells or supporting cells. Excess thyroid hormone is produced in the tumours.

Hyperthyroidism and Medication

Excessive iodine in some medications may cause oversecretion of thyroid hormones.

Hypothyroidism

Hypothyroidism occurs when there is a decrease in production of thyroid hormones. The decrease in thyroid hormones results in lowered basal metabolism. It may be a result of decreased pituitary stimulation of the thyroid gland or lack of hypothalamic thyroid-releasing factor. The most common occurrence in hypothyroidism is loss of thyroid tissue as a result of an autoimmune response or iodine deficiency. Hypothyroidism occurs most frequently in females over 50.

Symptoms of hypothyroidism include the following:

- Fatigue
- Weakness
- Depression

Congenital Hypothyroidism

In congenital hypothyroidism, the thyroid is nonfunctioning at birth. If untreated, it results in retardation of physical and mental growth.

Myxedema

Myxedema is a severe form of hypothyroidism that causes nonpitting edema throughout the body and thickening of facial features. Complications of this disease affect major organ systems. Myxedema coma results in cardiovascular collapse, electrolyte disturbances, respiratory depression, and cerebral hypoxia.

Thyroiditis

Thyroiditis is an inflammation of the thyroid gland. This inflammation may cause release of stored hormones, resulting in temporary hyperthyroidism of weeks or months.

Postpartum Thyroiditis

Postpartum thyroiditis is a temporary condition occurring in 5% to 9% of females postpartum.

Hashimoto's Thyroiditis

Hashimoto's thyroiditis is an autoimmune disease that is thought to be hereditary and results in primary hypothyroidism.

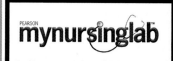
ABNORMAL FINDINGS

13

EYE

THE EYES ARE LOCATED IN THE ORBITAL cavities of the skull. Only the anterior aspect of the eye is exposed. The eyes are the sensory organs responsible for vision. Vision is a major mechanism for experiencing the world.

ANATOMY AND PHYSIOLOGY REVIEW

The eye is the structure through which light is gathered to produce vision. Layers and membranes serve several purposes. The accessory structures of the eye provide protection and are responsible for movement of the eye. Each anatomical structure is described in the following section.

Eye

The eye, commonly called the eyeball, is a fluid-filled sphere having a diameter of approximately 2.5 cm (1 in.). The eye receives light waves and transmits these waves to the brain for interpretation as visual images. Only a small portion of the eye is seen. Most of the eye is set into and protected by the bony orbit of the skull (see Figure 13.1).

The eye is composed of three layers: the sclera, the choroids, and the retina. The **sclera,** the outermost layer, is an extremely dense, hard, fibrous membrane that helps to maintain the shape of the eye. It is the white fibrous part of the eye that is seen anteriorly. Its primary function is to support and protect the structures of the eye (see Figure 13.2).

The **cornea** is the clear, transparent part of the sclera and forms the anterior one sixth of the eye. It is considered to be the window of the eye, allowing light to enter. The extensive nerve endings in the cornea are responsible for the blink reflex, increase the secretion of tears for protection, and are most sensitive to pain.

The **choroid,** the middle layer, is the vascular, pigmented layer of the eye. The **iris** is the circular, coloured, muscular aspect of this layer of the eye and is located in the anterior portion of the eye. The centre of the iris is opened and is called the pupil. The iris responds to light by making the pupil larger or smaller, thereby controlling the amount of light that enters the eye. A dim light will cause the iris to open, enlarging the pupil size (**mydriasis**). This increases the amount of light entering the eye, enhancing distance vision. A bright light causes the iris to respond by decreasing pupil size (**miosis**), thus decreasing the amount of light entering the eye, accommodating near vision. The third cranial nerve controls pupillary constriction and dilation. The parasympathetic branch of this nerve stimulates pupillary constriction while the sympathetic branch stimulates dilation of the pupil.

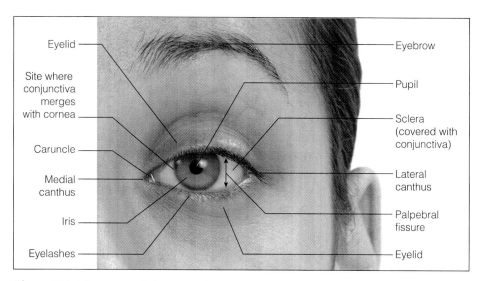

Figure 13.1 ● Structures of the external eye.

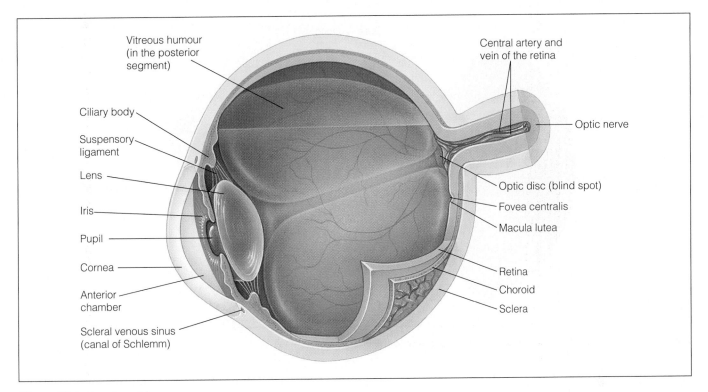

Vitreous humour (in the posterior segment)

Central artery and vein of the retina

Ciliary body

Suspensory ligament

Lens

Iris

Pupil

Cornea

Anterior chamber

Scleral venous sinus (canal of Schlemm)

Optic nerve

Optic disc (blind spot)

Fovea centralis

Macula lutea

Retina

Choroid

Sclera

Figure 13.2 ● Interior of the eye.

The third and innermost membrane, the **retina,** is the sensory portion of the eye. The retina, a direct extension of the optic nerve, helps to change light waves into neural impulses for interpretation as visual impulses by the brain. The retina contains many rods and cones. The rods function in dim light and are also considered to be peripheral vision receptors. The cones function in bright light, are central vision receptors, and provide colour to sight.

The **optic disc,** on the nasal aspect of the retina, is round with clear margins. It is usually creamy-yellow and is the point at which the optic nerve and retina meet. The colour of the disc and the retinal background differ according to skin colour. The colour is lighter in people with light skin and darker in individuals with dark skin. The centre of this disc, the physiological cup, is the point at which the vascular network enters the eye.

The **macula** is responsible for central vision. The macula, with its yellow, pitlike centre called the *fovea centralis,* appears as a hyperpigmented spot on the temporal aspect of the retina.

Refraction of the Eye

Light rays travel in a straight line. The light rays must change direction or refract as they pass from one source to another source for vision to occur. Each structure in the pathway of light has a different density. Several structures of the eye help with the deflection or refraction of the light rays. The structures responsible for refraction include the cornea, aqueous humour, crystalline lens, and vitreous humour.

Refraction allows the light rays to enter the eye and be aimed (reflected) to the correct part of the retina for most accurate vision. **Emmetropia** is the normal refractive condition of the

eye. **Myopia** (nearsightedness) is a condition in which the light rays focus in front of the retina. In **hyperopia** (farsightedness) the light rays focus behind the retina.

The **aqueous humour** is a clear, fluidlike substance found in the anterior segment of the eye that helps maintain ocular pressure. The aqueous humour is a refractory medium of the eye that is constantly being formed and is always flowing through the pupil and draining into the venous system. The **vitreous humour,** another refractory medium, is a clear gel located in the posterior segment of the eye. This gel helps maintain the intraocular pressure and the shape of the eye, and transmits light rays through the eye.

The **lens,** situated directly behind the pupil, is a biconvex (convex on both surfaces), transparent, and flexible structure. It separates the anterior and posterior segments of the eye. The ability of the lens to accommodate or change its shape permits light to focus properly on the retina and enhances fine focusing of images.

Visual Pathways

An object external to the body creates an image. Via light waves, this image is transported to the brain for interpretation as vision. Light waves must bend to focus correctly on the retina. The refractory structures—the cornea, aqueous humour, anterior and posterior chambers, lens, and vitreous humour—help bend the light waves onto the retina. This retinal image, via the nerve fibres, is conducted to the optic nerve (cranial nerve II). At the optic chiasm, the optic fibres of the nerves cross over and join the temporal fibres from the opposite eye. Optic tracts encircle the brain and the impulse is transmitted to the occipital lobe of the brain for interpretation (see Figure 13.3).

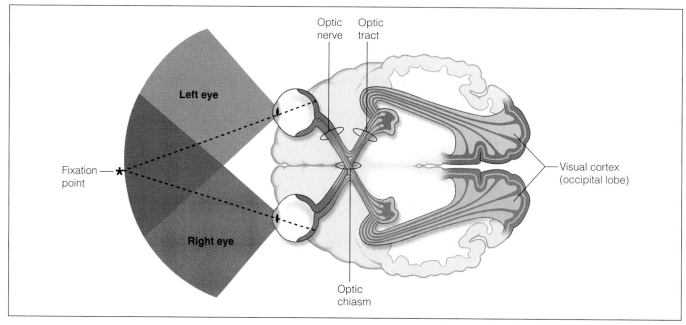

Figure 13.3 ● Visual fields of the eye and the visual pathway to the brain.

Accessory Structures of the Eye

The eye has several external accessory structures. The eyebrows are the coarse short hairs that are located on the lower portion of the forehead at the orbital margins. The primary function of the eyebrow is to protect the eye (Figure 13.1).

The eyelids, or **palpebrae,** are the movable folds of skin that cover and protect the eyes. The opening between the upper and lower eyelids is called the **palpebral fissure.** The eyelids meet medially and laterally to form the medial canthus and the lateral canthus. The meibomian glands, embedded in the eyelids, are modified sebaceous glands that produce an oily substance to help lubricate the eyes and eyelids. The eyelashes are hairs projecting from the eyelids. The large supply of nerve fibres helps support the blink reflex, thereby protecting the eye.

The conjunctiva, a thin mucous membrane, lines the interior of the eyelids and continues over the anterior portion of the eye, meeting the cornea but not covering it. The conjunctiva protects the eye by preventing foreign objects from entering the eye. The conjunctiva also produces a lubricating fluid that prevents the eyes from drying.

The lacrimal apparatus consists of the lacrimal glands and ducts. Lacrimal secretions, commonly called tears, are secreted and spread over the conjunctiva when blinking. The tears enter the lacrimal puncta and drain via the many ducts into the posterior nasal passage (see Figure 13.4).

Each eye has six extrinsic or extraocular muscles. They help hold the eye in place within the bony orbit. These muscles are the lateral rectus, medial rectus, superior rectus, inferior rectus, inferior oblique, and superior oblique (see Figure 13.5).

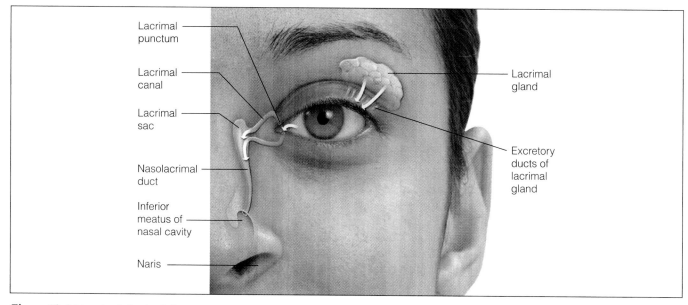

Figure 13.4 ● Lacrimal glands of the eye.

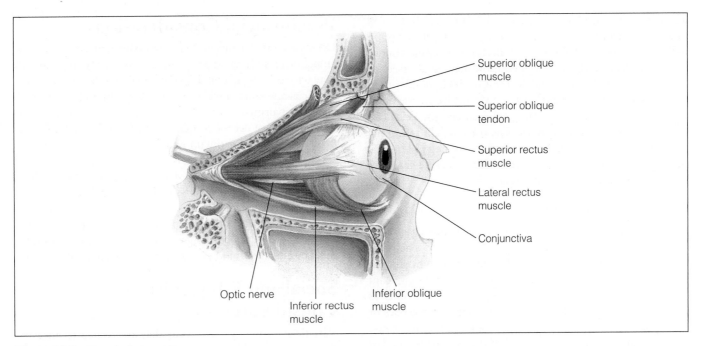

Figure 13.5 ● Extraocular muscles.

With the coordination of these muscles, the individual experiences one-image sight. These muscles are innervated by cranial nerves III, IV, and VI. Figure 13.6 depicts the correlation of eye movement with eye muscle and cranial nerve.

SPECIAL CONSIDERATIONS

Throughout the assessment process, the nurse gathers subjective and objective data about the client's state of health. By using critical thinking and the nursing process, the nurse identifies many factors to be considered when collecting the data. Vision and eye health are influenced by a number of factors, including age, developmental level, race, ethnicity, occupation, socioeconomics, and emotional well-being. The nurse must consider these factors when gathering subjective and objective data during a comprehensive health assessment.

Developmental Considerations

Comprehensive health assessment includes interpretation of findings in relation to normative values. The following sections describe normal variations in structures and functions of the eye for different age groups.

Infants and Children

At birth, the eyes of the neonate should be symmetrical. The pupils are equal and respond to light. The iris is generally brown in dark-skinned neonates, and grey-blue in light-skinned neonates. By about the third month of age, the colour of the eyes begins to change to its more permanent shade. Many times, the eyelids are edematous at birth. Little to no tears are present at birth, but they begin to appear by the fourth week. Binocular vision (vision in both eyes) begins to develop by 6 weeks of age. Before this time, neonates will attempt to fixate on

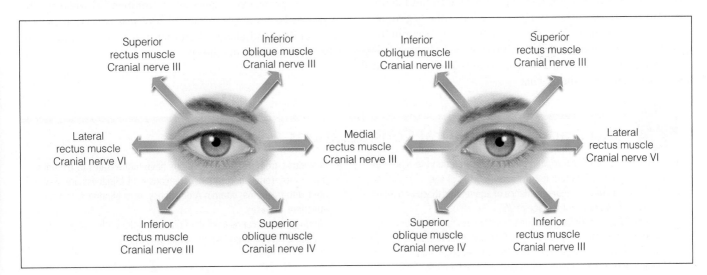

Figure 13.6 ● Eye movements with muscle and nerve coordination.

a bright or moving object. The eyes reach adult size by 8 years of age. The **red reflex,** a glowing red colour that fills the pupil as light from the ophthalmoscope reflects off the retina, should be elicited from birth. Peripheral vision may be assessed by using the confrontation visual field test in children older than 3 years of age. It is important to assess extraocular muscle function as early as possible in young children because delay can lead to permanent visual damage. The corneal light reflex, the Hirschberg test, can be used to determine symmetry of muscle function. Lateral deviations of the eye (disconjugate gaze) are normal findings until 4 months of age.

The Pregnant Female

The pregnant female may complain of dry eyes and may discontinue wearing contact lenses during her pregnancy. The pregnant client may also describe visual changes caused by shifting fluid in the cornea. These symptoms are usually not significant and disappear after childbirth. Changes in eyesight, such as refraction changes requiring a new prescription for glasses or contact lenses, blurriness, or distorted vision, can occur because of temporary changes in the shape of the eye during the last trimester of pregnancy and the first 6 weeks postpartum.

The Older Adult

By age 45, the lens of the eye loses elasticity, and the ciliary muscles become weaker, resulting in a decreased ability of the lens to change shape to accommodate for near vision. This condition is called **presbyopia.** The loss of fat from the orbit of the eye produces a drooping appearance. The lacrimal glands decrease tear production, and the client may complain of a burning sensation in the eyes. The cornea of the eye may appear cloudy, and the nurse may detect a deposit of white-yellow material around the cornea, called arcus senilis. This is a deposition of fat, but it is considered normal after age 45 to 50 and has no effect on vision. The pupillary light reflex is slower with age, and the pupils may be smaller in size.

Within the eye, the blood vessels are pale, and the nurse may detect small, round yellow dots scattered on the retina. These yellow dots do not interfere with vision. As the client ages, the lens continues to thicken and yellow, forming a dense area that reduces lens clarity. This condition is the beginning of a **cataract** formation. Macular degeneration can occur in the older client, resulting in a loss of central vision. The ophthalmoscopic examination may reveal narrowed blood vessels with a granular pigment in the macula.

Psychosocial Considerations

Decreased visual acuity and visual impairment can affect individuals across the age span. Children with vision impairments may have developmental delays and may require special assistive social and educational services into adulthood. Adults with vision impairments may lose some personal independence, may experience decreased quality of life, and may find it difficult to obtain or maintain employment. Visual impairment results in stress for individuals and families as they adapt to alterations in the activities of daily living and as they navigate the healthcare and social service systems for diagnosis, treatment, and assistance.

Eye contact with other people varies, especially during the communication process. Age, gender, and culture influence the type and amount of eye contact people make with others.

Social and Ethnocultural Considerations

Variations in the eye can occur that are related to ancestry. For example, people of Asian descent tend to have prominent epicanthic folds (a vertical fold of skin) covering the inner canthus of the eye. Dark-skinned individuals may have dark pigmented spots on the sclera, and their retinae may appear darker. People with light-coloured eyes typically have lighter retinae and better night vision but are more sensitive to bright sunlight and artificial light.

Excessive sun exposure without the use of sunglasses can promote cataract formation. A deficiency of vitamin A can cause night blindness. Some medications have side effects that cause excessive corneal dryness, vision changes, or increased intraocular pressure. When assessing a client who wears contact lenses, it is important to determine what type of contact lens is worn (hard versus soft, extended wear versus daily change) and evaluate the client's cleansing routine. Clients should be taught that makeup and applicators should be discarded after 3 months, and makeup should not be shared to reduce the risk of infection. Trauma or damage to the eye can occur in work, recreational, and social environments. Safety glasses or protective goggles are recommended when the eye is at risk. For example, protective eyewear is used in carpentry, welding, and chemical laboratories to prevent debris or splashes from entering the eye.

Social and Ethnocultural Considerations

- Prevalence rates of age-related macular degeneration are higher in white people than in other groups over 75 years of age.
- Black females have a higher incidence of age-related macular degeneration than males until the age of 75.
- Cataracts occur more frequently in white females than in other races.
- Glaucoma occurs more frequently in Blacks than in whites.
- The prevalence of myopia is related to national origin and ethnicity. Myopia occurs more frequently in industrialized nations.

- Individuals from developing nations have higher rates of blindness than those from other nations. The causes of blindness are associated with trachoma, vitamin A deficiency, river blindness, and other infectious diseases.
- Blindness can occur as a result of diabetic retinopathy. Rates of type 2 diabetes are higher in some ethnic groups.

GATHERING THE DATA

Health assessment of the eye includes the gathering of subjective and objective data. The subjective data are collected during the interview in which the professional nurse uses a variety of communication techniques to elicit general and specific information about the health of the eye. Health records combine subjective and objective data. The results of laboratory tests and radiological studies are important secondary sources of objective data. Physical assessment of the eye, during which objective data is collected, includes the technique of inspection, palpation, the application of specific tests of vision and structures of the eye, and the use of the ophthalmoscope to assess the inner eye.

HEALTH HISTORY

The health history for assessment of the eye concerns data related to the structures of the internal and external eye, and those data concerned with vision. The nurse will observe the client and listen for cues that relate to the status and function of the eye. The nurse may use closed or open-ended questions to obtain information. Follow-up bulleted questions or requests for descriptions are required to clarify data or to supply missing information. Follow-up questions are used to identify the source of problems, duration of difficulties, measures to alleviate problems, and cues about the client's knowledge of his or her own health and health practices.

The health history guides the physical assessment of the eye. The information obtained is considered in relation to norms and expectations about the function of the eye and structures of the eye. Therefore, the nurse must consider age, gender, race, culture, environment, health practices, past and current problems, and therapies when framing questions and using techniques to elicit information. To address all the factors when conducting a health history, specific questions related to disorders of the eye and function have been developed. These questions focus on the most common concerns or injuries associated with the eye; questions related to past health history; questions related to behaviours; questions that address environmental concerns; and those that are specific to clients according to age, including the pregnant female.

The nurse must consider the client's ability to participate in the health history interview and physical assessment of the eye. The ability to communicate is essential to the health history. If language barriers exist, a translator must be used. If the client is experiencing discomfort or anxiety, efforts to address those problems have priority over other aspects of health assessment. As the nurse gathers the data, she or he will shift the type of questions to direct questions that give the client room to explain or qualify. The mnemonic O-P-Q-R-S-T-U, which stands for onset (chronology), precipitating (or palliative), quality, region (or radiation), severity, timing, and understanding, will help

the learner remember the dimensions of the symptoms. The nurse will keep in mind that not all these qualifiers will apply to each symptom

HEALTH HISTORY QUESTIONS RATIONALES

The following sections provide sample questions and follow-up questions. Rationales for some questions are provided. The list of questions is not all-inclusive but rather represents the more common concern or injury questions required in a health history related to the eye. An example of using O-P-Q-R-S-T-U with pain is provided.

Questions Related to Common Concerns or Injuries

The most common concerns related to illness or injury of the eye are as follows:

- Pain
- Change in visual acuity
- Redness, swelling, drainage

1. **Pain**
   - Do you experience pain in your eyes? *If yes:*
   - When did you first notice the pain? How long does it last? *Onset (chronology)*
   - What makes the pain worse? What makes the pain better? *Precipitating (palliative)*

▶ Eye pain can be superficial, affecting the outer eye only, or deep and throbbing, possibly associated with glaucoma. Any sudden onset of eye pain should be referred immediately to a physician.

HEALTH HISTORY QUESTIONS	RATIONALES

- Would you describe the pain as sharp? dull? burning? *Quality*
- Does the pain radiate? Where? *Radiation*
- How would you rate the pain on a scale of 1 to 10, with 10 being the worst pain? *Severity*
- How often do you experience the pain? When does the pain occur? How long does it last? *Timing*
- What do you think is causing the pain? *Understanding*

2. **Change in visual acuity**
   - Have you noticed any change in your visual acuity?

▶ A sudden change in visual acuity may be related to trauma, whereas a slow change may be related to age or illness. Changes in vision may indicate problems with the cranial nerve II, III, IV, or VI, a brain tumour, increased intracranial pressure, or ocular disease.

   - Have you experienced blurred vision?

▶ Blurred vision can be an indication of a neurological, cardiovascular, or endocrine problem; a need for corrective lenses; or cataracts.

   - Do you ever experience double vision (diplopia)?

▶ Double vision can be caused by muscle or nerve complications and some medications.

   - Have you ever been bothered by floaters or spots in front of your eyes?

▶ Black dots or spots are known as floaters. Floaters are considered normal unless they obstruct vision.

3. **Redness, swelling, drainage**
   - Have you experienced any redness of the eyes?

▶ Redness of the eyes may be related to infection, inflammation, external irritants, such as a foreign body, or overuse.

   - Have you experienced any swelling of the eyes?

▶ Swelling in the eyes may be caused by an infection, inflammation, or foreign body.

   - Have you experienced any drainage from your eyes?

▶ Drainage may be related to an infection, inflammation, or a foreign body. Determine the characteristics of the drainage. Clear drainage is most likely tears and may be caused by a blocked tear duct or a foreign body. Purulent drainage indicates an infection or inflammation.

   - Describe any associated symptoms with the above indicators.

▶ A common associated symptom with redness, swelling, or drainage is itchy, burning eyes. Burning and itching of the eyes are often caused by altered tear production or allergies.

Questions Related to Past Health History

1. **Do you wear glasses or contact lenses?** *If yes:*
   - How long have you used glasses or contact lenses?
   - Describe your vision with and without the use of glasses or contact lenses.

▶ These questions elicit information about vision correction and the effectiveness of the correction.

2. **Do you have any eye diseases, such as glaucoma, cataracts, corneal injury, Horner's syndrome, or exophthalmos (bulging eyes)?** *If yes:*
   - When were you diagnosed with the problem?
   - Has the problem ever recurred? (*acute*)
   - How are you managing the disease now? (*chronic*)

▶ Give the client an opportunity to provide information about a specific eye disease or problem. If a diagnosed illness is identified, follow-up about the date of diagnosis, treatment, and outcomes is required. Data about each illness identified by the client are essential to an accurate health assessment. Illnesses can be classified as acute or chronic, and follow-up about each classification will differ.

HEALTH HISTORY QUESTIONS	RATIONALES

3. Have you or any member of your family been diagnosed with hypertension, diabetes, or glaucoma?

▶ This question may reveal information about diseases associated with genetic or familial predisposition. Each disease can lead to vision problems. Hypertension can cause arteriosclerosis of the retina. Diabetes can cause diabetic retinopathy (bleeding in the capillaries of the retina).

Questions Related to Behaviours

Healthcare behaviours include both health practices and health patterns. Health practices consist of following recommendations for disease prevention, including screening for risks, screening for early detection of problems, and immunization. Health patterns are habits or acts that affect the client's health. Health behaviours may also include seeking healthcare from healthcare providers who use alternative methods to diagnose and treat illness. Clients should be questioned in a nonjudgmental way and areas for health teaching should be identified.

1. What was the date of your last eye examination? What were the results of that examination?

Follow-up questions are required when a problem with vision or with the structures of the eye has been identified.

▶ These questions provide specific information about healthcare practices and identify any known visual problems.

Questions Related to the Environment

Environment refers to both internal and external environments. Questions related to the internal environment include all the previous questions and those associated with internal or physiological responses. Questions regarding the external environment include those related to home, work, or social environments.

Internal Environment

1. What medications are you taking?

2. Are you taking any medications specifically for the eyes?

▶ Some medications have side effects that involve the eye.

External Environment

The following questions deal with the physical environment of the client. That includes the indoor and outdoor environments of the home and the workplace, those encountered for social engagements, and any encountered during travel.

1. Have you been exposed to inhalants, such as dust, pollen, chemical fumes, or flying debris that caused eye irritation?

2. What were those irritants?

3. What was the effect on your eyes?

4. What have you done to remedy the eye problem?

5. What have you done to decrease the exposure to the irritant?

6. What kind of activities do you perform at work?

7. Do you need or wear safety glasses at work?

8. For how many hours in the workday are you using a computer?

9. What sports or hobbies do you participate in?

10. Do you routinely wear sunglasses when outside in bright light?

Follow-up questions should include all the questions previously mentioned that address symptoms and problems.

▶ Use of equipment at work or at home may require the use of safety glasses to prevent eye injury.

▶ Prolonged work under bright lights or at a computer screen can cause eyestrain.

▶ Some athletic activities put the client at risk for eye injury, and shields or masks are recommended to prevent or reduce the risk for injury.

GATHERING THE DATA

HEALTH HISTORY QUESTIONS	RATIONALES

Questions Related to Age

The health history must reflect the anatomical and physiological differences that exist along the age span.

Questions Regarding Infants and Children

1. Did the mother have any vaginal infections at the time of delivery?

   ▶ Vaginal infections in the mother can cause eye infections in the newborn.

2. Did the baby get eye ointment after birth?

3. Was the infant preterm or full term?

   ▶ If the infant was born preterm, resuscitation and oxygen may have been required, which can damage the eyes.

4. Does the infant look directly at you? Does the infant follow objects with the eyes?

   ▶ The infant may have crossed eyes or eyes that move in different directions normally until 4 months of age; after that, the findings may be associated with weakness of the eye muscles.

5. Do you have concerns about the child's ability to see? Does the school-age child like to sit at the front of the classroom?

   ▶ Poor eyesight may necessitate sitting at the front of the room.

6. Has the child had a vision examination? When was the last eye examination?
   • How often has the child's vision been checked?
   • By whom?
   • What were the results?

7. Does the child rub his or her eyes frequently?

   ▶ Rubbing of the eyes can be associated with infection, allergy, or vision problems. Some children rub their eyes when fatigued.

Question for the Pregnant Female

1. Have you had any changes in your eyesight during your pregnancy?

   ▶ Changes in vision should be referred to an ophthalmologist.

Questions for the Older Adult

1. Do you experience dryness or burning in your eyes?

   ▶ Dryness is usually due to decreased tear production, which occurs with aging.

2. Do you have problems seeing at night?

   ▶ Night blindness is associated with cataracts and some retinal diseases.

3. Do bright lights bother you?

   ▶ The lens of the eye thickens with aging; therefore, accommodation to light is not as rapid.

4. Are you routinely tested for glaucoma?

5. What was the date of your last eye examination?

GATHERING THE DATA

PHYSICAL ASSESSMENT

ASSESSMENT TECHNIQUES AND FINDINGS

Physical assessment of the eyes requires the use of inspection, palpation, and tests of the function of the eyes. The ophthalmoscope is used to assess the internal eye. During each assessment, the nurse is gathering data related to the client's vision, the internal and external structures, and functions of the eye. Inspection includes looking at the size, shape, and symmetry of the eye, eyelids, eyebrows, and eye movements. Knowledge of the norms and expectations related to the eye and vision according to age and development is essential in determining the meaning of the data.

In adults and children over 6 years of age, normal visual acuity is 20/20. Normal vision for children under 6 years of age varies. Further information about vision in children is included in Chapter 25 of this text. ⊙ Presbyopia, the inability to accommodate for near vision, is common in clients over the age of 45. The size, shape, and position of the eyes should be symmetrical. The sclerae are white, the cornea is clear, and the pupils are round and symmetrical and respond briskly to light. The eyebrows are located equally above the eyes; the eyelashes are full and everted. The eyes are moist, indicating tear production. The movements of the eye are smooth and symmetrical. On ophthalmoscopic examination, the red reflex is visible in each eye and the retinae are a uniform yellowish pink, with a sharply defined disc and visible vessels.

Physical assessment of the eyes follows an organized pattern. It begins with assessment of visual acuity and is followed by assessments of visual fields, muscle function, and external eye structures. The assessment of the eye concludes with the ophthalmoscopic examination.

EQUIPMENT

visual acuity charts (Snellen or E for distance vision, Rosenbaum for near vision)
cotton-tipped applicator
opaque card or eye cover
ophthalmoscope
penlight

HELPFUL HINTS

- Provide specific instructions about what is expected of the client. This includes telling the client clearly which eye to cover when conducting an assessment of visual acuity.
- The ability to read letters will determine the type of acuity chart to be used. Children and non-English-speaking clients can use the E chart or a chart with figures and images for visual acuity.
- An opaque card or eye cover is used for covering the eye in several assessments. The client must be instructed not to close or apply pressure to the covered eye.
- Several types of lighting are required. Visual acuity requires bright lighting, while the room is darkened to assess papillary responses and the internal eye.
- The room must allow the client to stand 6 m (20 ft.) from the Snellen chart or a special chart that accommodates a smaller room must be used.
- The assessment may be conducted with the client seated or standing. The nurse stands or sits at eye level with the client.
- Use routine practices.

TECHNIQUES AND NORMAL FINDINGS	ABNORMAL FINDINGS AND SPECIAL CONSIDERATIONS

TESTING VISUAL ACUITY

Two methods of reporting vision acuity are used. When metric acuity is used, normal vision is referred to as 6/6 vision (for 6 metres). The other, better-known system (and the one we will use in this book) reports normal vision acuity as 20/20 (for 20 ft.).

Distance Vision

1. Position the client.

   - Position the client exactly 6 m (20 ft.) from the Snellen chart. The client may be standing or seated. The chart should be at the client's eye level. The distance at which the person stands is based on the chart used. Most rooms don't have 6 m (20 ft.) of space available, so smaller charts are used that give the same

Techniques and Normal Findings

specifications from a shorter distance (such as letters that subtend the same angle at 3 m or 9 ft.). Normal vision is still reported as 20/20 when using these charts.

2. Instruct the client.

- Explain that you are testing distance vision. Explain that the client will read the letters from the top of the chart down to the smallest line of letters that the client can see, reading each line left to right. Explain that each line of the chart has a number that indicates what the client's vision is in relation to that of a person with normal vision (see Figure 13.7).

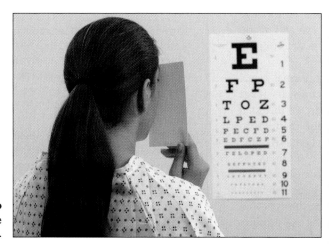

Figure 13.7 •
Testing distance vision.

Testing Distance Vision

1. Ask the client to cover one eye with the opaque card or eye cover. Tell the client to read, left to right, from the top of the chart down to the smallest line of letters that the client can see.

2. Ask the client to cover the other eye and to read from the top of the chart down to the smallest line of letters that the client can see.

3. Ask the client to read from the top of the chart down to the smallest line of letters that the client can see with both eyes uncovered.

4. If a client uses corrective lenses for distance vision, test first with eyeglasses or contact lenses. Then test without glasses or contact lenses.

- The results are recorded as a fraction. The numerator indicates the distance from the chart (6 m or 20 ft.). The denominator indicates the distance at which a person with normal vision can read the last line.

- The standard reference for vision is 20/20, but visual acuity can be sharper, such as 20/15 or 20/10. If a client's vision is 20/30, the client reads at 20 ft. what a person with normal vision reads at 30 ft. Observe while the client is reading the chart.

- If the client is unable to read more than one half of the letters on a line, record the number of the line above.

▶ Frowning, leaning forward, and squinting indicate visual or reading difficulties.

Inability to see objects at a distance is myopia. The larger the denominator, the worse the vision. Vision of 20/200 or worse in the better eye with correction is considered legal blindness.

PHYSICAL ASSESSMENT

TECHNIQUES AND NORMAL FINDINGS

The Snellen E Chart

The Snellen E chart has Es pointing in different directions (see Figure 13.8).

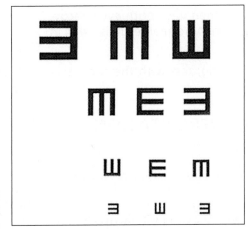

Figure 13.8 ●
E chart for testing distance vision.

- The Es become smaller row by row, from the top to the bottom of the chart. Numbers on each line correspond to the client's vision in relation to that of a person with normal distance vision reading the E chart.
- Repeat steps 1 to 4 as previously noted but ask the client to start at the top of the chart and to point in or state the direction in which the arms of the E open (right, left, up, or down) on each line until the client can no longer see the Es.
- Observe while the client is reading the chart.

Near Vision

1. Position the client.
   - The client is sitting with a Rosenbaum chart held at a distance of 35.5 cm (14 in.) from the eyes.

2. Instruct the client.
   - Explain that you are testing near vision and that the client will read the letters from the top of the card down to the smallest line the client can see. Tell the client to hold the card at the same distance throughout the test (see Figure 13.9). Explain that each line on the card corresponds to a number that indicates what the client's vision is in relation to that of a person with normal vision. The numbers may or may not be printed on the card.

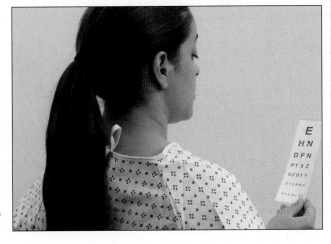

Figure 13.9 ●
Testing near vision.

TECHNIQUES AND NORMAL FINDINGS	ABNORMAL FINDINGS AND SPECIAL CONSIDERATIONS

Testing Near Vision

1. Ask the client to cover one eye with the opaque card or eye cover.

2. Repeat the test with the other eye and then with both eyes uncovered. The results are recorded as a fraction. A normal result is 14/14 in each eye.

3. If a client uses corrective lenses for reading, test with the corrective lenses.

▶ Inability to see objects at close range is called hyperopia. Presbyopia, the inability to accommodate for near vision, is common in people more than 45 years of age.

TESTING VISUAL FIELDS BY CONFRONTATION

1. Position the client.
   * The client should be sitting 0.5 to 1 m (2 to 3 ft.) from you and at eye level.

2. Instruct the client.
   * Explain that you are testing peripheral vision. The client will alternately cover an eye and must look directly into your open eye. A pen or penlight will be moved into the client's field of vision, sequentially and from four directions. The client is to indicate by saying "now" or "yes" when the object is first seen.

3. Ask the client to cover one eye with a card and look directly into your opposite eye.

4. Holding a penlight in one hand, extend your arm upward, and advance it in from the peripheral fields to the midline point, then from the nasal field toward the eye (see Figure 13.10).

▶ If the client is not able to see the object at the same time as the nurse does, the client may have some peripheral vision loss and should be evaluated further. This test assumes that the nurse has normal peripheral vision.

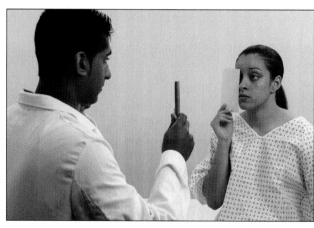

Figure 13.10 ●
Testing visual fields
by confrontation.

5. Be sure to keep the penlight equidistant between the client and yourself.

6. Ask the client to report when the object is first seen. Repeat the procedure upward, toward the nose, and downward. Then repeat the entire procedure with the other eye covered.

TESTING THE SIX CARDINAL FIELDS OF GAZE

1. Position the client.
   * The client is sitting in a comfortable position. You are at eye level with the client.

TECHNIQUES AND NORMAL FINDINGS	ABNORMAL FINDINGS AND SPECIAL CONSIDERATIONS

2. Instruct the client.
   - Explain that you will be testing eye movements and the muscles of the eye. Explain that the client must keep the head still while following a pen or penlight that you will move in several directions in front of the client's eyes.

3. Stand about 0.5 m (2 ft.) in front of the client.

4. First option: Use the letter H method.
   - Starting at midline, move the penlight to the extreme left, then straight up, then straight down.
   - Drop your hand. Position the penlight against the midline.
   - Now move the penlight to the extreme right, then straight up, then straight down (see Figure 13.11).

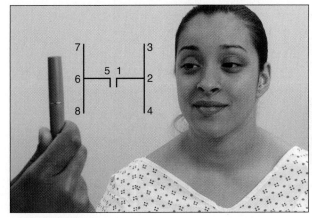

Figure 13.11 ●
Testing cardinal field of gaze.

5. Second option: Use the wagon wheel method.
   - Start at midline move the pen or light in the direction to form a star or wagon wheel.
   - Use random direction pattern to create the movement.
   - Always return the light or pen to the centre before changing direction (see Figure 13.12).

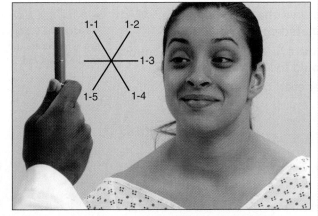

Figure 13.12 ●
Alternative method of testing cardinal field of gaze.

6. Assess the client's ability to follow your movements with the eyes (Figure 13.11). **Nystagmus,** rapid fluttering of the eyeball, can normally occur at completion of extreme lateral eye movement.

▶ If nystagmus occurs during testing, there could be a weakness in the extraocular muscles or cranial nerve III.

TECHNIQUES AND NORMAL FINDINGS	ABNORMAL FINDINGS AND SPECIAL CONSIDERATIONS

ASSESSMENT OF CORNEAL LIGHT REFLEX

1. **Position the client.**
   - You will sit at eye level with the client.
2. **Instruct the client.**
   - Explain that you are examining the cornea of the eyes. Instruct the client to stare straight ahead while you hold a penlight 30 cm (12 in.) from both eyes.
3. **Shine the light into the eyes from a distance of 30 cm (12 in.) (see Figure 13.13).**
   - The reflection of light should appear in the same spot on both pupils. This appears as a "twinkle" in the eye.

▶ If the reflection of light is not symmetrical, there could be a weakness in the extraocular muscles.

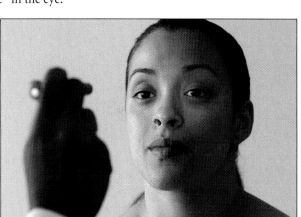

Figure 13.13 ●
Testing the corneal light reflex.

PERFORM THE COVER TEST

1. **Position the client.**
   - You should be sitting at eye level with the client.
2. **Instruct the client.**
   - Explain that this test determines the balance mechanism (fusion reflex) that keeps the eyes parallel. Explain that the client will look at a fixed point while covering each eye. You will observe the eyes.
3. **Cover one eye with a card and observe the uncovered eye, which should remain focused on the designated point.**
4. **Remove the card from the covered eye and observe the newly uncovered eye for movement. It should focus straight ahead.**
5. **Repeat the procedure with the other eye.**

▶ If there is a weakness in one of the eye muscles, the fusion reflex is blocked when one eye is covered and the weakness of the eye can be observed.

INSPECTION OF THE PUPILS

1. **Position the client.**
   - In this and all subsequent tests, you will sit at eye level with the client.
2. **Instruct the client.**
   - Explain that you will be looking at the client's eyes to assess the size and shape of the pupils.
3. **Inspect the pupils.**
   - The pupils should be round, equal in size and shape, and in the centre of the eye. These characteristics are controlled by cranial nerve III.

▶ Pupils that are not round and symmetrical may indicate previous ocular surgery, increased intracranial pressure, or cranial nerve pathology.

| TECHNIQUES AND NORMAL FINDINGS | ABNORMAL FINDINGS AND SPECIAL CONSIDERATIONS |

EVALUATION OF PUPILLARY RESPONSE

1. Instruct the client.
   - Explain that you are testing the pupil's response to light. Tell the client that the room light must be dimmed. Explain that you will shine a light directly at each eye and that the client must stare straight ahead.

2. Moving your penlight in from the client's side, shine light directly into one eye.

3. Observe the constriction in the illuminated pupil.
   - Also observe the simultaneous reaction (**consensual constriction**) of the other pupil.

TESTING FOR ACCOMMODATION OF PUPIL RESPONSE

1. Instruct the client.
   - Explain that you are testing muscles of the eye. Tell the client to shift the gaze from the far wall to an object held 10 to 12 cm (4 to 5 in.) from the client's nose.

2. Ask the client to stare straight ahead at a distant point.

3. Hold a penlight about 10 to 12 cm (4 to 5 in.) from the client's nose; then ask the client to shift the gaze from the distant point to the penlight.
   - The eyes should converge (turn inward) and the pupils should constrict as the eyes focus on the penlight. This pupillary change is **accommodation**, a change in size to adjust vision from far to near.
   - A normal response to pupillary testing is recorded as PERRLA (pupils equal, round, react to light, and accommodation).

TESTING OF THE CORNEAL REFLEX

1. Instruct the client.
   - Explain that you will be testing nerve stimulation to the cornea. Tell the client that you will be touching each eye gently and quickly with a wisp of cotton. The client will react by blinking the eyes. The client may experience tearing of the eyes.

2. Take a sterile cotton ball and twist it into a very thin strand.

3. By using a lateral approach, gently touch the cornea on the outer aspect of each eye (see Figure 13.14).

▶ If the illuminated pupil fails to constrict, there is a defect in the direct pupillary response. If the unilluminated pupil fails to constrict, there is a defect in the consensual response, controlled by cranial nerve III (oculomotor).

▶ Lack of **convergence** (turning inward of the eye) and failure of the pupils to constrict indicates dysfunction of cranial nerves III, IV, and VI.

▶ If one or both eyes fail to respond, there could be a problem with cranial nerve V, VII, or both, since cranial nerve V is sensory for this reflex, and cranial nerve VII is motor. Note that long-term use of contact lenses can diminish the corneal reflex.

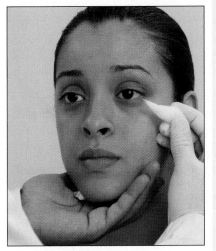

Figure 13.14 ●
Testing the corneal reflex.

TECHNIQUES AND NORMAL FINDINGS	ABNORMAL FINDINGS AND SPECIAL CONSIDERATIONS

4. Confirm that both eyes blink when either cornea is touched. Be sure not to touch the eyelashes or conjunctiva.

INSPECTION OF THE EXTERNAL EYE

1. Instruct the client.
   - Explain that you will be examining the client's eye. You will be looking at the client's eyes and touching them to see inside the lids. Explain that you will provide specific instructions before each test.

2. Stand directly in front of the client and focus on the external structures of the eye. The eyebrows should be symmetrical and the eyelashes similar in quantity and distribution. The eyebrows and eyelashes should be free of flakes and drainage.

3. With the client's eyes open, confirm that the distances between the palpebral fissures are equal. Confirm that the upper eyelid covers a small arc of the iris.

4. Confirm that the eyelids symmetrically cover the eyeballs when closed. The eyeball should be neither protruding nor sunken.

5. Gently separate the eyelids and ask the client to look up, down, and to each side. The conjunctiva should be moist and clear, with small blood vessels. The lens should be clear, and the sclera white. The irises should be round and both of the same colour, although irises of different colours can be a normal finding.

6. Inspect the cornea by shining a penlight from the side across the cornea. The cornea should be clear with no irregularities. The pupils should be round and equal in size (see Figure 13.15).

▶ Absence of the lateral third of the eyebrow is associated with hypothyroidism. Absent eyelashes may indicate pulling or plucking associated with obsessive-compulsive behaviour.

Ptosis (drooping of one eyelid) can be caused by a dysfunction of cranial nerve III (oculomotor). Eyes that protrude beyond the supraorbital ridge can indicate a thyroid disorder; however, this trait may be normal for the client. Edema of the eyelids can be caused by allergies, heart disease, or kidney disease. Inability to move the eyelids can indicate dysfunction of the nervous system, including facial nerve paralysis.

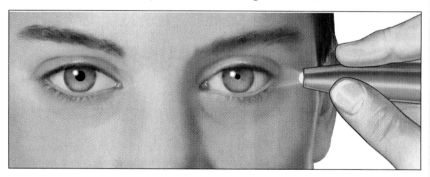

Figure 13.15 ● Inspecting the cornea.

PALPATION OF THE EYE

1. Ask the client to close both eyes.

2. Use the first two or three fingers to gently palpate the lacrimal sacs, the eyelids, and the eyeballs.

3. Confirm that there is no swelling or tenderness and that the eyeballs feel firm.

▶ Swelling may be a symptom of infection, cardiovascular problems, or renal problems.

▶ Less than firm eyeballs can be an indication of dehydration.

TECHNIQUES AND NORMAL FINDINGS	ABNORMAL FINDINGS AND SPECIAL CONSIDERATIONS

EXAMINATION OF THE CONJUNCTIVA AND SCLERA UNDER THE LOWER EYELID

1. Evert the lower eyelid by asking the client to look down, pressing the lower lid against the lower orbital rim, and then asking the client to look up (see Figure 13.16).

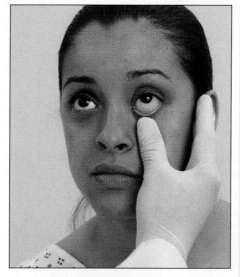

Figure 13.16 ●
Inspecting the conjunctiva of the lower lid.

• The conjunctiva should be pink with no tenderness or irregularities. If you find any abnormality, examine the conjunctiva under the upper eyelid.

▶ Inflammation and edema of the conjunctiva indicate an infection or a possible foreign body.

2. Ask the client to close the eyes.

3. Evert the upper eyelid by placing a cotton-tipped applicator against the upper lid (see Figure 13.17).

4. Grasp the eyelashes and pull the eyelid downward, forward, and up over the applicator (see Figure 13.18). Inspect the conjunctiva.

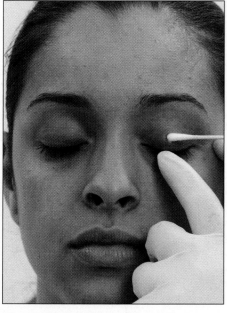

Figure 13.7 ● Step 1 of upper eyelid eversion.

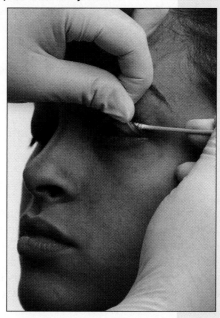

Figure 13.18 ● Step 2 of upper eyelid eversion.

PHYSICAL ASSESSMENT

TECHNIQUES AND NORMAL FINDINGS	ABNORMAL FINDINGS AND SPECIAL CONSIDERATIONS

5. Gently release and return the eyelid to the normal position when finished.

INSPECTION OF THE FUNDUS WITH THE OPHTHALMOSCOPE

1. Instruct the client.
   - Explain that you will be using the ophthalmoscope to look into the inner deep part of the eye (**fundus**) and that the lights in the room will be dimmed. Explain that the client must stare ahead at a fixed point while you move in front with the ophthalmoscope. Tell the client to maintain a fixed gaze, as if looking through you. Explain that you will place your hand on the client's head so you both remain stable. (Refer to Chapter 6 to review the parts of the ophthalmoscope. ⬭)

2. To examine the right eye, hold the ophthalmoscope in your right hand with the index finger on the lens wheel.

3. Begin with the lens on the 0 diopter. With the light on, place the ophthalmoscope over your right eye (see Figure 13.19).

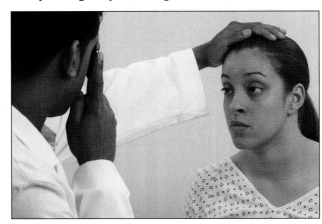

Figure 13.19 ● Approaching the client for the ophthalmoscopic exam.

4. Stand at a slight angle lateral to the client's line of vision.

5. Approach the client at about a 15-degree angle toward the client's nose.

6. Place your left hand on the client's shoulder or head.

7. Hold the ophthalmoscope against your head, directing the light into the client's pupil. Keep your other eye open.

8. Advance toward the client.

9. As you look into the client's pupil, you will see the red reflex, which is the reflection of the light off the retina. Remember to examine the client's right eye with your right eye, and the client's left eye with your left eye. At this point, you may need to adjust the lens wheel to bring the ocular structures into focus. Normally, you will see no shadows or dots interrupting the red reflex. If the light strays from the pupil, you will lose the red reflex. Adjust your angle until you see the red reflex again.

▶ Persistent absence of the red reflex may indicate a cataract, an opacity of the lens.

PHYSICAL ASSESSMENT

Techniques and Normal Findings

10. Keep advancing toward the client until the ophthalmoscope is almost touching the client's eyelashes (see Figure 13.20).

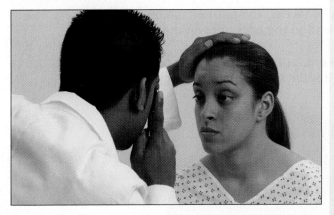

Figure 13.20 ●
Examining the eye by using the ophthalmoscope.

11. Rotate the diopter wheel if necessary to bring the ocular fundus into focus.

12. If the client's vision is myopic, you will need to rotate the wheel into the minus numbers (see Figure 13.21).

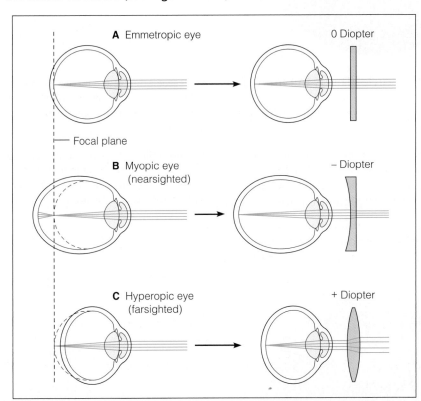

Figure 13.21 ● Use of diopter to adjust for problems of refraction. A. In the emmetropic (normal) eye, light is focused properly on the retina, and the 0 diopter is used. B. In the myopic eye, light from a distant source converges to a focal point before reaching the retina. Negative diopter numbers are used. C. In the hyperopic eye, light from a near source converges to a focal point past the retina. Positive diopter numbers are used.

TECHNIQUES AND NORMAL FINDINGS

ABNORMAL FINDINGS AND SPECIAL CONSIDERATIONS

13. If the client's vision is hyperopic, rotate the wheel into the plus numbers.

14. Begin to look for the optic disc by following the path of the blood vessels. As they grow larger, they lead to the optic disc on the nasal side of the retina (see Figure 13.22).

    The optic disc normally looks like a round or oval yellow-orange depression with a distinct margin. It is the site where the optic nerve and blood vessels exit the eye.

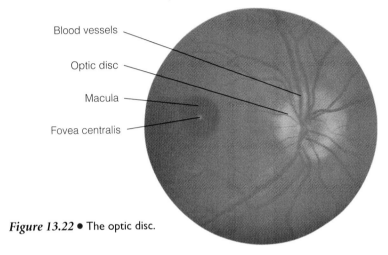

Figure 13.22 ● The optic disc.

15. Follow the vessels laterally to a darker circle. This is the macula, or area of central vision.

    The *fovea centralis*, a small white spot located in the centre of the macula, is the area of sharpest vision.

16. Systematically inspect these structures. A crescent shape around the margin of the optic disc is a normal finding. A *scleral crescent* is an absence of pigment in the choroid and is a dull white. A *pigment crescent*, which is black, is an accumulation of pigment in the choroid.

17. Use the optic disc as a clock face for documenting the position of a finding, and the diameter of the disc (DD) for noting its distance from the optic disc. For instance, "at 2:00, 2 DD from the disc" describes the finding in Figure 13.23.

▶ Degeneration of the macula is common in older adults and results in impaired central vision. It may be due to hemorrhages, cysts, or other alterations.

▶ Abnormalities of the retinal structures present as dark or opaque spots on the retina, an irregularly shaped optic disc, and lesions or hemorrhages on the fundus.

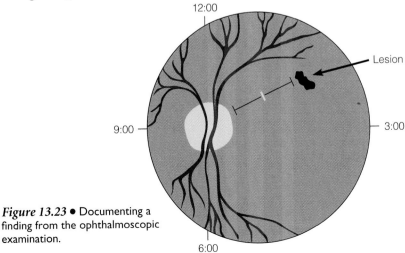

Figure 13.23 ● Documenting a finding from the ophthalmoscopic examination.

PHYSICAL ASSESSMENT

TECHNIQUES AND NORMAL FINDINGS	ABNORMAL FINDINGS AND SPECIAL CONSIDERATIONS
18. Trace the path of a paired artery and vein from the optic disc to the periphery in the four quadrants of the eyeball.	▶ An absence of major vessels in any of the four quadrants is an abnormal finding. Constricted arteries look smaller than two thirds the diameter of accompanying veins. Crossing of the vessels more than 2 DD away from the optic disc requires further evaluation.
19. Note the number of major vessels, colour, width, and any crossing of the vessels.	
20. Repeat the preceding procedure to examine the client's left eye by using your left hand and left eye.	▶ Extremely tortuous vessels also require further evaluation.

SAMPLE DOCUMENTATION

Subjective: No history of pain, change in visual acuity, or redness/swelling/drainage. Does not require corrective lenses. No personal or family history of eye disease or hypertension.

Objective: Eyebrows equal, no ptosis, eyeballs firm to palpation. PERRLA.

Vision: Snellen 20/20 both eyes. Rosenbaum 14/14 both eyes. Peripheral vision equal by confrontation. EOM intact by six cardinal fields, cover test, and symmetric corneal light reflex.

APPLICATION THROUGH CRITICAL THINKING

CASE STUDY

John Jerome is a 45-year-old Black male who made an appointment for an annual employment physical examination. Mr. Jerome completed a written questionnaire in preparation for his meeting with a healthcare professional. He checked "none" for all categories of family history of disease except diabetes. He indicated that he knew of no changes in his health since his last examination.

The following observations were made during the initial encounter with Mr. Jerome. A tall, Black male wearing eyeglasses entered the room. He turned his head to the left and right and looked about the room before sitting across from the examiner. The client had some redness in the sclera of both eyes. During the interview, the client revealed that his last eye examination occurred 6 months ago, and he received a prescription for new glasses. He stated that he was still having a problem with the new glasses and needed to have them checked. When asked to describe the problem, Mr. Jerome replied, "I just don't feel right with these glasses, and these are the second pair in a little over a year." He further stated, "I just think I am overworking my eyes lately. I need to rest them more

than ever and I have had some headaches. I thought the glasses would help, but it hasn't gotten better." The client denied any other problems. In response to inquiries about family history, he reported that his mother had diabetes but had no problems with her eyes. He didn't know of any other eye problems in his family, except his mother had told him that an aunt of hers had been blind for some time. He reiterated that his only problem of late had been "this thing with my glasses; otherwise I feel fine."

The physical examination revealed the following:

- Vital signs: B/P 128/84—P 88—RR 22
- Height 1.9 m (6′3″), weight 85 kg (188 lb.)
- Eyeball firm to palpation
- Moderately dilated pupils
- Cupping of the optic disc (an indication of glaucoma)

▶ Complete Documentation

The following information is summarized from the case study.

SUBJECTIVE DATA: Visit for annual employment physical examination. Negative family history except diabetes. No changes in health since last examination. Last eye examination 6 months ago—result prescription for new glasses. Stated he was having a problem with the new glasses. "I don't feel right with them." Stated, "I think I'm overworking my eyes lately. I thought the new glasses would help, but it hasn't gotten better." History of aunt with blindness.

OBJECTIVE DATA: Turns head to left and right and looked around room before sitting across from examiner. Scleral red-

ness bilaterally. Eyeball firm to palpation. Pupils moderate dilation. Cupping of optic disc. Height 1.9 m (6′3″), weight 85 kg (188 lb.), VS: B/P 128/84—P 88—RR 22.

ASSESSMENT FORM			
HISTORY	No	Yes	Describe
Visual disorder		X	*(glasses) see below—aunt blind*
Diabetes		X	*(mother)*
Hypertension	X		
Glaucoma	X		
Correction	*Eyeglasses—"I just don't feel right"*		
Last exam	*6 months ago*		
Other	*"Headache"*		
PHYSICAL			
VS	*BP 128/84—P 88—RR 22*		
	Ht. 1.9 m (6′3″) Wt. 85 kg (188 lb.)		
Eyeball	*Firm*		
Pupils	*Dilated*		
Optic disc	*Cupping*		

►Critical Thinking Questions

1. What conclusions would the nurse reach based on the data?
2. How was this conclusion formulated?
3. What information is missing?
4. Describe the priority for this client and the options that apply.
5. Create a plan to address the problem.

►Applying Nursing Diagnoses

1. *Disturbed visual sensory perception* is a nursing diagnosis in the NANDA-I taxonomy (see Appendix A ⬭). Identify the data in the case study for John Jerome that support this diagnosis.
2. *Anxiety* and *denial* are included as nursing diagnoses in the NANDA-I taxonomy (see Appendix A ⬭). Are there data in the case study to support these diagnoses? If so, identify the data.
3. Use the NANDA-I taxonomy in Appendix A to identify additional diagnoses for John Jerome. ⬭

► Prepare Teaching Plan

LEARNING NEED: The data in the case study revealed that Mr. Jerome was experiencing eye problems and had a family history of diabetes and blindness. Because of his history, he would be tested for diabetes and screened for diabetic retinopathy. His eye examination revealed cupping of the optic disc and slightly dilated pupils, both of which are associated with glaucoma. Blindness can occur with glaucoma and may have caused his aunt's blindness. Mr. Jerome will be referred for further evaluation of two suggested problems.

The case study provides data that are representative of risks, symptoms, and behaviours of many individuals. Therefore, the following teaching plan is based on the need to provide information to members of any community about glaucoma.

GOAL: The participants in this learning program will have increased awareness about glaucoma and follow recommendations for eye care.

OBJECTIVES: At the completion of this learning session, the participants will be able to do the following:

1. Discuss glaucoma.
2. Identify risk factors associated with glaucoma.
3. List the diagnostic tests for glaucoma.
4. Describe recommendations for eye care.

APPLICATION OF OBJECTIVE 2: Identify risk factors associated with glaucoma.

Content	Teaching Strategy and Rationale	Evaluation
• Black people: Glaucoma is six to eight times more common in Black people. • Age: Individuals over the age of 60 are six times as likely to get glaucoma as younger people. • Heredity: Individuals with a family history, especially immediate family, of glaucoma are at greater risk. Family history increases risk four to nine times. • Steroid use: Some evidence links glaucoma with steroid use. It is associated with high doses of steroids, for example, that would be used for severe asthma. • Eye injury: Blunt trauma, such as occurs with a blow to the head or blunt trauma to the eye in baseball or boxing, can cause glaucoma immediately or years later.	• Lecture • Discussion • Audiovisual materials • Printed materials Lecture is appropriate when disseminating information to large groups. Discussion allows participants to bring up concerns and to raise questions. Audiovisual materials, such as illustrations of the structures of the eye, reinforce verbal presentation. Printed material, especially to be taken away with learners, allows review, reinforcement, and reading at the learner's pace.	• Written examination. May use short answer, fill-in, or multiple-choice items or a combination of items. If these are short and easy to evaluate, the learner receives immediate feedback.

HEALTH PROMOTION ASSESSMENT TOOL

Social Determinants of Health	Level of Action	Action Strategies
Personal coping skills	Individual	**Develop personal skills** • Discuss the importance of yearly eye exams. • Encourage rest to avoid overworking eyes. • Explore the onset of headaches in terms of what triggers them and, depending on the triggers, discuss methods of coping or further assessments that would be warranted.
Health services	Individual	**Create supportive environments** • Provide referral to an ophthalmologist to assess Mr. Jerome's sclera redness, the cupping of the optic disk, and to double check the prescription for glasses he received 6 months ago. • Refer Mr. Jerome to his family physician for laboratory tests to rule out diabetes.

ABNORMAL FINDINGS

Abnormalities of the eye arise for a variety of reasons and can be associated with vision, eye movement, and the internal and external structures of the eye. The following sections address abnormal findings associated with the functions and structures of the eye.

Visual Acuity

Visual acuity is dependent on the ability of the eye to refract light rays and focus them on the retina. The shape of the eye is one determinant in the refractive and focusing processes of vision.

Emmetropia is the normal refractive condition of the eye in which light rays are brought into sharp focus on the retina (see Figure 13.24).

Myopia (nearsightedness) is generally inherited and occurs when the eye is longer than normal. As a result, light rays focus in front of the retina (see Figure 13.25).

Hyperopia (farsightedness) is also an inherited condition in which the eye is shorter than normal. In hyperopia the light rays focus behind the retina (see Figure 13.26).

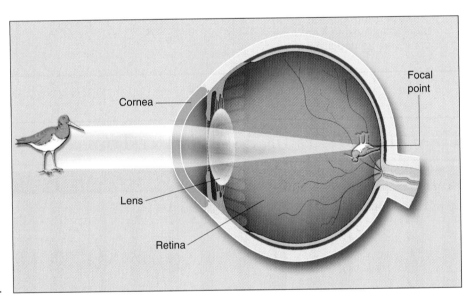

Figure 13.24 ● Emmetropia.

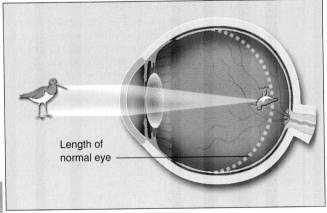

Figure 13.25 ● Myopia.

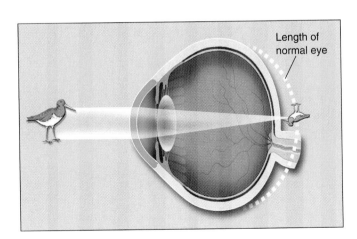

Figure 13.26 ● Hyperopia.

Astigmatism is often a familial condition in which the refraction of light is spread over a wide area rather than on a distinct point on the retina. In the normal eye, the cornea is round in shape, whereas in astigmatism the cornea curves more in one direction than another. As a result, light is refracted and focused on two focal points on or near the retina. Vision in astigmatism may be blurred or doubled (see Figure 13.27).

Presbyopia is an age-related condition in which the lens of the eye loses the ability to accommodate. As a result, light is focused behind the retina, and focus on near objects becomes difficult.

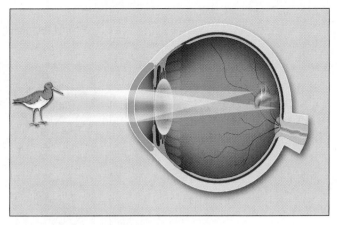

Figure 13.27 ● Astigmatism.

Visual Fields

The **visual field** refers to the total area in which objects can be seen in the periphery while the eye remains focused on a central point. Testing visual fields enables the examiner to detect and map losses in peripheral vision. The mapping aids in determination of the problem. Changes in visual fields accompany damage to the retina, lesions in the optic nerve or chiasm, increased intraocular pressure, and retinal vascular damage. The normal visual pathways and loss of visual fields in relation to the previously mentioned conditions are depicted in Figures 13.28 and 13.29, respectively.

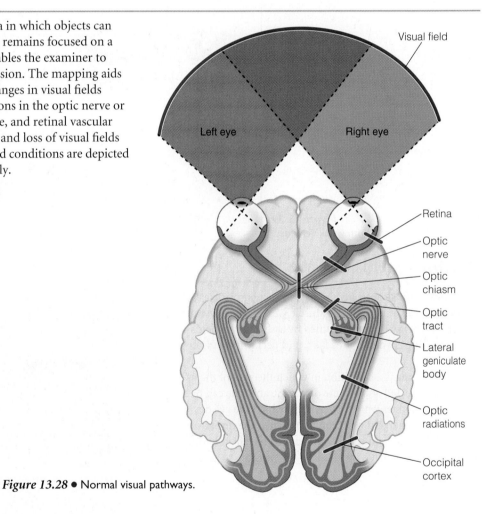

Figure 13.28 ● Normal visual pathways.

Retinal Damage

LEFT EYE   RIGHT EYE

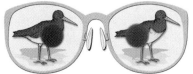

Blind spots—in localized damaged areas.

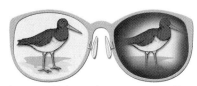

Increased intraocular pressure resulting in decreased peripheral vision.

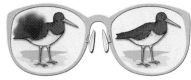

Retinal detachment—vision diminishes in affected area.

LEFT EYE   RIGHT EYE

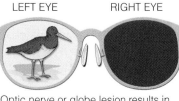

Optic nerve or globe lesion results in unilateral blindness.

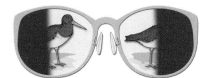

Optic chiasm lesion—results in bilateral heteronymous hemianopsia (loss of temporal visual fields).

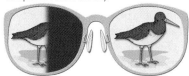

Lesion occurs in uncrossed fibres of optic chiasm resulting in left hemianopsia (nasal).

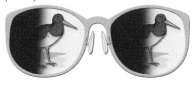

Right optic tract or optic radiation lesion resulting in loss of right nasal and left temporal fields. Homonymous hemianopsia.

Figure 13.29
Client's view with visual field loss.

Cardinal Fields of Gaze

Eye movement is controlled by six extraocular muscles and by cranial nerves III, IV, and VI. Muscle weakness or dysfunction of a cranial nerve can be identified by assessing the fields of gaze, assessing corneal light reflex, and performing the cover test.

Strabismus is a condition in which the axes of the eyes cannot be directed at the same object. Strabismus can be classified as convergent (esotropia) in which the eye deviates inward, and divergent (exotropia) in which the deviation is outward. In strabismus, light can be seen to reflect in different axes (see Figure 13.30).

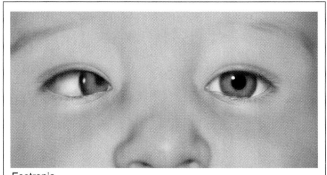

Esotropia

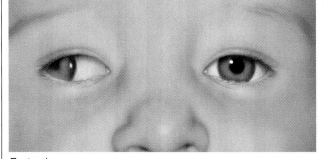

Exotropia

Figure 13.30 ● Strabismus.

Esophoria (inward turning of the eye) and **exophoria** (outward turning of the eye) are detected in the cover test. Esotropic findings are depicted in Figure 13.31.

Nonparallel eye movements and failure of the eyes to follow in a certain direction are indicative of problems with extraocular muscles or cranial nerves. Figure 13.32 provides details about the specific muscles and nerves associated with abnormal eye movement.

Figures 13.33 through 13.53 include information about abnormalities in pupillary response, structures of the external eye, and the fundus of the eye.

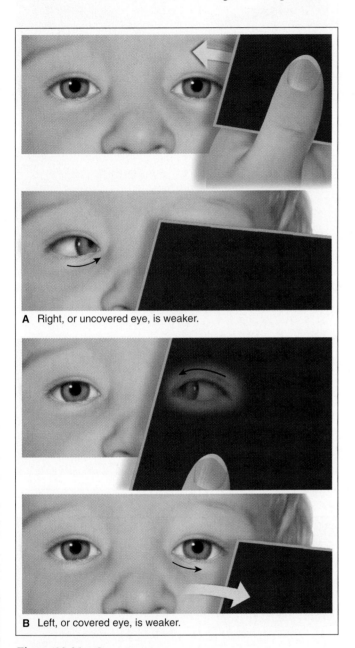

A Right, or uncovered eye, is weaker.

B Left, or covered eye, is weaker.

Figure 13.31 ● Cover test.

Disruption of Function		
Muscle	**Cranial Nerve**	**Results**
Superior rectus	Oculomotor	Inability to move eye upward or temporally
Superior oblique	Trochlear	Inability to move eye down or nasally
Lateral rectus	Abducens	Inability to move eye temporally
Inferior oblique	Oculomotor	Inability to move eye upward or temporally
Inferior rectus	Oculomotor	Inability to move eye downward or temporally
Medial rectus	Oculomotor	Inability to move eye nasally

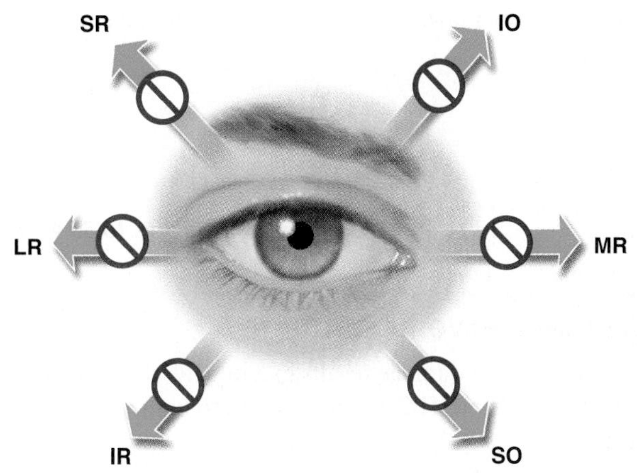

SR · IO · LR · MR · IR · SO

Figure 13.32 ● Extraocular muscle abnormalities.

Abnormal Pupillary Response

Adie's Pupil

Also known as tonic pupil, Adie's pupil is unilateral and slug-gish pupillary response (see Figure 13.33).

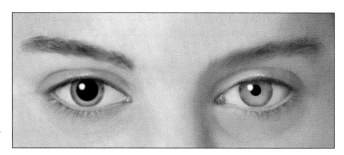

Figure 13.33 ●
Tonic pupil (Adie's pupil).

Argyll Robertson Pupils

Argyll Robertson pupils exist bilaterally and are small, irregu-lar, and nonreactive to light (see Figure 13.34). These occur with central nervous system disorders, including tumour, syphilis, and opioid use.

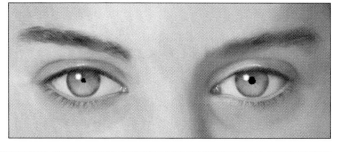

Figure 13.34 ●
Argyll Robertson pupils.

Anisocoria

Anisocoria is unequal pupillary size, which may be a normal finding or may indicate central nervous system disease (see Figure 13.35).

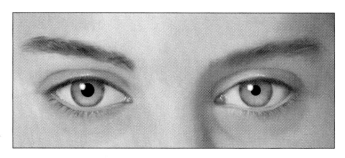

Figure 13.35 ● Anisocoria.

Cranial Nerve III Damage

Cranial nerve III damage results in a unilaterally dilated pupil (see Figure 13.36). There is no reaction to light. Ptosis may be seen.

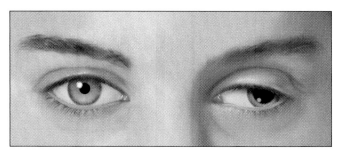

Figure 13.36 ●
Cranial nerve III damage.

Horner's Syndrome

Horner's syndrome is a result of blockage of sympathetic nerve stimulation. Findings include unilateral, small, regular pupil that is nonreactive to light (see Figure 13.37). Ptosis and anhidrosis (loss of sweating) of the same side accompany the pupillary signs.

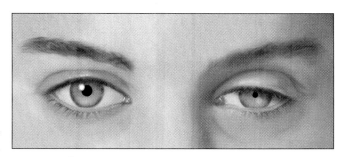

Figure 13.37 ●
Horner's syndrome.

ABNORMAL FINDINGS

Mydriasis

Mydriasis refers to fixed and dilated pupils (see Figure 13.38). This condition may occur with sympathetic nerve stimulation, glaucoma, central nervous system damage, or deep anaesthesia.

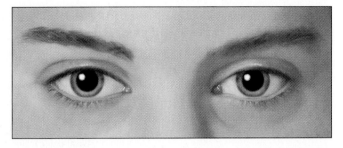

Figure 13.38 ● Mydriasis.

Miosis

Miosis refers to fixed and constricted pupils (see Figure 13.39). This condition may occur with the use of opioids, with damage to the pons, or as a result of treatment for glaucoma.

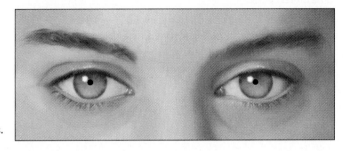

Figure 13.39 ● Miosis.

Monocular Blindness

Monocular blindness results in direct and consensual response to light directed in the normal eye and absence of response in either eye when light is directed in the blind eye (see Figure 13.40).

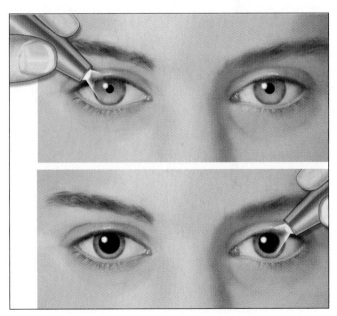

Figure 13.40 ●
Monocular blindness.

Abnormalities of the Structures of the External Eye

Acute Glaucoma

Acute glaucoma is a result of sudden increase in intraocular pressure resulting from blocked flow of fluid from the anterior chamber. The pupil is oval in shape and dilated (see Figure 13.41). There is circumcorneal redness. The cornea appears cloudy and steamy. Pain is sudden in onset and is accompanied by decrease in vision and halos around lights. Acute glaucoma requires immediate intervention.

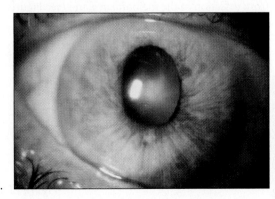

Figure 13.41 ● Acute glaucoma.

Basal Cell Carcinoma

Basal cell carcinoma has a papular appearance (see Figure 13.42). This form of cancer is usually seen on the lower lid and medial canthus.

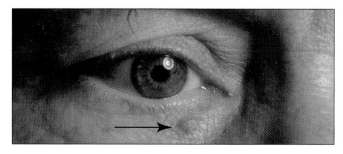

Figure 13.42 ●
Basal cell carcinoma.

Blepharitis

Blepharitis is inflammation of the eyelids (see Figure 13.43). Staphylococcal infection leads to red, scaly, and crusted lids. The eye burns, itches, and tears.

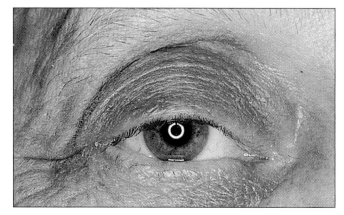

Figure 13.43 ● Blepharitis.

Cataract

A cataract is an opacity in the lens (see Figure 13.44). It usually occurs in aging.

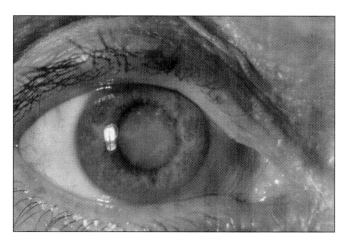

Figure 13.44 Cataract.

Chalazion

A chalazion is a firm, nontender nodule on the eyelid, arising from infection of the meibomian gland (see Figure 13.45). It is not painful unless inflamed.

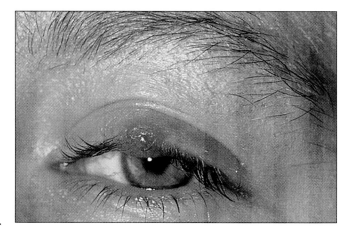

Figure 13.45 ● Chalazion.

Conjunctivitis

Conjunctivitis is an infection of the conjunctiva usually caused by bacteria or virus but may result from chemical exposure (see Figure 13.46).

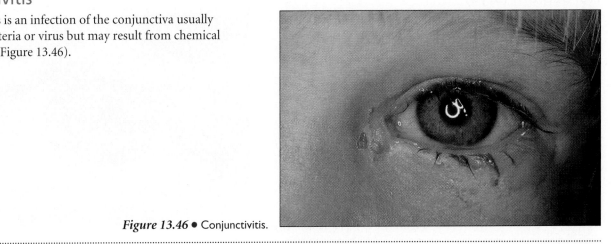

Figure 13.46 ● Conjunctivitis.

Ectropion

Ectropion is eversion of the lower eyelid caused by muscle weakness. The palpebral conjunctiva is exposed (see Figure 13.47).

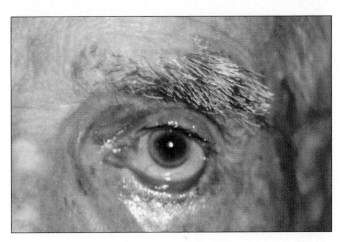

Figure 13.47 Ectropion.

Entropion

Entropion is inversion of the lid and lashes caused by muscle spasm of the eyelid (see Figure 13.48). Friction from lashes can cause corneal irritation.

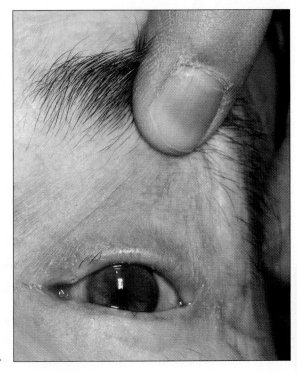

Figure 13.48 ● Entropion.

Hordeolum (Stye)

A hordeolum or stye is a result of a staphylococcal infection of hair follicles on the margin of the lids (see Figure 13.49). The affected eye is swollen, red, and painful.

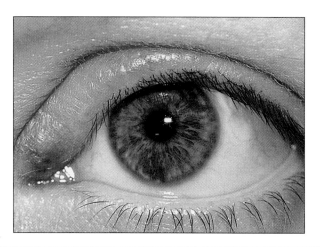

Figure 13.49 ● Hordeolum (stye).

Iritis

Iritis is a serious disorder characterized by redness around the iris and cornea (see Figure 13.50). The pupil is often irregular. Vision is decreased and the client experiences deep, aching pain.

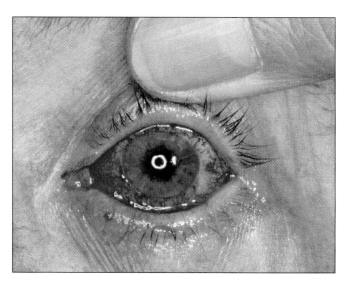

Figure 13.50 Iritis.

Periorbital Edema

Periorbital edema refers to swollen, puffy lids (see Figure 13.51). Periorbital edema occurs with crying, infection, and systemic problems including kidney failure, heart failure, and allergy.

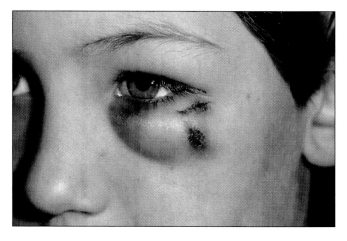

Figure 13.51 ● Periorbital edema.

Ptosis

Ptosis refers to drooping of the eyelid (Figure 13.36). This occurs with cranial nerve damage or systemic neuromuscular weakness.

Abnormalities of the Fundus

Diabetic Retinopathy

Diabetic retinopathy refers to the changes that occur in the retina and vasculature of the retina, including microaneurysms, hemorrhages, macular edema, and retinal exudates (see Figure 13.52).

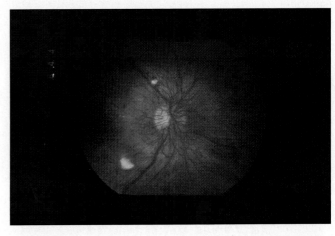

Figure 13.52 ●
Diabetic retinopathy.

Hypertensive Retinopathy

Hypertensive retinopathy refers to the changes in the retina and vasculature of the retina in response to elevations in blood pressure that accompany atherosclerosis, heart disease, and kidney disease. The changes include flame hemorrhages, nicking of vessels, and "cotton wool" spots that arise from infarction of the nerve fibres.

Macular Degeneration

Age-related macular degeneration (ARMD) is a degenerative condition of the macula, the central retina (see Figure 13.53). Central vision is lost gradually while peripheral vision remains intact. The eyes are affected at different rates.

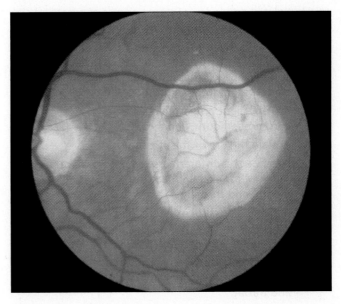

Figure 13.53 ●
Macular degeneration.

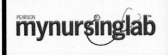
ABNORMAL FINDINGS

14

EARS, NOSE, MOUTH, AND THROAT

THE STRUCTURES OF THE EAR, NOSE, MOUTH, and throat are responsible for the senses of hearing, smell, and taste. Each of these body systems will be discussed in this chapter and again when describing the neurological assessment in Chapter 24. ⚭

ANATOMY AND PHYSIOLOGY REVIEW

The anatomical structures of the ear, nose, mouth, and throat include the internal and external ear, the nose and sinuses, the oral cavity, and the pharynx (throat). Each of the structures will be described in the following sections.

Ear

The ear is the sensory organ that functions in hearing and equilibrium. It is divided into the external, middle, and inner ear. The external portion, or what most people think of as the ear, is called the **auricle** or **pinna**. It has a shell of cartilage covered with skin that funnels sound into the meatus (opening) of the external auditory canal.

External Ear

Figure 14.1 depicts the surface anatomy of the external ear. The external large rim of the auricle is called the **helix**. The **tragus** is a stiff projection that protects the anterior meatus of the auditory canal. The **lobe** of the ear is a small flap of flesh at the inferior end of the auricle. The external auditory canal is about 2.5 cm (1 in.) in length, is S-shaped, and leads to the middle ear. It is lined with glands that secrete a yellow-brown wax called **cerumen**. These secretions lubricate and protect the ear. The functions of chewing and talking help move the cerumen in the canal. The mastoid process, part of the temporal bone of the skull, is adjacent to the cavity of the middle ear. It contains many air cells and is assessed with the ear. This process has no role in hearing or balance. The mastoid process may become infected following ear infections in the adult.

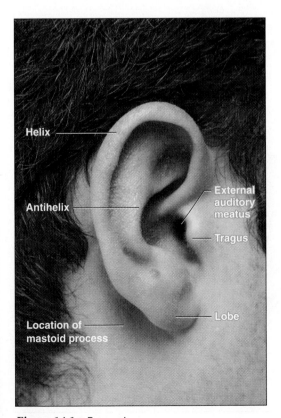

Figure 14.1 ● External ear.

Middle Ear

The external ear and middle ear are separated by the **tympanic membrane** or eardrum (see Figure 14.2). This thin, translucent membrane is pearly grey in colour and lies obliquely in the canal. Sound waves entering the auditory canal strike the membrane, causing it to vibrate. The vibrations are transferred to the **ossicles**, or bones of the middle ear: the malleus, the incus, and the stapes. The ossicles, in turn, transfer the vibration to the oval window of the inner ear. Note that the malleus projects inferiorly and laterally and can be seen through the translucent tympanic membrane when viewed with the otoscope. The **eustachian tube** or auditory tube connects the middle ear with the nasopharynx. This tube helps to equalize air pressure on both sides of the tympanic membrane. The middle ear functions to conduct sound vibrations from the external ear to the inner ear. It also protects the inner ear by reducing loud sound vibrations.

Inner Ear

The inner ear contains the bony labyrinth, which consists of a central cavity called the vestibule, three semicircular canals responsible for the sense of equilibrium, and the **cochlea**, a spiral chamber that contains the receptors for hearing. Impulses from the equilibrium receptors of the inner ear are sent via cranial nerve VIII to the brain. Responses are then initiated to activate the eyes and muscles of the body to maintain balance. The cochlea transmits sound vibrations to the auditory nerve (cranial nerve VIII), which in turn carries the impulse to the auditory cortex in the temporal lobe of the brain for interpretation as hearing.

The major functions of the ears are collecting and transporting sound vibrations to the brain and maintaining the sense of equilibrium.

Nose and Sinuses

The nose is a triangular projection of bone and cartilage situated midline on the face (see Figure 14.3). It is the only externally visible organ of the respiratory system. During inspiration, air enters the nasal cavity, where it is filtered, warmed, and moistened before it moves toward the trachea and lungs.

The nasal mucosa with its rich blood supply helps filter inspired air and has a redder appearance than the oral mucosa. Three turbinates (superior, middle, and inferior) project from the medial wall into each side of the nasal cavity. These bony projections, covered with nasal mucosa, add surface area for cleaning, moistening, and warming air entering the respiratory tract. Each side of the posterior nasal cavity opens into the nasopharynx (see Figure 14.4).

The olfactory cells located in the roof of the nasal cavity form filaments that connect to the olfactory nerve (cranial nerve I) and are responsible for the sense of smell.

The **paranasal sinuses** are mucous-membrane-lined, air-filled cavities that surround the nasal cavity and perform the same air-processing functions of filtration, moistening, and warming. The paranasal sinuses are named for the bones of the skull in which they are contained: sphenoid, frontal, ethmoid,

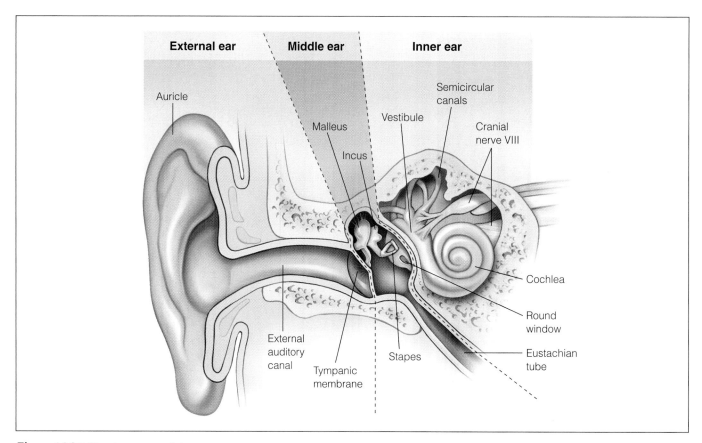

Figure 14.2 ● The three parts of the ear.

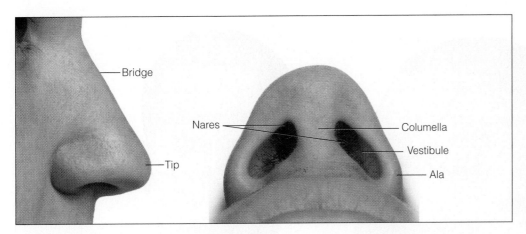

Figure 14.3 • The nose.

and maxillary. The frontal and maxillary sinuses are accessible to examination and are discussed later in this chapter (see Figure 14.5).

The major functions of the nose and sinuses are the following:

- Providing an airway for respiration
- Filtering, warming, and humidifying air flowing into the respiratory tract
- Providing resonance for the voice
- Housing the olfactory receptors

Mouth

The oral cavity is the beginning of the alimentary canal and digestive system (see Figure 14.6). The oral cavity is divided into two parts by the teeth: the vestibule and the mouth. The vestibule, the anterior and smaller of the two regions, is composed of the lips, the buccal mucosa, the outer surface of the gums and teeth, and the cheeks. At the posterior aspect of the teeth, the mouth is formed and includes the tongue, the hard and soft palate, the **uvula**, and the mandibular arch and maxillary arch.

The lips are folds of skin that cover the underlying muscle. They help keep food in place when chewing and play a role in speech. The cheeks form the side of the face and are continuous with the lips. Like the lips, the skin covers the underlying muscle. Both the lips and cheeks are lined internally with mucous membranes.

The gingivae or gums are bands of fibrous tissue that surround each tooth. The gums cover the mandibular and maxillary arches.

Thirty-two permanent teeth in the adult and 20 deciduous teeth in the child sit in the alveoli sockets of the mandible and maxilla (see Figure 14.7 on page 281). The enamel-covered crown is the visible portion of the tooth. The root, embedded in the jawbone, helps hold the tooth in place. Teeth are used for biting and chewing food.

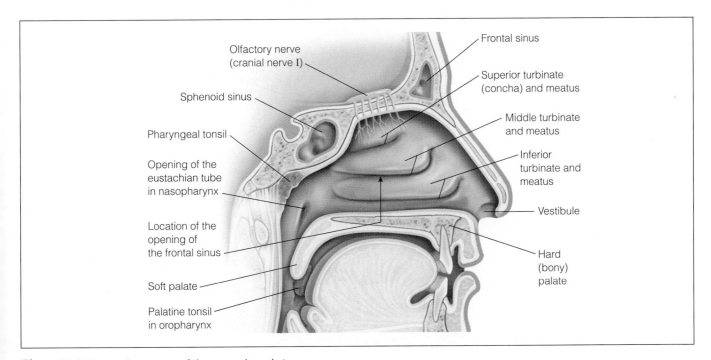

Figure 14.4 • Internal structure of the nose—lateral view.

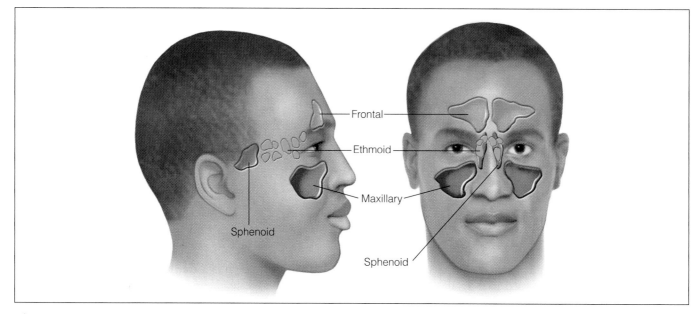

Figure 14.5 ● Nasal sinuses.

The tongue, the organ for taste, sits on the floor of the mouth. Its base sits on the hyoid bone. The anterior portion of the tongue is attached to the floor of the mouth by the frenulum. The ventral surface (undersurface) of the tongue is smooth with visible vessels. The dorsal (top) surface of the tongue is rough and supports the papillae. Papillae contain the taste buds and assist with moving food in the mouth. Taste buds are distributed throughout the tongue and are innervated by the facial and glossopharyngeal nerves (see Figure 14.8 on page 282). The tongue also assists with speech and swallowing. These actions are stimulated by the hypoglossal nerve (cranial nerve XII).

Hard and soft palates form the roof of the mouth. The **hard palate**, formed by bones, is the anterior portion of the roof of the mouth. The **soft palate**, formed by muscle, does not have a bony structure and is the posterior and somewhat mobile aspect of the roof of the mouth. The uvula hangs from the free edge of the soft palate. The uvula and soft palate move with swallowing, breathing, and phonation and are innervated by cranial nerves IX and X.

Parotid, submandibular, and sublingual salivary glands are responsible for the production of saliva (see Figure 14.9 on page 282). The parotid glands are situated anterior to the ear within the cheek. Saliva enters the mouth via Stensen's duct,

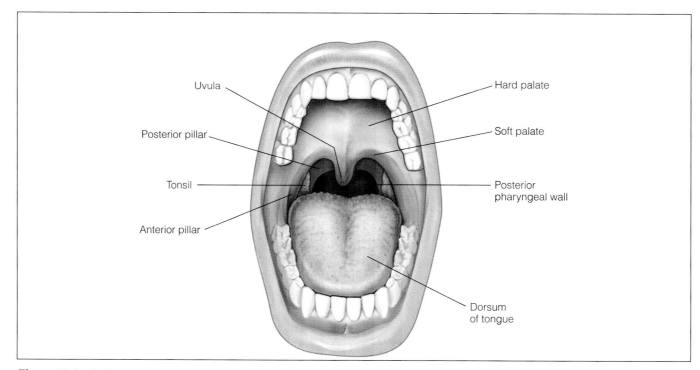

Figure 14.6 ● Oral cavity.

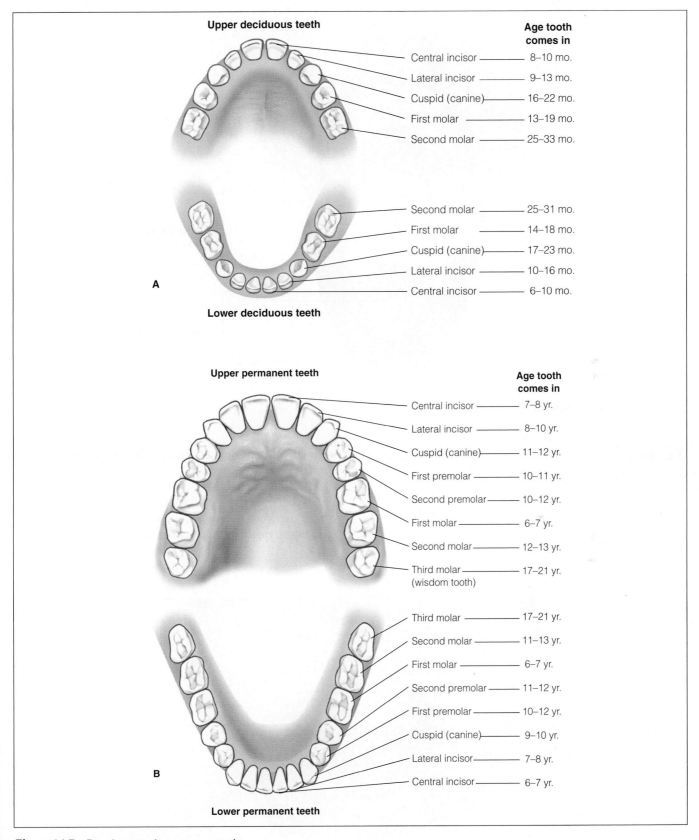

Figure 14.7 ● Deciduous and permanent teeth.

located in the buccal mucosa opposite the second upper molar. The submandibular glands sit beneath the mandible at the angle of the jaw. Saliva from these glands enters the mouth via Wharton's duct. The orifices of these ducts are on both sides of the frenulum on the floor of the mouth. The sublingual salivary glands, the smallest of the glands, are situated in the floor of the mouth and have many ducts that empty into the floor of the mouth.

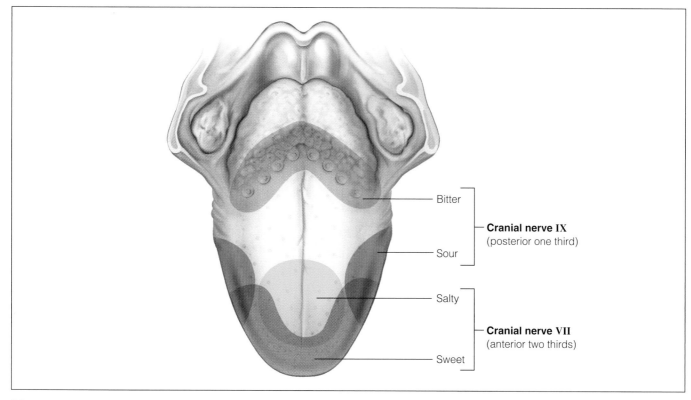

Figure 14.8 • Taste buds of the tongue.

Throat

The throat, known as the pharynx, connects the nose, mouth, larynx, and esophagus. The three sections of the throat are the nasopharynx (behind the nose), the oropharynx (behind the mouth), and the laryngopharynx (behind the larynx). The nasopharynx is behind the nose and above the soft palate. The adenoids and openings of the eustachian tubes are located in the nasopharynx.

The oropharynx is behind the mouth and below the nasopharynx. It extends to the epiglottis and serves as a passageway for air and food. The tonsils are located behind the pillars (palatopharyngeal folds) on either side.

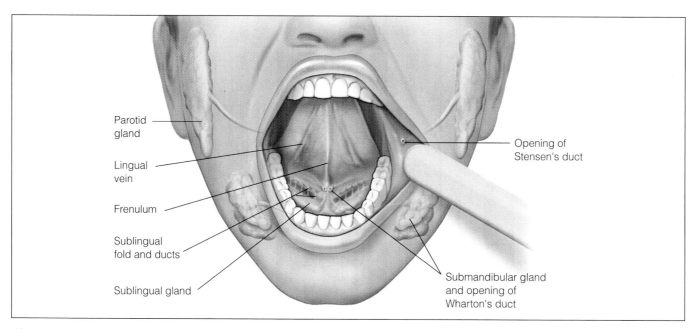

Figure 14.9 Salivary glands.

SPECIAL CONSIDERATIONS

The nurse must be aware that variations in findings from health assessment occur in relation to age, developmental level, race, ethnicity, work history, living conditions, socioeconomics, and emotional well-being. The following sections describe some factors to consider when collecting subjective and objective data.

Developmental Considerations

Changes in anatomy and physiology occur during growth and development. The ability to interpret data in relation to the normative values at various ages is important in the assessment process. Specific variations for different age groups are presented in the next sections.

Infants and Children

The infant's auditory canal is shorter than the adult's and has an upward curve, which persists until about 3 years of age. Children have a more horizontal auditory tube than adults, which leads to easier migration of organisms from infection in the throat to the middle ear. The nose of a child is too small to examine with a speculum. True development of the nose begins in the pubertal period with the development of secondary sex characteristics. Both sets of teeth develop before birth. Deciduous (baby) teeth begin to erupt between 6 months and 2 years of age. Eruption of permanent teeth begins at around age 6 and continues through adolescence. Salivation begins at 3 months of age. Drooling of saliva occurs for several months until swallowing saliva is learned.

The Pregnant Female

Changes in estrogen levels cause increased vascularity throughout the body in pregnancy. Vessel changes of the middle ear may cause a feeling of fullness or earaches. Hyperemia (increased blood flow) to the sinuses can cause rhinitis (inflammation of the nasal cavity) and epistaxis (nosebleed). The sense of smell is heightened in pregnancy. Edema of the vocal cords may cause hoarseness or deepening of the voice. Hyperemia of the throat can lead to an increase in snoring. Small blood vessels and connective tissue increase in the mouth. As a result, gingivitis or inflammation of the gums occurs in many females, which leads to bleeding and discomfort with brushing of the teeth and eating.

The Older Adult

The older adult may have coarse hairs at the opening of the auditory meatus. The ears may appear more prominent, because cartilage formation continues throughout life. The tympanic membrane becomes paler and thicker with aging. Assessment of hearing may reveal a loss of high-frequency tones, which is consistent with aging. Over time, this loss often progresses to lower-frequency sounds as well. Gradual hearing loss with age is called **presbycusis.**

As the adult ages, many changes occur inside the mouth. The lips and buccal mucosa of the mouth become thinner and less vascular. Gums are paler. The tongue develops more fissures, and motor function may become impaired, resulting in problems with swallowing. Senile tremors may cause slight protrusion of the tongue. A decreased sense of taste and smell may contribute to a decreased appetite and poor nutrition. Production of saliva may also decrease because of atrophy of the salivary glands or as a side effect of a medication. Gums begin to recede, and some tooth loss may occur because of osteoporosis. If teeth are lost, the remaining teeth may drift. Lesions of the mouth may develop from ill-fitting dentures.

Psychosocial Considerations

A client who is under a great deal of stress may be prone to mouth ulcers and lip biting. Tics (involuntary muscle spasms) and unconscious clenching of the jaw may indicate psychosocial disturbances. Relaxation techniques, such as meditation and guided imagery, may help relieve these stress-related behaviours.

Social and Ethnocultural Considerations

Dark-skinned clients may have darker cerumen, and their oral mucosa may be darker. White people tend to have more tooth decay and tooth loss than Black people. The size of the teeth varies with cultural ancestry. White people have the smallest teeth; Asians and Australian Aborigines have the largest.

A client's occupation may increase the risk for hearing loss. For example, construction workers, welders, groundskeepers, and musicians should be evaluated and use earplugs. Noise levels in the home may also need to be evaluated.

A client's socioeconomic status may affect the appearance and function of the structures of the mouth. For example, many clients do not have dental insurance and cannot afford regular dental care.

Social and Ethnocultural Considerations

- Otitis media occurs more frequently and with greater severity in children.
- Cerumen appears dry and grey to brown in Asians and Aboriginals.

- Cerumen appears moist and yellow-orange in Blacks and whites.
- Cleft lip and palate occur with greatest frequency in Asians and least often in Black people.

GATHERING THE DATA

Health assessment of the ears, nose, mouth, and throat includes gathering subjective and objective data. Recall that subjective data collection occurs during the client interview, before the actual physical assessment. During the interview the nurse uses a variety of communication techniques to elicit general and specific information about the state of health or illness of the client's ears, nose, mouth, and throat. Health records, the results of laboratory tests, and X-rays are important secondary sources to be reviewed and included in the data-gathering process. In physical assessment of the ears, nose, mouth, and throat, the techniques of inspection, palpation, and percussion will be used. Before proceeding, it may be helpful to review the information about each of the data-gathering processes and practise the techniques of health assessment. Some special equipment and assessments will be included—for example, the use of the otoscope.

HEALTH HISTORY

The health history concerns data related to the structures and functions of the ears, nose, mouth, and throat. Subjective data related to these structures are gathered during the health history. The nurse must be prepared to observe the client and listen for cues related to the functions of these structures. The nurse may use open-ended or closed questions to obtain information. Follow-up questions or requests for descriptions are required to clarify data or gather missing information. Follow-up questions identify the source of problems, duration of difficulties, and measures to alleviate problems. They also provide clues about the client's knowledge about his or her own health.

The health history guides the physical assessment of the ears, nose, mouth, and throat. The information is always considered in relation to normative parameters and expectations about function. Therefore, the nurse must consider age, gender, race, culture, environment, health practices, past and concurrent problems, and therapies when framing questions and using techniques to elicit information. To address all the factors when conducting a health history, specific questions related to the functions and disorders of the ear, nose, mouth, and throat have been developed. These questions focus on the most common concerns associated with illness or infections of the ear, nose, mouth, and throat; those related to habits or practices; questions that address the internal and external environment; and questions that are specific to clients according to age.

The nurse must consider the client's ability to participate in the health history interview and physical assessment of the ears, nose, mouth, and throat. If a client is experiencing pain, discomfort, or anxiety, attention must focus on relief of symptoms.

As the nurse gathers the data, she or he will shift the type of questions to direct questions that give the client room to explain or qualify. The mnemonic O-P-Q-R-S-T-U, which stands for onset (chronology), precipitating (or palliative), quality, region (or radiation), severity, timing, and understanding, will help the learner remember the dimensions of the symptoms. The nurse will keep in mind that not all these qualifiers will apply to each symptom.

HEALTH HISTORY QUESTIONS	RATIONALES

The following sections provide sample questions and follow-up questions. Rationales for some questions are provided. The list of questions is not all-inclusive but rather represents the more common concern or injury questions required in a health history related to the ears, nose, mouth, and throat. An example of using O-P-Q-R-S-T-U with pain is provided.

Questions Related to Common Concerns or Injuries

Questions Related to the Ear

The most common concerns related to the ear are as follows:
- Earache or pain
- Change in hearing
- Drainage
- Dizziness or vertigo

1. **Earache or pain**
   - Do you have an earache or experience pain in your ears? *If yes:*
   - When did you first notice the pain? How long does it last? *Onset (chronology)*

▶ Pain in one or both ears may be caused by a cold, an ear or sinus infection, trauma, dental problems, or cerumen blockage.

HEALTH HISTORY QUESTIONS	RATIONALES

- What makes the pain worse? What makes the pain better? *Precipitating (palliative)*
- Would you describe the pain as sharp? throbbing? burning? *Quality*
- Does the pain radiate? Where? *Radiation*
- How would you rate the pain on a scale of 1 to 10, with 10 being the worst pain? *Severity*
- How often do you experience the pain? Does it occur at specific times of the day or during certain activities? How long does it last? *Timing*
- What do you think is causing the pain? *Understanding*
- Where is the pain?

2. **Change in hearing**
   - Have you noticed any change in your hearing? If so, was the change gradual or sudden?

▶ A client's failure to respond to questions or frequent requests for the nurse to repeat questions may indicate a hearing loss. Hearing acuity decreases gradually with age. Any sudden loss of hearing should be investigated.

   - When was your last hearing test?

▶ Hearing tests should be conducted annually for children, middle adults, and older adults who live or work in noisy environments. Hearing loss in one ear could indicate an obstruction with cerumen or a ruptured tympanic membrane.

3. **Drainage**
   - Have you experienced any ear drainage?

▶ Ear drainage may indicate an infection. Bloody or purulent drainage could indicate **otitis media**, infection of the middle ear. Serous drainage could indicate allergic reaction. Clear drainage could be cerebral spinal fluid following trauma.

4. **Dizziness or vertigo**
   - Have you experienced any dizziness?

▶ These symptoms could indicate a problem with the inner ear, could be related to a neurological problem, or could be related to a medication.

Questions Related to the Nose and Sinuses

The most common concerns related to the nose and sinuses are as follows:

- Sinus pain
- Change in sense of smell
- Epistaxis (nosebleeds)
- Trauma

1. **Sinus pain**
   - Do you have any pain in your sinuses? *If yes:*
   - When did you first notice the pain? How long does it last? *Onset (chronology)*
   - What makes the pain worse? What makes the pain better? *Precipitating (palliative)*
   - Would you describe the pain as sharp? throbbing? aching? *Quality*
   - Does the pain radiate? Where? *Radiation*
   - How would you rate the pain on a scale of 1 to 10, with 10 being the worst pain? *Severity*
   - How often do you experience the pain? Does it occur at specific times of the day or during certain activities? How long does it last? *Timing*
   - What do you think is causing the pain? *Understanding*
   - Where is the pain?

▶ Pain in the sinuses may be related to sinusitis, nasal congestion, allergies, or a tooth infection.

GATHERING THE DATA

HEALTH HISTORY QUESTIONS	RATIONALES

2. Change in sense of smell
- Have you experienced any change in your sense of smell?

▶ Anosmia, the absence or loss of the sense of smell, may be neurological, hereditary, or caused by a deficiency of zinc in the diet.

3. Epistaxis (nosebleeds)
- Have you experienced any nosebleeds?

▶ Nosebleeds can occur as a result of trauma, excessive nose blowing, high blood pressure, overuse of nasal sprays, and certain blood disorders.

4. Trauma
- Have you ever had any nose injury?

▶ Trauma to the nose may cause nosebleeds and a deviated septum.

Questions Related to the Mouth and Throat

The most common concerns related to the mouth and throat are as follows:
- Sore throat
- Difficulty swallowing
- Sores or lesions
- Change in sense of taste

1. Sore throat
- Do you have a sore throat? *If yes:*
- When did you first notice the pain? How long does it last? *Onset (chronology)*
- What makes the pain worse? What makes the pain better? *Precipitating (palliative)*
- Would you describe the pain as sharp? dull? burning? *Quality*
- Does the pain radiate? Where? *Radiation*
- How would you rate the pain on a scale of 1 to 10, with 10 being the worst pain? *Severity*
- How often do you experience the pain? When does the pain occur? while eating? when swallowing? How long does it last? *Timing*
- What do you think is causing the pain? *Understanding*
- Where is the pain?

▶ A sore throat may be the result of irritation from sinus drainage, viral or bacterial infection, or the first sign of throat cancer.

2. Difficulty swallowing
- Do you have any problems swallowing?

▶ Dysphagia, or difficulty swallowing, may be due to a neurological or gastrointestinal problem, or it may be related to ill-fitting dentures or malocclusion (misalignment of the upper and lower teeth). Achalasia, a chronic difficulty in swallowing caused by constriction of the esophagus, may be related to anxiety or stress. Painful or difficult swallowing could be related to cancer of the throat or esophagus.

3. Sores or lesions
- Do you have any sores or lesions in your mouth or on your tongue?

▶ Lesions of the mouth or tongue may be cold sores or mouth ulcers. They may also accompany viral infections and gum infections. Some lesions may be caused by ill-fitting dentures. Any lesion of the mouth that does not heal should be evaluated for oral cancer.

4. Change in sense of taste
- Have you noticed a change in your sense of taste?

▶ Loss of the sense of taste commonly accompanies colds. A foul taste in the mouth may signal a gum infection or inadequate care of teeth or dentures. Smokers may experience a change in their sense of taste.

HEALTH HISTORY QUESTIONS	RATIONALES

Questions Related to Past Health History

1. **Do you have or have you ever had any ear diseases, such as Meniere's disease, vertigo, or acoustic neuroma?** *If yes:*
   - When were you diagnosed with the problem?
   - Has the problem ever recurred? *(acute)*
   - How are you managing the disease now? *(chronic)*

▶ Listing possible disease is a comprehensive and easy way to elicit information about all diagnoses related to the ear. The client has an opportunity to provide information about specific illnesses affecting the ears. If a diagnosed illness is identified, follow-up about the diagnosis, treatment, and outcomes is required. Data about each illness identified by the client are essential to an accurate health assessment. Illnesses are classified as acute or chronic, and follow-up regarding each classification will differ.

2. **Do you now have or have you had an ear infection?** *If yes:*
   - When were you diagnosed with the problem?
   - Has the problem ever recurred? *(acute)*
   - How are you managing the infection now? *(chronic)*

▶ If an infection is identified, follow-up about the date of infection, treatment, and outcomes is required. Data about each infection identified by the client are essential to an accurate health assessment. Infections can be classified as acute or chronic, and follow-up regarding each classification will differ.

Questions Related to Behaviours

Healthcare behaviours include both health practices and health patterns. Health practices consist of following recommendations for disease prevention, including screening for risks, screening for early detection of problems, and immunization. Health patterns are habits or acts that affect the client's health. Health behaviours may also include seeking healthcare from healthcare providers who use alternative methods to diagnose and treat illness. Clients should be questioned in a nonjudgmental way and areas for health teaching should be identified.

1. **How do you clean your ears?**

▶ Many people use cotton-tipped applicators to remove cerumen. This practice can cause trauma to the eardrum and cause cerumen to become impacted. Ear canals should never be cleaned. Cerumen moves to the outside naturally. Commercial cerumen removal products are available but should be used with the guidance of a healthcare provider.

2. **Do you either own or use a hearing aid?**

▶ Some clients have hearing aids but will not use them because of increased background noise, because of embarrassment, or because they cannot pay for the batteries for the hearing aid.

Questions Related to the Environment

Environment refers to both internal and external environments. Questions related to the internal environment include all the previous questions and those associated with internal or physiological responses. Questions regarding the external environment include those related to home, work, or social environments.

Internal Environment

1. **Are you taking any medications?** *If yes:*
   - What are they?
   - How often?

▶ Certain medicines affect the ears. Aspirin can cause tinnitus (ringing in the ears). Some antibiotics can cause hearing loss and dizziness.

HEALTH HISTORY QUESTIONS	RATIONALES

External Environment

The following questions deal with the physical environment of the client. That includes the indoor and outdoor environments of the home and the workplace, those encountered for social engagements, and any encountered during travel.

1. **Are you frequently exposed to loud noise?** *If yes:*
   - When?
   - How often?
   - Are protective devices available and do you use them?

▶ Long-term exposure to loud noise can result in hearing loss. Clients at risk are those with jobs in noisy factories; jobs at airports; jobs requiring the use of explosives, firearms, jackhammers, or other loud equipment; and jobs in nightclubs. Frequent exposure to loud music, either live or from stereos or headphones, can also contribute to hearing loss.

2. **Do you experience ear infections or irritations after swimming or being exposed to dust or smoke? If so, describe them.**

▶ Contaminated water left in the ear may cause **otitis externa**, swimmer's ear. Irritation of the ear after exposure to certain substances may indicate an allergy to such substances.

Questions Related to Age

The health history must reflect the anatomical and physiological differences that exist along the age span.

Questions Regarding Infants and Children

1. **Does the child have recurrent ear infections?** *If yes:*
   - How many ear infections has the child had in the last 6 months?
   - How were they treated?
   - Has the child had any ear surgery, such as insertion of ear tubes? If so, when?
   - What were the results?
   - Does the child attend daycare?

2. **Does the child tug at his or her ears?**

▶ Tugging at the ears can be an early sign of infection.

3. **Does the child respond to loud noises?**

▶ A lack of response could indicate hearing loss.

4. **If the child is over 6 months of age, does the child babble?**

▶ A child who does not babble may have a hearing impairment.

5. **Have you ever had the child's hearing tested?** *If yes:*
   - What were the results?

6. **Has the child had measles, mumps, or any disease with a high fever?**
   - Has the child been treated recently with any antibiotics, such as streptomycin or neomycin?

▶ High fevers and certain drugs can cause hearing loss.

7. **How do you clean the child's ears?**

▶ The nurse should ascertain whether the procedure is harmful, such as cleaning ears with cotton swabs, which may cause impacted cerumen.

8. **Does the child put objects into his or her nose?**

▶ Foreign objects can cause trauma to nasal tissues.

9. **Does the child frequently have drainage from the nose?**

▶ Frequent drainage can indicate an infection or allergies.

GATHERING THE DATA

HEALTH HISTORY QUESTIONS	RATIONALES
10. Does the child suck his or her thumb or a pacifier?	▶ These behaviours can interfere with alignment of secondary teeth.
11. When did the child's teeth begin to erupt?	▶ Late eruption of teeth could indicate delayed development.
12. Does the child go to bed with a bottle at night? *If yes:* • What is in the bottle?	▶ Frequent use of a bottle with milk or juice at night can cause tooth decay.
13. Does the child know how to brush teeth? • Does the child brush daily?	
14. How often does the child go to the dentist?	▶ Children should begin annual visits to the dentist between the ages of 3 and 4 years.
15. Is the child's drinking water fluoridated?	▶ Fluoride in the water supply helps prevent tooth decay.

Questions for the Pregnant Female

1. Have you ever experienced a humming in your ears?

▶ Humming in the ears during pregnancy may occur with hypertension associated with preeclampsia (a serious condition that can threaten maternal and fetal health).

2. Have you experienced an earache or a feeling of fullness in your ears?

▶ Changes in estrogen produce increased vascularity throughout the systems of the body during pregnancy. The vascularity may cause a feeling of fullness or an aching in the ears.

3. Have you had nosebleeds during your pregnancy? If so, how often?

▶ Nosebleeds and nasal congestion are common during pregnancy because of increased vascularity in the nasal passages.

Questions for the Older Adult

1. Do you wear a hearing aid? *If yes:*
   • Is it effective?
   • How often do you wear your hearing aid?

▶ Many older adults have a hearing loss but cannot adjust to using a hearing aid or cannot afford batteries for the hearing aid.

2. Do you have any difficulty operating the hearing aid?
   • How do you clean the hearing aid?

▶ Some clients forget to clean the tubes of the hearing aid periodically.

3. Are you able to chew all types of food?

▶ If teeth are missing or dentures fit improperly, the client may not be able to chew meat or certain vegetables, resulting in undernutrition.

4. Do you experience dryness in your mouth?

▶ Certain medications may cause dryness, which may interfere with the client's appetite or digestion.

5. Do you wear dentures?
   • If so, do they fit properly?

▶ Ill-fitting dentures can interfere with proper nutrition and can cause various problems in the mouth, such as lesions and bleeding gums.

PHYSICAL ASSESSMENT

ASSESSMENT TECHNIQUES AND FINDINGS

Physical assessment of the ears, nose, mouth, and throat requires the use of inspection, palpation, percussion, and transillumination of sinuses. In addition, special examination techniques include the use of the otoscope, tuning fork, and nasal speculum. These techniques are used to gather objective data. Knowledge of normal or expected findings is essential in determining the meaning of data as the nurse proceeds.

Adults have binaural hearing; the ears are symmetrical in size, shape, colour, and configuration. The external auditory canal is patent and free of drainage. The external ear and mastoid process are free of lesions, and the tragus is movable. Under otoscopic examination the external ear canal is open, nontender, and free of lesions, inflammation, and foreign substances. Cerumen, if present, is soft and in small amounts. The tympanic membrane is flat, grey, and translucent without lesions. The malleolar process and reflected light are visible on the tympanic membrane. The tympanic membrane flutters with the Valsalva manoeuvre. During hearing tests, air conduction is better than bone conduction. Adults are able to maintain balance.

The external nose is free of lesions, the nares are patent, and the mucosa of the nasal cavity is dark pink and smooth. The nasal septum is midline, straight, and intact. The sinuses are nontender and transilluminate. The lips are smooth, symmetrical, and lesion-free. The adult has 32 permanent teeth that are white with smooth edges. The tongue is mobile, is pink, and has papillae on the dorsum. The oral mucosa is pink, moist, and smooth. Salivary ducts are visible and not inflamed. The membranes and structures of the throat are pink and moist. The uvula is midline and, like the soft palate, rises when the client says "ah."

Physical assessment of the ears, nose, mouth, and throat follows an organized pattern. It begins with instruction of the client and proceeds through inspection, palpation, and otoscopic examination of the ears, followed by hearing assessment and the Romberg test. The nose is inspected and the internal aspect is visualized while using a speculum. The sinuses are palpated, percussed, and transilluminated. The assessment concludes with inspection of the external mouth, inspection of the internal structures of the mouth, and assessment of the throat.

EQUIPMENT

examination gown
nasal speculum
clean, nonsterile exam gloves
penlight
otoscope
gauze pads
tuning fork
tongue blade

HELPFUL HINTS

- Provide specific instructions about what is expected of the client. The nurse will state whether the head must be turned or the mouth opened.
- Consider the age of the client. Response to directions varies across the lifespan.
- Pay attention to nonverbal cues throughout the assessment.
- Hearing difficulties may affect the data-gathering process. Clarify problems and possible remedies before beginning the assessment. The client may use sign language, hearing aids, lip reading, or written communication.
- Explain the use of each piece of equipment throughout the assessment.
- Use routine practices.

TECHNIQUES AND NORMAL FINDINGS

ABNORMAL FINDINGS AND SPECIAL CONSIDERATIONS

EAR

1. **Position the client.**
   - The client should be in a sitting position. Lighting must be adequate to detect skin colour changes, discharge, and lesions.

2. **Instruct the client.**
   - Explain that you will be carrying out a variety of assessments of the ear. Tell the client you will be touching the ear areas, that it should not cause discomfort, and that any pain or discomfort should be reported.

TECHNIQUES AND NORMAL FINDINGS	ABNORMAL FINDINGS AND SPECIAL CONSIDERATIONS

3. Note that you will have begun to evaluate the client's hearing while taking the health history.

   • Did the client hear the questions you asked?

   • Did the client answer appropriately?

   • Generally, the formal evaluation of hearing is performed after otoscopic examination so that physical barriers to hearing, such as large amounts of cerumen, can be identified.

4. Inspect the external ear for symmetry, proportion, colour, and integrity.

   • Confirm that the external auditory meatus is patent with no drainage. The colour of the ear should match that of the surrounding area and the face, with no redness, nodules, swelling, or lesions.

▶ Any discharge, redness, or swelling may indicate an infection or allergy.

5. Palpate the auricle and push on the tragus (see Figure 14.10).

   • Confirm that there are no hard nodules, lesions, or swelling. The tragus should be movable.

   • This technique should not cause pain.

▶ Pain could be the result of an infection of the external ear (otitis externa). Pain could also indicate temporomandibular joint dysfunction with pressure on the tragus. Hard nodules (tophi) are uric acid crystal deposits, which are a sign of gout. Lesions accompanied by a history of long-term exposure to the sun may be cancerous.

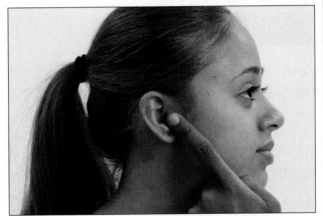

Figure 14.10
Palpating the tragus.

6. Palpate the mastoid process lying directly behind the ear (see Figure 14.11).

   • Confirm that there are no lesions, pain, or swelling.

▶ **Mastoiditis** is a complication of either a middle ear infection or a throat infection. Mastoiditis is very difficult to treat. It spreads easily to the brain since the mastoid area is separated from the brain by only a thin, bony plate.

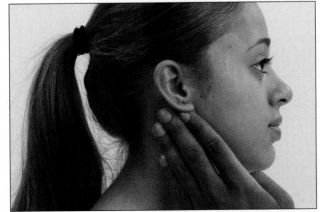

Figure 14.11 ●
Palpating the
mastoid process.

7. Inspect the auditory canal by using the otoscope.

   • For the best visualization, use the largest speculum that will fit into the auditory canal.

PHYSICAL ASSESSMENT

Techniques and Normal Findings

- Ask the client to tilt the head away from you toward the opposite shoulder.
- Hold the otoscope between the palm and first two fingers of the dominant hand. The handle may be positioned upward or downward (see Figure 14.13).
- Use your other hand to straighten the canal.
- In the adult client, pull the pinna up, back, and out to straighten the canal (see Figure 14.12).

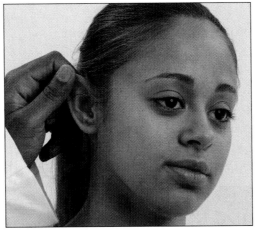

Figure 14.12 ●
Pulling the pinna to straighten the canal.

- Be sure to maintain this position until the speculum is removed.
- Instruct the client to tell you if any discomfort is experienced but not to move the head or suddenly pull away.

CLINICAL TIP

Use care when inserting the speculum of the otoscope into the ear. The inner two thirds of the ear are very sensitive, and pressing the speculum against either side of the auditory canal will cause pain.

- With the light on, use the upward or downward position of the handle to insert the speculum into the ear (see Figure 14.13). The external canal should be open and without tenderness, inflammation, lesions, growths, discharge, or foreign substances.
- Note the amount of cerumen that is present, the texture, and the colour.

▶If the ear canal is occluded with cerumen, it must be removed. Most cerumen can be removed with a cerumen spoon. If the cerumen is dry, the external canal should be irrigated by using a bulb syringe and a warmed solution of mineral oil and hydrogen peroxide, followed by warm water.

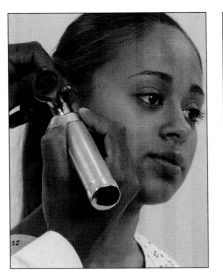
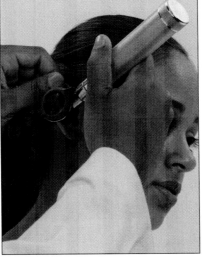

Figure 14.13 ● Two techniques for holding and inserting an otoscope.

PHYSICAL ASSESSMENT

| TECHNIQUES AND NORMAL FINDINGS | ABNORMAL FINDINGS AND SPECIAL CONSIDERATIONS |

8. **Examine the tympanic membrane by using the otoscope.**
   - The membrane should be flat, grey, and translucent with no scars (see Figure 14.14). A cone-shaped reflection of the otoscope light should be visible at the 5-o'clock position in the right ear and the 7-o'clock position in the left ear. The short process of the malleus should be seen as a shadow behind the tympanic membrane. The membrane should be intact.
   - If you cannot visualize the tympanic membrane, remove the otoscope, reposition the auricle, and reinsert the otoscope. Do not reposition the auricle with the otoscope in place.

▶ White patches on the tympanic membrane indicate scars from prior infections. If the membrane is yellow or reddish, it could indicate an infection of the middle ear. A bulging membrane may indicate increased pressure in the middle ear, whereas a retracted membrane may indicate a vacuum in the middle ear, caused by a blocked eustachian tube.

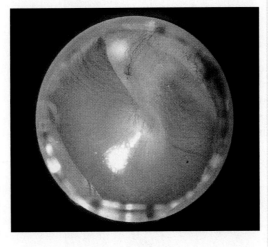

Figure 14.14 ●
Normal tympanic membrane with cone of light and process of malleus.

9. **While looking through the otoscope, instruct the client to perform the Valsalva manoeuvre.**
   - Have the tympanic membrane in clear view.
   - Ask the client to close the lips, pinch the nose, and gently blow the nose.
   - This manoeuvre lets you assess the mobility of the tympanic membrane and the patency of the eustachian tubes. The tympanic membrane should flutter toward the otoscope slightly as the client performs this manoeuvre.

▶ Rigidity of the tympanic membrane may be due to a variety of alterations and requires further evaluation.

CLINICAL TIP

An older client should not be asked to perform the Valsalva manoeuvre because it may result in dizziness. This manoeuvre is also dangerous if the client has an upper respiratory infection, because it could force pathogenic organisms into the middle ear.

10. **Perform the whisper test.**
    - This test evaluates hearing acuity for high-frequency sounds.
    - Ask the client to hold the heel of the hand over the left ear or to place one finger on the tragus to block the sound.
    - Cover your mouth so that the client cannot see your lips.
    - Standing at the client's side at a distance of 30 to 60 cm (1 to 2 ft.), whisper a simple phrase, such as "The weather is hot today." Ask the client to repeat the phrase. Then do the same procedure to test the right ear by using a different phrase. The client should be able to repeat the phrases correctly (see Figure 14.15).

▶ Inability to repeat the phrases may indicate a loss of the ability to hear high-frequency sounds.

TECHNIQUES AND NORMAL FINDINGS

ABNORMAL FINDINGS AND
SPECIAL CONSIDERATIONS

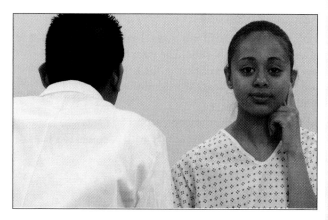

Figure 14.15 ●
Performing the
whisper test.

- Tuning forks are used to evaluate auditory acuity. The tines of the fork, when activated, produce sound waves. The frequency, or cycles per second (cps), is the expression used to describe the action of the instrument. A fork with 512 cps vibrates 512 times per second and is the size of choice for auditory evaluations. The tines are set into motion by squeezing, stroking, or lightly tapping against your hand. The fork must be held at the handle to prevent interference with the vibration of the tines (see Figure 14.16).

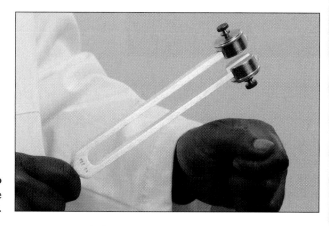

Figure 14.16 ●
Activating the
tuning fork.

- The following tests use a tuning fork primarily to evaluate conductive versus perceptive hearing loss. **Air conduction (AC)** is the transmission of sound through the tympanic membrane to the cochlea and auditory nerve. **Bone conduction (BC)** is the transmission of sound through the bones of the skull to the cochlea and auditory nerve.

11. Perform the Rinne test.

- The Rinne test compares air and bone conduction. Hold the tuning fork by the handle and gently strike the fork on the palm of your hand to set it vibrating.
- Place the base of the fork on the client's mastoid process (see Figure 14.17A).
- Ask the client to tell you when the sound is no longer heard.
- Note the number of seconds. Then immediately move the tines of the still-vibrating fork in front of the external auditory meatus. It should be 1 cm (about 0.5 in.) from the meatus.
- Ask the client to tell you again when the sound is no longer heard (see Figure 14.17B). Again note the number of seconds. Normally, the sound is heard twice as long by air conduction as by bone conduction after bone conduction stops. For example, a normal finding is AC 30 seconds, BC 15 seconds.

▶ If the client hears the bone-conducted sound as long as or longer than the air-conducted sound, the client may have some degree of conductive hearing loss.

Techniques and Normal Findings

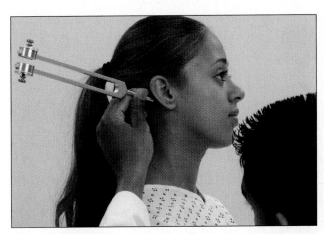

Figure 14.17A ● Rinne test. Bone conduction.

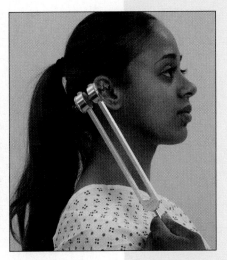

Figure 14.17B ● Rinne test. Air conduction.

12. Perform the Weber test.

- The Weber test uses bone conduction to evaluate hearing in a person who hears better in one ear than in the other. Hold the tuning fork by the handle and strike the fork on the palm of the hand. Place the base of the vibrating fork against the client's skull. The midline of the anterior portion of the frontal bone is used. The midline of the forehead is an alternative choice (see Figure 14.18).

▶ If the client hears the sound in one ear better than the other ear, the hearing loss may be due to either poor conduction or nerve damage. If the client has poor conduction in one ear, the sound is heard better in the impaired ear because the sound is being conducted directly through the bone to the ear, and the extraneous sounds in the environment are not being picked up. Conductive loss in one ear may be due to impacted cerumen, infection, or a perforated eardrum. If the client has a hearing loss due to nerve damage, the sound is referred to the better ear, in which the cochlea or auditory nerve is functioning better.

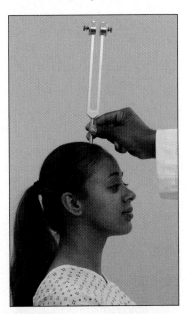

Figure 14.18 ●
Weber test.

- Ask the client if the sound is heard equally on both sides or better in one ear than the other. The normal response is bilaterally equal sound, which is recorded as "no lateralization." If the sound is lateralized, ask the client to tell you which ear hears the sound better.

▶ The abnormal findings are recorded as "sound lateralizes to (right or left) ear."

13. Perform the Romberg test.

- The Romberg test assesses equilibrium. Ask the client to stand with feet together and arms at the sides, first with eyes opened and then with eyes closed (see Figure 14.19).

Techniques and Normal Findings

ABNORMAL FINDINGS AND SPECIAL CONSIDERATIONS

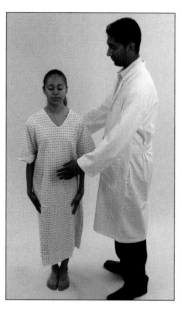

Figure 14.19 ●
Romberg test.

- Wait about 20 seconds. The person should be able to maintain this position, although some mild swaying may occur. Mild swaying is documented as a negative Romberg. It is important to stand nearby and prepare to support the client if a loss of balance occurs. Hearing and balance are functions of cranial nerve VIII and are discussed in Chapter 24. ⬭

▶ If the client is unable to maintain balance or needs to have the feet farther apart, there may be a problem with functioning of the vestibular apparatus.

NOSE AND SINUSES

Note: The sense of smell and function of cranial nerve I is evaluated with the neurological assessment presented in Chapter 24. ⬭

1. **Instruct the client.**
   - Explain that you will be looking at and touching the client's nose. Tell the client to inform you of any discomfort.

2. **Inspect the nose for symmetry, shape, skin lesions, or signs of infection.**
   - Confirm that the nose is straight, the nares are equal in size, the skin is intact, and no drainage is present (see Figure 14.20).

▶ If breathing is noisy or a discharge is present, the client may have an obstruction or an infection.

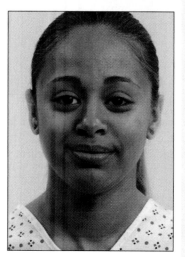

Figure 14.20 ●
Inspection of the nose.

TECHNIQUES AND NORMAL FINDINGS	ABNORMAL FINDINGS AND SPECIAL CONSIDERATIONS

3. **Test for patency.**
   - Press your finger on the client's nostril to occlude one naris, and ask the client to breathe through the opposite side.
   - Repeat with the other nostril.
   - The client should be able to breathe through each naris.

▶ If the client cannot breathe through each naris, severe inflammation or an obstruction may be present.

▶ Ineffective breathing patterns or mouth breathing may be related to nasal swelling or trauma.

4. **Palpate the external nose for tenderness, swelling, and stability.**
   - Use two fingers to palpate the nose.
   - Note the smoothness and stability of the underlying soft tissue and cartilage.

5. **Inspect the nasal cavity by using a nasal speculum.**
   - With your nondominant hand, stabilize the client's head. With the speculum in your dominant hand, insert the speculum with blades closed into the naris. Then separate the blades, dilating the naris (see Figure 14.21). The speculum should be in the dominant hand for better control at the time of insertion to avoid hitting the sensitive septum.

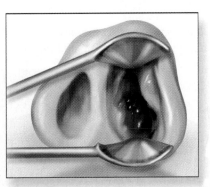
Figure 14.21 ●
Using the nasal speculum.

   - With the client's head erect, inspect the inferior turbinates (Figure 14.21).
   - With the client's head tilted back, inspect the middle meatus and middle turbinates. Mucosa should be dark pink and smooth, without swelling, discharge, bleeding, or foreign bodies. The septum should be midline, straight, and intact.
   - When finished with inspection, close the blades of the speculum and remove. Again, do not hit the sensitive septum.
   - Repeat on other side.

▶ If the mucosa is swollen and red, the client may have an upper respiratory infection. If mucosa is pale and boggy or swollen, the client may have chronic allergies. A *deviated septum* appears as an irregular lump in one nasal cavity. Slight deviations do not present problems for most clients. **Nasal polyps** are smooth, pale, benign growths found in many clients with chronic allergies.

6. **Palpate the sinuses.**
   - Begin by pressing your thumbs over the frontal sinuses below the superior orbital ridge. Palpate the maxillary sinuses below the zygomatic arches of the cheekbones (see Figures 14.22A and 14.22B).
   - Observe the client for signs of discomfort. Ask the client to inform you of pain.

▶ Tenderness on palpation may indicate chronic allergies or sinusitis.

PHYSICAL ASSESSMENT

TECHNIQUES AND NORMAL FINDINGS	ABNORMAL FINDINGS AND SPECIAL CONSIDERATIONS

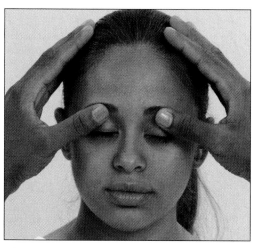

Figure 14.22A ● Palpating the frontal sinuses.

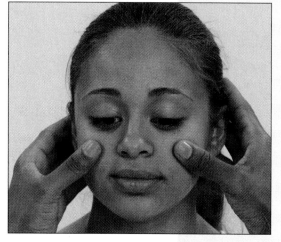

Figure 14.22B ● Palpating the maxillary sinuses.

7. **Percuss the sinuses.**
   - To determine if there is pain in the sinuses, directly percuss over the maxillary and frontal sinuses by lightly tapping with one finger (see Figures 14.23A and 14.23B).

▶ Pain may indicate sinus fullness, allergies, or infection.

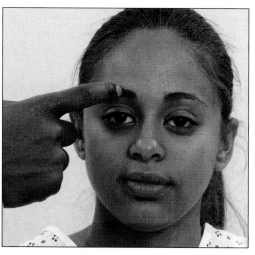

Figure 14.23A Percussion of frontal sinuses.

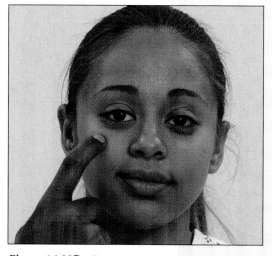

Figure 14.23B ● Percussion of maxillary sinuses.

8. **Transilluminate the sinuses.**
   - If you suspect a sinus infection, the maxillary and frontal sinuses may be transilluminated.
   - To transilluminate the frontal sinus, darken the room and hold a penlight under the superior orbit ridge against the frontal sinus area (see Figure 14.24A).
   - Cover the penlight with your hand. There should be a red glow over the frontal sinus area (see Figure 14.24B).
   - To test the maxillary sinus, place a clean penlight in the client's mouth and shine the light on one side of the hard palate, then on the other side.
   - There should be a red glow over the cheeks (see Figure 14.25A). Make sure the penlight is cleaned before using it again.

▶ If there is no red glow under the eyes, the sinuses may be inflamed.

Techniques and Normal Findings

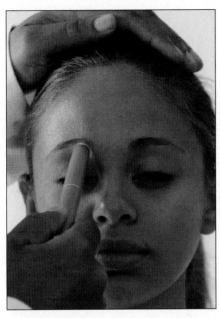

Figure 14.24A ● Transillumination of the frontal sinuses.

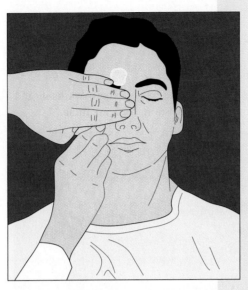

Figure 14.24B ● Observing transillumination of the frontal sinuses.

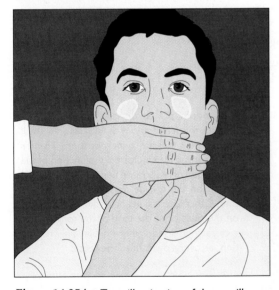

Figure 14.25A ● Transillumination of the maxillary sinuses.

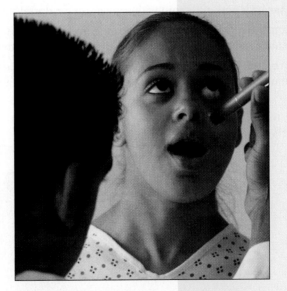

Figure 14.25B Transillumination of the maxillary sinuses by using alternative technique.

- An alternative technique is to place the penlight directly on the cheek and observe the glow of light on the hard palate (see Figure 14.25B).

MOUTH AND THROAT

Note: Be sure to wear clean, nonsterile examination gloves for this part of the assessment.

1. **Inspect and palpate the lips.**
   - Confirm that the lips are symmetrical, smooth, pink, moist, and without lesions. Makeup or lipstick should be removed.

▶ Lesions or blisters on the lips may be caused by the herpes simplex virus. These lesions are also known as **fever blisters** or **cold sores**. However, lesions must be evaluated for cancer, because cancer of the lip is the most common oral cancer. Pallor or cyanosis of the lips may indicate hypoxia.

PHYSICAL ASSESSMENT

Techniques and Normal Findings

2. Inspect the teeth.

   • Observe the client's dental hygiene. Ask the client to clench the teeth and smile while you observe occlusion.

   • Note dentures and caps at this time.

   • The teeth should be white, with smooth edges, and free of debris. Adults should have 32 permanent teeth (see Figure 14.26), if wisdom teeth are intact.

▶ Loose, painful, broken or misaligned teeth, malocclusion, and inflamed gums need further evaluation.

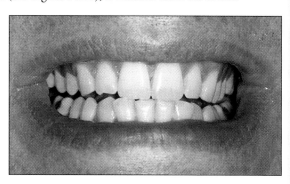

Figure 14.26 ●
Inspecting the teeth.

3. Inspect and palpate the buccal mucosa, gums, and tongue.

   • Look into the client's mouth under a strong light.

   • Confirm that the tongue is pink and moist with papillae on the dorsal surface.

   • Ask the client to touch the roof of the mouth with the tip of the tongue. The ventral surface should be smooth and pink. Palpate the area under the tongue.

   • Check for lesions or nodules. Use a gauze pad and grasp the client's tongue. Inspect for any lumps or nodules (see Figure 14.27). The tissue should be smooth.

   • Use a tongue blade to hold the tongue aside while you inspect the mucous lining of the mouth and the gums.

▶ A smooth, coated, or hairy tongue is usually related to dehydration or disease. A small tongue may indicate undernutrition. Tremor of the tongue may indicate a dysfunction of the hypoglossal nerve (cranial nerve XII). Persistent lesions on the tongue must be evaluated further. Cancerous lesions occur most commonly on the sides or at the base of the tongue. The gums are diseased if there is bleeding, retraction, or overgrowth onto the teeth.

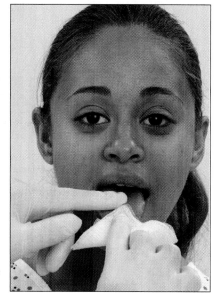

Figure 14.27
Palpating the tongue.

   • Confirm that these areas are pink, moist, smooth, and free of lesions.

   • Confirm the integrity of both the soft and the hard palate.

   • The sense of taste (cranial nerves VII and IX) and movement of the tongue (cranial nerve XII) are discussed in detail in Chapter 24. ∞

| TECHNIQUES AND NORMAL FINDINGS | ABNORMAL FINDINGS AND SPECIAL CONSIDERATIONS |

4. **Inspect the salivary glands.**

 - The salivary glands open into the mouth. Wharton's ducts (submandibular) open close to the lingual frenulum. Stensen's ducts (parotid) open opposite the second upper molars. Both ducts are visible, whereas the ducts of the sublingual glands are not visible.
 - Confirm that all salivary ducts are visible, with no pain, tenderness, swelling, or redness.
 - Touch the area close to the ducts with a sterile applicator, and confirm the flow of saliva.

▶ Pain or the lack of saliva can indicate infection or an obstruction.

5. **Inspect the throat.**

 - Use a tongue blade and penlight to inspect the throat (see Figure 14.28).

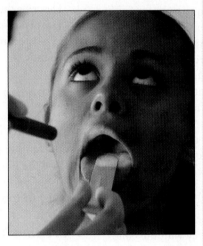

Figure 14.28 ●
Inspecting the throat.

 - Ask the client to open the mouth wide, tilt the head back, and say "aah." The uvula should rise in the midline.
 - Use the tongue blade to depress the middle of the arched tongue enough so that you can clearly visualize the throat but not so much that the client gags. Ask the client to say "aah" again.
 - Confirm the rising of the soft palate, which is a test for cranial nerve X.
 - Confirm that the tonsils, uvula, and posterior pharynx are pink and are without inflammation, swelling, or lesions. Observe the tonsils behind the anterior tonsillar pillar. They should be pink, with slight vascularity present. Tonsils may be partially or totally absent.
 - As you inspect the throat, note any mouth odours.
 - Discard the tongue blade.

▶ Viral pharyngitis may accompany a cold. Tonsils may be bright red and swollen and may have white spots on them.

▶ Clients with diabetic acidosis have a sweet, fruity breath. The breath of clients with kidney disease smells of ammonia.

SAMPLE DOCUMENTATION

Subjective: No history of earache, drainage, dizziness/vertigo, change in hearing, sinus pain, change in sense of smell, nosebleeds/epistaxis, trauma, sore throat, difficulty swallowing, change in sense of taste, sores, or lesions. No past history of diseases of the ear or ear infections.

Objective: *Ears:* Ears equal in size and shape. *Hearing:* Weber, no lateralization, Rinne, AC > BC, whisper test, client able to correctly repeat spoken words.

Nose: Nares patent, no alteration in sense of smell.

Mouth and throat: Gag reflex intact, uvula midline, no difficulty swallowing. Tongue midline, no tremors.

PHYSICAL ASSESSMENT

APPLICATION THROUGH CRITICAL THINKING

CASE STUDY

Harold Chandler is a 35-year-old executive in a computer firm who comes to the employees' wellness centre complaining of a marked loss of hearing in his left ear. He says that he woke up yesterday with a "feeling of fullness" in his left ear but no pain. He further relates that his 3-year-old daughter has a "bad cold and an earache," and he wonders if he has "the same thing." He denies any other symptoms of infection, has had no discharge from either ear, and is not taking any medicine at this time. He has not had an audiometric examination since his last physical 3 years ago. He further volunteers that he has just returned from a business trip to Europe and wonders whether the pressurized atmosphere of the airplane "created a problem with his hearing." Nurse Michael Andrews's assessment of Mr. Chandler reveals normal vital signs. His left ear's external canal is uniformly pink, with no redness, swelling, lesions, or discharge.

The Weber test reveals lateralization to the left ear. The otoscopic examination reveals a left ear impacted with brown-grey cerumen, and the tympanic membrane cannot be visualized. Examination of the right ear shows the external canal is uniformly pink with no redness, swelling, lesions, or discharge. During the otoscopic examination, the tympanic membrane is easily visualized. It is translucent and pearl-grey with the cone of light at the 5-o'clock position. No perforations are noted.

To visualize the tympanic membrane of the left ear, Mr. Andrews prepares a solution of mineral oil and hydrogen peroxide and instills the solution into the left ear canal to soften the cerumen. Then he irrigates the canal with warm water by using a bulb syringe. After Mr. Andrews completes the irrigation, Mr. Chandler is surprised to discover that his hearing has returned in his left ear. Now Mr. Andrews completes the otoscopic examination. He is able to visualize the tympanic membrane, which is translucent and pearl-grey with the cone of light at the 7-o'clock position. No perforations are noted.

To be sure that Mr. Chandler's hearing has been restored, Mr. Andrews performs a screening evaluation of his auditory function. He is able to hear a low whisper at 0.75 m (2 ft.). His Rinne test is positive, and his Weber test indicates equal lateralization.

►Complete Documentation

The following is sample documentation for Harold Chandler.

SUBJECTIVE DATA: 35-year-old c/o hearing loss (L) ear. Woke up yesterday with fullness, no pain (L) ear. His 3-year-old daughter has "bad cold and earache," wonders if he has the same. Denies signs of infection, no discharge, and no medication. Audiometric examination 3 years ago. Recent air travel, wonders if pressurized atmosphere created hearing problem.

OBJECTIVE DATA: Ears equal in size, shape. Tragus mobile, nontender bilaterally. Left ear canal pink, no redness, edema, lesions, discharge. Weber—lateralization to left. Otoscopic examination: Left ear impacted with brown-grey cerumen, no visualization tympanic membrane. Right ear canal pink, clear, no edema, tympanic membrane grey with no lesions.

►Critical Thinking Questions

1. Describe the application of critical thinking to the situation.
2. How was information clustered to guide decision making?
3. What recommendations should the nurse provide for this client?

►Applying Nursing Diagnoses

1. *Disturbed sensory perception* is a nursing diagnosis in the NANDA-I taxonomy. Do the data for Mr. Chandler support this diagnosis? If so, identify the data.
2. Use the NANDA-I taxonomy in Appendix A to develop a diagnosis for Mr. Chandler. ⚭ Identify the data required for the PES (problem, etiology, signs or symptoms) statement.

►Prepare Teaching Plan

LEARNING NEED: Mr. Chandler experienced a hearing problem and sought treatment because he was unsure of the cause. The data revealed his concern that the hearing loss and ear discomfort he experienced were from "a cold, like my daughter's" or "pressure changes during air travel." After examination, it was determined that the cause of Mr. Chandler's problem was impacted cerumen.

The case study provides data that are representative of symptoms and behaviours of a variety of hearing and ear problems. Individuals and groups could benefit from education about the ear, hearing loss, and care of the ear. The following teaching plan is intended for a group of learners and focuses on ear care.

GOAL: The participants will practise safe care of the ear.

OBJECTIVES: On completion of this educational session, the participants will be able to do the following:

1. Identify the structures of the ear.
2. Discuss common problems with the ear.
3. Describe measures for care of the ear.

ASSESSMENT FORM

EXTERNAL EAR:

Size	L = R	__x__ yes	_____ no			
Shape	L = R	__x__ yes	_____ no			
Lesions	L	_____ yes	__x__ no			
	R	_____ yes	__x__ no			
Tragus	L	Mobile __x__ yes	_____ no	Tender	__x__ no	_____ yes
	R	Mobile __x__ yes	_____ no	Tender	__x__ no	_____ yes
Meatus	L	Patent __x__ yes	_____ no	Discharge	__x__ no	_____ yes
	R	Patent __x__ yes	_____ no	Discharge	__x__ no	_____ yes

INTERNAL EAR:

Canal	L	Clear _____ yes	__x__ no	Impacted cerumen	
	R	Clear __x__ yes	_____ no		
Cerumen	L	Present _____ small	_____ medium	__x__ large	
	R	Present __x__ small	_____ medium	_____ large	
	L	Soft _____ yes	__x__ no	Colour Brown-grey	
	R	Soft __x__ yes	_____ no	Colour Orange	
Tympanic	L	Grey _____ yes	_____ no	(unknown)	
	R	Grey __x__ yes	_____ no		
	L	Lesions _____ no	_____ yes	(unknown)	
	R	Lesions __x__ no	_____ yes		
Weber	L = R	_____ yes	__x__ no	Lateralizes left	

Application of Objective 3: Describe measures for care of the ear.

Content	Teaching Strategy and Rationale	Evaluation

• *An old adage:* Never put anything smaller than your elbow in your ear.
 • Ear canals should never have to be cleaned. The cerumen moves to the outside naturally.
 • Sometimes, the cerumen is excreted in large amounts or it is not effectively cleared.
 • Do's and Do not's
   • Do consult your physician when you have ear symptoms.
   • Do follow the instructions for use of commercial earwax removal products.
   • Don't use cotton swabs, hair-pins, or paper clips to attempt to remove cerumen. You may perforate the eardrum or merely push the cerumen farther into the canal.
	• Lecture
	 • Discussion
	 • Audiovisual materials
	 • Printed materials
	
	 Lecture is appropriate when disseminating information to large groups.
	
	 Discussion allows participants to bring up concerns and to raise questions.
	
	 Audiovisual materials, such as illustrations of the structures of the ear, reinforce verbal presentation.
	
	 Printed material, especially to be taken away with learners, allows review, reinforcement, and reading at the learner's own pace.
		• Written examination. May use short answer, fill-in, or multiple-choice items or a combination of items.
		 • If these are short and easy to evaluate, the learner receives immediate feedback.

Circle **T** for true and **F** for false, fill in the blank, or select the correct answer(s) for the following statements:

1. The outer ear funnels sound.　　　　　　　　　　　T　　　F

2. Cerumen is made in the ear canal.　　　　　　　　　T　　　F

3. The eardrum separates the outer and inner ear.　　　T　　　F

4. The eustachian tube helps equalize pressure in the ear.　T　　　F

5. Structures of the ear regulate balance.　　　　　　　T　　　F

6. The purposes of cerumen are to _____ and _____ .

7. Hearing loss can occur in which of the following problems:
   a. infection
   b. neurological problems
   c. perforated eardrum
   d. cerumen buildup

8. The symptoms of cerumen blockage are _____
   _____ .

9. You should not use cotton swabs in the ear canal because _____
   _____ .

10. Always follow the directions when using _____ .

Health Promotion Assessment Tool

Social Determinants of Health	Level of Action	Action Strategies
Personal coping skills	Individual	**Develop personal skills** • Discuss the importance of yearly ear exams. • Discuss ear care and methods to avoid buildup and impaction of cerumen in ears. • Teach Mr. Chandler the signs and symptoms of ear infections.
Health services	Individual	Create supportive environments • Provide an audiometric examination.

ABNORMAL FINDINGS

Abnormal findings in the ears, nose, mouth, and throat include lesions, deformities, infectious processes, and dental problems. Figures 14.29 through 14.52 depict common abnormal findings in these structures.

Ear

Hemotympanum

Hemotympanum is a bluish tinge to the tympanic membrane, indicating the presence of blood in the middle ear (see Figure 14.29). It is usually caused by head trauma.

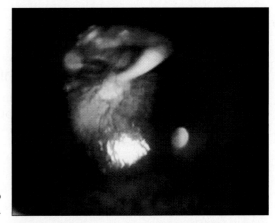

Figure 14.29 ●
Hemotympanum.

Otitis Externa

Otitis externa is infection of the outer ear, often called "swimmer's ear." Otitis externa causes redness and swelling of the auricle and ear canal (see Figure 14.30). Drainage is usually scanty. It may be accompanied by itching, fever, and enlarged lymph nodes.

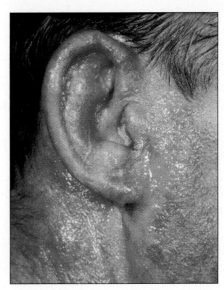

Figure 14.30 ●
Otitis externa.

Otitis Media

Otitis media is infection of the middle ear producing a red, bulging eardrum, fever, and hearing loss (see Figure 14.31). The otoscopic examination reveals absent light reflex. Otitis media is more common in children, whose auditory tubes are wider, shorter, and more horizontal than those of adults, thus allowing easier access for infections ascending from the pharynx.

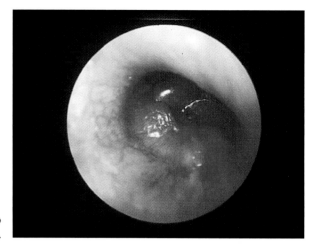

Figure 14.31 ●
Otitis media.

Perforation of the Tympanic Membrane

Perforation of the tympanic membrane is a rupturing of the eardrum caused by trauma or infection. During otoscopic inspection, the perforation may be seen as a dark spot on the eardrum (see Figure 14.32).

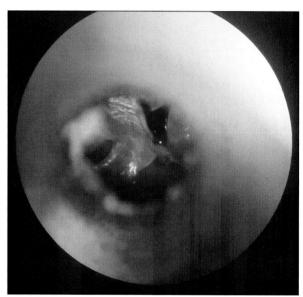

Figure 14.32
Perforation of tympanic membrane.

Scarred Tympanic Membrane

A scarred tympanic membrane is a condition in which the eardrum has white patches of scar tissue caused by repeated ear infections (see Figure 14.33).

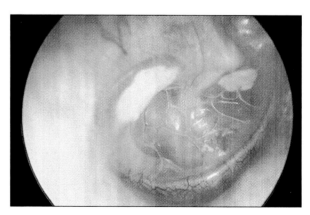

Figure 14.33 ●
Scarred tympanic membrane.

Tophi

Tophi are small white nodules on the helix or antihelix (see Figure 14.34). These nodules contain uric acid crystals and are a symptom of gout.

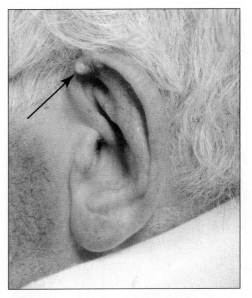

Figure 14.34 ●
Tophi.

Tympanostomy Tubes

Tympanostomy tubes are ear tubes inserted to relieve middle ear pressure and allow drainage from repeated middle ear infections (see Figure 14.35).

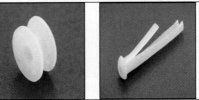

Figure 14.35
Tympanostomy tubes.

Nose and Sinuses

Epistaxis

Epistaxis is a nosebleed. This may follow trauma, such as a blow to the nose, or it may accompany another alteration in health, such as rhinitis, hypertension, or a blood coagulation disorder (see Figure 14.36).

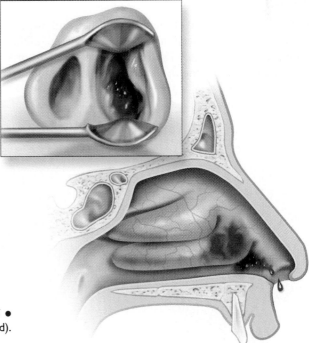

Figure 14.36 ●
Epistaxis (nosebleed).

Rhinitis

Rhinitis is a nasal inflammation usually caused by a viral infection or allergy. It is accompanied by a watery and often copious discharge, sneezing, and congestion (stuffy nose). Acute rhinitis (see Figure 14.37) is caused by a virus, whereas allergic rhinitis (see Figure 14.38) results from contact with allergens, such as pollen and dust.

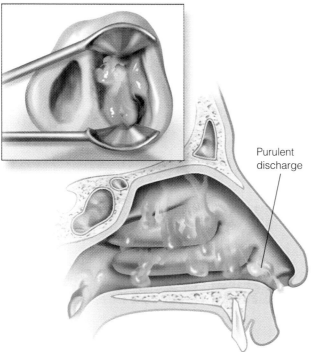

Figure 14.37 • Acute rhinitis.

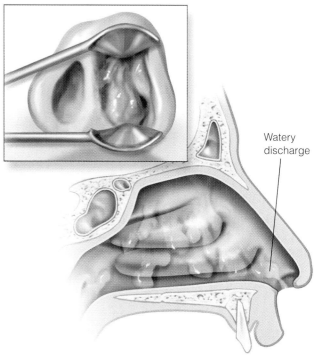

Watery discharge

Figure 14.38 • Allergic rhinitis.

Sinusitis

Sinusitis is inflammation of the sinuses, usually following an upper respiratory infection. It causes facial pain, inflammation, and discharge (see Figure 14.39). Fever, chills, or a dull, pulsating pain in the cheeks or teeth may accompany sinusitis.

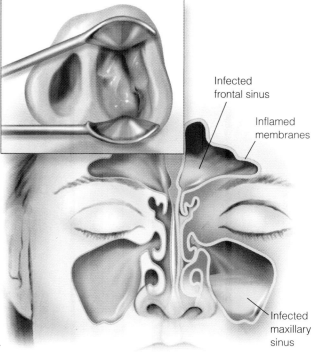

Infected frontal sinus

Inflamed membranes

Infected maxillary sinus

Figure 14.39 • Sinusitis.

Deviated Septum

A deviated septum is a slight ingrowth of the lower nasal septum (see Figure 14.40). When viewed with a nasal speculum, one nasal cavity appears to have an outgrowth or shelf.

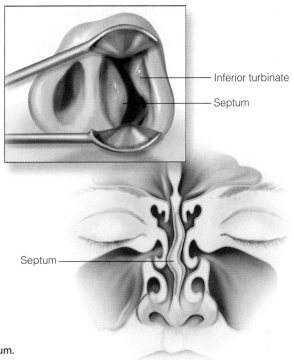

Inferior turbinate

Septum

Septum

Figure 14.40 ● Deviated septum.

Nasal Polyps

Nasal polyps are pale, round, firm, nonpainful overgrowth of nasal mucosa usually caused by chronic allergic rhinitis (see Figure 14.41).

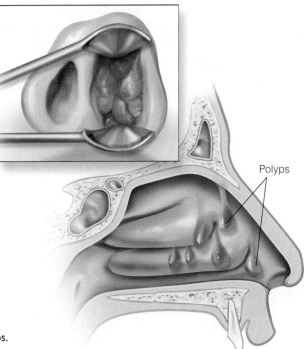

Polyps

Figure 14.41 ● Nasal polyps.

Perforated Septum

A perforated septum is a hole in the septum caused by chronic infection, trauma, or sniffing cocaine (see Figure 14.42). It can be detected by shining a penlight through the naris on the other side.

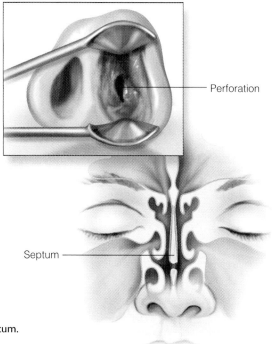

Figure 14.42 ● Perforated septum.

Mouth and Throat

Ankyloglossia

Ankyloglossia is a fixation of the tip of the tongue to the floor of the mouth because of a shortened lingual frenulum (see Figure 14.43). The condition is usually congenital and may be corrected surgically.

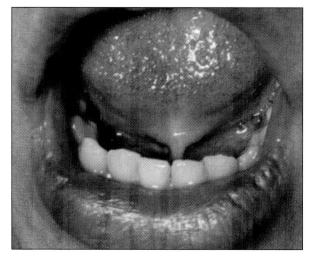

Figure 14.43 ● Ankyloglossia.

Aphthous Ulcers

Aphthous ulcers, commonly called *canker sores*, are small, round, white lesions occurring singularly or in clusters on the oral mucosa (see Figure 14.44). The lesions are acutely painful when they come in contact with the tongue, a toothbrush, or food. They commonly result from oral trauma, such as jabbing the side of the mouth with a toothbrush, but they are also associated with stress, exhaustion, and allergies to certain foods.

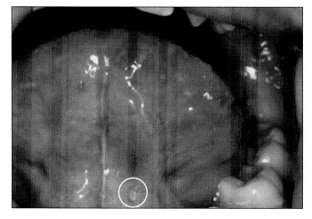

Figure 14.44 ● Aphthous ulcers.

Black Hairy Tongue

Black hairy tongue is a temporary condition caused by the inhibition of normal bacteria and the overgrowth of fungus on the papillae of the tongue (see Figure 14.45). It is usually associated with the use of antibiotics.

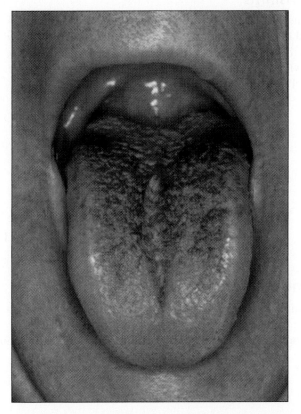

Figure 14.45 ●
Black hairy tongue.

Gingival Hyperplasia

Gingival hyperplasia is an enlargement of the gums (see Figure 14.46) frequently seen in pregnancy, in leukemia, or after prolonged use of phenytoin (Dilantin).

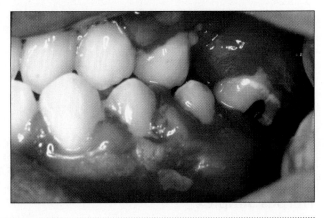

Figure 14.46 ●
Gingival hyperplasia.

Gingivitis

Gingivitis is inflammation of the gums (see Figure 14.47). It may be caused by poor dental hygiene or a deficiency of vitamin C. If left untreated, gingivitis may progress to periodontal disease and tooth loss.

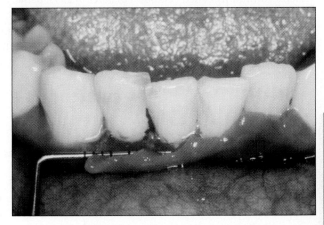

Figure 14.47 ●
Gingivitis.

Tonsillitis

Tonsillitis is inflammation of the tonsils. The throat is red and the tonsils are swollen and covered by white or yellow patches or exudate (see Figure 14.48). Lymph nodes in the cervical chain may be enlarged. Tonsillitis may be accompanied by a high fever.

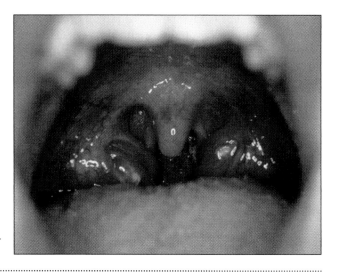

Figure 14.48 ● Tonsillitis.

Smooth Tongue

Smooth tongue is a condition occurring as a result of vitamin B and iron deficiency. The surface of the tongue is smooth and red, with a shiny appearance (see Figure 14.49).

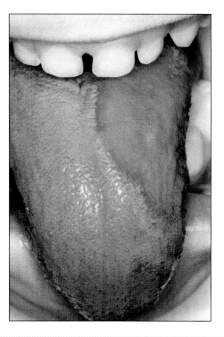

Figure 14.49 ●
Smooth, glossy tongue
(atrophic glossitis).

Herpes Simplex

Herpes simplex is a virus that is often accompanied by clear vesicles commonly called *cold sores* or *fever blisters,* usually at the junction of the skin and the lip (see Figure 14.50). The vesicles erupt, and then crust and heal within 2 weeks. They usually recur, especially after heavy exposure to bright sunlight (e.g., after a day at the beach).

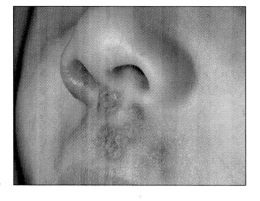

Figure 14.50 ● Herpes simplex.

Carcinoma

Oral cancers are most commonly found on the lower lip or the base (underside) of the tongue (see Figure 14.51). Cancer is suspected if a sore or lesion does not heal within a few weeks. Heavy smoking, especially pipe smoking, and chewing tobacco increase the risk of oral cancer, as does chronic heavy use of alcohol.

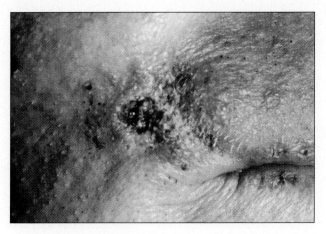

Figure 14.51 ● Carcinoma.

Leukoplakia

Leukoplakia is a whitish thickening of the mucous membrane in the mouth or tongue (see Figure 14.52). It cannot be scraped off. Most often associated with heavy smoking or drinking, it can be a precancerous condition.

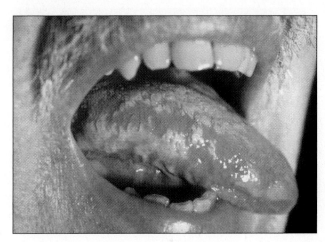

Figure 14.52 ● Leukoplakia.

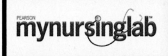

Visit the MyNursingLab website at http://www.pearsoned.ca/mynursinglab. This online homework and tutorial system puts you in control of your own learning with study and practice tools directly correlated to this chapter's content.

15

RESPIRATORY SYSTEM

THE PRIMARY RESPONSIBILITY OF THE RESPIRATORY SYSTEM is the exchange of gases in the body. Exchange of oxygen and carbon dioxide is essential to the homeostatic and hemodynamic process of the body. The intake of oxygen needed for metabolism and the release of carbon dioxide, which is the waste product of metabolism, occur with each respiratory cycle. This delicate balance of gas exchange is influenced by the nervous system, the cardiovascular system, and the musculoskeletal system. The central nervous system, influenced by the amount of gases in the blood, regulates the rate and depth of each respiratory cycle. The cardiovascular system is responsible for transporting the gases throughout the body. The musculoskeletal system provides the bones to protect the structures of the respiratory system, and the muscular activity allows for the rhythmic movement of the thoracic cavity. This coordinated movement with pressure changes in the thoracic cavity leads to the exchange of the oxygen and carbon dioxide.

Other responsibilities of the respiratory system are to maintain acid-base balance and assist with the production of vocal sounds. The amount of carbon dioxide in the blood directly influences the amount of carbonic acid and hydrogen ion concentration in the blood. The respiratory system responds to the needs of the body to either retain or excrete carbon dioxide. The production of vocal sounds occurs as air moves out of the lungs and passes over the vocal cords; the individual produces sounds commonly called speech.

Assessment of respiratory function is an integral aspect of the total client assessment performed by the nurse. Developmental and environmental factors are considered during assessment of the respiratory system. The nurse must be cognizant of factors that influence respiratory health as questions for the health history are formulated and physical assessment is performed.

ANATOMY AND PHYSIOLOGY REVIEW

The thorax, commonly called the chest, is a closed cavity of the body, containing structures needed for respirations. The thorax, or thoracic cavity, is surrounded by ribs and muscles and extends from the base of the neck to the diaphragm. It has three sections: the mediastinum and the right and left pleural cavities. The **mediastinum** contains the heart, trachea, esophagus, and major blood vessels of the body. Each pleural cavity contains a lung (see Figure 15.1).

The major structures of the respiratory system are situated in the thoracic cavity. The major function of the respiratory system is to supply the body with oxygen and expel carbon dioxide. Air moves in and out of the lungs with each **respiratory cycle**. A complete respiratory cycle consists of an inspiratory phase and an expiratory phase of breathing. The exchange of oxygen and carbon dioxide at the alveoli level of the lung is *external respiration*. Gases are transported from the lungs via the blood to the cells of the body. As the gases move across the systemic capillaries, exchange of oxygen and carbon dioxide occurs at the cellular level and *internal respiration* occurs.

The respiratory system consists of the upper and lower respiratory tracts. The structures of the upper respiratory tract consist of the nose, the mouth, the sinuses, the pharynx, the larynx, and a portion of the trachea. The lower respiratory tract includes the distal portion of the trachea, bronchi, and lungs. Pleural membranes, the muscles of respiration, and the mediastinum complete the lower respiratory tract.

The anatomy and physiology review and assessment of the structures of the upper respiratory tract were discussed in Chapter 12. ⬭ Before proceeding, it may be helpful to review this information.

Lower Respiratory Tract

The lower respiratory tract includes the trachea, bronchi, and lungs. Additional structures of the pleural membranes, the mediastinum, and the muscles of respiration are also discussed at this time. Consideration must be given to all structures during the assessment process.

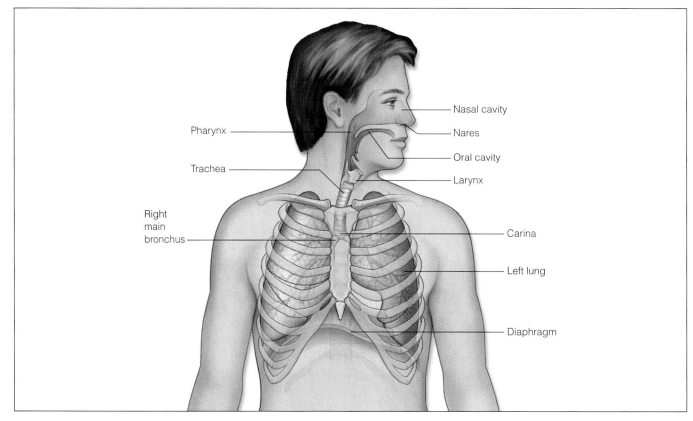

Figure 15.1 ● Anatomy of the respiratory system.

Trachea

The trachea, located in the mediastinum, descends from the larynx in the neck to the main bronchi at the distal point. It is approximately 10 to 12 cm (4 in.) long and 2.5 cm (1 in.) in diameter. The trachea is a very flexible and mobile structure, bifurcating anteriorly at about the sternal angle and posteriorly at about the vertebrae T_3 to T_5. The trachea contains 16 to 20 rings of hyaline cartilage. These C-shaped rings help maintain the shape of the trachea and prevent its collapse during inspiration and expiration. Just above the point of bifurcation, the last tracheal cartilage, known as the carina, is expanded. The carina separates the openings of the two main bronchi. The trachea, like other structures of the respiratory tract, is lined with a mucus-producing membrane that traps dust, bacteria, and other foreign bodies. This membrane at the level of the carina is most sensitive to foreign substances. Coughing and cilia, hairlike projections of the membrane, help sweep debris toward the mouth for removal.

Bronchi

Anteriorly, the trachea bifurcates at about the level of the sternal angle, forming the right and left main bronchi (see Figure 15.2). The right main bronchus is shorter, wider, and more vertical than the left bronchus; therefore, aspirated objects are more likely to enter the right lung. The bronchi continue to divide within each lobe of the lung. The terminal bronchioles are less than 0.5 mm (0.2 in.) in diameter. The bronchi and the many branches continue to warm and moisten air as it moves along the respiratory tract to the alveoli in the lungs.

Lungs

The lungs are cone-shaped, elastic, spongy, air-filled structures that are situated in the pleural cavities of the thorax on either side of the mediastinum (see Figure 15.3). The apex of each lung is 2 to 4 cm (1 to 1.5 in.) above the inner third of the clavicle, and the base of each lung is at the level of the diaphragm. The left lung has two lobes (upper and lower) and tends to be longer and narrower than the right lung. The left lung accommodates the heart at the medial surface. The oblique fissure separates the two lobes of this lung. The right lung has three lobes (upper, middle, and lower) and is slightly larger, wider, and shorter than the left lung. The horizontal and oblique fissures separate the lobes of the right lung. Within each lung, the numerous terminal bronchioles branch into the alveolar ducts, which lead into alveolar sacs and alveoli. The single-layered cells of the alveoli permit simple diffusion and gas exchanges to occur (see Figure 15.4 on page 318).

Pleural Membranes

The pleura is a thin, double-layered, serous membrane that lines each pleural cavity. The parietal membrane lines the superior aspect of the diaphragm and the thoracic wall. The visceral membrane covers the outer surface of the lung. A pleural fluid produced by these membranes acts as a lubricant, allowing the lung to glide during the respiratory cycle of inspiration and expiration. The surface tension created by the fluid and the negative pressure between the membranes helps keep the lungs expanded. As the negative pressure changes, a person is able to move air into and out of the lungs.

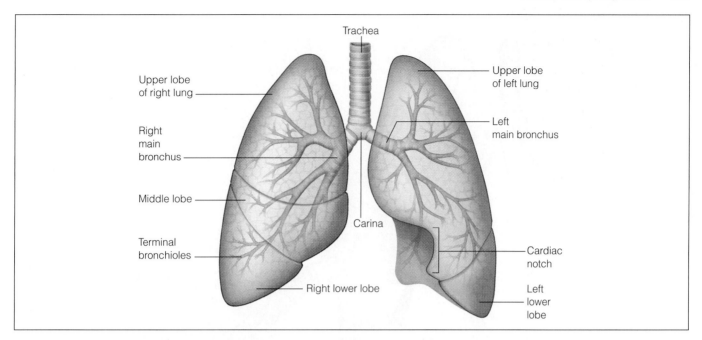

Figure 15.2 • Respiratory passages.

Mediastinum

The mediastinum is the middle section of the thoracic cavity and is surrounded by the right and left pleural cavities. The mediastinum contains the heart, the trachea, the esophagus, the proximal portion of the right and left main bronchi, and the great vessels of the body.

Respiratory Process

Respiratory process is a general term that encompasses the structures and activities of respiration. The respiratory process is dependent on the muscles of the thorax, the structures of the thoracic cage, and the ability of air to move in and out of the body.

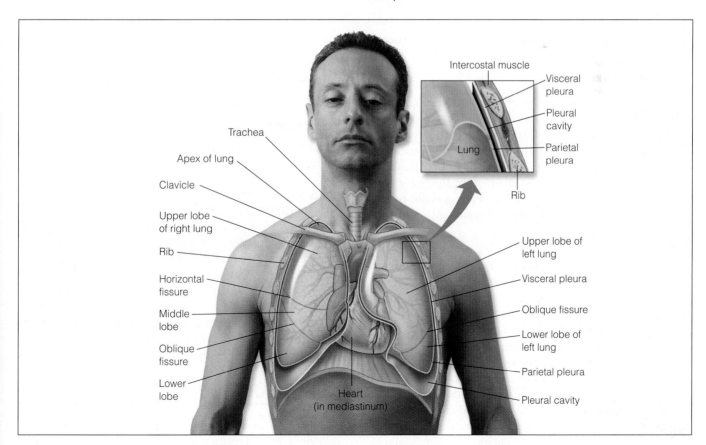

Figure 15.3 • Anterior view of thorax and lungs.

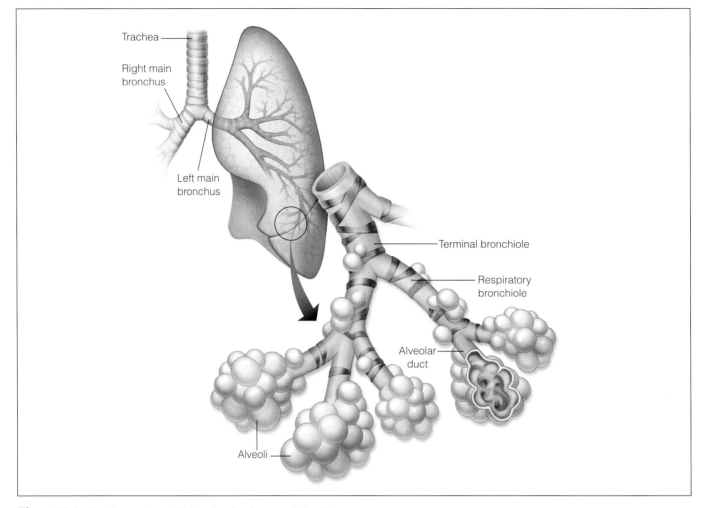

Figure 15.4 ● Respiratory bronchioles, alveolar ducts, and alveoli.

Muscles of Respiration

The muscles of the thoracic cage (internal and external inter-costal) and the diaphragm assist in the breathing process. The synergistic action of these muscle groups aids in the respiratory cycle of inspiration and expiration. The accessory muscles of the neck (trapezius, scalene, and sternocleidomastoid), abdo-men (rectus), and chest (pectorals) will assist the respiratory cycle as necessary. The accessory muscles play a major role in the respiratory cycle during distress and pathology.

Thoracic Cage

The thoracic cage consists of bones, cartilage, and muscles of the thorax. The sternum (breastbone) is located in the anterior midline of the thorax. The vertebrae are located at the dorsal or posterior aspect of the thorax. The 12 pairs of ribs circle the body, form the lateral aspects of the thorax, and are attached to the vertebrae and sternum. Anteriorly, the first seven pairs of true ribs articulate directly to the sternum. The cartilage of ribs 8, 9, and 10 articulates with the cartilage of rib 7, whereas the pairs of 11 and 12 are free floating and do not articulate anteriorly. The costal cartilage and external intercostal muscles help to complete the thoracic cage. This bony cage helps protect the many vital organs of the pleura and mediastinum, supports the shoulders and upper extremities, and helps support many muscles of the upper part of the body.

Respiratory Cycle

Respiratory cycle, respirations, and *breathing* are terms used interchangeably to indicate the movement of air in and out of the body. Breathing consists of two phases: inspiration and expiration, thus, the term *respiratory cycle.* Inspiration is con-sidered to be the active aspect of the respiratory cycle. For air to enter the body, respiratory muscles contract, the chest expands, alveolar pressure decreases, and the negative intrapleural pres-sure increases. These combined activities allow air to enter the expanded lungs. During expiration, the passive phase of the process, the activities reverse themselves, the lungs recoil, and air leaves the body. The regular, even-depth, rhythmic pattern of inspiration and expiration describes **eupnea**: normal breath-ing. A change in this pattern, producing shortness of breath or difficulty in breathing, is **dyspnea**.

LANDMARKS

Identification and location of **landmarks** helps the nurse develop a mental picture of the structures being assessed.

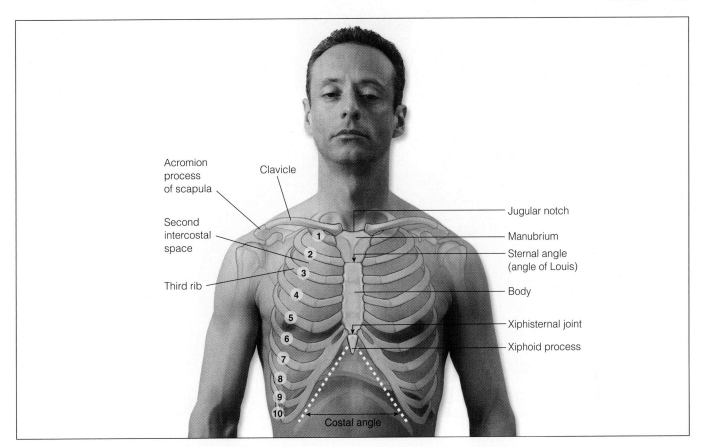

Figure 15.5 ● Landmarks of the anterior thorax, anterior view.

Thoracic reference points and specific anatomical structures are used as landmarks (see Figure 15.5). They help provide an exact location for the assessment findings and an accurate orientation for documentation of findings. Landmark identification for the thorax includes bony structures, horizontal and vertical lines, and the division of the thorax.

The thorax may be divided into two or three sections for assessment. Two sections include the anterior and posterior thorax, while three sections include the anterior, lateral, and posterior aspects. This text uses the former option: The lateral areas are incorporated into the anterior and posterior sections. The bony structures include the sternum, clavicles, ribs, and vertebrae. At the horizontal plane, the landmarks are the clavicles, the ribs, and the corresponding intercostal spaces. Anteriorly, the vertical lines start at the sternum and are strategically drawn parallel to this structure. Posteriorly, the vertical lines start at the vertebral column and additional lines are drawn parallel to this reference point.

The first bony landmark to be considered is the sternum, commonly called the breastbone. It is a flat, elongated bone located in the midline of the anterior thoracic cage and consists of three parts: the manubrium, body, and xiphoid process. The clavicles and some of the pairs of ribs articulate with the sternum. The **manubrium** is the superior portion of the sternum. The depression at the superior border is called the suprasternal notch or jugular notch. This becomes a primary landmark used to identify and locate other landmarks. The manubrium joins the body of the sternum. As these structures meet, a

horizontal ridge is formed, referred to as the sternal angle or **angle of Louis**. The second rib and the second intercostal space are at this level of the sternum. The sternum terminates at the xiphoid process. This process and the inferior borders of the seventh ribs form a triangle referred to as the costal angle. The inferior border of the ribs and the costal angle help identify the level of the diaphragm, the base of the lungs, and the separation of the thoracic cavity from the abdomen (Figure 15.5).

The clavicles are long, slender, curved bones that articulate with the manubrium at the medial aspect. The lateral aspects help form the shoulder joint with the acromion of the scapula. The clavicles act as a shock absorber, protecting the upper portion of the thoracic cage and the delicate underlying structures. Lung tissue will be assessed above and below the clavicles. Findings above the clavicle are considered supraclavicular, while findings below the clavicle are infraclavicular.

The 12 pairs of ribs are another bony landmark used in respiratory assessment. The ribs circle the body and help form horizontal reference points. Posteriorly, each rib attaches to a thoracic vertebra. The ribs curve downward and forward as they become anterior. Bilaterally, the first seven ribs attach to the sternum and are called true ribs. Ribs 8, 9, and 10 attach to cartilage of the superior rib, while ribs 11 and 12 are free floating anteriorly. A number identifies each rib. Each intercostal space, the space between the ribs, takes the number of the superior rib. The first rib and the first intercostal space, being obscured by the clavicle, are not palpable. Anteriorly, ribs 2 to 7 and the corresponding

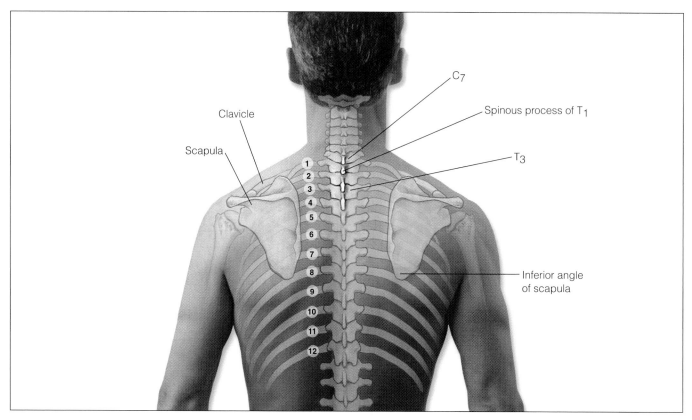

Figure 15.6 ●; Landmarks: Posterior thorax.

intercostal spaces are easily palpated along the sternal border. Posteriorly, the ribs are best palpated and counted close to the vertebral column. Each rib and intercostal space form a horizontal line used as a landmark.

The vertebral column is located at the midline of the posterior portion of the thoracic cage. Twelve vertebrae are thoracic, and a pair of ribs articulates with each. The vertebral column contributes to the vertical lines to be discussed later in this chapter. The seventh cervical vertebra (C_7) is most visible at the base of the neck. The much larger spinous process contributes to the uniqueness of the vertebrae. This prominent vertebra (C_7) is used to count and locate other spinous processes. When two spinous processes are equally prominent, they are C_7 and T_1 (see Figure 15.6).

Five imaginary vertical lines are identified on the anterior aspect of the thoracic cage (see Figure 15.7). These lines are the sternal line, the right and left midclavicular lines, and the right and left anterior axillary lines. The sternal or midsternal line (SL) starts at the sternal notch and descends through the xiphoid process. It divides the sternum in half and ultimately identifies the right and left thoracic cage. The right and left midclavicular lines are parallel to the sternal line. The midclavicular line begins at the midpoint of the clavicle and descends to the level of the twelfth rib. The nipples of the breast are slightly lateral to this line. This line subdivides the right and left thoracic cage into two equal parts. The anterior axillary line (AAL) is another line drawn parallel to the sternal line. It begins at the anterior fold of the axillae and descends along the anterior lateral aspect of the thoracic cage to the twelfth rib.

Five imaginary lines are located on the posterior aspect of the thoracic cage (see Figure 15.8). The vertebral line, the right and left scapular lines, and the right and left posterior axillary lines are used as landmarks on the posterior aspect of the thoracic cage. The vertebral or midspinous line commences at C_7 and descends through the spinous process of each thoracic vertebra. It divides the vertebral column in half, forming the posterior right and left thoracic cage.

The scapular line, parallel to the vertebral line, is drawn from the inferior angle of the scapula to the level of the twelfth rib. This line subdivides the right and left thoracic cage into two equal parts. The posterior axillary line (PAL) is parallel to the vertebral line. It starts at the posterior axillary fold and descends along the lateral aspect of the thoracic cage to the twelfth rib.

The lateral aspect of the thoracic cage is the third section to be considered. Three imaginary lines are identified in this section (see Figure 15.9 on page 322). They are the anterior, posterior, and midaxillary lines. Two of these lines, the anterior and posterior lines, have been described. The midaxillary line is parallel and equidistant to the anterior and posterior axillary lines. This line descends from the middle of the axillae to the level of the twelfth rib. It forms the frontal plane dividing the thorax into the anterior and posterior portions.

The described landmarks serve as a reference point for internal structures of the respiratory system. Recall that the trachea bifurcates, forming the right and left main bronchus. Anteriorly, this occurs at the level of the angle of Louis or sternal angle. Posteriorly, this bifurcation occurs between the third and fifth thoracic vertebrae.

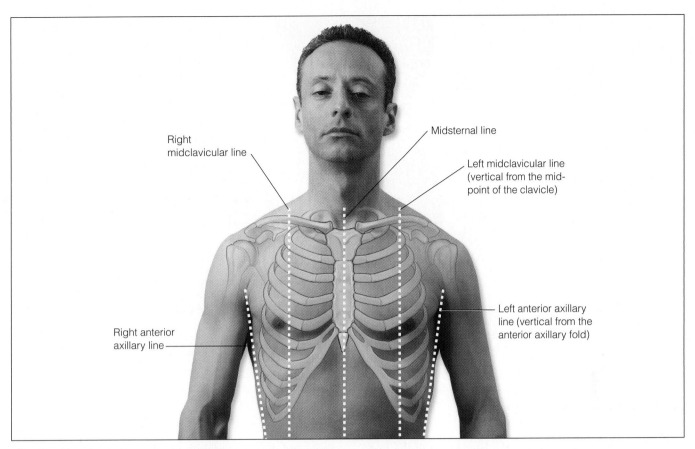

Right midclavicular line

Midsternal line

Left midclavicular line (vertical from the mid-point of the clavicle)

Right anterior axillary line

Left anterior axillary line (vertical from the anterior axillary fold)

Figure 15.7 ● Lines of the anterior thorax.

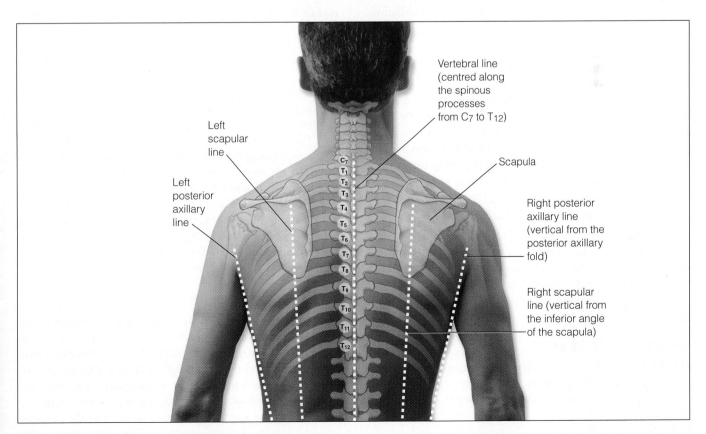

Vertebral line (centred along the spinous processes from C7 to T12)

Left scapular line

Scapula

Left posterior axillary line

Right posterior axillary line (vertical from the posterior axillary fold)

Right scapular line (vertical from the inferior angle of the scapula)

Figure 15.8 ● Lines of the posterior thorax.

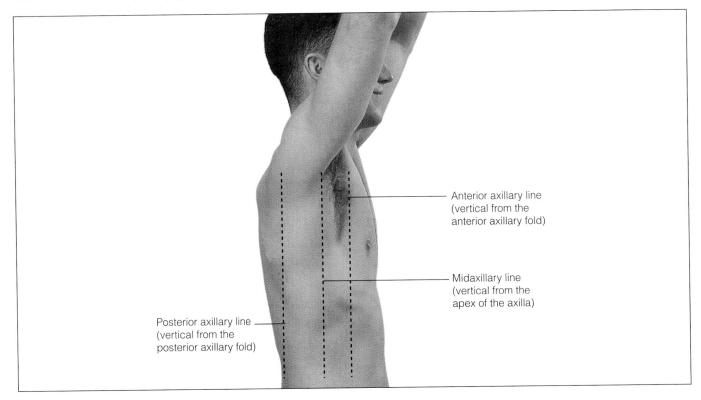

Figure 15.9 ● Lines of the lateral thorax.

The clavicle, the scapula, and the lateral base of the neck form a triangle at the superior aspect of the thorax. This triangle, also known as Krönig's area, will be used for palpation of muscles and lymph nodes and for percussion and auscultation of the apex and the lungs.

SPECIAL CONSIDERATIONS

Throughout the assessment process, the nurse gathers subjective and objective data about the client's state of health. By using critical thinking and the nursing process, the nurse identifies many factors to be considered when collecting the data, including age, developmental level, work history, living conditions, socioeconomic status, and emotional wellness.

Developmental Considerations

Growth and development are dynamic processes that describe change over time. The collection of data and interpretation of findings in relation to normative values is important. These data will reflect the growth and developmental stages of the individual. The following discussion presents specific variations for different age groups.

Infants and Children

During fetal development, respirations are passive and gas exchange occurs at the placenta. At birth, rapid changes occur in the respiratory system as fetal circulation closes. One significant change that occurs is a marked increase in pulmonary blood flow. Other changes include the closure of the foramen ovale and ductus arteriosus and the increase in chest expansion. Gaseous exchanges now take place via the respiratory system and atmosphere. During the first several hours of extrauterine life, the respiratory rate of the newborn is rapid (40 to 80 per minute) and irregular. During the neonatal and infant period, the respiratory rate decreases and becomes more regular. By 5 years of age, the respiratory rate is about 35 breaths per minute.

At birth, the circumference of the chest is slightly less than the circumference of the head. During childhood, chest circumference exceeds head size by about 5 to 7 cm (2 to 3 in.). The chest is usually round, with the lateral and anterior-posterior diameters being almost equal. Bony structures of the chest are more prominent during infancy since skin and musculature are thin. Neonates have a respiratory rate and depth likely to be irregular. At this age, breathing involves use of abdominal muscles; therefore, inspection of the abdomen will yield a more accurate respiratory rate. Abdominal breathing continues during childhood until about 5 to 7 years of age. Costal breathing is the expected pattern after 7 years of age.

The Pregnant Female

The hormonal changes of pregnancy and the growing fetus produce changes in the respiratory system of the pregnant female. The ligaments of the thorax relax, the horizontal diameter expands, and the costal angle increases. At rest, the diaphragm rises into the chest to accommodate the fetus and respirations are diaphragmatic. Shortness of breath (dyspnea), especially in the last trimester, are common as the maternal and fetal demand for oxygen increases. Throughout pregnancy, the total oxygen consumption can increase by 20% and the maternal respiratory rate increases approximately two breaths per minute. Maternal hyperventilation occurs because of the increase in minute ventilation that exceeds the increase in oxygen consumption.

The Older Adult

As individuals age, body functions change. Many activities of the respiratory system demonstrate a decrease in efficiency. The lungs lose their elasticity, the skeletal muscles begin to weaken, and bones lose their density. As a result, it becomes more difficult for the older adult to expand the thoracic cage and take a deep breath. The diameters of the thoracic cage change. The appearance of a barrel chest and calcification of cartilage may contribute to the decrease in thoracic excursion. Thus, the older adult inhales and exhales smaller amounts of air. There is less oxygen for body use, and more carbon dioxide is retained. This is related to the loss of elasticity of the alveoli. The older adult also experiences an increase in residual volume and hypoventilation. Weakening of the chest muscles hinders the older adult's ability to cough. Dry mucous membranes decrease cilia in the system, and the inability to cough compromises airway clearance.

Rate of respirations in the older adult is slightly higher than in the middle-aged adult. The older adult has a shallower respiratory cycle because of the decreased vital capacity. Auscultatory sounds may be less audible because of the decreased pulmonary function. The trapping of air in the alveoli will produce a sound of hyperresonance on percussion.

The older adult may tire more easily and may need frequent rest periods during the assessment process. Deep mouth breathing during auscultation may increase the fatigue of the older adult. As with any client, the nurse must prevent hyperventilation at this time.

Psychosocial Considerations

Stress, anxiety, pain, and fatigue may exacerbate respiratory problems. Clients experiencing acute or chronic respiratory problems will have a physiological alteration with gas exchange. These changes can limit or restrict the individual's ability to independently perform the activities of daily living and to participate in activities, exercise, and sports. This limitation may contribute to social isolation, changes role activities, lowers self-esteem, and increases the dependency factor with support systems.

Certain drugs, such as bronchodilators, are used in the treatment of respiratory conditions and may cause the hands to tremble visibly. The nurse should not confuse this sign with nervousness. Even mild respiratory distress is frightening for the client and family. Proceeding in a calm and reassuring manner helps reduce the client's fear. Parents of young children who have experienced severe asthmatic attacks in the past may be extremely anxious any time the child develops a cold, seasonal allergy, or any other respiratory problem. A calm and careful assessment of the current health status helps to decrease the anxiety level of all involved individuals.

Social and Ethnocultural Considerations

Race, ethnicity, and socioeconomic status are significant factors in respiratory health. The incidence of respiratory diseases, such as tuberculosis, asthma, chronic obstructive pulmonary disease, and obstructive sleep apnea, is greater in poor rural populations and in recent immigrant groups. Thorough assessment of the respiratory system is best accomplished when the client is disrobed and the surfaces of the anterior and posterior chest can be visualized, touched, and auscultated. Some cultural or religious practices, including the wearing or prohibition of removal of symbolic icons, jewellery, undergarments, or clothing, may interfere with physical examination. Additionally, the requirement of a same-sex examiner or the presence of a companion during the assessment is an issue that the nurse must address. Careful questioning of the client, with the assistance of a translator when necessary, during the interview will allow for clarification, negotiation, and decision making about the assessment process.

Clients with allergies or asthma should be encouraged to explore the possibility of allergens in their work or home environment. For example, pets, dust, and moulds are common allergens found in the home. Second-hand smoke in the home or work environment can also lead to respiratory distress. Research has established a link between exposure to second-hand smoke and the development of lung cancer.

In some industries, workers may be exposed to substances that are hazardous to their respiratory health, such as caustic fumes, fungi, asbestos, coal tar, nickel, silver, textile fibres, chromate, and vinyl chlorides. All these substances are known carcinogens. Exposure to large amounts of dust in a granary or mine may lead to the development of silicosis. Coal miners are susceptible to pneumoconiosis, a form of black lung disease. People working in an office building may need to be concerned with air conditioners and forced air heat. The ducts of the cooling and heating systems can carry airborne organisms, increasing the risk for respiratory infections.

The geographic location of an individual's environment also influences respiratory health. Factors to be considered are temperature, moisture, altitude, and pollution. A cold environment encourages vasoconstriction and ultimately a decreased need for oxygen. An environment with increased moisture or humidity has heavy air. Individuals will tire easily, increasing the need for oxygen. As the altitude increases, the partial pressure of oxygen decreases. The individual must adapt by increasing the rate and depth of the respiratory cycle. Air pollution with smog, industrial wastes, or exhaust fumes contributes to respiratory problems in all people.

Factors within the home and social environment will influence respiratory health. Forced air heating or wood heating are very drying to the membranes of the body. Individuals are encouraged to add moisture or use a humidifier to keep the air moist and support respiratory health. In the hot, humid, hazy days of summer, an air conditioner or dehumidifier may be necessary to reduce the moisture in the air. Second-hand smoke, foods, dust, pets, and stress will also contribute to respiratory changes.

Social and Ethnocultural Considerations

- In the past 50 years more women have started smoking, which has resulted in an increased prevalence of such diseases as lung cancer and chronic obstructive pulmonary disease (COPD) among females. COPD is now being reported more in women than in men under age 75.
- Lung cancer has become a major health issue for women. Both the incidence and the mortality rates among older women are increasing, in contrast to the decreases seen among older men.
- Asthma rates continue to climb. The prevalence of self-reported asthma is higher among women than men and is increasing for both sexes. Children in urban areas and from lower socioeconomic groups have a higher incidence of asthma.
- Although Canada's overall tuberculosis (TB) rate is low, the rate of TB remains high in Canadian-born Aboriginal peoples and in people who were born in countries with a high incidence of TB. Poverty and overcrowding have long been associated with TB—therefore, others at risk are the residents of long-term-care and correctional facilities.
- Overall, influenza and pneumonia remain major contributors to deaths and hospitalization among older adults. Together, they are the leading cause of death from infectious disease in Canada.
- Sleep disorders are associated with reduced quality of life, decreased cardiovascular health, and increased healthcare use, accidents, and mortality. Since obesity is a risk factor for sleep apnea, efforts to promote healthy weights may help prevent this disease.
- The nurse must consider linguistic and cultural factors to avoid miscommunication and misinterpretation of information about diagnoses when caring for some immigrant populations.

GATHERING THE DATA

Respiratory health assessment includes the gathering of subjective and objective data. Recall that subjective data collection occurs during the client interview, before the actual physical assessment. During the interview the nurse uses a variety of communication techniques to elicit general and specific information about the client's state of respiratory health or illness. Health records, the results of laboratory tests, and X-rays are important secondary sources to be reviewed and included in the data-gathering process. In physical assessment of the respiratory system, the techniques of inspection, palpation, percussion, and auscultation will be used. Before proceeding, it may be helpful to review the information about each of the data-gathering processes and practise the techniques of health assessment.

HEALTH HISTORY

The health history for the respiratory system concerns data related to the structures and functions of that system. Subjective data related to respiratory status are gathered during the health history. The nurse must be prepared to observe the client and listen for cues related to the function of the respiratory system. The nurse may use open-ended or closed questions to obtain information. Often a number of follow-up questions or requests for descriptions are required to clarify data or gather missing information. The subjective data collected and the questions asked during the health history will provide information to help meet the goal of promoting respiratory health. Follow-up questions are intended to identify the source of problems, the duration of difficulties, and measures to alleviate problems. Follow-up questions also provide clues about the client's knowledge of his or her own health.

The health history guides the physical assessment of the respiratory system. The information is always considered in relation to norms and expectations about respiratory function. Therefore, the nurse must consider age, gender, race, culture, environment, health practices, past and concurrent problems, and therapies when framing questions and using techniques to elicit information. To address all the factors when conducting a health history, specific questions related to respiratory status and function have been developed. These questions focus on the most common concerns or injuries associated with the respiratory system; questions related to past health history; questions related to behaviours; questions that address environmental concerns; and those that are specific to clients according to age, including the pregnant female.

The nurse must consider the client's ability to participate in the health history interview and physical assessment of the respiratory system. If a client is experiencing dyspnea, cyanosis, difficulty with speech, and the anxiety that accompanies any of these problems, attention must focus on relief of symptoms and restoration of oxygenation.

As the nurse gathers the data, she or he will shift the type of questions to direct questions that give the client room to explain or qualify. The mnemonic O-P-Q-R-S-T-U, which stands for onset (chronology), precipitating (or palliative), quality, region (or radiation), severity, timing, and understanding, will help the learner remember the dimensions of the symptoms. The nurse will keep in mind that not all these qualifiers will apply to each symptom.

HEALTH HISTORY QUESTIONS

RATIONALES

The following sections provide sample questions and follow-up questions. Rationales for some questions are provided. The list of questions is not all-inclusive but rather represents the more common concern or injury questions required in a health history related to the respiratory system. An example of using O-P-Q-R-S-T-U with cough is provided.

Questions Related to Common Concerns or Injuries

The most common concerns related to illness or injury of the respiratory system are as follows:

- Cough
- Dyspnea or shortness of breath (SOB)
- Orthopnea
- Pain

1. **Cough**
   - Do you have a cough? *If yes:*
   - When did you first start coughing and how long does it last? *Onset (chronology)*
   - What makes the cough worse? What makes the cough better? *Precipitating (palliative)*
   - Describe your cough. Is it dry, hacking, hoarse, moist, barking? Are you coughing up mucus or phlegm? Describe the characteristics of the mucus: colour, consistency or thickness, odour, changes in the characteristics. *Quality*
   - Does the cough cause discomfort anywhere else? *Radiation*
   - How would you rate the cough on a scale of 1 to 10, with 10 being the worst cough? *Severity*
   - How often do you experience the cough? Does the cough occur at a certain time of day? *Timing*
   - What do you think is causing the cough? *Understanding*

► This question helps the nurse determine if the problem is current, experienced in the past only, or chronic.

► The type of cough may be a symptom associated with a specific disease or problem. For example, wet or moist coughs are most often associated with lung infection.

► The colour and odour of any mucus or phlegm (sputum) are associated with specific diseases or problems. For example, rust-coloured mucus is associated with tuberculosis, while green or yellow mucus often signals lung infection.

2. **Dyspnea or shortness of breath (SOB)**
   - Do you experience difficulty breathing? *If yes:*
   - What provokes the SOB and what makes it better?
   - How would you rate the SOB on a scale of 1 to 10, with 10 being the worst SOB?
   - Are there associated symptoms? cough? chest pain? change in skin colour?
   - Is the SOB brought on by activity? If yes, assess the amount of activity, such as walking a block or climbing 10 steps.

3. **Orthopnea**
   - Do you experience difficulty breathing when you lie down? *If yes:*
   - When you sleep do you lie down flat, prop yourself up with pillows, or sit up?
   - How many pillows do you use?
   - How long have you slept like this?

► The norm is for a client to sleep fully reclined with a pillow. The number of pillows for propping up should be determined. Clients who must prop themselves up or sit up while sleeping may have orthopnea, that is, dyspnea when lying down. It is important to determine if the propping up or sitting up is simply a preference or because of breathing problems or some other cause.

4. **Pain**
   - Do you experience pain in your chest? *If yes:*
   - When did you first notice the pain? How long does it last?
   - What makes the pain worse? What makes the pain better?
   - Would you describe the pain as sharp? dull? achy?
   - Where is the pain located? Does the pain radiate?
   - How would you rate the pain on a scale of 1 to 10, with 10 being the worst pain? Does the pain affect your breathing or any other functions?
   - How often do you experience the pain? When does the pain occur, with a cough, all day long? How long does it last?
   - What do you think is causing the pain?

► Chest pain may be related to cardiac or respiratory problems.

GATHERING THE DATA

HEALTH HISTORY QUESTIONS	RATIONALES

Questions Related to Past Health History

1. **History of respiratory infections**
   - Do you, or does anyone in your family, have a history of recurring or chronic respiratory infections, such as allergies, asthma, COPD, emphysema, pneumonia, or recurrent or frequents colds? *If yes:*
   - When were you or your family member diagnosed with the problem?
   - Has the problem ever recurred? *(acute)*
   - How are you managing the problem now? *(chronic)*
   - Does your respiratory infection affect your ability to carry out your activities of daily living?
   - Have you discussed this with a healthcare professional? If so, what treatment was recommended and did it help?

▶ This question may reveal information about respiratory diseases associated with familial or genetic predisposition. Follow-up is required to obtain details about specific problems and their occurrence, treatment, and outcomes.

▶ The client has an opportunity to provide information about specific respiratory illnesses. If a diagnosed illness or infection is identified, follow-up about the date of diagnosis or infection, treatment, and outcomes is required. Data about each illness or infection identified by the client are essential to an accurate health assessment. Illnesses and infections can be classified as acute or chronic, and follow-up regarding each classification will differ.

Questions Related to Behaviours

Healthcare behaviours include both health practices and health patterns. Health practices consist of following recommendations for disease prevention, including screening for risks, screening for early detection of problems, and immunization. Health patterns are habits or acts that affect the client's health. Health behaviours may also include seeking healthcare from healthcare providers who use alternative methods to diagnose and treat illness. Clients should be questioned in a nonjudgmental way and areas for health teaching should be identified.

1. **Do you or have you ever smoked tobacco?** *If yes:*
   - What type of tobacco product do or did you smoke?
   - How much of the product do or did you smoke?
   - When did you start smoking?
   - When did you stop smoking?
   - Have you tried to stop smoking?
   - Do you have any symptoms related to smoking?

   - Are you exposed to second-hand smoke at home or in your workplace?

▶ Smoking tobacco products is associated with respiratory diseases, including emphysema and lung cancer. Tobacco products include cigarettes, cigars, and pipe tobacco.

▶ If the client exhibits or affirms that respiratory symptoms exist, the nurse should ask questions for any associated symptoms, as previously described.

2. **Do you or have you ever inhaled marijuana, herbal products, or chemical preparations?** *If yes:*
   - Do you smoke or inhale marijuana, other herbal products, or chemical preparations, such as glue or spray paint or street drugs? Have you done so in the past? (For those clients who state they have inhaled substances in the past, ask, "When did you stop using the substance?")
   - What is the substance you inhale?
   - How much do you use?
   - How often do you inhale the substance?

▶ Inhalation of marijuana, herbal substances, or chemicals may result in respiratory problems associated with incidental or continuous irritation of the linings of the respiratory organs.

3. **Have you received immunization for respiratory illnesses, such as flu or pneumonia?** *If yes:*
   - What immunizations have you had?
   - When was each given? Were there any adverse effects?
   - When was your last chest X-ray and TB test?

▶ Immunization status and a reduction in the risk of infection from flu or pneumonia are important for preventing lung problems.

HEALTH HISTORY QUESTIONS	RATIONALES

4. Do you take any over-the-counter or prescription medications?

▶ The answer establishes the client's self-care behaviours.

5. Do you exercise regularly?

▶ The answer establishes the client's self-care behaviours.

Questions Related to the Environment

Environment refers to both internal and external environments. Questions related to the internal environment include all the previous questions and those associated with internal or physiological responses. Questions regarding the external environment include those related to home, work, or social environments.

External Environment

The following questions deal with the physical environment of the client. That includes the indoor and outdoor environments of the home and the workplace, those encountered for social engagements, and any encountered during travel.

1. **Do you have any allergies?** *If yes:*
   * Do those allergies affect respiratory function?
   * What is or was your respiratory response to the allergens?
   * Have you discussed this with a healthcare professional? If so, what treatment was recommended and did it help?

▶ Allergies often result in respiratory problems, including asthma and bronchitis. It is important to determine if specific allergens have been identified and if the client uses appropriate measures to address the problems. Remedies may include avoidance of the allergen.

2. **Are you now or have you ever been exposed to respiratory irritants (gases, fumes, dust, lint, smoke, chemical exhaust)? If so, were the irritants identified?**
   * Where are or were the irritants? in the home, in the workplace, in the community, or outside of the community?
   * What is or was your respiratory response to irritants?
   * Have you discussed this with a healthcare professional? If so, what treatment was recommended and did it help?

▶ Irritants, pollutants, and chemicals in the environment can result in acute and chronic respiratory disease (i.e., mesothelioma, asbestosis, and psittacosis). Acute and chronic problems with respiratory function can have devastating effects on the ability to function. Identification of the place of exposure or possible exposure through travel, military, or employment service may assist in identifying probable causes for new or ongoing respiratory problems.

Questions Related to Age

The health history must reflect the anatomical and physiological differences that exist along the age span.

Questions Regarding Infants and Children

1. **Is the child taking solid foods?**
   * When were they started?
   * What types of food are taken?
   * Does the child have difficulty chewing or swallowing?

▶ Introduction of solid foods puts infants at risk for aspiration.

2. **How many colds has the child had in the past 12 months?**
   * What was the course of the cold?

▶ Children may experience as many as six uncomplicated respiratory infections in a year. More than this number of complicated infections may indicate chronic disease.

3. **Has the child been immunized against respiratory illnesses?**
   * What immunization did your child have?
   * When was it given?
   * Were there any adverse effects?

▶ This question identifies risk reduction and assists in discrimination of symptoms when they occur. Infants are at greater risk for complications from flu and pneumonia.

GATHERING THE DATA

HEALTH HISTORY QUESTIONS	RATIONALES

Questions for the Pregnant Female

1. **Do you experience any shortness of breath or dyspnea?**
   - When does it occur?
   - How long have you experienced this?
   - Have you sought a remedy?

▶ The enlarged uterus puts pressure on the diaphragm and can decrease lung expansion, which may result in shortness of breath.

Questions for the Older Adult

1. **Describe any changes in breathing you have experienced.**
2. **Have you had any difficulty performing activities that you once found easy?**
3. **Do you find that you are more tired than you have been in the past?**

▶ Older adults may experience symptoms associated with reduced oxygenation as a result of changes in posture and muscle strength that may contribute to reduced lung expansion. Fatigue may be associated with anemia and other chronic problems, such as COPD, asthma, and cancer.

4. **Have you received any immunization for respiratory illnesses?**
   - What immunization did you receive?
   - When was it given?
   - Were there any adverse effects?

▶ Older adults are at greater risk for flu and pneumonia.

PHYSICAL ASSESSMENT

ASSESSMENT TECHNIQUES AND FINDINGS

Physical assessment of the respiratory system requires the use of inspection, palpation, percussion, and auscultation. During each of the procedures, the nurse is gathering data related to the client's breathing and level of oxygenation. The nurse inspects skin colour, structures of the thoracic cavity, chest configuration, and respiratory rate, rhythm, and effort. Knowledge of norms or expected findings is essential in determining the meaning of the data as the nurse proceeds.

Adults normally breathe at a rate of 12 to 20 breaths per minute. Infants and children have higher rates—up to 40 breaths per minute in newborns. The respiratory cycle includes full inspiration and expiration. The ratio of the length of inspiration to expiration is about 1:2 (I:E). Breathing should be even, regular, and coordinated. Chest movement should be uniform; the structures of the thorax should be aligned and the thorax should be symmetrical. The sternum is midline and flat. The costal angle is less than 90 degrees in an adult. The vertebrae are midline and follow the pattern of cervical, thoracic, and lumbar curves. The anterior to posterior diameter of the chest should be half of the lateral diameter. Pink skin or pink undertones indicate normal oxygenation. Assessment for a pink tongue or pink oral mucous membranes may be required in dark-skinned individuals. The colour of the skin of the thorax should be consistent with that of the rest of the body.

See Box 15.1 for normal and abnormal respiration patterns, Box 15.2 for normal chest configurations, and Box 15.3 for abnormal chest configurations.

Physical assessment of the respiratory system follows an organized pattern. It begins with a client survey followed by inspection of the anterior thorax and complete assessment of the posterior thorax. The assessment ends with palpation, percussion, and auscultation of the anterior thorax. The nurse includes the anterior, posterior, and lateral aspects of the thorax when conducting each assessment.

EQUIPMENT

examination gown and drape	stethoscope	tissues
examination gloves	skin marker	face mask
examination light	metric ruler	

HELPFUL HINTS

- Provide an environment that is comfortable and private.
- Explain each step of the procedure.
- Provide specific instructions about what is expected of the client, such as whether deep or regular breathing will be required.
- Tell client the purpose of each procedure and when and if discomfort will accompany any examination.
- Pay attention to nonverbal cues that may indicate discomfort and ask the client to indicate if he or she experiences any difficulties or discomforts.
- An organized and professional approach goes a long way toward putting the client at ease.

BOX 15.1	Normal and Abnormal Respiratory Rates and Patterns

Normal Findings

Eupnea

Even depth
Regular pattern
Inspiration = Expiration
Occasional sigh

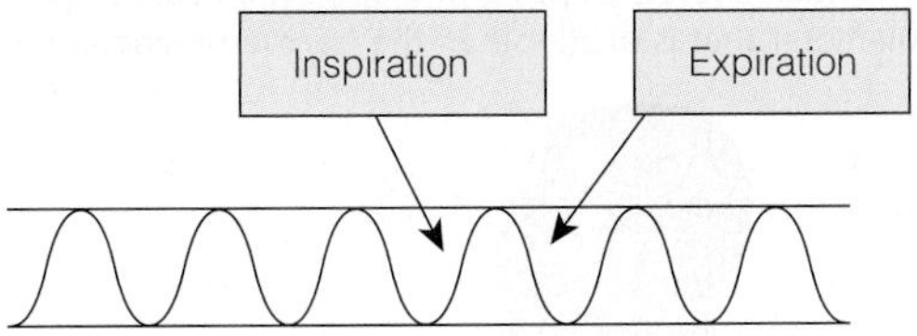

Eupnea with sigh

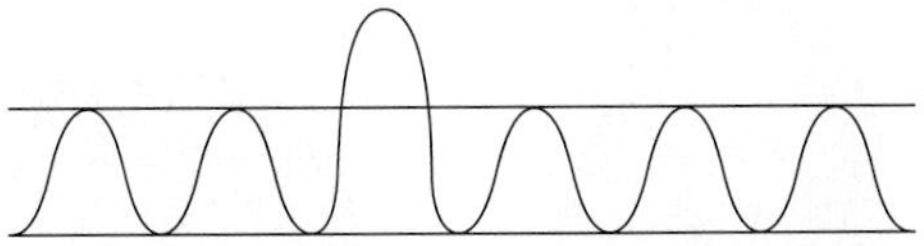

Abnormal Findings

Tachypnea

Rapid, shallow respirations
Rate >24
Precipitating factors: fever, fear, exercise, respiratory insufficiency, pleuritic pain, alkalosis, pneumonia

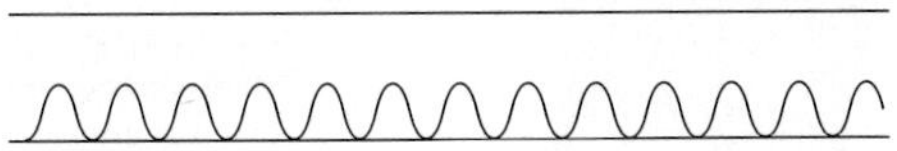

Bradypnea

Slow, regular respirations
Rate <10
Precipitating factors: diabetic coma, drug-induced respiratory depression, increased intracranial pressure

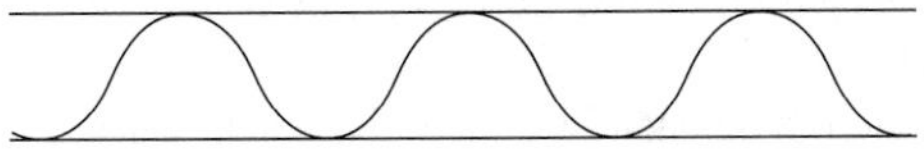

Hyperventilation

Rapid, deep respirations
Rate >24
Precipitating factors: extreme exertion, fear, diabetic ketoacidosis (Kussmaul's), hypoxia, salicylate overdose, hypoglycemia

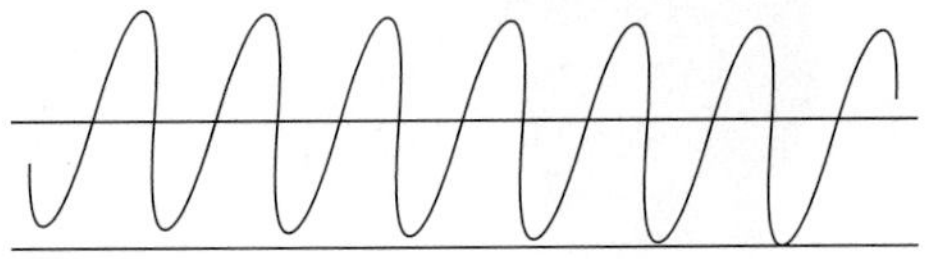

Hypoventilation

Irregular, shallow respirations
Rate <10
Precipitating factors: narcotic overdose, anaesthetics, prolonged bed rest, chest splinting

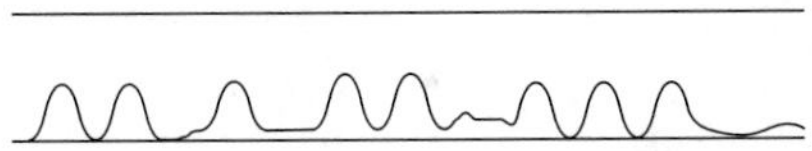

Cheyne-Stokes

Periods of deep breathing alternating with periods of apnea
Regular pattern
Precipitating factors: normal children and aging, heart failure, uremia, brain damage, drug-induced respiratory depression

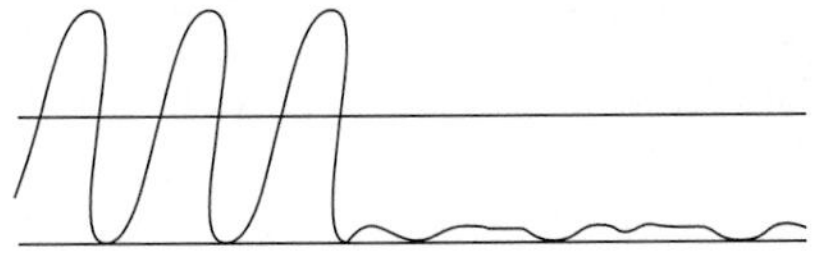

Biot's (Ataic) Respirations

Shallow, deep respirations with periods of apnea
Irregular pattern
Precipitating factors: respiratory depression, brain damage

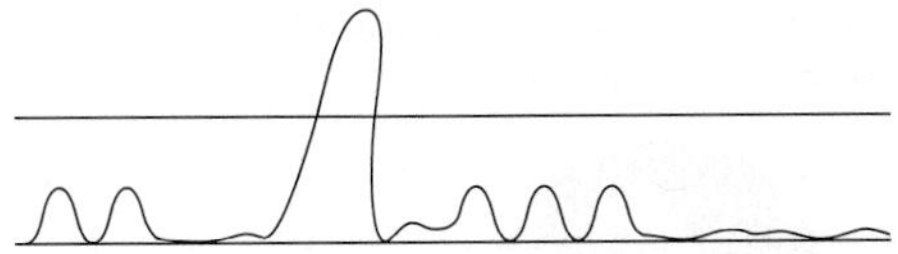

Sighing

Frequent sighs
Precipitating factors: hyperventilation syndrome, nervousness
Causes: dyspnea, dizziness

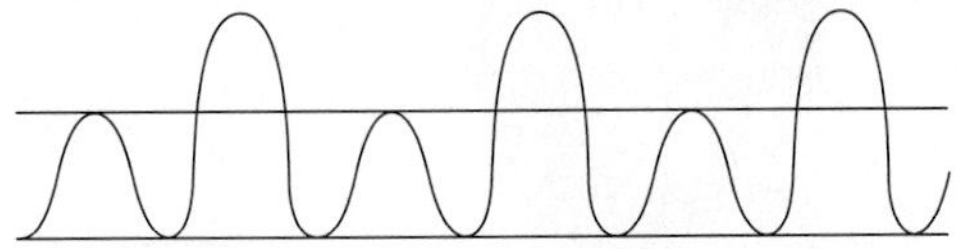

Obstructive Breathing

Prolonged expiration
Precipitating factors: COPD, asthma, chronic bronchitis

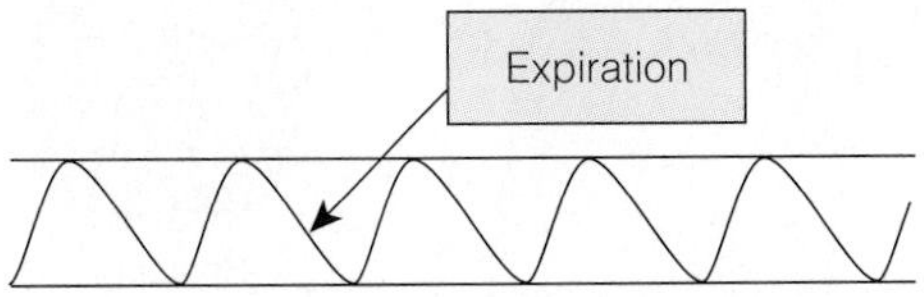

Prolonged expiration

PHYSICAL ASSESSMENT

BOX 15.2	Normal Chest Configurations

Adult

The adult chest is elliptical in shape with an anteroposterior diameter that is smaller than the transverse diameter in a 1:2 ratio.

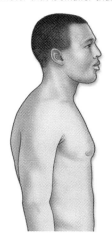
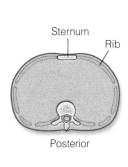

Sternum
Rib
Posterior

Child

The chest of a child is of adult proportion by age 6.

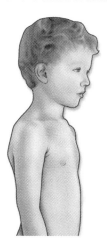
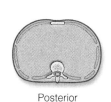

Posterior

Infant

The infant chest is rounded in shape with equal lateral and anteroposterior diameters.

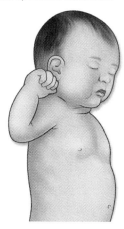

Posterior

BOX 15.3	Abormal Chest Configurations

Barrel Chest

The anteroposterior diameter is equal to the transverse diameter, and the ribs are horizontal. A barrel chest accompanies COPD and may occur normally with aging.

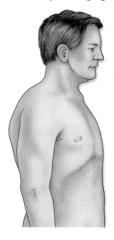
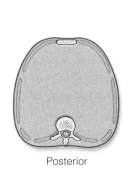

Posterior

Funnel Chest (Pectus Excavatum)

This is a congenital deformity characterized by depression of the sternum and adjacent costal cartilage. All or part of the sternum may be involved but predominant depression is at the lower portion where the body meets the xiphoid process.

If the condition is severe, chest compression may interfere with respiration. Murmurs may be present with cardiac compression.

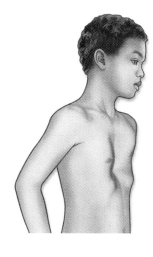
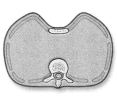

Posterior

BOX 15.3 | **Abormal Chest Configurations** *(continued)*

Scoliosis

Scoliosis is a condition in which there is lateral curvature and rotation of the thoracic and lumbar spine. It occurs more frequently in females. Scoliosis may result in elevation of the shoulder and pelvis.

Deviation greater than 45° may cause distortion of the lung, which results in decreased lung volume or difficulty in interpretation of findings from physical assessment.

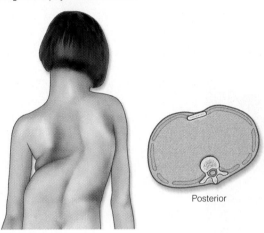

Posterior

Kyphosis

Kyphosis is exaggerated posterior curvature of the thoracic spine. It is associated with aging. Severe kyphosis may decrease lung expansion and increase cardiac problems.

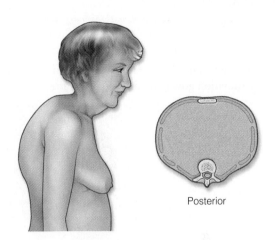

Posterior

Pigeon Chest (Pectus Carinatum)

This congenital deformity is characterized by forward displacement of the sternum with depression of the adjacent costal cartilage. This condition generally requires no treatment.

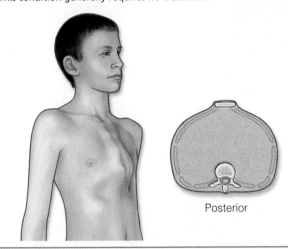

Posterior

TECHNIQUES AND NORMAL FINDINGS

SURVEY

A quick survey enables the nurse to identify any immediate problem and the client's ability to participate in the assessment.

Inspect the overall appearance, posture, and position of the client. Note the skin colour and respiratory effort.

CLINICAL TIP

Individuals experiencing pain and dyspnea, who are restless, anxious, and unable to follow directions, may need immediate medical assistance.

ABNORMAL FINDINGS AND SPECIAL CONSIDERATIONS

▶ Clients experiencing anxiety may demonstrate pallor and shallow breathing. Acknowledgment of the problem and discussion of the procedures often provide some relief. If a client is in obvious respiratory distress, the problem must be addressed. The client may require referral to a healthcare provider or emergency care facility.

▶ Circumoral cyanosis (blue colour around the mouth) may be present in clients with respiratory distress or hypoxia.

TECHNIQUES AND NORMAL FINDINGS	ABNORMAL FINDINGS AND SPECIAL CONSIDERATIONS

INSPECTION OF THE ANTERIOR THORAX

CLINICAL TIP
Be sensitive to the client's privacy, and limit exposure of body parts.

1. **Position the client.**
   - The client should be in a sitting position with clothing removed except for an examination gown and drape (see Figure 15.10).

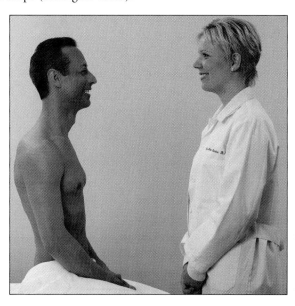

Figure 15.10 • Client positioned and draped for examination.

   - Stand in front of the client. Lighting must be adequate to detect colour differences, lesions, and chest movement.

2. **Instruct the client.**
   - Explain that you are going to be looking at the client's chest structures. Tell the client to breathe normally.

3. **Observe skin colour.**
   - Skin colour varies among individuals, but pink undertones indicate normal oxygenation. Skin colour of the thorax should be consistent with that of the rest of the body.

   ▶ Pigments and levels of oxygenation influence skin colour. Pallor, cyanosis, rubor, erythema, or greyness requires further evaluation.

4. **Inspect the structures of the thorax.**
   - The clavicles should be at the same height. The sternum should be midline. The costal angle should be less than 90 degrees.

   ▶ Misalignment of clavicles may be caused by deviations in the vertebral column, such as scoliosis. Increase in the costal angle in an adult may indicate COPD. The thorax of children is rounder than that of adults.

5. **Inspect for symmetry.**
   - The structures of the chest and chest movement should be symmetrical.

   ▶ Asymmetry may indicate postural problems or underlying respiratory dysfunction.

6. **Inspect chest configuration.**
   - The adult transverse diameter is approximately twice that of the anteroposterior diameter (AP:T = 1:2).

   ▶ A change in the ratio requires further evaluation. Remember: older adults may have a decreased ratio.

| TECHNIQUES AND NORMAL FINDINGS | ABNORMAL FINDINGS AND SPECIAL CONSIDERATIONS |

7. Count the respiratory rate.

- Count the number of respiratory cycles per minute. Normal adult respiratory rate is 12 to 20.
- Observe chest movement.
- Observe the muscles of the chest and neck, including the intercostal muscles and sternocleidomastoids.
- Do not tell the client that you are counting respirations—it may alter the normal breathing pattern.
- Respirations should be even and smooth. Chest movement should be symmetrical.
- Males tend to breathe abdominally.
- Females breathe more costally.

▶ Intercostal muscle retraction and prominent sternocleidomastoids may be seen in respiratory distress.

INSPECTION OF THE POSTERIOR THORAX

1. Instruct the client.

- Explain to the client that you will be performing several assessments and that you will provide instructions as you move from one step to the next. Tell the client to try to relax and breathe normally to begin the examination.

2. Observe skin colour.

- Skin colour of the posterior thorax should be consistent with that of the rest of the body.

3. Inspect the structures of the posterior thorax.

- The height of the scapulae should be even; the vertebrae should be midline.

▶ Lateral deviation of the spine and elevation of one scapula is indicative of scoliosis.

4. Inspect for symmetry.

- The structures of the chest and chest movement should be symmetrical.

▶ Asymmetry may indicate postural problems or underlying respiratory problems.

5. Observe respirations.

- Respirations should be smooth and even.

PALPATION OF THE POSTERIOR THORAX

1. Instruct the client.

- Explain that you will be touching the client's back to determine if there are any areas of tenderness. Tell the client to breathe normally during this part of the examination and to tell you if pain or discomfort is felt at any area.

▶ Pain may occur with inflammation of fibrous tissue or underlying structures, such as the pleura. Crepitus is a crunching feeling under the skin caused by air leaking into subcutaneous tissue.

2. Lightly palpate the posterior thorax.

- Use the fingerpads to lightly palpate the posterior thorax. Include the entire thorax by starting at the areas above each scapula and move from side to side to below the twelfth rib and laterally to the midaxillary line on each side (see Figure 15.11).
- Assess muscle mass.
- Assess for growths, nodules, and masses.
- Assess for tenderness.
- Muscle mass should be firm and underlying tissue smooth. The chest should be free of lesions or masses. The area should be nontender to palpation.

TECHNIQUES AND NORMAL FINDINGS	ABNORMAL FINDINGS AND SPECIAL CONSIDERATIONS

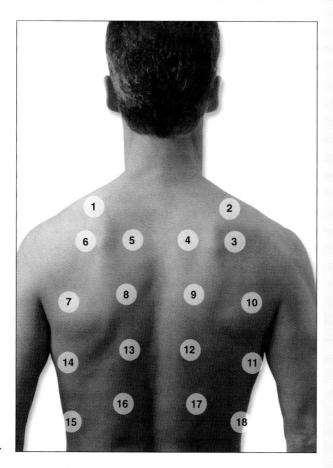

Figure 15.11 ●
Pattern for palpating
the posterior thorax.

3. **Palpate and count ribs and intercostal spaces.**

   - Instruct the client to flex the neck, round the shoulders, and lean forward. Tell the client you will be applying light pressure to the spine and rib areas. Instruct the client to breathe normally and to tell you of pain or discomfort.

   - When the neck is flexed, the spinous process of C_7 is most prominent. When two spinous processes are equally prominent, they are C_7 and T_1. Use the fingerpads to palpate each spinous process. The spinous processes should form a straight line. Further assessment is discussed in Chapter 23. ⬭ Move to the left and right to identify ribs and intercostal spaces from C_7 through T_{12}.

   ▶ Lateral deviation of the thoracic spinous processes indicates a scoliosis.

4. **Palpate for respiratory expansion.**

   - Explain that you will be assessing the movement of the chest during breathing by placing your hands on the lower chest and asking the client to take a deep breath.

   - Place the palmar surface of your hands, with thumbs close to the vertebrae, on the chest at the level of T_{10}. Pinch up some skin between your thumbs. Ask the client to take a deep breath (see Figure 15.12).

   - The movement and pressure of the chest against your hands should feel smooth and even. Your thumbs should move away from the spine and the skin should move smoothly as the chest moves with inspiration.

   ▶ Unilateral decrease or delay in expansion may indicate underlying fibrotic or obstructive lung disease or may result from splinting associated with pleural pain or pneumothorax.

PHYSICAL ASSESSMENT

TECHNIQUES AND NORMAL FINDINGS	ABNORMAL FINDINGS AND SPECIAL CONSIDERATIONS

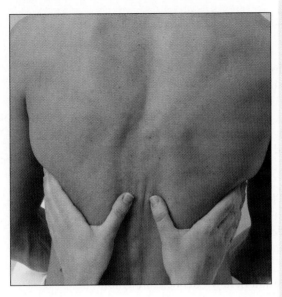

Figure 15.12 ● Palpation for respiratory expansion.

5. Palpate for tactile fremitus.

- **Fremitus** is the palpable vibration on the chest wall when the client speaks. Fremitus is strongest over the trachea, diminishes over the bronchi, and becomes almost nonexistent over the alveoli of the lungs.

- Explain that you will be feeling for vibrations on the chest while the client speaks. Tell the client you will be placing your hands on various areas of the chest while he or she repeats "ninety-nine" or "one, two, three" in a clear, loud voice.

- Use the ulnar surface of the hand or the palmar surface of the hand at the base of the metacarpophalangeal joints when palpating. Palpate and compare symmetrical areas of the lungs by moving from side to side from apices to bases. Using one hand to palpate for fremitus is believed to increase accuracy of findings. Two-handed methods may, however, increase speed and facilitate identification of asymmetry (see Figure 15.13).

▶ Decreased or absent fremitus may result from a soft voice, from a very thick chest wall, or from underlying diseases including COPD, pleural effusion, fibrosis, or tumour. Increased fremitus occurs with fluid in the lungs or in infection.

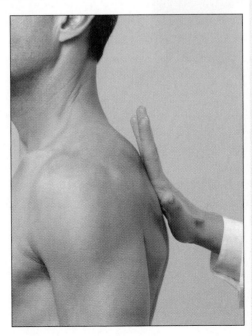

Figure 15.13 ● Palpation for tactile fremitus by using metacarpophalangeal joint area.

PHYSICAL ASSESSMENT

| TECHNIQUES AND NORMAL FINDINGS | ABNORMAL FINDINGS AND SPECIAL CONSIDERATIONS |

PERCUSSION OF THE POSTERIOR THORAX

1. Visualize the landmarks.

   • Observe the posterior thorax and visualize the horizontal and vertical lines, the level of the diaphragm, and the fissures of the lungs.

2. Recall the expected findings.

   • Percussion allows assessment of underlying structures. The usual sound in the thorax is **resonance**, a long, low-pitched hollow sound.

   ▶ An unexpected finding would be hyper-resonance, which is heard in conditions of overinflation of the lungs, as in emphysema, or with pneumothorax.

3. Instruct the client.

   • Explain to the client that you will be tapping on the chest in a variety of areas.

   • Tell the client to breathe normally through this examination. Ask the client to lean forward and round the shoulders. This position moves the scapulae laterally, permitting more area at the upper vertebral borders, and widens the intercostal spaces for percussion.

   • Position the client so that your arms are almost fully extended throughout the percussion.

4. Percuss the lungs.

   • Place the pleximeter in the intercostal space parallel to the ribs during percussion. Standing slightly to the side of the client allows the pleximeter finger to lie more firmly on the chest as you move through all thoracic areas.

   • Percuss the apex of the left lung, and then the apex of the right lung. Percuss from side to side, comparing sounds in the intercostal spaces as you percuss to the bases of the lungs and laterally to each midaxillary line (see Figure 15.14).

   ▶ Percussion will yield dull sounds over solidified or fluid-filled areas, as may exist in pleural effusion. Percussion over bone will yield flat sounds. Be sure to check that finger placement is correct.

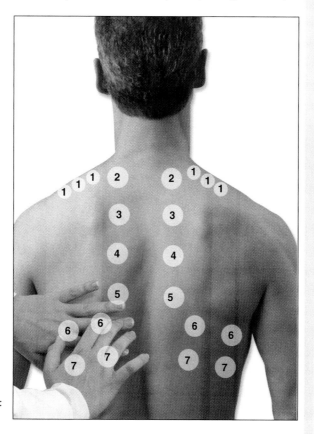

Figure 15.14 ●
Pattern for percussion: Posterior thorax.

TECHNIQUES AND NORMAL FINDINGS	ABNORMAL FINDINGS AND SPECIAL CONSIDERATIONS

5. **Percuss for movement of the diaphragmatic excursion.**

- This assessment requires the use of a skin marker and a ruler. The client remains in the position previously described for percussion. Explain that you will be doing more tapping on the chest and at two points you will ask the client to exhale and inhale. Determine the level of the diaphragm during quiet respiration by placing the pleximeter finger above the expected level of diaphragmatic **dullness** (T_7 or T_8) at the midscapular line. Percuss in steps downward until dullness replaces resonance on both sides of the chest. Mark those areas. These marks should be at approximately the level of T_{10}.

- The marks should be parallel.

- Measure diaphragmatic movement by asking the client to fully exhale. Starting at the previous skin marking on the left chest, percuss upward from dullness to resonance. Mark that area. Then ask the client to inhale fully and hold it as you begin to percuss from the level of the diaphragm downward, moving from resonance to dullness. Mark that area and repeat on the right side of the chest. Use the ruler to measure the difference between the marks for exhalation and inhalation (see Figure 15.15).

▶ An asymmetrical diaphragm may indicate diaphragmatic paralysis or pleural effusion of the elevated side.

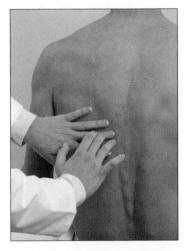

Figure 15.15A ● Diaphragmatic movement, percussion.

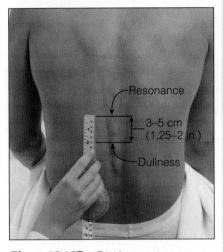

Resonance

3–5 cm (1.25–2 in.)

Dullness

Figure 15.15B ● Diaphragmatic movement, measurement.

- The distance between the marks should be 3 to 5 cm (1.25 to 2 in.) and even on each side. The right side may be 1 to 2 cm (0.5 to 1 in.) higher because of the location of the liver.

- Anticipate a greater distance on a physically fit client.

▶ Shortened excursion indicates that the lungs are not fully expanding. Pain or abdominal pressure can inhibit full expansion. The diaphragmatic movement is shortened in client's with emphysema, atelectasis (a collapsed lung), or respiratory depression.

AUSCULTATION OF THE POSTERIOR THORAX

Auscultation of the respiratory system refers to listening to the sounds of breathing through the stethoscope. The sounds are produced by air moving through the airways. Sounds change as the airway size changes or with the presence of fluid or mucus.

The pattern for auscultation of the respiratory system is the same as that for percussion (see Figure 15.16).

▶ Auscultation through clothing or coarse chest hair may produce deceptive sounds. Thick, coarse chest hair may be matted with a damp cloth or lotion to prevent interference with auscultation.

TECHNIQUES AND NORMAL FINDINGS

ABNORMAL FINDINGS AND SPECIAL CONSIDERATIONS

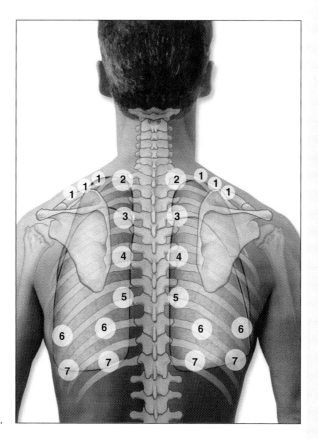

Figure 15.16 ●
Pattern for ausculta-
tion: Posterior thorax.

Use the diaphragm of the stethoscope and listen through the full respiratory cycle. When auscultating, classify each sound according to intensity, location, pitch, duration, and characteristic.

CLINICAL TIP

It is important to monitor the client's breathing to prevent hyperventilation.

Four normal breath sounds are heard during respiratory auscultation. **Tracheal sounds** are harsh, high-pitched sounds heard over the trachea when the client inhales and exhales. **Bronchial sounds** are loud, high-pitched sounds heard next to the trachea and are longer on exhalation. **Bronchovesicular sounds** are medium in loudness and pitch. They are heard between the scapula, posteriorly and next to the sternum, and anteriorly on inhalation and exhalation. **Vesicular sounds** are soft and low-pitched and heard over the remainder of the lungs. Vesicular sounds are longer on inhalation than exhalation (see Table 15.1). Only the bronchovesicular and vesicular sounds can be auscultated on the posterior thorax (see Figure 15.17).

TABLE 15.1	Normal Breath Sounds		
SOUND	LOCATION	RATIO INSPIRATION TO EXPIRATION	QUALITY
Tracheal	Over trachea	I < E	Harsh, high-pitched
Bronchial	Next to trachea	I < E	Loud, high-pitched
Bronchovesicular	Sternal border between scapula	I = E	Medium loudness, medium pitch
Vesicular	Remainder of lungs	I > E	Soft, low-pitched

PHYSICAL ASSESSMENT

TECHNIQUES AND NORMAL FINDINGS

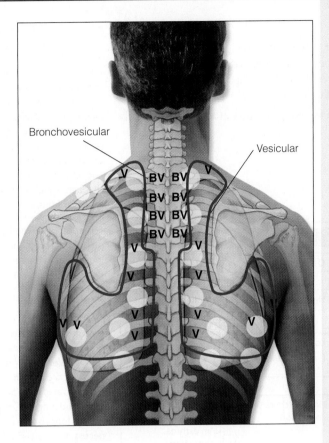

Figure 15.17 ●
Auscultatory sounds:
Posterior thorax.

1. **Instruct the client.**
   - Explain that you will be listening to the client's breathing by using the stethoscope.
   - The client will be in the same position as during percussion. Ask the client to breathe deeply through the mouth each time the stethoscope is placed on a new spot. Tell the client to let you know if he or she is becoming tired or short of breath and if so you will stop and allow time to rest.

2. **Visualize the landmarks.**
   - Visualize the landmarks as you did before percussing the posterior thorax.

3. **Auscultate for tracheal sounds.**
   - Auscultate at the vertebral line superior to C_7.

4. **Auscultate for bronchial sounds.**
   - Start at the vertebral line at C_7 and move the stethoscope down toward T_3. The sound will be bronchial.

5. **Auscultate for bronchovesicular sounds.**
   - The right and left primary bronchi are located at the level of T_3 and T_5. Auscultate at the right and left of the vertebrae at those levels. The breath sounds will be bronchovesicular.

TECHNIQUES AND NORMAL FINDINGS

ABNORMAL FINDINGS AND SPECIAL CONSIDERATIONS

6. Auscultate for vesicular sounds.
   - Auscultate the lungs by following the pattern used for percussion. Move the stethoscope from side to side while comparing sounds. Start at the apices and move to the bases of the lungs and laterally to the midaxillary line. The breath sounds over most of the posterior surface are vesicular.
   - While auscultating the thorax, you are assessing air entry at all levels, especially the lower lobes.

▶ Auscultation of diminished but normal breath sounds in both lungs may indicate emphysema, atelectasis, bronchospasm, or shallow breathing. Breath sounds heard in just one lung indicate pleural effusion, pneumothorax, tumour, or mucus plugs in the airways in the other lung. Finding bronchial or bronchovesicular sounds in areas where normally vesicular sounds are heard indicates that alveoli and small bronchioles are affected by fluid or exudate. Fluid and exudate decrease the movement of air through small airways and result in loss of vesicular sounds.

▶ Added or adventitious sounds are superimposed on normal breath sounds and often are indicative of underlying airway problems or diseases of the cardiovascular or respiratory systems.

Adventitious sounds are classified as discontinuous or continuous. Discontinuous sounds are crackles, which are intermittent, nonmusical, and brief. These sounds are commonly referred to as **rales**. Fine rales or fine crackles are soft, high-pitched, and very brief. Coarse rales or crackles are louder, lower in pitch, and longer. Continuous sounds are musical and longer than rales or crackles but do not necessarily persist through the entire respiratory cycle. The two types are wheezes or sibilant wheezes and rhonchi (sonorous wheezes). **Wheezes** (sibilant) are high-pitched with a shrill quality. **Rhonchi** are low-pitched with a snoring quality (see Table 15.2).

TABLE 15.2	Adventitious Sounds		
SOUND	**OCCURRENCE**	**QUALITY**	**CAUSES**
Rales or Crackles			
Fine	End inspiration, don't clear with cough	High-pitched, short, crackling	Collapsed or fluid-filled alveoli open
Coarse	End inspiration, don't clear with cough	Loud, moist, low-pitched, bubbling	
Ronchi			
Wheezes (sibilant)	Expiration Inspiration when severe	High-pitched, continuous	Blocked airflow as in asthma, infection, foreign body obstruction
Ronchi (sonorous)	Expiration/ inspiration Change or disappear with cough	Low-pitched, continuous, snoring, rattling	Fluid-blocked airways
Stridor	Inspiration	Loud, high-pitched crowing heard without stethoscope	Obstructed upper airway
Friction rub	Inhalation/ exhalation	Low-pitched grating, rubbing	Pleural inflammation

ASSESSMENT OF VOICE SOUNDS

Assessment of voice sounds is completed only when a pathology is suspected and is not part of the routine exam. The spoken voice can be heard over the chest wall. The sound is produced by vibrations as the client speaks.

1. Instruct the client.
   - The client will remain in the same position as for percussion and auscultation. Explain that you will be listening to the chest while the client says certain words, letters, or numbers.

2. Auscultation of voice sounds.
   - Use the same pattern for evaluating voice sounds as for auscultation of the lungs. This sequence will be followed for three different findings.

Techniques and Normal Findings

- **Bronchophony.** Ask the client to say "ninety-nine" each time you place the stethoscope on the chest. In normal lung tissue the sound will be muffled.
- **Egophony.** Ask the client to say "E" each time you place the stethoscope on the chest. In normal lung tissue you should hear "eeeeee" through the stethoscope.
- **Whispered pectoriloquy.** Ask the client to whisper "one, two, three" each time you place the stethoscope on the chest. In normal lung tissue the sound will be faint, almost indistinguishable.
- Voice sounds are heard as muffled sounds in the normal lung.

▶ The words sound loud and more distinct over areas of lung consolidation.

▶ The "E" sounds like "aaaaay" over areas of lung consolidation.

▶ The numbers sound loud and clear over areas of lung consolidation.

ASSESSMENT OF THE ANTERIOR THORAX

Inspection of the anterior thorax was conducted before the entire assessment of the posterior thorax. That assessment included a survey and inspection of chest structures, skin colour, and respiratory rate and pattern.

PALPATION OF THE ANTERIOR THORAX

1. **Position the client.**
   - The client is usually in a supine position for palpation, percussion, and auscultation of the anterior thorax. If the client is experiencing discomfort or dyspnea, a sitting position may be used, or the client may be in a Fowler's position. The breasts of female clients normally flatten when in a supine position. Large and pendulous breasts may have to be moved to perform a complete assessment. Explain this to the client and inform her that she may move and lift her own breasts if that will make her more comfortable.

2. **Instruct the client.**
   - Explain to the client that you will be performing several assessments and that you will continue to provide explanations as you move from one assessment to the next. Tell the client to breathe normally throughout this initial examination and to tell you if pain or discomfort is felt at any area.

3. **Palpate the sternum, ribs, and intercostal spaces.**
   - Locate the suprasternal notch; palpate downward to the sternal angle (angle of Louis), where the manubrium meets the body of the sternum. Palpate laterally to the left and right to locate the second rib and second intercostal space. Continue palpating the sternum to the xiphoid process and to the left and right of the sternum to count the ribs.
   - The sternum should feel flat except for the ridge of the sternal angle and should taper to the xiphoid. The ribs should feel smooth, and the spacing of ribs and intercostal spaces should be symmetrical.

4. **Palpate the trachea.**
   - Explain to the client that you will be palpating the neck to check the position of the trachea. The trachea is normally midline; it can be shifted to one side or the other depending on the underlying pathology.

▶ Tracheal displacement is the result of masses in the neck or mediastinum, pneumothorax, fibrosis, pleural effusion, or atelectasis.

5. **Lightly palpate the anterior thorax.**
   - Use the fingerpads to lightly palpate the anterior thorax. Include the entire thorax by starting at the areas above each clavicle and move from side to side to below the costal angle and laterally to the midaxillary line (see Figure 15.18).

TECHNIQUES AND NORMAL FINDINGS

ABNORMAL FINDINGS AND
SPECIAL CONSIDERATIONS

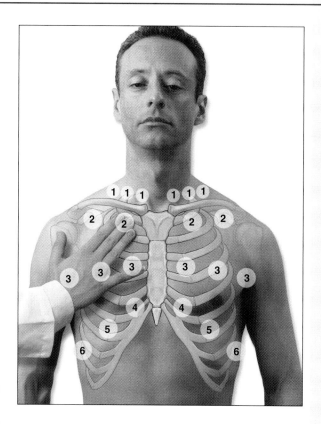

Figure 15.18 ●
Pattern for palpation:
Anterior thorax.

- Assess muscle mass.
- Assess for growths, nodules, and masses.
- Assess for tenderness.
- Muscle mass should be firm and underlying tissue smooth. The chest should be free of lesions or masses. The area should be nontender to palpation.

6. **Palpate for respiratory expansion.**
   - Explain that you will be assessing movement of the chest during breathing by placing your hands on the lower chest and asking the client to take a breath.
   - Place the palmar surface of your hands along each costal margin with thumbs close to the midsternal line. Pinch up some skin between your thumbs. Ask the client to take a deep breath (see Figure 15.19).
   - The movement of the chest beneath your hands should feel smooth and even. Your thumbs should move apart and the skin move smoothly as the chest expands with inspiration.

7. **Palpate for tactile fremitus.**
   - Explain that you will be feeling for vibrations on the chest wall while the client speaks. Explain that you will be placing your hands on various areas of the chest while the client repeats "ninety-nine" or "one, two, three" in a clear, loud voice.
   - Use the ulnar surface of the hand or the palmar surface of the hand at the base of the metacarpophalangeal joints when palpating for fremitus. Palpate and compare symmetrical areas of the lungs by moving from side to side from apices to bases (see Figure 15.20). Displace female breasts as required.
   - Fremitus normally diminishes as you move from large to small airways and is decreased or absent over the precordium.

▶ Pain may occur with inflammation of fibrous tissue or underlying structures. Crepitus may be felt if there is air in the subcutaneous tissue.

▶ Unilateral decrease or delay in expansion may indicate fibrotic or obstructive lung disease or may result from splinting associated with pleural pain.

▶ Absent or decreased fremitus in other areas may result from underlying diseases including emphysema, pleural effusion, or fibrosis.

| TECHNIQUES AND NORMAL FINDINGS | ABNORMAL FINDINGS AND SPECIAL CONSIDERATIONS |

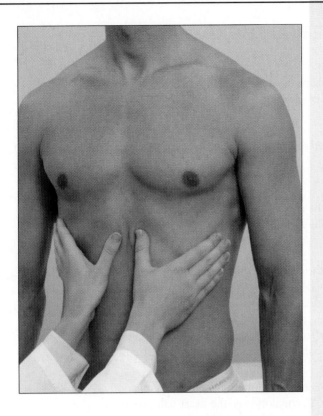

Figure 15.19 ●
Palpation for respiratory
expansion: Anterior view.

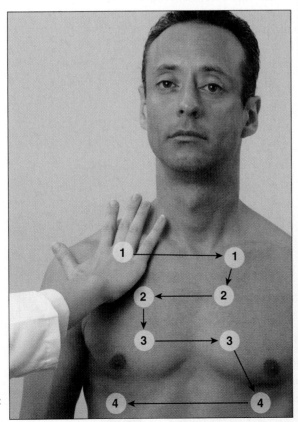

Figure 15.20
Palpation for tactile fremitus:
Anterior thorax.

TECHNIQUES AND NORMAL FINDINGS	ABNORMAL FINDINGS AND SPECIAL CONSIDERATIONS

PERCUSSION OF THE ANTERIOR THORAX

1. Visualize the landmarks.
   - Observe the anterior thorax and visualize the horizontal and vertical lines, the level of the diaphragm, and the lobes of the lungs.

2. Recall the expected findings.
   - Percussion allows assessment of underlying structures. The usual sound in the thorax is resonance.

   ▶ An unexpected sound would be hyperresonance, which is heard in conditions of overinflation of the lungs.

3. Instruct the client.
   - Explain that you will be tapping on the client's chest in a variety of areas. Tell the client to breathe normally throughout this examination.

4. Percuss the lungs.
   - Begin at the apices of the lungs. Ask the client to turn the head to the opposite side of percussion to increase the size of the surface required for placing your pleximeter finger and to avoid interference from the clavicle. Move to the chest wall and place the pleximeter in the intercostal space parallel to the ribs during percussion. Percuss the anterior chest from side to side, comparing sounds, in the intercostal spaces. Percuss to the bases and laterally to the midaxillary line (see Figure 15.21).

   ▶ Percussion of the anterior thorax will yield dull sounds over solidified or fluid-filled areas, as may exist in pleural effusion, consolidation, or tumour.

   - Percussion over bone or organs will yield flat or dull sounds. Avoid percussion over the clavicles, sternum, and ribs. Percussion over the heart will produce dullness to the left of the sternum from the third to fifth intercostal spaces. Percuss the left lung lateral to the midclavicular line. Percussion sounds in the lower left thorax change from resonance to tympany over the gastric air bubble. Percussion sounds in the right lower thorax change from resonance to dullness at the upper liver border.

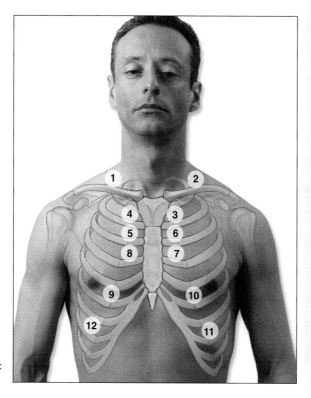

Figure 15.21 ●
Pattern for percussion:
Anterior thorax.

| TECHNIQUES AND NORMAL FINDINGS | ABNORMAL FINDINGS AND SPECIAL CONSIDERATIONS |

AUSCULTATION OF THE ANTERIOR THORAX

Auscultation is used to identify and discriminate between normal and adventitious breath sounds. Listen to the full respiratory cycle with each placement of the stethoscope (see Figure 15.22).

1. **Instruct the client.**
   - Explain that you will be listening to the client's breathing with the stethoscope. Ask the client to breathe deeply through the mouth each time the stethoscope is placed on the chest and to let you know if he or she is becoming short of breath or tired.

2. **Auscultate the trachea.**
   - Place the stethoscope over the trachea, above the suprasternal notch. You will hear tracheal breath sounds. Move the stethoscope to the left, then the right side of the trachea, just above each sternoclavicular joint. You will hear bronchial breath sounds.

3. **Auscultate the apices.**
   - Place the stethoscope in the triangular areas just superior to each clavicle. You will hear vesicular sounds.

4. **Auscultate the bronchi.**
   - The bronchi are auscultated at the second and third intercostal spaces at the left and right sternal borders. You will hear bronchovesicular sounds.

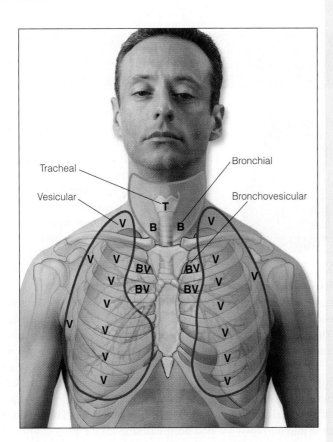

Figure 15.22 ●
Auscultatory sounds:
Anterior thorax.

TECHNIQUES AND NORMAL FINDINGS	ABNORMAL FINDINGS AND SPECIAL CONSIDERATIONS

5. Auscultate the lungs.

- Auscultate the lungs by following the pattern for percussion. Move the stethoscope from side to side as you compare sounds. Move down to the sixth intercostal space and laterally to the midaxillary line. You will hear vesicular sounds.

6. Interpret the findings.

- Refer to the descriptions and interpretations of normal and adventitious breath sounds described in auscultation of the posterior thorax (see pages 338 and 340).

SAMPLE DOCUMENTATION

Subjective: Client reports no history of cough, chest pain, dyspnea/shortness of breath, orthopnea, allergies, or Hx of resp disease. No exposure to toxins or respiratory irritants at home or at work. Nonsmoker, yearly flu shot, TB immunization up to date, and last chest X-ray 5 years ago.

Objective: *Inspection:* RR 20, chest movement symmetrical, general colour pink, no cyanosis or pallor, no signs of respiratory distress, no nasal flaring, pursed lip breathing, or use of accessory muscles. AP:T diameter 1:2.

Palpation: No tenderness, masses, or bulges on the thorax, thoracic expansion and tactile fremitus equal bilaterally, trachea midline.

Percussion: Resonance over lung tissue and diaphragmatic excursion 6 cm bilaterally.

Auscultation: Lung fields clear and no adventitious sounds.

APPLICATION THROUGH CRITICAL THINKING

CASE STUDY

Janet Noseworthy, a 14-year-old female, has been seen regularly in the clinic for chronic asthma. Today, Janet's mother has accompanied her for a checkup. Janet has required two visits to the emergency room (ER) for severe wheezing in the month since her last clinic visit.

The physical assessment revealed that the client was in no distress and breath sounds were clear. Her vital signs were B/P 126/82—P 84—RR 20. Her skin was warm, dry, and pink. Janet could speak clearly and seemed relaxed.

During the interview the nurse learned that the client has been following her prescribed treatments and has done well except for the two ER visits.

The nurse learned that each ER visit occurred after school hours. The client experienced severe shortness of breath and wheezing that was unrelieved by rest or use of her inhalers. ER treatment consisted of injection of epinephrine and administration of oxygen, IV fluids, Benadryl, and steroids. Each ER

visit lasted approximately 6 hours. The client's breathing was restored to nearly normal at discharge and she was given a prescription for a course of prednisone.

When asked if she could identify any precipitating factors, Janet replied, "I know they happened on days that we had gym, but I don't usually have a problem with that." The nurse asked if she had any changes in her routines, activities, or environments. She said, "No, not that I can think of." Her mother stated, "We're so upset. She's been out twice this month." The client then added, "Yes, I hate to have to miss school and get behind and now my friend and I have to work twice as hard as before to get our project done."

The nurse asked about the project and the client said, "We are working on an art project—collecting materials and doing a thing on textures. It's pretty cool. We collected old clothes from a second-hand store and a garage sale and we've been cutting them up sort of in a collage." The nurse asked if the work on the project coincided with her recent attacks. The client said, "Gee, I don't know, I never thought about it." Her mother stated, "Oh, we never even thought about that, but on both days, she had been working on the project after school with her friend and really got bad as the evening wore on."

ASSESSMENT FORM

REASON FOR VISIT

Scheduled monthly checkup

HISTORY

Chronic asthma, follows prescribed treatment

Two recent ER visits R/T severe wheezing

Epinephrine, IV, Benadryl, steroids—6 h stay

Discharges—prednisone—recovery—resume normal routine

Episodes R/T work with "old" clothes for school project.

ASSESSMENT

BP: 126/82   P 84   RR 20

Skin: Pink, warm, dry

Lungs: Clear—all fields

Affect: Relaxed

Speech: Clear

▶ Complete Documentation

The following is a sample documentation from assessment of Janet Noseworthy.

SUBJECTIVE DATA: Visit to clinic for a checkup, 14-year-old female with asthma. Required two ER visits for severe wheezing in month since last clinic visit. Following prescribed treatments. Doing well except ER visits. ER visits occurred on school days when client had gym, but usually no problem with physical activity. ER visits associated with work on art project—a textile collage from old clothes. Wheezing started after work on project and increased in severity requiring epinephrine, IV, Benadryl, and steroids. Client is discharged with course of oral steroids after each visit. Resumed normal treatment and activity after episodes.

OBJECTIVE DATA: Breath sounds clear. Skin warm, dry, and pink. Clear speech, relaxed. VS: B/P 126/82—P 84—RR 20.

▶ Critical Thinking Questions

1. Describe the nurse's thoughts and actions as the nurse applies the steps of the critical thinking process in this situation.
2. In interpreting the data, how would they be clustered?
3. What are the options that could be developed for this 14-year-old and her mother?

▶ Applying Nursing Diagnoses

1. Identify two NANDA-I nursing diagnoses (see Appendix A ⟨⟩) that could be derived from the data in this case study.
2. Are the data in the case study supportive of the diagnosis *ineffective breathing pattern*? Provide examples of the definition, defining characteristics, and risks or related factors of the diagnoses.

▶ Prepare Teaching Plan

LEARNING NEED: Data reveal two episodes of respiratory distress following the construction of a textile collage for a school project. Janet needs to learn more about environmental allergens as causing her respiratory distress.

GOAL: Janet will decrease the number of acute respiratory distress episodes.

OBJECTIVES: At the end of the lesson, Janet will be able to do the following:
1. Identify locations of known allergens in her environment.
2. Identify strategies to decrease her exposure to allergens.

APPLICATION OF OBJECTIVE 2: Identify strategies to decrease her exposure to allergens (cognitive).		
Content	**Teaching Strategy**	**Evaluation**
You have been able to recall your allergens and have identified environmental placement. Now you need to look for alternatives to prevent future exposure and distress. Alternative strategies could include the following: • Work in a well-ventilated area. • Plan all activities to decrease exposure to allergens. • Use clean and dry materials. • Select other substances for texture: wood, stone, plastic. Wash material before handling. • Read all labels to be sure allergens are not in the product being used. • Use objects that are allergen-free.	• One-to-one discussion to provide recall and reinforcement of learner's knowledge. • Printed material to provide review and reinforcement of material.	Name three alternative strategies to be used when completing the school project.

Health Promotion Assessment Tool

Social Determinants of Health	Level of Action	Action Strategies
Physical environment	Individual and family	**Develop personal skills** • Teach Janet and her mother about common asthma triggers that could be present on used clothing (e.g., animal hair, dust mites, or mildew).
Physical environment	Family	**Create supportive environments** • Inspect and wash all used clothes from the Salvation Army or other sources before Janet handles them.
Physical environment	Community: Patients and families who use the services of the asthma clinic and local hospital ER department	**Reorient health services** • Assess the extent of the problem within the asthma clinic population and people seeking services from the ER. Are others experiencing asthma attacks following exposure to used clothing? • Analyze the data. If this is a reoccurring issue within the community, it may warrant taking broader community-based preventive action. • Determine the best messages to help asthma patients avoid exposure to possible asthma triggers. • Develop warning posters on potential asthma triggers to display in the asthma clinic and local ER waiting room and give asthma patients tear-off sheets with the prevention messages.

Abnormal Findings

Respiratory Disorders

Asthma

A chronic hyperreactive condition resulting in bronchospasm, mucosal edema, and increased mucus secretion. Usually occurs in response to inhaled irritants or allergens (see Figure 15.23).

Inspection: Dyspnea, increased respiratory rate, use of accessory muscles, anxiety, audible wheeze, prolonged expiration.

Palpation: Decreased tactile fremitus.

Percussion: Resonance. Hyperresonance when chronic.

Auscultation: Breath sounds obscured by wheezes. Decreased voice sounds. In severe asthma, air movement may be so limited that no breath sounds are heard.

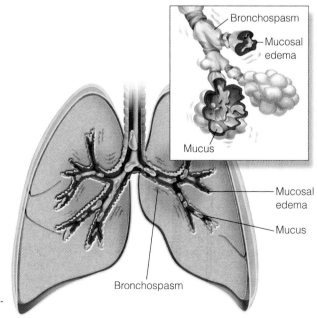

Figure 15.23 • Asthma.

Atelectasis

A condition in which there is an obstruction of airflow. The alveoli or an entire lung may collapse from airway obstruction, such as a mucus plug, lack of surfactant, or a compressed chest wall (see Figure 15.24).

Inspection: Decreased lung expansion on the affected side, increased respiratory rate, dyspnea, cyanosis. If severe, the trachea shifts to the affected side.

Palpation: Lack of tactile fremitus.

Percussion: Dullness over the affected area.

Auscultation: Decreased or absent breath sounds and voice sounds.

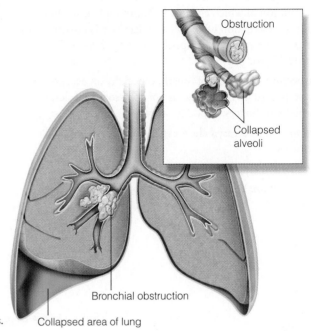

Figure 15.24 ● Atelectasis.

Chronic Bronchitis

Chronic inflammation of the tracheobronchial tree leads to increased mucus production and blocked airways. A productive cough is present (see Figure 15.25).

Inspection: Dyspnea, chronic productive cough, tachypnea, use of accessory muscles.

Palpation: Normal tactile fremitus.

Percussion: Resonance.

Auscultation: Wheezes and rhonchi may be present.

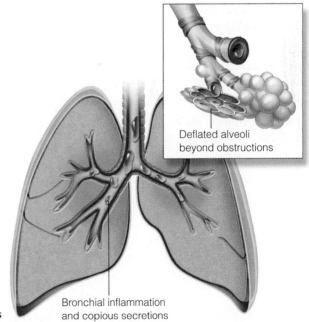

Figure 15.25 ● Chronic bronchitis

Emphysema

A condition in which chronic inflammation of the lungs leads to destruction of alveoli and decreased elasticity of the lungs. As a result, air is trapped and lungs hyperinflate (see Figure 15.26).

Inspection: Shortness of breath, especially on exertion, barrel chest, pursed lip breathing, use of accessory muscles, cyanosis, clubbing of fingers, tripod posture.

Palpation: Decreased chest expansion, decreased tactile fremitus.

Percussion: Hyperresonance.

Auscultation: Decreased vesicular sounds and possible wheeze.

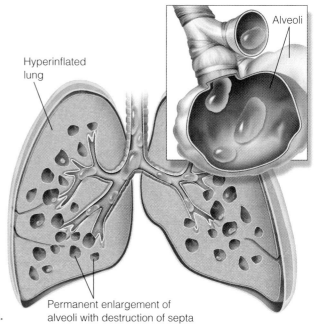

Figure 15.26 ● Emphysema.

Lobar Pneumonia

An infection causes fluid, bacteria, and cellular debris to fill the alveoli (see Figure 15.27).

Inspection: Tachypnea, productive cough, chills.

Palpation: Increased tactile fremitus. Decreased chest expansion of the affected side.

Percussion: Dullness over the affected area.

Auscultation: Bronchophony, egophony, whispered pectoriloquy. Bronchial breath sounds and crackles.

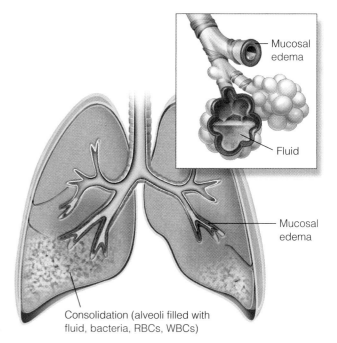

Figure 15.27 ● Lobar pneumonia.

Pleural Effusion

In this condition, fluid accumulates in the pleural space (see Figure 15.28).

Inspection: Dyspnea. In severe effusion, tracheal shift to the unaffected side.

Palpation: Decreased tactile fremitus and chest expansion on the affected side.

Percussion: Dullness over the fluid.

Auscultation: Breath sounds and voice sounds decreased or absent. Possible pleural rub.

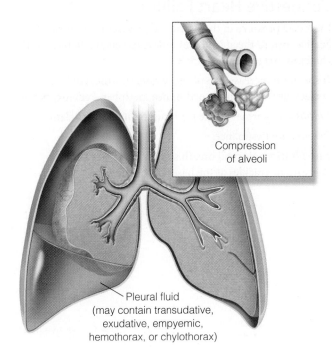

Compression of alveoli

Pleural fluid (may contain transudative, exudative, empyemic, hemothorax, or chylothorax)

Figure 15.28 ● Pleural effusion.

Pneumothorax

A condition in which air moves into the pleural space and causes partial or complete collapse of the lung. Pneumothorax can be spontaneous, traumatic, or tension (see Figure 15.29).

Inspection: Tachypnea, decreased expansion of the chest wall on the affected side, tracheal shift to the unaffected side.

Palpation: Decreased tactile fremitus.

Percussion: Hyperresonance.

Auscultation: Breath sounds and voice sounds are decreased or absent.

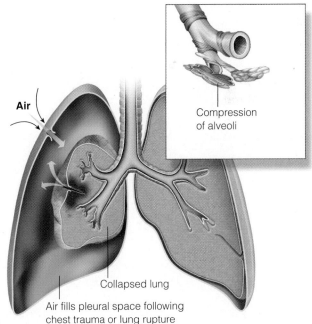

Air

Compression of alveoli

Collapsed lung

Air fills pleural space following chest trauma or lung rupture

Figure 15.29 ● Pneumothorax.

Congestive Heart Failure

Increased pressure in the pulmonary veins causes interstitial edema around the alveoli and may cause edema of the bronchial mucosa (see Figure 15.30).

Inspection: Increased respiratory rate, shortness of breath (especially on exertion), orthopnea, peripheral edema, pallor.

Palpation: Normal tactile fremitus. Skin cool and clammy.

Percussion: Resonance.

Auscultation: Normal breath sounds and voice sounds. Wheezes or crackles at the bases of the lungs.

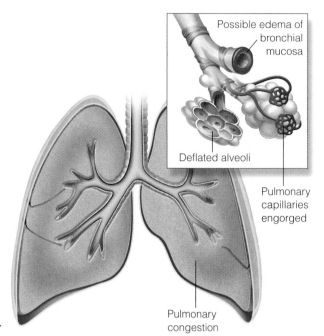

Possible edema of bronchial mucosa

Deflated alveoli

Pulmonary capillaries engorged

Pulmonary congestion

Figure 15.30 ● Congestive heart failure.

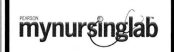

16

BREASTS AND AXILLAE

CHAPTER OBJECTIVES

On completion of this chapter, you will be able to

1. Relate knowledge of anatomy and physiology to the physical examination of a client.
2. Identify landmarks that guide assessment of the breasts and axillae.
3. Relate knowledge of the principles of communication to the health history interview.
4. Conduct a health history interview that represents a comprehensive account of the client's physical and psychosocial health status in relation to the breasts and axillae.
5. Explain client preparation for assessment of the breasts and axillae.
6. Describe the different assessment techniques required for examination of the breasts and axillae.
7. Perform a physical examination of a client's breasts and axillae by using appropriate equipment and assessment techniques.
8. Differentiate between normal and abnormal findings in assessment of the breasts and axillae.
9. Describe developmental, psychosocial, ethnocultural, and environmental variations in assessment techniques and findings in relation to the breasts and axillae.
10. Apply critical thinking in selected situations related to assessment of the breasts and axillae.
11. Document findings of the breast and axillary examination by using appropriate terminology.

CHAPTER OUTLINE

ACCORDING TO THE CANADIAN CANCER SOCIETY (2009), breast cancer is the most common cancer among Canadian women. In 2009, it was estimated that 22 700 women would be diagnosed with breast cancer and 5400 would die of it. On average, 437 Canadian women every week are diagnosed with breast cancer, and every week 104 die. One in 9 women will develop breast cancer, and 1 in 28 will die of it. Although these statistics appear discouraging, breast cancer mortality has declined overall and for each age group since the 1990s, largely because of mammography screening and improved treatments for breast cancer. The use of screening programs that detect tumours before they become clinically apparent is beneficial, and a thorough breast examination is a part of that screening process (see Table 16.1 for screening guidelines).

The assessment of the breasts and axillae begins with a thorough health history. During the health history, the nurse gathers additional information by asking pertinent questions relating to the client's general health and breast and lymph nodes in particular. The physical assessment of the breasts may be incorporated into the total body assessment, along with the heart and lung assessment, when the client is sitting and again when supine. Although the majority of the material in this chapter assumes that the client is female, it was estimated that 180 men would be diagnosed with breast cancer in 2009 and 50 would die of it (Canadian Cancer Society, 2009). It is important to incorporate assessment of the male client's breasts during the physical assessment, usually when assessing the thorax.

Accurate knowledge of the structure and function of the breasts and lymphatic system is necessary to carry out the assessment activities related to the breasts and axillae. It is also important that the nurse understand the interrelationships of the various body systems that contribute to this region. For example, the musculoskeletal system supports the overlying integument, and the lymphatic system drains the region. In addition, while performing the assessment, the nurse must keep in mind the normal variations for the client's developmental stage. An understanding and acceptance of different individuals' feelings, beliefs, and practices regarding the breasts and breast care are also essential.

ANATOMY AND PHYSIOLOGY REVIEW

The breasts are located on the anterior chest and supported by muscles and ligaments. The breast includes the areola and nipple, as well as the glandular, adipose, and fibrous tissue. A system of lymph nodes drains lymph from the breasts and axillae. These tissues and structures are described in the following paragraphs.

Breasts

The breasts are paired mammary glands located on the anterior chest wall. Breast tissue extends from the second or third rib to the sixth or seventh rib and from the sternal margin to the midaxillary line, depending on body shape and size (see Figure 16.1). The

TABLE 16.1	Breast Cancer Screening Guidelines
IF YOU ARE	**YOU SHOULD**
40 to 49	Have a clinical breast examination by a trained healthcare professional at least every 2 years.
	Talk to your doctor about your risk of breast cancer, along with the benefits and risks of mammography.
50 to 69	Have a clinical breast examination by a trained healthcare professional at least every 2 years.
	Have a mammogram every 2 years.
70 or older	Talk to your doctor about how often you should be tested for breast cancer.

Source: Canadian Cancer Society. (2009). *Breast cancer.* Retrieved from http://www.cancer.ca/Ontario/Prevention/Get%20 screened/Early%20detection%20and%20screening%20for%20breast%20cancer.aspx?sc_lang=en&r=1

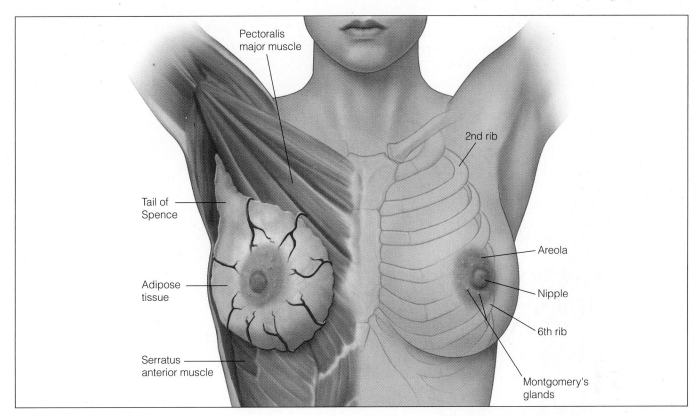

Pectoralis
major muscle

2nd rib

Tail of
Spence

Areola

Adipose
tissue

Nipple

6th rib

Serratus
anterior muscle

Montgomery's
glands

Figure 16.1 • Anatomy of the breast.

breasts lie anterior to the pectoralis major and serratus anterior muscles. The nipple is centrally located within a circular pigmented field of wrinkled skin called the **areola**.

The surface of the areola is speckled with tiny sebaceous glands known as **Montgomery's glands** (or Montgomery's tubercles; see Figure 16.2). Hair follicles are normally seen around the periphery of the areola. Commonly, breast tissue extends superiolaterally into the axilla as the **axillary tail** (tail of Spence). The internal and lateral thoracic arteries and cutaneous branches of the posterior intercostal arteries provide an abundant supply of blood to the breasts.

Breasts are composed of glandular, fibrous, and adipose (fat) tissue. The glandular tissue is arranged into 15 to 20 lobes per breast that radiate from the nipple (see Figure 16.3). Each lobe is composed of 20 to 40 lobules that contain the **acini cells** (or alveoli) that produce milk. These cells empty into the lactiferous ducts, which carry milk from each lobe to the nipple. The fibrous tissue provides support for the glandular tissue. **Suspensory ligaments** (Cooper's ligaments) extend from the connective tissue layer through the breast and attach to the fascia underlying the breast. Subcutaneous and retromammary adipose tissue make up the remainder of the breast. The proportions of these three components vary with age, the general state of the client's health, menstrual cycle, pregnancy, lactation, and other factors. Supernumerary nipples or breast tissue may be present along the **mammary ridge**, or "milk line," which extends from each axilla to the groin (see Figure 16.4). Usually this tissue atrophies during development, but occasionally a nipple persists and is visible. It needs to be differentiated from a mole (see Figure 16.5). For the purpose of documenting

assessment findings, the breast is divided into four quadrants, defined by a vertical line and a horizontal line that intersect at the nipple (see Figure 16.6 on page 357). The location of clinical findings may be described according to clock positions, for example, at the 2-o'clock position, 5 cm (2 in.) from the nipple. The male breast is composed of a small nipple and flat areola. These are superior to a thin disc of undeveloped breast tissue that may not be distinguishable from the surrounding tissues. The major functions of the female breasts include producing, storing, and supplying milk for the process of lactation. Breasts also provide a mechanism for sexual arousal.

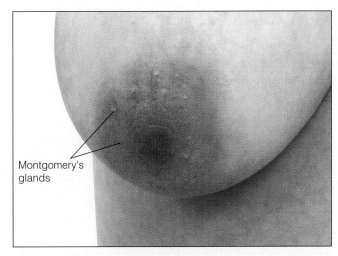

Montgomery's
glands

Figure 16.2 • Montgomery's glands.

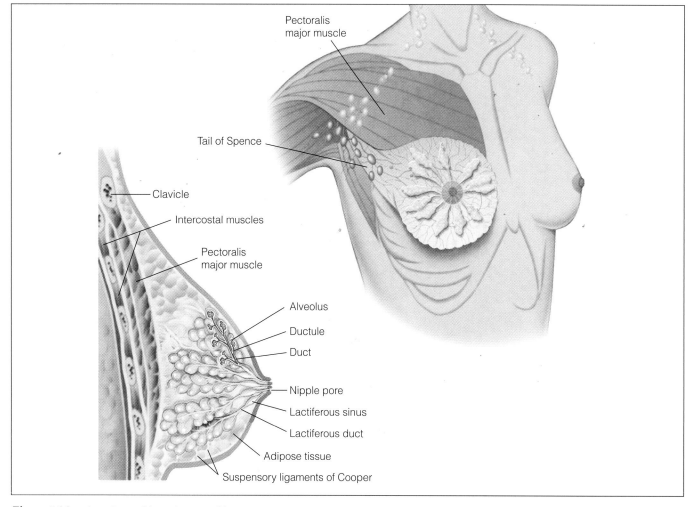

Figure 16.3 ● Anterior and lateral views of breast anatomy.

Axillae and Lymph Nodes

A complex system of lymph nodes drains lymph from the breasts and axillae and returns it to the blood. Superficial lymph nodes drain the skin, and deep lymph nodes drain the mammary lobules. Figure 16.7 depicts the groups of nodes that drain the breasts and axillae.

The lymph nodes are usually nonpalpable. The following nodes are palpated during the assessment.

1. Internal mammary nodes
2. Supraclavicular nodes
3. Subclavicular (infraclavicular) nodes

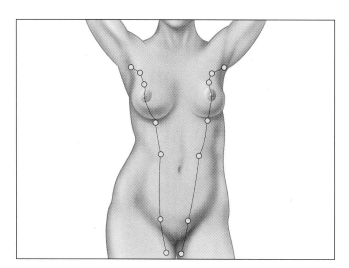

Figure 16.4 ● Mammary ridge.

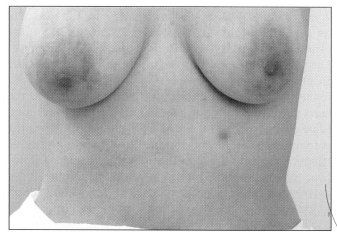

Figure 16.5 ● Supernumerary nipple.

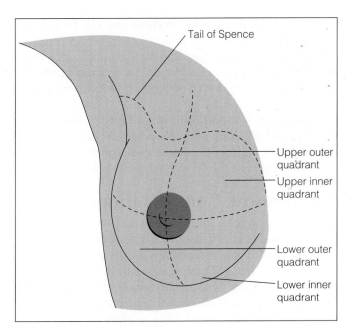

Figure 16.6 ● Breast quadrants.

4. Interpectoral nodes
5. Central axillary nodes
6. Brachial (lateral axillary) nodes
7. Subscapular (posterior axillary) nodes
8. Anterior pectoral (anterior axillary) nodes

The internal mammary nodes drain toward the abdomen and the opposite breast. Most of the lymph from the rest of the breast drains toward the axilla and subclavicular region. Thus, a cancerous lesion can spread via the lymphatic system to the subclavicular nodes, into deep channels within the chest or abdomen, and even to the opposite breast. The male breast has

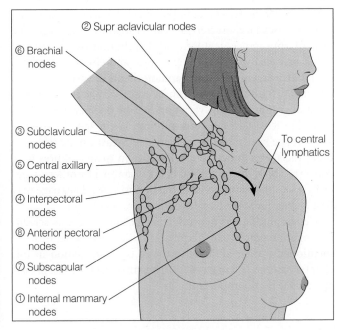

Figure 16.7 ● Lymphatic drainage of the breast.

the same potential and needs to be examined as well. The major functions of the lymphatic system include returning water and proteins from the interstitial spaces to the blood, thus helping to maintain blood osmotic pressure and body fluid balance. It also helps filter out microorganisms and other body debris.

Muscles of the Chest Wall

The major muscles of the chest wall, which support the breast and contribute to its shape, are the pectoralis major and serratus anterior muscles (Figure 16.1). The overall contour of the breasts is determined by the suspensory ligaments, which provide support. The major function of the muscles of the chest wall is to support breast and lymphatic tissue.

SPECIAL CONSIDERATIONS

Age, developmental level, race, ethnicity, work history, living conditions, socioeconomics, and emotional well-being are among the factors that influence breast health. These factors must be considered when collecting subjective and objective data during the comprehensive health assessment. The nurse applies critical thinking to assess the client's state of health and to identify the factors that may influence breast health.

The Male Breast

Men have breast tissue just as women do, and they can develop breast cancer. In Canada, less than 1% of all breast cancer occurs in men (Canadian Cancer Society, 2009). Breast cancer is most commonly diagnosed in men over 60 years of age but can be found in men of all ages. As such, examination of the breast should be performed on all men, and assessment techniques are discussed further in this chapter.

Developmental Considerations

Growth and development are dynamic processes that describe change over time. The following discussion presents specific variations of the breasts for different age groups.

Infants and Children

The breast tissue of newborns is sometimes swollen because of the hyperestrogenism of pregnancy. Some infants may produce a thin discharge called "witch's milk." This secretion subsides as the infant's body eliminates maternal hormones.

Breast tissue starts to enlarge in females with the onset of puberty, usually between the ages of 9 and 13. At first there is only a bud around the nipple and areola, which may be tender initially. The ductile system matures, extensive fat deposits occur, and the areola and nipples grow and become pigmented. These changes are correlated with an increased level of estrogen and progesterone in the body as sexual maturity progresses. Growth of the breasts is not necessarily steady or symmetrical, which may be frustrating or embarrassing to some girls. Because a female's primary sexual organs cannot be observed, breast development provides visual confirmation that the adolescent is becoming a woman. For the developing adolescent, her breasts are a visible symbol of her feminine identity and an important part of her body image and self-esteem. The nurse can reassure girls that the rate of breast tissue growth depends on changing hormone levels and is uniquely individual, as are the eventual size and shape of the breasts.

Benign fibroadenomas in adolescent females are not uncommon. The nurse should reassure the girl and her parents or caregivers that no correlation has been established between fibroadenomas and malignant cancers. In most cases, only one fibroadenoma is found. Occasionally, there are several detected and they sometimes occur in both breasts. Fibroadenomas vary in size and may grow over time but do not become malignant. The cause of fibroadenomas is unknown.

Adolescent males may experience temporary breast enlargement, called **gynecomastia,** in one or both breasts. It is usually self-limiting and resolves spontaneously. Another concern to adolescent males is transient masses beneath one areola or both. These "breast buds" usually disappear within a year of onset.

The Pregnant Female

During pregnancy, breast tissue enlarges as glandular and ductal tissue increases in preparation for lactation. During the second month of pregnancy, nipples and areolae darken and enlarge. The degree of pigmentation varies with complexion. Nipples may leak **colostrum** in the month before childbirth. As breast tissue enlarges, venous networks may be more pronounced.

During pregnancy breast tissue will be firmer, larger, and possibly tender. Most breasts have a normal pattern of lumpiness or nodularity caused by the complex milk gland structure of the breasts and the effects female hormones have on these glands. The areolae and nipples are usually darker.

The Older Adult

More time may be required for the health history of an older client. Many people have a difficult time talking about something as private as the breasts, and older adults may be even less comfortable with this topic. They may be modest and self-conscious, or they may feel that the nurse is too young to understand. There may also be cultural taboos about such private matters. The nurse should acknowledge that talking about the breasts may be somewhat uncomfortable but explain that sharing this information will promote the client's health.

Older adults may have limited range of motion. If so, the client should be asked to raise her arms to a height that does not cause discomfort. Because the older adult may have failing eyesight, pamphlets and handouts with large print should be provided.

As menopause approaches, glandular tissue decreases and is replaced by fatty tissue. The lobular texture of glandular tissue is replaced by a finer, granular texture. Breasts are less firm and tend to be more pendulous. As the suspensory ligaments relax, breast tissue hangs more loosely from the chest wall. The nipples become smaller and flatter and lose some erectile ability. The mammary ridge thickens and can be palpated more easily.

Gynecomastia may occur in older adult males as a result of hormonal changes caused by disease or medication. The nurse must be sensitive to possible embarrassment during the exam.

Most women who develop breast cancer have no risk factors other than simply being a woman and getting older (especially being over 50). Older adults should speak with their healthcare provider about their risk factors and breast-health screening.

Psychosocial Considerations

A client's overall sense of self-esteem may be reflected in the way she feels about her breasts. In fact, some women may view their breasts as a badge of femininity. Media portrayal of idealized images of "perfect" breasts, especially by advertisers, may increase this feeling. Thus, clients whose breasts are smaller or larger than average, clients with asymmetrical breasts, and clients who have had a mastectomy or other breast surgery or trauma are at an increased risk for body image disturbance, self-esteem disturbance, and dysfunctional grieving.

Some women may not seek medical attention after discovering a breast lump. This behaviour may be related to anxiety and fear of cancer or surgery, a body image change, or a change in significant relationships. Other factors may include denial, feelings of powerlessness, or a lack of knowledge about breast disorders. During the assessment of the breasts and axillae, the nurse needs to encourage the client to share her fears and concerns. Research indicates that a high-fat diet especially after menopause may increase a female's risk of developing breast cancer. Excessive alcohol intake has also been implicated.

Social and Ethnocultural Considerations

The nurse must be aware of variations in breast development related to ethnicity. For example, Black females may develop secondary sexual characteristics earlier than white females. The time of appearance, texture, and distribution of axillary and pubic hair also vary according to race and ethnicity. Feelings of embarrassment may differ among clients of various cultural or religious groups. Breast cancer rates vary across different cultural groups, but this variation may be due partly to differences in diet or alcohol consumption. White females over 40 years of age have a higher incidence of breast cancer than any other racial or ethnic groups. Females in many cultures have concerns about disrobing and being examined by others, especially when the examiner is of the opposite sex. Language may be a barrier for some females of immigrant cultures.

Geographic factors may influence a client's access to screening mammography and regular physical examinations. As mentioned earlier, although most of the information in this chapter assumes a female client, assessment of the male breasts and axillae is also important.

GATHERING THE DATA

Breast health assessment includes the gathering of subjective and objective data. Subjective data collection occurs during the client interview, before the actual physical assessment. During the interview the nurse uses a variety of communication techniques to elicit general and specific information about the client's state of breast health or illness. Health records, the results of laboratory tests, mammography, and other diagnostic imaging are important secondary sources to be reviewed and included in the data-gathering process. During physical assessment of the breasts and axillae, the techniques of inspection and palpation will be used. Before proceeding, it may be helpful to review the information about each of the data-gathering processes and practise the techniques of health assessment.

HEALTH HISTORY

The health history for the breasts and axillae concerns data related to the structures and functions of the breasts and lymphatic system. Subjective data related to breast health are gathered during the health history. The nurse must be prepared to observe the client and listen for cues related to the breasts and axillae. The nurse may use open-ended or closed questions to obtain information. Often a number of follow-up questions or requests for descriptions are required to clarify data or gather missing information. Follow-up questions are aimed at identifying the source of problems, duration of difficulties, measures to alleviate problems, and clues about the client's knowledge of his or her own health. The subjective data collected and the questions asked during the health history provide information to help meet the goals of improving breast health and preventing and controlling breast disease.

The health history guides physical assessment of the breasts and axillae. The information is always considered in relation to norms and expectations about breast and lymphatic function. Therefore, the nurse must consider age, gender, race, culture, environment, and health practices, as well as past and concurrent problems and therapies, when framing questions and using techniques to elicit information. To address all the factors when conducting a health history, specific questions related to the breasts and axillae examination have been developed. These questions focus on the most common concerns or injuries associated with the breasts and axillae examination; questions related to past health history; questions related to behaviours; questions that address environmental concerns; and those that are specific to clients according to age, including the pregnant female.

The nurse must consider the client's ability to participate in the health history and physical assessment of the breasts and axillae. If a client is experiencing discomfort, pain, or anxiety related to the breast, attention must focus on relief of the problems.

As the nurse gathers the data, she or he will shift the type of questions to direct questions that give the client room to explain or qualify. The mnemonic O-P-Q-R-S-T-U, which stands for onset (chronology), precipitating (or palliative), quality, region (or radiation), severity, timing, and understanding, will help the learner remember the dimensions of the symptoms. The nurse will keep in mind that not all these qualifiers will apply to each symptom.

HEALTH HISTORY QUESTIONS

RATIONALES

The following sections provide sample questions and follow-up questions. Rationales for some questions are provided. The list of questions is not all-inclusive but rather represents the more common concern or injury questions required in a health history related to the breasts and axillae system. An example of using O-P-Q-R-S-T-U with pain is provided.

Questions Related to Common Concerns or Injuries

The most common concerns related to illness or injury of the breast and axillae are as follows:

- Pain
- Mass or swelling
- Nipple changes and discharge
- Changes in skin over the breast

HEALTH HISTORY QUESTIONS	RATIONALES

GATHERING THE DATA

1. **Pain**
   - Are you having any pain at this time? *If yes:*
   - When did you first notice the pain? How long does it last? Have you experienced any trauma to the breast? *Onset (chronology)*
   - What makes the pain worse? better? *Precipitating (palliative)*
   - Can you describe the pain? Is it sharp? dull? burning? *Quality*
   - Where is the pain located? Does the pain radiate? Is it in both breasts? *Radiation*
   - How often do you experience the pain? How would you rate the pain on a scale of 1 to 10, with 10 being the worst pain? *Severity*
   - Is the pain associated with changes in nipple size? nipple discharge? breast mass? menstrual cycle? *Timing*
   - What do you think is causing the pain? *Understanding*

▶ Pain is not typically found in breast cancer. Rapid growing cysts may be painful. Trauma, such as that from contact sports or automobile accidents, can cause bruising of the breast.

2. **Mass or swelling**
   - Have you noticed any changes in breast size, symmetry, shape, or colour? *If yes:*

   - When did you first notice the change?
   - Is there any pain associated with the mass or changes?

▶ A lump may indicate a benign cyst, a fibroadenoma, fatty necrosis, or a malignant tumour.

▶ A lump or swelling that coincides with the menstrual or premenstrual cycle is common. "Lumpy breasts" occurring monthly before the onset of menses and resolving at the end of menstruation may be due to a benign condition called physiological nodularity.

   - Is there any discharge associated with the mass or changes?

▶ Discharge associated with a breast mass is suggestive of a neoplasm.

3. **Nipple changes and discharge**
   - Have you noticed any changes in nipple and areola characteristics? *If yes:*
   - Describe the changes.

▶ Eczematous changes of the skin of the nipple and areola may indicate mammary Paget's disease, a rare form of breast cancer.

   - Have you noticed any nipple discharge? *If yes:*
   - Is it from one or both nipples?

▶ Unilateral discharge is suggestive of benign breast disease, an intraductal papilloma, or cancer.

   - Describe the discharge.

▶ Nipple discharge resulting from medication is usually clear. A bloody drainage is always a concern and needs to be further evaluated, especially in the presence of a lump.

   - Are these changes or discharge associated with a breast mass? nipple retraction? breast tenderness?

4. **Changes in skin over the breast**
   - Have you noticed any changes in the skin characteristics over the breast?

▶ Dimpling of the skin or retraction of the nipple suggests cancer.

Questions Related to Past Health History

1. **History of breast cancer**
   - Have you ever had any breast disease, such as cancer, fibrocystic breast disease, benign breast disease, or fibroadenoma?

▶ A history of breast cancer poses the risk of recurrence. Both fibroadenoma and the general lumpiness of fibrocystic breast disease need to be differentiated from cancer.

   - Have you had cancer in any other region of your body, such as the uterus, ovaries, or colon?

▶ A history of these cancers increases the risk for breast cancer.

HEALTH HISTORY QUESTIONS	RATIONALES

- Has your mother or sister had breast cancer?

▶ If the client's mother or sister had breast cancer, the client is at greater risk, especially if the cancer occurred before menopause.

- Has one of your grandmothers or an aunt had breast cancer?

▶ If the client's grandmother or aunt had breast cancer, the client is at slightly greater risk.

Questions Related to Behaviours

Healthcare behaviours include both health practices and health patterns. Health practices consist of following recommendations for disease prevention, including screening for risks, screening for early detection of problems, and immunization. Health patterns are habits or acts that affect the client's health. Health behaviours may also include seeking healthcare from healthcare providers who use alternative methods to diagnose and treat illness. Clients should be questioned in a nonjudgmental way and areas for health teaching should be identified.

1. **Do you exercise?**
   - If so, describe your routine.
   - What kind of bra do you wear when you exercise?

▶ Firm support of breast tissue is recommended during exercise to prevent loss of tissue elasticity.

2. **Have you ever had a mammogram?**
   - If so, when was your most recent one?

3. **Do you see your healthcare provider regularly for a physical examination?**

▶ Clinical breast exams are an important part of breast cancer screening.

Questions Related to the Environment

Environment refers to both internal and external environments. Questions related to the internal environment include all the previous questions and those associated with internal or physiological responses. Questions regarding the external environment include those related to home, work, or social environments.

Internal Environment

1. **What medications are you presently taking?**

▶ Hormone replacement therapy is associated with an increased risk of cancer. Females taking these drugs need to be monitored carefully.

2. **How do you feel about your breasts?**

▶ Answers to this question may reveal a body image disturbance, self-esteem disturbance, dysfunctional grieving (in a female who has had a mastectomy), or ineffective breastfeeding (in a lactating female).

3. **How old were you when you started to menstruate?**

▶ Clients with a history of menarche before age 12 are at greater risk for breast cancer.

4. **Do you have children?** *If yes:*
   - How old were you when they were born?

▶ Females who have never had children or who had their first child after age 30 are at greater risk for breast cancer.

5. **Have you gone through menopause?**
   - If so, at what age?
   - Were there any residual problems?

▶ Females who undergo menopause after the age of 55 are at greater risk for breast cancer. Postmenopausal weight gain may increase risk of breast cancer. After menopause, decreased estrogen levels may result in decreased firmness of breast tissue. The client should be reassured that this is normal.

GATHERING THE DATA

HEALTH HISTORY QUESTIONS	RATIONALES
6. **Have you been treated with hormone therapy during or since menopause?**	▶ Combined hormone replacement therapy places clients at increased risk for breast cancer.
7. **Describe your weight from childhood up until now.** • Describe your dietary intake.	▶ Obesity is considered a predisposing factor in breast cancer.

External Environment

The following questions deal with the physical environment of the client. That includes the indoor and outdoor environments of the home and the workplace, those encountered for social engagements, and any encountered during travel.

1. **Have you been exposed to any environmental carcinogens, such as benzene or asbestos, or to excessive radiation, such as frequent repeated X-rays?**	▶ Such exposures increase the risk of breast cancer.

Questions Related to Age

The health history must reflect the anatomical and physiological differences that exist along the age span.

Questions Regarding Preadolescents

1. **Have you noticed any changes in the size or shape of your breasts?** • If so, tell me about these changes.	▶ Growth of the breasts is not necessarily steady or symmetrical. This fact may be frustrating or embarrassing to some girls. The nurse should, if appropriate, reassure the client that her breast development is normal.
2. **How do you feel about your breasts and the way they are changing?**	▶ Breast development provides visual confirmation that the pubescent female is becoming a woman. For the developing pubescent female, her breasts are a visible symbol of her feminine identity and an important part of her body image and self-esteem. Girls should be reassured that the rate of growth of breast tissue depends on changing hormone levels and is uniquely individual, as are the eventual size and shape of the breasts. The nurse can reassure males that breast enlargement is generally temporary and occurs in response to hormonal changes.

Questions for the Pregnant Female

1. **What changes in your breasts have you noticed since your last examination?**	▶ The breasts continue to change throughout pregnancy. Some expected changes are increased size, sense of fullness or tingling, prominent veins, darkened areolae, and a more erect nipple. Colostrum, a thick, yellowish discharge, may be expressed from the breasts in the final weeks of pregnancy. The client should be reassured that all these changes are normal.

Questions for the Older Adult

All the preceding questions apply to the menopausal and postmenopausal client.

▶ It is important to obtain information from the older client because the incidence of breast cancer and mortality rates increase with age.

PHYSICAL ASSESSMENT

ASSESSMENT TECHNIQUES AND FINDINGS

Physical assessment of the breasts and axillae requires the use of inspection and palpation. During each of the procedures, the nurse is gathering data related to the breasts and axillae. Inspection includes looking at skin colour, structures of the breast, and the appearance of the axillae. Knowledge of norms or expected findings is essential in determining the meaning of the data.

Adult breasts are generally symmetrical, although one breast is typically slightly larger than the other. The areolae should be round or oval and nearly equal in size. The nipples are the same colour as the areolae. The nipples are in the centre of the breast, point outward and upward, and are free of discharge, ulcerations, and crust. The breasts should move away from the chest wall symmetrically and with ease. The texture of the skin is smooth and the breast tissue is slightly granular. The axillae are clean and hair is present or removed. The skin is moist. Lymph nodes are nonpalpable.

Physical assessment of the breasts and axillae follows an organized pattern. It begins with a client survey, followed by inspection of the breasts while the client assumes a variety of positions. Palpation includes the entire surface of each breast, including the tail of Spence, and the lymph nodes of the axillae.

EQUIPMENT

examination gown and drape
clean, nonsterile examination gloves
small pillow or rolled towel
metric ruler

HELPFUL HINTS

* Provide an environment that is warm, comfortable, and private to relieve client anxiety.
* Provide specific instructions to the client; state whether the client must sit, stand, or lie down during a procedure.
* Exposure of the breasts is uncomfortable for many females. Use draping techniques to maintain the client's dignity.
* Explore cultural and language barriers at the onset of the interaction.
* Nonsterile examination gloves may be required to prevent infection when clients have lesions or drainage in and around the breasts.
* Use routine practices.

TECHNIQUES AND NORMAL FINDINGS

ABNORMAL FINDINGS AND SPECIAL CONSIDERATIONS

INSPECTION OF THE BREAST

1. **Instruct the client.**
   * Explain to the client that you will be examining her breasts in a variety of ways. First, you will have the client sit and then assume several positions that move the breasts away from the chest wall so that differences in size, shape, symmetry, contour, and colour can be detected. Inform the client that she will then lie down and you will examine each breast by palpating the breast tissue and nipple. Also be sure to examine her axillae. Explain the purpose of each examination in terms the client will understand. Tell the client that none of the examinations should be painful; however, she must inform you of any tenderness or discomfort as the examination proceeds.

2. **Position the client.**
   * The client should sit comfortably and erect, with the gown at the waist so both breasts are exposed (see Figure 16.8).

PHYSICAL ASSESSMENT

<table>
<tr><td>

TECHNIQUES AND NORMAL FINDINGS

</td><td>

ABNORMAL FINDINGS AND SPECIAL CONSIDERATIONS

</td></tr>
</table>

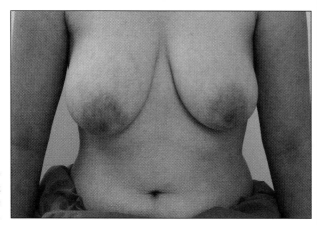

Figure 16.8 ● The client is seated at the beginning of the breast examination.

3. Inspect and compare size and symmetry of the breasts.
   - One breast may normally be slightly larger than the other.

▶ Obvious masses, flattening of the breast in one area, dimpling, or recent increase in the size of one breast may indicate abnormal growth or inflammation.

4. Inspect for skin colour.
   - Colour should be consistent with the rest of the body. Observe for thickening, tautness, redness, rash, or ulceration.

▶ Inflamed skin is red and warm. Edema from blocked lymphatic drainage in advanced cancer causes an "orange peel" appearance called **peau d'orange** (see Figure 16.9).

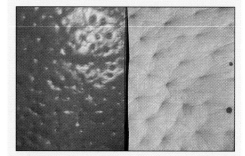

Figure 16.9 ● Left, orange peel; Right, peau d'orange sign.

▶ Pronounced unilateral venous patterns may indicate increased blood flow to a malignancy.

5. Inspect for venous patterns.
   - Venous patterns are the same bilaterally. Venous patterns may be more predominant in pregnancy or obesity.

6. Inspect for moles or other markings.
   - Moles that are unchanged, nontender, and longstanding are of no concern. Striae that are present in pregnancy or after recent weight loss or gain may appear purple. Striae become silvery white over time.

▶ Moles that have changed or appear suddenly require further evaluation. A mole along the milk line may be a supernumerary nipple (Figure 16.5).

7. Inspect the areolae.
   - The areolae are normally round or oval and almost equal in size. Areolae are pink in light-skinned people and brown in dark-skinned people. The areolae darken in pregnancy.

▶ Peau d'orange associated with cancer may be first seen on the areolae. Redness and fissures may develop with breastfeeding.

PHYSICAL ASSESSMENT

| TECHNIQUES AND NORMAL FINDINGS | ABNORMAL FINDINGS AND SPECIAL CONSIDERATIONS |

8. Inspect the nipples.

- Nipples are normally the same colour as the areolae and are equal in size and shape. Nipples are generally everted but may be flat or inverted. Nipples should point in the same direction outward and slightly upward. Nipples should be free of cracks, crust, erosions, ulcerations, pigment changes, or discharge.

▶ Recent retraction or inversion of a nipple or change in the direction of the nipple is suggestive of malignancy. Discharge requires cytological examination. A red, scaly eczema-like area over the nipple could indicate mammary Paget's disease, a rare type of breast cancer. The area may exude fluid, scale, or crust (see Figure 16.10).

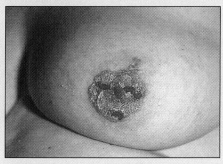

Figure 16.10 ● Mammary Paget's disease of the nipple.

9. Observe the breasts for shape, surface characteristics, and bilateral pull of suspensory ligaments.

- Ask the client to assume the following positions while you continue to inspect the breasts.

10. Inspect with the client's arms over the head (see Figure 16.11).

▶ Dimpling of the skin over a mass is usually a visible sign of breast cancer. Dimpling is accentuated in this position. Variations in contour and symmetry may also indicate breast cancer.

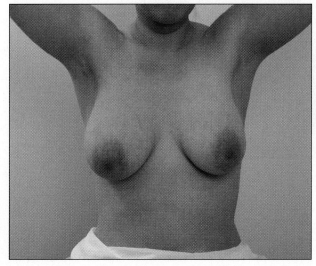

Figure 16.11 ● Inspection of the breasts with the client's arms above her head.

TECHNIQUES AND NORMAL FINDINGS

ABNORMAL FINDINGS AND SPECIAL CONSIDERATIONS

11. Inspect with the client's hands pressed against her waist (see Figure 16.12).

▶ Tightening of the pectoral muscles may help to accentuate dimpling.

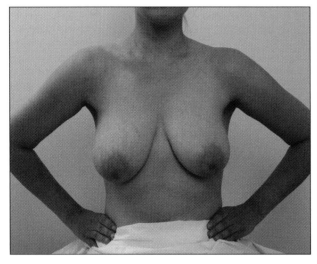

Figure 16.12 ● Inspection of the breasts with the client's hands pressed against her waist.

12. Inspect with the client's hands pressed together at the level of the waist (see Figure 16.13).

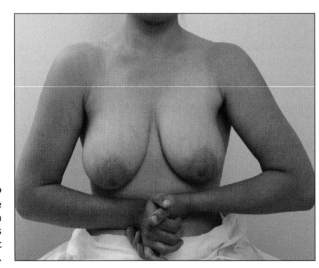

Figure 16.13 ● Inspection of the breasts with the client's hands pressed together at the level of her waist.

TECHNIQUES AND NORMAL FINDINGS	ABNORMAL FINDINGS AND SPECIAL CONSIDERATIONS

13. Inspect with the client leaning forward from the waist (see Figure 16.14).
   - The breasts normally fall freely and evenly from the chest.

▶ Breast cancer should be suspected if the breasts do not fall freely from the chest.

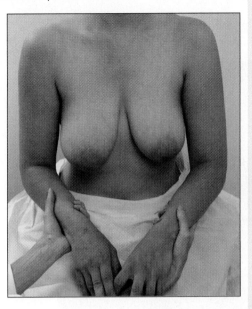

Figure 16.14 ● Assisting the client to lean forward for inspection.

PALPATION OF THE BREAST

1. **Position the client.**
   - Ask the client to lie down. Cover the breast that is not being examined. Place a small pillow or rolled towel under the shoulder of the side to be palpated and position the client's arm over her head. This manoeuvre flattens the breast tissue over the chest wall.

2. **Instruct the client.**
   - Explain that you will be touching the entire breast and nipple. Tell the client to inform you of any discomfort or tenderness.

3. **Palpate skin texture.**
   - Skin texture should be smooth, with uninterrupted contour.

▶ Thickening of the skin suggests an underlying carcinoma.

4. **Palpate the breast.**
   - Use the fingerpads of the first three fingers in a slightly rotary motion to press the breast tissue against the chest wall. Be sure to palpate the entire breast. Several patterns can be used, but the most common is the concentric circle pattern (see Figure 16.15).

▶ The incidence of breast cancers is highest in the upper outer quadrant, including the axillary tail. Masses in the tail must be distinguished from enlarged lymph nodes.

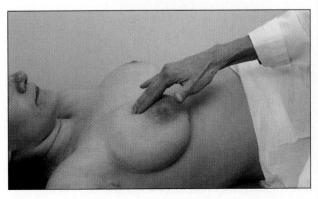

Figure 16.15 ●
Palpating the breast.

<table>
<tr><td>

TECHNIQUES AND NORMAL FINDINGS

</td><td>

ABNORMAL FINDINGS AND
SPECIAL CONSIDERATIONS

</td></tr>
</table>

- Start at the periphery of the breast and palpate in small circles until you reach the nipple. Try not to lift the fingerpads off the breast as you move from one area to another.

- An alternative pattern used during palpation is the back and forth technique (see Figure 16.16).

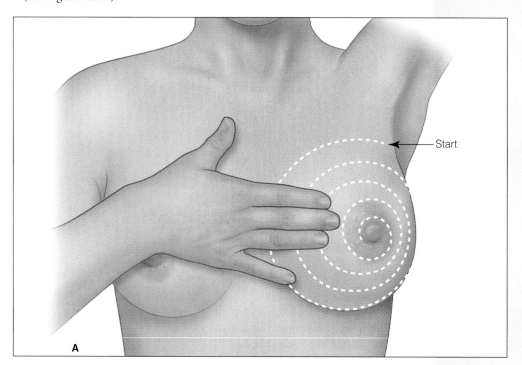

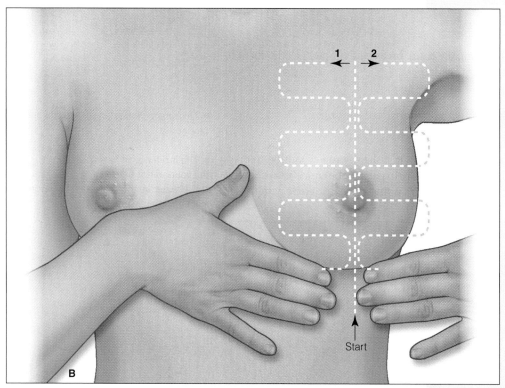

Figure 16.16 ● Alternative patterns for palpation. A. Concentric circles. B. Back and forth technique.

| TECHNIQUES AND NORMAL FINDINGS | ABNORMAL FINDINGS AND SPECIAL CONSIDERATIONS |

- Palpation then continues into the tail of Spence (see Figure 16.18).

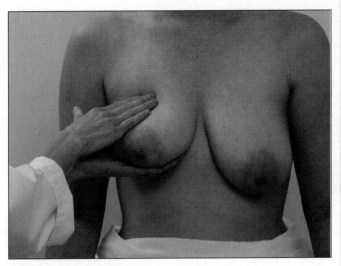

Figure 16.17 ● Palpating a pendulous breast.

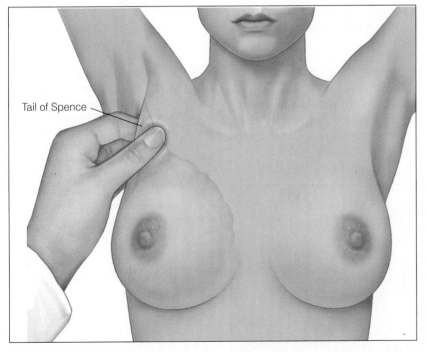

Tail of Spence

Figure 16.18 ● Palpating the tail of Spence.

5. **Palpate the nipple and areolae.**
   - Compress the tissue between the thumb and forefinger (see Figure 16.19) to observe for drainage. Confirm that the nipple is free of discharge, that it is non-tender, and that the areola is free of masses.

TECHNIQUES AND NORMAL FINDINGS	ABNORMAL FINDINGS AND SPECIAL CONSIDERATIONS

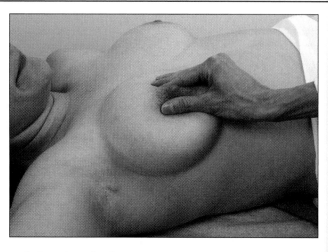

Figure 16.19 ●
Palpating the nipple.

• Repeat steps 1 through 5 on the other breast.

EXAMINATION OF THE AXILLAE

1. Instruct the client.

   • Explain that you will be examining the axillae by looking and palpating. Tell the client that she will sit for this examination and you will support the arm while palpating with the other hand. Explain that relaxation will make the examination more comfortable. Tell the client to inform you of any discomfort.

2. Position the client.

   • Ask the client or assist the client to assume a sitting position. Flex the arm at the elbow and support it on your arm. Note the presence of axillary hair. Confirm that the axilla is free of redness, rashes, lumps, or lesions. With the palmar surface of your fingers, reach deep into the axilla (see Figure 16.20). Gently palpate the anterior border of the axilla (anterior or subpectoral nodes), the central aspect along the rib cage (central nodes), the posterior border (subscapular or posterior nodes), and along the inner aspect of the upper arm (lateral nodes).

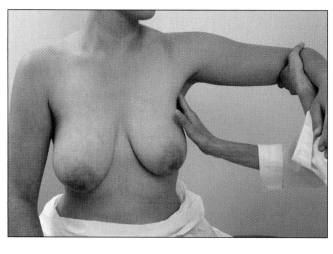

Figure 16.20 ●
Palpating the axilla.
Note that the nurse
is supporting
the woman's arm
with her own
nondominant arm.

INSPECTION OF THE MALE BREAST

1. Instruct the client.

   • Explain all aspects of the procedure and the purpose for each part of the examination.

▶ Lactation not associated with childbearing is called **galactorrhea.** It occurs most commonly with endocrine disorders or medications, including some antidepressants and antihypertensives.

Unilateral discharge from the nipple is suggestive of benign breast disease, an intraductal papilloma, or cancer.

▶ Infections of the breast, arm, and hand cause enlargement and tenderness of the axillary lymph nodes. Hard, fixed nodes are suggestive of cancer or lymphoma. Clients who have had a wide local excision (removal of tumour and narrow margin of normal tissue) or mastectomy (removal of tumour and extensive areas of surrounding tissue) need to be examined carefully. The remaining tissue on the chest wall should be palpated as it would be for nonsurgical clients.

TECHNIQUES AND NORMAL FINDINGS	ABNORMAL FINDINGS AND SPECIAL CONSIDERATIONS

2. Position the client.
   - The client is in the sitting position with the gown at the waist.

3. Inspect the male breasts.
   - Observe that breasts are flat and free of lumps or lesions.

PALPATION OF THE MALE BREAST AND AXILLAE

1. Position the client.
   - Place the client in a supine position.

2. Instruct the client.
   - Explain that you will be using the pads of your fingers to gently palpate the breast area. Instruct the client to report any discomfort.

3. Palpate the male breasts.
   - Using the fingerpads of the first three fingers, gently palpate the breast tissue, using concentric circles until you reach the nipple. The male breast feels like a thin disc of tissue under a flat nipple and areola (see Figure 16.21).

▶ Gynecomastia (breast enlargement in males) is a temporary condition seen in infants, at puberty, and in older males. In older males it may accompany hormonal treatment for prostate cancer. Breast cancer in the male is usually identified as a hard nodule fixed to the nipple and underlying tissue. Nipple discharge may be present.

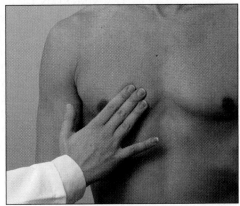

Figure 16.21 ●
Palpation of the male breast.

4. Palpate the nipple.
   - Compress the nipple between your thumb and forefinger.
   - The nipple should be free of discharge.

5. Repeat on the other breast.

6. Palpate the axillae.
   - Palpate axillary nodes in the male as you would for the female.

PHYSICAL ASSESSMENT

SAMPLE DOCUMENTATION

Subjective: 51-year-old female presents to clinic. Denies pain or tenderness of breasts. No breast lumps or discharge reported. No redness, lesions, or swelling noted. Denies any trauma to breasts and has never had breast surgery. Personal and family history negative for breast disease. No previous mammograms. Smoker, half a pack per day. Social drinker. No medications.

Objective: Breasts large, symmetrical. No redness or lesions noted on breasts or axillae. Areola everted. No dimpling noted with range of motion. No masses on palpation of breasts, tail of Spence, and axillae. Nontender. Nipples free of discharge.

APPLICATION THROUGH CRITICAL THINKING

CASE STUDY

The following information was gathered during a comprehensive health assessment of Carol Jenkins, a 29-year-old female.

The client stated that she has had breast tenderness associated with her periods for most of her adult life. The tenderness has increased over the past several months. Her breasts seem swollen and heavy, and what used to hurt in the outer portion of the breast has changed to discomfort all over. The physical examination revealed round, tender, mobile masses with smooth borders in all quadrants. The nipples are everted, round, and free of lesions. The breasts are symmetrical in shape and contour.

ASSESSMENT FORM

REASON FOR VISIT
Increasing breast tenderness over past several months.

Findings

Breasts: *Symmetrical shape, contour*

Nipples: *Round, everted, no lesions*

Palpation: *Round mobile masses, smooth borders—*

  all quadrants

▶ Complete Documentation

The following is sample documentation for Carol Jenkins.

SUBJECTIVE DATA: Breast tenderness "with periods" for most of her adult life. Tenderness increasing over past several months. Breasts seem "swollen and heavy." Discomfort in outer breast now "discomfort all over."

OBJECTIVE DATA: Round, mobile masses with smooth borders in all quadrants bilaterally. Nipples everted, round, free of lesions. Breasts symmetrical in shape and contour.

▶ Critical Thinking Questions

1. What is most likely the cause of the client's symptoms?
2. Identify several differential diagnoses.
3. What information is required to validate the diagnoses?
4. What recommendations should the nurse make for this client?

▶ Applying Nursing Diagnoses

1. *Pain (chronic)* is a nursing diagnosis in the NANDA-I taxonomy. Do the data for Carol Jenkins support this diagnosis? If so, provide supporting data.
2. Identify additional nursing diagnoses from the NANDA-I taxonomy (see Appendix A ⚭) for Carol Jenkins. Identify the data that support the PES (problem, etiology, signs or symptoms) statements.

▶ Prepare Teaching Plan

LEARNING NEED: The data from the case study reveal that Carol Jenkins is concerned about her breast discomfort. Her symptoms indicate benign (fibrocystic) breast disease. Education about this disorder and methods to monitor breast health will be provided to this client.

The case study provides data that are representative of concerns about breast disease, especially cancer, of many individuals. Therefore, the following teaching plan is based on the need to provide information to members of any community about measures to detect breast cancer.

GOAL: The participants in this learning program will have increased awareness of recommendations for screening for breast cancer.

OBJECTIVES: At the completion of this learning session, the participants will be able to do the following:

1. Identify the recommended schedule for breast cancer screening.
2. Describe methods for breast cancer screening.

Application of Objective 1: Identify the recommended schedule for breast cancer screening.

Content	Teaching Strategy	Evaluation
• Breast awareness. • Clinical examination by a health-care provider every 3 years between the ages of 20 and 40. • Clinical breast examination by a healthcare provider every 2 years for women 41 to 49. • Over 50 years of age, annual clinical examination. • Mammogram first at age 50. After age 50, mammogram every 1 to 2 years.	• Lecture • Discussion • Audiovisual materials • Printed materials Lecture is appropriate when disseminating information to large groups. Discussion allows participants to bring up concerns and to raise questions. Audiovisual materials, such as illustrations of the breast and techniques, reinforce verbal presentation. Printed material, especially to be taken away with learners, allows review, reinforcement, and reading at the learner's pace.	• Written examination. May use short answer, fill-in, or multiple-choice items, or a combination of items. If these are short and easy to evaluate, the learner receives immediate feedback.

HEALTH PROMOTION ASSESSMENT TOOL

Social Determinants of Health	Level of Action	Action Strategies
Personal coping skills	Individual	**Develop personal skills** • Discuss the importance of continuing breast self-examinations. • Discuss with Ms. Jenkins expected changes in her breasts that may be associated with her periods and how what she is experiencing may be similar or different. • Discuss methods of managing discomfort in her breasts. • Assess breast support needs and style of bra worn. Refer Ms. Jenkins to a bra-fitting specialist, if needed. • Discuss the changes that occur in breasts during pregnancy.
Health services	Individual	**Create supportive environments** • Provide a pregnancy test to rule out pregnancy. • Provide a referral to a physician to further investigate the round, tender, mobile masses with smooth borders in all quadrants.

ABNORMAL FINDINGS

Some of the problems identified during the physical assessment are entirely within the realm of nursing and are addressed with appropriate nursing interventions. Some problems, however, require collaborative management. Benign breast disease, fibroadenoma, intraductal papilloma, mammary duct ectasia, and breast cancer are the most common breast conditions that will challenge the nurse and the rest of the healthcare team. These common abnormalities are discussed in this section.

Benign Breast Disease

One of the most common benign breast problems is benign breast disease (also called fibrocystic breast disease). It is typically first seen in females in their 20s and is characterized by lumps, breast pain or tenderness, and nipple discharge. These symptoms are a result of *fibrosis,* a thickening of the normal breast tissue, which may be accompanied by cyst formation. Usually located in the upper outer quadrant, the cysts probably are a result of fluctuating hormones in the body that cause excessive cell growth in the ducts and lobules and inhibit the draining of normal secretions. The breasts usually become painful just before the onset of menses, and pain resolves at the end of menstruation. On palpation, the masses feel soft, well demarcated, and freely movable; they are almost always bilateral (see Figure 16.22). Discharge from the nipples may be clear, straw coloured, milky, or green. This is a disease of the reproductive years, and symptoms usually resolve after menopause because of a lack of estrogen.

Benign breast disease is not usually clinically significant, and there is no direct link between fibrocystic tissue changes and the incidence of cancer. In some cases, however, it may result in ductal hyperplasia and dysplasia, which may eventually develop into noninvasive intraductal, lobular, or intraepithelial carcinoma. The hyperplasia and dysplasia can lead to an invasive carcinoma. Additionally, the presence of nodular tissue in the breast makes the early detection of malignant nodules more challenging. The physician monitors fibrocystic breast disease through periodic mammography and determines if an aspiration or biopsy is necessary.

Pharmacological hormones and diuretics may be used in medical management to relieve symptoms. Some studies suggest that limiting caffeine may help relieve symptoms, but the evidence is inconclusive. The nurse might suggest that the female client try eliminating caffeine, especially in the premenstrual time, and determine for herself if this action brings relief. The nurse may also suggest decreasing salt intake and taking mild analgesics. Wearing a supportive bra decreases discomfort. The nurse reinforces the need for regular mammography and physical examination.

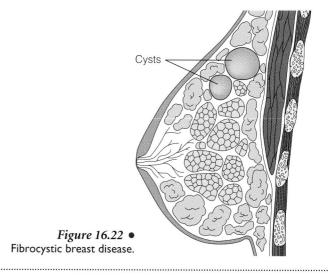

Figure 16.22 ●
Fibrocystic breast disease.

Fibroadenoma

Fibroadenoma is a common benign tumour of the glandular tissue of the breast. It is most common in females in their teens and early 20s. Its development in adolescents appears to be linked to breast hypertrophy, which may occur during the growth spurt of puberty. Fibroadenomas are well-defined, round, firm tumours, about 1 to 5 cm (0.5 to 2 in.) in diameter, which can be moved freely within the breast tissue (see Figure 16.23). They usually occur as a single tumour near the nipple or in the upper outer quadrant. Because they are asymptomatic, they are often not discovered until direct examination. Careful observation over time is the usual treatment. Biopsy or excision of the lump, performed on an outpatient basis, is indicated if the findings are inconclusive. No relationship has been established between fibroadenomas and malignant neoplasms.

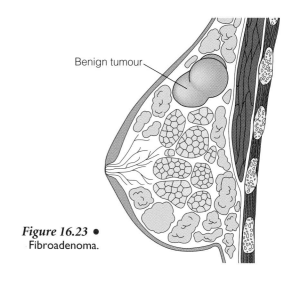

Figure 16.23 ●
Fibroadenoma.

Intraductal Papilloma

Intraductal papillomas (see Figure 16.24) are tiny growths of epithelial cells that project into the lumen of the lactiferous ducts. These growths are fragile, and even minimal trauma causes leakage of blood or serum into the involved duct and subsequent discharge. Intraductal papillomas are the primary cause of nipple discharge in females who are not pregnant or lactating. They are more commonly found in menopausal females but may occur at any age.

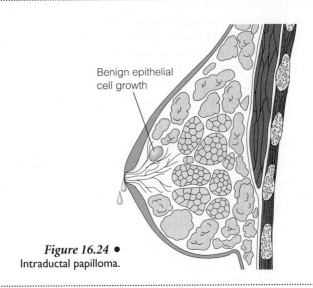

Benign epithelial cell growth

Figure 16.24 ●
Intraductal papilloma.

Mammary Duct Ectasia

Mammary duct ectasia (see Figure 16.25) is an inflammation of the lactiferous ducts behind the nipple. As cellular debris and fluid collect in the involved ducts, they become enlarged and form a palpable, painful mass. A thick, sticky discharge from the nipple is common. Because there may be some nipple retraction, a careful assessment is required to distinguish the condition from breast cancer. Although the disorder is painful, it is not associated with cancer and usually resolves spontaneously.

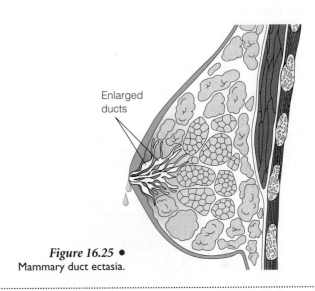

Enlarged ducts

Figure 16.25 ●
Mammary duct ectasia.

Carcinoma of the Breast

The common signs of carcinoma of the breast (see Figure 16.26) include the following:

- *Dimpling of the skin over the tumour caused by a retraction or pulling inward of breast tissue.* This results primarily from tissue fibrosis. Retraction is also caused by fat necrosis and mammary duct ectasia (described in the previous section).
- *Deviation of the breast or nipple from its normal alignment.* Deviation is also caused by retraction. The nipple typically deviates toward the underlying cancer.
- *Nipple retraction.* The nipple flattens or even turns inward. Retraction is also caused by tissue fibrosis.
- *Irregular shape of one breast as compared with the other, such as a flattening of one quadrant.* Irregularity of shape is also caused by retraction.
- *Edema, which may result in a peau d'orange appearance, especially near the nipple.* Edema is caused by blockage of the lymphatic ducts that normally drain the breast.
- *Discharge, which may be bloody or clear.* The screening examination and studies for breast cancer are physical examination

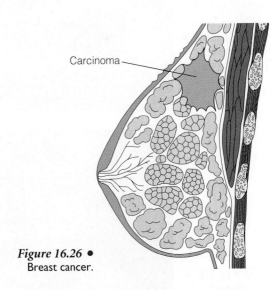

Carcinoma

Figure 16.26 ●
Breast cancer.

and mammography. A positive diagnosis of cancer is made by histological examination following an open or closed (needle) biopsy. The tumour is then staged to determine characteristics of the tumour, nodal involvement, and the presence or absence of distant metastasis. The outcome of this staging determines which protocol is used for treatment. Treatment may consist of surgery, radiation therapy, chemotherapy, or a combination of these modalities.

Performing a breast self-examination (BSE) as a means of detecting breast cancer is no longer promoted. In 2006, the Society of Obstetricians and Gynaecologists of Canada recommended that BSE not be used as a screening technique. The Canadian Cancer Society agreed in 2007. Researchers have been unable to find evidence that BSE reduces mortality from breast cancer. This being said, women should be encouraged to know what is normal for them (see Box 16.1), be informed

---

BOX 16.1 | TEACHING BREAST SELF-EXAMINATION

Although breast self-examination is no longer promoted, the nurse should be able to teach it to any client who asks. For some women, performing a monthly examination in a systematic way gives them a feeling of control over their own health. The formal method of checking the breasts is set out below.

1. Teach the client to observe her breasts in front of a mirror and in good lighting. Tell her to observe her breasts in four positions:
   - With her arms relaxed and at her sides
   - With her arms lifted over her head
   - With her hands pressed against her hips
   - With her hands pressed together at the waist, leaning forward

Instruct her to look at each breast individually, and then to compare them. She should observe for any visible abnormalities, such as lumps, dimpling, deviation, recent nipple retraction, irregular shape, edema, discharge, or asymmetry.

2. Teach the client to palpate both breasts while standing or sitting, with one hand behind her head (see Figure 16.27A). Tell her that many women palpate their breasts in the shower because water and soap make the skin slippery and easier to palpate. Show the client how to use the pads of her fingers to palpate all areas of her breast. To ensure all areas are palpated, the client may want to use the concentric circles technique (see Figure 16.27B). Tell her to press the breast tissue gently against the chest wall and to be sure to palpate the axillary tail.
3. Instruct the client to palpate her breasts again while lying down, as described in step 2. Suggest that she place a folded towel under the shoulder and back on the side to be palpated. The arm on the examining side should be over her head, with the hand under the head (see Figure 16.27C).
4. Teach the client to palpate the areolae and nipples next. Show her how to compress the nipple to check for discharge (see Figure 16.27D).

If a woman will not be performing a regular self-examination of her breasts, she should be taught to be aware of what is normal for her own breasts. The Canadian Cancer Society (2010) recommends that women spend time looking at and feeling their breasts, and that includes all breast tissue: the nipples, under the armpits, and up to the collarbone.

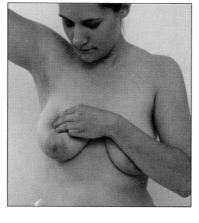

Figure 16.27A ● Breast awareness. A. The female palpates her breasts while standing or sitting upright.

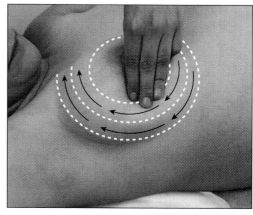

Figure 16.27B ● Breast awareness. B. The concentric circles approach.

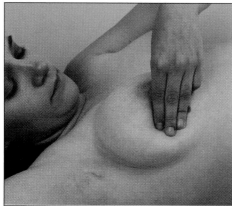

Figure 16.27C ● Breast awareness. C. The female client palpates her breasts while lying down.

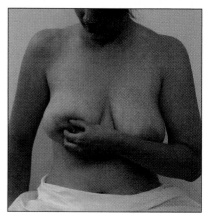

Figure 16.27D ● Breast awareness. D. The woman palpates her nipples.

of early symptoms of breast cancer, and promptly report any changes or concerns. It is encouraging to note that a recent study by Jelinski, Maxwell, Onysko, and Bancej (2005) showed that not recommending BSE is unlikely to influence mammography participation.

Abnormalities of the Male Breast

Male breast tissue is similar to that of the female. Therefore, changes in relation to hormone secretion and disease occur. The following sections describe abnormalities in the male breast.

Gynecomastia

Gynecomastia is enlargement of the breast tissue in the male. This change can occur at birth in response to maternal hormones. Additionally, at the onset of puberty more than 30% of males have enlargement of one or both breasts in response to hormonal changes. This can be a cause of embarrassment or shame if it occurs before puberty. Gynecomastia may also occur in males over 50 because of pituitary or testicular tumours and in males taking estrogenic medication for prostate cancer. Gynecomastia may occur in cirrhosis of the liver and with adrenal and thyroid diseases (see Figure 16.28).

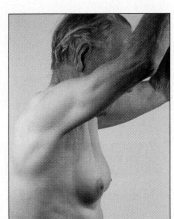

Figure 16.28 ●
Gynecomastia.

Carcinoma

Male breast cancer is rare. Less than 1% of all breast cancer occurs in men. Predisposing factors include radiation exposure, cirrhosis, and estrogen medications. Increased rates have been seen in males with a familial history of breast cancer in primary female relatives (see Figure 16.29).

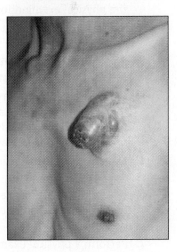

Figure 16.29 ●
Carcinoma of the breast.

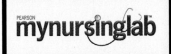

Visit the MyNursingLab website at http://www.pearsoned.ca/mynursinglab. This online homework and tutorial system puts you in control of your own learning with study and practice tools directly correlated to this chapter's content.

17

CARDIOVASCULAR SYSTEM

THE CARDIOVASCULAR SYSTEM CIRCULATES BLOOD CONTINUOUSLY throughout the body to deliver oxygen and nutrients to the body's organs and tissues and to dispose of their excreted wastes. The health of the cardiovascular system may be promoted throughout the lifespan by means of self-care habits, such as eating a low-fat diet, exercising, and not smoking. Still, the delicate balance of this system is vulnerable to stress, trauma, and a variety of pathological mechanisms that may impair its ability to function. Inadequate tissue perfusion results in both a diminished supply of nutrients necessary for metabolic functions and a buildup of metabolic wastes.

To perform an accurate cardiovascular assessment, a solid understanding of cardiovascular anatomy and physiology, reviewed in the next section, is necessary. By asking appropriate questions during the health history, the nurse uncovers clues to the client's health status and any cardiovascular problems. Assessment of the client's psychosocial health, self-care habits, family, culture, and environment is a major part of the health history. It is important for the nurse to keep these findings in mind while conducting the physical assessment and to recognize that the health of the cardiovascular system affects and is affected by the health of all other body systems.

During the physical assessment, the nurse assesses and evaluates the sometimes ambiguous cues of actual and potential cardiac disease. A plan of collaborative or independent nursing care is then developed. Finally, the nurse plays a key role in teaching the healthy client the facts about preventing cardiovascular disease. For the client with cardiovascular disease, the nurse provides teaching to promote optimum health according to the client's individual needs.

ANATOMY AND PHYSIOLOGY REVIEW

The cardiovascular system is composed of the heart and the vascular system. The heart includes the cardiac muscle, atria, ventricles, valves, coronary arteries, cardiac veins, electrical conducting structures, and cardiac nerves. The vascular system is composed of the blood vessels of the body: the arteries, arterioles, veins, venules, and capillaries. In this chapter, only the coronary blood vessels are considered in detail. The peripheral vascular system is discussed in Chapter 18. ⬯ The major functions of the cardiovascular system are transporting nutrients and oxygen to the body, removing wastes and carbon dioxide, and maintaining adequate perfusion of organs and tissues.

Pericardium

The **pericardium** is a thin sac composed of a fibroserous material that surrounds the heart (see Figure 17.1). Its tougher outer layer, called the *fibrous pericardium*, protects the heart and anchors it to the adjacent structures such as the diaphragm and great vessels. The inner layer is called the *serous pericardium*. The pericardium is also composed of two layers: parietal and visceral. The parietal layer is the outer layer. The **visceral layer of pericardium** is the inner layer, which lines the surface of the heart. Fluid between the fibrous and serous pericardium lubricates the layers and allows for a gliding motion between them with each heartbeat.

Heart

The **heart** is an intricately designed pump composed of a meticulous network of synchronized structures. It lies behind the sternum and typically extends from the second rib to the fifth intercostal space (see Figure 17.2). The heart sits obliquely within the thoracic cavity between the lungs and above the diaphragm in an area called the **mediastinal space**. Ventrally, the right side of the heart is more forward than the left. The heartbeat is most easily palpated over the apex; thus, this point is referred to as the point of maximum impulse (PMI).

The heart is approximately 12.5 cm (5 in.) long, 9 cm (3.5 in.) across, and 6 cm (2.5 in.) thick. It is slightly larger than a clenched fist. The heart of the female typically is smaller and weighs less than the heart of the male.

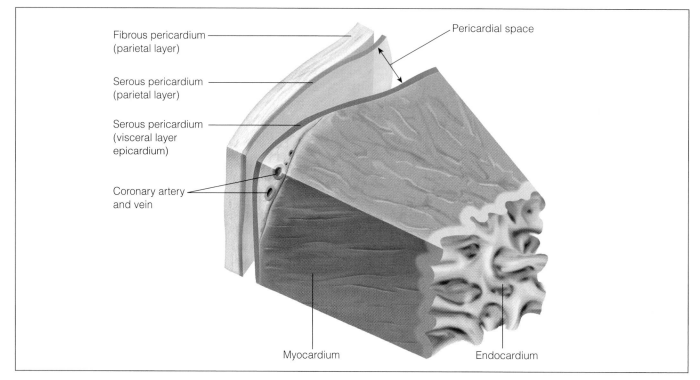

Figure 17.1 ● Layers of the heart.

Heart Wall

The heart wall is composed of three layers: epicardium, myocardium, and endocardium (Figure 17.1). The outer layer, called the **epicardium**, is anatomically identical to the visceral pericardium. The **myocardium** is the thick, muscular layer. It is made up of bundles of cardiac muscle fibres reinforced by a branching network of connective tissue fibres called the fibrous skeleton of the heart. The innermost layer is the **endocardium**,

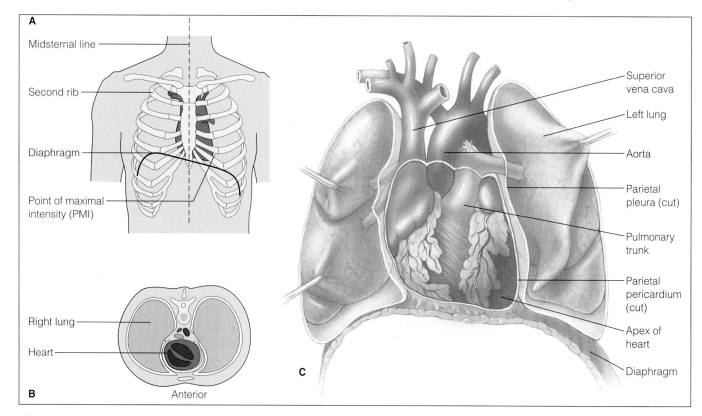

Figure 17.2 ● Location of the heart in the mediastinum of the thorax. *A.* Relationship of the heart to the sternum, ribs, and diaphragm. *B.* Cross-sectional view showing relative position of the heart in the thorax. *C.* Relationship of the heart and great vessels to the lungs.

a smooth layer that provides an inner lining for the chambers of the heart. The endocardium is continuous with the linings of the blood vessels that enter and leave the cardiac chambers.

Cardiac muscle is quite different from skeletal muscle. The muscle cells are shorter, interconnected, branched structures. Mitochondria, the cell's energy-producing organelles, make up about 25% of cardiac muscle fibres versus only about 2% of skeletal muscle fibres. This higher ratio is related to the much higher energy requirements of cardiac muscle. Unlike the independently functioning fibres of skeletal muscle, the fibres of cardiac muscle are interconnected by special junctions that provide for the conduction of impulses across the entire myocardium. This property allows the heart to contract as a single unit.

Heart Chambers

The heart is composed of four chambers: two smaller superior chambers called atria, and two larger inferior chambers called ventricles (see Figure 17.3). One atrium is located on the right side of the heart and one on the left side. These serve as receiving chambers for blood returning to the heart from the major blood vessels of the body. The atria then pump the blood into the right and left ventricles, which lie directly below them. The ventricles also are located on each side of the heart. They eject blood into the vessels leaving the heart. A longitudinal partition separates the heart chambers. The *interatrial septum* separates the two atria, and the *interventricular septum* divides the ventricles.

RIGHT ATRIUM. The **right atrium** is a thin-walled chamber located above and slightly to the right of the right ventricle. It forms the right border of the heart. Deoxygenated venous blood from the systemic circulation enters the right atrium via the inferior and superior venae cavae (two main structures of the venous system) and the coronary sinus. The blood is then ejected from the right atrium through the tricuspid valve into the right ventricle.

RIGHT VENTRICLE. The **right ventricle** is shaped like a triangle and forms much of the anterior or sternocostal surface of the heart. After receiving deoxygenated blood from the right atrium, the right ventricle ejects it through the trunk of the pulmonary arteries so that the blood can be oxygenated within the lungs. Its wall is much thinner than that of the left ventricle, reflecting the relative low vascular pressure in the vessels of the lungs.

LEFT ATRIUM. The **left atrium** forms the posterior aspect of the heart. Its muscular structure is slightly thicker than that of the right atrium. It receives oxygenated blood from the pulmonary vasculature via the pulmonary veins. From here, the blood is pumped into the left ventricle.

LEFT VENTRICLE. The **left ventricle** is located behind the right ventricle and forms the left border of the heart. The left ventricle, which is egg shaped, is the most muscular chamber of the heart. The thick wall of ventricular muscle permits the pumping of blood into the aorta against high systemic vascular resistance. This causes the left ventricle to develop more mass

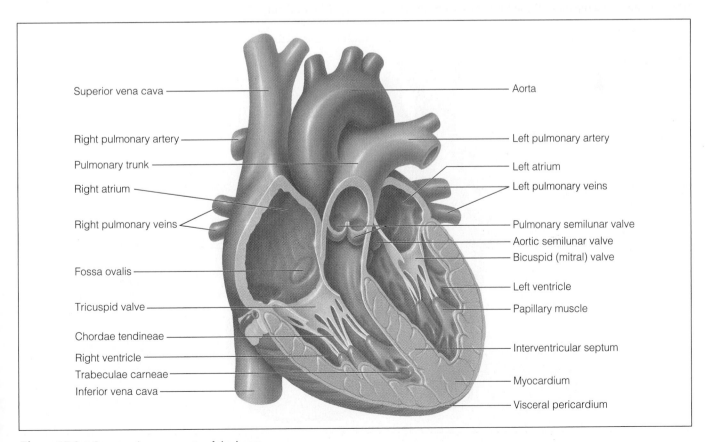

Figure 17.3 • Structural components of the heart.

than the right ventricle. The left ventricle of a female has about 10% less mass compared with that of a male.

Valves

The valves of the heart are structures through which blood is ejected either from one chamber to another or from a chamber into a blood vessel. The flow of blood in a healthy individual with competent valves is mostly unidirectional. When valves are diseased, forward blood flow is restricted, resulting in regurgitation (backflow) of blood into the chambers of the heart. The regurgitation is assessed as murmurs. Valves are classified by their location as either atrioventricular or semilunar.

Atroventricular Valves

The **atrioventricular (AV) valves** separate the atria from the ventricles. The tricuspid valve lies between the right atrium and the right ventricle, whereas the thicker mitral (bicuspid) valve lies between the left atrium and left ventricle.

The AV valves open as a direct result of atrial contraction and the concomitant buildup of pressure within the atria. This pressure forces the valvular leaflets to open. When the ventricles contract, the increased ventricular pressure forces the valvular leaflets shut, thus preventing the blood from flowing back into the atria.

Semilunar Valves

The **semilunar valves** separate the ventricles from the vascular system. The pulmonary semilunar valve separates the right ventricle from the trunk of the pulmonary arteries, and the aortic semilunar valve separates the left ventricle from the aorta.

The semilunar valves open in response to rising pressure within the contracting ventricles. When the pressure is great enough, the cusps open, allowing blood to be ejected into either the pulmonary trunk or the aorta. On relaxation of the ventricles, the valves close, allowing for ventricular filling and preventing backflow into the chambers.

Heart Sounds

Closure of the valves of the heart gives rise to heart sounds (see Figure 17.4). Normal heart sounds include S_1 and S_2. These are heard as the *lub-dub* of the heart when auscultated over the precordium, the area of the chest that lies over the heart. The first heart sound, S_1 (*lub*), is heard when the AV valves close. Closure of these valves occurs when the ventricles have been filled. The second heart sound, S_2 (*dub*), occurs when the aortic and pulmonic valves close. These semilunar valves close when the ventricles have emptied their blood into the aorta and pulmonary arteries.

The heart sounds are associated with the contraction and relaxation phases of the heart. **Systole** refers to the phase of ventricular contraction. In the systolic phase, the ventricles have been filled and then contract to expel blood into the aorta and pulmonary arteries. Systole begins with the closure of the AV valves (S_1) and ends with the closure of the aortic and pulmonic valves (S_2).

Diastole refers to the phase of ventricular relaxation. In the diastolic phase, the ventricles relax and are filled as the atria contract. Diastole begins with the closure of the aortic and pulmonic valves (S_2) and ends with the closure of the AV valves (S_1) (see Figure 17.5).

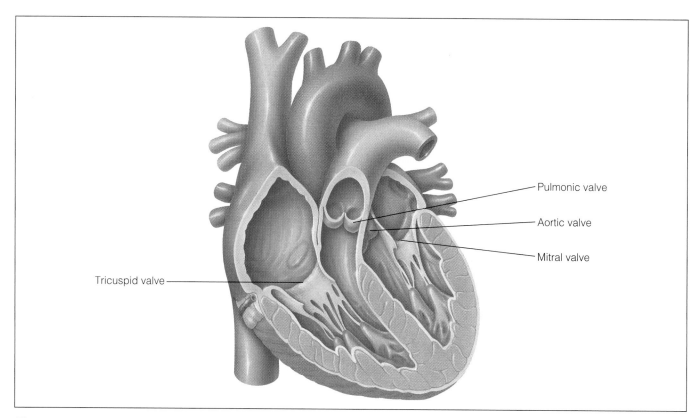

Figure 17.4 ● Valves of the heart.

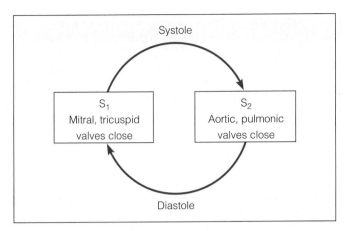

Figure 17.5 • Heart sounds in systole and diastole.

Splitting of S_2 occurs toward the end of inspiration in some individuals. This results from a slight difference in the time in which the semilunar valves close. The increase in intrathoracic pressure during inspiration is a normal splitting of S_2. The aortic valve closes slightly faster than the pulmonic valve. As a result, a split sound is heard (instead of *dub*, one hears *t-dub*). The valves close at the same time during expiration, and the sound of S_2 is *dub*.

Two other heart sounds that may be present in some healthy individuals are S_3 and S_4. S_3 may be heard in children, in young adults, or in pregnant females in their third trimester. It is heard after S_2 and is termed a *ventricular gallop*. When the AV valves open, blood flow into the ventricles may cause vibrations. These vibrations create the S_3 sound during diastole. The S_4 may also be heard in children, well-conditioned athletes, and even healthy older adults without cardiac disease. It is caused by atrial contraction and ejection of blood into the ventricles in late diastole. S_4 is heard before S_1 and is termed an *atrial gallop*. S_3 and S_4 may be associated with pathological conditions, such as myocardial infarction (MI) or heart failure.

Heart sounds are interpreted according to the characteristics of pitch, duration, intensity, phase, and location on the precordium. Table 17.1 provides information about the characteristics of heart sounds.

Additional Heart Sounds

The valves of the heart open without sound unless the tissue has been damaged. Clicks and snaps may be heard in clients with valvular disease. An opening snap may be heard in mitral stenosis. Ejection clicks occur in damaged pulmonic and aortic valves, and nonejection clicks are heard in prolapse of the mitral valve.

Friction rubs result from inflammation of the pericardial sac. The surfaces of the parietal and visceral layers of the pericardium cannot slide smoothly and produce the rubbing or grating sound.

Heart murmurs are harsh blowing sounds caused by disruption of blood flow into the heart, between the chambers of the heart, or from the heart into the pulmonary or aortic systems. Methods to distinguish heart murmurs are provided in Table 17.2 in the Abnormal Findings section.

Coronary Arteries

The word *coronary* comes from the Latin word meaning crown, which accurately describes this extensive network of arteries supplying the heart (see Figure 17.6 on page 385). The coronary arteries are visible initially on the external surface of the heart but descend deep into the myocardial tissue layers. Their function is to transport blood, bringing nutrients and oxygen to the myocardial muscle. The coronary arteries fill during diastole.

The main coronary arteries are the left main coronary artery, the right coronary artery, the left anterior descending coronary artery, and the circumflex coronary artery. These arteries and those that branch from them may vary in size and configuration among individuals. The coronary arteries are located above the aortic valve. The right and left main coronary arteries originate from the aorta and then diverge to provide blood to different surfaces. Atherosclerotic plaque in these arteries and in their branches contributes significantly to the development of ischemic and injury processes and the potential for death.

Cardiac Veins

The venous system of the heart is composed of the great cardiac vein, oblique vein, anterior cardiac vein, small cardiac vein, middle cardiac vein, cordis minimae veins, and posterior cardiac vein. The great cardiac vein serves as the tributary for the majority of venous blood drainage and empties into the coronary sinus. The small venae cordis minimae drain into the cardiac chambers.

Cardiac Conduction System

The heart has its own conduction system, which can initiate an electrical charge and transmit that charge via cardiac muscle fibres throughout the myocardial tissue. This electrical charge stimulates the heart to contract, causing the propulsion of blood throughout the heart chambers and vascular system. The main structures of the **cardiac conduction system** are the sinoatrial node (SA node), the intra-atrial conducting pathways, the atrioventricular node (AV node), the bundle of His, the right and left bundle branches, and the Purkinje fibres (see Figure 17.7 on page 386).

Sinoatrial Node

The **sinoatrial (SA) node** initiates the electrical impulse. For this reason, it has been called the pacemaker of the heart. The SA node is located at the junction of the superior vena cava and right atrium. The autonomic nervous system feeds into the SA node and can influence it to either speed up or slow down the discharge of electrical current. In the healthy individual, the SA node discharges an average of 60 to 100 times a minute.

Intra-atrial Conduction Pathway

These loosely organized conducting fibres assist in the propagation of the electrical current emitted from the SA node through the right and left atrium. The network is composed of three main pathways: anterior, middle, and posterior.

TABLE 17.1 | Characteristics of Heart Sounds

HEART SOUNDS			CARDIAC CYCLE TIMING	AUSCULTATION SITE	POSITION	PITCH
S_1 S_2 LUB — dub		S_1	Start of systole	Best at apex with diaphragm	Position does not affect the sound	High
S_1 S_2 lub — DUB		S_2	End of systole	Both at 2nd ICS; pulmonary component best at LSB; aortic component best at RSB with diaphragm	Sitting or supine	High
S_1 S_2 T		Split S_1	Beginning of systole	If normal, at 2nd ICS, LSB; abnormal if heard at apex	Better heard in the supine position	High
S_1 S_2		Fixed Split S_2	End of systole	Both at 2nd ICS; pulmonary component best at LSB; aortic component best at RSB with diaphragm	Better heard in the supine position	High
Expiration S_1 S_2 $P_2 A_2$		Paradoxical Split S_2	End of systole	Both at 2nd ICS; pulmonary component best at LSB; aortic component best at RSB with diaphragm	Better heard in the supine position	High
Expiration S_1 S_2 Inspiration S_1 S_2		Wide Split S_2	End of systole	Both at 2nd ICS; pulmonary component best at LSB; aortic component best at RSB with diaphragm	Better heard in the supine position	High
S_1 S_2 S_3		S_3	Early diastole right after S_2	Apex with the bell	Auscultated better in left lateral position or supine	Low
S_1 S_2 S_4		S_4	Late diastole right before S_1	Apex with the bell	Auscultated in almost a left lateral position or supine	Low

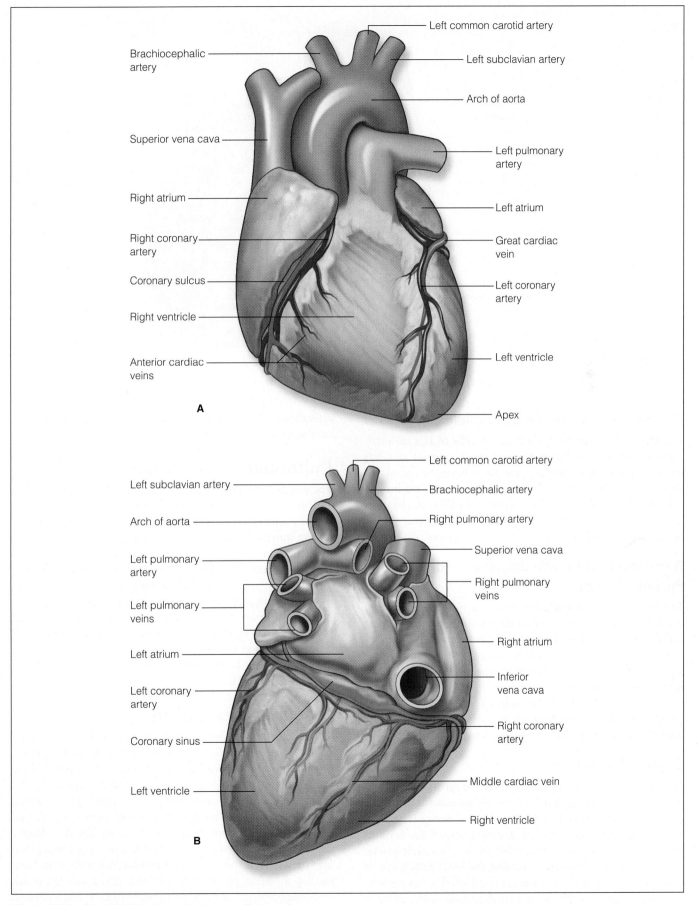

Figure 17.6 ● Vessels of the heart. A. Anterior. B. Posterior.

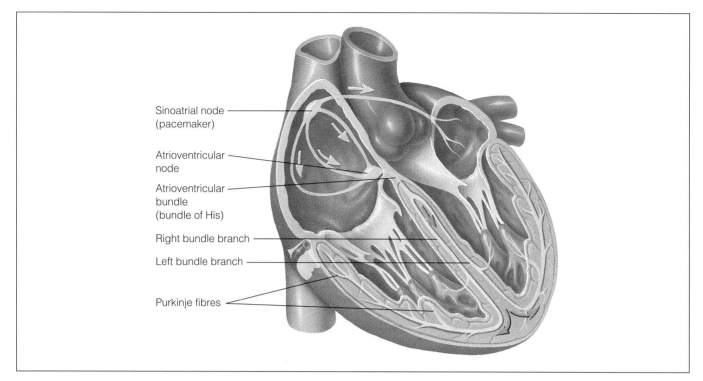

Sinoatrial node
(pacemaker)

Atrioventricular
node

Atrioventricular
bundle
(bundle of His)

Right bundle branch

Left bundle branch

Purkinje fibres

Figure 17.7 ● Conduction system of the heart.

Atrioventricular Node and Bundle of His

The **atrioventricular (AV) node** and **bundle of His** are intricately connected and function to receive the current that has finished spreading throughout the atria. Here the impulse is slowed for about 0.1 seconds before it passes onto the bundle branches. The AV node is also capable of initiating electrical impulses in the event of SA node failure. The intrinsic rate of firing is slower and averages about 60 per minute.

Right and Left Bundle Branches and Purkinje Fibres

The right and left **bundle branches** are like expressways of conducting fibres that spread the electrical current through the ventricular myocardial tissue. Arising from the right and left bundle branches are the **Purkinje fibres**. These fibres fan out and penetrate into the myocardial tissue to spread the current into the tissues themselves.

The bundle branches are also capable of initiating electrical charges in case both the SA node and the AV node fail. Their intrinsic rate averages 40 to 60 per minute.

Cardiac Nerves

Just as an extensive network of vessels transports oxygen and nutrients to the myocardial tissue and removes waste products, an equally important network of autonomic nerves is present. Both sympathetic nervous fibres and parasympathetic nervous fibres interact with the myocardial tissue. The sympathetic fibres stimulate the heart, increasing the heart rate, force of contraction, and dilation of the coronary arteries. Conversely, the parasympathetic fibres, such as the vagus nerve, exercise the opposite effect. The central nervous system influences the activation and interaction of these nerves through the information supplied by the cardiac plexus.

Pulmonary Circulation

The vessels of the pulmonary circulation include arteries, veins, and an expansive network of pulmonary capillaries. This vascular system carries deoxygenated blood to the lungs, where carbon dioxide is exchanged for oxygen. Deoxygenated blood from the veins of the body enters this network by passing into the right atrium. It is then ejected through the tricuspid valve into the right ventricle and passes through the pulmonic valve into the pulmonary artery and pulmonary circulation. The pulmonary artery is the only artery to carry unoxygenated blood. After going through the pulmonary capillary network, oxygenated blood returns to the left atrium via the pulmonary veins (see Figure 17.8). Pulmonary veins are the only veins to carry oxygenated blood.

Systemic Circulation

The vessels of the systemic circulation also include arteries, veins, and capillaries. This vascular system supplies freshly oxygenated blood to the body's periphery and returns deoxygenated blood to the pulmonary circuit. The arteries of the systemic circulation are composed of elastic tissue and smooth muscle, which allows their walls to stretch during systole. During systole, the elasticity of the walls propels the blood forward into the systemic circulation. The left ventricle propels freshly oxygenated blood into the aorta. As the blood moves toward the body periphery, the major arteries of the body subdivide into arterioles, which carry the nutrients and oxygen to the smallest blood vessels of the body: the capillaries. Oxygen and nutrients are exchanged

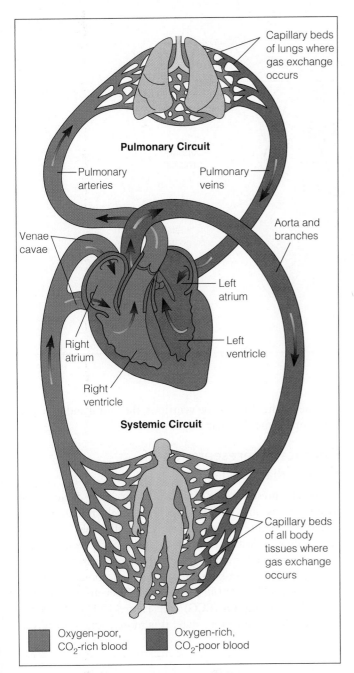

Pulmonary Circuit

Capillary beds of lungs where gas exchange occurs

Pulmonary arteries

Pulmonary veins

Aorta and branches

Venae cavae

Left atrium

Right atrium

Left ventricle

Right ventricle

Systemic Circuit

Capillary beds of all body tissues where gas exchange occurs

Oxygen-poor, CO_2-rich blood

Oxygen-rich, CO_2-poor blood

Figure 17.8 • Pulmonary and systemic circulation. The left side of the heart pumps oxygenated blood (shown in red) into the arteries of the systemic circulation, which provides oxygen and nutrients to the cells. Deoxygenated blood (shown in blue) returns via the venous system into the right side of the heart, where it is transported to the pulmonary arterial system to be reoxygenated.

in the capillaries for carbon dioxide and metabolites, which are then carried into the venules, and then the veins, and finally the superior and inferior venae cavae, which carry the deoxygenated blood into the right atrium of the heart (Figure 17.8).

Landmarks for Cardiovascular Assessment

Landmarks for assessing the cardiovascular system include the sternum, clavicles, and ribs. By correlating assessment findings

with the overlying body landmarks, the nurse may gain vital information concerning underlying pathological mechanisms. Many landmarks identified during the respiratory assessment are also used when performing a cardiac assessment. These include the sternum and the second through fifth intercostal spaces. It may be helpful to review the landmarks in Chapter 15 before proceeding. ⬭

The **sternum** is the flat, narrow centre bone of the upper anterior chest (see Figure 17.9). The adult sternum has three sections: the upper sternum is called the manubrium, the middle part is the body, and the inferior piece is the xiphoid process. The average sternal length in an adult is 18 cm (7 in.). During cardiovascular assessment, the sternum is used as a vertical landmark, and the angle of Louis is used to locate the second intercostal space.

The clavicles are bones that attach at the top of the manubrium of the sternum above the first rib (Figure 17.9). The midclavicular line (MCL) is used as a landmark for cardiovascular assessment.

The 12 pairs of ribs are flat, arched bones that form the thoracic cage. Between each rib is an intercostal space (ICS). The first ICS lies between the first and the second rib, and each remaining ICS is numbered successively (Figure 17.9). The intercostal spaces, horizontal landmarks for cardiac assessment, are used to locate the base of the heart and the apex of the heart, and to auscultate the valvular sounds. The second ICS is located by feeling the angle of Louis, sliding the finger laterally to the second rib, and then sliding the finger down below the rib to the intercostal space. Each succeeding ICS is located by sliding the finger over the rib into the ICS. Additional landmarks are identified later in this chapter.

Cardiac Cycle

The **cardiac cycle** describes the events of one complete heartbeat—that is, the contraction and relaxation of the atria and ventricles. A healthy individual's heart averages about 72 beats per minute (bpm); thus, the average time for each cardiac cycle to be completed is 0.8 seconds. Synchrony between the mechanical and electrical events of the cycle is imperative. Any interruption in this balance affects the ability of the heart to provide oxygen and nutrients to the body. Significant disruptions in synchrony can be fatal.

Electrical and Mechanical Events

The cardiac cycle can be divided into three periods (see Figure 17.10): ventricular filling, ventricular systole, and isovolumetric relaxation.

VENTRICULAR FILLING. This is the start of the cardiac cycle. Blood enters passively into the ventricles from the atria. About 70% of the blood that eventually ends up in the ventricles enters at this time. As this blood is entering the ventricles, the atria are stimulated to contract by the electrical current emanating from the SA node. Another 30% volume of blood exits the atria into the ventricles. This extra 30% volume is termed the *atrial kick.*

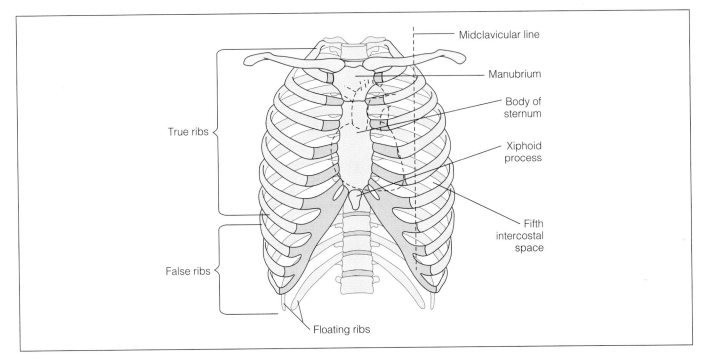

Figure 17.9 ● Landmarks for cardiovascular assessment.

VENTRICULAR SYSTOLE. The electrical current stimulates the ventricles, and they respond by contracting. The force of contraction increases the pressure within both ventricles. The mitral and tricuspid valves respond to this increased pressure by snapping shut (S_1). The ventricular pressure continues to increase until it causes the aortic and pulmonic valves to open. Blood rushes out of the ventricles into the systemic and pulmonary circulation.

ISOVOLUMETRIC RELAXATION. Once the majority of blood is ejected, the pressure in the aorta and pulmonary artery becomes higher than in the ventricles, causing the aortic and pulmonic valves to shut (S_2). During ventricular systole, the atria have been filling with blood returning from the systemic and pulmonary circulation. When the pressure in the atria

becomes higher than in the ventricles, the mitral and tricuspid valves open, and the cycle begins again.

Electrical Representation of the Cardiac Cycle

Electrical representations of the cardiac cycle are documented by deflections on recording paper. A straight horizontal line means the absence of electrical activity. Deflections representing the flow of electrical current toward or away from an electrode record the timing of the electrical events in the cardiac cycle. The terms describing the electrical deflections are *P wave*, *PR interval*, *QRS interval*, and *T wave*. They are recorded as an **electrocardiogram (ECG)** (see Figure 17.11). When the cardiac cell is in a resting state, it is more positively charged

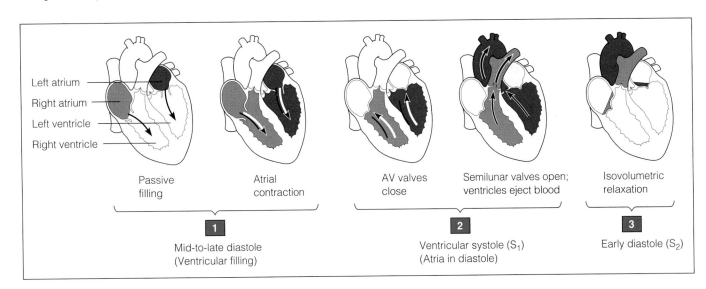

Figure 17.10 ● The cardiac cycle.

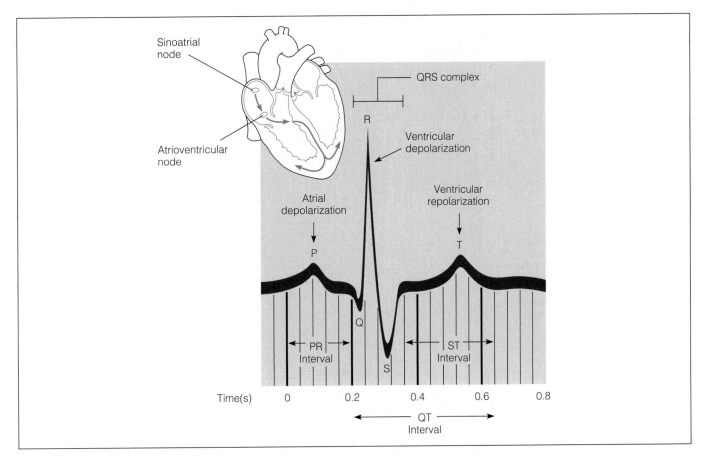

Figure 17.11 ● Electrocardiogram wave.

on the outside of the cell and more negatively charged on the inside of the cell. This spread of electrical current, called *depolarization*, causes the inside of the cardiac cell to become more positively charged. Depolarization occurs when the electrical current normally initiated in the SA node spreads across the atria. Contraction of the atria follows after stimulation by the electrical current. After contraction, the cardiac cells experience *repolarization*, during which the inside of the cell returns to its more negatively charged state. The same process occurs in the ventricles.

P WAVE. The P wave represents part of atrial depolarization. The pacemaker of the heart, the SA node, emits an electrical charge that initially spreads throughout the right and left atria. As a result of the electrical stimulation, the myocardial cells contract. The initial P wave deflection is caused by the initiation of the electrical current and atrial response to the current. It lasts an average 0.08 seconds.

PR INTERVAL. The PR interval represents the time needed for the electrical current to travel across both atria and arrive at the AV node. The normal PR interval averages 0.12 to 0.20 seconds.

QRS INTERVAL. The QRS interval represents ventricular depolarization. Atrial repolarization is hidden in the QRS interval. The ventricular myocardial cells also respond to the spread of electrical current by becoming more positively charged. This change in polarity is ventricular depolarization. The QRS interval should be 0.08 to 0.11 seconds.

T WAVE. The T wave represents ventricular repolarization. Once the ventricular myocardial cells have been stimulated by the electrical current and contract, they return to their original electrical potential state. This change in polarity is repolarization. The atria also repolarize, but it is not recorded because it occurs at the same time as ventricular repolarization; therefore, the QRS covers it.

QT INTERVAL. The QT interval represents the period from the beginning of ventricular depolarization to the moment of repolarization. Thus, it represents ventricular contraction. Electrical events in the heart occur slightly ahead of the mechanical events. Figure 17.12 illustrates the events of the cardiac cycle in relation to heart sounds, pressure waves, and the ECG.

Measurements of Cardiac Function

When the heart is functioning at optimal level, the synchrony of the events of the cardiac cycle produces an outflow of blood with oxygen and nutrients to every cell in the body. The terms that describe the effectiveness of the action of the cardiac cycle are stroke volume, cardiac output, and cardiac index.

Stroke volume describes the amount of blood that is ejected with every heartbeat. Normal stroke volume is 55 to 100 mL/beat. The formula for calculating stroke volume is

Stroke volume = Cardiac output/Heart rate for 1 minute

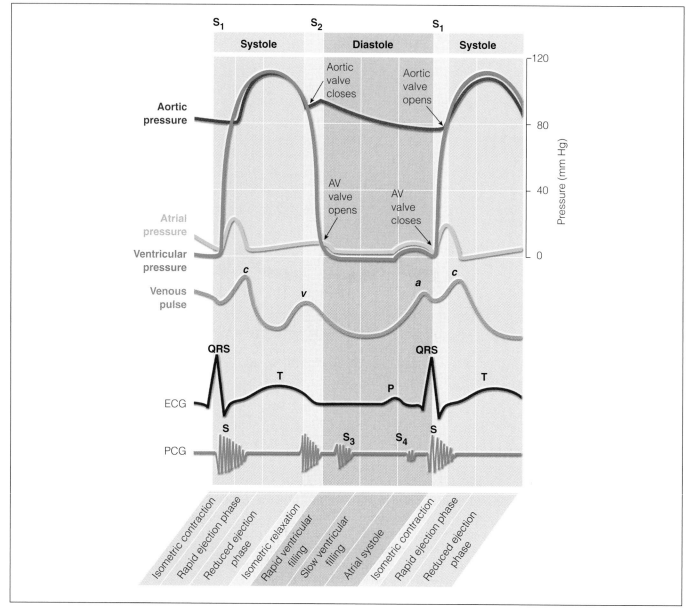

Figure 17.12 ● Events of the cardiac cycle.

Cardiac output describes the amount of blood ejected from the left ventricle in 1 minute. Normal adult cardiac output is 4 to 8 L/min. The formula for calculating cardiac output is

Cardiac output = Stroke volume × Heart rate for 1 minute

The cardiac index is a valuable diagnostic measurement of the effectiveness of the pumping action of the heart. The cardiac index takes into consideration the individual's weight, which is a significant factor in judging the effectiveness of the pumping action. For example, suppose a cardiac output of 4 is obtained for two clients: an older female who weighs 60 kg (130 lb.) and a middle-aged male who weighs 130 kg (285 lb.). The female's cardiac index is significantly higher than that of the male, whose pumping effectiveness is significantly compromised. The formula for calculating cardiac index is

Cardiac index = Cardiac output/Body surface area

The body surface area (BSA) measurement is obtained and determined from published tables.

Two strong forces influence pumping action: preload and afterload. Preload is influenced by the volume of the blood in the ventricles and relates to the length of ventricular fibre stretch at the end of diastole. The Frank-Starling law states that an increasingly greater contractile ability is provided with greater stretching of the ventricular muscle fibres. Thus, the greater the stretch, the greater the contractile force, and the greater the volume of blood ejected with each contraction. Afterload is the amount of stress or tension present in the ventricular wall during systole. It is interrelated to the pressure in the aorta, because the pressure in the ventricular wall must be greater than that in the aorta and pulmonary trunk for the semilunar valves to open (see Figure 17.13).

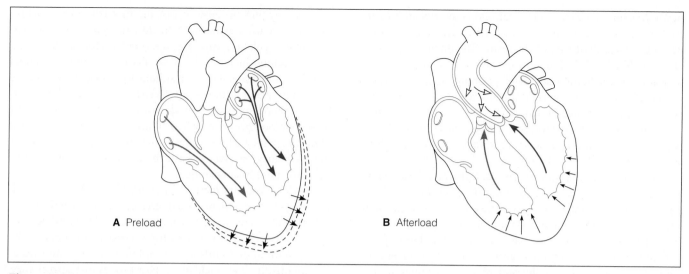

Figure 17.13 • A. Preload is related to the amount of blood and stretching of the ventricular myocardial fibres.
B. Afterload is the pressure that the ventricles must overcome in order to open the aortic and pulmonic valvular cusps.

SPECIAL CONSIDERATIONS

Many factors influence the client's health status, including age, developmental level, race, ethnicity, work history, living conditions, socioeconomics, and emotional well-being. Each factor must be addressed while gathering subjective and objective data during comprehensive health assessment.

Developmental Considerations

Anatomy and physiology change as individuals grow and develop. It is important to understand these normal changes when interpreting findings in health assessment. Variations in the cardiovascular system for different age groups are presented in the following sections.

Infants and Children

During development, the fetus receives its nutrients and oxygen from its mother. The lungs are nonfunctional, and oxygen is carried in blood from the placenta to the right side of the heart. The majority of this blood passes through the foramen ovale to the left side of the heart, then into the aorta to enter the systemic circulation. The *foramen ovale* is a passageway for blood between the right and left atria. The rest of the blood passes through the pulmonary artery and ductus arteriosus and enters the aorta (see Figure 17.14). The *ductus arteriosus* is an opening between the pulmonary artery and the descending aorta.

Inflation of the lungs at birth causes the pulmonary vasculature to dilate. Oxygenation occurs for the first time within the

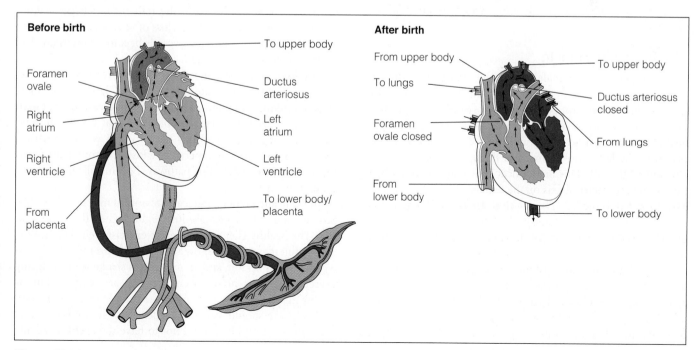

Figure 17.14 • Location of the main structures and vessels present in the fetal and postpartal cardiovascular anatomy.

newborn's lungs. The foramen ovale closes shortly after birth because of increased pulmonary vascular return and decreased pressure in the right side of the heart. The ductus arteriosus closes within 24 to 46 hours in response to multiple physiological events, including decreased pulmonary resistance and decreased pressure in the right atrium versus increased pressure in the left atrium. Murmurs may be auscultated if these openings remain patent. However, if a ventricular septal defect is present, the murmur it causes may not be auscultated until the 4th to 6th week after delivery.

The infant's arterial pressure rises at birth, and the systemic vascular resistance increases significantly when the umbilical cord is cut. Over time, the left ventricle increases in size and mass as it works to pump blood into the aorta against increasingly elevating systemic vascular resistance. The blood pressure of the full-term infant may average 70/50 mm Hg, and 10 mm Hg less in both systolic and diastolic readings in the preterm newborn. For more information, see Table 25.1 in Chapter 25. ◯◯ Weight significantly influences blood pressure.

The heart rate of the newborn initially may be as high as 175 to 180 bpm. Over the first 6 to 8 hours, it gradually decreases to an average of 115 to 120 bpm. Stimulation that causes crying, screaming, or coughing may cause the heart rate to rise temporarily to 180 bpm.

A newborn's cardiovascular system undergoes tremendous changes at birth and during the first several days of life. The infant should be easily aroused and alert. The skin should demonstrate perfusion, with pink quality in the nail beds, mucous membranes, and conjunctiva regardless of the baby's race. Precordial bulging and chest deformities, such as pigeon chest and barrel chest, are of concern.

The nurse should use a small diaphragm and bell with an infant or a child for optimal auscultation of heart sounds. Pathological murmurs of a congenital cause include patent ductus arteriosus, tetralogy of Fallot, and septal defects. A complete assessment of infants and children is provided in Chapter 25. ◯◯

The Pregnant Female

During pregnancy, a female's body undergoes phenomenal adaptations, especially in the cardiovascular system. Usually these adaptations do not place her life at risk; however, if preexisting cardiovascular or other disease is present, the female's health may be significantly compromised. The heart is displaced to the left and upward, and the apex is pushed laterally and to the left. This anatomical shift may be seen when examining the electrical axis on the female's 12-lead ECG. The axis is rotated to the left. The physical strength of the female's abdominal muscles, the shape of the fetus, the gestational age, and the structural anatomy of the uterus influence the extent of this shift.

The cardiovascular system undergoes many physiological changes during pregnancy. Blood volume may increase as much as 30% to 50%. Red blood cell genesis is dramatically stimulated, and plasma volume increases by as much as 50%. Plasma albumin, conversely, decreases. Cardiac output

increases by 30% to 50% in just the first trimester. Dilation of surface veins, together with the low resistance of the uteroplacental circulation, increases the venous return to the heart. Stroke volume increases by 30%. Because of the substantial increase in volume and the resultant increased workload, the heart may appear as much as 10% larger on chest radiography. Systolic blood pressure may decrease by 2 to 3 mm Hg and diastolic blood pressure by 5 to 10 mm Hg during the first half of the pregnancy. These values return to their previous levels as the pregnancy progresses. Last, the great vessels may become more tortuous in appearance.

Resting pulse may increase by about 10 to 15 bpm, although not every client experiences this increase. Because of the increased volume, preexisting murmurs may become louder. Murmurs may even be auscultated for the first time. Systolic murmurs are the most common (90% incidence), and diastolic murmurs occur less frequently (20% incidence). Heart tones may also change: the S_1 may split, and a prominent S_3 may be heard.

The position of the client can influence the cardiovascular dynamic state. Cardiac output may decrease when she lies on her back because of compression of the vena cava and aorta. The brachial pressure is highest when the client is sitting and then decreases when she is supine. Pressure is lowest when she is in the lateral recumbent position. Monitoring a client's blood pressure and pattern of the pressures is crucial. A blood pressure of 140/90 or greater may indicate preeclampsia and needs further assessment and monitoring. A complete assessment of the pregnant female is provided in Chapter 26. ◯◯

The Older Adult

In the older adult, the heart may stay the same size, enlarge, or atrophy. During normal aging in the absence of disease, the heart walls may thicken to some extent. The left atrium may increase in size over time. Significant enlargement of the left ventricle can be attributed to the influence of hypertension. Aging can also contribute to the loss of ventricular compliance as the cardiac valves and large vessels become more rigid. The aorta may dilate and lengthen.

Physiologically, systolic blood pressure may increase; however, resting heart rate may show no significant change. Diastolic filling time and pressure may increase to maintain a cardiac output adequate for physiological needs. On auscultation, the older client may have an S_4. Last, the electrical conduction system may experience a loss of automaticity when the SA node and conducting pathways become fibrotic and lose cellular integrity.

In the healthy older adult, cardiac output may remain stable. Stroke volume may increase just slightly when the client is at rest. The healthy client may tolerate exercise well. The healthy older adult may actually show a decreased heart rate, maximum oxygen consumption, and an increase in stroke volume during exercise. A client who has been physically active most of his or her life may have twice the work capacity of a client who has not.

The nurse should assess the older client in a position that is comfortable and be careful not to have the client make any quick movements, such as suddenly sitting, standing up, or lying down after standing or sitting. Systolic murmurs become more common as people age, especially because of aortic stenosis. These murmurs are usually best auscultated in the aortic area or base of the heart. Nonphysiological murmurs are not normal findings. However, an S_4 sound is a common finding in older adults who do not have identified cardiovascular disease. In individuals with heart disease, however, an S_4 is a pathological finding. The nurse must be mindful of the presence of any other heart sounds beyond S_1 and S_2 or any change in characteristics of preexisting heart sounds. The physician should be informed of any significant findings. Chapter 27 describes a complete assessment of the older adult. ∞

Psychosocial Considerations

Stress causes an individual to experience longer periods of sympathetic stimulation, which increases the workload on the heart. Systemic vascular resistance may be elevated for longer periods, especially in situations of excessive stress. An individual who exhibits type A behaviour may be driven to succeed, to excel, and to be the best regardless of the cost. For many years, type A behaviour has been thought to contribute to the development of heart disease. Counselling, relaxation, yoga, meditation, and biofeedback techniques are usually helpful to reduce stress levels.

Social and Ethnocultural Considerations

Individuals whose blood-related parents, aunts, uncles, or siblings demonstrate atherosclerotic heart disease before the age of 50 are considered at risk for diabetes, hypertension, or high lipid levels.

In some cultures, heavier individuals are considered healthier than those who are leaner. The selection and preparation of food may also reflect cultural influences. The use of lard and other forms of saturated fat is common in some cultures and may contribute to the development of hypertension and diabetes. Cardiovascular disease contributes to a significant percentage of deaths in individuals from most cultural backgrounds. The correlation of diet and heritage is also significant, as demonstrated by the low incidence of heart disease in Japanese individuals adhering to a traditional Japanese diet and the increasing incidence of heart disease in Japanese individuals who have adopted a Western diet of red meat and saturated fats.

Some data suggest that a low socioeconomic bracket is correlated with a higher incidence of hypertension, especially among adult females. The correlation may exist between this situation and the effect of stress related to lower incomes, limited exercise, diets containing saturated fats, or lack of access to quality healthcare.

Diet is one factor that may significantly influence the development of cardiovascular disease. Intake of fat, especially saturated fat, contributes significantly to cardiovascular disease. "Couch potato" is a popular term that describes a lifestyle of inactivity. Studies on individuals who perform continuous aerobic exercise for at least 30 to 45 minutes at least three times a week have shown a significant correlation to a slower progression of atherosclerosis. Exercise also helps to diffuse the effects of stress and, in most individuals, provides a feeling of relaxation. Smoking is a well-known contributor to the development of cardiovascular disease; in fact, it is one of the most devastating. The chemicals inhaled in cigarette smoke alter and injure the linings of the arteries, especially in areas of bifurcation (division into branches). Inhalation of passive smoke is also detrimental to the cardiovascular system.

Cocaine, especially crack cocaine, causes increased oxygen demands on the heart. Ventricular ectopy, electrical impulses that originate in the ventricles and cause early contraction of the ventricles, has been linked to cocaine use. Coronary artery spasm, myocardial infarction, malignant hypertension, and ruptured aorta also have been attributed to cocaine.

Alcoholism is associated with the development of many cardiovascular complications, such as cardiomyopathy (discussed later in the chapter). Alcohol consumption may also cause ventricular ectopy, which contributes to decreased cardiac output and may be life threatening.

Social and Ethnocultural Considerations

- Hypertension, a risk factor for coronary heart disease, occurs more frequently in Aboriginal and Black people and those of South Asian descent.
- Diabetes is a risk factor for cardiovascular disease. Groups with higher incidence of diabetes should be routinely assessed for cardiovascular disease.
- Smoking contributes to cardiovascular disease.

- White females between the ages of 65 and 74 years have a higher incidence of cardiovascular disease than Black females.
- Black people with heart failure have higher mortality rates than white people with the same disease.
- High serum cholesterol levels increase the risk for heart disease. White people have higher serum cholesterol levels than Black people.

GATHERING THE DATA

Cardiovascular assessment includes the gathering of subjective and objective data. Subjective data collection occurs during the client interview, before the actual physical assessment. During the interview the nurse uses a variety of communication techniques to elicit general and specific information about the client's state of cardiovascular health or illness. Health records, the results of laboratory tests, cardiograms, and other tests are important secondary sources to be reviewed and included in the data-gathering process. In physical assessment of the cardiovascular system, the techniques of inspection, palpation, percussion, and auscultation will be used. Before proceeding, it may be helpful to review the information about each of the data-gathering processes and practise the techniques of health assessment.

HEALTH HISTORY

The health history for the cardiovascular system concerns data related to the structures and functions of that system. Subjective data related to cardiac status are gathered during the health history. The nurse must be prepared to observe the client and listen for cues related to the function of the cardiovascular system. The nurse may use open-ended or closed questions to obtain information. Often a number of follow-up questions or requests for descriptions are required to clarify data or gather missing information.

The health history guides the physical assessment of the cardiovascular system. The information is always considered in relation to normal parameters and expectations about cardiovascular function. Therefore, the nurse must consider age, gender, race, culture, environment, health practices, past and concurrent problems, and therapies when framing questions and using techniques to elicit information.

To address all the factors when conducting a health history, specific questions related to cardiovascular status and function have been developed. These questions focus on the most common concerns or injuries associated with the cardiovascular system; questions related to past health history; questions related to behaviours; questions that address environmental concerns; and those that are specific to clients according to age, including the pregnant female.

As the nurse gathers the data, she or he will shift the type of questions to direct questions that give the client room to explain or qualify. The mnemonic O-P-Q-R-S-T-U, which stands for onset (chronology), precipitating (or palliative), quality, region (or radiation), severity, timing, and understanding, will help the learner remember the dimensions of the symptoms. The nurse will keep in mind that not all these qualifiers will apply to each symptom.

<table>
<tr><td>

HEALTH HISTORY QUESTIONS

</td><td>

RATIONALES

</td></tr>
</table>

The following sections provide sample questions and follow-up questions. Rationales for some questions are provided. The list of questions is not all-inclusive but rather represents the more common concern or injury questions required in a health history related to the cardiovascular system. An example of using O-P-Q-R-S-T-U with pain is provided.

Questions Related to Common Concerns or Injuries

The most common concerns related to illness or injury of the cardiovascular system are as follows:

- Chest pain
- Fatigue or activity intolerance
- Syncope (fainting) and dizziness
- Dyspnea
- Peripheral edema
- Nocturia
- Palpitations or arrhythmias

HEALTH HISTORY QUESTIONS

RATIONALES

1. **Chest pain**
   * Are you experiencing any chest pain at this time? *If yes:*
   * When did you first notice the pain? How long does it last? *Onset (chronology)*
   * What makes the pain worse? What makes the pain better? *Precipitating (palliative)*

   ▶ The nurse should look for activity, emotion, stress, or drugs as a precipitating factor. However, heart symptoms may have no precipitating factors.

   * Can you describe the pain? sharp? dull? burning? crushing? aching? *Quality* The description of the quality offers clues to the potential origin of the disease, especially when chest pain is present.
   * Where is the pain located? Does the pain radiate? *Region (radiation)*

   ▶ If the symptom or one of the symptoms is chest discomfort, the client should be asked to show the nurse the location on the body. Often, the client identifies chest discomfort of cardiac origin by placing a clenched fist over the precordium. When the client points one or more fingers to a limited area on the chest wall, it is generally more indicative of pain of a pulmonary or muscular origin. Females may experience less severe cardiac pain over the precordium, back pain, or fatigue.

   * How often do you experience the pain? Does the pain occur at rest? with physical activity? with stress? when moving your arms? How would you rate the pain on a scale of 1 to 10, with 10 being the worst pain? *Severity*
   * Is the pain associated with nausea or vomiting? sweating? shortness of breath? coughing? palpitations? fever? leg pain? *Timing*
   * What do you think is causing the pain? *Understanding*

2. **Fatigue or activity intolerance**
   * Do you experience fatigue or activity intolerance? *If yes:*
   * When does it start and how long does it last?
   * Are there specific times of the day when you feel tired?

   ▶ Compromised cardiac output may lead to fatigue, which manifests during the evening or late in the day.

   * Is the fatigue relieved by rest?
   * Does is it affect your activities of daily living?

   ▶ Inability to carry out or perform personal or work-related activities can be indicative of problems in the cardiovascular system.

3. **Syncope (fainting) and dizziness**
   * Do you experience dizziness or fainting? *If yes:*

   ▶ Dizziness and fainting can occur as a result of decreased blood flow to the brain, which may be related to inadequate cardiovascular function. However, dizziness may also be due to inner ear infections or other pathology.

   * Does it occur at a particular time of the day?
   * Did you lose consciousness?
   * What were you doing just before you felt dizzy? Were you lying down? sitting? standing?
   * Were there any other symptoms accompanying the fainting, such as nausea? chest pain? confusion? palpitations? difficulty breathing?

   ▶ Orthostatic hypotension is a common cause of episodes of feeling dizzy or even fainting.

4. **Dyspnea**
   * Do you experience difficulty breathing (shortness of breath)? *If yes:*

   ▶ Dyspnea (shortness of breath or SOB) may result from a variety of factors related to a compromised cardiovascular system, such as coronary artery disease, congestive heart failure, pulmonary dysfunction, and myocardial infarction. Dyspnea can be categorized as mild, moderate, or extreme. It can occur during rest or sleep.

GATHERING THE DATA

HEALTH HISTORY QUESTIONS

RATIONALES

- What provokes the SOB and what makes it better?
- Does the SOB occur at rest? Is the SOB brought on by activity? If yes, assess the amount of activity (i.e., walking a block, climbing 10 steps).
- Are there associated symptoms? cough? dizziness?
- When do you feel short of breath (i.e., at night, on awakening)?

5. **Peripheral edema**
   - Do you experience swelling in your legs, ankles, and feet? *If yes:*

   ▶ Edema in the lower extremities represents right-sided heart failure.

   - When did you first notice the swelling?
   - Is the swelling in one or both legs?

   ▶ Unilateral swelling may be related to a problem with the peripheral vascular system.

   - Is the swelling worse at a particular time of the day?
   - Does it disappear after a night's rest? Does elevating your legs help reduce the swelling?

6. **Nocturia**
   - Do you have the urge to urinate at night? *If yes:*

   ▶ Increased urination during the night is associated with heart failure. Fluid that has been retained in the legs is reabsorbed when lying down.

   - How many times do you wake up during the night to urinate?

7. **Palpitations or arrhythmias**
   - Have you experienced pounding or racing sensations in your chest, throat, or neck? *If yes:*

   ▶ Palpitations and arrhythmias are a result of disturbances in the heart rhythm, often because of cardiovascular disease, compromised cardiac output, or heart failure.

   - Does it feel like your heart skips a beat or stops beating?

Questions Related to Past Health History

1. **Have you ever been diagnosed with a cardiovascular disease?** *If yes:*

   ▶ If a diagnosed illness is identified, follow-up about the date of diagnosis, treatment, and outcomes is required. Data about each illness identified by the client are essential to an accurate health assessment. Illnesses can be classified as acute or chronic, and follow-up regarding each classification will differ.

   - When were you diagnosed with the problem?
   - Has the problem ever recurred? *(acute)*
   - How are you managing the disease now? *(chronic)*
   - Does your cardiovascular illness affect your ability to carry out your activities of daily living?
   - Have you discussed this with a healthcare professional? If so, what treatment was recommended and did it help?

   ▶ Inability to carry out or perform personal or work-related activities can also be indicative of problems in the cardiovascular system.

2. **Do you have hypertension, diabetes, or a thyroid disorder?**
   Some medical conditions, such as diabetes, hypertension, or thyroid dysfunction, can contribute to cardiovascular problems.

3. **Do you have a family history of cardiovascular problem or disease?** *If yes:*

   ▶ This question may reveal information about cardiovascular disease associated with familial predisposition. Follow-up is required to obtain details about specific problems, reoccurrence, treatment, and outcomes.

   - What is the disease or problem?
   - Who in the family has been affected by this problem?
   - What was the outcome?

HEALTH HISTORY QUESTIONS	RATIONALES

Questions Related to Behaviours

Healthcare behaviours include both health practices and health patterns. Health practices consist of following recommendations for disease prevention, including screening for risks, screening for early detection of problems, and immunization. Health patterns are habits or acts that affect the client's health. Health behaviours may also include seeking healthcare from healthcare providers who use alternative methods to diagnose and treat illness. Clients should be questioned in a nonjudgmental way and areas for health teaching should be identified.

1. **Have you ever had a diagnostic test, such as an electrocardiogram, stress test, or echocardiogram for a cardiovascular problem?**

   ▶ The client has the opportunity to provide information about diagnostic testing related to cardiovascular problems.

2. **Describe your diet.**

   ▶ Diet is one of the key interventions that a client can control when working to minimize the effects of aging, slow the progression of disease, or maintain optimum health while experiencing cardiovascular disease.

   - What types of foods do you eat? How often? How much?
   - How much daily fibre do you consume?
   - Have you tried to lose weight? If so, describe type of diet, duration of the diet, and diet supplements you take.

   ▶ Supplementing the diet with vitamins under proper supervision may be beneficial. A poorly informed client may ingest an unbalanced proportion of supplements and compromise a healthy state. The nurse must be alert if the client has been dieting to reduce weight. Many diets deplete valuable electrolytes and subject the client to potential complications. Muscle wasting may occur if the diet is deficient in protein. Lack of protein may compromise cardiac function.

3. **Do you smoke or are you currently exposed to second-hand smoke? How long have you smoked?** *If yes:*

   ▶ Smoking has been linked to hypertension and is strongly suspected of contributing to injury in the walls of arteries, thus accelerating the development of atherosclerotic plaques. It is believed that the chemical contained in the cigarette smoke injures the inner wall of arterial vessels, thus contributing to the subsequent development of a coronary artery plaque.

   - How many packs a day?
   - If you are exposed to second-hand smoke, where and for how long each day?

4. **Do you take any drugs (over the counter or illicit) or drink alcohol?**

   ▶ Substance abuse, especially of cocaine, is associated with coronary artery spasm and potential of ischemia or injury of myocardial tissue.

GATHERING THE DATA

HEALTH HISTORY QUESTIONS	RATIONALES

5. **Do you exercise regularly If so, please describe your physical activity.**

▶ The benefits of exercise are well documented, yet the type, duration, and frequency of the exercise regimen produce variable results. It is important for the client to have a basic understanding of the benefits of aerobic versus nonaerobic exercise. Studies suggest that regular aerobic exercise, approximately 30 to 60 minutes per day, can lessen the risk of developing hypertension, high cholesterol, and obesity, all contributing factors to heart disease and stroke (Heart and Stroke Foundation, 2010). Have the client describe the type of activity and the duration, as the time required to reap the benefits of exercise is dependent on the level of intensity.

Questions Related to the Environment

Environment refers to both internal and external environments. Questions related to the internal environment include all the previous questions and those associated with internal or physiological responses. Questions regarding the external environment include those related to home, work, or social environments.

Internal Environment

1. **What medications do you take?**

▶ It is important to assess the client's knowledge, compliance, and ability to administer medication accurately, whether ordered by a physician or not. Medication actions may vary depending on the mix of medications, diet, and additional supplementation.

2. **Are you experiencing any side effects that you think may be related to medications?**

3. **How would you describe your personality?**

▶ Having a type A personality is often associated with heart disease. It is not so much the behaviours as the effect of constant sympathetic stimulation on the cardiovascular system and the constant stress and drain on the rejuvenation process after a stressful event that may contribute to decompensation and increase vulnerability to disease processes. Excessive stress, no matter what the client's personality type, is a risk factor for cardiovascular disease.

- How many hours do you work in a typical week? Do you work on weekends?
- Describe the major stressors in your life.
- What do you do to relieve stress?

The nurse should ask the female client the following questions.

4. **Do you take oral contraceptives?**

▶ If the client is over 35, takes oral contraceptives containing high doses of synthetic estrogen and progesterone, and smokes, the risk of developing cardiovascular disease increases significantly.

5. **Are you still menstruating?** *If no:*

▶ The decreased levels of estrogen associated with menopause increase a women's risk of developing heart disease. By age 65, a woman's risk is the same as a man's (Canadian Women's Health Network, 2006).

- At what age did menopause start?

HEALTH HISTORY QUESTIONS	RATIONALES

External Environment

The following questions deal with the physical environment of the client. That includes the indoor and outdoor environments of the home and the workplace, those encountered for social engagements, and any encountered during travel.

1. **What is your present occupation?**

   ▶ Jobs with long hours, stress, deadlines, and tension are thought to contribute to the development of cardiovascular disease.

2. **Have you been exposed to any chemicals or other hazardous substances?**

   ▶ Such exposure may correlate to stress, alterations in eating habits and exercise habits, recreational drug use, and alterations in sleep patterns.

Questions Related to Age

The health history must reflect the anatomical and physiological differences that exist along the age span.

Questions Regarding Infants and Children

If you are talking to the child's mother, ask the following questions:

1. **What was the pregnancy with this child like?**

2. **Did you experience any complications during pregnancy?**

   ▶ Complications during pregnancy may contribute to malformations in the infant or child.

3. **Did you smoke, take drugs, or drink alcohol during pregnancy?**

   ▶ Cigarettes, recreational drugs, such as cocaine, and alcohol may have significant effects on the development of the fetal cardiovascular system, especially in the first trimester.

For all caregivers or parents, ask the following questions:

4. **Does the infant take a long time to feed?** *If yes:*
   • Does the infant seem tired after eating?

   ▶ Fatigue can be related to congenital heart disease. It is especially noticeable during feeding.

   • Does the infant ever become short of breath?

5. **What is the child's energy level like?**

   ▶ Reduced energy levels and easy fatigability may suggest underlying cardiovascular abnormalities, such as atrial septal defect or large ventricular septal defect.

   • Does the child tire easily?
   • Does the child ever become short of breath?

6. **Does the child have symptoms of joint pain, headaches, fever, or respiratory infections?**

   ▶ Rheumatic fever may follow a respiratory infection with group A beta-hemolytic *streptococcus pyogenes* (strep throat) and produce symptoms of fever, swollen and painful joints, and headaches.

7. **Do you feel that the infant or child is gaining weight and growing at a normal pace?**

   ▶ Failure to grow is associated with congenital heart disease, such as ventricular septal defect.

Questions for the Pregnant Female

1. **Do you have any history of heart disease?**

   ▶ The changes of pregnancy can place the client with preexisting heart disease at risk.

HEALTH HISTORY QUESTIONS	RATIONALES
2. Do you have a history of hypertension? Has hypertension been apparent during this pregnancy?	▶ Hypertension is a symptom of preeclampsia and places the mother and infant at risk.
3. Have you experienced headaches or dizziness?	▶ Headaches and dizziness are associated with hypertension and preeclampsia. Preeclampsia can also be accompanied by chest pain, visual changes, and abdominal pain.
4. Have you observed any swelling on your face and hands?	▶ Swelling can indicate a preeclamptic condition.

Questions for the Older Adult

All the questions listed in the general section can offer significant data. In addition to the routine questions, the nurse should ask the following ones.

1. Have you noticed any change in your ability to concentrate, remember things, or perform simple mental tasks?	▶ In the older adult, a change in mental capacity suggests inadequate perfusion and can be seen in clients with myocardial ischemia and infarction or increasingly severe congestive heart failure.
2. Have you experienced any reactions to medications you are currently taking?	▶ Many cardiovascular medications interact with medications for other diseases and may increase or reduce their effects.

PHYSICAL ASSESSMENT

ASSESSMENT TECHNIQUES AND FINDINGS

Physical assessment of the cardiovascular system requires the use of inspection, palpation, percussion, and auscultation. During each of the procedures, the nurse is gathering objective data related to the function of the heart as determined by the heart rate and the quality and characteristics of the heart sounds. In addition, the nurse observes for signs of appropriate cardiac function in relation to oxygen perfusion by assessing skin colour and temperature, abnormal pulsations, and the characteristics of the client's respiratory effort. Knowledge of normal parameters and expected findings is essential in determining the meaning of the data during a physical health assessment.

Adults have uniform skin colour on the face, trunk, and extremities. The eyes are symmetrical. The periorbital area is flat, and the eyes do not bulge. The sclera of the eye should be white, the cornea clear, and the conjunctiva pink. The lips should be smooth and noncyanotic. The head should be steady and the skull proportional to the face. The earlobe should be smooth and without creases. The jugular veins are not visible when the chest is upright. Further, the jugular veins distend only 3 cm (1 in.) above the sternal angle when the client is at a 45-degree angle. Carotid pulsations are visible bilaterally. The fingers should be round and even with flat pink nails. The respiratory pattern is even, regular, and unlaboured. Intercostal spaces and clavicles are visible; chest veins are evenly distributed and flat; no bulges or masses are visible. Pulsations over the pericardium are absent; however, aortic pulsations in the epigastric area are visible in thin clients. The lower extremities are of uniform colour and temperature, with even hair distribution. The skeleton should be free of deformity and the neck and extremities in proportion to the torso. Palpation over the pericardium reveals slight vibration at the apical area only. Carotid pulses are palpable and equal in intensity. Dullness to percussion should extend to the midclavicular line at the fifth intercostal space. S_2 is louder than S_1 at the aortic and pulmonic auscultatory areas. S_1 and S_2 are heard equally at Erb's point (third left intercostal space). S_1 is louder than S_2 at the tricuspid and apical areas. Murmurs are absent. The carotid pulse is synchronous with the apical pulse.

Physical assessment of the cardiovascular system follows an organized pattern. It begins with inspection of the client's head and neck, including eyes, ears, lips, face, skull, and neck vessels. The upper extremities, chest, abdomen, and lower extremities are also inspected. Palpation includes the precordium and carotid pulses. Percussion of the chest is conducted to determine the cardiac borders. Auscultation includes the heart in five areas with the diaphragm and the bell of the stethoscope. The carotid arteries and the apical pulse are auscultated.

PHYSICAL ASSESSMENT

EQUIPMENT

examination gown
metric rulers
examination drape
Doppler
stethoscope
lamp

HELPFUL HINTS

- Provide specific instructions throughout the assessment. Explain what is expected of the client and state that he or she will be able to breathe regularly throughout the examination.
- Assessment of the heart will require several position changes. The nurse should assist the client if necessary, allow time for movement if the client is uncomfortable, and explain the purpose of the position change.
- The nurse's hands and the stethoscope should be warmed before beginning the examination.
- The room should be quiet so that subtle sounds can be heard.
- Provide adequate draping to prevent unnecessary exposure of the female breasts.
- Use routine practices.

TECHNIQUES AND NORMAL FINDINGS	ABNORMAL FINDINGS AND SPECIAL CONSIDERATIONS

INSPECTION

1. **Instruct the client.**
   - Explain that you will be looking at the head, neck, and extremities to provide clues to cardiac function.
   - Explain that you will ask the client to sit up and lie down as part of the examination and that you will provide specific instructions and assistance as required throughout the examination. Explain that you will be touching the neck and chest, as well as tapping on the chest and listening with the stethoscope. Tell the client that none of the procedures should cause discomfort but assure the client that you will stop any time if discomfort occurs or the examination is causing fatigue.

2. **Position the client.**
   - Begin the examination with the client seated upright with the chest exposed (see Figure 17.15).

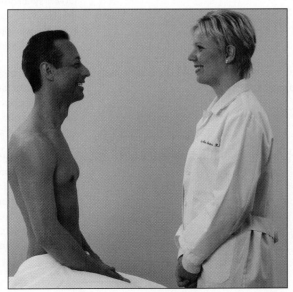

Figure 17.15 ●
The client is positioned for the examination.

TECHNIQUES AND NORMAL FINDINGS	ABNORMAL FINDINGS AND SPECIAL CONSIDERATIONS

3. Inspect the client's face, lips, ears, and scalp.

- These structures can provide valuable clues to the client's cardiovascular health. Begin with the facial skin. The skin colour should be uniform.

    ▶ Flushed skin may indicate rheumatic heart disease or the presence of a fever. Greyish undertones are often seen in clients with coronary artery disease or those in shock. A ruddy colour may indicate *polycythemia*, a condition in which there is a significantly increased number of red blood cells, or *Cushing's syndrome*, which is excessive secretion of adrenocorticotropic hormone (ACTH) by the pituitary gland.

- Examine the eyes and the tissue surrounding the eyes (periorbital area). The eyes should be uniform and not have a protruding appearance.

    ▶ Protruding eyes are seen in *hyperthyroidism*. In hyperthyroidism, excessive hormone secretion results in high cardiac output, a tendency toward tachycardia (rapid heart rate), and potential for congestive heart failure.

- The periorbital area should be relatively flat. No puffiness should be present.

    ▶ Periorbital puffiness may result from fluid retention (edema) or valvular disease.

- The sclera should be whitish. The cornea should be without an *arcus*, which is a ringlike structure.

    ▶ A blue sclera is often associated with **Marfan's syndrome**, a degenerative disease of the connective tissue, which over time may cause the ascending aorta to either dilate or dissect, leading to abrupt death. An arcus in a young person may indicate hypercholesterolemia; however, in Black people an arcus may be normal.

- The conjunctiva should be pinkish. The eyelid should be smooth. For information on how to examine the conjunctiva, see Chapter 13. ∞

    ▶ **Xanthelasma** are yellowish cholesterol deposits seen on the eyelids and are indicative of premature atherosclerosis.

- Inspect the lips. They should be uniform in colour without any underlying tinge of blue. The buccal mucosa, gums, and tongue are also inspected for cyanosis.

    ▶ Blue-tinged lips may indicate cyanosis, which is often a late sign of inadequate tissue perfusion.

- Assess the general appearance of the face. It should be uniform and flat.

    ▶ Clients with *Down syndrome* may exhibit a large protruding tongue, low-set ears, and an underdeveloped mandible. Children with Down syndrome often have congenital heart disease. Wide-set eyes may be seen in a child with *Noonan syndrome*, which is accompanied by pulmonic stenosis (narrowing).

- Examine the head. Look first for the ability of the client to hold the head steady. Rhythmic head bobbing should not be present.

    ▶ Head bobbing up and down in synchrony with the heartbeat is characteristic of severe aortic regurgitation. This bobbing is created by the pulsatile waves of regurgitated blood, which reverberate upward toward the head.

- Assess the structure of the skull and the proportion of the skull to the face.

    ▶ A protruding skull is seen in *Paget's disease of bone*, a rare disease characterized by localized loss of calcium from the bone and replacement with a porous bone formation, which leads to distorted, thickened contours. Paget's disease of bone is also characterized by a high cardiac output, which may lead to heart failure.

TECHNIQUES AND NORMAL FINDINGS	ABNORMAL FINDINGS AND SPECIAL CONSIDERATIONS

- Examine the client's earlobes. The earlobes should be relatively smooth without the presence of creases unless an injury has been sustained.

▶ Bilateral earlobe creases, especially in the young adult, are often associated with coronary artery disease.

4. **Inspect the jugular veins.**

- Examination of the jugular veins can provide essential information about the client's central venous pressure and the heart's pumping efficiency.

- Elevate the head of the examination table to 30 to 45 degrees, and adjust the gooseneck lamp to cast shadows on the client's neck. Tangential lighting is effective in visualizing the jugular vessels.

- Remove the pillow from under the client's head.

- Be sure that the client's head is turned slightly away from the side you are examining. Look for the external and internal jugular veins.

- Note that the jugular veins are not normally visible when the client sits upright. The external jugular vein is located over the sternocleidomastoid muscle. The internal jugular vein, which is the best indicator of central venous pressure, is located behind this muscle, medial to the external jugular and lateral to the carotid artery.

- If you are able to visualize the jugular veins, measure their distance superior to the clavicle. (Be sure not to confuse the carotid pulse with pulsations of the jugular veins.) The carotid pulse is lateral to the trachea. If jugular vein pulsations are visible, palpate the client's radial pulse and determine if these pulsations coincide with the palpated radial pulse.

▶ Obvious pulsations that are present during inspiration and expiration and coincide with the arterial pulse are commonly seen with severe congestive heart failure.

- Place one metric ruler, zero side down, vertically at the angle of Louis. Place a second metric ruler horizontally at a 90-degree angle to the first ruler. One end of this ruler should be at the angle of Louis and the other end in the jugular area on the lateral aspect of the neck (see Figure 17.16).

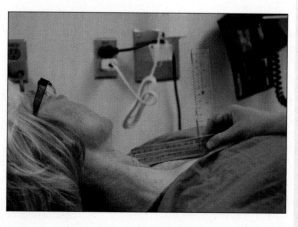

Figure 17.16 ●
Assessment of central
venous pressure.

- Inspect the neck for distension of the jugular veins. Raise the lateral portion of the horizontal ruler until it is at the top of the height of the distension, and measure the height of the jugular pulsation from the vertical ruler.

▶ Distension of the neck veins indicates elevation of central venous pressure commonly seen with right-sided congestive heart failure, fluid overload, or pressure on the superior vena cava.

- The jugular veins normally distend less than 3 cm (1 in.) above the sternal angle (Figure 17.16). You need to measure the distension only on one side.

5. **Inspect the carotid arteries.**

- The carotid arteries are located lateral to the client's trachea in a groove that is medial to the sternocleidomastoid muscle.

Techniques and Normal Findings	Abnormal Findings and Special Considerations

- Put the pillow under the client's head. With the client lying at a 45-degree angle, using tangential lighting, inspect the carotid arteries for pulsations. Pulsations should be visible bilaterally.

▶ Bounding pulses are not normal findings and may indicate fever. The absence of a pulsation may indicate an obstruction either internal or external to the artery.

- When you finish, help the client back to an upright sitting position.

6. Inspect the client's hands and fingers.

- Confirm that the fingertips are rounded and even. The fingernails should be relatively pink, with white crescents at the base of each nail.

▶ Fingertips and nails that are clubbed bilaterally are characteristic of congenital heart disease. Clubbing may be associated with cyanosis or long-term tobacco smoking. Thin red lines or splinter hemorrhages in the nail beds are associated with **infective endocarditis** (see Figure 17.17), a condition caused by bacterial infiltration of the lining of the heart's chambers.

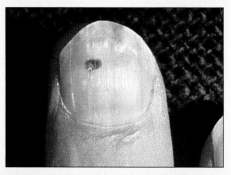

Figure 17.17 ● Splinter hemorrhage.

- Assess for Marfan's syndrome. Ask the client to make a fist by wrapping the fingers over the thumb. You can also assess for this syndrome by having the client wrap the thumb and little finger around the opposite wrist.

▶ If the thumb is readily visible outside the clenched fist or if the little finger extends at least 1 cm (0.5 in.) beyond the thumb when around the wrist, Marfan's syndrome should be suspected.

7. Inspect the client's chest.

- Observe the respiratory pattern, which should be even, regular, and unlaboured, with no retractions.

▶ Respiratory distress may be precipitated by various disorders. Pulmonary edema is often a severe complication of cardiovascular disease.

- Observe the veins on the chest, which should be evenly distributed and relatively flat.

▶ Dilated, distended veins on the chest indicate an obstructive process, as seen with obstruction of the superior vena cava.

- Inspect the entire chest for bulges and masses. The intercostal spaces and clavicles should be even.

▶ Bulges are abnormal and may indicate obstructions or aneurysms. Masses may indicate obstructions or presence of tumours.

- Inspect the entire chest for pulsations. Observe the client first in an upright position and then at a 30-degree angle, which is a low- to mid-Fowler's position. In particular, observe for pulsations over the five key landmarks (see Figure 17.18).

▶ If the entire *precordium* (anterior chest) pulsates and shakes with every heartbeat, extreme valvular regurgitation or shunting may be present.

- Start by observing the right sternal border (RSB), second ICS. Next, observe the left sternal border (LSB), second ICS.

▶ Pulsations present in the LSB, second ICS, indicate pulmonary artery dilation or excessive blood flow.

- Then observe the LSB, third to fifth ICS.

▶ Pulsations present in the LSB, third to fifth ICS, may indicate right ventricular overload.

Techniques and Normal Findings

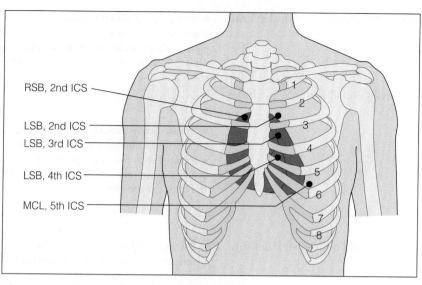

Figure 17.18 ● Landmarks in precordial assessments.

- Move on to the apex: fifth ICS, midclavicular line (MCL).
- Finish with the epigastric area, below the xiphoid process.
- Confirm that the apical impulse or *point of maximum impulse* (PMI) is located at the fifth ICS in the left MCL.

▶ If left ventricular hypertrophy is present, the PMI is displaced laterally from the fifth ICS, LMCL.

- Inspect the entire chest for heaves or lifts while the client is sitting upright and again with the client at a 30-degree angle.

▶ A heave or lift found in the LSB, third to fifth ICS, may indicate right ventricular hypertrophy or respiratory disease, such as pulmonary hypertension.

- *Heaves* or *lifts* are forceful risings of the landmark area.
- In particular, make sure you observe over the five key landmarks previously listed.

8. **Inspect the client's abdomen.**
   - Have the client lie flat, if possible.
   - Be mindful of any discomfort or difficulty in breathing.
   - Look for pulsations in the abdominal area over the areas where the major arteries are located. These sites include the following:

▶ Pulsations may be visible in lean clients. These are usually normal if seen in the epigastric area. Peristaltic waves may also be seen in thin individuals. They must not be confused with vascular pulsations. Prominent pulsations that are located in areas outside of the gastric area and are readily visible may be potentially life threatening.

   - The *aorta*, which is located superior to the umbilicus to the left of the midline.
   - The *left renal artery*, which is located to the left of the umbilicus in the left upper quadrant.
   - The *right renal artery*, which is located to the right of the umbilicus in the right upper quadrant.
   - The *right iliac artery*, which is located to the right of the umbilicus in the right lower quadrant.

TECHNIQUES AND NORMAL FINDINGS	ABNORMAL FINDINGS AND SPECIAL CONSIDERATIONS

- The *left iliac artery*, which is located to the left of the umbilicus in the left lower quadrant.

▶ Abnormal pulsations usually indicate the presence of aortic aneurysm, which is a ballooning caused by a weakness in the walls of arteries. These findings require immediate physician referral.

- Chapter 19 of this text reviews abdominal arteries and abdominal quadrants. ⚭

- Note the pattern of fat distribution.

▶ Males usually deposit fat in the abdominal area. This distribution pattern is thought to be associated with the development of coronary artery disease. Females usually deposit fat in the buttocks and thighs.

9. **Inspect the client's legs.**
   - Help the client to a sitting position.
   - Inspect the legs for skin colour. The skin colour should be even and uniform.

▶ Patches of lighter colour may indicate compromised circulation. Mottling indicates severe hemodynamic compromise.

   - Inspect the legs for hair distribution. The distribution should be even without bare patches devoid of hair.

▶ Patchy hair distribution is often a sign of circulatory compromise that has occurred over time. The client should be asked if the hair distribution on the legs has changed over time.

10. **Inspect the client's skeletal structure.**
    - Ask the client to stand.
    - Observe the skeletal structure, which should be free of deformities.

▶ *Scoliosis* is associated with a prolapsed mitral valve.

    - Observe the neck and extremities, which should be in proportion to the torso.

▶ A client who is tall and thin with an elongated neck and extremities should be evaluated further for the presence of Marfan's syndrome.

PALPATION

Palpate the chest in six areas. Palpate each area with the client exhaling and with the client holding the breath (if the client is able to do so). Note that palpation may be performed with the client sitting upright, reclining at a 45-degree or 30-degree angle, or lying flat. Start by palpating with the client sitting upright and then in the lowest position that the client can comfortably tolerate (see Figure 17.19).

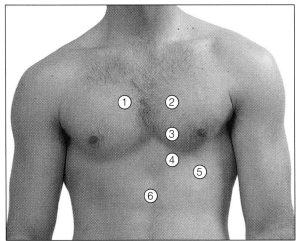

Figure 17.19 ●
Landmarks for palpation
of the chest.

| TECHNIQUES AND NORMAL FINDINGS | ABNORMAL FINDINGS AND SPECIAL CONSIDERATIONS |

1. **Palpate the chest.**
   - Place your right hand over the RSB, second ICS. Palpate with the base of your fingers.
   - You should not feel any pulsation, heave, or vibratory sensation against your palm in this location.

   ▶ Pulsations or heaves in the RSB, second ICS, indicate the presence of ascending aortic enlargement or aneurysm, aortic stenosis, or systemic hypertension.

   - Place your hand on the LSB, second ICS.
   - You should not feel any pulsation, heave, or vibratory sensation against your palm in this location except in some very thin clients who are nervous about the examination.

   ▶ Pulsations or heaves in the LSB, second ICS, are associated with pulmonary hypertension, pulmonary stenosis, right ventricular enlargement, atrial septal defect, enlarged left atrium, and large posterior left ventricular aneurysm.

   - Move your hand to the LSB, third then fourth ICS. No pulsations, heaves, or vibratory sensations should be felt.

   ▶ Pulsations or heaves over the LSB, third or fourth ICS, may indicate right ventricular enlargement or pressure overload on this ventricle, pulmonary stenosis, or pulmonary hypertension.

   - Place your right hand over the apex: MCL, fifth ICS.

   ▶ The presence of a heave, which is a forceful thrust over the fifth ICS, MCL, indicates the potential presence of increased right ventricular stroke volume or pressure and mild to moderate aortic regurgitation. If vibration is felt in a downward and lateral position from where the normal PMI should be palpated, or if it can be palpated in an area greater than 1 cm (0.5 in.) in diameter, these conditions may be present: left ventricular hypertrophy, severe left ventricular volume overload, or severe aortic regurgitation.

   - When palpating over the MCL, fifth ICS, you should feel a soft vibration, a tapping sensation, with each heartbeat. The vibration felt in this location should be isolated to an area no more than 1 cm (0.5 in.) in diameter.
   - Palpate the epigastric area, below the xiphoid process.

   ▶ The presence of heaves or thrills in the sub-xiphoid area suggests the presence of elevated right ventricular volume or pressure overload. **Thrills** are soft vibratory sensations best assessed with either the fingertips or the palm flattened on the chest.

   - Repeat the palpation technique, with the client at either a 30-degree angle or lying flat.

   > **CLINICAL TIP**
   > *Some clients are unable to lie flat. The client should be placed in the lowest angle that is comfortably tolerated. It is necessary to be alert to any physical distress experienced by the client during examination and stop activity immediately if distress is experienced.*

   - Palpation with the client lying flat normally reveals either no pulsation or very faint taps in a very localized area. No thrills, heaves, or lifts should be palpated in any of the five locations.

2. **Palpate the client's carotid pulses.**
   - The carotid artery is located in the groove between the trachea and sterno-cleidomastoid muscle beneath the angle of the jaw.

PHYSICAL ASSESSMENT

TECHNIQUES AND NORMAL FINDINGS

ABNORMAL FINDINGS AND SPECIAL CONSIDERATIONS

- It is important to palpate carotid pulses to assess their presence, strength, and equality. The client may remain supine, or you may help the client to sit upright.
- Ask the client to look straight ahead and keep the neck straight (see Figure 17.20).
- Palpate each carotid pulse separately. Normal findings bilaterally should demonstrate equality in intensity and regular pattern. The pulses should be strong but not bounding. If the pulse is difficult to palpate, ask the client to turn the head slightly to the examining side.

▶ Diminished or absent carotid pulses may be found in clients with carotid disease or dissecting ascending aneurysm. Absence of both pulses indicates *asystole* (absent heart rate). If the client is in critical care and has an arterial line, a printout of the arterial waveform should be obtained.

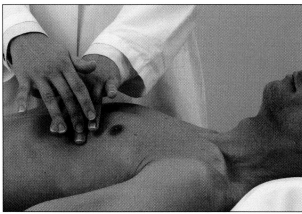

Figure 17.20 ●
Palpating the
carotid artery.

CLINICAL TIP

The carotid pulses must never be palpated simultaneously since this may obstruct blood flow to the brain.

PERCUSSION

1. **Percuss the client's chest to determine the cardiac border.**
   - Help the client to a reclining position at the lowest angle the client can tolerate.
   - Place the middle finger of your nondominant hand (pleximeter) in the fifth ICS at the left anterior axillary line.
   - Tap this finger at the distal phalanx by using the plexor of your dominant hand (see Figure 17.21). You should hear resonance because you are over lung tissue.
   - Continue to percuss in the fifth ICS toward the left MCL and the LSB. The sound will change to dullness as you percuss over the heart.
   - Repeat the previous percussion technique in the third ICS and the second ICS on the left side of the thorax. The sound of resonance heard over the lung should change to dullness over the heart.

▶ Percussion of the heart is not normally performed during a regular physical examination of the cardiovascular system. If cardiac enlargement is suspected an X-ray provides the most accurate information about the size of the client's heart.

▶ An enlarged heart emits a dull sound on percussion over a larger area than a heart of normal size. An X-ray film of the chest provides the most accurate information about the size of the client's heart.

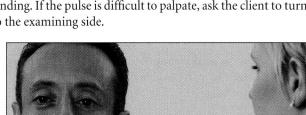

Figure 17.21 ●
Percussing the chest.

Techniques and Normal Findings	Abnormal Findings and Special Considerations

AUSCULTATION

The position of the client affects objective data collected from auscultatory examination. A full examination includes auscultation with the client sitting upright, leaning forward when upright, supine, and in the left lateral position. Have the client breathe normally initially. If you recognize the presence of abnormal sounds, have the client slow down the respirations so that you may listen to the effects of inspirations and expiratory efforts on the heart sounds. You may want to have some clients perform a forced expiration. When preparing to auscultate a child's chest, you may want to let the child listen to the parent's heart sounds with the stethoscope to reduce or prevent fear of this unfamiliar object. Use a stethoscope with a smaller bell and diaphragm when you examine a child.

1. **Auscultate the client's chest with the diaphragm of the stethoscope.**
   - Start the auscultation with the client sitting upright.
   - Move the stethoscope slowly across the chest and listen over each of the five key landmarks (see Figure 17.22).
   - Listen over the RSB, second ICS.
   - In this location, the S_2 sound should be louder than the S_1 sound, because this site is over the aortic valve.
   - Listen over the LSB, second ICS.
   - Also in this location the S_2 sound should be louder than the S_1 sound, because this site is over the pulmonic valve.
   - Listen over the LSB, third ICS, also called Erb's point.
   - You should hear both the S_1 and S_2 heart tones, relatively equal in intensity.
   - Listen at the LSB at the fourth ICS.
   - In this location the S_1 sound should be louder than the S_2 sound, because the closure of the tricuspid valve is best auscultated here.
   - Listen over the apex: fifth ICS, LMCL.
   - In this location the S_1 sound should also be louder than the S_2 sound, because the closure of the mitral valve is best auscultated here.

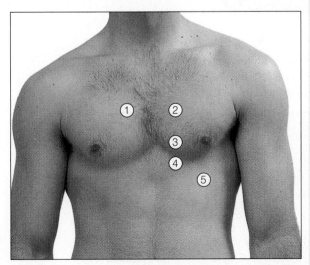

Figure 17.22 ●
Auscultating the chest over five key landmarks.

TECHNIQUES AND NORMAL FINDINGS	ABNORMAL FINDINGS AND SPECIAL CONSIDERATIONS

2. Auscultate the client's chest with the bell of the stethoscope.
   - Place the bell of the stethoscope lightly on each of the five key landmark positions shown with step 1.

   ▶ Low-pitched sounds are best auscultated with light application of the bell. Such sounds as S_3, S_4, murmurs (originating from stenotic valves), and gallops are best heard with the bell.

   - Listen for softer sounds over the five landmarks. Start with the bell and listen for the S_3 and S_4 sounds. Then listen for murmurs.

3. Auscultate the carotid arteries.
   - Listen with the diaphragm and bell of the stethoscope. Have the client hold the breath briefly. You may hear heart tones. This finding is normal.

   ▶ A **bruit**, a loud blowing sound, is an abnormal finding. It is most often associated with a narrowing or stricture of the carotid artery, usually associated with atherosclerotic plaque.

   - You should not hear any turbulent sounds, like murmurs.

4. Compare the apical pulse with a carotid pulse.
   - Auscultate the apical pulse.

   ▶ An apical pulse greater than the carotid rate indicates a pulse deficit. The rate, rhythm, and regularity must be evaluated.

   - Simultaneously palpate a carotid pulse.
   - Compare the findings. The two pulses should be synchronous. The carotid artery is used because it is closest to the heart and most accessible (see Figure 17.23).

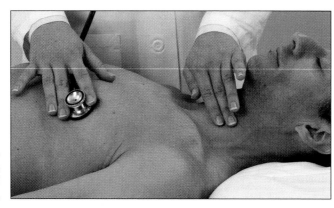

Figure 17.23 ●
Comparing the carotid and apical pulses.

5. Repeat the auscultation of the client's chest.
   - This time have the client lean forward, then lie supine, and finally lie in the left lateral position. Remember, not all clients will be able to tolerate all positions. In such cases, do not perform the technique (see Figure 17.24A–C).

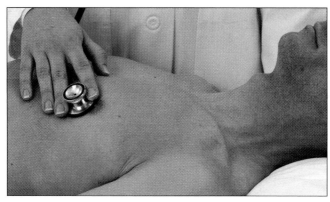

Figure 17.24A ●
Positions for auscultation of the heart. A. Supine.

Techniques and Normal Findings

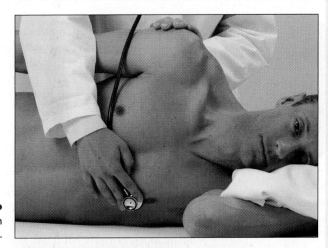

Figure 17.24B • Positions for auscultation of the heart. B. Lateral.

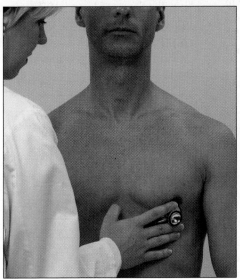

Figure 17.24C • Positions for auscultation of the heart. C. Sitting.

SAMPLE DOCUMENTATION

Subjective: No history of chest pain, fatigue/activity intolerance, fainting (syncope) or dizziness, peripheral edema, nocturia, or palpitations/arrhythmias. No history of CVS disease, diabetes, hypertension, or thyroid problems. Exercises regularly, relaxed individual, denies excess stress, and eats a healthful diet that includes the four food groups. Nonsmoker, drinks 3 glasses of wine each week, no nonprescription or illicit drug use.

Objective: *Inspection:* General colour uniform and pink. No nail clubbing. Extremities warm to touch and dry with no lesions. No visible bulges or masses on the anterior thorax. JVP < 2 cm.

Palpation: Apical heart rate at 78 bpm and regular. Apical impulse scarcely visible at 5th ICS, LMCL. Carotid pulse consistent with apical pulse. No palpable thrills. Peripheral pulses equal bilaterally +2.

Auscultation: S_1 loudest at apex and S_2 loudest at base.

APPLICATION THROUGH CRITICAL THINKING

CASE STUDY

Jason Chabar, a 56-year-old Black male, presents to the emergency room (ER) with a history of hypertension and type 1 diabetes mellitus, which he controls with diet and insulin injections. He smokes one pack of cigarettes daily and drinks three to four beers each night. He was recently laid off from an auto manufacturing plant where he had worked for 17 years. The Chabars are having trouble making mortgage and car payments. Today, when taking his morning walk, Mr. Chabar fatigued quickly, had difficulty catching his breath, felt a little nauseated, and experienced some unusual tingling in his left arm. Mr. Chabar states that his wife noticed that he was back from his walk early and saw that he did not look right. He felt it was not something to worry about. "It will go away if I rest," he said. His wife insisted that he go to the hospital.

First, the nurse must gather objective and subjective data to determine whether Mr. Chabar is in acute distress. The nurse will look for chest pain, pallor or cyanosis, respiratory effort, vital signs changes, and anxiety. If any of these are present, the nurse's goal is to maintain oxygen perfusion.

The nurse knows that hypertension and diabetes are risk factors for cardiovascular disease and that the symptoms of nausea, breathlessness, and numbness in the arm are indicators of a myocardial infarction (MI).

The nurse must avoid assumptions without evidence. For instance, the nurse might assume that the client has not followed his diabetes treatment regimen and is affected by hyperglycemia or hypoglycemia, that the client's medications have been ineffective or his hypertension has not been monitored, or that some event of a psychological nature gave rise to the client's symptoms.

The nurse begins the assessment by using an organized approach. The physical assessment reveals that Mr. Chabar is diaphoretic and his skin is grey-tinged, especially around the eyes. His vital signs are B/P 89/52—P 102—RR 34.

Mr. Chabar is in acute distress. Rapid interpretation of data is required. His skin colour suggests altered tissue perfusion.

He is hypotensive and tachycardic, and has an elevated respiratory rate. All the findings are indicative of an acute cardiovascular problem.

The goal is to restore tissue perfusion and prevent further systemic compromise.

Mr. Chabar is placed on a cardiac monitor, and administration of O$_2$ via nasal cannula is begun. Atropine as ordered by the ER physician is administered.

Following the atropine administration, the client's B/P is 110/70 and heart rate (HR) is 70.

Mr. Chabar occasionally rubs his chest and shakes his left arm but denies pain. He has occasional belching and states, "This is all probably from something I ate or an insulin reaction. I'd like to go home."

Mr. Chabar is to be admitted to the hospital and will go to the coronary care unit (CCU).

▶ Complete Documentation

The following is sample documentation for Jason Chabar.

SUBJECTIVE DATA: History of hypertension and type 1 diabetes, controlled with diet and insulin. Fatigued quickly during morning walk, difficulty catching his breath, nausea, unusual tingling in left arm. He felt it was nothing to worry about and "it will go away if I rest." Wife stated Mr. Chabar came home from walk "early" and he "did not look right."

OBJECTIVE DATA: 56-year-old Black male. Diaphoresis, grey-tinged skin, especially around eyes. VS: B/P 89/52—P 102—RR 34.

ASSESSMENT FORM

Chief Complaint: *Fatigue, difficulty breathing during walk, nausea, tingling left arm.*

History: *Hypertension, diabetes (type 1)—control diet, insulin, smokes, consumes 3-4 beers per day.*

Vital Signs: *B/P 89/52—P 102—RR 34*

Skin: *Diaphoresis, grey (especially eyes)*

▶ Critical Thinking Questions

1. What additional information will be required to formulate a plan of care for Mr. Chabar in the CCU?
2. How should the nurse interpret the client's desire "to go home" and statement that "This is all probably from something I ate or an insulin reaction"?
3. What evidence has been provided or is required to support or refute the possible assumptions about Mr. Chabar?
4. Explain the following conclusions about the client's physical condition:
   a. Decreased cardiac output
   b. Impaired gas exchange
   c. Fatigue
   d. Nausea

▶ Applying Nursing Diagnoses

1. *Cardiac output, decreased* is a nursing diagnosis in the NANDA-I taxonomy (see Appendix A). ⊂⊃ Do the data

in the case study support this diagnosis? If so, identify the supportive data.

2. *Pain, acute; tissue perfusion, ineffective;* and *anxiety* are diagnoses in the NANDA-I taxonomy. Do the data in the case study support these diagnoses? If so, identify the supporting data.

3. Use the data in the case study to develop additional nursing diagnoses. Identify the data to support the PES (problem, etiology, signs or symptoms) statement.

Prepare Teaching Plan

LEARNING NEED: Mr. Chabar has an increased risk for heart disease because he is Black, has been diagnosed with hypertension and diabetes, smokes, and consumes more than two alcoholic drinks per day. His symptoms include those that are typical in MI. He was reluctant to seek medical care, but at his wife's insistence, he received care shortly after the onset of symptoms.

The documentation for Mr. Chabar indicates that he will be admitted to the CCU for care of his acute cardiovascular problem. The symptoms suggest that Mr. Chabar suffered an MI.

While in the CCU, he will receive information about his condition and requirements for his posthospital healthcare regimen.

The case study provides data that are representative of risks, symptoms, and behaviours of many individuals. Therefore, the following teaching plan is based on the need to provide information to members of any community about MI and the importance of immediate care when symptoms arise.

GOAL: Participants will seek healthcare to promote cardiovascular health.

OBJECTIVES: On completion of this learning session, the participants will be able to do the following:

1. Describe MI.
2. Discuss risk factors for MI.
3. Describe symptoms of MI.
4. Identify lifesaving procedures.

Application of Objective 2: Discuss risk factors for an MI.		
Content	**Teaching Strategy**	**Evaluation**
Risk factors • Race: Black people have higher risk • Gender: males are at greater risk • High blood pressure • Diabetes • Family history • Aging • High cholesterol • Cigarette smoking • Stress • Obesity • Sedentary lifestyle	• Lecture • Discussion • Slides • Printed materials Lecture is appropriate when disseminating information to large groups. Discussion encourages learner participation and allows for questions and answers. Audiovisual materials, such as pictures and slides, provide visual reinforcement of information. Printed material can be used by the learner during and after the session to review materials.	• Written examination.

HEALTH PROMOTION ASSESSMENT TOOL

Social Determinants of Health	Level of Action	Action Strategies
Income and social support	Individual and family	**Create supportive environments** • Assist Mr. Chabar and his wife to identify social support that could help with their most immediate financial worries. These could include accessing bank services (to explore the feasibility of temporarily delaying mortgage payments), employment insurance, city social services, and consulting with the hospital social worker.
Social support networks	Family	**Create supportive environments** • Assess Mr. Chabar's social support networks like friends, and explore cardiology support groups. • Validate Mrs. Chabar's actions related to her insisting her husband seek appropriate healthcare. • Include Mrs. Chabar in teaching sessions with her husband to recognize signs and symptoms of health concerns (cardiac, diabetes), side effects of medications, and prevention strategies.
Personal coping skills	Individual	**Develop personal skills** • Commend Mr. Chabar for his commitment to exercise. • Refer Mr. Chabar to the above-mentioned financial services to address one of his major stressors.
		• Assess what a meaningful quality of life would look like for Mr. Chabar. Ask him what changes he would like to make to feel healthier. Assist him to develop a plan to address those changes. • Provide resources to support Mr. Chabar's level of readiness for behavioural change (example resources could include tobacco cessation programs and the Canadian Diabetes Association).

ABNORMAL FINDINGS

Abnormal findings in the cardiovascular system include murmurs (see Table 17.2, at the end of the section), diseases of the myocardium and pumping capacity, valvular heart disease, septal defects, congenital heart disease, and electrical rhythm disturbances.

Diseases of the Myocardium and Pumping Capacity of the Heart

Myocardial Ischemia

Ischemia is a common problem in which the oxygen needs of the body are heightened, thus increasing the work of the heart. Unfortunately, the oxygen needs of the heart are not met as it works harder, and an ischemic process ensues. Ischemia is usually due to the presence of atherosclerotic plaque. A blood clot may be associated with the plaque.

Myocardial Infarction

During infarction, complete disruption of oxygen and nutrient flow to the myocardial tissue occurs in the area below a total occlusion. Infarction leads to the death of the myocardial tissue unless flow of blood is reestablished.

Congestive Heart Disease

Congestive heart disease is the inability of the heart to produce a sufficient pumping effort. Most commonly, both right-sided and left-sided heart failure are present. Left-sided heart failure causes blood to back up into the pulmonary system and results in pulmonary edema. Right-sided heart failure causes backup of the blood into the systemic circulation and leads to distended neck veins, liver congestion, and peripheral edema.

Ventricular Hypertrophy

Ventricular hypertrophy occurs in response to pumping against high pressures. Right ventricular hypertrophy occurs with pulmonary hypertension, congenital heart disease, pulmonary disease, pulmonary stenosis, and right ventricular infarction.

Left ventricular hypertrophy occurs in the presence of systemic hypertension, congenital heart disease, aortic stenosis, or myocardial infarction to the left ventricle.

Valvular Disease

Valvular Heart Disease

Disease of the valves denotes either narrowing (stenosis) of the valve leaflets or incompetence (regurgitation) of these same leaflets. Valvular disease may be caused by rheumatic fever, congenital defects, myocardial infarction, and normal aging.

Mitral Stenosis

Mitral stenosis is a narrowing of the left mitral valve (see Figure 17.25).

Etiology: Rheumatic fever or cardiac infection.

Findings: Murmur heard at the apical area with the client in left lateral position.

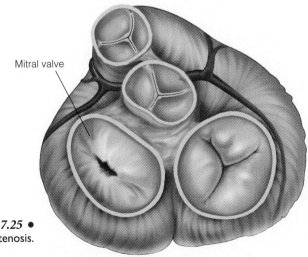

Mitral valve

Figure 17.25 ●
Mitral stenosis.

Aortic Stenosis

Aortic stenosis is a narrowing of the aortic valve (see Figure 17.26).

Etiology: Congenital bicuspid valves, rheumatic heart disease, atherosclerosis.

Findings: Murmur at aortic area, RSB, second ICS.

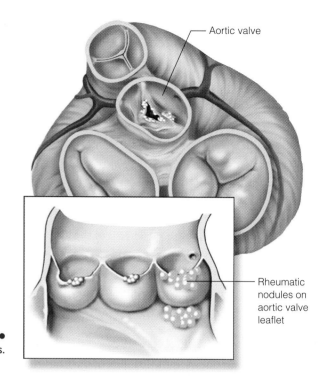

Aortic valve

Rheumatic nodules on aortic valve leaflet

Figure 17.26 ●
Aortic stenosis.

Mitral Regurgitation

Mitral regurgitation is the backflow of blood from the left ventricle into the left atrium (see Figure 17.27).

Etiology: Rheumatic fever, myocardial infarction, rupture of chordae tendineae.

Findings: Murmur at apex. Sound is transmitted to left axillae.

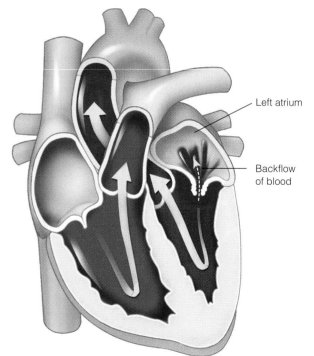

Left atrium

Backflow of blood

Figure 17.27 ●
Mitral regurgitation.

Pulmonic Stenosis

Pulmonic stenosis is narrowing of the opening between the pulmonary artery and the right ventricle (see Figure 17.28).

Etiology: Congenital.

Findings: Murmur at pulmonic area radiates to neck. Thrill in left second and third ICS.

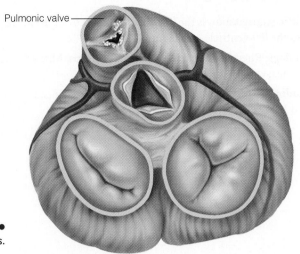

Pulmonic valve

Figure 17.28 ●
Pulmonic stenosis.

Tricuspid Stenosis

Tricuspid stenosis is narrowing or stricture of the tricuspid value of the heart (see Figure 17.29).

Etiology: Rheumatic heart disease, congenital defect, right atrial myxoma.

Findings: Murmur heard with the bell of the stethoscope over the tricuspid area.

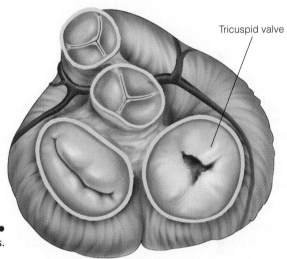

Tricuspid valve

Figure 17.29 ●
Tricuspid stenosis.

Mitral Valve Prolapse

Mitral valve prolapse is redundancy of the mitral valve leaflets so they prolapse into the left atrium (see Figure 17.30).

Etiology: May occur with pectus excavatum, often unknown.

Findings: Left lower sternal border in upright position.

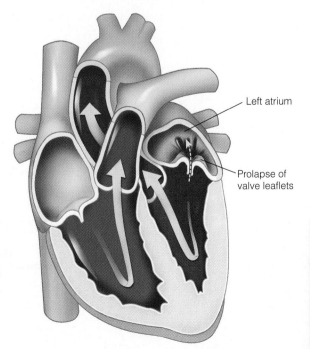

Left atrium

Prolapse of
valve leaflets

Figure 17.30 ●
Mitral valve prolapse.

Aortic Regurgitation

Aortic regurgitation is the backflow of blood from the aorta into the left ventricle (see Figure 17.31).

Etiology: Rheumatic heart disease, endocarditis, Marfan's syndrome, syphilis.

Findings: Murmur with client leaning forward. Click in second ICS.

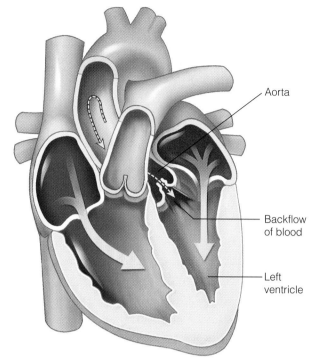

Figure 17.31 •
Aortic regurgitation.

Septal Defects

An atrial septal defect is an opening between the right and left atria, whereas a ventricular septal defect is an opening between the right and left ventricles. Both of these septal defects may result from congenital heart disease and myocardial infarction.

Ventricular Septal Defect

Regurgitation occurs through the defect resulting in a holosystolic murmur (see Figure 17.32). The murmur is loud, coarse, high-pitched, and heard at the LSB, third to fifth ICS.

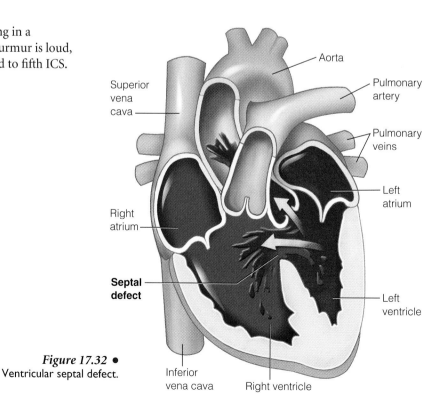

Figure 17.32 •
Ventricular septal defect.

Atrial Septal Defect

Regurgitation occurs through the defect resulting in a harsh, loud, high-pitched murmur heard at the LSB, second ICS (see Figure 17.33).

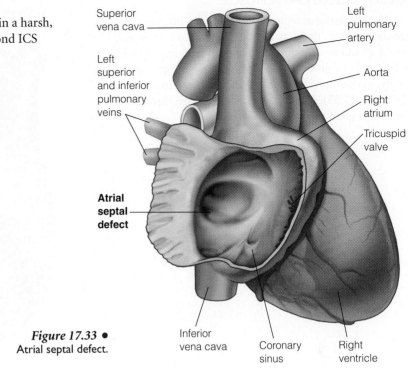

Figure 17.33 ●
Atrial septal defect.

Congenital Heart Disease

Congenital heart disease comes in many forms, which are related to developmental defects. Most often valves and septal structures are affected.

Coarctation of the Aorta

In this condition, the aorta is severely narrowed in the region inferior to the left subclavian artery (see Figure 17.34). The narrowing restricts blood flow from the left ventricle into the aorta and out into the systemic circulation, thus contributing to the development of congestive heart failure in the newborn. It can be surgically treated.

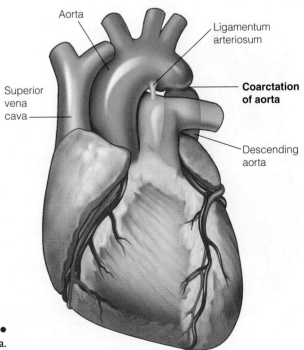

Figure 17.34 ●
Coarctation of the aorta.

Patent Ductus Arteriosus

The ductus arteriosus is an opening between the aorta and pulmonary artery that is present in the fetus. This opening should spontaneously close permanently between 24 and 48 hours after delivery. If this closure does not occur completely, a condition called patent ductus arteriosus exists (see Figure 17.35). It may be treated medically, through pharmacological therapy, and surgically.

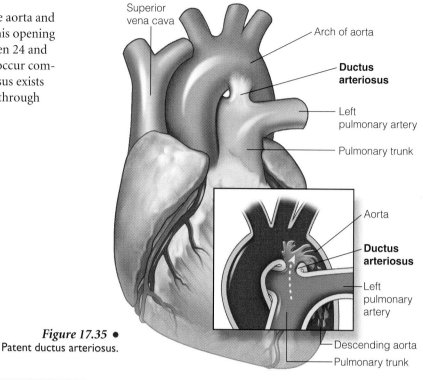

Figure 17.35 ●
Patent ductus arteriosus.

Tetralogy of Fallot

Tetralogy of Fallot involves four cardiac defects: dextroposition of the aorta, pulmonary stenosis, right ventricular hypertrophy, and ventricular septal defect (see Figure 17.36). This condition is life threatening for the newborn but can be treated surgically.

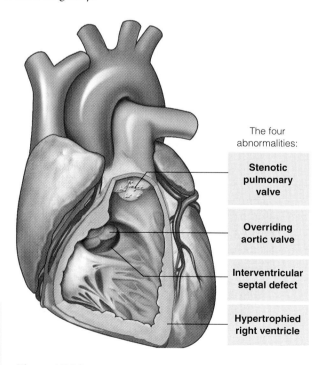

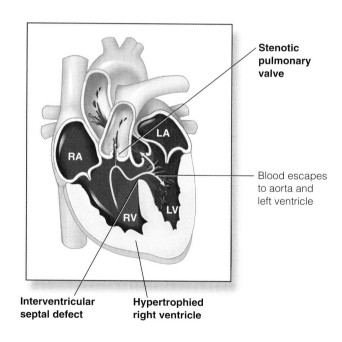

Figure 17.36 ● Tetralogy of Fallot.

Electrical Rhythm Disturbances

Rhythm disturbances are a common occurrence. Lethal dysrhythmias, such as ventricular tachycardia and ventricular fibrillation, are common complications of myocardial ischemia, myocardial infarction, and cardiomegaly. Heart blocks, such as first-degree atrioventricular block and second-degree atrioventricular heart block type 1, rarely compromise hemodynamic stability. However, second-degree atrioventricular heart block type 2 and third-degree atrioventricular heart block can significantly compromise hemodynamic stability, especially in the presence of myocardial infarction. Young individuals, mostly males, may suffer from tachycardias when extraconducting structures are present. These may be fatal in some cases.

Ventricular Tachycardia

Ventricle tachycardia is rapid, regular heartbeat as high as 200 bpm (see Figure 17.37).

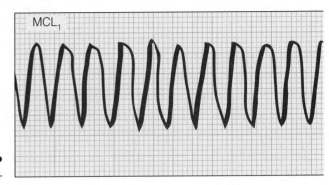

Figure 17.37 ●
Ventricular tachycardia.

Ventricular Fibrillation

Ventricular fibrillation is total absence of regular heart rhythm (see Figure 17.38).

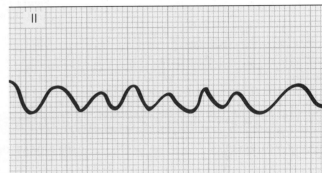

Figure 17.38 ●
Ventricular fibrillation.

Heart Block

Slow heart rate can be as low as 20 to 40 bpm (see Figure 17.39). Conduction between the atria and ventricles is disrupted.

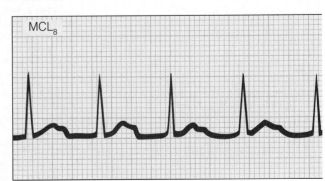

Figure 17.39 ●
Heart block.

Atrial Flutter

The atrial rate can be as high as 200 bpm and exceeds the ventricular response and rate (see Figure 17.40).

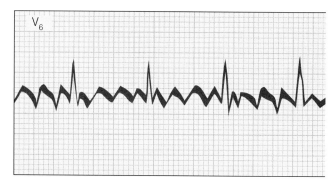

Figure 17.40 ●
Atrial flutter.

Atrial Fibrillation

Atrial fibrillation is dysrhythmic atrial contraction with no regularity or pattern (see Figure 17.41).

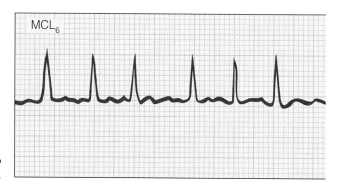

Figure 17.41 ●
Atrial fibrillation.

TABLE 17.2	Distinguishing Heart Murmurs
ASK YOURSELF	**INFORMATION**
1. How loud is the murmur?	Murmurs are graded on a rather subjective scale of 1 to 6: ● Grade 1: Barely audible with stethoscope; often considered physiological not pathological. Requires concentration and a quiet environment. ● Grade 2: Very soft but distinctly audible. ● Grade 3: Moderately loud; no thrill or thrusting motion is associated with the murmur. ● Grade 4: Distinctly loud; in addition to a palpable thrill. ● Grade 5: Very loud; can actually hear with part of the diaphragm of the stethoscope off the chest; palpable thrust and thrill present. ● Grade 6: Loudest; can hear with the diaphragm off the chest; visible thrill and thrust.
2. Where does it occur in the cardiac cycle: systole, diastole, or both?	Location in cardiac cycle ● Systole: early systole, midsystole, late systole ● Diastole: early diastole, mid-diastole, late diastole ● Both
3a. Is the sound continuous throughout systole, diastole, or only heard for part of the cycle?	Duration of murmur ● Continuous through systole only ● Continuous through diastole only ● Continuous through systole and diastole *Systolic murmurs* may be of two types: ● Midsystolic: Murmur is heard after S_1 and stops before S_2. ● Pansystolic or holosystolic: Murmur begins with S_1 and stops at S_2. *Diastolic murmurs* may be one of three types: ● Early diastolic: Murmur auscultated immediately after S_2 and then stops. There is a gap where this murmur stops and S_1 is heard. ● Mid-diastolic: Murmur begins a short time after S_2 and stops well before S_1 is auscultated. ● Late diastolic: This murmur starts well after S_2 and stops immediately before S_1 is heard.

TABLE 17.2	Distinguishing Heart Murmurs *(continued)*

ASK YOURSELF	INFORMATION
3b. What does the configuration of the sound look like? *Potential configurations:* S₁ ▬▬▬ S₂ **Pansytolic/holosystolic:** S₁ ▬▬ S₂ ▬▬ S₁ **Continuous** S₁ ▬▬ S₂ **Crescendo (systolic represented)**	S₂ ◄▬ S₁ **Decrescento (diastolic represented)** S₁ ◄▬► S₂ **Crescendo decrescendo (systole represented)** S₂ ▬▬ S₁ **Rumble**
4. What is the quality of the sound of the murmur?	• Blowing • Harsh • Musical • Raspy • Rumbling
5. What is the pitch or frequency of the sound?	• Low • Medium • High
6. In which landmark(s) do you best hear the murmur?	Use the five landmarks for auscultation: • Pulmonic areas 1 and 2 • Aortic area • Tricuspid area • Mitral area • Apex
7. Does it radiate?	• To the throat? • To the axilla?
8. Is there any change in pattern with respirations?	• Increases or decreases with inspiration? • Increases or decreases with expiration?
9. Is it associated with variations in heart sounds?	• Associated with split S₁? • Associated with split S₂? • Associated with S₃? • Associated with S₄? • Associated with a click or an ejection sound?
10. Does the intensity of the murmur change with position?	• Increases or decreases with squatting? • Increases or decreases with client in the left lateral position? (Do not have the client perform the Valsalva manoeuvre or any abrupt positional changes, because some clients do not tolerate position changes well.)

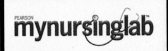

18

PERIPHERAL VASCULAR SYSTEM

THE PERIPHERAL VASCULAR SYSTEM IS MADE UP OF THE BLOOD VESSELS of the body. Together with the heart and the lymphatic vessels, they make up the body's circulatory system, which transports blood and lymph throughout the body. This chapter discusses assessment of the 96 500 km (60 000 mi.) network of veins and arteries that make up the peripheral vascular system, as well as the peripheral lymphatic vessels.

The vascular system plays a key role in the development of heart disease, one of the leading causes of death. People with high blood pressure have an increased risk of developing heart disease and stroke. Hypertension, the "silent killer," produces many physiological changes before any symptoms are experienced. This characteristic has tended to undermine efforts at treatment.

The nurse's efforts must be directed at prevention of problems of the circulatory system and promotion of a healthful way of life. A client's psychosocial health, self-care practices, and factors related to the client's family, culture, and environment all influence vascular health.

ANATOMY AND PHYSIOLOGY REVIEW

The peripheral vascular system is composed of arteries, veins, and lymphatics. Each of these will be described in the following sections.

Arteries

The **arteries** of the peripheral vascular system receive oxygen-rich blood from the heart and carry it to the organs and tissues of the body. The pumping heart (ventricular systole) creates a high-pressure wave or **pulse** that causes the arteries to expand and contract. This pulse propels the blood through the vessels and is palpable in arteries near the skin or over a bony surface. The thickness and elasticity of arterial walls help them to withstand these constant waves of pressure and to propel the blood to the body periphery. The thickness or viscosity of blood, the heart rate or cardiac output, and the ability of the vessels to expand and contract influence the arterial pulse. It is described as a smooth wave with a forceful ascending portion that domes and becomes less forceful as it descends. (Review Chapter 17 for more detailed information. ⟳)

In the arm, the pulsations of the *brachial artery* can be palpated in the antecubital region. The divisions of the brachial artery, the *radial* and *ulnar arteries,* can be palpated for pulsations over the anterior wrist. The major arteries of the arm are shown in Figure 18.1.

In the leg, the pulsations of the femoral artery can be palpated inferior to the inguinal ligament, about halfway between the anterior superior iliac spine and the symphysis pubis. The *femoral artery* continues down the thigh and becomes the *popliteal artery* as it passes behind the knee. Pulsations of the popliteal artery are palpable over the popliteal region. Below the knee, the popliteal artery divides into the anterior and posterior tibial arteries. The *anterior tibial artery* travels to the dorsum of the foot, and its pulsation can be felt just lateral to the prominent extensor tendon of the big toe close to the ankle. This pulse is known as the dorsalis pedis. Pulsations of the *posterior tibial artery* can be felt where it passes behind the medial malleolus of the ankle. The major arteries of the leg are illustrated in Figure 18.2.

The movement of blood through the systemic arterial system occurs in waves that cause two types of pressure. The blood pressure has two distinct parts: a systolic pressure and a diastolic pressure. The systolic pressure occurs during cardiac systole or ventricular contraction. It is the force of the blood that is exerted on the arterial wall during this cardiac action. The diastolic pressure occurs during cardiac diastole or ventricular relaxation. It is the force of the blood on the arterial wall during ventricular filling. Blood pressure is influenced by age, sympathoadrenal activity, blood volume, and ability of the vessels to contract and dilate. Blood pressure was discussed in greater detail in Chapter 7. ⟳

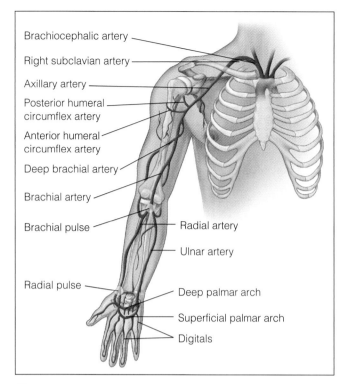

Figure 18.1 ● Main arteries of the arm.

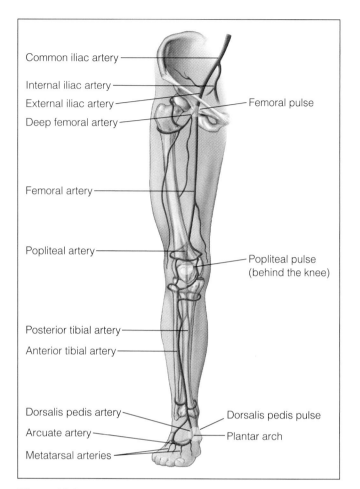

Figure 18.2 ● Main arteries of the leg.

Veins

The **veins** of the systemic circulation deliver deoxygenated blood from the body periphery back to the heart. Veins have thinner walls and a larger diameter than arteries and are able to stretch and dilate to facilitate venous return. Venous return is assisted by contraction of skeletal muscles during such activities as walking and by pressure changes related to inspiration and expiration. In addition, veins have one-way intraluminal valves that close tightly when filled to prevent backflow. Thus, venous blood flows only toward the heart. Problems with the lumen or valves of the leg veins can lead to *stasis,* or pooling of blood in the veins of the lower extremities.

The femoral and the popliteal veins are deep veins of the legs and carry about 90% of the venous return from the legs. The great and small saphenous veins are superficial veins that are not as well supported as the deep veins by surrounding tissues and therefore are more susceptible to venous stasis. The major veins of the leg are depicted in Figure 18.3.

Capillaries

Exchanges of gases and nutrients between the arterial and venous systems are conducted within beds of **capillaries,** the smallest vessels of the circulatory system. Blood pressure in the arterial end of the capillary bed forces fluid out across the capillary membrane and into the body tissues.

Lymphatic System

The lymphatic system consists of the vast network of vessels, fluid, various tissue, and organs throughout the body. These vessels help transport escaped fluid back to the vascular system.

The lymphoid organs have a major role in the body's defences and the immune system. These structures help fight infection and provide the individual with immunocompetence. The spleen, tonsils, and thymus gland are examples of lymphoid organs.

The **lymphatic vessels** form their own circulatory system in which their collected fluid flows to the heart. The vessels extend from the capillaries of their system to the two main lymphatic trunks. The *right lymphatic duct* collects lymph from the right upper extremity, which is the right side of the thorax and head. The *thoracic duct* collects lymph from the remaining part of the body. The thoracic duct responds to the protein and fluid pressure at the capillary end of the vessels that help keep the lymph properly circulated. During circulation, as blood continues through the capillary bed toward the smallest veins, called *venules,* more fluid leaves the capillaries than can be absorbed by the veins. The lymphatic system retrieves this excess fluid, called **lymph**, from the tissue spaces and carries it to the lymph nodes throughout the body. **Lymph nodes** are clumps of tissue located along the lymphatic vessels, either deep or superficially in the body. The lymph nodes usually are covered and protected by connective tissue and are therefore not palpable. Some of the more superficial nodes are located in the neck, the axillary region, and the inguinal region. Deeper clusters are located in the abdomen and thoracic cavity. The

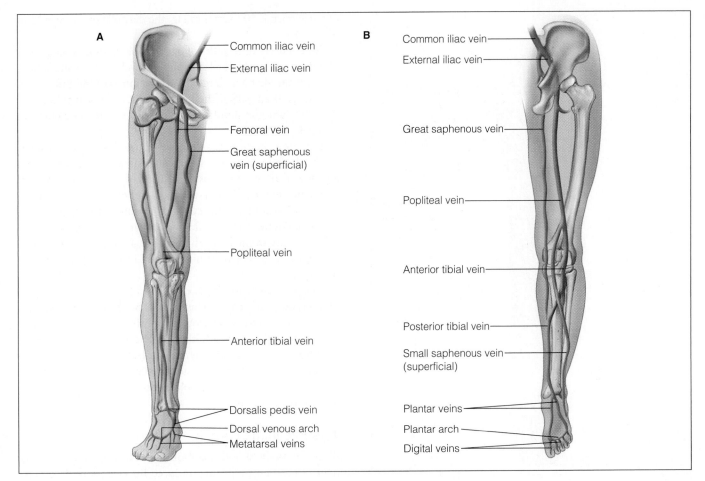

A
Common iliac vein
External iliac vein
Femoral vein
Great saphenous vein (superficial)
Popliteal vein
Anterior tibial vein
Dorsalis pedis vein
Dorsal venous arch
Metatarsal veins

B
Common iliac vein
External iliac vein
Great saphenous vein
Popliteal vein
Anterior tibial vein
Posterior tibial vein
Small saphenous vein (superficial)
Plantar veins
Plantar arch
Digital veins

Figure 18.3 • The main veins of the leg. A. Anterior view. B. Posterior view.

lymph nodes filter lymph fluid, removing any pathogens before the fluid is returned to the bloodstream.

The **epitrochlear node,** located on the medial surface of the arm above the elbow, drains the ulnar surface of the forearm and the third, fourth, and fifth digits. The nodes in the axilla of the arm drain the rest of the arm. The major lymph nodes of the arm are shown in Figure 18.4.

The legs have two sets of superficial inguinal nodes, a vertical group and a horizontal group. The vertical group is located close to the saphenous vein and drains that area of the leg. The horizontal group of nodes is found below the inguinal ligament. These nodes drain the skin of the abdominal wall, the external genitals, the anal canal, and the gluteal area. The major lymph nodes of the leg are illustrated in Figure 18.5.

The functions of the peripheral vascular system are the following:

- Delivering oxygen and nutrients to tissues of the body
- Transporting carbon dioxide and other waste products from the tissues for excretion
- Removing pathogens from the body fluid by filtering lymph

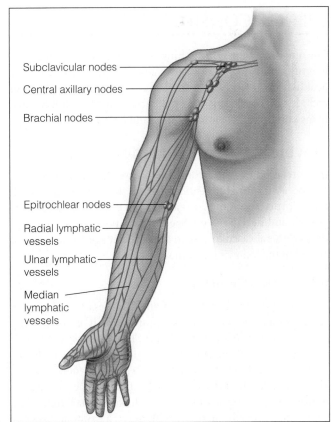

Subclavicular nodes
Central axillary nodes
Brachial nodes
Epitrochlear nodes
Radial lymphatic vessels
Ulnar lymphatic vessels
Median lymphatic vessels

Figure 18.4 • Main lymph nodes of the arm.

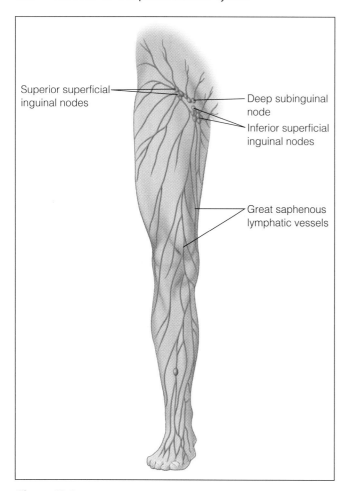

Figure 18.5 ● Main lymph nodes of the leg.

SPECIAL CONSIDERATIONS

The nurse must use critical thinking and the nursing process to identify factors to consider when conducting a comprehensive health assessment. Factors that affect the client's health status include age, developmental level, race, ethnicity, work history, living conditions, socioeconomics, and emotional well-being.

Developmental Considerations

Interpretation of data from health assessment is dependent on the ability to differentiate normal from abnormal findings. Normal variations in anatomy and physiology occur with growth and development. Specific variations associated with the peripheral vascular system for different age groups are discussed in the following sections.

Infants and Children

Assessing the blood pressure of an infant less than 1 year of age is difficult without special equipment. It is usually not necessary if the infant is moving well and the skin colour is good. However, if the child is lethargic and tires easily during feeding or the skin becomes cyanotic when the infant cries, the blood pressure should be measured with a Doppler flowmeter. A newborn's blood pressure is much lower than that of an adult and gradually increases with age. The systolic pressure

of a newborn is 50 to 80 mm Hg; the diastolic pressure is 25 to 55 mm Hg.

All children 18 months of age and older should have their blood pressure evaluated during their well-child examination. The cuff should be no larger than two thirds of the child's arm or smaller than half of the length of the child's arm between the elbow and the shoulder. Pediatric blood pressure cuffs are available.

In young children, the blood pressure should be measured on the thigh to rule out a significant difference between upper and lower extremity pressure. Such a difference in pressure could indicate coarctation (a narrowing) of the aorta. In a baby less than 1 year of age, the systolic pressure in the thigh should equal that of the arm. A child over 1 year of age will have a systolic pressure in the thigh that is 10 to 40 mm Hg higher than that in the arm. The diastolic pressure in the thigh equals that in the arm.

The pulse increases if the child has a fever. For every degree of fever, the pulse may increase 8 to 10 beats per minute (bpm). The lymphatic system develops rapidly from birth until puberty and then subsides in adulthood. The presence of enlarged lymph nodes in a child may not indicate illness. However, if an infection is present, the nodes may enlarge considerably. Chapter 25 describes a complete assessment of infants, children, and adolescents. ∞

The Pregnant Female

Blood pressure should be monitored throughout the pregnancy to test for pregnancy-induced hypertension. Blood volume during pregnancy almost doubles. In the second trimester, blood pressure may decrease because of the dilation of the peripheral vessels. However, blood pressure usually returns to the prepregnancy level by the third trimester. If the client has a history of hypertension before her pregnancy, the blood pressure may increase dramatically during the third trimester, posing the threat of cerebral hemorrhage. Pressure from the uterus on the lower extremities can obstruct venous return and lead to hypotension when the client is lying on her back, or it can cause edema, **varicosities** (distended veins) of the leg, and hemorrhoids. Chapter 26 describes a complete assessment of the pregnant female. ∞

The Older Adult

The aging process causes arteriosclerosis or calcification of the walls of the blood vessels. The arterial walls lose elasticity and become more rigid. This increase in peripheral vascular resistance results in increased blood pressure. The enlargement of calf veins can pose the risk of blood clots in leg veins. However, the amount of circulatory inadequacy at any given age is not predictable. The aging process may not cause any symptoms in some older clients.

Most hypertension is asymptomatic, but a severe elevation may produce a headache, epistaxis (nosebleed), shortness of breath, or chest pain. When evaluating the various arterial pulses, the nurse should keep in mind that the heart rate slows with the aging process. Some persons may normally have a rate of 50 bpm; however, the client should be evaluated if the pulse is below 60 bpm. Likewise, it is common for older clients to manifest irregular pulses often with occasional pauses or extra beats. Again, any client with an irregular pulse should be referred for further examination. Chapter 27 describes a complete assessment of the older adult. ∞

Psychosocial Considerations

Stress is among the factors that contribute to development of hypertension. Work-related stress has often been associated with hypertension. Stress can result from the rigors of everyday life in a complex and ever-changing world. Globalization and resulting economic fluctuations, spread of disease, and terrorist threats have created a stressful environment. An individual's response to stress can determine the risk of developing hypertension in response to stress.

Social and Environmental Considerations

The incidence of hypertension is greater among some ethnic groups; however, the nurse must conduct a complete assessment regarding factors that influence hypertension (e.g., traditional diets, smoking). Obesity is a risk factor for hypertension and is on the rise in Canada. This factor must also be investigated.

Risk factors for varicose veins include Irish and German descent, a family history of varicosities, a sedentary lifestyle, obesity, and multiple pregnancies.

Clients whose jobs require them to stand for most of the day, such as hairdressers and cashiers, are at greater risk for developing varicose veins. Desk jobs that require sitting for prolonged periods also contribute to venous stasis and varicose veins.

Social and Ethnocultural Considerations

- Skin colour variations across ethnic groups may affect assessment of circulation. The nurse must use skin temperature, capillary refill, and pulse characteristics when pink undertones are not easily detected.
- Diabetes increases the risk for peripheral vascular disease and is increasing in prevalence among certain groups. Ask about a personal or familial history of diabetes.

- Obesity is a risk factor for hypertension and peripheral vascular disease. Obesity is increasing in all groups at all ages.
- Smoking increases the risk for hypertension and peripheral vascular disease. Ask about a history of smoking.

GATHERING THE DATA

HEALTH HISTORY

Health assessment of the peripheral vascular system includes gathering subjective and objective data. During the interview the nurse uses a variety of communication techniques to elicit general and specific information about the client's state of health or illness. Health records and the results of laboratory tests are important secondary sources to be reviewed and included in the data-gathering process. In physical assessment of the peripheral vascular system, the techniques of inspection, palpation, and auscultation will be used. Before proceeding, it may be helpful to review the information about each of the data-gathering processes and practise the techniques of health assessment.

The health history for the peripheral vascular system concerns data related to the structures and functions of that system. Subjective data are gathered during the health history. The nurse must be prepared to observe the client and listen for cues related to the functions of the systems. The nurse may use closed or open-ended questions to obtain information. Often a number of follow-up questions or requests for descriptions are required to clarify data or gather missing information.

The health history guides the physical assessment of the peripheral vascular system. The information is always considered in relation to normal parameters and expectations. Therefore, the nurse must consider age, gender, race, culture, environment, health practices, past and concurrent problems, and therapies when framing questions and using techniques to elicit information. To address all the factors when conducting a health history, specific questions related to the peripheral vascular status and function have been developed. These questions focus on the most common concerns or injuries associated with the peripheral vascular system; questions related to past health history; questions related to behaviours; questions that address environmental concerns; and those that are specific to clients according to age, including the pregnant female.

The nurse must consider the client's ability to participate in the health history and physical assessment. If a client is experiencing pain or anxiety, attention must focus on relief of symptoms.

As the nurse gathers the data, she or he will shift the type of questions to direct questions that give the client room to explain or qualify. The mnemonic O-P-Q-R-S-T-U, which stands for onset (chronology), precipitating (or palliative), quality, region (or radiation), severity, timing, and understanding, will help the learner remember the dimensions of the symptoms. The nurse will keep in mind that not all these qualifiers will apply to each symptom.

HEALTH HISTORY QUESTIONS	RATIONALES

The following sections provide sample questions and follow-up questions. Rationales for some questions are provided. The list of questions is not all-inclusive but rather represents the more common concern or injury questions required in a health history related to the peripheral vascular system. An example of using O-P-Q-R-S-T-U with pain is provided.

Questions Related to Common Concerns or Injuries

The most common symptoms related to peripheral vascular illness or injury are as follows:

- Pain
- Edema (swelling)
- Skin changes in the extremities
- Temperature changes in the extremities
- Numbness and tingling

1. **Pain**
   - Are you having any leg pain or cramps at this time? *If yes:*

   ▶ Pain associated with **arterial insufficiency** (inadequate circulation in the arterial system, usually caused by the buildup of fatty plaque or calcification of the arterial wall) is usually described as gnawing, sharp, or stabbing and increases with exercise. Pain is relieved with the cessation of movement and when legs are dangling. Pain is most commonly in the calf of the leg but may also be present in the lower leg or top of the foot. **Venous insufficiency** (inadequate circulation in the venous system, usually caused by incompetent valves in deep veins or a blood clot in the veins) is described as aching or a feeling of fullness. It intensifies with prolonged standing or sitting in one position. Swelling and varicosities in the legs may also be present. The condition is relieved by elevating the legs or by walking.

   - When did you first notice the pain? How long does it last? *Onset (chronology)*
   - What makes the pain worse? What makes the pain better? *Precipitating (palliative)*
   - Can you describe the pain? It is sharp? dull? burning? cramping? *Quality*
   - Where is the pain located? Does the pain radiate? *Region (radiation)*
   - How often do you experience the pain? Does the pain affect your activities of daily living? How would you rate the pain on a scale of 1 to 10, with 10 being the worst pain? *Severity*
   - Is the pain associated with walking? Does it occur at rest? *Timing*
   - What do you think is causing the pain? *Understanding*

2. **Edema (swelling)**
   - Have you noticed any swelling or shiny skin, particularly on your legs?

   ▶ Obstruction to lymphatic flow, incompetent valves, and decreased osmotic pressure in the capillaries results in peripheral edema.

   - When did the swelling start? Does it get better or worse during the day?
   - What relieves the swelling?
   - Do you have any swollen glands? If so, where in your body?

   ▶ Enlarged lymph nodes are associated with an infectious process in the body.

HEALTH HISTORY QUESTIONS	RATIONALES

3. Skin changes in the extremities
- Have you noticed any skin changes on your arms and legs?

▶ Changes in skin texture and swelling are sometimes caused by fluid leaking into tissue spaces because of incompetent valves in veins.

- Has your skin been pale or blue?

▶ Colour changes may indicate pallor (arterial insufficiency) or cyanosis (venous insufficiency).

- Have you noticed skin changes, such as sores or ulcers, on your legs?

▶ Leg ulcers are an indication of chronic arterial or venous problems.

- Does your skin look shiny or feel tight?

▶ Peripheral arterial insufficiency can cause hair loss or skin changes.

4. Temperature changes in the extremities
- Have you noticed any change in temperature in your arms and legs, such as extreme coolness or heat?

▶ Extreme coolness may indicate arterial insufficiency. Extreme heat may indicate a blood clot.

5. Numbness and tingling
- Have you noticed any numbness and tingling in your extremities?

▶ Numbness and tingling indicates decreased circulation.

Questions Related to Past Health History

1. Have you ever been diagnosed with a peripheral vascular disease, such as hypertension, atherosclerosis, Raynaud's disease, varicose veins, or thrombophlebitis? *If yes:*
- When were you diagnosed with the problem?
- Has the problem ever recurred? *(acute)*
- How are you managing the disease now? *(chronic)*

▶ If a diagnosis of an illness is identified, follow-up about the date of the diagnosis, treatment, and outcomes is required. Data about each illness identified by the client are essential to an accurate health assessment. Illnesses can be classified as acute or chronic, and follow-up regarding each classification will differ.

- Does you peripheral vascular illness affect your ability to carry out your activities of daily living?
- Have you discussed this with a healthcare professional? If so, what treatment was recommended and did it help?

▶ Inability to carry out or perform personal or work-related activities can be indicative of problems in the peripheral vascular system.

2. Is there anyone in your family who has a history of peripheral vascular diseases or problems, such as hypertension (high blood pressure)? If so, what was it?

▶ This question may reveal information about peripheral vascular diseases associated with familial or genetic predisposition.

3. For male clients: Have you experienced any difficulty in achieving an erection?

▶ Impotence may occur as a result of a diminished arterial flow to the pelvic arteries. This condition is a common finding in peripheral vascular disease and is not always reported because of client embarrassment.

Questions Related to Behaviours

Healthcare behaviours include both health practices and health patterns. Health practices consist of following recommendations for disease prevention, including screening for risks, screening for early detection of problems, and immunization. Health patterns are habits or acts that affect the client's health. Health behaviours may also include seeking healthcare from healthcare providers who use alternative methods to diagnose and treat illness. Clients should be questioned in a nonjudgmental way and areas for health teaching should be identified.

1. Do you smoke?

▶ Nicotine is a vasoconstrictor and aggravates peripheral vascular disease.

HEALTH HISTORY QUESTIONS	RATIONALES

2. Have you tried to quit? Are there any factors that have affected your success with this?

3. Do you exercise regularly? Describe your exercise routine.

Questions Related to the Environment

Environment refers to both internal and external environments. Questions related to the internal environment include all the previous questions and those associated with internal or physiological responses. Questions regarding the external environment include those related to home, work, or social environments.

Internal Environment

1. What medications do you take?

▶ Contraceptive medications have been associated with blood clots in the peripheral vascular system.

2. Are you experiencing any side effects related to the medication?

3. Are you now or have you ever experienced anxiety or upset?

▶ Anxiety or situations of emotion affect the sympathetic nervous system, producing hormonal responses that affect vascular function.

External Environment

The following question deals with the physical environment of the client. That includes the indoor and outdoor environments of the home and the workplace, those encountered for social engagements, and any encountered during travel.

1. Describe your daily activities.

▶ A sedentary lifestyle and prolonged periods of sitting or standing at work or in the home can promote peripheral vascular problems, varicosities, or problems associated with venous stasis.

Questions Related to Age

The health history must reflect the anatomical and physiological differences that exist along the age span.

Questions Regarding Infants and Children

1. Has the infant become lethargic?

▶ Lethargy is one sign of hypertension or hypoxemia associated with vascular disease.

2. Has the child had blood pressure screening?

▶ All children 18 months of age and older should have their blood pressure evaluated during their well-child examination. They should be screened again between 4 and 5 years of age, and then during the school-age years only if the child is at risk for high blood pressure. During adolescence, children should be screened every second year.

3. Does the child have any enlarged lymph nodes?

▶ Enlarged lymph nodes in a child may not indicate illness. However, in infection considerable enlargement is found.

Questions for the Pregnant Female

1. Have you had your blood pressure monitored?

▶ Monitoring can reduce risks for pregnancy-induced hypertension.

2. Are you experiencing swelling on the face, hands, or legs?

▶ Pitting edema in the lower extremities is common in pregnancy, especially at the end of the day and into the third trimester.

Questions for the Older Adult

No additional questions for the older adult are required.

GATHERING THE DATA

PHYSICAL ASSESSMENT

ASSESSMENT TECHNIQUES AND FINDINGS

Physical assessment of the peripheral vascular and lymphatic systems requires the use of inspection, palpation, auscultation, and assessment of blood pressure. During each aspect of the assessment, the nurse is gathering objective data about circulation. Inspection includes looking at skin colour, appearance of superficial vasculature, and shape and size of the extremities and nails. Palpation of pulses and auscultation of blood pressure and arteries provide information about vascular status. Knowledge of normal parameters and expected findings is essential in determining the meaning of the data as the physical assessment is performed.

The adult has a normal systolic blood pressure of less than 120 and diastolic blood pressure below 80. The carotid pulses are palpable, symmetrical, and synchronous with S_1 of the heart. Auscultation of carotid arteries yields a soft sound, occasionally with transmission of heart sounds, but absence of bruits. The upper extremities should be of equal size and warm, with pink undertones and no edema. Capillary refill should occur in less than 2 seconds. The brachial and radial arteries should be equal in rate and symmetrical in amplitude. The epitrochlear nodes are not palpable. The lower extremities are warm and equal in size, the colour is consistent with the rest of the body, hair is evenly distributed, and the extremities have no edema, lesions, or varicosities. The inguinal nodes are nonpalpable. The femoral, popliteal, posterior tibial, and dorsalis pedis pulses are equal and symmetrical in rate and amplitude. The toenails are pink and without clubbing.

Physical assessment of the peripheral vascular and lymphatic systems proceeds in an organized pattern. Blood pressure is assessed in upper and lower extremities. A cephalocaudal pattern for assessment of the vascular and lymphatic system begins with the carotid arteries and follows through inspection of the upper and lower extremities and palpation of pulses and lymph nodes within them. Additional assessment techniques include the **Allen test** to determine patency of the radial and ulnar arteries, the **manual compression test** to determine the length of varicose veins, and the Trendelenburg test to evaluate valve competence when varicosities are present.

EQUIPMENT

examination gown	tourniquet
Doppler	stethoscope
sphygmomanometer	

HELPFUL HINTS

- The client should wear an examination gown, but undergarments may remain in place.
- The client should remove watches and jewellery that may interfere with assessment.
- Socks and stockings should be removed.
- The client will sit, stand, and lie in a supine position during various aspects of the assessment. The nurse should provide assistance and support when required and ensure that the client's respiratory effort will not be affected by moving about or when lying flat.
- Use routine precautions.

TECHNIQUES AND NORMAL FINDINGS	ABNORMAL FINDINGS AND SPECIAL CONSIDERATIONS

BLOOD PRESSURE

1. **Instruct the client.**

- Explain that you will be assessing blood pressure in the arms and legs. Tell the client you will inflate the cuff twice for each location. The first time you will only touch a pulse area, and the second time you will use the stethoscope. Tell the client to breathe normally and relax the extremity. The only discomfort should occur when the cuff is fully inflated and will be relieved as the cuff deflates. Tell the client to report any other problems.

- Ask the client to remain still and not to speak during the auscultation, as you will not hear well when the stethoscope is in place for the blood pressure reading.

- Explain that you will take the blood pressure while the client is sitting and then when lying down. The readings will be compared.

Techniques and Normal Findings	Abnormal Findings and Special Considerations

2. Position the client.

- Place the client in a sitting position on the examination table (see Figure 18.6).

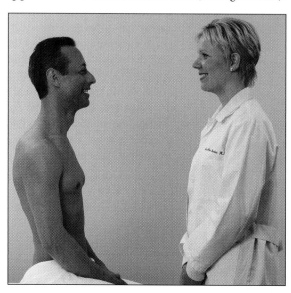

Figure 18.6 ●
The client is positioned
for the examination.

- Take the blood pressure in both arms. Assess the palpable systolic pressure (see Figure 18.7A and page 117 for details).

▶ Assessing the palpable systolic pressure helps to avoid an inaccuracy caused by auscultatory gap when auscultating blood pressure.

> **CLINICAL TIP**
> *Always ask the client about any medical conditions, such as an arteriovenous (A-V) fistula or a mastectomy, that preclude having blood pressure taken in both arms.*

- Auscultate the blood pressure (see Figure 18.7B).

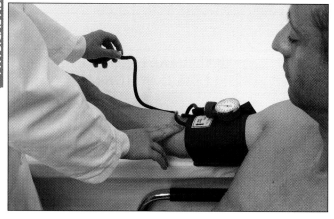

Figure 18.7A ● Blood pressure measurements. A. Palpable blood pressure.

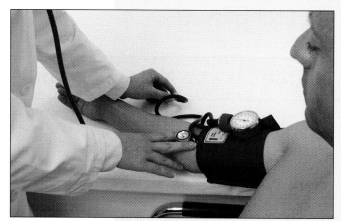

Figure 18.7B ● Blood pressure measurements. B. Auscultation of blood pressure.

- The blood pressure normally does not vary more than 5 to 10 mm Hg in each arm.

▶ A difference of 10 mm Hg or more between the arms may indicate an obstruction of arterial flow to one arm.

- The Canadian Hypertension Education Program (2009) has created guidelines regarding the interpretation of blood pressure measurements (Table 18.1). The

▶ A systolic reading below 90 or a diastolic reading under 60 may be an early indication of shock, which requires immediate medical attention.

| TECHNIQUES AND NORMAL FINDINGS | ABNORMAL FINDINGS AND SPECIAL CONSIDERATIONS |

diagnosis of hypertension is made after a series of visits, not with only one or two measurements.

TABLE 18.1	Canadian Hypertension Education Program Blood Pressure Guidelines for Adults	
CLASSIFICATION	**SYSTOLIC B/P (MM HG)**	**DIASTOLIC B/P (MM HG)**
Normal	<120	and <80
High-normal	130–139	85–89
Hypertension (1st visit)	>200	120
Hypertension (2nd visit)	140–190	110 *and* medical condition from list
		or B/P ≥ 180/110
Hypertension (3rd visit)	160–197	100–109

Source: Compiled by author based on Canadian Hypertension Education Program (2009).

3. Assist the client to a supine position.

4. Take the blood pressure in both arms, if possible.
   - Pressures are lower when taken in the supine position.
   - Standards for blood pressure are set for clients in the sitting position.

5. Take the blood pressure in both legs.
   - The blood pressure in the popliteal artery is usually 10 to 40 mm Hg higher than that in the brachial artery.

CAROTID ARTERIES

1. Inspect the neck for carotid pulsations.
   - With the client in a supine position, inspect the neck from the hyoid bone to the clavicles. Bilateral pulsations will be seen between the trachea and sternocleidomastoid muscle. They may not be visible in individuals with obesity.

2. Palpate the carotid pulses.
   - Place the pads of your first two or three fingers on the client's neck between the trachea and the sternocleidomastoid muscle, just below the angle of the jaw (see Figure 18.8).

▶ It is important to document the client's position for each assessment of blood pressure.

▶ The absence of pulsation may indicate internal or external obstruction.

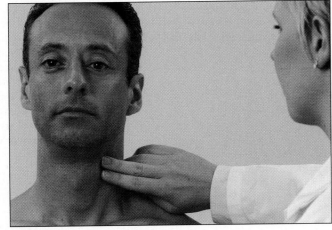

Figure 18.8 ●
Palpating the
carotid artery.

TECHNIQUES AND NORMAL FINDINGS

ABNORMAL FINDINGS AND SPECIAL CONSIDERATIONS

- Ask the client to turn the head slightly toward your hand to relax the sterno-cleidomastoid muscle.

- Palpate firmly but not so hard that you occlude the artery.

- Palpate one side of the neck at a time. If you are having difficulty finding the pulse, try varying the pressure of your fingers, feeling carefully below the angle.

▶ If both carotid arteries are palpated at the same time, the result can be a drop in blood pressure or a reduction in the pulse rate, from the stimulation of baroreceptors.

- Note the rate, rhythm, amplitude, and symmetry of the carotid pulses. Compare this rate to the apical pulse.

▶ A rate of more than 90 bpm is considered abnormal unless the client is anxious or has recently been exercising or smoking. A rate below 60 is also considered abnormal.

However, some athletes have a resting pulse as low as 50 bpm. An irregular rhythm or a pulse with extra beats or missed beats is considered abnormal. An exaggerated pulse or a weak, thready pulse is abnormal. A discrepancy between the two carotid pulses is abnormal.

3. Auscultate the carotid pulses.

- Use the diaphragm of the stethoscope to auscultate each carotid artery high in the neck, inferior to the angle of the jaw, and medial to the sternocleidomastoid muscle. Ask the client to hold his or her breath for several seconds to decrease tracheal sounds. You may need to have the client turn the head slightly to the side not being examined.

- Repeat the procedure by using the bell of the stethoscope.

CLINICAL TIP

It is important not to put pressure on the bell of the stethoscope as this may occlude the sounds in the blood vessel.

- While auscultating, you should hear a very quiet sound. Normal heart sounds could be transmitted to the neck, but there should be no swishing sounds.

▶ A swishing sound indicates the presence of a **bruit**, an obstruction causing turbulence, such as a narrowing of the vessel caused by the buildup of cholesterol.

An increased cardiac output, such as that seen in hyperthyroidism or anemia, also will produce a bruit.

ARMS

1. Assess the hands.

- Take the client's hands in your hands. Note the colour of skin and nail beds, the temperature and texture of the skin, and the presence of any lesions or swelling. Look at the fingers and nails from the side and observe the angle of the nail base. The angle should be about 160 degrees.

▶ Flattening of the angle of the nail and **clubbing** (enlargement of the tips of the fingers) is a sign of oxygen deprivation in the extremities. Clients with chronic hypoxia (oxygen deprivation) may have rounding of the tip of the finger described as "turkey drumsticks." The nail may feel spongy instead of firm, and there may be a blue discolouration of the nail.

Colour changes to skin may be due to peripheral vasospasm or vasoconstriction (i.e., Raynaud's disease).

- Assess the skin colour of the arms. Skin colour should match the skin tone of the rest of the body.

TECHNIQUES AND NORMAL FINDINGS	ABNORMAL FINDINGS AND SPECIAL CONSIDERATIONS

2. **Determine the ankle-brachial index (ABI).**

- The ankle-brachial index (ABI) is a noninvasive test for peripheral vascular disease (Canadian Cardiovascular Society, 2005). The systolic blood pressure in the brachial, posterior tibial, and dorsalis pedis arteries is measured by Doppler. To determine the systolic pressure in the lower extremity, apply an adult-sized cuff above the ankle and obtain a reading in either the posterior tibial or the dorsalis pedis artery. Divide this number by the systolic reading from the brachial artery.
- See Table 18.2 for guidelines on ABI readings.

TABLE 18.2	Ankle-Brachial Index (ABI)
ABI	**WHAT IT MEANS**
>1.2	Abnormal vessel hardening from peripheral vascular disease*
1.0–1.2	Within normal limits
0.9–1.0	Acceptable
0.8–0.9	Mild (some) arterial blockage or disease
0.5–0.8	Moderate arterial blockage or disease
<0.5	Severe arterial blockage or disease

Source: Compiled by author from Canadian Cardiovascular Society (2005).
*ABI is known to be unreliable with clients who have arterial calcification.

3. **Observe for capillary refill in both hands.**

- Holding one of the client's hands in your hand, apply pressure to one of the client's fingernails for 5 seconds.
- The area under pressure should turn pale. Release the pressure and note how rapidly the normal colour returns.
- In a healthy client, the colour should return in less than 1 to 2 seconds.
- Repeat the procedure for the other hand.

▶ A delayed capillary refill could indicate decreased cardiac output or constriction of the peripheral vessels. However, cigarette smoking, anemia, or cold temperatures can also cause delayed capillary refill.

4. **Place both arms together and compare their size.**

- They should be nearly equal in size.

▶ **Edema** (increased accumulation of fluid) in the arms could indicate an obstruction of the lymphatic system.

5. **Palpate the radial pulse.**

- The radial pulses are found on the ventral and medial side of each wrist. Ask the client to extend one hand, palm up.
- Palpate with two fingers over the radial bone (see Figure 18.9).

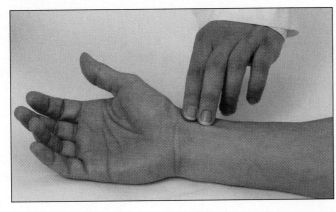

Figure 18.9 ●
Palpating the radial pulse.

TECHNIQUES AND NORMAL FINDINGS

ABNORMAL FINDINGS AND SPECIAL CONSIDERATIONS

- Repeat the procedure for the other arm. Note the rate, rhythm, amplitude, and symmetry of the pulses.
- Characteristics of peripheral pulses are included in Box 18.1.

▶ It is not necessary to palpate the ulnar pulses, located medial to the ulna on the flexor surface of the wrist. They are deeper than the radial pulses and are difficult to palpate.

BOX 18.1	Assessing Peripheral Pulses

Assess peripheral pulses by palpating with gentle pressure over the artery. Use the pads of your first three fingers.

Note the following characteristics:
- Rate—the number of beats per minute
- Rhythm—the regularity of the beats
- Symmetry—pulses on both sides of body should be similar
- Amplitude—the strength of the beat, assessed on a scale of 0 to 4:
  4 = Bounding
  3 = Increased
  2 = Normal
  1 = Weak
  0 = Absent or nonpalpable

6. **Palpate both brachial pulses.**
   - The brachial pulses are found just medial to the biceps tendon.

▶ If any pulses are difficult to palpate, a Doppler flowmeter should be used. When positioned over a patent artery, this device emits sound waves as the blood moves through the artery.

   - Ask the client to extend the arm.
   - Palpate over the brachial artery just superior to the antecubital region (see Figure 18.10).
   - Repeat the procedure for the other arm.
   - Note the rate, rhythm, amplitude, and symmetry of the pulses.
   - Grade the amplitude on the 4-point scale as before.

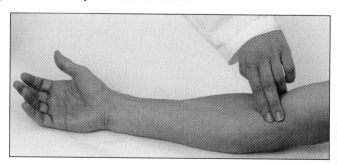

Figure 18.10 ●
Palpating the
brachial pulse.

7. **Perform the Allen test.**
   - If you suspect an obstruction or insufficiency of an artery in the arm, the Allen test may determine the patency of the radial and ulnar arteries.
   - Ask the client to place the hands on the knees with palms up.
   - Compress the radial arteries of both wrists with your thumbs.
   - Ask the client to open and close his or her fist several times.
   - While you are still compressing the radial arteries, ask the client to open his or her hands.
   - The palms should become pink immediately, indicating patent ulnar arteries.

▶ If normal colour does not return, the ulnar arteries may be occluded.

TECHNIQUES AND NORMAL FINDINGS	ABNORMAL FINDINGS AND SPECIAL CONSIDERATIONS

- Next, occlude the ulnar arteries and repeat the same procedure to test the patency of the radial arteries (see Figure 18.11).

▶ If normal colour does not return, the radial arteries may be occluded.

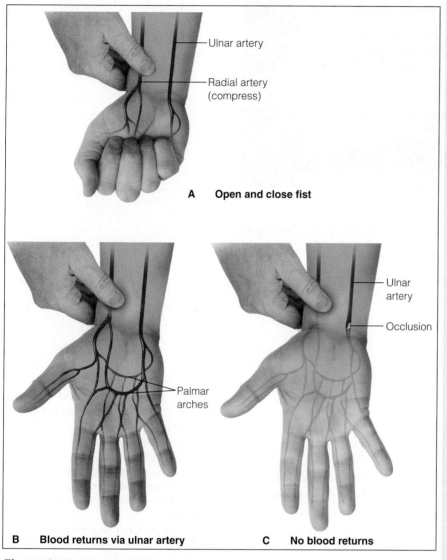

Ulnar artery

Radial artery (compress)

A   Open and close fist

Palmar arches

Ulnar artery

Occlusion

B   Blood returns via ulnar artery

C   No blood returns

Figure 18.11 ● The Allen test.

8. **Palpate the epitrochlear lymph node in each arm.**

- The epitrochlear node drains the forearm and the third, fourth, and fifth fingers.
- Hold the client's right hand in your right hand. With your left hand, reach behind the elbow to the groove between the biceps and triceps muscles (see Figure 18.12).
- Note the size and consistency of the node. Normally, it is not palpable or is barely palpable.
- Repeat the procedure for the left arm.

▶ An enlarged node may indicate an infection in the hand or forearm.

TECHNIQUES AND NORMAL FINDINGS	ABNORMAL FINDINGS AND SPECIAL CONSIDERATIONS

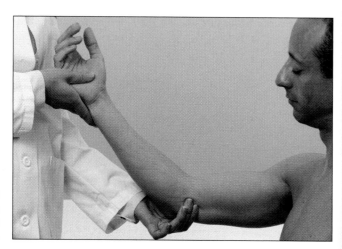

Figure 18.12 ●
Palpating the epitrochlear lymph node.

9. **Palpate the axillary lymph nodes.**

- With the palmar surface of your fingers, reach deep into the axilla. Gently palpate the anterior border of the axilla (anterior or subpectoral nodes), the central aspect along the rib cage (central nodes), the posterior border (subscapular/posterior nodes), and along the inner aspect of the upper arm (lateral nodes). Refer to Figure 16.20 for a depiction of palpating the axillary lymph nodes.

LEGS

1. **Inspect both legs.**

- Observe skin colour, hair distribution, and any skin lesions.

- Skin colour should match the skin tone of the rest of the body. Hair is normally present on the legs.
- If the hair has been removed, there is still usually hair on the dorsal surface of the great toes. Hair growth should be symmetrical. The skin should be intact with no lesions.

▶ If peripheral vessels are constricted, the skin will be paler than the rest of the body. If the vessels are dilated, the skin will have a reddish tone.

▶ A rusty discolouration over the anterior tibial surface with the skin intact is associated with decreased arterial circulation. The characteristic colour stems from blood leaking out of a vessel with decreased capacity for it to be reabsorbed.

If skin lesions or ulcerations are present, the size and location should be noted. Ulcers occurring as a result of arterial deficit tend to occur on pressure points, such as tips of toes and lateral malleoli. Venous ulcers occur at medial malleoli because of fragile tissue with poor drainage.

If any blackened tissue is discovered, the client must be referred to a physician immediately. The presence of blackened tissue can indicate tissue death (necrosis).

2. **Compare the size of both legs.**

- Both legs should be symmetrical in size. If the legs are unequal in size, measure the circumference of each leg at the widest point. It is important to measure each leg at the same point.

▶ A discrepancy in the size of the legs could indicate an accumulation of fluid (edema) resulting from increased pressure in the capillaries or an obstruction of a lymph vessel. Unequal size of the legs could also indicate a blood clot in the deep vessels of the leg.

| TECHNIQUES AND NORMAL FINDINGS | ABNORMAL FINDINGS AND SPECIAL CONSIDERATIONS |

3. Palpate the legs for temperature.
   - Palpate from the feet up the legs, using the dorsal surface of your hands.
   - Note any discrepancies.
   - The skin should be the same temperature on both legs.

▶ If the peripheral vessels are constricted, the skin will feel cool. If the peripheral vessels are dilated, the skin will feel warm. A difference in the temperature of the feet may be a sign of arterial insufficiency.

4. Assess the legs for the presence of superficial veins.
   - With the client in a sitting position and legs dangling from the examination table, inspect the legs.

▶ Varicosities (distended veins) frequently occur in the anterolateral aspect of the thigh and lower leg or on the posterolateral aspect of the calf. These bulging veins do not disappear when legs are elevated. Varicose veins are dilated but have a diminished blood flow and an increased intravenous pressure. An incompetent valve, a weakness in the vein wall, or an obstruction in a proximal vein causes varicosities.

   - Now ask the client to elevate the legs.
   - The veins may appear as nodular bulges when the legs are in the dependent position, but any bulges should disappear when the legs are elevated.
   - Palpate the veins for tenderness or phlebitis (inflammation).

5. Perform the manual compression test.
   - If varicose veins are present, you can determine the length of the varicose vein and the competency of its valves with the manual compression test.
   - Ask the client to stand.
   - With the fingers of one hand, palpate the lower part of the varicose vein.
   - Keeping that hand on the vein, compress the vein firmly at least 15 to 20 cm (6 to 8 in.) higher with the fingers of your other hand (see Figure 18.13).

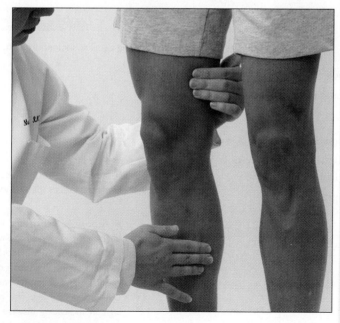

Figure 18.13 ● Performing the manual compression test.

   - You will not feel any pulsation beneath your lower fingers if the valves of the varicose vein are still competent.

▶ If the valves are incompetent, a pulse in the vein will be felt between your two hands.

TECHNIQUES AND NORMAL FINDINGS	ABNORMAL FINDINGS AND SPECIAL CONSIDERATIONS

6. **Perform the Trendelenburg test.**

- A second test to evaluate valve competence in the presence of varicosities is the Trendelenburg test.
- Assist the client to a supine position.
- Elevate the leg to 90 degrees until the venous blood has drained from the leg.
- Place a tourniquet around the upper thigh (see Figure 18.14A).
- Help the client to stand.
- Watch for filling of the venous system (see Figure 18.14B).

▶ A rapid filling of the superficial veins from above indicates incompetent valves.

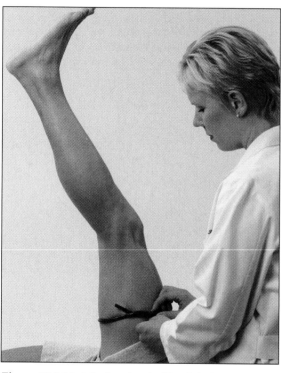

Figure 18.14A ● Performing the Trendelenburg test.
A. Applying tourniquet.

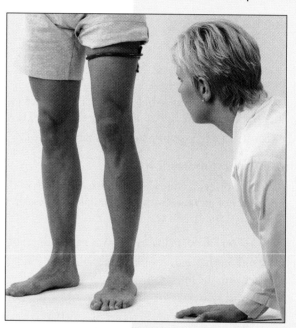

Figure 18.14B ● Performing the Trendelenburg test.
B. Watching for filling.

- The saphenous vein should fill from below in about 30 to 35 seconds.
- After the client has been standing for 20 to 30 seconds, remove the tourniquet and note whether the varicose veins fill from above.
- Competent valves prevent sudden retrograde filling.

▶ A sudden filling of superficial veins after removing the tourniquet indicates backward filling past incompetent valves.

7. **Test for Homans' sign.***

▶ A positive **Homans' sign** could indicate a blood clot in one of the deep veins of the leg. However, a positive Homans' sign could also indicate an inflammation of one of the superficial leg veins or an inflammation of one of the tendons of the leg. The reliability of Homans' sign in indicating disease has been shown to be inconsistent. Follow-up studies, such as a venous Doppler examination, may be required to identify the presence of a clot in the deep veins of the leg.

> **CLINICAL TIP**
>
> *Some facilities may still use the Homans' sign test to assess for deep vein thrombosis (DVT); however, this test has been found to have low sensitivity in predicting the presence of a clot. Look for colour changes, warmth, and increase in calf circumference as other means to assess for DVT.*

- Assist the client to a supine position.
- Flex the client's knee about 5 degrees.
- Now sharply dorsiflex the client's foot (see Figure 18.15).
- Ask whether the client feels calf pain.

*Caution should be taken when performing this test. If a deep vein thrombosis is suspected, performing the Homan's test or any type of massage should be avoided.

Techniques and Normal Findings

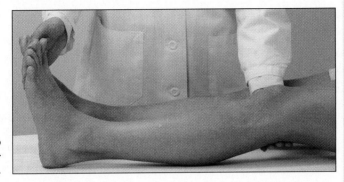

Figure 18.15 ●
Testing for
Homans' sign.

- This manoeuvre exerts pressure on the posterior tibial vein and should not cause pain.

8. **Palpate the inguinal lymph nodes.**
   - Move the client's gown aside over the inguinal region. Palpate over the top of the medial thigh (see Figure 18.16).
   - If the nodes can be palpated, they should be movable and not tender.
   - Repeat the procedure for the other leg.

▶ Lymph nodes that are larger than 1 cm (0.5 in.) or are tender may be an indication of an infection in the legs.

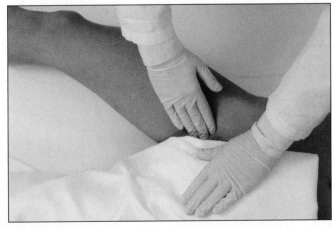

Figure 18.16 ●
Palpating the
inguinal lymph
nodes.

9. **Palpate both femoral pulses.**
   - The femoral pulses are inferior and medial to the inguinal ligament.

   - Ask the client to flex the knee and externally rotate the hip. Palpate over the femoral artery (see Figure 18.17).

▶ If it is not possible to palpate the femoral pulse, an artery may be occluded.

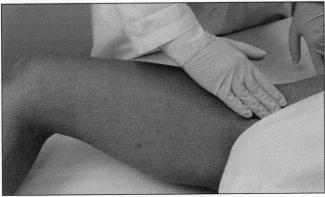

Figure 18.17 ●
Palpating the
femoral artery.

TECHNIQUES AND NORMAL FINDINGS	ABNORMAL FINDINGS AND SPECIAL CONSIDERATIONS

- The femoral artery is deep, and you may need to place one hand on top of the other to locate the pulse. Repeat the procedure for the other leg.
- Note the rate, rhythm, amplitude, and symmetry of the pulses.
- Grade the amplitude on the 4-point scale.

10. Palpate both popliteal pulses.

- The pulsations of the popliteal artery can be palpated deep in the popliteal fossa lateral to the midline.
- Ask the client to flex the knee and relax the leg.
- Palpate the popliteal pulse.
- If you cannot locate the pulse, ask the client to roll onto the abdomen and flex the knee (see Figure 18.18).
- Palpate deeply for the pulse.
- Repeat the procedure for the other leg.
- Note the rate, rhythm, amplitude, and symmetry of the pulses.
- Grade the amplitude on the 4-point scale.

► If the popliteal pulse cannot be palpated, an artery may be occluded. However, it can also be normal not to be able to palpate this pulse.

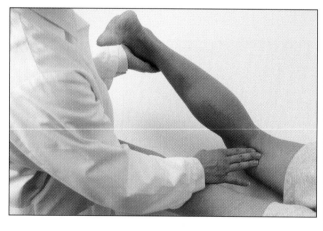

Figure 18.18 ●
Palpating the
popliteal pulse.

11. Palpate both dorsalis pedis pulses.

- The dorsalis pedis pulses may be felt on the medial side of the dorsum of the foot.

► Edema in the foot will make palpation difficult.

- Palpate the pulse lateral to the extensor tendon of the great toe (see Figure 18.19).

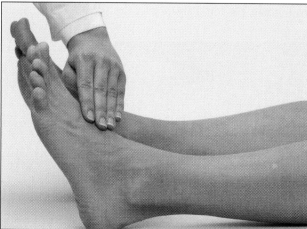

Figure 18.19 ●
Palpating the
dorsalis pedis pulse.

TECHNIQUES AND NORMAL FINDINGS	ABNORMAL FINDINGS AND SPECIAL CONSIDERATIONS

- Use light pressure.
- Repeat the procedure for the other foot.
- Note the rate, rhythm, amplitude, and symmetry of the pulses.
- Grade the amplitude on the 4-point scale.

12. Palpate both posterior tibial pulses.

- The posterior tibial pulses may be palpated behind and slightly inferior to the medial malleolus of the ankle, in the groove between the malleolus and the Achilles tendon.

- Palpate the pulse by curving your fingers around the medial malleolus (see Figure 18.20).

- Repeat the procedure for the other foot. Note the rate, rhythm, amplitude, and symmetry of the pulses.

- Grade the amplitude on the 4-point scale.

▶ If it is not possible to palpate the posterior tibial pulse, an artery may be occluded. If the client has edematous ankles, this pulse may be difficult to palpate.

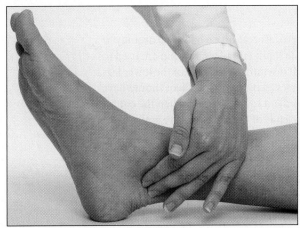

Figure 18.20 ●
Palpating the posterior tibial pulse.

13. Assess for arterial supply to the lower legs and feet.

- If you suspect an arterial deficiency, test for arterial supply to the lower extremities. Ask the client to remain supine.

- Elevate the client's legs 30 cm (12 in.) above the heart.

- Ask the client to move the feet up and down at the ankles for 60 seconds to drain the venous blood (see Figure 18.21).

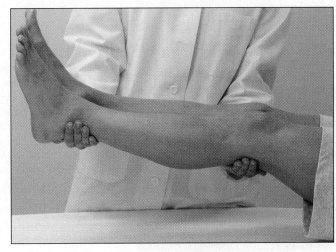

Figure 18.21 ●
Testing the arterial supply to the lower extremities.

TECHNIQUES AND NORMAL FINDINGS	ABNORMAL FINDINGS AND SPECIAL CONSIDERATIONS

- The skin will be blanched in colour because only arterial blood is present.
- Now ask the client to sit up and dangle the feet.
- Compare the colour of both feet.
- The original colour should return in about 10 seconds.

▶ Marked pallor of the elevated extremities may indicate arterial insufficiency. A marked bluish-red colour of the dependent feet occurs with severe arterial insufficiency. This colour is due to a lack of oxygenated blood to the area, which leads to a loss of vasomotor tone and venous stasis.

- The superficial veins in the feet should fill in about 15 seconds.
- The feet of a dark-skinned person may be difficult to evaluate, but the soles of the feet should reflect a change in colour.

▶ Delayed filling of the superficial veins of the feet also could indicate arterial insufficiency. Motor loss may occur with arterial insufficiency.

Sensory loss may occur with arterial insufficiency.

14. Test the lower legs for muscle strength.

- With the client in a sitting position, instruct the client to extend each knee while you apply opposing force. Instruct the client to flex the knees again. The client should be able to perform the movement against resistance. The strength of the muscles in both legs is equal. Testing of muscle strength is discussed in greater detail in Chapter 23. ⬭

15. Test the lower legs for sensation.

- Use a cotton wisp, lightly applied to symmetrical areas on each lower extremity to assess light touch. The rounded end and the sharp end of a safety pin are used to assess pain sensation. The ends are applied to symmetrical areas of the lower legs in a random pattern of sharp and dull to assess sensation. The client should have eyes closed during the assessment. Ask the client to state "now" when the cotton wisp is felt, and "sharp" or "dull" when the ends of the safety pin are applied.
- The client should sense touch and pain. Testing for sensation is discussed in greater detail in Chapter 24. ⬭

16. Check for edema of the legs.

- Press the skin for at least 5 seconds over the tibia, behind the medial malleolus, and over the dorsum of each foot (see Figure 18.22).

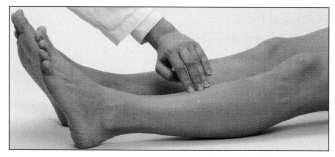

Figure 18.22 ●
Palpating for edema over the tibia.

- Look for a depression in the skin (called pitting edema) caused by the pressure of your fingers (see Figure 18.23).

▶ Pitting edema can be related to a failure of the right side of the heart or an obstruction of the lymphatic system. Edema in only one leg may indicate an occlusion of a large vein in the leg. Diminished arterial flow thickens toenails, which often become yellow and loosely attached to the nail bed. Clients with diabetes often acquire fungal and bacterial infections of the nail because of increased glucose collecting in the skin under the nail.

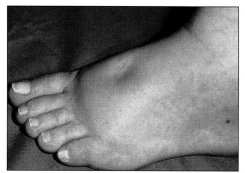

Figure 18.23 ●
Pitting edema of the lower extremities.

TECHNIQUES AND NORMAL FINDINGS	ABNORMAL FINDINGS AND SPECIAL CONSIDERATIONS

- If edema is present, you should grade it on a scale of 1+ (mild) to 4+ (severe) (see Figure 18.24).

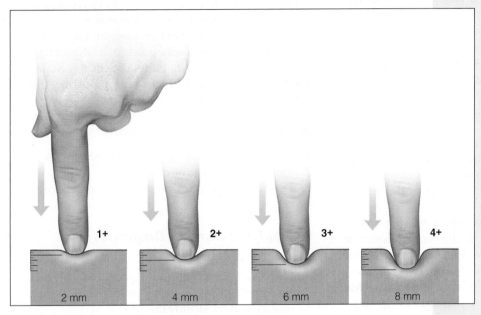

Figure 18.24 ● Grading pitting edema.

17. Inspect the toenails for colour and thickness.

- Nails should be pink and not thickened. Clubbing should not be present.

SAMPLE DOCUMENTATION

Subjective: *No history of leg pain or cramps. No changes in skin colour to extremities. No lesions or swelling present to legs, no lymphadenopathy. Denies smoking or ETOH abuse. Takes acetaminophen for occasional headache.*

Objective: *Upper extremities uniform in colour, warm to touch. Brachial and radial pulses regular 2+. No edema or lymphadenopathy. Lower extremities uniform in colour, warm to touch. No superficial veins visible. Femoral pulse regular 2+, popliteal regular 1+, dorsalis pedis and posterior tibialis regular 2+. No edema present.*

PHYSICAL ASSESSMENT

APPLICATION THROUGH CRITICAL THINKING

CASE STUDY

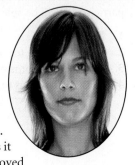

Jenny Battaglia, a 26-year-old female, is seen in the emergency department (ED) for pain in her lower legs. The client states that she has had pain in her calves for about 48 hours, starting when she got home from vacation. She does not recall any injury. She says it started like cramping but has not improved with rest or taking Tylenol. She thinks there is a little swelling and some tenderness.

The nurse knows that an organized approach to data collection is essential. Further, every effort must be made to get a comprehensive picture of the situation and to avoid missing pieces of information that will guide decision making for the client.

The approach to care of the client will be determined by the client's condition. When a client is in acute distress—for example, with dyspnea, with a bleeding injury, in shock, or in severe pain—data gathering focuses on the immediate problem and its resolution.

Ms. Battaglia is uncomfortable but does not appear to be in acute distress and denies severe discomfort. She states, "I'm a little nervous. I've never really been sick and have only been in the emergency department once before for a couple of stitches when I was 10." The nurse tells Ms. Battaglia that they will begin an examination to determine the cause of her problem.

The assessment reveals the following: A thin female client who is suntanned and without pink undertone to her skin. BP 116/64 (R) arm, sitting, pulse 88, 3+. Upper extremities symmetrical in size, no edema, radial and brachial pulses equal, regular. Lower extremities, edema, rubor (redness) bilateral posterior lower legs, warm and tender to touch. Pulses present, equal, 3+.

The nurse considers the data and determines that Ms. Battaglia is not in acute distress. However, rubor and edema in lower extremities suggest a vascular problem. The nurse decides to continue the health assessment by further interview for missing subjective information.

The interview reveals that Ms. Battaglia has no personal or family history of vascular problems, cardiovascular disease, or diabetes. She is not married and lives with her boyfriend. She takes Aspirin or Tylenol occasionally for headaches or menstrual cramps. She has no allergies. She is para 0 gravida 0, LMP 2 weeks before ED visit, regular menses, has taken birth control pills for 3 years.

The nurse asks Ms. Battaglia several questions about the leg pain. The client states it is 5 to 7 on a scale of 1 to 10 and continuous. Nothing she has done has relieved the pain. It started 48 hours ago "at the end of my vacation" and wakes her at night.

The nurse asks if travel was involved in the vacation. Ms. Battaglia says, "Yes, we flew to Aruba for 6 days. That's how I got a tan. We had a great time and I was feeling rested, ready to go back to work, and looked forward to seeing family and friends." Further questions reveal that the flight was 6 hours and Ms. Battaglia "slept almost all the way back, I never really moved."

The data suggest to the nurse that Ms. Battaglia has deep vein thrombosis (DVT). Ms. Battaglia is admitted to a medical unit. She will be on bed rest and receive anticoagulation.

► Complete Documentation

The following is a sample narrative complete documentation for Jenny Battaglia.

SUBJECTIVE DATA: Pain in lower legs for about 48 h. Started when she got home from vacation. No recall of injury. Started as cramping, no improvement with rest or Tylenol. She thinks there is some swelling and tenderness. "A little nervous." No personal or family history of vascular problems, cardiac disease, or diabetes. Single, lives with boyfriend. Tylenol or Aspirin occasionally for headache or menstrual cramps. No allergies. Gravida 0, Para 0, LMP 2 weeks before ED visit, regular menses. Oral contraceptives for 3 years. Air travel—flight of 6 h—Jenny slept almost all the time.

OBJECTIVE DATA: Suntanned, without pink undertone. Vital signs: BP 116/64 right, sitting. Radial pulse 88, 3+, T 37.4°C (99.20°F). Pain: 5 to 7 on a scale of 1 to 10, continuous, wakes at night. Upper extremities symmetrical in size, no edema, warm brachial and radial pulses = regular. Cap refill 2 sec L & R. Extremities—below knees, posterior bilateral rubor, edema 1+, warm, tender to touch. Pulses present, 3+. No lesions, no visible superficial vessels. Feet warm, no edema. Toenails—polish—unable to assess.

► Critical Thinking Questions

1. Identify the data that suggest the presence of DVT.
2. How would the data be clustered?
3. Describe the areas for client education derived from this case study.

► Applying Nursing Diagnoses

1. *Tissue perfusion, ineffective* is a nursing diagnosis in the NANDA-I taxonomy (see Appendix A ⊗). Does the case study for Ms. Battaglia provide data to support this diagnosis? If so, identify the data.
2. Explain your analysis of the data in the case study to formulate additional diagnoses.
3. Provide PES (problem, etiology, signs or symptoms) statements for additional diagnoses for Ms. Battaglia.

► Prepare Teaching Plan

LEARNING NEED: The data in the case study reveal that Ms. Battaglia is at risk for development of DVT because she is using oral contraceptives and has experienced recent air travel. Her symptoms are typical for DVT. She will be admitted for treatment of DVT and will receive education regarding her treatment regimen and follow-up care.

The case study provides data that are representative of risks, symptoms, and behaviours of many individuals. Therefore, the following teaching plan is based on the need to provide information to members of any community about DVT.

GOAL: The participants in this learning program will have increased awareness of risk factors and strategies to prevent DVT.

OBJECTIVES: At the completion of this learning session, the participants will be able to do the following:

1. Describe DVT.
2. Identify risk factors associated with DVT.
3. List the symptoms of DVT.
4. Discuss strategies to prevent DVT.

ASSESSMENT FORM

EXAM	FINDINGS

Peripheral Vascular System

Blood Pressure

	Sitting	Standing	Supine
Left	118/66	114/64	114/60
Right	120/70	118/68	116/66

Upper Extremity

Skin

Left: Colour _Pink_   Temperature _Warm_

Right: Colour _Pink_   Temperature _Warm_

Capillary Refill   Left ___<2 sec___   Right ___<2 sec___

Arm Size   Left = Right ✓

Edema

Left   0 ✓   1+ _____   2+ _____   3+ _____   4+ _____

Right   0 ✓   1+ _____   2+ _____   3+ _____   4+ _____

Pulses

Radial	Rate	80	Rhythm	Regular	Amplitude	2+
Ulnar	Rate	80	Rhythm	Regular	Amplitude	2+
Brachial	Rate	80	Rhythm	Regular	Amplitude	2+

Lower Extremity

Skin

Legs   Left: Colour _Rubor_   Temperature _Warm_

Right: Colour _Rubor_   Temperature _Warm_

Feet   Left: Colour _Pink_   Temperature _Warm_

Right: Colour _Pink_   Temperature _Warm_

Leg Size   Left = Right ___✓___ yes _____ no _____

Edema

Legs   Left   0 _____   1+ ✓   2+ _____   3+ _____   4+ _____

Right   0 _____   1+ ✓   2+ _____   3+ _____   4+ _____

Feet   Left   0 ✓   1+ _____   2+ _____   3+ _____   4+ _____

Right   0 ✓   1+ _____   2+ _____   3+ _____   4+ _____

Superficial Veins   Left ___Not visible_____

Right ___Not visible_____

Lesions   Left ___0_____

Right ___0_____

Homans' Sign   Left _____ + ___✓___ - Right _____ + ___✓___ -

Toenails   Left _unable to assess_   Right _unable to assess_

Pulses

Femoral	Rate	82	Rhythm	Regular	Amplitude	3+
Popliteal	Rate	82	Rhythm	Regular	Amplitude	3+
Posterior Tibial	Rate	82	Rhythm	Regular	Amplitude	3+
Dorsalis Pedis	Rate	82	Rhythm	Regular	Amplitude	3+

Application of Objective 2: Identify risk factors associated with DVT.

Content	Teaching Strategy	Evaluation
<ul><li>Age: over 40</li><li>Family history of clotting disorder or DVT</li><li>Circulation problems</li><li>Obesity</li><li>Cancer treatment</li><li>Pregnancy or recent birth</li><li>Oral contraception or hormone therapy</li><li>Immobility<ol><li>Sitting for long periods during auto or air travel</li><li>Illness</li><li>Recent surgery</li><li>Trauma</li></ol></li><li>Smoking</li><li>Dehydration</li></ul>	<ul><li>Lecture</li><li>Discussion</li><li>Audiovisual materials</li><li>Printed materials</li></ul>Lecture is appropriate when disseminating information to large groups. Discussion allows participants to bring up concerns and to raise questions. Audiovisual materials, such as illustrations of the vascular system and techniques, reinforce verbal presentation. Printed material, especially to be taken away with learners, allows review, reinforcement, and reading at the learner's pace.	<ul><li>Written examination.</li></ul>May use short answer, fill-in, or multiple-choice items or a combination of items. If these are short and easy to evaluate, the learner receives immediate feedback.

HEALTH PROMOTION ASSESSMENT TOOL

Social Determinants of Health	Level of Action	Action Strategies
Physical environment	Individual	Develop personal skills <ul><li>Assess Ms. Battaglia's knowledge of factors that contribute to deep vein thrombosis.</li><li>Assess her readiness to learn in relation to her current anxiety level.</li><li>Educate her on prevention of deep vein thrombosis and early recognition of signs and symptoms to prevent future DVT.</li></ul>

ABNORMAL FINDINGS

Findings from physical assessment of the peripheral vascular and lymphatic systems include normal and abnormal pulses (see Table 18.3) and common alterations of the peripheral vascular and lymphatic systems as shown in Figures 18.25 through 18.31.

TABLE 18.3 | Normal and Abnormal Pulses

NAME OF PULSE	CHARACTERISTICS	ARTERIAL WAVEFORM PATTERN	CONTRIBUTINWG CONDITIONS
Normal	• Regular, even in intensity		• None
Absent	• No palpable pulse, no waveform		• Arterial line disconnected • Cardiac arrest
Weak or thready	• Intensity of pulse is +1 • May wax and wane • May be difficult to find		• Shock • Severe peripheral vascular disease
Bounding	• Intensity of pulse is +4 • Very easy to observe in arterial locations near surface of skin • Very easy to palpate and difficult to obliterate with pressure from fingertips		• Hyperdynamic states, such as is seen with hyperthyroidism, exercise, anxiety; vasodilation seen in high cardiac output syndromes • May be due to normal aging secondary to arterial wall stiffening • Aortic regurgitation • Anemia
Bisferiens	• Has two systolic peaks with a dip in between • Easier to detect in the carotid location • In the case of hypertrophic obstructive cardiomyopathy only one systolic peak palpated, but waveform demonstrates double systolic peak		• Aortic regurgitation • Combination of aortic regurgitation and stenosis • Hypertrophic obstructive cardiomyopathy
Pulsus alternans	• Alternating strong and weak pulses • Equal interval between each pulse		• Aortic regurgitation • Terminal left ventricular heart failure • Systemic hypertension
Pulsus bigeminus	• Alternating strong and weak pulses, but the weak pulse comes in early after the strong pulse		• Regular bigeminal dysrhythmias, such as PVCs and PACs
Pulsus paradoxus	• Reduced intensity of pulse during inspiration versus expiration	Expiration Inspiration	• Cardiac tamponade • Acute pulmonary embolus • Pericarditis • May be present in clients with chronic lung disease • Hypovolemic shock • Pregnancy
Water-hammer and Corrigan's pulse	• Rapid systolic upstroke and no dicrotic notch secondary to rapid drop		• Aortic regurgitation
Unequal	• Difference in intensity or amplitude between right and left pulses	Right femoral Left femoral	• Dissecting aneurysm (location of aneurysm determines where the difference in amplitude is felt)

Arterial Insufficiency

Arterial insufficiency results in diminished or absent pulses; cool, shiny skin; absence of hair on toes; pallor on elevation, red colour when dependent; and deep muscle pain, usually in the calf or lower leg aggravated by activity and elevation of the limb. Pain is quickly relieved by rest. Ulcers caused by arterial insufficiency are usually seen on the toes or areas of trauma of the feet or lateral malleolus (see Figure 18.25). The ulcer is pale, with well-defined edges and no bleeding.

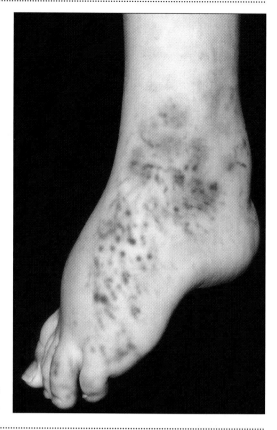

Figure 18.25 ●
Arterial insufficiency.

Arterial Aneurysm

Arterial aneurysm is a bulging or dilation caused by a weakness in the wall of an artery (see Figure 18.26). It can occur in the aorta and abdominal, renal, or femoral arteries. Aneurysms can sometimes be detected by a characteristic bruit over the artery; however, if they are located deep in the abdomen, they can be difficult to discover.

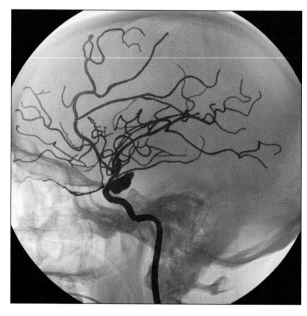

Figure 18.26 ●
Arterial aneurysm.

Venous Insufficiency

In venous insufficiency the temperature of skin is normal, but edema is usually present and is accompanied by a feeling of fullness in the legs. Skin around the ankles may be thickened and have a brown discolouration (see Figure 18.27). Discomfort is aggravated by prolonged standing or sitting and is relieved by rest but only after several hours. Ulcers related to venous insufficiency are often found on the medial malleolus and are characterized by bleeding and uneven edges. There is minimal pain associated with the ulcer, and the skin surrounding the ulcer is coarse.

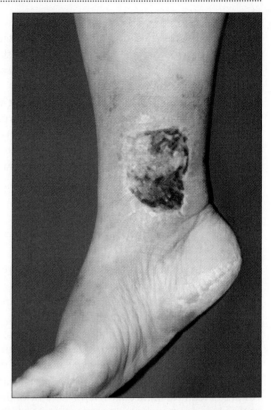

Figure 18.27 ●
Venous insufficiency.

Varicose Veins

Varicose veins are veins that have become dilated and have a diminished rate of blood flow and increased intravenous pressure (see Figure 18.28). The condition may be the result of incompetent valves that permit the reflux of blood or an obstruction of a proximal vein.

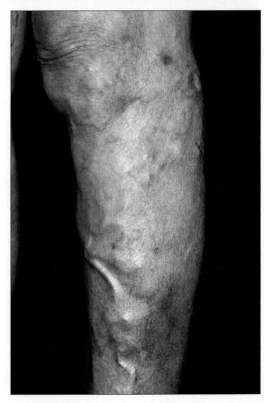

Figure 18.28 ●
Varicose veins.

Raynaud's Disease

Raynaud's disease is a condition in which the arterioles in the fingers develop spasms, causing intermittent skin pallor or cyanosis and then rubor (red colour). The spasms may last from minutes to hours, occurring bilaterally. The client may describe numbness or pain during the pallor or cyanotic state, and burning or throbbing pain during the rubor. This condition is seen most commonly in young, otherwise healthy females, frequently secondary to connective tissue disease, drug intoxication, pulmonary hypertension, or trauma (see Figure 18.29).

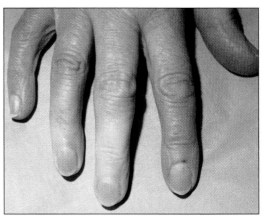

Figure 18.29 ●
Raynaud's disease.

Deep Vein Thrombosis

Deep vein thrombosis is the occlusion of a deep vein, such as in the femoral or pelvic circulation, by a blood clot. There may be no symptoms or the client may describe intense, sharp pain along the iliac vessels, in the popliteal space, or in the calf muscles. Pain may increase with sharp dorsiflexion of the foot (Homans' sign), but this manoeuvre is not absolutely reliable for diagnosis. There may also be slight swelling of the leg, some edema, low-grade fever, and tachycardia (rapid heartbeat). This condition requires immediate referral because of the danger of the clot migrating to the lung, resulting in a pulmonary embolism (see Figure 18.30).

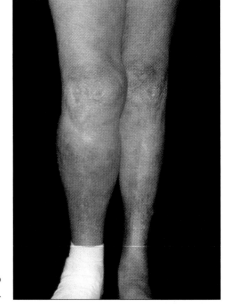

Figure 18.30 ●
Deep vein thrombosis.

Lymphedema

Lymphedema is unilateral swelling associated with an obstruction in lymph nodes (see Figure 18.31).

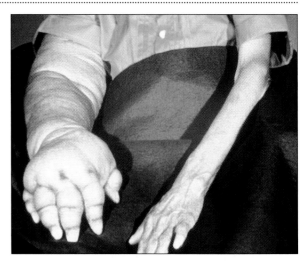

Figure 18.31 ●
Lymphedema.

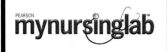

ABNORMAL FINDINGS

19

ABDOMEN

The **abdomen** is not a system unto itself. It is the largest cavity of the body and contains many organs and structures that belong to various systems of the body. For example, the liver, gallbladder, and stomach belong to the digestive system. The kidneys, ureters, and bladder belong to the urinary system. These structures and many others are assessed when performing an abdominal assessment. The primary focus of this chapter is the assessment of the structures of the digestive system.

The primary responsibility of the digestive system is to take in, break down, and absorb nutrients to be used by all cells of the body. The ability to perform these functions is influenced by the health of many other body systems. The parasympathetic fibres of the nervous system increase digestion while the sympathetic fibres inhibit the process. The respiratory system provides oxygen needed for the metabolic processes and removes the carbon dioxide created by metabolism. The hormones of the endocrine system help regulate digestion and the metabolic processes.

Abnormalities of the gastrointestinal system can include colorectal cancer, hepatitis, and food-borne illnesses. Health-related goals in these focus areas are to reduce deaths from colorectal cancer, to decrease the number of food-borne infections, to decrease anaphylaxis from foods, and to reduce the number of cases of hepatitis A, B, and C.

ANATOMY AND PHYSIOLOGY REVIEW

The abdomen is composed of the alimentary canal, the intestines, accessory digestive organs, the urinary system, the spleen, and reproductive organs. Each of these structures or systems will be discussed in the sections that follow.

Abdomen

The abdomen is situated in the anterior region of the body. It is inferior to the diaphragm of the respiratory system and superior to the pelvic floor. The abdominal muscles, the intercostal margins, and the pelvis form the anterior borders of the abdomen. The vertebral column and the lumbar muscles form the posterior borders of the abdomen.

The anatomy and physiology review of the abdomen has a two-point focus. The primary focus is the gastrointestinal system, and the secondary focus is the abdominal structures of other systems. The gastrointestinal system consists of the alimentary canal and the accessory organs of the digestive system. The **alimentary canal**, a continuous, hollow, muscular tube, begins at the mouth and terminates at the anus. The accessory organs include the teeth, salivary glands, liver, gallbladder, and pancreas (see Figure 19.1).

The anatomy, physiology, and assessment of the mouth, teeth, tongue, salivary glands, and pharynx are discussed in Chapter 14 of this text. ⬭ Before proceeding with the assessment of the abdomen, it may be helpful to review the information in that chapter.

Alimentary Canal

The alimentary canal is the continuous hollow tube extending from the mouth to the anus. The boundaries include the mouth, pharynx, esophagus, stomach, small and large intestines, rectum, and anus.

Esophagus

The esophagus, a collapsible tube, connects the pharynx to the stomach. Approximately 25 cm (10 in.) in length, it passes through the mediastinum and diaphragm to meet the stomach at the cardiac sphincter. The primary function of the esophagus is to propel food and fluid from the mouth to the stomach.

Stomach

The stomach extends from the esophagus at the cardiac sphincter to the duodenum at the pyloric sphincter. Located in the left side of the upper abdomen, the stomach is directly inferior to the diaphragm. The diameter and volume of the stomach are directly related

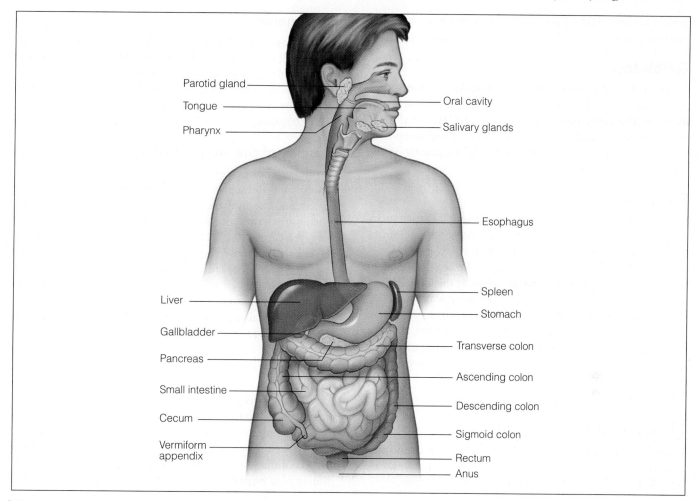

Figure 19.1 ● Organs of the alimentary canal and related accessory organs.

to the food it contains. Food mixes with digestive juices in the stomach and becomes chyme before entering the small intestine. The primary function of the stomach is the chemical and mechanical breakdown of food.

Small Intestine

The small intestine is the body's primary digestive and absorptive organ. Approximately 6 to 7 m (18 to 21 ft.) long, it has three subdivisions. The first segment, the duodenum, meets the stomach at the pyloric sphincter and extends to the middle region, called the jejunum. The ileum extends from the jejunum to the ileocecal valve at the cecum of the large intestine. Intestinal juices, bile from the liver and gallbladder and pancreatic enzymes, mix with the chyme to promote digestion and facilitate the absorption of nutrients. The primary functions of the small intestine are the continuing chemical breakdown of food and the absorption of digested foods.

Large Intestine

The last portion of the alimentary canal is the large intestine, which extends from the ileocecal valve to the anus. The large intestine is approximately 1.5 m (5 to 5.5 ft.) long. It consists of the cecum, ascending colon, transverse colon, descending colon, sigmoid colon, rectum, and anus. The vermiform

appendix is attached to the large intestines at the cecum. The appendix contains masses of lymphoid tissue that make only a minor contribution to immunity; however, when inflamed, the appendix causes significant health problems. The large intestine is wider and shorter than the small intestine. It is on the periphery of the abdominal cavity, surrounding the small intestine and other structures. The main functions of the large intestine are absorbing water from indigestible food residue and eliminating the residue in the form of feces.

Accessory Digestive Organs

The **accessory digestive organs**—the liver, gallbladder, and pancreas—contribute to the digestive process of foods. These structures connect to the alimentary canal by ducts.

Liver

The largest gland of the body, the liver is located in the right upper portion of the abdominal cavity, directly inferior to the diaphragm, and extends into the left side of the abdomen. The lower portion of the rib cage protects the liver, which makes only the lower border of the liver palpable. The only digestive function of the liver is the production and secretion of bile for fat emulsification. It has a major role in the metabolism of proteins, fats, and carbohydrates. The liver has the ability to store some vitamins, produce substances for coagulation of blood, produce antibodies, and detoxify harmful substances.

Gallbladder

Chiefly a storage organ for bile, the gallbladder, a thin-walled sac, is nestled in a shallow depression on the ventral surface of the liver. The gallbladder releases stored bile into the duodenum when stimulated and thus promotes the emulsification of fats. The main functions of the gallbladder are storing of bile and assisting in the digestion of fats.

Pancreas

An accessory digestive organ, the pancreas is a triangular-shaped gland located in the left upper portion of the abdomen. The head of the pancreas is nestled in the C curve of the duodenum, and the body and tail of the pancreas lie deep to the left of the stomach and extend toward the spleen at the lateral aspect of the abdomen. The pancreas is an endocrine and exocrine gland. As an endocrine gland, it secretes insulin, an important factor in carbohydrate metabolism. As an exocrine gland, it releases pancreatic juice, which contains a broad spectrum of enzymes that mixes with bile in the duodenum. The main function of the pancreas is assisting with the digestion of proteins, fats, and carbohydrates.

Other Related Structures

Some structures located in the abdomen have no connection to the digestive process. They are part of other systems and are considered with the general assessment of the abdomen.

Peritoneum

The **peritoneum** is a thin, double layer of serous membrane in the abdominal cavity. The visceral peritoneum covers the external surface of most digestive organs. The parietal peritoneum lines the walls of the abdominal cavity. The serous fluid secreted by the membranes helps lubricate the surface of the organs, allowing motion of structures without friction.

Muscles of the Abdominal Wall

Having no bony reinforcements, the anterior and lateral abdominal walls depend on the musculature for support and protection. The four pairs of abdominal muscles, when well toned, support and protect the abdominal viscera most effectively (see Figure 19.2). The muscle groups include the rectus abdominis, external oblique, internal oblique, and transverse abdominis. Secondary functions of these muscle groups include lateral flexion, rotation, and anterior flexion of the trunk. Simultaneous contraction of the muscle groups increases intra-abdominal pressure by compressing the abdominal wall. Weakness in the muscular structure will produce herniation of structures.

Aorta

As the descending aorta passes through the diaphragm and enters the abdominal cavity, it becomes the abdominal aorta. This penetration occurs at the T_{12} level of the vertebral column, slightly to the left of the midline of the body. The abdominal aorta continues to the L_4 level of the vertebral column, where it bifurcates to form the right and left common iliac arteries. The

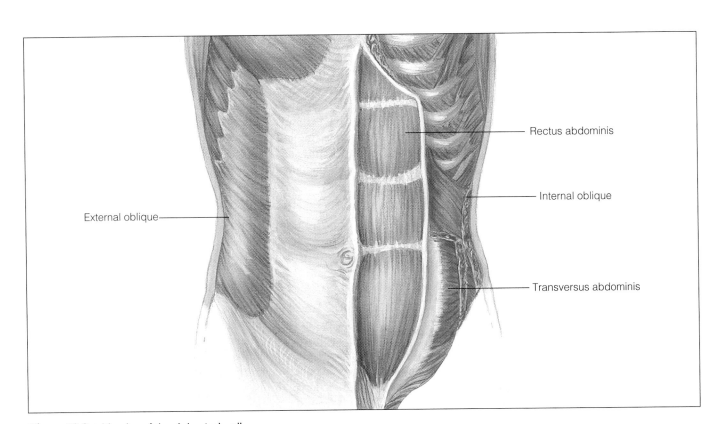

External oblique

Rectus abdominis

Internal oblique

Transversus abdominis

Figure 19.2 ● Muscles of the abdominal wall.

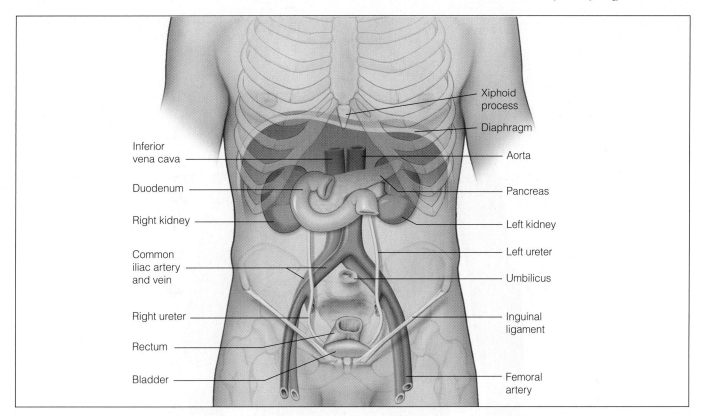

Figure 19.3 • Abdominal vasculature and deep structures.

Labels (clockwise):
- Xiphoid process
- Diaphragm
- Aorta
- Pancreas
- Left kidney
- Left ureter
- Umbilicus
- Inguinal ligament
- Femoral artery
- Bladder
- Rectum
- Right ureter
- Common iliac artery and vein
- Right kidney
- Duodenum
- Inferior vena cava

many branches of the abdominal aorta serve all the parietal and visceral structures (see Figure 19.3).

Kidneys, Ureters, and Bladder

The kidneys lie within the abdomen, behind the peritoneum. Responsible for the filtration of nitrogenous wastes and the production of urine, the kidneys are protected by the lower ribs. The slender tubelike structures that carry the urine from the kidneys to the bladder are the ureters. The urinary bladder, a smooth, collapsible muscular sac, is located in the pelvis of the abdominal cavity. The primary function of the bladder is to store urine until it can be released. As the bladder fills with urine, it may rise above the symphysis pubis into the abdominal cavity. Assessment of the kidneys, ureters, and bladder is discussed in Chapter 20 of this text. ⬭

Spleen

The spleen, the largest of the lymphoid organs, is located in the left upper portion of the abdomen directly inferior to the diaphragm. Surrounded by a fibrous capsule, the spleen provides a site for lymphocyte proliferation and immune surveillance and response. It filters and cleanses blood, destroying worn-out red blood cells and returning their breakdown products to the liver.

Reproductive Organs

In the female, the uterus, fallopian tubes, and ovaries are in the pelvic portion of the abdominal cavity. In the male, the prostate gland surrounds the urethra just below the bladder.

The assessment of these structures is discussed in Chapters 21 and 22 of this text. ⬭

Landmarks

Reference points and anatomical structures need to be identified when assessing the abdomen. Defined landmarks help to identify specific underlying structures and provide a source for description and recording of findings. Landmarks for the abdomen include the xiphoid process, umbilicus, costal margin, iliac crests, and pubic bone.

Mapping is the process of dividing the abdomen into quadrants or regions for the purpose of examination. To obtain the four quadrants, the nurse extends the midsternal line from the xiphoid process through the umbilicus to the pubic bone and then draws a horizontal line perpendicular to the first line, through the umbilicus. These two perpendicular lines form four equal quadrants of the abdomen, as illustrated in Figure 19.4. The quadrants are simply named right upper quadrant (RUQ), right lower quadrant (RLQ), left upper quadrant (LUQ), and left lower quadrant (LLQ).

The second mapping method divides the abdomen into nine regions. To obtain these abdominal regions, one extends the right and left midclavicular lines to the groin and then draws a horizontal line across the lowest edge of the costal margin. The final step is to draw another horizontal line at the level of the iliac crests. The abdomen has now been divided into nine regions as shown in Figure 19.5. The names of the regions are right hypochondriac, epigastric, left hypochondriac, right lumbar, umbilical, left lumbar, right inguinal, hypogastric or pubic, and left inguinal.

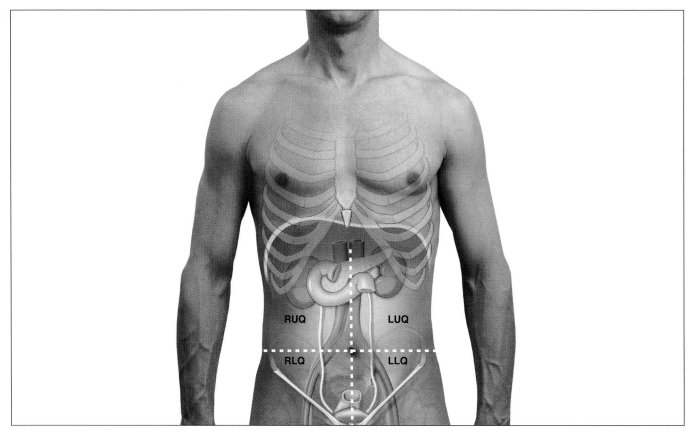

Figure 19.4 ● Mapping of the abdomen into four quadrants.

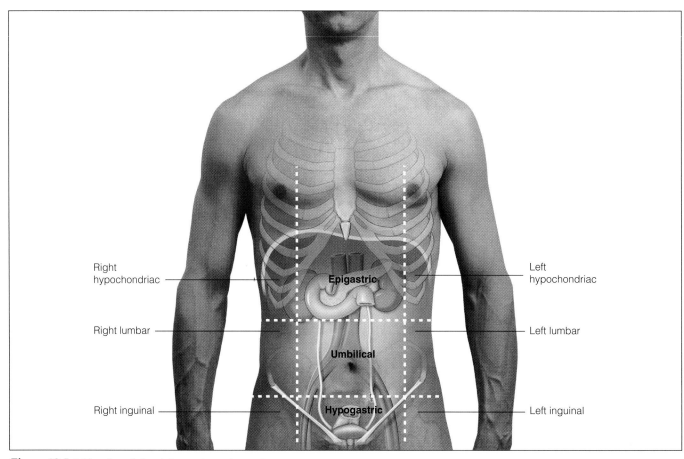

Figure 19.5 ● Mapping of the abdomen into nine regions.

Of the two methods described, the quadrant method is more commonly used. When using the quadrant method, it is important to pay attention to structures that are in the midline of the abdomen and do not belong to any specific quadrant. These structures include the abdominal aorta, urinary bladder, and uterus.

The nurse should select one mapping method and use it consistently. Once a method has been selected, the nurse visualizes the underlying structures before proceeding (see Figure 19.6). The gallbladder sits in the upper right quadrant of the abdomen inferior to the liver and lateral to the right midclavicular line (MCL). The kidneys are posterior to the abdominal contents

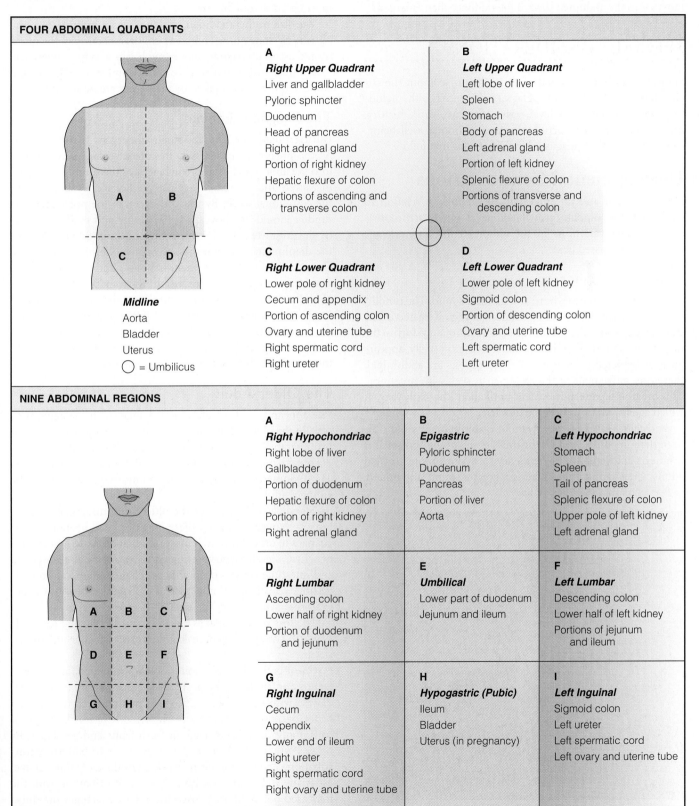

FOUR ABDOMINAL QUADRANTS

A
Right Upper Quadrant
Liver and gallbladder
Pyloric sphincter
Duodenum
Head of pancreas
Right adrenal gland
Portion of right kidney
Hepatic flexure of colon
Portions of ascending and
   transverse colon

B
Left Upper Quadrant
Left lobe of liver
Spleen
Stomach
Body of pancreas
Left adrenal gland
Portion of left kidney
Splenic flexure of colon
Portions of transverse and
   descending colon

C
Right Lower Quadrant
Lower pole of right kidney
Cecum and appendix
Portion of ascending colon
Ovary and uterine tube
Right spermatic cord
Right ureter

D
Left Lower Quadrant
Lower pole of left kidney
Sigmoid colon
Portion of descending colon
Ovary and uterine tube
Left spermatic cord
Left ureter

Midline
Aorta
Bladder
Uterus
◯ = Umbilicus

NINE ABDOMINAL REGIONS

A
Right Hypochondriac
Right lobe of liver
Gallbladder
Portion of duodenum
Hepatic flexure of colon
Portion of right kidney
Right adrenal gland

B
Epigastric
Pyloric sphincter
Duodenum
Pancreas
Portion of liver
Aorta

C
Left Hypochondriac
Stomach
Spleen
Tail of pancreas
Splenic flexure of colon
Upper pole of left kidney
Left adrenal gland

D
Right Lumbar
Ascending colon
Lower half of right kidney
Portion of duodenum
   and jejunum

E
Umbilical
Lower part of duodenum
Jejunum and ileum

F
Left Lumbar
Descending colon
Lower half of left kidney
Portions of jejunum
   and ileum

G
Right Inguinal
Cecum
Appendix
Lower end of ileum
Right ureter
Right spermatic cord
Right ovary and uterine tube

H
Hypogastric (Pubic)
Ileum
Bladder
Uterus (in pregnancy)

I
Left Inguinal
Sigmoid colon
Left ureter
Left spermatic cord
Left ovary and uterine tube

Figure 19.6 ● Upper torso: Organs of the four abdominal quadrants. Lower torso: Organs of the nine abdominal regions.

and situated in the retroperitoneal space, protected by the eleventh and twelfth pairs of ribs. The costovertebral angle is formed as the ribs articulate with the vertebra. The liver displaces the right kidney, thus making the lower pole palpable. The spleen, part of the lymphatic system, is at the level of the tenth rib lateral to the left midaxillary line. The lower pole moves into the abdomen toward the midline when enlarged.

SPECIAL CONSIDERATIONS

Subjective and objective data inform the nurse about the client's health status. A variety of factors influence health, including age, developmental level, race, ethnicity, work history, living conditions, socioeconomics, and emotional well-being. These factors will be discussed in the sections that follow.

Developmental Considerations

Data collection and interpretation of findings in relation to changes that accompany growth and development are important. Expected variations in the abdomen for different age groups are discussed next.

Infants and Children

The abdomen of the newborn and infant is round. The umbilical cord, containing two arteries and one vein, is ligated at the time of delivery. The stump dries and ultimately forms the umbilicus. The toddler has a characteristic potbelly appearance, as depicted in Figure 19.7. Respirations are abdominal; therefore, movement of the abdomen is seen with breathing. This breathing pattern is evident until about the sixth year, at which age respirations become thoracic.

Peristaltic waves are usually more visible in infants and children than in adults because the muscle wall of the abdomen is thinner. Children have the tendency to swallow more air than adults when eating, thus creating a greater sound of tympany

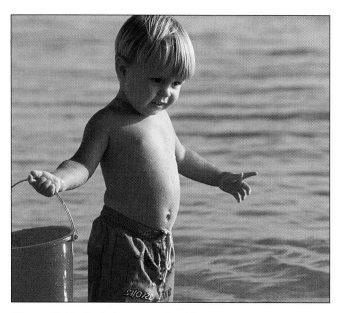

Figure 19.7 • Potbelly stance of toddler.

when percussion is performed. The area of tympany on the right side of the abdomen is smaller because the liver is larger in children.

Congenital disorders, such as cleft lip, cleft palate, esophageal atresia, pyloric stenosis, and hernias, influence the nutritional status, growth, and development of the child and therefore must be assessed with care.

The size of the abdomen at all ages is an indication of the nutritional state of the child. For children of all ages, the nurse should ascertain feeding and eating habits and food tolerance. Symptoms, such as nausea, vomiting, and skin rashes of the child, and the actions taken by the parent are important.

The Pregnant Female

During pregnancy, the abdomen undergoes many changes. As the pregnancy progresses, the uterus enlarges and moves into the abdominal cavity. The height of the fundus should be measured and compared against predictable levels based on the gestational week. By the 14th week of the pregnancy, the fundus should be above the pubic bone and easily palpable. By the 36th week, the fundus is high in the abdomen, close to the diaphragm, and compresses many abdominal structures. Constipation, flatulence, hemorrhoids, and frequent voiding are common problems resulting from the displacement of abdominal organs and pressure from the uterus. Changing levels of hormones decrease peristaltic activity leading to a decrease in bowel sounds. Acid indigestion or heartburn, nausea, vomiting, and constipation are additional problems with the gastrointestinal system during pregnancy.

The Older Adult

The appearance of the abdomen changes with the aging process. In the older adult, the abdomen may be more rounded or protuberant because of increased adipose tissue distribution, decreased muscle tone, and reduced fibroconnective tissue. The abdomen tends to be softer and more relaxed than in the younger adult.

The digestive system of the older adult undergoes characteristic changes; however, these may not be as pronounced as changes in other body systems. A gradual decrease in secretion of saliva, digestive enzymes, peristalsis, intestinal absorption, and intestinal activity occurs. These changes may lead to indigestion, constipation, and gastroesophageal reflux and could exacerbate any existing changes or disease.

The loss of teeth makes chewing and swallowing food difficult. Ill-fitting, broken, or lost dentures also alter nutritional status.

Constipation is a common problem with older adults. Many factors contribute to the problem of constipation. Periodontal disease with the subsequent loss of natural teeth is one such factor because the inability to chew foods results in a diet of soft, nonfibrous foods. Lack of fresh fruits and vegetables or other sources of bulk or fibre contributes to the pattern of constipation. The older adult may self-limit the daily fluid intake, especially water, to decrease frequency of urination, with the increased potential for constipation. Other changes the nurse should anticipate with this age group are dry mouth, delayed esophageal and gastric emptying, decreased gastric acid production, and decreased liver size.

Psychosocial Considerations

High stress levels may cause or aggravate abdominal problems. Gastritis, gastric or duodenal ulcers, and ulcerative colitis are several examples of stress-related problems.

Self-perception may have a subtle influence on the client's weight. Clients who perceive themselves as naturally thin may show greater dedication to restricting their caloric intake and exercising to maintain that self-image. Conversely, clients who perceive themselves as naturally fat may overeat and avoid exercise, feeling that there is nothing they can do to alter their weight.

Surgical scars may alter an individual's body image. Gastrointestinal surgery may require a colostomy, which might be a temporary or permanent change. Many adults consider "wearing a bag" a significant limitation, causing embarrassment and anxiety. This often leads to depression and withdrawal.

Social and Ethnocultural Considerations

Culture, customs, family, and religious practices influence the foods clients choose to eat. Certain foods may be prescribed in certain cultures or religions; however, a healthful diet usually can be achieved even with significant food restrictions. Clients used to a diet of meat and potatoes may not fully appreciate the value of fresh fruits and vegetables.

The financial security of the client also has an impact on eating habits. In some areas, certain foods may not be available year-round or may be much more costly than in other areas. For example, fresh fruits and vegetables typically increase in price in many northern regions in winter months. Unfortunately, highly processed foods are often cheaper but lower in fibre and nutrients than their fresh counterparts.

Social and Ethnocultural Considerations

- Liver disease is a medical problem known to be associated with excessive alcohol use. Liver problems include hepatitis, fatty liver, and cirrhosis. The problem of alcohol-related liver disease increases with age. Assess the amount of alcohol consumption for all clients by using the CAGE questionnaire (Chapters 2 and 27).
- Alcohol- and drug-related diseases (i.e., liver disease) occur more frequently in populations marginalized by poverty and other social and historical factors.
- Certain gender differences are recognized in the substance use literature. Men consume larger quantities of alcohol and drink more often than women at all ages; by contrast, women may be at greater risk of becoming dependent on prescription drugs.
- The types of foods eaten and the ways in which food is prepared is influenced by culture. Many gastrointestinal health problems (e.g., cholelithiasis) are associated with high cholesterol and obesity.
- In assessing for abdominal health problems, consider such factors as diet, exercise, smoking, and substance use. In providing education, consider such issues as the language spoken, literacy level, income and occupation, and social supports, in addition to age, class, gender, family history, ethnicity, and culture.
- The nurse must be sensitive to personal or cultural issues about disrobing for an abdominal assessment.
- Females may require the presence of another female during physical assessment of the abdomen, especially when the examiner is not of the same sex.

GATHERING THE DATA

Health assessment of the abdomen includes the gathering of subjective and objective data. Subjective data collection occurs during the client interview, before the actual physical assessment. During the interview the nurse uses a variety of communication techniques to elicit general and specific information about the client's state of abdominal health or illness. Health records, the results of laboratory tests, and radiological studies are important secondary sources to be reviewed and included in the data-gathering process.

During physical assessment of the abdomen, four techniques of physical assessment will be used. However, the order of the techniques changes to inspection, auscultation, percussion, and palpation. Auscultation is performed after inspection. This order prevents augmentation or disturbance of abdom-inal sounds that could occur from percussion and palpation. Percussion and palpation could influence peristaltic activity, thereby changing the findings on auscultation. The diaphragm of the stethoscope should be used when auscultating for bowel sounds. The nurse should not apply heavy pressure to the diaphragm since this could influence peristaltic activity and ultimately the natural sounds of the intestinal activity. The bell is used when auscultating the aorta and other arteries.

HEALTH HISTORY

The health history for assessment of the abdomen concerns data related to the structures and functions of organs within the abdomen. Subjective data related to the status and function of the structures within the abdomen are gathered during the health history. The nurse must be prepared to observe the client and listen for cues related to the function of the organs and systems within the abdomen. The nurse may use open-ended or closed questions to obtain information. Often a number of follow-up questions or requests for descriptions are required to clarify data or gather missing information.

The health history guides the physical assessment of the abdomen. The information is always considered in relation to norms and expectations about the function of organs and systems within the abdomen. Therefore, the nurse must consider age, gender, race, culture, environment, health practices, past and concurrent problems, and therapies when framing questions and using techniques to elicit information.

To address all the factors when conducting a health history, specific questions related to the abdominal status and function have been developed. These questions focus on the most common concerns or injuries associated with the abdominal system; questions related to past health history; questions related to

behaviours; questions that address environmental concerns; and those that are specific to clients according to age, including the pregnant female.

The nurse must consider the client's ability to participate in the health history and physical assessment of the abdomen. If a client is experiencing pain, cramping, problems with elimination (including frequency or urgency), difficulty swallowing, nausea and vomiting, or the anxiety that accompanies any of these problems, attention must focus on identification of immediate problems and relief of symptoms.

As the nurse gathers the data, she or he will shift the type of questions to direct questions that give the client room to explain or qualify. The mnemonic O-P-Q-R-S-T-U, which stands for onset (chronology), precipitating (or palliative), quality, region (or radiation), severity, timing, and understanding, will help the learner remember the dimensions of the symptoms. The nurse will keep in mind that not all these qualifiers will apply to each symptom.

HEALTH HISTORY QUESTIONS	RATIONALES

The following sections provide sample questions and follow-up questions. Rationales for some questions are provided. The list of questions is not all-inclusive but rather represents the more common concern or injury questions required in a health history related to the abdomen. An example of using O-P-Q-R-S-T-U with pain is provided.

Questions Related to Common Concerns or Injuries

The most common concerns related to illness or injury of the abdomen are as follows:

- Pain
- Nausea and vomiting
- Changes in bowel habits
- Changes in eating patterns or weight
- Abdominal distension

1. **Pain**
   - Are you having any abdominal pain at this time? *If yes:*
   - When did you first notice the pain? How long does it last? *Onset (chronology)*
   - What makes the pain worse? What makes the pain better? *Precipitating (palliative)*
   - Can you describe the pain? Is it sharp? dull? burning? cramping? *Quality*
   - Where is the pain located? Does the pain radiate? *Region (radiation)*

   - How often do you experience the pain? Does the pain affect your breathing or any other functions? How would you rate the pain on a scale of 1 to 10, with 10 being the worst pain? *Severity*
   - Is the pain associated with nausea? vomiting? sweating? constipation? diarrhea? bloody stools? abdominal distension? fever? chills? eating? *Timing*
   - What do you think is causing the pain? *Understanding*

2. **Nausea and vomiting**
   - Do you have nausea or vomiting?
   - How often are you nauseated?

▶ Pain could indicate cardiac disease, ulcers, cholecystitis, renal calculi, diverticulitis, urinary cystitis, or ectopic pregnancy.

HEALTH HISTORY QUESTIONS	RATIONALES

- Is there a difference in the nausea at different times of the day?
- Is the nausea accompanied by burning, indigestion, or bloating?
- Do you vomit when you experience the nausea?

▶ Vomiting can be related to a variety of pathological conditions, such as food poisoning, ulcers, varices of the esophagus, hepatitis, and the beginning of an intestinal obstruction. Medications, prescribed and over the counter, may contribute to or cause vomiting.

- How often do you vomit?
- What is the colour of the vomitus? amount?

▶ The colour and odour of vomitus may be associated with specific diseases or problems. For example, brown vomitus with a fecal odour can indicate an intestinal obstruction.

- Do you notice any unusual foul odour to the vomitus?
- Is the nausea or vomiting associated with abdominal pain? constipation? diarrhea? change in the colour of your stools? fever?

▶ Pain may occur because of associated muscle pain when vomiting or may be indicative of an underlying abdominal disease. Follow-up elicits details that assist in the data analysis.

- How frequently do you experience nausea or vomiting?
- What do you do to relieve the symptoms?
- Do you know what is causing the nausea or vomiting?

If the client is a woman, ask:
- When was your last period?

3. **Changes in bowel habits**
   - Have you experienced any changes in your elimination pattern or in your stool?
   - What kind of change has occurred in your elimination pattern or stool?

▶ These questions provide initial information about bowel functioning. The nurse determines if the client has an established pattern for bowel elimination. If the client indicates that there has been a change in the pattern of elimination or in the characteristics of the stool, follow-up questions are indicated. Tarry stool indicates bleeding in the upper part of the gastrointestinal tract. A clay colour indicates lack of bile in the stool.

- When did the change begin?
- Do you suffer from diarrhea or constipation?
- How long have you had diarrhea or constipation?
- When does the diarrhea or constipation occur?
- Do you have periods of diarrhea alternating with constipation?
- How many bowel movements do you have a day? What is the colour of the stool? What is the consistency?

▶ Dark, tarry stool indicates bleeding, usually in the upper or middle part of the intestinal tract. Frank (bright red) blood usually indicates lower tract bleeding or hemorrhoids.

- Can you identify anything you believe may have caused the change in your elimination pattern?
- What have you done about the problem?

4. **Changes in eating patterns or weight**
   - Has your appetite changed in the last 24 hours? in the last month? in the last year?

▶ These questions elicit basic information about the client's eating habits. In addition, appetite change can be indicative of underlying physical and psychological problems. If a change has occurred, it is important to find the client's perception of the change and to identify factors that may have contributed to the change.

HEALTH HISTORY QUESTIONS

RATIONALES

- How much have you had to eat or drink in the last 24 hours?

▶ In addition to obtaining data about weight, the nurse is building on the nutritional data already collected. The nurse is establishing the client's dietary patterns, paying special attention to overconsumption and underconsumption.

- Is this a typical eating pattern for you?
- Are there any foods that you cannot eat?
- Do you have any difficulty chewing or swallowing your food?
- Do you wear dentures? Do you have crowns?

▶ Ill-fitting dentures, failure to wear them, and missing or diseased teeth make chewing and swallowing difficult. Disorders of the throat and esophagus can also make swallowing difficult.

- What is your weight? Has your weight changed?

▶ Weight loss or gain can accompany physical and psychological problems. Dietary consumption is one of the leading factors in weight control. The nurse should determine if weight gain is associated with a decrease in activity, changes in metabolic rates, hormonal factors, or fluid retention. Psychological problems may cause an individual to overconsume or underconsume foods. Weight loss may be an appropriate or desired outcome for some individuals. The nurse must determine if the weight loss was purposeful. Weight loss can accompany problems associated with diabetes, hyperthyroidism, and some cancers.

- Over what period of time did the weight change occur?

▶ This question provides information about meeting nutritional requirements and input about diet and nutrition, which may contribute to obesity or problems with weight loss.

- What do you believe has contributed to your weight change?

5. **Abdominal distension**
   - Do you have feelings of bloating or increased gas?
   - For how long have you noticed your abdomen feeling distended?
   - Is the distension related to eating?

▶ Some foods (broccoli, cauliflower, figs, etc.) and lactose intolerance will cause this feeling. Some medications are constipating. Severe bloating and gas can be indicative of abdominal pathology.

- Is the distension lessened by passing gas from above or below?

Questions Related to Past Health History

1. **Have you ever been diagnosed with an abdominal illness, such as cholecystitis (inflammation of the gallbladder), cholelithiasis (gallstones), ulcers, diverticulosis, cirrhosis, rectal bleeding, or hepatitis?** *If yes:*

▶ If a diagnosis of an illness is identified, follow-up about the date of the diagnosis, treatment, and outcomes is required. Data about each illness identified by the client are essential to an accurate health assessment. Illnesses can be classified as acute or chronic, and follow-up regarding each classification will differ.

- When were you diagnosed with the problem?
- Has the problem ever recurred? *(acute)*
- How are you managing the illness now? *(chronic)*
- Does your abdominal illness affect your ability to carry out your activities of daily living?

▶ Inability to carry out or perform personal or work-related activities can be indicative of problems in the abdominal system.

HEALTH HISTORY QUESTIONS	RATIONALES

- Have you discussed this with a healthcare professional? If so, what treatment was recommended and did it help?

2. **Is there anyone in your family who has had an abdominal disease or problem? If so, what was it?**

▶ This question may reveal information about abdominal diseases associated with familial or genetic predisposition.

Questions Related to Behaviours

Healthcare behaviours include both health practices and health patterns. Health practices consist of following recommendations for disease prevention, including screening for risks, screening for early detection of problems, and immunization. Health patterns are habits or acts that affect the client's health. Health behaviours may also include seeking healthcare from healthcare providers who use alternative methods to diagnose and treat illness. Clients should be questioned in a nonjudgmental way and areas for health teaching should be identified.

1. **How much coffee, tea, cola, alcoholic beverages, and chocolate do you consume in a 24-hour period?**

▶ Caffeine and alcohol irritate the gastrointestinal system and can contribute to ulcers and irritable bowel syndrome.

2. **How much physical activity do you get in a typical week?**
   - Is there anything that you can think of that affects your ability to exercise?

3. **Do you take antacids or laxatives?**

Questions Related to the Environment

Environment refers to both internal and external environments. Questions related to the internal environment include all the previous questions and those associated with internal or physiological responses. Questions regarding the external environment include those related to home, work, or social environments.

Internal Environment

1. **How would you describe your stress level?**
   - Do you think you are coping well?

▶ Prolonged stress is linked to gastrointestinal disease.

2. **Could your coping skills be better?**

External Environment

The following questions deal with the physical environment of the client. That includes the indoor and outdoor environments of the home and the workplace, those encountered for social engagements, and any encountered during travel.

1. **Do you work with any chemical irritants?**
   - Exposure to benzene, lead, or nickel may lead to gastric irritation. Excessive exposure to chemical hepatotoxins, such as carbon tetrachloride, may lead to postnecrotic cirrhosis.

2. **Have you recently done any travelling?**

▶ Water purification and food storage methods vary in different regions and different countries. Exposure to food-borne or water-borne microorganisms can lead to gastroenteritis, hepatitis, diarrhea, or parasite infestation.

3. **Where did you travel?**

Questions Related to Age

The health history must reflect the anatomical and physiological differences that exist along the age span.

GATHERING THE DATA

HEALTH HISTORY QUESTIONS	RATIONALES

Questions Regarding Infants and Children

1. Is the baby breastfed or bottle-fed?

2. Does the baby tolerate the feeding?

3. How frequently does the baby eat?

4. Have you recently started the baby on any new foods?

5. Is the baby colicky? What do you do to relieve the colic?

6. What and how much does the toddler eat?

  ▶ Eating habits, patterns, and preferences established in the early years of life are likely to have a lasting effect.

7. What does the child eat?

8. Does the child bring a lunch and snack to school or buy them at school?

9. When at home, how often does the child snack, and what are the snacks?

Questions for the Pregnant Female

1. Are you experiencing any nausea or vomiting?

  ▶ Nausea is common during early pregnancy and may be due to changing hormone levels and changes in carbohydrate metabolism. Fatigue is also a factor. Vomiting is less common. If it occurs more than once a day or for a prolonged period, the client should be referred to a physician.

2. Are you experiencing any elimination problems, such as constipation?

3. Are you experiencing heartburn or flatulence?

  ▶ Heartburn (regurgitation of gastric contents into the esophagus) is primarily caused by displacement of the stomach by the enlarging uterus. Flatulence results from the decreased gastrointestinal motility, common during pregnancy, and pressure on the large intestine from the growing uterus.

Questions for the Older Adult

1. Are you ever incontinent of feces?

  ▶ Muscle tone decreases with age, and the older adult may lose sphincter control.

2. How often are you constipated?

  ▶ Constipation is a common problem with older adults. Influencing factors include decreased peristaltic activity, decreased desire to eat, and self-limited fluid intake.

3. Do you take laxatives? How often?

  ▶ To help relieve constipation, some older clients take over-the-counter laxatives. With prolonged use, laxatives can become habit forming.

4. How many foods containing fibre or roughage do you eat during a typical day?

  ▶ Older adults tend to have diets low in fibre or roughage. Loss of natural teeth and ill-fitting dentures make chewing difficult.

5. How much fluid do you drink in a typical day?

6. Are you able to get to the store for groceries?

  ▶ Responses to questions 6 and 7 help determine mobility patterns, availability of food, and social isolation at mealtimes.

7. Do you eat alone or with someone?

PHYSICAL ASSESSMENT

ASSESSMENT TECHNIQUES AND FINDINGS

Physical assessment of the abdomen requires the use of inspection, auscultation, percussion, and palpation. This order differs from that of physical assessment of other systems. The nurse should remember to auscultate after inspection. Delaying percussion and palpation prevents disturbance of the normal bowel sounds. During each procedure, the nurse is gathering data related to problems with underlying abdominal organs and structures. Inspection includes looking at skin colour, structures of the abdomen, abdominal contour, pulsations, and abdominal movements. Knowledge of normative values or expected findings is essential in determining the meaning of the data as the physical assessment is performed.

The skin of the abdomen should be consistent with the skin of the rest of the body. The umbilicus should be midline in an abdomen that may be round, flat, convex, or protuberant. The abdomen should be symmetrical and free of bulges. Pulsations and wavelike movements below the xiphoid process are normal in thin adults.

Physical assessment of the abdomen follows an organized pattern. It begins with a client survey, followed by inspection, auscultation, percussion, and palpation of the abdomen. The lateral aspects of the abdomen are included when conducting each assessment.

> **EQUIPMENT**
>
> examination gown and drape
> skin marker
> clean, nonsterile examination gloves
> metric ruler
>
> examination light
> tissues
> stethoscope
> tape measure

> **HELPFUL HINTS**
> - Provide an environment that is warm and comfortable.
> - Encourage the client to void before the examination.
> - Provide instructions about what is expected of the client, such as taking several deep breaths to relax abdominal muscles.
> - Pay attention to nonverbal cues that may indicate discomfort. Facial gestures, legs flexed at the knees, and abdominal guarding with the hands are all indices of discomfort.
> - When a client is experiencing abdominal pain, examine that area last.
> - Stand on the right side of the client, unless otherwise indicated, because the liver and right kidney are in the right side of the abdomen.
> - Maintain the dignity of the client through appropriate draping techniques.
> - Use routine practices.

| TECHNIQUES AND NORMAL FINDINGS | ABNORMAL FINDINGS AND SPECIAL CONSIDERATIONS |

SURVEY

A quick survey of the client enables the nurse to identify any immediate problems as well as the client's ability to participate in the assessment.

▶ Clients experiencing anxiety may demonstrate pallor and shallow breathing. They may be diaphoretic and use their hands to guard their abdomen.

Inspect the overall appearance, posture, and position of the client. Observe for signs of pain or discomfort and signs of anxiety or distress.

▶ Acknowledgment of the problem and a discussion of the procedures often provide some relief. If the client is experiencing severe pain or discomfort, the problem must be addressed and a complete abdominal assessment may need to be delayed.

INSPECTION OF THE ABDOMEN

1. Position the client.
   - The client should be in a supine position with a small pillow placed beneath the head and knees. Drape the examination gown over the chest, exposing the abdomen. Place the drape at the symphysis pubis, covering the client's pubic area and legs (see Figure 19.8).

▶ These measures relax the abdominal musculature and prevent unnecessary exposure of the client.

PHYSICAL ASSESSMENT

TECHNIQUES AND NORMAL FINDINGS	ABNORMAL FINDINGS AND SPECIAL CONSIDERATIONS

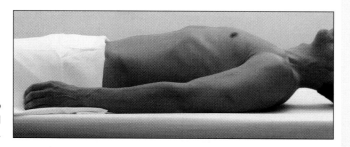

Figure 19.8 •
Client positioned and draped.

- Stand at the right side of the client. Lighting must be adequate to detect colour differences, lesions, and movements of the abdomen.

2. **Instruct the client.**
- Explain that you will be looking at the client's abdomen. Tell the client to breathe normally.

▶ If the client is guarding the abdomen, demonstrated by posture or breathing, the client should be asked to take several deep breaths. This assists in relaxation of abdominal musculature.

3. **Map the abdomen.**
- Visualize the imaginary horizontal and vertical lines delineating the abdominal quadrants and regions as identified in Figures 19.4 and 19.5.
- Visualize the underlying structures as identified in Figure 19.6.

4. **Determine the contour of the abdomen.**
- Observe the profile of the abdomen between the costal margins and the symphysis pubis.

▶ A protuberant abdomen is normal in pregnancy. It may indicate obesity or ascites (abnormal collection of fluid in the peritoneal cavity) in a nonpregnant client.

- The abdominal profile should be viewed at eye level. You may need to sit or kneel to observe the abdominal profile (see Figure 19.9).

5. **Observe the position of the umbilicus.**
- The umbilicus is normally in the centre of the abdomen. It may be inverted or protruding. The umbilicus should be clean and free of inflammation or drainage.

▶ A protruding or displaced umbilicus is a normal variation in pregnant females. In the nonpregnant adult, it could indicate an abdominal mass or distended urinary bladder. Inflammation or drainage may indicate an infection or complication from recent laparoscopic surgery. A displaced or protruding umbilicus may be a sign of a hernia in a child.

6. **Observe skin colour.**
- The abdominal skin should be consistent in colour and lustre with the skin of the rest of the body. The skin is smooth, moist, and free of lesions.

▶ Taut, glistening skin could indicate ascites.

7. **Observe the location and characteristics of lesions, scars, and abdominal markings.**

▶ **Striae**, commonly called stretch marks, are silvery, shiny, irregular markings on the skin. These are seen in obesity, pregnancy, and ascites.

Scars indicate previous surgery or trauma and the possibility of underlying adhesions. The location of all lesions must be documented as baseline data and for determination of change in future assessment.

- Such lesions as macules, moles, and freckles are considered normal findings.

PHYSICAL ASSESSMENT

<table>
<tr><td>

TECHNIQUES AND NORMAL FINDINGS

</td><td>

</td></tr>
</table>

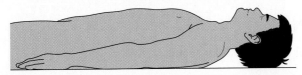

Flat. A straight horizontal line is observed from the costal margin to the symphysis pubis. This contour is common in a thin person.

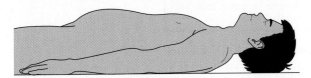

Rounded. Sometimes called a convex abdomen. The horizontal line is now curved outward, indicating an increase in abodominal fat or a decrease in muscle tone. This contour is considered a normal variation in the toddler and the pregnant female.

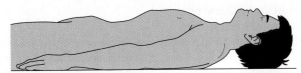

Scaphoid. Sometimes called a concave abdomen. The horizontal line now curves towards the vertebral column, giving the abodominal a sunken appearance. In the adult, this contour is seen in the very thin person.

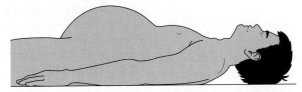

Protuberant. Similiar to the rounded abdomen, only greater. This contour is anticipated in pregnancy. It is also seen in the adult with obesity, ascites, and other conditions.

Figure 19.9 ● Contour of the abdomen *(continued).*

8. **Observe the abdomen for symmetry, bulging, or masses.**
   - First observe the abdomen while standing at the client's side. Second, observe the abdomen while standing at the foot of the examination table. Compare the right and left sides. The sides should appear symmetrical in shape, size, and contour.
   - Third, return to the client's side and use a tangential light across the abdomen. No shadows should appear.
   - Observe the abdomen from eye level, by sitting or kneeling, and shine the light across the abdomen. The abdomen should appear symmetrical without bulges or masses.
   - You may repeat all the assessments above while asking the client to take a deep breath and raise the head off the pillow.

9. **Observe the abdominal wall for movement.**
   - Movements can include pulsations or peristaltic waves. In thin clients it is normal to observe a pulsation of the abdominal aorta below the xiphoid process. The observation of peristaltic waves in thin clients is normal.

▶ Asymmetry may indicate masses, adhesions, or strictures of underlying structures.

▶ Shadows may indicate bulges or masses.

▶ Bulges could indicate tumours, cysts, or hernias.

▶ Deep breathing and head raising accentuate masses.

▶ Marked pulsations could indicate aortic aneurysm or increased pulse pressure. Increased peristaltic activity could indicate gastroenteritis or an obstructive process.

PHYSICAL ASSESSMENT

TECHNIQUES AND NORMAL FINDINGS	ABNORMAL FINDINGS AND SPECIAL CONSIDERATIONS

AUSCULTATION OF THE ABDOMEN

Auscultation of the abdomen refers to listening to bowel sounds, vascular sounds, and friction rubs through the stethoscope.

> **CLINICAL TIP**
>
> *It is important to auscultate before percussing and palpating, because the latter techniques could alter peristaltic action.*

The pattern for auscultation of bowel sounds is to begin in the RLQ and then proceed through each remaining quadrant. The diaphragm of the stethoscope is used to auscultate bowel sounds. The pattern for auscultation of vascular sounds is to begin at the midline below the xiphoid process for the aorta and to proceed from side to side over renal, iliac, and femoral arteries. The bell of the stethoscope is used to auscultate vascular sounds.

The pattern for auscultation for friction rubs is to begin in the RLQ and proceed through each of the remaining quadrants and to listen over the liver and spleen.

The normal bowel sounds heard on auscultation of the abdomen are irregular, high-pitched, gurgling sounds.

Normal bowel sounds occur from 5 to 30 times per minute. Borborygmi (stomach growling) refers to more frequent sounds heard in clients who have not eaten in a few hours.

Auscultation of the normal abdomen will not produce vascular sounds or friction rubs.

▶ Hyperactive bowel sounds are loud, high-pitched, and rushing. They may occur more frequently with gastroenteritis or diarrhea.

1. **Instruct the client.**
   - Explain that you will be listening to the client's abdomen with the stethoscope. The client will be in the supine position. Tell the client to breathe normally. Explain that you will be moving the stethoscope around the client's abdomen and stopping to listen when the stethoscope is placed down. Inform the client that this will cause no discomfort.

▶ Vascular sounds include bruits and venous hum. A **bruit** is pulsatile and blowing. A venous hum is soft, continuous, and low-pitched. **Friction rub** refers to a rough, grating sound caused by the rubbing together of organs or an organ rubbing on the peritoneum.

2. **Auscultate for bowel sounds.**
   - Use the diaphragm of the stethoscope. Start in the RLQ and move through the other quadrants. Note the character and frequency of the sounds. Count the sounds for at least 60 seconds (see Figure 19.10).

▶ Hyperactive sounds are common in gastro-enteritis and diarrhea. Hypoactive sounds are common following abdominal surgery and occur in end-stage intestinal obstruction. Absence of bowel sounds may indicate paralytic ileus.

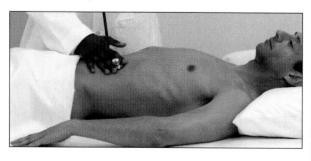

Figure 19.10 ● Auscultating the abdomen for bowel sounds.

   - Normal bowel sounds are irregular, gurgling, and high-pitched. They occur from 5 to 30 times per minute. Borborygmi is a normal finding.

▶ Clients with paralytic ileus or intestinal obstruction require immediate attention.

> **CLINICAL TIP**
>
> *It may be difficult for the novice nurse to hear bowel sounds in some clients. All four quadrants are auscultated for a total of at least 5 minutes before documenting absent bowel sounds.*

TECHNIQUES AND NORMAL FINDINGS	ABNORMAL FINDINGS AND SPECIAL CONSIDERATIONS

3. Auscultate for vascular sounds.

- Use the bell of the stethoscope. Listen at the midline below the xiphoid process for aortic sounds. Move the stethoscope from side to side as you listen over the renal, iliac, and femoral arteries (see Figure 19.11).

▶ Bruits heard during systole and diastole may indicate arterial occlusion.

A venous hum usually indicates increased portal tension.

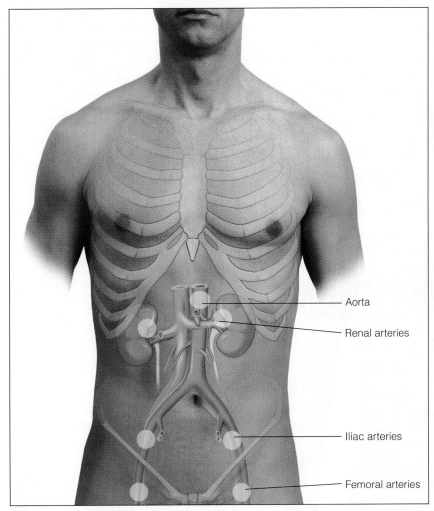

Aorta

Renal arteries

Iliac arteries

Femoral arteries

Figure 19.11 ● Auscultatory areas for vascular sounds.

4. Auscultate for friction rubs.

- Auscultate the abdomen, listening for a coarse, grating sound. Listen carefully over the liver and spleen. Friction rubs are not normally heard.

PERCUSSION OF THE ABDOMEN

1. Visualize the landmarks.

- Observe the abdomen and visualize the horizontal and vertical lines. Visualize the organs and underlying structures of the abdomen.

2. Recall the expected findings.

- Percussion allows you to assess underlying structures. The normal sounds heard over the abdomen are tympany, a loud, hollow sound; and dullness, a short, high-pitched sound heard over solid organs and the distended bladder.

▶ Hyperresonance is louder than tympany and is heard over air-filled or distended intestines. Flat sounds are short and abrupt and heard over bone. Correct placement of the fingers is important.

PHYSICAL ASSESSMENT

TECHNIQUES AND NORMAL FINDINGS	ABNORMAL FINDINGS AND SPECIAL CONSIDERATIONS

3. **Instruct the client.**
   - Explain that you will be tapping on the client's abdomen in a variety of areas.
   - Tell the client to breathe normally through this examination. If muscle tension is detected, ask the client to take several deep breaths.

4. **Percuss the abdomen.**
   - Place your pleximeter finger on the abdomen during the examination. Review the technique of percussion in Chapter 6. ⃝⃝ Start in the RLQ and percuss through all the remaining quadrants (see Figure 19.12).

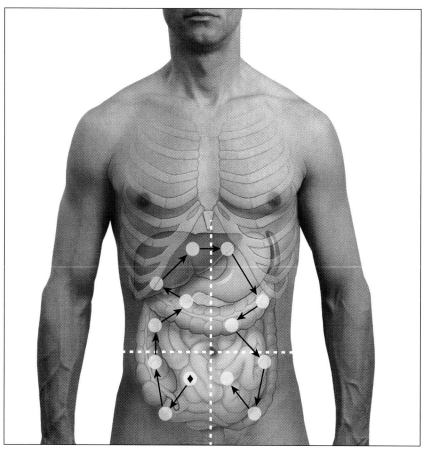

Figure 19.12 ● Percussion pattern for abdomen.

   - Percussion over the abdomen produces tympany. Tympany is more pronounced over the gastric bubble. Dullness is heard over the liver and spleen.

PERCUSSION OF THE LIVER

Percuss the liver to determine the upper and lower borders at the anterior axillary line, midclavicular line, and midsternal line. Measure the distance between marks drawn to identify the borders.

1. **Instruct the client.**
   - Explain that you will be tapping the client's abdomen and chest on the right side. Explain that you will be making marks on the abdomen and using a ruler to measure the marks in order to evaluate the size of the liver. Tell the client to remain relaxed and that there should be no discomfort during this assessment.

▶ Dullness may indicate an enlarged uterus, distended urinary bladder, or ascites. Dullness in the LLQ may indicate the presence of stool in the colon. It is important to ask when the client last had a bowel movement.

| TECHNIQUES AND NORMAL FINDINGS | ABNORMAL FINDINGS AND SPECIAL CONSIDERATIONS |

2. Percuss the liver.

- Begin percussion at the level of the umbilicus and move toward the rib cage along the extended right MCL (see Figure 19.13).

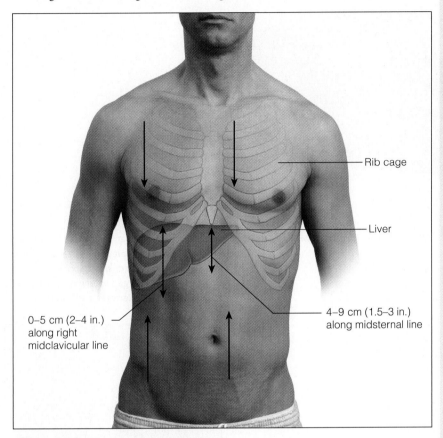

Rib cage

Liver

0–5 cm (2–4 in.) along right midclavicular line

4–9 cm (1.5–3 in.) along midsternal line

Figure 19.13 ● Percussion pattern for liver.

- The first sound you should hear is tympany. When the sound changes to dullness, you have identified the lower border of the liver. Mark the point with a skin-marking pen. The lower border is normally at the costal margin.
- Percuss downward from the fourth intercostal space along the right MCL. The first sound you should hear is resonance because you are over the lung. Percuss downward until the sound changes to dullness. This is the upper border of the liver. Mark the point with a pen. The upper border should be at the level of the sixth intercostal space.
- Measure the distance between the two points. The upper and lower borders should be no more than 10 cm (4 in.) apart. This distance is called the *liver span*.

▶ Dullness below the costal margin suggests liver enlargement or downward displacement because of respiratory disease. Dullness above the fifth or sixth intercostal space could indicate an enlarged liver (hepatomegaly) or displacement upward because of ascites or a mass.

PERCUSSION OF THE SPLEEN

The spleen is located in the left side of the abdomen. Percussion is conducted to identify enlargement of the organ.

1. Instruct the client.

- Explain that you will be tapping on the left side of the client's abdomen to examine the spleen. Tell the client to continue to relax, taking deep breaths if required.

| TECHNIQUES AND NORMAL FINDINGS | ABNORMAL FINDINGS AND SPECIAL CONSIDERATIONS |

2. Percuss the spleen.

- Percuss the abdomen on the left side posterior to the midaxillary line (see Figure 19.14).

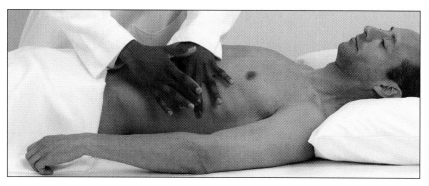

Figure 19.14 ● Percussing the spleen.

- A small area of splenic dullness will usually be heard from the sixth to tenth intercostal spaces.

▶ Splenic dullness at the left anterior axillary line indicates splenomegaly, an enlarged spleen. The dull percussion sound is identifiable before an enlarged spleen is palpable. The spleen enlarges anteriorly and inferiorly (see Figure 19.15).

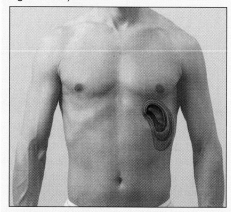

Figure 19.15 ● Splenic enlargement.

PALPATION OF THE ABDOMEN

Palpation of the abdomen is conducted to determine organ size and placement, muscle tightness or guarding, masses, tenderness, and the presence of fluid. This is performed after auscultation to avoid changing the natural sounds and movements of the abdomen. Identify painful areas and palpate these areas last.

You will use both light and deep palpation.

1. Instruct the client.

- Explain that you will be touching the client's abdomen with your hands. Explain that you are going to use light touch and then slight pressure to explore the abdomen. Instruct the client to inform you of any discomfort. Observe the client's facial expression for signs of pain. Also watch for the tendency to guard the abdomen with the hands, or to flex the knees.

- Instruct the client to take several deep breaths to relax the muscles of the abdomen.

▶ Muscle tightness or guarding may indicate abdominal pain. Guarding is involuntary contraction of abdominal muscles associated with peritonitis.

▶ Abdominal pain from an organ is often experienced as referred pain—that is, pain felt on the surface of the abdomen or back.

| TECHNIQUES AND NORMAL FINDINGS | ABNORMAL FINDINGS AND SPECIAL CONSIDERATIONS |

2. **Lightly palpate the abdomen.**
   - Place the palmar surface of your hand on the abdomen and extend your fingers. Lightly press into the abdomen with your fingers (see Figure 19.16).

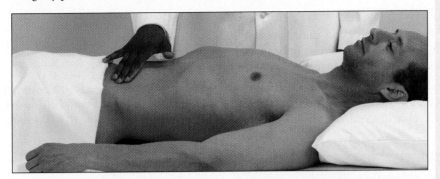

Figure 19.16 ● Light palpation of abdomen.

   - Move your hand over the four quadrants by lifting your hand and then placing it in another area. Do not drag or slide your hand over the surface of the skin.
   - The abdomen should be soft, smooth, nontender, and pain-free.

3. **Deeply palpate the abdomen.**
   - Proceed as for light palpation, described in the previous step. Exert pressure with your hand to depress the abdomen about 4 to 5 cm (2 in.).
   - Palpate all four quadrants in an organized sequence.

   ▶ Masses, tumours, or obstructions may be palpated.

   - In an obese client or a client with an enlarged abdomen, use a bimanual technique. Place the fingers of your nondominant hand over your dominant hand (see Figure 19.17).

   ▶ In the pregnant female the uterus is palpable. The height of the fundus varies according to the week of gestation.

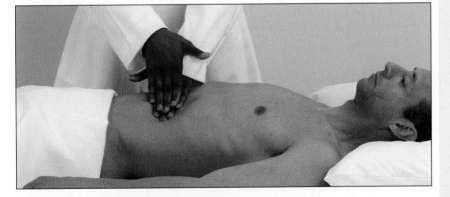

Figure 19.17 ● Deep palpation of abdomen.

   - Identify the size of the underlying organs and any masses for tenderness. The pancreas is nonpalpable because of its size and location.

   ▶ A mass in the LLQ may be stool in the colon. A vaguely palpable sensation of fullness in the epigastric region may be pancreatic in origin.

PALPATION OF THE LIVER

The liver is palpated to detect enlargement, pain, and consistency.

1. **Instruct the client.**
   - Explain that you will be using your hands to palpate the client's liver. Explain that you will place one hand under the ribs in the back and ask the client to

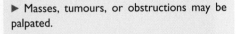

PHYSICAL ASSESSMENT

TECHNIQUES AND NORMAL FINDINGS

take a deep breath while you apply slight pressure in an upward motion under the ribs on the client's right side. Instruct the client to tell you of any pain and observe the client for cues of discomfort.

2. **Palpate the liver.**

   - Stand on the right side of the client. Place your left hand under the lower portion of the ribs (ribs eleven and twelve). Tell the client to relax into your left hand. Lift the rib cage with your left hand.

   - Place your right hand into the abdomen by using an inward and upward thrust at the costal margin (see Figure 19.18). Ask the client to take a deep breath. The descent of the diaphragm will cause the liver to descend, and the lower border will meet your right hand.

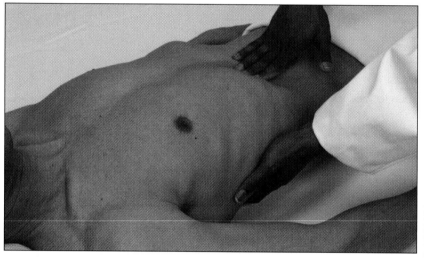

Figure 19.18 ● Palpating the liver.

   - Normally, the liver is nonpalpable, except in thin clients. If you feel the lower border of the liver it will be smooth, firm, and nontender.

PALPATION OF THE SPLEEN

The spleen is palpated to detect enlargement. Careful palpation is required because the spleen is fragile and sensitive.

1. **Instruct the client.**

   - Explain that you will be touching the client with both hands to palpate the spleen. Explain that you will be lifting the client slightly with your left hand while applying slight pressure with your fingers under the ribs on the left side. Instruct the client to inform you of any pain or discomfort.

2. **Palpate the spleen.**

   - Stand on the client's right side. Place your left hand under the lower border of the rib cage on the left side and elevate the rib cage. This moves the spleen anteriorly. Press the fingers of your right hand into the left costal margin area of the client (see Figure 19.19).

   - Ask the client to take a slow, deep breath. As the diaphragm descends, the spleen moves forward to the fingertips of your right hand. The spleen is normally not palpable.

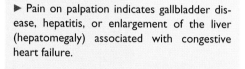
▶ Pain on palpation indicates gallbladder disease, hepatitis, or enlargement of the liver (hepatomegaly) associated with congestive heart failure.

▶ Nodules occur with cirrhosis or metastatic carcinoma.

▶ Splenomegaly, enlargement of the spleen, occurs in acute infections, such as mononucleosis. The enlarged spleen is palpable.

TECHNIQUES AND NORMAL FINDINGS	ABNORMAL FINDINGS AND SPECIAL CONSIDERATIONS

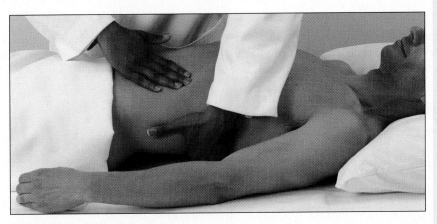

Figure 19.19 ● Palpating the spleen.

ADDITIONAL PROCEDURES

1. **Palpate the aorta for pulsations.**
   - Use your fingertips to press deeply and firmly in the upper abdomen to the left of midline below the xiphoid process.
   - The average adult aorta is 3 cm (1 in.) wide.

2. **Palpate for rebound tenderness (Blumberg's sign).**

   - With the client in a supine position, hold your hand at a 90-degree angle to the abdominal wall in an area of no pain or discomfort. Press deeply into the abdomen, using a slow, steady movement.
   - Rapidly remove your fingers from the client's abdomen (see Figure 19.20).
   - Ask if the client feels any pain. Normally, the client feels the pressure but no pain.

▶ Obesity and masses make palpation of the aorta difficult.

▶ The widened aorta may indicate aneurysm.

▶ The experience of sharp stabbing pain as the compressed area returns to a noncompressed state is known as **Blumberg's sign**. This finding occurs in peritoneal irritation and requires immediate medical attention. Pain referred to McBurney's point (2.5 to 5 cm or 1 to 2 in. above the anterosuperior iliac spine, on a line between the ileum and the umbilicus) on palpation of the left lower abdomen is Rovsing's sign, suggestive of peritoneal irritation in appendicitis.

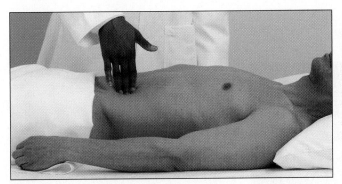
A

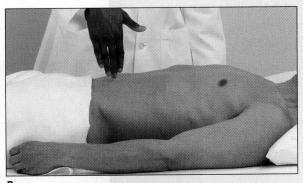
B

Figure 19.20 ● Palpating for rebound tenderness. A. Applying pressure. B. Rapid release of pressure.

Techniques and Normal Findings

Abnormal Findings and Special Considerations

3. Percuss the abdomen for ascites.

   - **Ascites** is an abnormal collection of fluid in the peritoneal cavity. With the client in a supine position, percuss at the midline to elicit tympany. Continue to percuss in lateral directions away from the midline and listen for dullness (see Figure 19.21).

   ▶ Ascites is found in congestive heart failure, cirrhosis, renal failure, and in many types of cancer.

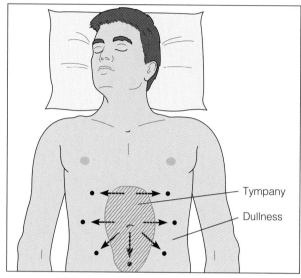

Figure 19.21 ●
Percussion pattern for ascites.

Tympany
Dullness

   - Mark the skin, identifying possible levels of fluid.

   - An alternative method, called *shifting dullness,* is to position the client on the right or left side. Percuss the abdomen. Because fluid settles, anticipate tympany at a superior level and dullness at lower levels (see Figure 19.22).

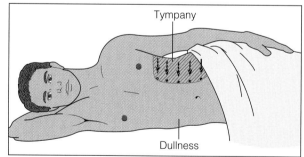

Tympany

Figure 19.22 ●
Percussion pattern for ascites.

Dullness

   - If ascites is suspected, measure the abdominal girth with a tape measure.

4. Perform the liver scratch test.

   - The liver scratch test is used as an alternative or to confirm the results of a percussed liver span (see Figure 19.23).

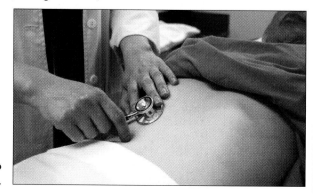

Figure 19.23 ●
Liver scratch test.

PHYSICAL ASSESSMENT

TECHNIQUES AND NORMAL FINDINGS	ABNORMAL FINDINGS AND SPECIAL CONSIDERATIONS

- Place the diaphragm of the stethoscope over the upper margin of the liver.
- Lightly scratch the skin over the lower abdomen and move upward until the sound is magnified by the mass of the liver.
- This point is the lower margin of the liver.

5. **Test for psoas sign.**
   - Perform this test when lower abdominal pain is present and you suspect appendicitis.
   - With the client in a supine position, place your right hand just above the level of the client's right knee. Ask the client to raise the leg to meet your hand. Flexion of the hip causes contraction of the psoas muscle (see Figure 19.24).

▶ Pain during this manoeuvre is indicative of irritation of the psoas muscle and is associated with peritoneal inflammation or appendicitis.

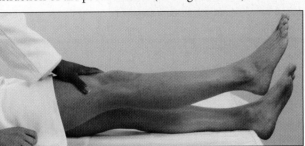

Figure 19.24 ●
Psoas sign.

- Normally there is no abdominal pain associated with this manoeuvre.

6. **Conduct the obturator test.**
   - While the client is supine, flex the client's thigh at the hip.
   - Bend the client's knee and rotate the leg internally and externally at the hip, as shown in Figure 19.25.

▶ This test causes pain if there is an inflammatory process adjacent to the obturator muscle.

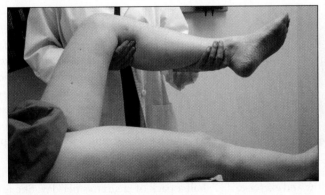

Figure 19.25 ●
The obturator test.

7. **Test for Murphy's sign.**
   - While palpating the liver, ask the client to take a deep breath. The diaphragm descends, pushing the liver and gallbladder toward your hand. In a healthy client, liver palpation is painless.

▶ Sharp abdominal pain and the need to halt the examination is a positive Murphy's sign. This occurs in clients with cholecystitis (inflammation of the gallbladder).

8. **Test for costovertebral tenderness.**
   - Perform this test with the client seated.
   - Make a fist and gently tap the area overlying the posterior costovertebral angle on each side (see Figure 19.26). In a healthy client, the percussion is painless.

▶ Clients with pyelonephritis (kidney infection) usually have extreme pain even on slight percussion of these areas.

TECHNIQUES AND NORMAL FINDINGS	ABNORMAL FINDINGS AND SPECIAL CONSIDERATIONS

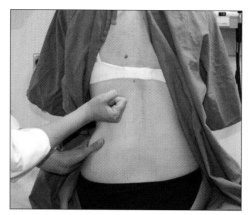

Figure 19.26 ●
Testing for costovertebral
tenderness.

SAMPLE DOCUMENTATION

Subjective: No complaints of nausea or vomiting, no loss of appetite. BM once a day, formed. Nonsmoker, drinks ETOH 1–2/week. No meds. Past medical hx and family hx unremarkable. No allergies.

Objective: Abdomen flat. Umbilicus midline. No masses visible. Bowel sounds present in all 4 quadrants. No bruits heard. Tympany heard in all 4 quadrants. Liver span 8 cm. No pain to light or deep palpation.

APPLICATION THROUGH CRITICAL THINKING

CASE STUDY

Bernice Flett is a 45-year-old Aboriginal woman who presents to the clinic with complaints of abdominal pain. She has been seen for abdominal pain twice in the last two months; however, she states that the pain is increasing. She is a G4P4, ages ranging between 18 and 9 years. She states that since having her children, she has gained more than 50 kg (110 lb.) and finds it difficult to find time to eat healthy and exercise. She works at a local community office as a receptionist.

While interviewing Ms. Flett, she tells you that her appetite is good, but since the pain began last night, her appetite has decreased significantly. She states that this is common for her when she has these "attacks." She has had a gradual weight increase over the past several years and states that "I just can't find time to eat right and exercise." Her bowel movements are regular, but she has noticed that they are greyer than usual. She has had no increase in gas or bloating, and no one else in her household is experiencing these same problems. She has previously been healthy and her past medical history is unremarkable.

When the nurse asks Ms. Flett to recall what she was doing when the pain occurred, Ms. Flett states that it began approximately 1 hour after eating supper. Her family had a typical supper of fried chicken, potatoes and gravy, and peas and carrots. Ms. Flett started feeling nauseated about an hour after supper and lay down. There was no emesis associated with this. About 15 minutes later, she started experiencing pain in the right upper quadrant of her abdomen and describes the pain as "sharp and burning." She rates the pain as a 7 on a scale of 1 to 10.

Ms. Flett states that she does not drink alcohol and smokes half a pack of cigarettes per day. She is particularly concerned about her illness and the impact it has on her work and her family. She tells you that her husband works long hours in construction, and in addition to her job, she provides for all her family's needs. She states, "My children will not be taken care of if I can't do this for them." She has some family support but does not want to impose on them.

The physical examination reveals vital signs of B/P 138/87—P 96—RR 22—T 37.7°C (99.9°F). The skin is slightly diaphoretic, warm, and pale. The abdomen is protuberant and soft. Bowel sounds are present in all four quadrants, and no vascular sounds are present. There is no tenderness on palpation of the left upper, left lower, or right lower quadrant. Guarding and pain are present in the right upper quadrant, and there is a positive Murphy's sign. The plan for this client is to begin antispasmodic medications for pain. Monitor for pain relief. Health teaching is required regarding diet and cholelithiasis. Schedule a follow-up appointment in two weeks or sooner if symptoms worsen.

S—*Periodic, upper right abdominal pain for several months, getting worse*

Regular BM—colour grey when pain comes

No interest in food

Gain of 50 kg (110 lb.) after kids

Pain occurs 1–2 h after eating dinner

Pain sharp

Nervous about pain and what it might mean for family

O—**Pallor**

Skin slightly diaphoretic, warm, pale

VS: B/P 138/87—P 96—RR 22—T 37.7°C (99.9°F)

Abdomen soft, nontender, BS present 4 Qs, guarding and pain upper right quadrant; positive Murphy sign.

A—*Increasing late p.m. upper abdominal pain over several months. Nervous, bilary colic*

P—*Begin antispas, p docs*

Teaching: diet and cholelithiasis

Monitor pain relief

Schedule follow-up appointment

▶ Complete Documentation

The following is sample documentation for Bernice Flett.

SUBJECTIVE DATA: Episodic pain to the right upper quadrant over the past two months. Described as "burning" and "sharp." Pain occurs after eating high-fat meal. Associated nausea, no vomiting. Rest used to relieve pain but no longer effective. Fifty kg gradual weight gain over several years. No ETOH use, smoker. Concerned about being unavailable to family when she is ill.

OBJECTIVE DATA: B/P 138/87—P 96—RR 22—T 37.7°C. Skin warm, clammy. Abdomen protuberant, soft. Bowel sounds present in all 4 quadrants, guarding to RUQ, positive Murphy's sign.

ASSESSMENT: RUQ pain associated with fatty meals 2 months.

PLAN: Begin antispasmodic medications for pain. Monitor for pain relief. Health teaching re: diet and cholelithiasis. Schedule

follow-up appointment in two weeks or sooner if symptoms worsen.

▶ Critical Thinking Questions

1. What data suggest the likelihood of cholelithiasis?
2. How would the data be clustered to formulate nursing diagnoses?
3. Discuss education strategies to promote, maintain, or restore the client's health.

▶ Applying Nursing Diagnoses

1. *Pain, acute* is a diagnosis in the NANDA-I taxonomy. Do the data for Bernice Flett support this diagnosis? If so, how?
2. *Nutrition, imbalanced: More than body requirements* is a diagnosis in the NANDA-I taxonomy. Do the data for Bernice Flett support this diagnosis? If so, how?
3. Refer to the NANDA-I taxonomy in Appendix A to formulate additional nursing diagnoses for Ms. Flett. ∞

▶ Prepare Teaching Plan

LEARNING NEED: Ms. Flett sought healthcare for acute pain that was previously resolved with rest. That strategy is no longer effective. The data reveal a multiparous, obese woman with an active household and little time for healthy eating or physical activity. The pain occurs after eating high-fat meals. Her pain is described as "sharp" and "burning" and is located in her right upper quadrant. Following the interview and physical examination, the plan of care included antispasmodic medications and a likely diagnosis of cholelithiasis. A follow-up appointment has been scheduled.

The case study provided data that are consistent with a diagnosis of cholelithiasis. Diet, exercise, lifestyle, gender, and parity are all contributing factors in this situation. Some of these are not modifiable, but understanding the modifiable factors would benefit individuals at risk of developing cholelithiasis, biliary colic, and cholecystitis. The following teaching plan is intended for individuals of any community about cholelithiasis.

GOAL: The participants in this learning program will have increased awareness of factors associated with cholelithiasis and strategies to prevent it from occurring.

OBJECTIVES: On the completion of this learning session, the participants will be able to do the following:

1. Describe cholelithiasis.
2. Identify factors associated with cholelithiasis.
3. List the symptoms of cholelithiasis.
4. Relate lifestyle to cholelithiasis.
5. Discuss strategies to prevent cholelithiasis.

Application of Objective 4: Relate lifestyle to cholelithiasis.

Content	Teaching Strategy	Evaluation
• Cholelithiasis attacks can be prevented by lifestyle changes. • High-fat diets are a primary cause of cholelithiasis. • Obesity is a risk factor for cholelithiasis. • People with alcoholic cirrhosis are susceptible to cholelithiasis. • Symptoms can often be alleviated through diet and exercise. If symptoms are not treated or worsen, surgical intervention may be required.	• Lecture • Discussion • Audiovisual materials • Printed materials Lecture is appropriate when disseminating information to large groups. Discussion allows participants to bring up concerns and to raise questions. Audiovisual materials, such as illustrations of the gastrointestinal system reinforce verbal presentation. Printed material, especially to be taken away with learners, allows review, reinforcement, and reading at the learner's pace.	• Written examination. May use short answer, fill-in, or multiple-choice items, or a combination of items. If these are short and easy to evaluate, the learner receives immediate feedback. • Question-and-answer period. With small groups, can prompt discussion. Provides immediate feedback.

HEALTH PROMOTION ASSESSMENT TOOL

Social Determinants of Health	Level of Action	Action Strategies
Personal coping skills	Individual	**Develop personal skills** • Together with Ms. Flett, assess what behavioural changes she would be most interested in making to improve her health. Weigh the pros and cons of each suggested change, including available supports for her to attain success and potential barriers. • Complete a diet assessment of food likes and dislikes, culturally acceptable/desired foods and eating patterns, and explore the role food plays in her life and family eating patterns. Refer Ms. Flett to a nutritionist/dietician. • Explore the role tobacco use has in Ms. Flett's life and assess her readiness to quit smoking to improve her health. Where does she smoke, when does she smoke, does she smoke alone or with others, does anyone else in her household smoke, and how many times has she tried to quit (include details such as how long she remained tobacco free and any withdrawal symptoms)? Based on her answers, refer her to appropriate local tobacco cessation supports and resources. The Canadian Cancer Society may be one such resource: http://www.ncic.cancer.ca.
Work and working conditions and social support networks	Individual, family, and community	**Create supportive environments** • Ms. Flett's working conditions are sedentary. She could explore manageable options for physical exercise, such as walking at lunch hour with a co-worker. • Explore healthy activities she can engage in with her children to further increase her exercise level.
Social support networks	Family and community	**Create supportive environments** • Assess who in Ms. Flett's extended family may be willing to offer support and what

Health Promotion Assessment Tool (continued)

Social Determinants of Health	Level of Action	Action Strategies
		support might be available. What barriers have prevented her from seeking support? What does "imposing" on her family mean to Ms. Flett? Is there an opportunity to develop a reciprocal supportive arrangement that would not be seen as an imposition but as mutually beneficial? • Explore her beliefs and practices regarding division of household tasks, including the roles of children in helping out. Is there an opportunity to engage her children in helping with household tasks?

Abnormal Findings

Abnormal findings in the abdomen occur in association with general health and in illness. For example, protrusion of the abdomen is seen in obese individuals and in pregnancy. Abdominal hernias are often seen in otherwise healthy adults and children. Untreated hernias, however, can lead to obstructive intestinal complications that give rise to acute symptoms and serious health problems. Further, alterations of the gastrointestinal tract include nutritional problems, eating disorders, cancers, ulcers, and inflammatory and infectious processes.

For accurate diagnosis in many abdominal and gastrointestinal problems, the health history and physical assessment are accompanied by observations of products of elimination and require diagnostic testing. Diagnostic testing includes laboratory studies of blood, urine, and feces, as well as radiographic and magnetic resonance imaging (MRI). In appendicitis, for example, physical findings include facial expressions demonstrating pain, abdominal guarding, tenderness to palpation at McBurney's point, RLQ rebound tenderness, and a positive Rovsing's sign (pain in the RLQ on palpation of the LLQ). Diagnosis is confirmed by an elevation in the white blood cell count and a flat-plate abdominal X-ray. Abnormal findings from abdominal assessment are presented in the following sections.

Abnormal Abdominal Sounds

When conducting an abdominal assessment, the nurse auscultates for bowel sounds and for vascular sounds. Table 19.1 includes information for interpretation of abnormal abdominal sounds.

TABLE 19.1	Abnormal Abdominal Sounds	
SOUND	**LOCATION**	**CAUSATIVE FACTORS**
Bowel sounds		
Hyperactive sounds	Any quadrant	Gastroenteritis, diarrhea
Hyperactive sounds followed by absence of sound	Any quadrant	Paralytic ileus
High-pitched sounds with cramping	Any quadrant	Intestinal obstruction
Vascular sounds		
Systolic bruit (blowing)	Midline below xiphoid	Aortic arterial obstruction
	Left and right lower costal borders at clavicular line	Stenosis of renal arteries
	Left and right abdomen at clavicular line between umbilicus and anterior iliac spine	Stenosis of iliac arteries
	Venous hum (continuous tone)	Epigastrium and around umbilicus
Portal hypertension		
Rubbing		
Friction rub (harsh, grating)	Left and right upper quadrants, over liver and spleen	Tumour or inflammation of organ

Abdominal Pain

Pain is associated with acute and chronic conditions that affect the digestive organs and abdominal structures. Table 19.2 provides information about several disorders that cause abdominal pain. Disruption of function of the abdominal structures may result in referred pain. **Referred pain** is located where the development of structures occurred in the fetus. Figure 19.27 includes referred cutaneous pain areas in the female. Referred pain in males often includes referred pain in the scrotum caused by appendicitis or renal colic.

TABLE 19.2	Pain in Common Abdominal Disorders		
DISORDER	**DEFINITION**	**PAIN CHARACTERISTICS**	**PRECIPITATING FACTORS**
Appendicitis	Acute inflammation of vermiform appendix	Epigastric and periumbilical Localizes to RLQ Sudden onset	Obstruction (fecal stone, adhesions)
Cholecystitis	Acute or chronic inflammation of wall of gallbladder	RUQ, radiates to right scapula Sudden onset	Fatty meals, obstruction of duct in cholelithiasis
Diverticulitis	Inflammation of diverticula	Cramping LLQ Radiates to back	Ingestion of fibre-rich diet, stress (outpouches of mucosa through intestinal wall)
Duodenal ulcer	Breaks in mucosa of duodenum	Aching, gnawing, epigastric	Stress, use of NSAIDs, *H. pylori*
Ectopic pregnancy	Implantation of blastocyte outside of the uterus, generally in the fallopian tube	Fullness in the rectal area Abdominal cramping, unilateral pain	Tubal damage, pelvic infection, hormonal disorders
Gastritis	Inflammation of mucosal lining of the stomach (acute and chronic)	Epigastric pain	Acute: NSAIDs, alcohol abuse, stress, infection Chronic: *H. pylori,* autoimmune responses
Gastroesophageal reflux disease (GERD)	Backflow of gastric acid to the esophagus	Heartburn, chest pain	Food intake, lying down after meals
Intestinal obstruction	Blockage of normal movement of bowel contents	Small intestine: aching Large intestine: spasmodic pain Neurogenic: diffuse abdominal discomfort Mechanical: colicky pain associated with distension	Mechanical: physical block from impaction, hernia, volvulus Neurogenic: manipulation of bowel during surgery, peritoneal irritation
Irritable bowel syndrome (spastic colon)	Problems with GI motility	LLQ accompanied by diarrhea or constipation or alternating between them Pain increases after eating and decreases after bowel movement	Stress, intolerated foods, caffeine, lactose intolerance, alcohol, familial linkage
Pancreatitis	Inflammation of the pancreas	Upper abdominal, knifelike, deep epigastric or umbilical area pain	Ductal obstruction, alcohol abuse, use of acetaminophen, infection

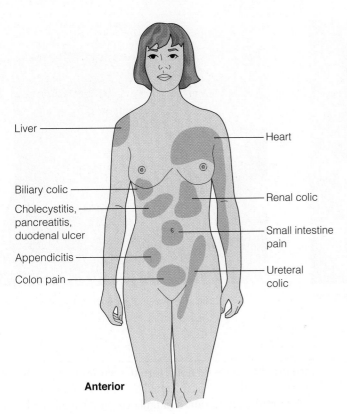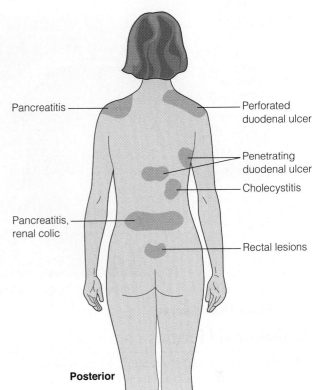

Liver
Heart
Biliary colic
Cholecystitis, pancreatitis, duodenal ulcer
Appendicitis
Colon pain
Renal colic
Small intestine pain
Ureteral colic

Anterior

Pancreatitis
Perforated duodenal ulcer
Penetrating duodenal ulcer
Cholecystitis
Pancreatitis, renal colic
Rectal lesions

Posterior

Figure 19.27 ● Referred cutaneous pain areas.

Abdominal Distension

Abdominal distension occurs for a variety of reasons, including obesity, gaseous distension, tumour, and ascites. Each of these is described in the sections that follow.

Obesity

Distension or protuberance of the abdomen occurs in obesity. The increase in the size of the abdomen is caused by a thick-ened abdominal wall and fat deposited in the mesentery and omentum. Percussion produces normal tympanic sounds.

Gaseous Distension

Gaseous distension of the abdomen is a result of increased production of gas in the intestines, which occurs with the ingestion of some foods. Gaseous distension is also associated with altered peristalsis in which gas cannot move through the intestines. This type of distension is seen in paralytic ileus and intestinal obstruction. Gaseous distension can be localized or generalized. Percussion produces tympany over a large area.

Tumour

The presence of an abdominal tumour produces abdominal distension. The abdomen is firm to palpation and dull to percussion. This type of distension is common in ovarian and uterine tumours.

Ascites

Ascites is the accumulation of fluid in the abdomen (see Figure 19.28). The abdomen becomes protuberant with bulging flanks. Fluid descends with gravity, resulting in dullness to percussion in the lower abdomen. Ascites may also be assessed by placing the client in a lateral position and observing fluid shift to the dependent side. Ascites occurs in cirrhosis, congestive heart failure (CHF), nephrosis, peritonitis, and neoplastic diseases.

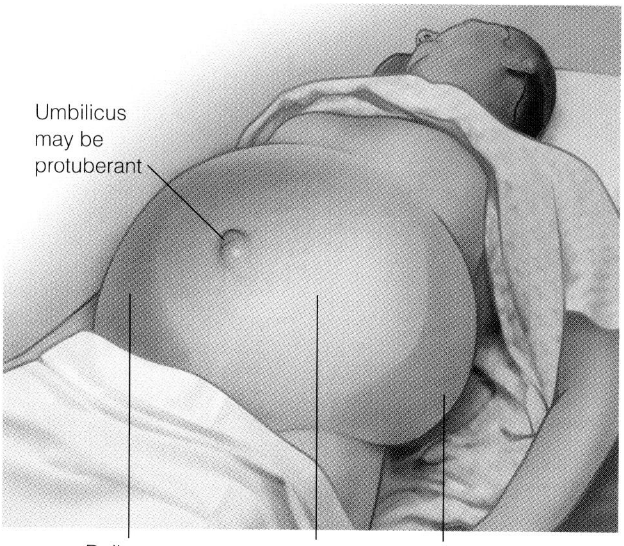

Umbilicus
may be
protuberant

Dullness   Tympany   Bulging flank with fluid

Fluid level   Tympany   Dullness

Figure 19.28 ● Ascites.

Abdominal Hernias

A **hernia**, commonly called a rupture, is a protrusion of an organ or structure through an abnormal opening or weakened area in a body wall. The abdominal wall is the most common site of hernias. This weakening could be congenital or acquired. If the protruding or displaced abdominal contents return to their normal position when the client relaxes, the hernia is said to be reducible or reduced. When the displaced or pro-

truding structures do not return to their normal position, the hernia is said to be incarcerated or nonreducible. An incarcerated hernia can become strangulated. In strangulated hernias, the blood supply to the displaced abdominal contents is compromised. The strangulated visceral contents can become gangrenous. Overstretched rectus muscles with weakened fascia cause an umbilical hernia.

Umbilical Hernia

An *umbilical hernia* occurs at the umbilicus (see Figure 19.29). The abdominal rectus muscle separates or weakens, allowing abdominal structures, usually the intestines, to push through and come closer to the skin. Umbilical hernias are more common in children than in adults.

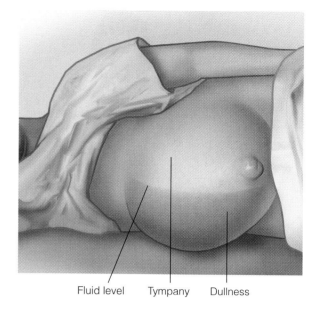

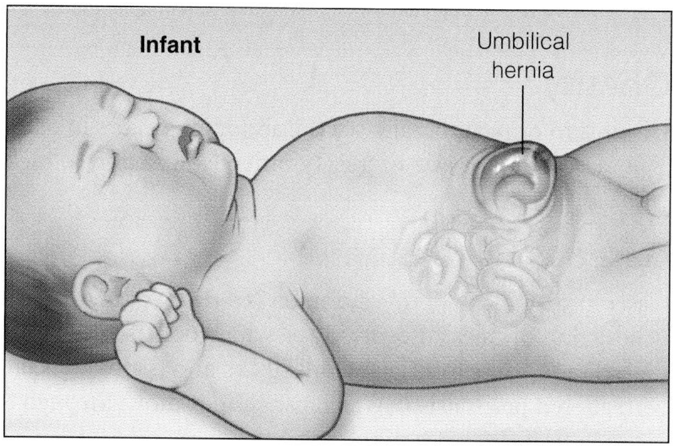

Figure 19.29 ●
Umbilical hernia.

Ventral (Incisional) Hernias

A *ventral hernia* is also known as an incisional hernia because it occurs at the site of an incision (see Figure 19.30). The incision weakens the muscle, and the abdominal structures move closer to the skin. Causes include obesity, repeated surgeries, infection during the postoperative period, impaired wound healing, and poor nutrition.

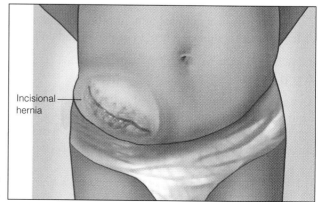

Figure 19.30 ●
Ventral hernia.

Hiatal Hernia

A *hiatal hernia* is due to a weakening in the diaphragm that allows a portion of the stomach and the esophagus to move into the thoracic cavity. This hernia is classified as sliding or rolling and is more common in adults than children. Abdominal hernias are illustrated in Figure 19.31.

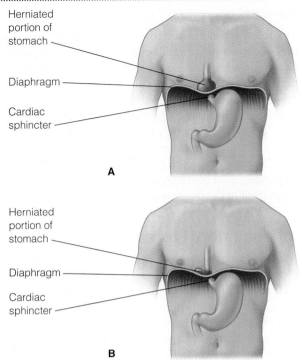

Herniated portion of stomach

Diaphragm

Cardiac sphincter

A

Herniated portion of stomach

Diaphragm

Cardiac sphincter

B

Figure 19.31 ●
Abdominal hernias. A. Sliding hiatal hernia. B. Rolling hiatal hernia.

Alterations of the Gastrointestinal Tract

Alterations of the gastrointestinal tract include nutritional problems, eating disorders, cancers, and inflammatory diseases. These alterations are described in the following sections.

Nutritional Problems

Nutritional problems include malnutrition, obesity, and overweight. **Malnutrition** is an imbalance, whether a deficit or an excess, of the required nutrients of a balanced diet. *Undernutrition* denotes inadequate intake of the nutrients needed to maintain optimal body functioning. *Overnutrition* is an excessive intake of nutrients, either as food or as food supplements. For example, overnutrition of vitamin A can lead to toxicity symptoms, such as nausea and vomiting. Both undernutrition and overnutrition are forms of malnutrition.

The Public Health Agency of Canada and the World Health Organization use a weight-classification system based on the body mass index (BMI) for evaluating overweight and obesity among adults. **Overweight** is determined as a BMI of 25.0 to 29.9. A BMI of 30.0 or more is considered **obesity.** As the BMI increases, the risk of developing health problems also increases.

Eating Disorders

An eating disorder is a condition in which a person's current intake of food differs significantly from that person's normal intake. Eating disorders typically result from an attempt to lose weight; however, the attempt to lose weight may be a misguided response to psychosocial problems.

Anorexia nervosa is a complex psychosocial problem characterized by a severely restricted intake of nutrients and a low body weight. The anorexic typically experiences intense fear of gaining weight or becoming fat, feels fat even when emaciated, and refuses to maintain body weight over a minimal normal weight for age and height. Many anorexics experi-

ence constipation, gastrointestinal bloating or distension, nausea, and abdominal pain.

Bulimia nervosa is an eating disorder characterized by binge eating and purging or another compensatory mechanism to prevent weight gain. Typically, the bulimic consumes large portions of high-calorie food, typically about 4000 calories at one time. The individual then tries to compensate and prevent weight gain by vomiting; by using laxatives, enemas, diuretics, or diet pills; or by overexercising. Many bulimics experience tooth decay, dehydration, laxative dependence, and rectal bleeding.

Cancers

Colorectal cancer is a malignant lesion involving any part of the large intestine, sigmoid colon, or rectum. Predisposing factors include poor dietary habits and chronic constipation. Signs and symptoms vary according to the location of the growth. A change in bowel habits or patterns is a characteristic with any location. In many cases, when an intestinal obstruction occurs, surgery is required and the client may need a permanent colostomy.

Cancer of the esophagus is a malignant growth of the esophagus, most common in males over 50 years of age. The lower third of the esophagus is most commonly involved.

Clients commonly complain of weight loss, **dysphagia** (difficulty swallowing), and odynophagia (pain on swallowing). Alcohol abuse, smoking, and poor oral hygiene appear to be predisposing factors.

Cancer of the stomach is a malignant growth of the stomach. The cancerous lesions are found most frequently in the distal third of the stomach. The disease is often in the advanced stages before a diagnosis is made. Dietary habits seem to be an influencing factor. Weight loss, nausea, vomiting, abdominal pain, abdominal distension, and some bleeding are the common complaints of the client.

Inflammatory Processes

Ulcerative colitis is a recurrent inflammatory process causing ulcer formation in the lower portions of the large intestine and rectum. This condition is common in adolescents and young adults. The distribution of the inflammatory process is diffuse. The ulcerative areas abscess and later become necrotic. Diarrhea, abdominal pain, and cramping with weight loss are common symptoms of the disease process.

Esophagitis is an inflammatory process of the esophagus. It is caused by a variety of irritants. The more common causes include smoking, alcohol abuse, reflux of gastric contents, and ingestion of extremely hot or cold foods and liquids.

Peritonitis is a local or generalized inflammatory process of the peritoneal membrane of the abdomen. The precipitant can be an infectious process (pelvic inflammatory disease), perforation of an organ (ruptured duodenal ulcer), internal bleeding (ruptured ectopic pregnancy), or trauma (stab wound to abdomen).

Hepatitis is an inflammatory process of the liver. Its causes include viruses, bacteria, chemicals, and drugs. Types of hepatitis include the following:

- *Hepatitis A virus* (HAV) is transmitted via enteric routes (feces or oral routes).
- *Hepatitis E virus* (HEV) is a non-A, non-B type transmitted enterically. HEV is most common in people who travel to India, Africa, Asia, and Central America.

Crohn's disease is a chronic inflammatory process of the ileum. It is sometimes called regional ileitis, which is a misnomer because it can involve any part of the lower intestinal tract. Crohn's disease is characterized by "skipped" sections of involvement. It is most common in young adults and usually has an insidious onset. The inflammation involves all layers of the intestinal mucosa. Transverse fissures develop in the bowel, producing a characteristic cobblestone appearance.

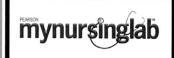

20

URINARY SYSTEM

THE URINARY SYSTEM IS COMPOSED OF THE KIDNEYS, ureters, bladder, and urethra. The **glomeruli** (tufts of capillaries) of the kidneys filter more than 1 L (1 qt.) of fluid each minute. As a result, wastes, toxins, and foreign matter are removed from the blood. The urinary system acts through the kidneys to prevent the accumulation of nitrogenous wastes, promotes fluid and electrolyte balance, assists in maintenance of blood pressure, and contributes to erythropoiesis (development of mature red blood cells).

The organs of the urinary system are distributed among the retroperitoneal space, abdomen, and genitals. Assessment of the urinary system is incorporated into assessment of the abdomen and reproductive systems. Urinary function is interdependent with other body systems. In addition, psychosocial and developmental factors affect the function of the urinary system.

ANATOMY AND PHYSIOLOGY REVIEW

The structures of the urinary system include the kidneys, ureters, urinary bladder, urethra, and renal vasculature (blood vessels). Each of the structures will be described in the sections that follow.

Kidneys

The **kidneys** are bean-shaped organs located in the retroperitoneal space on either side of the vertebral column. Extending from the level of the twelfth thoracic vertebra to the third lumbar vertebra, the upper portion of the kidneys is protected by the lower rib cage. The right kidney is displaced downward by the liver and sits slightly lower than the left kidney. A layer of fat cushions each kidney, and the kidney itself is surrounded by tissue called the renal capsule (see Figure 20.1). Each adult kidney weighs approximately 150 g (5 oz.) and is 11 to 13 cm (4 to 5 in.) long, 5 to 7 cm (2 to 3 in.) wide, and 2.5 to 3 cm (1 in.) thick. The superior part of the kidney is referred to as the upper pole, whereas the inferior surface is called the lower pole.

The inner portion of the kidney is called the *renal medulla.* The renal **medulla** is composed of structures called pyramids and calyces. The pyramids are wedgelike structures made up of bundles of urine-collecting tubules. At their apex, the pyramids have papillae that are enclosed by cuplike structures called calyces. The calyces collect urine and transport it into the renal pelvis, which is the funnel-shaped superior end of the ureter (see Figure 20.2).

The outer portion of each kidney is called the renal **cortex.** It is composed of more than 1 million nephrons, which form urine. The first part of each nephron is the renal corpuscle, which consists of a tuft of capillaries called a glomerulus. These glomeruli begin the filtration of the blood. Larger blood components, such as red blood cells and larger proteins, are separated from most of the fluid, which passes into the glomerular capsule (or Bowman's capsule). The filtrate then moves into a proximal convoluted tubule, then into the loop of Henle, and finally into a distal convoluted tubule, from which it is collected as urine by a collecting tubule. Along the way, some of the filtrate is resorbed, along with electrolytes and chemicals, such as glucose, potassium, phosphate, and sodium. Each collecting tubule guides the urine from several nephrons out into the renal pyramids and calyces, and from there through the renal pelvis and into the ureters.

The major functions of the kidneys are the following:

- Eliminating nitrogenous waste products, toxins, excess ions, and drugs through urine
- Regulating the volume and chemical makeup of the blood
- Maintaining balance between water and salts, and acids and bases
- Producing renin, an enzyme that assists in the regulation of blood pressure
- Producing the hormone erythropoietin, which stimulates production of red blood cells in the bone marrow
- Assisting in the metabolism of vitamin D

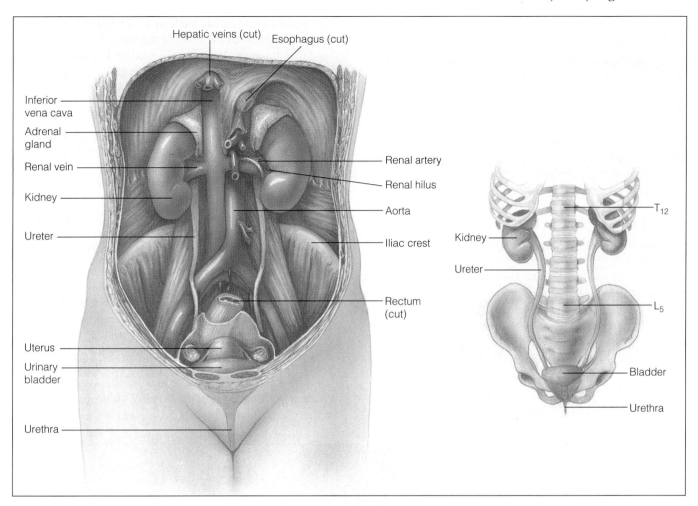

Figure 20.1 ● The urinary system. A. Anterior view of the urinary organs of a female. B. Relationship of the kidneys to the vertebrae.

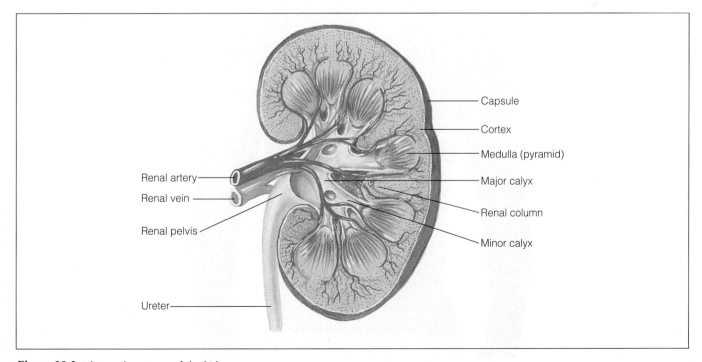

Figure 20.2 ● Internal anatomy of the kidney.

Renal Arteries

The kidneys require a tremendous amount of oxygen and nutrients and receive about 25% of the cardiac output. Although not part of the urinary system, an extensive network of arteries intertwines within the renal network. These arteries include renal arteries, arcuate arteries, interlobular arteries, afferent arteries, and efferent arterioles. The major function of the renal arteries is providing a rich supply of blood (approximately 1200 mL or 40 fl.oz. per minute when an individual is at rest) to the kidneys.

Ureters

The **ureters** are mucous-membrane-lined narrow tubes approximately 25 to 30 cm (10 to 12 in.) long and 6 to 12 mm (0.25 to 0.5 in.) wide. As the ureter leaves the kidney, it travels downward behind the peritoneum to the posterior wall of the urinary bladder. The major function of the ureters is transporting urine from the kidney to the urinary bladder.

Urinary Bladder

The urinary bladder is a hollow, muscular, collapsible pouch that acts as a reservoir for urine. It lies on the pelvic floor in the retroperitoneal space. The bladder is composed of two parts: the rounded muscular sac made up of the detrusor muscle and the portion between the body of the bladder and the urethra known as the neck. In males, the bladder lies anterior to the rectum, and the neck of the bladder is encircled by the prostate gland of the male reproductive system. In females, the bladder lies anterior to the vagina and uterus. As urine accumulates, the fundus, the superior wall of the bladder, ascends in the abdominal cavity and assumes a rounded shape that is palpable. When moderately filled (500 mL or 17 fl.oz.), the bladder is approximately 12.5 cm (5 in.) long. When larger amounts of urine are present, the bladder becomes distended and rises above the symphysis pubis.

The major functions of the urinary bladder are storing urine temporarily and contracting to release urine during micturition.

Urethra

The **urethra** is a mucous-membrane-lined tube that transports urine from the urinary bladder to the exterior. In females, the urethra is approximately 3 to 4 cm (1.5 in.) long and lies along the anterior wall of the vagina. The female urethra terminates in the external urethral orifice or meatus, which lies between the clitoris and the vagina. The male urethra is approximately 20 cm (8 in.) long and runs the length of the penis. It terminates in the external urethral orifice in the glans penis. In addition to

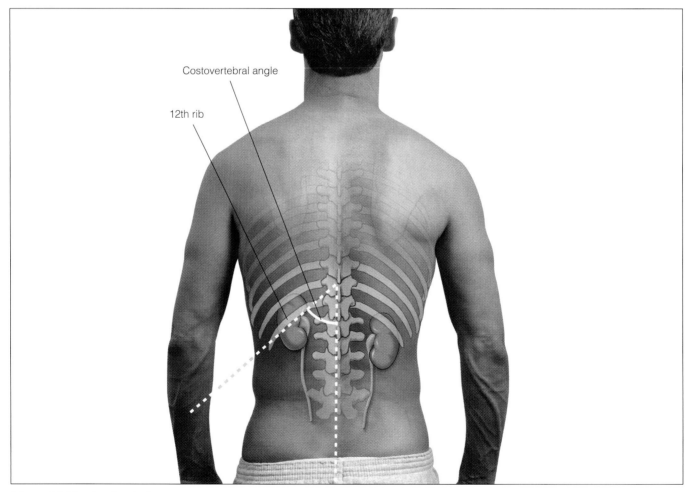

Figure 20.3A ● Landmarks for urinary assessment. A. The costovertebral angle.

providing a passageway for urine, the male urethra also carries semen outside of the body. Because the female urethra is short and its meatus lies close to the anus, it can become contaminated with bacteria more readily than the male urethra. A more detailed review of the penis, prostate gland, and male and female external genitalia is presented in Chapters 21 and 22. ⊙ The major function of the urethra is providing a passage for the elimination of urine.

Landmarks

During assessment of the urinary system, the nurse uses three landmarks to locate and palpate the kidneys and urinary bladder. These landmarks are the costovertebral angle, the rectus abdominis muscle, and the symphysis pubis. The **costovertebral angle (CVA)** is the area on the lower back formed by the vertebral column and the downward curve of the last posterior rib as depicted in Figure 20.3A. It is an important anatomical landmark because the lower poles of the kidney and ureter lie below this surface. The rectus abdominis muscles are a longitudinal pair of muscles that extend from the pubis to the rib cage on either side of the midline as illustrated in Figure 20.3B. These muscles are used as guidelines for positioning the hands when palpating the kidneys through the abdominal wall. The symphysis pubis is the joint formed by the union of the two pubic bones by cartilage at the midline of the body (Figure 20.3B).

The bladder is cradled under the symphysis pubis. When the bladder is full, the nurse is able to palpate it as it rises above the symphysis pubis.

SPECIAL CONSIDERATIONS

The client's health status is influenced by a number of factors, including age, developmental level, race, ethnicity, work history, living conditions, socioeconomics, and emotional health. During a comprehensive health assessment, effective communication and critical thinking enable the nurse to identify the ways in which one or more factors influence the client's health, beliefs, and practices.

Developmental Considerations

Changes in anatomical structures and functions occur as a normal part of growth and development. Knowledge of normal, age-related variations in findings from health assessment is essential in interpreting data and planning care for clients. Specific variations in the urinary system for different age groups are presented in the sections that follow.

Infants and Children

Renal blood flow increases with a significant allotment to the renal medulla at birth. The glomerular filtration rate also

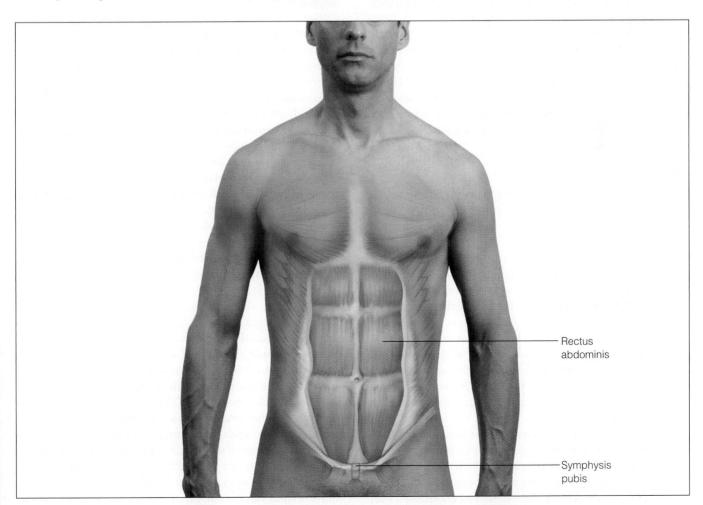

Rectus abdominis

Symphysis pubis

Figure 20.3B ● Landmarks for urinary assessment. B. The rectus abdominis muscles and the symphysis pubis.

increases at birth, compared with the fetal filtration rate, and continues to increase until the first or second year of life. The fluid and electrolyte balance in an infant or child is fragile. Illnesses that cause dehydration, loss of fluids, or lack of fluid intake may rapidly lead to metabolic acidosis and fluid imbalance. Serious, chronic dysfunction of this system may impair the child's growth and development.

It is important to consider the health practices of the family when the genital areas are unclean in infants or children of any age. Presence of a diaper rash is a clue that the nurse should explore the family's hygiene practices; however, diaper rash is often difficult to control, and supportive teaching is indicated.

The nurse examines infants for anomalies, such as scrotal edema, undescended testes, and noncentral placement of the urinary meatus. Bedwetting is a difficult problem for both the child and the family and may influence the child's relationship with the family. The child's confidence and social development may also be affected by bedwetting. Bedwetting is not generally considered problematic unless the child has no daytime dryness after 4 years of age or no nighttime dryness after 6 years of age.

The Pregnant Female

During the first trimester, the enlarging uterus presses against the bladder, increasing the frequency of urination. Frequency decreases during the second trimester and then recurs during the third trimester as the presenting part of the fetus descends into the pelvis and again presses on the bladder.

During pregnancy, the amount of urine produced increases, causing the client to feel the need to urinate more frequently. There is also a tendency for the urine to test positive for sugar. In the postpartum period, edema and hyperemia of the bladder mucosa cause decreased sensation and contribute to overdistension of the bladder. Incomplete emptying of the bladder often accompanies this condition, increasing the client's susceptibility to urinary tract infection.

The Older Adult

The effects of aging take their toll on the kidneys. The weight of the kidneys may drop by as much as 30%, particularly in the renal cortex. Renal blood flow and perfusion gradually decrease. The capillary system in the glomeruli atrophies. Although the vasculature in the renal medulla remains relatively well preserved, the arcuate and interlobular arteries may become distorted, resulting in a tortuous configuration. All structures of the renal cortex and the renal medulla experience some degree of decline, especially the nephrons. About 30% to 50% of the glomeruli degenerate because of fibrosis, hyalinization (accumulation of glassy tissue), and fat deposition. All these factors contribute to the loss of filtration surface area in the glomerular capillary tufts by the age of 75. Creatinine clearance decreases slowly after 40 years of age, as does the ability to concentrate and dilute urine.

The older client's decreased sensation of thirst and resultant decreased intake of water relates directly to the body's compensatory response of concentrating urine. However, antidiuretic hormone is not as effective as in a younger client; thus, concentrations and activity of renin and aldosterone are reduced with advanced age by as much as 30% to 50%. This combination of circumstances places the older client at risk for hyperkalemia (high level of potassium in the blood).

The older adult also has a reduced capacity to produce ammonia, which interacts with acids. Reduced ability to clear medications and acids, along with reduced ability to resorb bicarbonate and glucose, makes the older client more susceptible to toxicity related to medications, the effects of respiratory or metabolic acidosis, increased concentrations of glucose in the urine, and the loss of fluids.

Urinary elimination becomes a major concern as an individual advances in age and significant changes in urinary and bladder function begin to occur. Major changes in both males and females include urinary retention leading to more urinary infections; involuntary bladder contractions resulting in urgency, frequency, and incontinence; decreased bladder capacity causing frequent voiding; and weakening of the urinary sphincters causing urgency and incontinence.

Nocturia (nighttime urination) is another major concern of older persons, especially males. When an older person is at rest in a horizontal position, the heart is able to pump blood through the kidneys more efficiently, facilitating the excretion of urine. This factor, combined with weakened bladder and urethral muscles, contributes to nocturnal micturition. Other causes of nocturia, such as urinary infection, hyperglycemia (too much glucose in the blood), medication use, and stool impactions, should not be ruled out.

Benign prostatic hypertrophy (hyperplasia) is a common cause of urinary retention and obstruction in males. As males age, the prostate gland enlarges, encroaching on the urethra. Unrecognized urinary tract obstruction from an enlarged prostate results in damage to the upper urinary tract.

Postmenopausal females experience a decrease in estrogen, which affects the strength of the pubic muscles and may lead to urine leakage, reduced acidity in the lower urinary tract, and urinary tract infections.

The nurse should allow older clients with urinary tract problems extra time to explain their concerns. Quite often, older adults have difficulty talking about bladder or bowel concerns because they consider the subject too personal. Additionally, some clients may find it distasteful to discuss elimination with anyone of the opposite sex. It is helpful to use the terms with which the client is comfortable and familiar.

When assessing an individual who experiences incontinence, the nurse should ask about the client's ability to get to the washroom. Many clients who are diagnosed as incontinent simply cannot get to the washroom on time because of other age-related conditions, such as arthritis, strokes, or blindness. Whenever possible, the nurse should observe clients in their own settings to determine what disabilities or environmental barriers (e.g., stairs, distance) hinder the ability to function.

The physical assessment of the older person is similar to that of any other adult. Because the abdominal musculature of older persons tends to be more flaccid than that of younger adults, less pressure is used during deep palpation. The kidneys of the older client are more difficult to palpate abdominally because the mass of the adrenal cortex decreases with age. The nurse should omit blunt percussion in a frail older person. Palpation of the costovertebral angles and flanks can be used instead to reveal any pain or tenderness. A digital examination of the prostate gland is generally included as part of the urinary assessment in older males. Palpation of the urethra through the anterior vaginal wall is recommended for all older females.

Psychosocial Considerations

Clients experiencing incontinence are at increased risk for social isolation, self-esteem disturbance, and other psychosocial problems. A stressful lifestyle may contribute to chronic urinary tract infections. Stasis of urine and resultant infection may occur when a client feels "too busy" to empty the bladder as needed. Urinary tract infections in females can also result from sexual trauma, sexual intercourse with a new partner, or coital frequency. The nurse should consider the possibility of sexual abuse in a child or an adolescent who presents with a urinary tract infection.

Social and Ethnocultural Considerations

When considering the influence of culture on a client's health-care practices, the nurse must be open-minded and sensitive to the specific values and beliefs of the client without passing judgment. Not all individuals adhere to the norms, values, and practices of their culture. Consideration for the client's privacy and modesty is essential when obtaining subjective and objective data regarding urinary elimination. Though not every client is embarrassed by these components of assessment, many individuals experience considerable uneasiness. It is essential to afford the client as much privacy and dignity as possible. Some individuals will not disrobe or allow a physical examination by anyone of the opposite sex. Other clients will not allow a sample of their body fluids to be taken and examined by strangers.

Clients with hypertension or diabetes mellitus are especially vulnerable to kidney damage if they do not follow a strict medication and diet regimen. The nurse can help all clients maintain optimal health by providing information on diet, prevention of hypertension, and the importance of compliance with medication regimens.

Renal **calculi** (stones) occur with greater frequency in some ethnic populations, as well as in populations that live in areas where the mineral content of water is high. A thorough history must be conducted to determine if the individual is at risk of developing stones. Hypertension is a risk factor for chronic kidney disease. Hypertension is associated with a number of factors, including diet, exercise, substance use, diabetes, age, and gender. Hypertension and chronic kidney disease are highly prevalent diseases that tend to occur more frequently among disadvantaged populations. A significant proportion of Aboriginal people live in poverty, which is associated with high rates of chronic kidney disease and risk factors, such as hypertension. Improvement of the socioeconomic status of Aboriginal people will likely reduce chronic kidney disease in this group.

Information obtained during the health history may identify whether the client is taking herbal remedies prescribed by a healer. The nurse should obtain as complete information about the remedies as possible.

Social and Ethnocultural Considerations

- Hypertension and chronic kidney disease are highly prevalent diseases that tend to occur more frequently among disadvantaged populations.
- Diabetes is a risk factor for urinary tract infection and chronic kidney disease.
- It is important to consider many factors when providing education regarding diet, exercise, and substance use, including language spoken, literacy level, income and occupation, and social supports, in addition to age, gender, family history, ethnicity, and culture. However, it is also important to remember that the ability of a client to modify behaviour is dependent on the client's personal and social contexts.
- The nurse needs to consider that the functions of the urinary system are considered private by many people.
- Certain medications can affect the colour or amount of urine that is produced. Urine is often used to assess kidney function.

GATHERING THE DATA

Assessment of the health of the urinary system includes gathering subjective and objective data. Subjective data collection occurs during the client interview, before the actual physical assessment. During the interview the nurse uses a variety of communication techniques to elicit general and specific information about the client's state of health or illness. Health records and the results of laboratory tests are important secondary sources to be reviewed and included in the data-gathering process. During physical assessment of the urinary system, the techniques of inspection, palpation, percussion, and auscultation will be used to collect objective data.

HEALTH HISTORY

The health history for the urinary system concerns data related to the structures and functions of that system. Subjective data are gathered during the health history. The nurse must be prepared to observe the client and listen for cues related to the functions of the urinary system. The nurse may use open-ended or closed questions to obtain information. Often a number of follow-up questions or requests for descriptions are required to clarify data or gather missing information. Follow-up questions are aimed at identifying the source of problems, duration of difficulties, measures to alleviate problems, and clues about the client's knowledge of his or her own health.

Discussion of the urinary system may be difficult for some clients because it is considered a private matter. The nurse should try to use the terms used by the client in referring to parts of the body and urination.

The health history guides the physical assessment of the urinary system. The information is always considered in relation to norms and expectations about the function of the urinary system. Therefore, the nurse must consider age, gender, race, culture, environment, health practices, past and concurrent problems, and therapies when framing questions and using techniques to elicit information. To address all the factors when conducting a health history, specific questions related to

urinary status and function have been developed. These questions focus on the most common concerns or injuries associated with the urinary system; questions related to past health history; questions related to behaviours; questions that address environmental concerns; and those that are specific to clients according to age, including the pregnant female.

The nurse must consider the client's ability to participate in the health history and physical assessment of the urinary system. If a client is experiencing pain, urgency, incontinence, or the anxiety that accompanies any of these problems, attention must focus on relief of symptoms.

As the nurse gathers the data, she or he will shift the type of questions to direct questions that give the client room to explain or qualify. The mnemonic O-P-Q-R-S-T-U, which stands for onset (chronology), precipitating (or palliative), quality, region (or radiation), severity, timing, and understanding, will help the learner remember the dimensions of the symptoms. The nurse will keep in mind that not all these qualifiers will apply to each symptom.

HEALTH HISTORY QUESTIONS	RATIONALES

The following sections provide sample questions and follow-up questions. Rationales for some questions are provided. The list of questions is not all-inclusive but rather represents the more common concern or injury questions required in a health history related to the urinary system. An example of using O-P-Q-R-S-T-U with pain is provided.

Questions Related to Common Concerns or Injuries

The most common concerns related to illness or injury of the urinary system are as follows:

- Pain
- Dysuria
- Frequency, urgency, or hesitancy with urination
- Nocturia
- Changes in urine colour and quality

1. **Pain**
   - Are you having any abdominal pain at this time? *If yes:*

     ▶ Gradual enlargement of an organ (e.g., from a tumour) is typically painless. Other types of pain involving the urinary system may indicate infection or inflammation.

   - When did you first notice the pain? How long does it last? Does it occur before, during, or after urination? *Onset (chronology)*

     ▶ Painful urination may indicate the presence of an infective process.

   - What makes the pain worse? What makes the pain better? *Precipitating (palliative)*
   - Can you describe the pain? Is it constant? sharp? dull? burning? cramping? *Quality*
   - Where is the pain located? Does the pain radiate to any other area of your body? Where? *Radiation*

     ▶ Back or abdominal pain often accompanies renal disease.

   - How often do you experience the pain? Does the pain affect your breathing or any other functions? How would you rate the pain on a scale of 1 to 10, with 10 being the worst pain? *Severity*

HEALTH HISTORY QUESTIONS

RATIONALES

- Is the pain associated with nausea? vomiting? sweating? abdominal distension? fever? chills? eating? changes in colour of urine? burning on urination? *Timing*
- What do you think is causing the pain? *Understanding*

2. Dysuria

- Do you have burning with urination? *If yes:*
- Does the burning occur before, during, or after urination?
- How long have you been experiencing burning on urination?
- Have you noticed any changes with your urine?

▶ Dysuria (painful urination) is frequently associated with inflammation or infection of the lower urinary tract. It is typically accompanied by suprapubic pain, frequency, and urgency.

3. Frequency, urgency, or hesitancy with urination
Frequency

- Have you experienced any change in the frequency of urination? *If yes:*
- How much do you pass each time you urinate? (Note: The nurse may use terms familiar to the client, such as *pass water,* when asking about urination.)

▶ Many factors influence the number of times and amount that a client voids. Among these are the size of the bladder, amount of fluid intake, type of fluid or solid intake, and medications. An adult may void five or six times per day in amounts averaging 100 to 400 mL (3.5 to 13.5 fl.oz.). A child may void more frequently in smaller amounts. The key is to determine the client's normal patterns.

- Have you had any of the following changes: urinating less often or urinating less fluid?

▶ Changes in urinary elimination patterns signal fluid retention, which may indicate heart failure, kidney failure, or improper nutritional intake. Other considerations include obstructions, infections, and endocrine disorders.

- When you urinate, do you feel you are able to empty your bladder completely?

▶ The feeling of being unable to empty the bladder may indicate the client is retaining urine or developing increased residual urine, which may contribute to the development of infection.

Urgency

- Have you experienced any change in your sense of urgency with urination? *If yes:*
- Are you always able to control when you are going to urinate?
- If not, do you have to hurry to the bathroom as soon as you feel the urge to urinate?

▶ Urgency and stress incontinence may be caused by an infection, an inflammatory process, or the loss of muscle control over urination, such as after the vaginal delivery of a child or vaginal hysterectomy.

- Have you ever had an "accident" and wet yourself?
- Have you ever urinated by accident when you have coughed, sneezed, or lifted a heavy object?

Hesitation

- Have you experienced any hesitancy with urination? *If yes:*
- Do you have difficulty starting the stream?
- Does the stream flow continuously, or does it start and stop?

▶ Urine flow that starts and stops may signify the presence of prostate disease in the male.

- Do you need to strain or push during urination to empty your bladder completely?

HEALTH HISTORY QUESTIONS	RATIONALES

- If you have urinary problems, have they caused you embarrassment or anxiety?

▶ These are important considerations, as embarrassment or anxiety may affect the clients' ability to function in other parts of their lives.

- Have your urinary problems affected your social, personal, or sexual relationships?

4. **Nocturia**
   - Do you ever have to get up at night to urinate? *If yes:*

▶ Nocturia may indicate the presence of aging changes in the older adult, cardiovascular disease, diuretic therapy, or habit. Nocturia can be influenced by the amount and timing of fluid intake.

   - How many times per night?
   - Is there any predictable pattern?
   - Describe your fluid intake for a day.

5. **Changes in urine colour and quality**
   - Have you noted any change in the colour or odour of your urine? *If yes:*
   - Is your urine clear? What colour is it?

▶ Colour changes offer clues to the presence of infection, kidney stones, or neoplasm.

   - Have you noticed any cloudiness in your urine?

▶ Changes in urine colour or cloudiness can be associated with infection, including sexually transmitted infections, or other diseases.

   - Do you ever have red urine?

▶ Hematuria (blood in the urine) should be investigated to determine whether the blood is present before, during, or after urination. Hematuria is a significant finding and warrants additional follow-up.

   - Have you seen any clots in the urine?
   - Is the red urine associated with anything, such as flank pain? burning on urination? weight loss? weight gain?
   - When did the change in urine colour start? Had you been doing anything different before then, such as strenuous activity?
   - Are you taking any medications?

▶ Some medications can change the colour of the urine.

   - Do you eat beets often?

▶ Some foods, especially beets, can change the colour of the urine.

Questions Related to Past Health History

1. **History of abdominal disease or problems**
   - Is there anyone in your family who has been diagnosed with a disease of the kidneys or bladder? If so, what was it?
   - Have you ever been diagnosed with a disease of the kidney or bladder? If so, what was it? When?
   - Has the problem ever recurred? *(acute)*
   - How are you managing the disease now? *(chronic)*
   - Do you now have or have you had an infection in the urinary system?

▶ If an infection is identified, follow-up about the date of infection, treatment, and outcomes is required. Data about each infection identified by the client are essential to an accurate health assessment. Infections can be classified as acute or chronic, and follow-up regarding each classification will differ.

   - An alternative to the previous question is to list possible urinary system infections, such as cystitis (inflammation of the bladder), pyelonephritis (inflammation of the kidney), and prostatitis (inflammation of the prostate gland), and ask the client to respond yes or no as each is stated.

▶ This alternative is a comprehensive and easy way to elicit information about all urinary system infections. Follow-up would be carried out for each identified infection, as in the previous question.

HEALTH HISTORY QUESTIONS	RATIONALES

- Have you ever had surgery on the urinary system?
- Do you have any of these problems: high blood pressure, diabetes, frequent bladder infections, kidney stones?

▶ High blood pressure can contribute to the development of renal disease. Diabetes can significantly contribute to the development of renal disease. Infections can be caused by inadequate fluid intake, inadequate hygiene, and structural anomalies. In some clients this is an infrequent situation; in others it is a common malady. Kidney stones may be an isolated event or a recurring condition. Parathyroid disorders and any condition that causes an increase in blood calcium may contribute to the formation of kidney stones.

- Do you have any of these neurological diseases: multiple sclerosis, Parkinson's disease, a spinal cord injury, stroke?

▶ These conditions contribute to the retention and stasis of urine, thus placing the client at risk for chronic urinary infections.

- Do you have any history of cardiovascular disease?

▶ Hypertension, in particular, may significantly contribute to the development of renal failure.

- Have you had influenza, a skin infection, a respiratory tract infection, or other infection recently?

▶ If the infection was untreated, the client may be at risk for developing a renal infection.

Questions Related to Behaviours

Healthcare behaviours include both health practices and health patterns. Health practices consist of following recommendations for disease prevention, including screening for risks, screening for early detection of problems, and immunization. Health patterns are habits or acts that affect the client's health. Health behaviours may also include seeking healthcare from healthcare providers who use alternative methods to diagnose and treat illness. Clients should be questioned in a nonjudgmental way and areas for health teaching should be identified.

1. **Describe your diet. Be sure to include fluid intake.**

▶ Such questions as these may provide information regarding the client's hydration status, allergic reaction to food, and retention of fluid.

2. **Do you smoke or are you exposed to second-hand smoke? How much and for how long?**

▶ Smoking has been linked to hypertension, which over time may contribute to the development of renal failure.

3. **Do you use recreational drugs? What type? How often?**

▶ Substance abuse over time may lead to kidney failure, inadequate nutrition and hydration, and susceptibility to infection.

4. **How often do you have intercourse? Do you urinate after intercourse?**

▶ Some clients have a tendency to develop urinary tract infections if they do not urinate after intercourse.

5. *For female clients, ask:* **How do you cleanse yourself after urination or a bowel movement?**

▶ Cleansing materials, such as bubble bath, sprays, and powders, may increase the incidence of urinary tract infections. Improper cleansing methods after elimination may also lead to infection.

Questions Related to the Environment

Environment refers to both internal and external environments. Questions related to the internal environment include all the previous questions and those associated with internal or physiological responses. Questions regarding the external environment include those related to home, work, or social environments.

GATHERING THE DATA

HEALTH HISTORY QUESTIONS	RATIONALES

Internal Environment

1. **What medications do you currently take?**

▶ It is important to know the client's compliance with the medication regimen. If the client has not completed a regimen of antibiotic therapy to clear a urinary tract infection, kidney infection, or sexually transmitted infection, the infection may persist.

2. **Do you take any vitamins, protein powders, or dietary supplements? How much and how often?**

▶ Excessive ingestion of some substances can contribute to the development of renal disorders.

External Environment

The following questions deal with the physical environment of the client. That includes the indoor and outdoor environments of the home and the workplace, those encountered for social engagements, and any encountered during travel.

1. **Do you live or work in an industry that exposes you to toxic chemicals?**

▶ This exposure may contribute to the development of cancer of the urinary system.

2. **Have you recently done any travelling?**

▶ The client may have been exposed to bacterial, viral, or fungal agents that affect renal function.

Questions Related to Age

The health history must reflect the anatomical and physiological differences that exist along the age span.

Questions Regarding Infants and Children

1. **Has the child ever been diagnosed with a kidney disorder?**

▶ Some disorders, such as infections, are easily treated and do not recur; others, such as glomerulonephritis, may be chronic.

2. **Has the child had hearing problems?**

▶ The ears and kidneys develop at the same time in utero. Congenital deafness is associated with renal disease.

3. **Have you ever observed any unusual shape or structure in the child's genital anatomy?**

▶ Parents may report abnormally shaped external genitals, as seen in hypospadias (placement of the urinary meatus on the underside of the penis) and epispadias (placement of the urinary meatus on the top side of the penis). In children with exstrophy of the bladder, the lower urinary tract is visible.

4. **Has the child ever had problems with involuntary urination?**

▶ **Enuresis** is involuntary urination after age 4. If it occurs at night, it is termed nocturnal enuresis after age 6. This condition may have extensive impact on the social, mental, and physical well-being of the family and child.

5. **Has the child decreased play activity?**

▶ Loss of interest in play may signal fatigue, which may be associated with renal failure.

6. **Are you changing the baby's diaper more or less than before?**

▶ There are a variety of contributors to changes in elimination patterns, but renal failure, dehydration, overhydration, diet changes, obstruction, and stress can contribute to a change in normal pattern.

Questions for the Pregnant Female

1. **Have you noticed any changes in your urinary pattern?**

▶ Often, the developing fetus places increasing pressure on the mother's bladder, causing urinary urgency. As a result, the client voids more often, in smaller amounts.

GATHERING THE DATA

TECHNIQUES AND NORMAL FINDINGS

RATIONALES

2. **Have you noticed unusual swelling in your ankles, feet, fingers, or wrists? Do have frequent headaches?**

▶ These signs may be associated with pregnancy-induced hypertension and preeclampsia.

Questions for the Older Adult

1. **Have you noticed any unusual swelling in your ankles, feet, fingers, or wrists?**

▶ Swelling may be indicative of congestive heart failure. Weight gain, fatigue, activity intolerance, and shortness of breath may be associated with the swelling.

2. *If the client is male, ask:* **Have you noticed voiding in small amounts, feeling the need to void more frequently than in the past, or difficulty initiating the stream of urine?**

▶ These symptoms may be due to an enlarged prostate.

PHYSICAL ASSESSMENT

ASSESSMENT TECHNIQUES AND FINDINGS

The urinary physical assessment is typically done concurrently with the abdominal examination. Physical assessment of the urinary system includes the use of inspection, palpation, percussion, and auscultation. The skills are used to gather information about the function of the urinary system. Knowledge of normal parameters and expected findings is essential in determining the meaning of the data as the nurse performs the physical assessment.

Adult skin is moist and supple with pink undertones. The abdomen is symmetrical and free of lesions, bruises, and swelling. The renal arteries are without bruits. The costovertebral angle and flanks are symmetrical, even in colour, and nontender to palpation and percussion. The kidneys are not enlarged; they are rounded, smooth, firm, and nontender. The bladder is nonpalpable, and percussion reveals tympany above the symphysis pubis.

Physical assessment of the urinary system follows an organized pattern. It begins with a survey of the client's general appearance followed by inspection of the abdomen. The renal arteries are auscultated and then the costovertebral angles and flank areas are inspected, palpated, and percussed. The kidneys are palpated. Bladder size is determined by palpation and percussion of the lower abdomen.

> **EQUIPMENT**
> examination gown and drape
> stethoscope
> clean, nonsterile examination gloves
> specimen container

> **HELPFUL HINTS**
> - Have the client empty the bladder before the examination and collect a urine specimen at that time.
> - Provide clear instructions for specimen collection and provide privacy.
> - Males and females respond in a variety of ways when exposed for examination of private areas. Use appropriate draping to maintain the dignity of the client.
> - Explain each step of the procedures and tell the client to report any discomfort or difficulty.
> - Use routine practices.

TECHNIQUES AND NORMAL FINDINGS

ABNORMAL FINDINGS AND SPECIAL CONSIDERATIONS

GENERAL SURVEY

A quick survey of the client enables the nurse to identify any immediate problem as well as the client's ability to participate in the assessment.

1. **Instruct the client.**
   - Explain that you will be looking, listening, touching, and tapping on parts of the abdomen. Tell the client you will explain each procedure as it occurs. Tell the client to report any discomfort and that you will stop the examination if the procedure is uncomfortable.

TECHNIQUES AND NORMAL FINDINGS	ABNORMAL FINDINGS AND SPECIAL CONSIDERATIONS

2. Position the client.

- Begin the examination with the client in a supine position with the abdomen exposed from the nipple line to the pubis (see Figure 20.4).

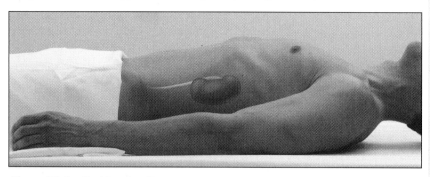

Figure 20.4 ● Position the client.

3. Assess the general appearance.

- Assess general appearance and inspect the client's skin for colour, hydration status, scales, masses, indentations, or scars.
- The client should not show signs of acute distress and should be mentally alert and oriented.

▶ Clients with kidney disorders frequently look tired and complain of fatigue. If a kidney disorder is suspected, it is important to look for signs of circulatory overload (pulmonary edema) or peripheral edema (puffy face or fingers), or indications of pruritus (scratch marks on the skin).

Azotemia (elevated nitrogenous wastes in the blood) contributes to mental confusion.

4. Inspect the abdomen for colour, contour, symmetry, and distension.

- It may be helpful to stand at the foot of the exam table and inspect the abdomen from there (see Figure 20.5).

▶ A distended bladder may be visible in the suprapubic area, indicating the need to void and perhaps the inability to do so.

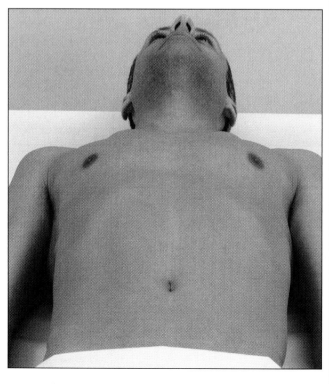

Figure 20.5 ●
Inspecting the abdomen from the foot of the exam table.

| TECHNIQUES AND NORMAL FINDINGS | ABNORMAL FINDINGS AND SPECIAL CONSIDERATIONS |

- Note that visual inspection of the suprapubic area may confirm the presence or absence of a distended bladder.

▶ Many diseases can contribute to abdominal distension. These include renal conditions, such as polycystic kidney disease; enlarged kidneys, as seen in acute pyelonephritis (kidney inflammation); ascites (accumulation of fluid) caused by hepatic disease; and displacement of abdominal organs. Pressure from the abdominal contents on the diaphragm may alter the client's breathing pattern.

- Normally, the client's abdomen is not distended, is relatively symmetrical, and is free of bruises, masses, and swellings. (A complete discussion of abdominal assessment is provided in Chapter 19. ⟳)

5. **Auscultate the right and left renal arteries to assess circulatory sounds.**
   - Gently place the bell of the stethoscope over the extended midclavicular line (MCL) on either side of the abdominal aorta, which is located above the level of the umbilicus (see Figure 20.6).

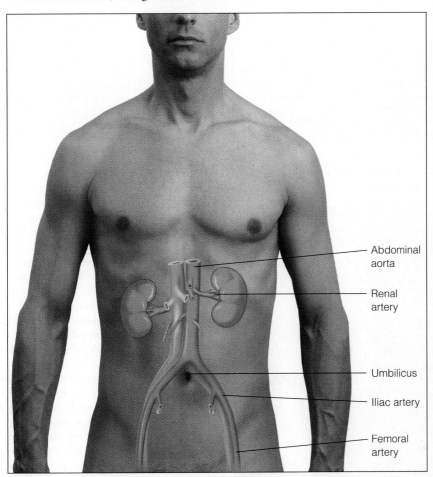

Abdominal aorta

Renal artery

Umbilicus

Iliac artery

Femoral artery

Figure 20.6 ● Auscultating the renal arteries.

- Be sure to auscultate both the right and the left sides, and over the epigastric and umbilical areas.
- In most cases, no sounds are heard; however, an upper abdominal bruit is occasionally heard in young adults and is considered normal. On a thin adult, renal artery pulsation may be auscultated.

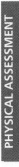

PHYSICAL ASSESSMENT

TECHNIQUES AND NORMAL FINDINGS	ABNORMAL FINDINGS AND SPECIAL CONSIDERATIONS

THE KIDNEYS AND FLANKS

1. Position the client.
   - Place the client in a sitting position facing away from you with the client's back exposed.

2. Inspect the left and right costovertebral angles for colour and symmetry.
   - The colour should be consistent with the rest of the back.

   ▶ A protrusion or elevation over a costovertebral angle occurs when the kidney is grossly enlarged or when a mass is present.

3. Inspect the flanks (the side areas between the hips and the ribs) for colour and symmetry.
   - The costovertebral angles and flanks should be symmetrical and even in colour.

   ▶ This finding must be carefully correlated to other diagnostic cues as the assessment proceeds. If ecchymosis (bruising) is present (Grey Turner's sign), there may be other signs of trauma, such as blunt force trauma, penetrating wounds, or lacerations.

> **CLINICAL TIP**
>
> *Do not percuss or palpate the client who reports pain or discomfort in the pelvic region. Do not percuss or palpate the kidney if a tumour of the kidney, such as a neuroblastoma or Wilms' tumour, is suspected. Palpation increases intra-abdominal pressure, which may contribute to intraperitoneal spreading of this neuroblastoma. Deep palpation should be performed only by experienced practitioners.*

4. Gently palpate the area over the left costovertebral angle (see Figure 20.7).
   - Watch the reaction and ask the client to describe any sensation the palpation causes. Normally, the client expresses no discomfort.

   ▶ Pain, discomfort, or tenderness from an enlarged or diseased kidney may occur over the costovertebral angle, flank, and abdomen. When questioned, the client complains of a dull, steady ache. This type of pain is associated with polycystic formation, pyelonephritis, and other disorders that cause kidney enlargement. In the client with polycystic kidney disease, a sharp, sudden, intermittent pain may mean that a cyst in the kidney has ruptured. If the costovertebral angle is tender, red, and warm, and the client is experiencing chills, fever, nausea, and vomiting, the underlying kidney could be inflamed or infected.

   The pain caused by calculi (stones) in the kidney or upper ureter is unique and different in character, severity, and duration from that caused by kidney enlargement. This pain occurs as calculi travel from the kidney to the ureters and the urinary bladder.

   Some clients experience no pain, and others feel excruciating pain. A stationary stone causes a dull, aching pain. As stones travel down the urinary tract, spasms occur. These spasms produce sharp, intermittent, colicky pain (often accompanied by chills, fever, nausea, and vomiting) that radiates from the flanks to the lower quadrants of the abdomen, and in some cases, the upper thigh and scrotum or labium.

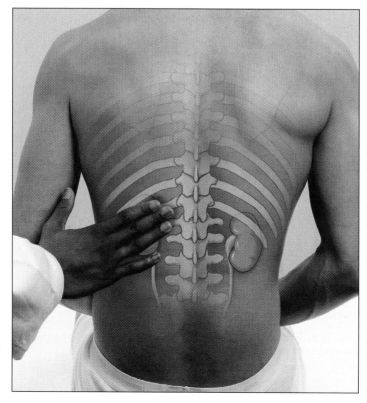

Figure 20.7 ●
Palpating the costovertebral angle.

| TECHNIQUES AND NORMAL FINDINGS | ABNORMAL FINDINGS AND SPECIAL CONSIDERATIONS |

If the client reports severe pain, **hematuria** (blood in the urine) or **oliguria** (diminished volume of urine), and nausea and vomiting, it is important to be alert for hydroureter, a frequent complication that occurs when a renal calculus moves into the ureter. The calculus blocks and dilates the ureter, causing spasms and severe pain. Hydroureter can lead to shock, infection, and impaired renal function. If the nurse suspects hydroureter or obstruction at any point in the urinary tract, medical collaboration must be sought immediately.

5. Use blunt or indirect percussion to further assess the kidneys.
   - Place your left palm flat over the left costovertebral angle.
   - Thump the back of your left hand with the ulnar surface of your right fist, causing a gentle thud over the costovertebral angle (see Figure 20.8).

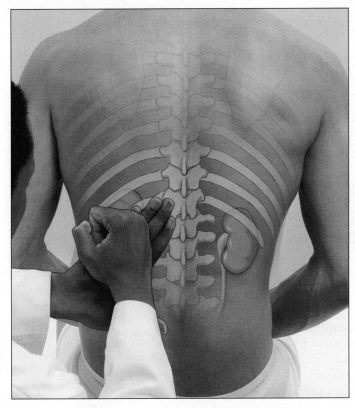

Figure 20.8 ● Blunt percussion over the left costovertebral angle.

   - Repeat the procedure on the right side. Ask the client to describe the sensation as you examine each side.

   ▶ Pain or discomfort during and after blunt percussion suggests kidney disease. This finding is correlated with other assessment findings.

   - The client should feel no pain or tenderness with pressure or percussion.

THE LEFT KIDNEY

1. Attempt to palpate the lower pole of the left kidney.
   - Although it is not usually palpable, attempt to palpate the lower pole of the kidney for size, contour, consistency, and sensation. Note that the rib cage obscures the upper poles.

   ▶ When enlargement occurs in the presence of such conditions as neoplasms and polycystic disease, the kidneys may be palpable. Otherwise, they are rarely palpable.

Techniques and Normal Findings

Abnormal Findings and Special Considerations

CLINICAL TIP

Because deep kidney palpation can cause tissue trauma, novice nurses should not attempt either deep palpation or capture of the kidney unless supervised by an experienced nurse or nurse practitioner. Deep kidney palpation should not be done in clients who have had a recent kidney transplant or an abdominal aortic aneurysm.

- Position the client in a supine position. All palpation should be performed from the client's right side.
- While standing on the client's right side, reach over the client and place your left hand between the posterior rib cage and the iliac crest (the left flank).
- Place your right hand on the left upper quadrant of the abdomen lateral and parallel to the left rectus muscle, just below the costal margin.
- Instruct the client to take a deep breath. As the client inhales, lift the client's left flank with your left hand and press deeply with your right hand (approximately 4 cm or 1.5 in.) to attempt to palpate the lower pole of the kidney (see Figure 20.9).

▶ Care must be taken not to mistake an enlarged spleen for an enlarged left kidney. An enlarged kidney feels smooth and rounded, whereas an enlarged spleen feels sharper, with a more delineated edge.

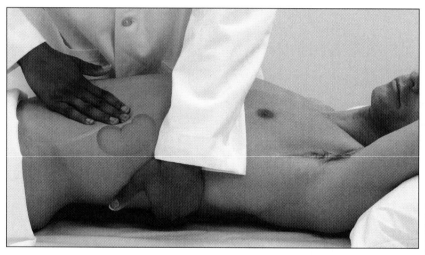

Figure 20.9 ● Palpating the left kidney.

2. Attempt to capture the left kidney.

- Because of its position deep in the retroperitoneal space, the left kidney is not normally palpable. The capture manoeuvre may enable you to palpate it. This manoeuvre is possible because the kidneys descend during inspiration and slide back into their normal position during exhalation.
- Standing on the client's right side, place your left hand under the client's back to elevate the flank as before. Place your right hand on the left upper quadrant of the abdomen lateral and parallel to the left rectus muscle, with the fingertips just below the left costal margin. Instruct the client to take a deep breath and hold it. As the client inhales, attempt to capture the kidney between your two hands. Ask the client to exhale slowly and then to briefly hold the breath. At the same time, slowly release the pressure of your fingers.
- As the client exhales, you will feel the captured kidney move back into its previous position. The kidney surface should be rounded, smooth, firm, and nontender.

▶ An enlarged palpable kidney could be painful for the client. This suggests a tumour, a cyst, or hydronephrosis (distension of the kidney with urine, often caused by a blockage).

| TECHNIQUES AND NORMAL FINDINGS | ABNORMAL FINDINGS AND SPECIAL CONSIDERATIONS |

THE RIGHT KIDNEY

1. **Attempt to palpate the lower pole of the right kidney.**
   - Standing on the client's right side, place your left hand under the back parallel to the right twelfth rib (about halfway between the costal margin and iliac crest), with your fingertips reaching for the costovertebral angle. Place your right hand on the right upper quadrant of the abdomen, lateral to the right rectus muscle and just below the right costal margin.
   - Instruct the client to take a deep breath. As the client inhales, lift the flank with your left hand and use deep palpation to feel for the lower pole of the kidney.

2. **Attempt to capture the right kidney.**
   - Place your left hand under the client's right flank.
   - Place your right hand on the right upper quadrant of the abdomen with the fingertips lateral and parallel to the right rectus muscle, just below the right costal margin.

   ▶ It is important not to mistake an enlarged liver for an enlarged right kidney. An enlarged kidney feels smooth and rounded, whereas an enlarged liver is closer to the midline and has a more distinct border. Polycystic kidney disease or carcinoma should be suspected when there is gross enlargement of the kidney. The kidneys may be two or three times their normal size in clients with polycystic disease.

   - Instruct the client to take a deep breath and hold it. As the client inhales, attempt to capture the kidney between your two hands.
   - Ask the client to exhale slowly and then to briefly hold the breath. At the same time, slowly release the pressure of your fingers.
   - As the client exhales, you will feel the captured kidney move back into its previous position. The kidney surface should be rounded, smooth, firm, and nontender.
   - The lower pole of the right kidney is palpable in some individuals, especially in thin, relaxed females. If palpable, the lower pole of the kidney has a smooth, firm, uninterrupted surface.
   - During the capture manoeuvre, some clients describe a nonpainful sensation as the kidney slides between the nurse's fingers back into its normal position.

THE URINARY BLADDER

1. **Palpate the bladder to determine symmetry, location, size, and sensation.**
   - Use light palpation over the lower portion of the abdomen. The abdomen should be soft.

   ▶ A distended bladder feels smooth, round, and taut. An asymmetrical contour or nodular surface suggests abnormal growth that should be correlated with other findings. In males with urethral obstruction caused by hypertrophy (growth caused by enlargement in the size of cells) or hyperplasia (growth caused by an increase in the number of cells) of the prostate, the bladder is enlarged.

   - Use deep palpation to locate the fundus (base) of the bladder, approximately 5 to 7 cm (2 to 2.5 in.) below the umbilicus in the lower abdomen. Once you have located the fundus of the bladder, continue to palpate, outlining the shape and contour (see Figure 20.10).

PHYSICAL ASSESSMENT

TECHNIQUES AND NORMAL FINDINGS	ABNORMAL FINDINGS AND SPECIAL CONSIDERATIONS

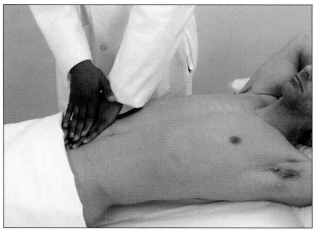

Figure 20.10 ●
Palpating the bladder.

- Slide your fingers over the surface of the bladder and continue palpating to determine smoothness and continuity.
- The surface of the bladder should feel smooth and uninterrupted. An empty bladder is usually not palpable. When the bladder is moderately full, it should be firm, smooth, symmetrical, and nontender. As the bladder fills, the fundus can reach the level of the umbilicus. A full bladder is firm and buoyant.

2. **Percuss the bladder to determine its location and degree of fullness.**

> **CLINICAL TIP**
> *If the bladder is distended with urine and the client is unable to void, assess the bladder with a bladder scanner (if available) for urinary retention. Alternatively, obtain an order to catheterize the client. Reduce the contents of the bladder slowly to prevent atony (lack of muscle tone) of the bladder wall.*

- Begin with direct percussion of the bladder over the suprapubic area.
- Move your fingers upward toward the umbilicus as you continue to percuss. A full bladder produces a dull tone on percussion. Continue percussing upward toward the umbilicus until no more dull tones are heard. The point at which dull tones cease is the upper margin of the bladder.
- Some practitioners conclude the assessment of the urinary system with the inspection and palpation of the penis and urethral meatus in the male client or the inspection of the urethral meatus in the female client. Other practitioners consider these structures with the assessment of the genitalia. These techniques are discussed in Chapters 21 and 22. ∞

SAMPLE DOCUMENTATION

Subjective:　No complaint of abdominal pain or burning with voiding. No changes in frequency of urination or amount of urine passed. Does not experience any sense of urgency with voiding. No change in colour of urine. Occasionally up at night to void but attributes this to drinking water before bedtime. No past history of surgery to the urinary system, no cardiac medical history, normotensive. No meds, allergic to sulpha drugs: experiences hives.

Objective:　Skin moist and even in colour. Abdomen, flank, and costovertebral angle symmetrical. Renal arteries without bruits. Kidneys and bladder nonpalpable. Client denies any costovertebral angle tenderness. Tympany present over symphysis pubis

PHYSICAL ASSESSMENT

APPLICATION THROUGH CRITICAL THINKING

CASE STUDY

Ms. Sadie Basset is a 52-year-old Black female who arrives at the woman's health clinic complaining of itching, burning, and frequency of urination. She tells Louise Lo, RN, "I feel like I have to go to the bathroom every 10 minutes. I'm just miserable. I'm burning all the time, and I have tenderness here." (She points to her lower abdominal area.) Ms. Basset states that sometimes she feels a sharp abdominal pain and a sudden urge to urinate. On a few of these occasions, she has had difficulty getting to the bathroom on time and has even had a few "accidents." Ms. Lo asks if Ms. Basset has any illnesses. Ms. Basset reports that she was diagnosed with diabetes mellitus a few weeks ago.

After the interview, Ms. Lo performs a physical examination. Blood pressure is 106/82, pulse 68, respirations 20, and temperature 38.4°C (101.2°F). Abdomen is flat and soft. Bowel sounds are active and present in all four quadrants. The client complains of tenderness over the suprapubic area on palpation. The urinary meatus is red and edematous with no apparent discharge. Induration of the urinary meatus is noted on palpation of the anterior vaginal wall. The urinary stream is strong and steady. The urine is dark yellow with a hint of blood. It is cloudy and has a strong, foul odour.

Ms. Lo determines that there are four targets of concern for Ms. Basset: urge incontinence, pain, elevated temperature, and lack of knowledge.

ASSESSMENT FORM

Chief Complaint: *Frequent urination—urinary, urgency*

                     Pain lower abdomen.

History: *Diabetes—diagnosed 2 weeks ago.*

Vital Signs: *B/P 106/82—P 68—RR 20—T 38.4°F*

Abdomen: *Soft, flat BS + X4. Tender over suprapublic area.*

External Genitalia: *Meatus red, no edema, no discharge,*

                     indurated.

Urine: *Urinary stream strong and steady. Dark, cloudy, strong,*

                     foul odor, Hematest positive.

▶ Complete Documentation

The following is sample documentation for Sadie Basset.

SUBJECTIVE DATA: Complains of itching, burning, and frequency of urination. "I feel like I'm going to the bathroom every 10 minutes. I'm just miserable. I'm burning all the time and I have tenderness here" (points to lower abdomen). Sometimes feels a sharp abdominal pain and sudden urge to urinate. Occasional difficulty getting to bathroom and a few "accidents." Diagnosed with diabetes 2 weeks ago.

OBJECTIVE DATA: VS: B/P 106/82—P 68—RR 20. Temperature 38.4°C. Abdomen flat, soft. Bowel sounds present all quadrants. Tenderness over suprapubic area on palpation. Urinary meatus red, edematous, no discharge. Induration of meatus. Urinary stream strong, steady. Urine dark yellow, cloudy, strong, foul odour, urine dip positive for blood.

▶ Critical Thinking Questions

1. Identify the data that support Ms. Lo's targets of concern.
2. What additional missing data are required to determine treatment for this client?
3. Describe a plan of nursing care for Ms. Basset.

▶ Applying Nursing Diagnoses

1. *Impaired urinary elimination* is a nursing diagnosis in the NANDA-I taxonomy (see Appendix A). Do the data from the case study for Sadie Basset support this diagnosis? If so, identify the data to support the diagnosis.
2. *Knowledge, deficiency* is a diagnosis in the NANDA-I taxonomy. Do the data in the case study support this diagnosis? If so, identify the data to support the diagnosis.
3. Refer to the NANDA-I taxonomy to formulate additional nursing diagnoses for Sadie Basset.

▶ Prepare Teaching Plan

LEARNING NEED: Sadie Basset has been newly diagnosed with diabetes and has frequent, painful urination and lower abdominal pain. Her urine is dark, cloudy, and foul smelling with a hint of blood. The data indicate that she has a urinary tract infection. Diabetes increases the risk for development of urinary tract infection. Therefore, the nurse has a twofold responsibility. First, the nurse must ascertain Ms. Basset's ability to adhere to the prescribed regimen for diabetes. Second, in the presence of this acute problem, the nurse must address this client's need to learn about urinary tract infections.

GOAL: Sadie Basset will reduce her risk for further episodes of urinary tract infections.

OBJECTIVES: On completion of this learning experience, Sadie Basset will be able to do the following:

1. Describe urinary tract infections.
2. Identify factors that contribute to the development of urinary tract infections.
3. Describe measures to prevent urinary tract infections.

Application of Objective 3: Describe measures to prevent urinary tract infections.

Content	Teaching Strategy	Evaluation
• Follow the prescribed diabetic regimen. • Report changes in blood glucose readings. • Drink six to eight glasses of water daily. • Urinate as soon as you feel the urge. Do not wait. • Clean the genital area from front to back to prevent organisms from the rectal area from entering the vagina or urethra. • Shower rather than bathe in a tub. • Avoid irritation of the urethra that can occur with douching, vaginal sprays, perfumed soaps, and bubble bath. Avoid wet clothing. • Avoid tight clothing and pantyhose without cotton linings. • Clean the genital area before and after intercourse. • Urinate after intercourse.	• One-on-one discussion Permits repetition and introduction of sensitive information.	• Verbal questioning in which Ms. Basset describes the eight measures to prevent urinary tract infections.

HEALTH PROMOTION ASSESSMENT TOOL

Social Determinants of Health	Level of Action	Action Strategies
Personal coping skills	Individual	**Develop personal skills** • Assess Ms. Basset's knowledge and comfort with daily management of her diabetes and explore her interest in joining a diabetic support group, since future UTI prevention will be facilitated through blood sugar level control. • Assess her understanding and ability to practise healthy hygiene within the context of her living and working conditions, including accessibility of washroom facilities during working hours. • Assess her understanding and ability to adhere to a diabetic diet. Refer her to a dietician, if required, and support any diet modifications she has already made. • Assess her physical activities on a daily and weekly basis, and encourage physical activity and exercise on a daily basis. Educate Ms. Basset on the general health benefits of physical activity and exercise, including benefits for blood sugar control.

ABNORMAL FINDINGS

Common alterations of the urinary system include bladder cancer, kidney and urinary tract infections, calculi, tumours, renal failure, and changes in urinary elimination. Each of these alterations will be discussed in the sections that follow.

Bladder Cancer

Seen later in life, bladder cancer occurs more frequently in males than in females. Smoking has been linked to this disease.

The client may be asymptomatic or have hematuria, flank pain, and frequent urination.

Glomerulonephritis

This entity is an inflammation of the glomerulus. The key clinical manifestations are hematuria with red blood cell casts

and proteinuria (protein in the urine).

Renal Calculi

Calculi are stones that block the urinary tract. They are usually composed of calcium, struvite, or a combination of magnesium, ammonium, phosphate, and uric acid. Pain is the primary symptom. The pain may radiate and is variable in

location and severity. Other symptoms include spasms, nausea, vomiting, pain on urination, frequency and urgency of urination, and gross hematuria.

Renal Tumour

Renal tumours may be either benign or malignant, with malignant being more common. Research has shown an association between renal tumours and smoking. The key manifestations

of renal tumours are hematuria, flank pain, weight loss, and palpable mass in the flank.

Renal Failure

Renal failure may be acute or it may progress to a chronic state. Acute renal failure that does not progress to a chronic state includes three stages: oliguria, diuresis (very large production of urine), and recovery. Other symptoms include fluid retention, hyperkalemia, hyperphosphatemia (elevated levels of phosphorus in the blood), nausea, and vomiting. Uremia

(blood poisoning from a buildup of substances normally excreted in the urine) is the classic hallmark of chronic renal failure. Anorexia, nausea, vomiting, mentation changes, uremic frost, pruritus (itchiness), weight loss, fatigue, and edema are common symptoms of uremia.

Urinary Tract Infection

Bacteria cause urinary tract infections. The bladder is the most common site of the infection, which results in inflammation of the bladder called cystitis; however, infection may include the kidneys. Clients may be asymptomatic, but the classic symp-

toms include urgency, frequency, dribbling, pain on urination, and suprapubic or lower back pain. Hematuria, as well as cloudy and foul-smelling urine, may accompany the other signs.

Changes in Urinary Elimination

The following are examples of alterations in urinary elimination:

Dysreflexia affects clients with spinal cord injuries at level T_7 or higher. Bladder distension causes a sympathetic response that can trigger a potentially life-threatening hypertensive crisis.

Incontinence is the inability to retain urine. If this is the client's problem, the nurse must determine which of the five types of incontinence is present.

- *Functional incontinence* occurs when the client is unable to reach the toilet in time because of environmental, psychosocial, or physical factors.
- *Reflex incontinence* occurs in clients with spinal cord damage and urine is involuntarily lost.
- *Stress incontinence,* involuntary urination, occurs when intra-abdominal pressure is increased during coughing, sneezing, or straining. Aging changes may also contribute to stress incontinence.
- *Urge incontinence* may be caused by consuming a significant volume of fluids over a relatively short period of time. Urge incontinence may also be due to diminished bladder capacity.
- *Total incontinence* is related to a neurological condition.

Urinary retention is a chronic state in which the client cannot empty his or her bladder. In most cases, the client voids small amounts of overflow urine when the bladder reaches its greatest capacity.

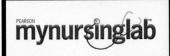

ABNORMAL FINDINGS

21

MALE REPRODUCTIVE SYSTEM

THE MALE REPRODUCTIVE SYSTEM PRODUCES HORMONES, which affect physical development and sexual behaviour. The reproductive organs in males provide for sexual pleasure and the production of offspring. The structures of the male reproductive system produce the male sex hormones and produce and transport sperm (the male reproductive cells) and protective fluid (semen) for the deposition of sperm within the female reproductive tract. Many factors, including psychosocial health, self-care habits, family, culture, and environment, affect reproductive health. Therefore, the nurse must consider these factors while conducting the interview and physical assessment. The nurse must have a thorough understanding of the constituents of a healthy reproductive system and consider the relationship of other body systems to the reproductive system.

During the physical assessment, the nurse will assess and evaluate the occasional ambiguous cues of actual and potential reproductive disease and the variety of contributors to the development of pathology. The nurse documents and communicates the findings to the other members of the healthcare team. Additionally, the nurse has a key role in teaching the client how to establish and maintain reproductive wellness. The goal of client education is the promotion of optimum health according to the client's individual needs.

ANATOMY AND PHYSIOLOGY REVIEW

The male reproductive system includes the penis, scrotum, testes, spermatic cord, duct system, accessory glands, and inguinal and perianal areas. These will be described in the sections that follow.

Male Reproductive System

The male reproductive system is divided anatomically into external and internal genital organs. The penis and scrotum, the two external organs, are easily inspected and palpated. Only some of the internal structures are palpable. A basic understanding of anatomical structure and function is fundamental to performing assessment techniques correctly and safely. Figure 21.1 illustrates the gross anatomy of the male reproductive system.

Some of the male reproductive organs serve dual roles as part of the reproductive system and the urinary system. As part of the urinary system, the male genitals serve as a passageway for expelling urine. The functions of the male reproductive system are manufacturing and protecting sperm for fertilization, transporting sperm to the female vagina, regulating hormonal production of and secretion of male sex hormones, and providing sexual pleasure.

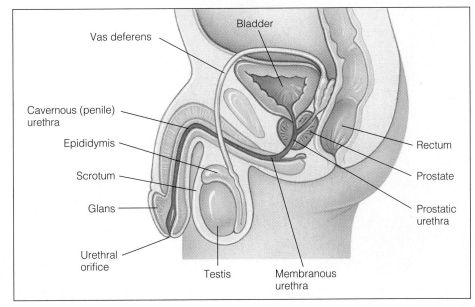

Figure 21.1 ● Gross anatomy of the male reproductive organs.

Scrotum

The **scrotum** is a loosely hanging, pliable, pear-shaped pouch of darkly pigmented skin that is located behind the penis. It houses the testes, which produce sperm. Spermatogenesis (sperm production) requires an environment in which the temperature is slightly lower than core body temperature; thus, the scrotum hangs outside the abdominopelvic cavity and is usually about (3°C or 5.5°F) cooler than core body temperature. A vertical septum within the scrotum divides it into two sections, each containing a testis, epididymis, vas deferens, and spermatic cord, as well as other functional structures (see Figure 21.2 and Figure 21.3).

Pubic hair scantily covers the scrotum. It is visibly asymmetrical, with the left side extending lower than the right, because the left spermatic cord is longer.

Below the scrotal surface lie two muscles, the cremaster muscle and the dartos muscle, which play a protective role in sperm production and viability. In cold temperatures, the dartos muscle wrinkles the scrotal skin, whereas the cremaster muscle contracts, causing the testes to elevate toward the body. Warmer temperatures cause the reverse reaction. The testes also become more wrinkled and contract toward the body during sexual arousal.

The major functions of the scrotum are protecting the testes, epididymides, and part of the spermatic cord, and protecting sperm production and viability through the maintenance of an appropriate surface temperature.

Testes

The **testes** are two firm, rubbery, olive-shaped structures that measure 4 to 5 cm (1.5 to 2 in.) long and 2 to 2.5 cm (1 in.) wide. They manufacture sperm and are thus the primary male sex organs. Each testis has two coats, the outer tunica vaginalis and the inner tunica albuginea, that separate it from the scrotal wall. Within each testis are the seminiferous tubules that produce sperm, and Leydig's cells that produce testosterone. Testosterone plays a significant role in sperm production and the development of male sexual characteristics. The testes receive their blood supply from the testicular arteries. The testicular veins not only remove deoxygenated blood from the testes but also form a network called the pampiniform plexus (Figure 21.2). This plays a crucial supportive role in regulating the temperature in the testes by cooling arterial blood before it passes into the testes. The major functions of the testes are producing spermatozoa and secreting testosterone.

Spermatic Cord

The **spermatic cord** is composed of fibrous connective tissue. Its purpose is to form a protective sheath around the nerves, blood vessels, lymphatic structures, and muscle fibres associated with the scrotum (Figure 21.2).

Duct System

The duct system plays a crucial role in the transportation of sperm. The three structures composing the duct system are the epididymis, the ductus deferens, and the urethra (Figure 21.2 and Figure 21.3).

Epididymis

Positioned on top of and just posterior to each testicle is a comma- or crescent-shaped **epididymis**, which is palpable on physical examination. It is actually a long, coiled tube, about

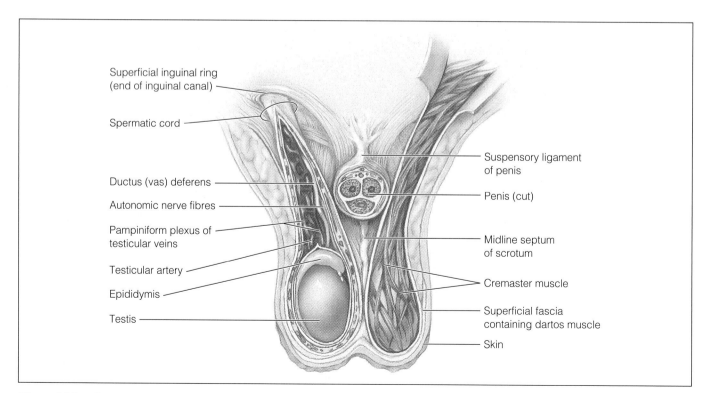

Figure 21.2 ● Contents of the scrotum, anterior view.

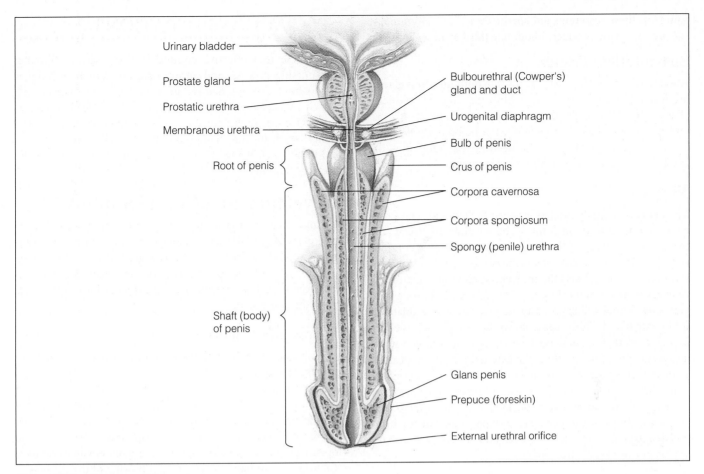

Figure 21.3 • Structure of the penis.

5.5 to 6 m (18 to 19.5 ft.) in length, which forms the beginning of the male duct system. Once the immature sperm have been produced in the testes, they are transported into the epididymis, where they mature and become mobile. During orgasm, forceful contraction of muscles in this structure propels the sperm into the ductus deferens. The major functions of the epididymis are storing sperm as they mature and transporting sperm to the ductus deferens.

Ductus Deferens

Also known as the vas deferens, this tubular structure stretches from the end of the epididymis to the ejaculatory duct. Extending about 46 cm (18 in.) long, the tube runs through the inguinal canal, on the backside of the bladder, and to the ejaculatory duct as it enters into the prostate gland. Mature sperm remain in the ductus deferens until ready for transport. The major functions of the ductus deferens are serving as an excretory duct in the transport of sperm and serving as a reservoir for mature sperm.

Urethra

The **urethra** serves as a conduit for the transportation of both urine and semen to the outside of the body. It is composed of three sections: the prostatic urethra, the membranous urethra, and the spongy (penile) urethra (Figure 21.3).

Accessory Glands

The accessory glands play a crucial role in the formation of semen. These glands include the seminal vesicles, the prostate gland, and the bulbourethral gland.

Seminal Vesicles

The **seminal vesicles** are a pair of saclike glands, 7.5 cm (3 in.) long, located between the bladder and rectum. These vesicles are the source of 60% of the semen produced. Semen, a thick yellow fluid, is composed of a high concentration of fructose, amino acids, prostaglandins, ascorbic acid, and fibrinogen. It is secreted into the ejaculatory duct, where it mixes with sperm, which has been propelled from the ductus deferens. Semen nourishes and dilutes the sperm, enhancing its motility. Seminal fluid is propelled from the ejaculatory duct into the prostatic urethra.

Prostate Gland

The **prostate gland** borders the urethra near the lower part of the bladder. About the size of a chestnut (2 cm or 1 in.), it is partially palpable through the front wall of the rectum because it lies just anterior to the rectum (Figure 21.1). The prostate is composed of glandular structures that continuously secrete a milky, alkaline solution. During sexual intercourse, glandular activity increases, and the alkaline secretions flow into the urethra. Because sperm motility is reduced in an acidic environment, these secretions aid sperm transport. Additionally, the prostate gland produces about one third of all semen.

Bulbourethral Glands

Also referred to as Cowper's glands, the **bulbourethral glands** are located below the prostate within the urethral sphincter (Figure 21.3). These glands are small (4.5 to 5 mm or 0.2 in.) and round. Just before ejaculation, the bulbourethral glands secrete a clear mucus into the urethra that lubricates the urethra and increases its alkaline environment.

Penis

The **penis** is centrally located between the left and right groin areas and lies directly in front of the scrotum. Internally, the penile shaft consists of the penile urethra and three columns of highly vascular, erectile tissue: the two dorsolateral columns (corpora cavernosa) and the midventral column surrounding or encasing the urethra (Figure 21.3). The penis contracts and elongates during sexual arousal when its vasculature dilates as it fills with blood. This process allows the penis to become firm and erect so that it can deposit sperm into the female vagina. The distal end of the urethra (the external meatus) appears as a small opening centrally located on the glans of the penis, the cone-shaped distal end of the organ. In uncircumcised males, the glans is covered by a layer of skin called the foreskin. The major functions of the penis are serving as an exit for urine and as a passageway for sperm to exit and be deposited into the vagina during sexual intercourse.

Inguinal Areas

The inguinal areas are located laterally to the pubic region over the iliac region or the upper part of the hip bone. Within this area are the inguinal ligaments and the inguinal canals, which lie above the inguinal ligaments. The inguinal canals are associated with the abdominal muscles and actually represent a potential weak link in the abdominopelvic wall. When a separation of the abdominal muscle exists, the weak points of these canals afford an area for the protrusion of the intestine into the groin region. This protrusion is called an **inguinal hernia**. Table 21.1 describes types, characteristics, and signs and symptoms of inguinal hernias.

Perianal Area

The **anus** is the terminal end of the gastrointestinal system. The anal canal is between 2 and 4 cm (1 and 1.5 in.) long, opens onto the perineum at the midpoint of the gluteal folds, and has internal and external muscles. The external muscles are skeletal muscles, which form the part of the anal sphincter that voluntarily controls evacuation of stool. Above the anus is the rectum with the prostate gland in close proximity to the anterior surface of the rectum. Mucosa of the anus is moist, darkly pigmented, and hairless. Lying between the scrotum and the anus is the **perineum**, which has a smooth surface and is free of lesions.

SPECIAL CONSIDERATIONS

The nurse uses effective communication, critical thinking, the nursing process, and appropriate assessment techniques throughout a comprehensive assessment process to determine the client's health status. Health status is influenced by a number of factors, including age, developmental level, race, ethnicity, work history, living conditions, socioeconomics, and emotional well-being. These factors will be described in the sections that follow.

Developmental Considerations

Changes in anatomy and physiological function occur as normal parts of growth and development. The accurate interpretation of findings from assessment is dependent on knowledge of the expected variations across the age span. The sections that follow address specific age-related variations in the male reproductive system.

Infants and Children

The male newborn's genitals should be clearly evident and not ambiguous. If there is ambiguity, referral for genetic counselling is indicated. The penis may vary in size but averages about 2.5 cm (1 in.) in length and is slender. The urethral meatus should be in the centre of the glans. If the opening is located on the underside of the glans, **hypospadias** is present. If the opening is on the superior aspect of the glans, **epispadias** exists. *Chordee,* a tight band of skin, causes bowing of the penis. The penis appears to have a C shape. This is associated with epispadias and hypospadias. The foreskin may be somewhat tight and not retractable until 2 or 3 years of age. If it is still tight after this time, **phimosis** exists. Cultural values and religious beliefs may determine whether the family or caregiver circumcises the child. The family requires teaching about either maintaining the cleanliness of the uncircumcised penis or caring for the penis in the days following a circumcision.

The male infant's scrotum should be consistent in colour with other body parts. It should seem oversized in comparison with the penis. This proportion changes as the infant grows. If the scrotum is enlarged and filled with fluid, a hydrocele may be present. The testes should be palpable and are about 2 cm (1 in.) in diameter at birth. Undescended testes, called cryptorchidism, is a common finding, especially if the infant is preterm. The testes should descend spontaneously within the first year of life. If both testes do not descend, the male will be infertile and will be at a greater risk for testicular cancer. Enlargement of the testes in adolescence indicates the presence of a tumour. Testes smaller than 1.5 to 2.0 cm (0.75 to 1.0 in.) may indicate adrenal hyperplasia.

The onset of puberty in the male child occurs between 10 and 15 years of age. At this time, under the influence of elevating levels of testosterone, the male child begins to develop adult sexual characteristics. The testes and scrotum enlarge. Pubic, facial, and axillary hair develops. The penis begins to elongate, and the testes begin to produce mature sperm. The male child will experience unexpected erections and nocturnal emissions (wet dreams). Open, supportive communication is essential at this time. The nurse can show male children pictures of the sexual maturation of genitals to demonstrate that their development is normal. Table 21.2 includes Tanner's staging for evaluating sexual maturity. The male child often displays a fascination with his genitals. Masturbation and exploration of the genitals are usual practices in infants, toddlers, and preschoolers. Males may express curiosity in comparing their genitals with those of other children, both male and female, in preschool and school ages.

Precocious puberty is an endocrine disorder characterized by the development of adult male characteristics in males under age 10. It includes dense pubic hair, penile enlargement, and enlargement of the testes. Precocious puberty may be idiopathic or caused by a genetic trait, lesions in the pituitary gland or hypothalamus, or testicular tumours. Referral to an endocrinologist may be required for definitive diagnosis.

It is important to assess not only the physical development of the male child's sexual organs but also the presence of abnormalities, such as infection, tumours, and hernias. Assessment is completed by using the same methods as described for the adult male.

It is essential to assess for sexual molestation in male children. Some signs of sexual molestation are trauma, depression, eating disorders, and bruising, swelling, and inflammation in the genital and anal areas. Additionally, the male child may appear withdrawn. Often the male child will deny the experience.

Adolescents often express interest in the changes related to puberty. The desire to explore sexual relationships and sexual contact, from kissing and fondling to intercourse, may be intense. Thus, adolescents need counselling on relationship issues, birth control, protection against sexually transmitted infections

TABLE 21.1 | Inguinal Hernias

TYPE OF HERNIA	CHARACTERISTICS	SIGNS AND SYMPTOMS
Direct hernia	Extrusion of abdominal intestine into inguinal ring. Bulging occurs in the area around the pubis. Abdominal intestine may remain within the inguinal canal or extrude past the external ring.	Most often is painless. Appears as a swelling. During palpation, have the client cough. You will feel pressure against the side of your finger.
Indirect hernia	Abdominal intestine may remain within the inguinal canal or extrude past the external ring. Most common type of hernia. Located within the femoral canal.	Appears as a swelling. During palpation, have the client cough. You will feel pressure against your fingertip. Palpate a soft mass.
Femoral hernia	Bulge occurs over the area of the femoral artery. The right femoral artery is affected more frequently than the left. Lowest incidence of all three hernias.	May not be painful; however, once strangulation occurs, pain is severe.

TABLE 21.2	Maturation Stages in the Male
Stage 1	Preadolescent, hair present is no different from that on abdomen. Testes, scrotum, and penis are the same size and shape as in young child.
Stage 2	Pubic hair slightly pigmented, longer, straight hair, often still downy, usually at base of penis, sometimes on scrotum; enlargement of scrotum and testes.
Stage 3	Pubic hair dark, definitely pigmented, curly pubic hair around base of penis; enlargement of penis, especially in length, further enlargement of testes, descent of scrotum.
Stage 4	Pubic hair definitely adult in type but not in extent, spread no further than inguinal fold. Continued enlargement of penis and sculpturing of glans, increased pigmentation of scrotum.
Stage 5	Hair spread to medial surface of thighs in adult distribution. Adult stage, scrotum ample, penis reaching nearly to bottom of scrotum.

(STIs), and delaying sexual activity. An adolescent may be concerned about or confused by an attraction to individuals of the same sex. It is important to provide open communication so that the adolescent may express concerns.

The Older Adult

The older male client experiences the following changes to the external genitals. Pubic hair thins and greys, the prostate gland enlarges, the size of the penis and testes may diminish, the scrotum hangs lower, and the testes are softer to palpation. Sperm production decreases in middle age; however, the older male may remain able to contribute viable sperm and father children throughout his lifespan.

Sexual function and ability change as well. Testosterone production decreases, resulting in diminished libido. Sexual response is often slower and not as intense. The older male may be slower to achieve erection yet may be able to maintain the erection longer. Ejaculation can be less forceful and last for a shorter time, and less semen may be ejaculated.

Even though older male adults can achieve sexual gratification and participate in a satisfying sexual relationship, a decrease in sexual drive may contribute to the client's withdrawing from sexual experiences and relationships. The following factors are known to influence sexual drive:

- Chronic or acute diseases
- Certain medications
- Loss of spouse or significant other
- Loss of privacy
- Depression
- Fatigue
- Any stressful situation
- Use of alcohol or illicit drugs

Psychosocial Considerations

Fatigue, depression, and stress can decrease sexual desire in a client of any age. Grief over the loss of a relationship, whether because of separation, divorce, or death, can have long-term effects on a client's willingness to seek new relationships. Feelings of betrayal—for example, when a partner becomes intimate with another person—can have the same effect.

Past or recent trauma, as from childhood abuse, physical assault, and sexual assault, whether or not penetration occurred, may have a significant impact on a client's ability to enjoy a sexual relationship. This may be true even if the trauma is completely repressed.

A male's body image may be affected by his perception of his penis size in relation to that of other males. Some males fear that they are too small to satisfy a female sexually. Caring and sensitive teaching is needed to help the client understand that variations in penis size are normal and that little correlation exists between penis size and a partner's sexual satisfaction.

Males who have had a surgical sterilization procedure may feel suddenly freed from the worry of unwanted pregnancy and experience an increase in sexual desire, or they may suddenly feel less masculine than before the surgery and withdraw from sexual relationships.

Social and Ethnocultural Considerations

Some cultures and religions have specific beliefs or encourage specific behaviours related to circumcision and sexual practices. For example, the Jewish religion requires the child to be circumcised by the eighth day of life by a trained person, called a mohel. Muslims practise circumcision but not necessarily on the eighth day of life. In addition, many religions forbid premarital sex. When assessing clients, the nurse must never assume that clients share all the beliefs or follow all the practices of their own religious or cultural group or those of the nurse.

Testicular cancer is the most common type of cancer in males between the ages of 15 and 49; thus, even adolescent males should perform a monthly testicular self-examination (see Box 21.1). Prostate cancer is the second-leading cause of cancer-related deaths in males. Screening for prostate-specific antigen (PSA) and an annual prostate exam after the age of 50 is essential. Prostate cancer is more common in Black males. The signs of the condition are not usually noticeable until the prostatic cancer is advanced. The signs are usually confounding because benign prostatic disease presents with similar symptoms. These signs are dribbling, retention of urine, difficulty initiating the urinary stream, and cystitis. Risk factors include a family history of prostatic cancer, smoking, and age.

Adults living in overcrowded conditions may feel that their lack of privacy inhibits their ability to experience sexual gratification. Today, one or more grandparents or older relatives may live with their adult child, and sexual expression and gratification may be compromised for all the adults in the family.

Sexual, physical, or verbal abuse among family members may cause significant sexual dysfunction. Some family members may be aware of the experience but be unwilling or unable to stop the perpetrators or help the victims.

Negative family reactions to an individual's sexual orientation and lifestyle choices can constrain a person's ability and willingness to find a sexual partner and maintain a satisfying sexual relationship. The family's influence may be so strong that individuals choose partners acceptable to the family but who do not meet their own needs or desires. This can have a negative emotional and physical impact on the individuals.

Several environmental and occupational exposures have been linked to birth defects, decreased libido, diminished sperm count, and abnormal sperm morphology. In dealing with males in their reproductive stages, or with those who express complaints of decreased libido, a thorough investigation of their workplace and occupational exposures should be conducted.

BOX 21.1	**Testicular Self-Examination**

Testicular cancer has no early warning signs. Thus, males should perform a testicular self-exam monthly, beginning in adolescence. Describe to the client how to perform the exam:

- The best time to perform the exam is in the shower or bath, since the heat and steam will warm your hands and the water will help your hands to glide over the skin surface. If your hands are cold, a reflex response will occur, causing your testicles to move up against your body. They will then be more difficult for you to feel.
- Feel each testicle by applying gentle pressure with your thumb, index, and middle fingers. If your testicle hurts while you feel it, you are pressing too hard.
- The contour of the testicle should be smooth, rounded, and firm.
- You will feel the epididymis on top of and behind each testicle.
- You should not feel any distinct lumps or areas of hardness, nor should your testicle be enlarged. If any of these signs are present, make an appointment with your physician immediately.

Social and Ethnocultural Considerations

- The risk of prostate cancer is highest after age 60 to 65.
- Risk of prostate or testicular cancer is higher for those males with a family history.
- Prostate cancer occurs more frequently in Black men.
- The risk of bladder cancer is highest for men over 65 and testicular cancer is highest for men 15 to 49 years of age.
- Bladder cancer occurs more frequently in whites and is lowest for Asians.
- Exposure to certain industrial chemicals (especially dyes and arsenic) places a person at higher risk for bladder cancer.
- Treatment with certain medications, such as cyclophosphamide (used to treat cancer and some other conditions), places a person at higher risk for bladder cancer.
- Circumcision is required in some religions and preferred in many cultures.
- In many cultures and religions, physical examination by a healthcare provider of the opposite sex is prohibited.

- Discussion of sexual activity and reproductive function is unacceptable in many cultures.
- Fifty-three percent of same-sex married spouses in Canada are men. The healthcare needs of this group may vary from those of heterosexual men.

Sources: Canadian Cancer Society. (2009). *Causes of testicular cancer.* Retrieved from **http://www.cancer.ca/Ontario/About cancer/Types of cancer/ Causes of testicular cancer.aspx?sc_lang=en&r=; Canadian Cancer Society. (2009b).** *Causes of bladder cancer.* **Retrieved from http://www. cancer.ca/Canada-wide/About%20cancer/Types%20of%20cancer/ Causes%20of%20bladder%20cancer.aspx?sc_lang=en; Canadian Cancer Society. (2009).** *Causes of prostate cancer.* **Retrieved from http:/ /www.cancer.ca/canada-wide/about%20cancer/types%20of%20can-cer/what%20is%20prostate%20cancer.aspx?sc_lang=en; Statistics Canada. (2009).** *Gay pride... by the numbers.* **Retrieved from http:// www42.statcan.ca/smr08/smr08_118-eng.htm**

GATHERING THE DATA

Health assessment of the male reproductive system includes gathering subjective and objective data. Subjective data collection occurs during the client interview, before the actual physical assessment. During the interview the nurse uses a variety of communication techniques to elicit general and specific information about the client's state of health or illness. Health records, the results of laboratory tests, and X-rays are important secondary sources to be reviewed and included in the data-gathering process. During physical assessment of the male reproductive system, the techniques of inspection and palpation will be used.

HEALTH HISTORY

The health history for the male reproductive system concerns data related to the structures and functions of this body system. Subjective data related to the status of the reproductive system is gathered during the health history. The nurse must be prepared to observe the client and listen for cues related to the function of this body system. The nurse may use open-ended or closed questions to obtain information. Often, a number of follow-up questions or requests for descriptions are required to clarify data or gather missing information. Follow-up questions are aimed at identifying the source of problems, duration of difficulties, measures to alleviate problems, and clues about the client's knowledge of his own health.

Because of the dual functions of some of the male reproductive structures, some of the data gathered during the focused interview will relate to the status of the urinary system and to the reproductive system. Some commonly reported problems are those related to altered patterns of voiding, the presence of masses or lesions, unusual discharge, pain and tenderness, changes in sexual functioning, contact with a sexual partner who may have an STI, and infertility. Examination of the anus and rectum is included in examination of the male reproductive system. Related problems include hemorrhoids, fissures, and infectious processes.

Nurses need to understand their own feelings and comfort about various aspects of sexuality to be efficient in gathering data. It is essential for the nurse to put aside personal beliefs and values about sexual practices and focus in a culturally competent and nonjudgmental manner on gathering data to determine the health status of the male client.

During the health history, the nurse will need to create an atmosphere that facilitates open communication and comfort for the client. Male clients commonly experience anxiety, fear, and embarrassment when the nurse requests information about a topic that, in most clients' minds, is very personal. These emotions may be expressed either verbally or nonverbally. With this in mind, the nurse should approach the client in as nonthreatening a manner as possible and assure the male client that the information provided and the results of the physical examination will remain confidential. Furthermore, the nurse should be aware of personal behaviours that may hinder effective communication. The nurse should sit down with the male client to convey that it is important to spend time discussing the client's concerns. The nurse's verbal and nonverbal communication should convey a nonjudgmental attitude while requesting only the information needed to assess the client's health status. It is a good idea to begin with questions that are the least threatening and have the least sexual connotation, because the information the nurse gathers may reveal some abnormality that may threaten sexual activity and health. A conversational approach with the use of open-ended statements may be helpful, especially with male adolescents. As the client provides information, the male client's choice of terminology can serve as a guide in deciding which terms would be most appropriate to use. When discussing any sensitive or controversial topic, it is always best to start with a general statement that opens the door for male clients to express their thoughts.

The health history guides the physical assessment of the male reproductive system. The information is always considered in relation to normal parameters and expectations about the function of the system. Therefore, the nurse must consider age, gender, race, culture, environment, health practices, past and concurrent problems, and therapies when framing questions and using techniques to elicit information. To address all the factors when conducting a health history, specific questions related to reproductive status and function have been developed. These questions focus on the most common concerns or injuries associated with the male reproductive system; questions related to past health history; questions related to behaviours; questions that address environmental concerns; and those that are specific to clients according to age.

The nurse must consider the client's ability to participate in the health history and physical assessment of the male reproductive system. If a client is experiencing discomfort or anxiety, the nurse should focus on relief of symptoms.

As the nurse gathers the data, she or he will shift the type of questions to direct questions that give the client room to explain or qualify. The mnemonic O-P-Q-R-S-T-U, which stands for onset (chronology), precipitating (or palliative), quality, region (or radiation), severity, timing, and understanding, will help the learner remember the dimensions of the symptoms. The nurse will keep in mind that not all these qualifiers will apply to each symptom.

HEALTH HISTORY QUESTIONS	RATIONALES

Questions Related to Common Concerns or Injuries

The sections that follow provide sample questions and follow-up questions. Rationales for some questions are provided. The list of questions is not all-inclusive but rather represents the more common concern or injury questions required in a health history related to the male reproductive system. An example of using O-P-Q-R-S-T-U with pain is provided.

The most common concerns related to illness or injury of the male reproductive system are as follows:

- Pain
- Penile discharge
- Penile lesions
- Genital rashes
- Scrotal enlargement
- Groin mass or swelling
- Erectile dysfunction
- Infertility

1. **Pain**
   - Are you having any pain at this time? *If yes:*
   - When did you first notice the pain? How long does it last? *Onset (chronology)*

   ▶ This question helps the nurse determine if the problem is current, experienced in the past only, or chronic.

   - What makes the pain worse? better? *Precipitating (palliative)*
   - Can you describe the pain? It is sharp? dull? burning? *Quality*

   ▶ Testicular torsion may cause excruciating acute pain in the testicular area. Often, the affected testicle will be higher in the scrotal sac than the unaffected testicle. A dull, aching pain is a common symptom of **epididymitis** (inflammation of the epididymis), a common infection in males.

   - Where is the pain located? Does the pain radiate? *Radiation*
   - How often do you experience the pain? How would you rate the pain on a scale of 1 to 10, with 10 being the worst pain? *Severity*
   - Is the pain associated with nausea? vomiting? abdominal distension? fever? chills? burning on urination? *Timing*
   - What do you think is causing the pain? *Understanding*

2. **Penile discharge**
   - Have you noticed any unusual discharge from your penis? *If yes:*

   ▶ Discharge characteristics may indicate whether an infectious process is occurring.

   - What colour? odour? amount?
   - When did you first notice the discharge?
   - Is there any burning or pain with the discharge?
   - Are you sexually active? *If yes,* What kind of sexual activities do you engage in? with men, women, or both? with one or more partners?

   ▶ Questions about types of sexual activities provide information related to risk for STIs.

   - Have you engaged in any sexual activities that would put you at risk of contracting a sexually transmitted infection?

   ▶ Engaging in unprotected intercourse while not in a monogamous relationship is considered a risk for contracting STIs, such as herpes, gonorrhea, syphilis, and chlamydia. It also puts the client as risk for contracting HIV and hepatitis B and C.

3. **Penile lesions**
   - When did you first notice the lesions?

   ▶ A history regarding the lesions should alert the nurse to the possibility of venereal disease.

HEALTH HISTORY QUESTIONS	RATIONALES

4. **Genital rashes**
   - Is there any itching or pain associated with the rash?
   - Is the rash located on any other part of your body?

▶ Male genital rashes are very common. Contact dermatitis, psoriasis, and fixed drug reactions have all been linked to genital rashes so it is important for the nurse to conduct a complete history.

5. **Scrotal enlargement**
   - When did you first notice the enlargement?
   - Exactly where is it?
   - Is it painful?

▶ Most of the time, enlargement is unilateral.

6. **Groin mass or swelling**
   - When did you first notice this?
   - Is it painful?
   - Does it change in size with any type of movement?
   - Have you ever had a hernia?

▶ Hernias are the most common reason for groin swelling and can often be reduced by lying down.

7. **Erectile dysfunction**
   - Are you sexually active? If so, how would you describe your sexual relationships?

▶ These questions may prompt the male client to discuss any concerns about reproductive health.

   - Are there any obstacles to your ability to achieve sexual satisfaction?

▶ Causes of inability to achieve sexual satisfaction include fear of acquiring an STI, fear of being unable to satisfy the partner, fear of pregnancy, confusion regarding sexual orientation, unwillingness to participate in sexual activities enjoyed by the partner, job stress, financial considerations, crowded living conditions, loss of partner, or history of sexual trauma.

   - Have you noticed a change in your sex drive recently? Can you associate the change with anything in particular?

▶ This may be indicative of some physical or psychological problems that need follow-up. Often, clients can relate a decrease in sex drive with stress, illness, drug therapy, or some other factor.

   - Are you able to be sexually aroused?

▶ A variety of factors may influence an individual's ability to become sexually aroused. These include use of prescribed or illicit drugs, disorders of the nervous system, diabetes, stress, and fear (e.g., of intimacy, inability to satisfy a partner, or acquiring an STI).

   - Are you able to achieve and maintain an erection?

▶ The ability to achieve an erection depends on both physiological factors and state of mind.

   - When you have an erection, is the shaft of the penis straight or crooked?

▶ **Peyronie's disease** causes the shaft of the penis to be crooked during an erection.

   - Are you able to achieve orgasm?

▶ Premature ejaculation is defined by some researchers as orgasm immediately after, or even before, penetration. It may also be defined as ejaculation before the male's sexual partner reaches orgasm in more than half the male's sexual experiences. It is often a devastating disorder that may severely compromise sexual relationships. The client can learn techniques to delay ejaculation.

8. **Infertility**

GATHERING THE DATA

HEALTH HISTORY QUESTIONS	RATIONALES

- Do you have children? *If yes,* How many?
- *If not,* Have you tried to have children?
- How long have you been trying?

▶ The couple is not considered possibly infertile unless they have been unable to conceive for a year.

- How often do you and your partner have intercourse?

▶ For couples attempting to become pregnant, it is important to engage in intercourse routinely, two to three times a week. Although nurses do not treat infertility, they may be involved in teaching the client about certain measures that may be helpful for determining the optimal time for intercourse. Concerns about infertility can produce great anxiety for many couples.

Questions Related to Past Health History

1. **Have you ever had mumps?**

▶ Mumps occurring after puberty has been linked to sterility in males.

Questions Related to Behaviours

Healthcare behaviours include both health practices and health patterns. Health practices consist of following recommendations for disease prevention, including screening for risks, screening for early detection of problems, and immunization. Health patterns are habits or acts that affect the client's health. Health behaviours may also include seeking healthcare from healthcare providers who use alternative methods to diagnose and treat illness. Clients should be questioned in a nonjudgmental way and areas for health teaching should be identified.

1. *For clients who are sexually active:*
    - What type of contraception do you use?

▶ This question helps determine the client's knowledge of the product being used and practices around contraception.

    - Would you like to know more about the use of contraceptives?

▶ This is a very important question to ask adolescents who shy away from talking about sexual practices but have said that they are sexually active.

2. **Do you check your genitals on a routine basis?**

▶ Self-examination of the genitals should be performed at least monthly for early detection of changes that need follow-up. Teaching may be indicated if the client is not performing self-examination. Refer to Box 21.1.

3. **How do you protect yourself from sexually transmitted infections, including HIV?**

▶ Abstinence is the only 100% effective protection against STIs. Latex condoms offer significant protection, especially when treated with spermicide; however, they are not 100% effective.

4. **Do you drink alcohol? If so, how many drinks per week do you consume?**

▶ Alcoholism has been linked to impotence. Additionally, intake of alcoholic beverages can contribute to an individual taking chances, such as failing to use condoms, and can affect fertility.

5. **Do you use recreational drugs? If so, what type and how much?**

▶ Taken in sufficient amounts, some drugs, such as marijuana and opiates, may decrease libido and lead to impotence. Drug use may also contribute to failure to use protection against STIs.

GATHERING THE DATA

HEALTH HISTORY QUESTIONS	RATIONALES

Questions Related to the Environment

Environment refers to both internal and external environments. Questions related to the internal environment include all the previous questions and those associated with internal or physiological responses. Questions regarding the external environment include those related to home, work, or social environments.

Internal Environment

1. **Do you know if your mother received diethylstilbestrol (DES) treatment during pregnancy?**

▶ Some reports indicate that sons of DES mothers have higher than average rates of genitourinary problems, such as hypospadias, infertility, and undescended or enlarged testicles. They may be at risk for testicular cancer and have low sperm counts. Physician referral is indicated if the client's response is yes.

2. **Do you take any prescribed or over-the-counter medications, home remedies, herbal or cultural medicines, or dietary supplements?**

▶ Medications, herbs, dietary supplements, and home remedies can alter, enhance, or interfere with one another in terms of therapeutics and can result in side effects affecting reproductive functioning. For example, saw palmetto is used to improve prostate health. Herbal testosterone products, such as nettle root, are also available.

External Environment

The following questions deal with the physical environment of the client. That includes the indoor and outdoor environments of the home and the workplace, those encountered for social engagements, and any encountered during travel.

1. **Have you been exposed to lead, chemicals, or toxins in the environment?**

▶ Lead exposure may result in decreased libido and sperm abnormalities.

2. **Do you use protective equipment when engaged in work or athletic activities?**

▶ The use of protective equipment, including athletic supports and cups, reduces the incidence of testicular damage.

Questions Related to Age

The health history must reflect the anatomical and physiological differences that exist along the age span.

Questions Regarding Infants and Children

1. **Have you noticed any redness, swelling, or discharge that is discoloured or foul smelling in the child's genital areas?**

▶ These symptoms may indicate inflammatory processes or infection.

2. **Have you noticed any asymmetry, lumps, or masses in the infant's genitals?** *If the parent or caregiver answers yes:*
   - Where are they?
   - Are they movable?
   - Hard or soft?
   - Does touching the mass elicit a pain response from the child?

▶ These symptoms may indicate the development of an obstructive process, hydrocele, or inguinal hernia.

3. **Has the child complained of itching, burning, or swelling in the genital area?**

▶ These symptoms may indicate the presence of pinworms or infections such as yeast infections.

HEALTH HISTORY QUESTIONS	RATIONALES

The nurse should ask the preschool child, school-age child, or adolescent the following questions:

1. **Has anyone ever touched you where you didn't want him or her to? Where?**
   (The nurse may want to have the child point to a picture.)

2. **Has anyone ever asked you to touch him or her where you didn't want to? (If the child answers yes, the child may be sexually abused. The nurse should try to obtain additional information by asking the following questions but remember to be sensitive.)**

3. **Where did he or she ask you to touch him or her?**

4. **Who touched you? How many times did this happen? Who knows about this?**

▶ The nurse must try to determine exactly what the person did to the child. Has there been more than touching? Has any other form of sexual contact occurred? The child may feel responsible for the situation and not want to discuss it. The abuser is most often a parent or relative. The nurse should assure the child that he has not been bad and that it helps to talk to an adult about it. Referral should be made to a specialist immediately for sexual abuse examination. Careful documentation is required. Information may be considered forensic evidence. Nurses have the legal duty to report all suspected cases of child abuse to the local police or child welfare agency.

Questions Regarding Adolescents

Many of the questions the nurse asks male adolescents are similar to those the nurse would ask male adults. It is important to explore adolescents' feelings and concerns regarding their sexual development—for instance, concerns about wet dreams. The male adolescent should be reassured that these changes are normal. Some adolescents may be confused about their feelings of sexual attraction to the opposite or same sex. The nurse should ask open-ended questions and assure the male adolescent that all such feelings are normal.

Whether or not a male adolescent admits to being sexually active, the nurse should offer information on teenage pregnancy, birth control, and protection against STIs. Some teenagers may be fearful that the nurse will relay this information to their parents. The nurse should reinforce that all information is confidential, except in situations of sexual abuse.

1. **Are you having sex with anyone now?**

▶ Use of gender-neutral terms prevents value judgments about sexual orientation, which allows clients to define what sex is to them. Many teens think anything that does not involve vaginal penetration is not sex. The nurse should stress that oral sex and other acts are indeed sexual activity.

Questions for the Older Adult

The questions for older male adults are the same as those for younger male adults. In addition, the nurse should explore whether older clients perceive any changes in their sexuality related to advancing age. For example, an older male may find he needs more time to achieve erection. The older adult can be reassured that these changes are normal and do not necessarily indicate disease.

PHYSICAL ASSESSMENT

ASSESSMENT TECHNIQUES AND FINDINGS

The adult male has clean, evenly distributed pubic hair in a diamond pattern, thinning as it extends toward the umbilicus. The penis is free of hair and is of a size appropriate to the stage of development. The skin is of darker pigment than the rest of the body and loose over a flaccid penis. The dorsal vein is midline on the shaft of the penis. The glans penis is smooth and free of lesions or discharge. The urinary meatus is in the centre of the tip of the penis. The scrotum is pear shaped with wrinkled, loose skin and is lower on the left side. The inguinal areas are flat. The penis and scrotum are nontender to palpation. The testes are mobile, smooth, elastic, and solid. The spermatic cord is palpable, smooth, and resilient. The inguinal canal is free of masses or lumps. The anus is darkly pigmented and the perianal area is smooth. The bulbourethral gland is smooth and lesion-free, and the prostate gland is nontender, smooth, and firm.

Physical assessment of the male reproductive system follows an organized pattern. It begins with inspection and palpation of the external genitalia. This is followed by inspection of the perianal area, palpation of the bulbourethral and prostate glands via rectal examination, and examination of stool for occult blood.

> **EQUIPMENT**
>
> examination gown and drape
> clean, nonsterile examination gloves
> examination light
> flashlight
> lubricant
> slides and swabs to obtain a specimen of abnormal discharge
> occult blood test

> **HELPFUL HINTS**
>
> * Provide an environment that is warm and private.
> * Explain each step in the procedure and provide specific instructions about what is expected of the client. For example, the nurse should state whether the client will be expected to sit, stand, or bear down during an assessment.
> * Males from puberty through adulthood respond in a variety of ways when the genitals are exposed for examination. It is imperative to maintain the client's dignity throughout the assessment.
> * Explore cultural issues and seek remedies for concerns at the onset of the interaction.
> * Use routine practices.

TECHNIQUES AND NORMAL FINDINGS	ABNORMAL FINDINGS AND SPECIAL CONSIDERATIONS

INSPECTION

1. Instruct the client.
   * Have the male client empty his bladder and bowel before the examination.
   * Explain to the client that you will be looking at and touching his genitals and pubic area. Tell him that the assessment should not cause physical discomfort. However, he must tell you of pain or discomfort at any point during the examination.
   * Reassure the client that anxiety and embarrassment are normal. Explain that relaxation and focus on instructions will make the assessment easier. If the client experiences an erection during the examination, explain that this is normal and has no sexual connotation.

2. Position the client.
   * The client stands in front of the examiner for the first part of the assessment.

3. Position yourself on a stool sitting in front of the client.

4. Inspect the pubic hair.

TECHNIQUES AND NORMAL FINDINGS	ABNORMAL FINDINGS AND SPECIAL CONSIDERATIONS

- Observe the pubic hair for normal distribution, amount, texture, and cleanliness (see Figure 21.4).

▶ The amount, distribution, and texture of pubic hair vary according to the client's age and race. Absent or extremely sparse hair in the pubic area may be indicative of sexual underdevelopment (Table 21.2). The pubic hair of older adult males may be grey and thinning. Men may have different hair patterns because of waxing or other grooming practices. Confirm the use of these practices with the client.

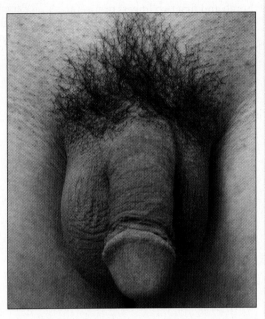

Figure 21.4 ●
Inspecting the pubic hair.

- Confirm that pubic hair is distributed heavily at the symphysis pubis in a diamond- or triangular-shaped pattern, thinning out as it extends toward the umbilicus. The hair will thin as it reaches the inner thigh area and over the scrotum. Hair should be absent on the penis.
- If the client has complained of itching in his pubic area, comb through the pubic hair with two or three fingers.
- Confirm the absence of small bluish-grey spots, or nits (eggs), at the base of the pubic hairs.

▶ These signs indicate the presence of crab or pubic lice. Marks may be visible from persistent scratching to relieve the intense itching crabs cause.

5. **Inspect the penis.**
   - Inspect the penis size, pigmentation, glans, location of the dorsal vein, and the urethral meatus.
   - Start by confirming that the penis size is appropriate for the stage of development of the client. In adult males, penis size varies.

▶ Penis size varies according to the developmental stage of the client (Table 21.2).

   - Note the pigmentation of the penis.
   - Pigmentation should be evenly distributed over the penis. The colour depends on the client's race but will be slightly darker than the colour of the skin over the rest of his body.

▶ Pigmentation of the penis of males with lighter complexions ranges from pink to light brown. In dark-skinned clients, the penis is light to dark brown.

   - Assess the looseness of the skin over the shaft of the penis. The skin should be loose over the flaccid penis.
   - Confirm that the dorsal vein is midline on the shaft.
   - Inspect the glans penis. It should be smooth and free of lesions or discharge. No redness or inflammation should be present. **Smegma**, a white, cheeselike substance, may be present. This finding is considered normal.

▶ Discharge or lesions may indicate the presence of infective diseases, such as *herpes, genital warts, or syphilis,* or may indicate cancer. If discharge is present, the substance should be cultured. Consistency, colour, and odour are noted.

PHYSICAL ASSESSMENT

| TECHNIQUES AND NORMAL FINDINGS | ABNORMAL FINDINGS AND SPECIAL CONSIDERATIONS |

- If the client is uncircumcised, either ask the client to pull the foreskin back or do so yourself. To retract the foreskin, gently pull the skin down over the penile shaft from the side of the glans using the thumb and first two fingers or forefinger (see Figure 21.5).

▶ Phimosis is a condition in which the foreskin is so tight that it cannot be retracted.

Paraphimosis describes a condition in which the foreskin, once retracted, becomes so tight that it cannot be moved back over the glans.

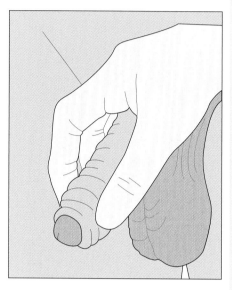

Figure 21.5 ●
Retracting the foreskin.

- Gently move the foreskin back into place over the glans. The foreskin should move smoothly.

▶ Immediate assistance must be sought if the foreskin cannot be retracted. Prolonged constriction of the vessels can obstruct blood flow and lead to tissue damage or necrosis.

6. Assess the position of the urinary meatus.

- The meatus should be located in the centre of the tip of the penis (see Figure 21.6).

▶ In rare cases, the urinary meatus is located on the upper side of the glans (*epispadias*) or the under side of the glans (*hypospadias*). These conditions are usually corrected surgically shortly after birth.

A pinpoint appearance to the urinary meatus is indicative of **urethral stricture**.

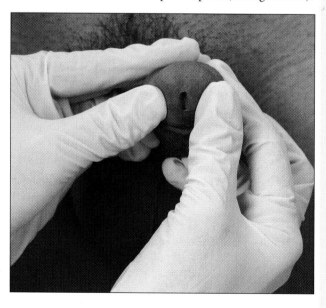

Figure 21.6 ●
Assessing the position of the urinary meatus.

7. Inspect the scrotum.

- Ask the client to hold his penis up so that the scrotum is fully exposed (see Figure 21.7). Optionally, you may hold the penis up by letting it rest on the back of your nondominant hand.

PHYSICAL ASSESSMENT

TECHNIQUES AND NORMAL FINDINGS	ABNORMAL FINDINGS AND SPECIAL CONSIDERATIONS

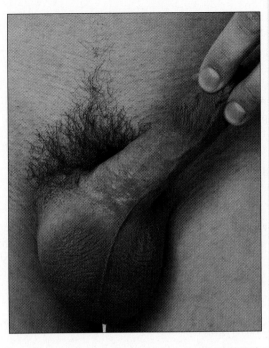

Figure 21.7 ●
Inspecting the scrotum.

- Observe the shape of the scrotum and how it hangs. It should be pear shaped, with the left side hanging lower than the right.

  ▶ An appearance of flatness could suggest testicular abnormality. Older adult males may have a pendulous, sagging scrotal sac.

- Inspect the front and back of the scrotum. The skin should be wrinkled, loosely fitting over its internal structures. Note any swelling, redness, distended veins, and lesions. If swelling is present, note if it is unilateral or bilateral.

  ▶ Scrotal swelling and inflammation could suggest problems, such as **orchitis** (inflammation of the testicles), *epididymitis* (inflammation of the epididymis), *scrotal edema* (an accumulation of fluid in the scrotum), *scrotal hernia,* or *testicular torsion* (twisting of the testicle onto the spermatic cord). Swelling and inflammation may also be seen in renal, cardiovascular, and other systemic disorders.

- If you detect a mass, you may want to perform transillumination.

  ▶ Note any area where the light does not transilluminate. Light will not penetrate a mass. Masses may indicate *testicular tumour,* **spermatocele** (a cyst located in the epididymis), or other conditions.

- In a darkened room, place a lighted flashlight behind the area in which the abnormal mass was palpated (see Figure 21.8).

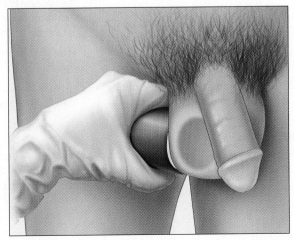

Figure 21.8 ●
Transilluminating the scrotum.

TECHNIQUES AND NORMAL FINDINGS

ABNORMAL FINDINGS AND SPECIAL CONSIDERATIONS

- Note that the light shines through the scrotum with a red glow. The testicle shows up as a nontransparent oval structure.
- Repeat these steps on the other side and compare the results.

8. Inspect the inguinal area.

- The inguinal area should be flat. This may be difficult to confirm if the client is overweight. Even in the presence of adipose tissue, the contour of the inguinal area should be consistent with the rest of the body. Lymph nodes are present in this location, but not normally visible.
- Inspect both the right and the left inguinal areas with the client breathing normally.
- Have the client hold his breath and bear down as if having a bowel movement.
- Observe for any evidence of lumps or masses. The contour of the inguinal areas should remain even.

▶ Masses or lumps may be related to the presence of an inguinal hernia or cancer within the reproductive, abdominal, urinary, lymphatic, and other systems.

PALPATION

1. Palpate the penis.

- Place the glans between your thumb and forefinger.
- Gently compress the glans, allowing the meatus to gape open (see Figure 21.9). The meatus should be pink, patent, and free of discharge.

▶ The client may be hesitant to verbalize pain when palpation is performed. It is important to watch for nonverbal facial and body gestures.
   A *urethral stricture* is suspected if the meatus is only about the size of a pinpoint.
   Signs of *urethritis* include redness and edema around the glans and foreskin, eversion of urethral mucosa, and drainage. If urethritis is suspected, the client should be asked if he experiences itching and tenderness around the meatus and painful urination. If drainage is present, observe for colour, consistency, odour, and amount. Obtain a specimen if indicated. Suspect a gonococcal infection (gonorrhea) if the drainage is profuse and thick, purulent, and greenish yellow.
   Consider inflammation or infection higher up in the urinary tract if redness, edema, and discharge are visible around the urethral opening, because the mucous membrane in the urethra is continuous with the mucous membrane in the rest of the tract.

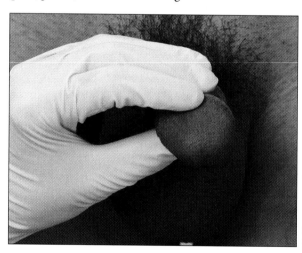

Figure 21.9 ●
Palpating the penis.

- Note any discharge or tenderness.

- Continue gentle palpation and compression up the entire shaft of the penis.

▶ Be alert for any lesions, masses, swelling, or nodules.

▶ Note characteristics of any abnormal findings. Culture any discharge.

2. Palpate the scrotum.

- Ask the client to hold his penis up to expose the scrotum.
- Gently palpate the left and then the right scrotal sacs (see Figure 21.10). Each scrotal sac should be nontender, soft, and boggy. The structures within the sacs should move easily with your palpation.

▶ Assess shape, size, consistency, location, and mobility of any masses. If the client expresses pain, lift the scrotum. If the pain is relieved, the client may have epididymitis, inflammation of the epididymis.

PHYSICAL ASSESSMENT

TECHNIQUES AND NORMAL FINDINGS	ABNORMAL FINDINGS AND SPECIAL CONSIDERATIONS

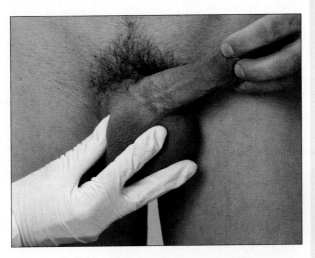

Figure 21.10 •
Palpating the scrotum.

- Note any tenderness, swelling, masses, lesions, or nodules.

CLINICAL TIP
Do not pinch or squeeze any mass, lesion, or other structure.

---

3. **Palpate the testes.**
   - Be sure that your hands are warm.

   - Approach each testis from the bottom of the scrotal sac, and gently rotate it between your thumb and fingertips (see Figure 21.11). Each testis should be nontender, oval shaped, walnut-sized, smooth, elastic, and solid.

▶ The **cremasteric reflex** may cause the testicles to migrate upward temporarily. Cold hands, a cold room, or the stimulus of touch could cause this response.

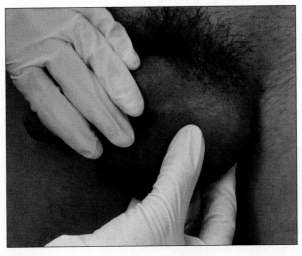

Figure 21.11 •
Palpating the testes.

4. **Palpate the epididymis.**
   - Slide your fingertips around to the posterior side of each testicle to find the epididymis, a small, crescent-shaped structure.

▶ In some clients, the epididymis may be palpated on the front surface of each testis.

TECHNIQUES AND NORMAL FINDINGS	ABNORMAL FINDINGS AND SPECIAL CONSIDERATIONS

5. Palpate the spermatic cord.

- Slide your fingers up just above the testicle, feeling for a vertical, ropelike structure about 3 mm (0.1 in.) wide.

▶ A cord that is hard, beaded, or nodular could indicate the presence of a varicosity or varicocele. A **varicocele** is a distended cord and is a common cause of male infertility. On palpation, it may feel like a "bag of worms."

- Do not squeeze or pinch. Trace the cord up to the external inguinal ring by using a gentle rotating motion.
- Gently grasp the cord between your thumb and index finger (see Figure 21.12).

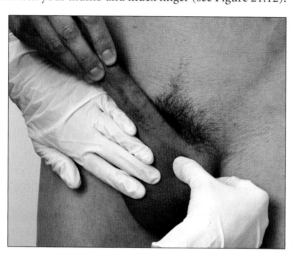

Figure 21.12 ●
Palpating the spermatic cord.

- The cord should feel thin, smooth, nontender to palpation, and resilient.

6. Palpate the inguinal region.

- Start by preparing the client for palpation in the right inguinal area.
- Ask the client to shift his balance so that his weight is on his left leg.
- Place your right index finger in the upper corner of the right scrotum.
- Slowly palpate the spermatic cord up and slightly to the client's left.
- Allow the client's scrotal skin to fold over your index finger as you palpate.
- Proceed until you feel an opening that feels like a triangular slit. This is the external ring of the inguinal canal. Attempt to gently glide your finger into this opening (see Figure 21.13).

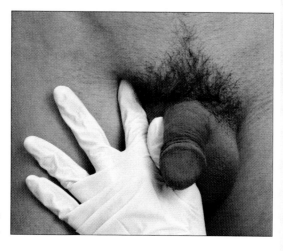

Figure 21.13 ●
Palpating the inguinal canal.

Techniques and Normal Findings

> **CLINICAL TIP**
> *If you cannot insert your finger with gentle pressure, do not force your finger into the opening.*

- If the opening has admitted your finger, ask the client to either cough or bear down.
- Palpate for masses or lumps.
- Repeat this procedure by palpating the client's left inguinal area. Use your left index finger when performing the palpation.

▶ An *inguinal hernia* feels like a bulge or mass.

A *direct inguinal hernia* can be palpated in the area of the external ring of the inguinal ligament. It will be felt either right at the external ring opening or just behind it.

An *indirect inguinal hernia* is more common, especially in younger males. It is located deeper in the inguinal canal than the direct inguinal hernia. It can pass into the scrotum, whereas a direct inguinal hernia rarely protrudes into the scrotum.

It is also possible that a *femoral hernia* may be present. It is more commonly found in the right inguinal area and near the inguinal ligament. Table 21.1 illustrates these three types of hernias. If the client displays an acute bulge with tenderness, pain, nausea, or vomiting, he may have a strangulated hernia. Help him to lie down and request immediate assistance from a physician.

7. **Palpate the inguinal lymph chain.**
   - Use the pads of your first three fingers to palpate the inguinal lymph nodes.
   - Confirm that nodes are nonpalpable and the area is nontender (see Figure 21.14).

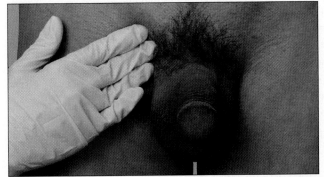

Figure 21.14 ●
Palpating the inguinal lymph nodes.

- Occasionally some of the inguinal lymph nodes are palpable. They are usually less than 0.5 cm (0.25 in.) in size, spongy, movable, and nontender.

▶ It is important to assess if a node is larger than 0.5 cm (0.25 in.) or if multiple nodes are present. Tenderness in this area suggests infection of the scrotum, penis, or groin area.

8. **Inspect the perianal area.**
   - Reposition the client. Ask the client to turn and face the table and bend over at the waist. The client can rest his arms on the table (see Figure 21.15).
   - If the client is unable to tolerate this position, he may lie on his left side on the examination table with both knees flexed.

TECHNIQUES AND NORMAL FINDINGS

ABNORMAL FINDINGS AND SPECIAL CONSIDERATIONS

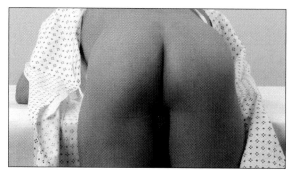

Figure 21.15 ●
Positioning for assessment
of internal structures.

- Inspect the sacrococcygeal and perianal areas. The skin should be smooth and without lesions.

▶ Tufts of hair or dimpling at the sacrococcygeal area are associated with pilonidal cysts. Rashes, redness, excoriation, or inflammation in the perianal area can signal infection or parasitic infestation.

9. Palpate the sacrococcygeal and perianal areas.
- The areas should be nontender and without palpable masses.

▶ Tenderness, mass, or inflammation may indicate a pilonidal cyst, an anal abscess, a fissure, or pruritus.

10. Inspect the anus.
- Spread the buttocks apart. Visualize the anus. The skin is darker and coarse. The area should be free of lesions.
- Ask the client to bear down. The tissue stretches, but there are no bulges or discharge.

▶ Lesions may include skin tags, warts, hemorrhoids, or fissures.

▶ Fistulas, fissures, internal hemorrhoids, or rectal prolapse are more easily detected when the client bears down.

11. Palpate the bulbourethral gland and the prostate gland.
- Lubricate the index finger of your dominant hand with lubricating gel.
- Tell the client that you are going to insert your finger into his rectum to palpate his prostate gland. Explain that the insertion may cause him to feel as if he needs to have a bowel movement. Tell him that this technique should not cause pain but to inform you immediately if it does.
- Place the index finger of your dominant hand against the anal opening (see Figure 21.16). Be sure that your finger is slightly bent and not forming a right angle to the buttocks. If you insert your index finger at a right angle to the buttocks, the client may experience pain.

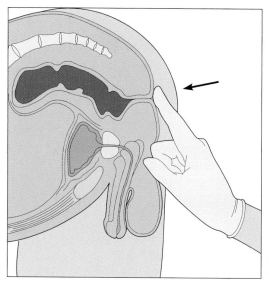

Figure 21.16 ●
Placing the finger against
the anal opening.

| TECHNIQUES AND NORMAL FINDINGS | ABNORMAL FINDINGS AND SPECIAL CONSIDERATIONS |

- Apply gentle pressure as you insert your bent finger into the anus (see Figure 21.17).

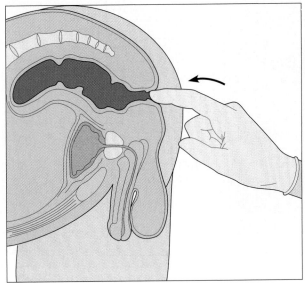

Figure 21.17 •
Inserting the finger
into the anus.

- As the sphincter muscle tightens, stop inserting your finger.
- Resume as the sphincter muscle relaxes.
- Press your right thumb gently against the perianal area.
- Palpate the bulbourethral gland by pressing your index finger gently toward your thumb (see Figure 21.18). This should not cause the client to feel pain or tenderness. No swelling or masses should be felt.

▶ If the bulbourethral gland is inflamed, the client may feel pain on palpation. Referral for further examination is warranted.

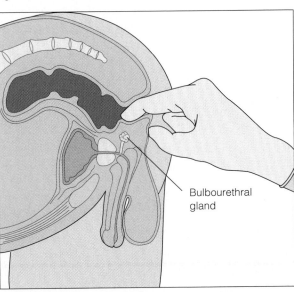

Bulbourethral
gland

Figure 21.18 •
Palpating the
bulbourethral gland.

- Release the pressure between your index finger and thumb. Continue to insert your index finger gently (see Figure 21.19).
- Palpate the posterior surface of the prostate gland.
- Confirm that it is smooth, firm, even somewhat rubbery, nontender, and extends out no more than 1 cm (0.5 in.) into the rectal area.
- Remove your finger slowly and gently.

▶ Note tenderness, masses, nodules, hardness, or softness. Nodules are characteristic of *prostate cancer.* Tenderness indicates inflammation.

TECHNIQUES AND NORMAL FINDINGS

ABNORMAL FINDINGS AND SPECIAL CONSIDERATIONS

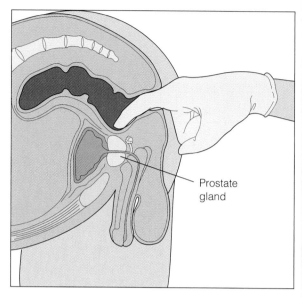

Figure 21.19 ●
Palpating the
prostate gland.

12. Examine the stool.

- Inspect feces remaining on the gloved finger. Feces is normally brown and soft.

▶ Rectal bleeding is suspected when bright red blood is on the surface of the stool. Feces mixed with bright red blood is associated with bleeding above the rectum. Black, tarry stool is associated with upper gastrointestinal tract bleeding.

- Test feces for occult blood. Normally, the test is negative. A positive test may signal the presence of occult blood but may occur if red meat was eaten within 3 days of the test.
- Remove your gloves.
- Wash your hands.
- Help the client to a comfortable position.
- Give the client tissues to wipe the perianal area.

SAMPLE DOCUMENTATION

Subjective: 27-year-old male presents to clinic for routine check. No concerns with urination, sexual function, or ejaculation. Urine clear amber, no discharge. Stable, monogamous relationship, uses condoms. Nonsmoker, nondrinker. No meds, no allergies.

Objective: Genital area free of rednwess or lesions. No masses or tenderness on palpation to shaft, glands, or scrotum. Testes ovoid, nontender. No abnormalities detected with transillumination. No bulges in inguinal canal, no lymphadenopathy. Prostate surface smooth, nontender.

APPLICATION THROUGH CRITICAL THINKING

CASE STUDY

James Lewis is a 24-year-old male who is seen in the clinic for "pain in the groin." During the interview the client states, "I have a soreness in my groin area on both sides." Mr. Lewis denies any trauma to the area, states he has not done any heavy lifting or been involved in athletic activities or "working out." He reports that he is in good health. He does not take any medications except vitamins and occasionally some non-Aspirin product for a headache. He denies nausea, vomiting, diarrhea, or fever. He has no pain in his legs or back. He tells the nurse his appetite is okay but he is tired. He thinks his fatigue is because he's been "a little worried about this problem and really having a hard time deciding to come in for help."

When asked about the onset of the problem, Mr. Lewis explains that he "started feeling some achiness about a week ago." When asked if he has ever experienced these feelings before, he replies, "No." He is then asked to describe or discuss any other symptoms. He looks away, shifts in his chair, and then says, "Well, I have had some burning when I pass urine, and it's kind of cloudy."

Mr. Lewis tells the nurse that he is sexually active and is not in a monogamous relationship. He generally avoids using condoms because "I've known these girls for a long time."

The physical examination yields the following information: B/P 128/86—P 96—RR 20—T 37°C (98.6°F). His colour is pale, and the skin is moist and warm. External genitalia are intact, without lesions or erythema. There is lymphadenopathy in bilateral groin areas. Compression of the glans yields milky discharge. A smear of urethral discharge is obtained and returns positive for both gonococcal and chlamydia. He is treated with a 7-day regimen of oral antibiotics and STI contact tracing is completed.

The nurse recommends a single-dose treatment for gonorrhea and an oral regimen for chlamydia. A urine specimen will be obtained and submitted with the urethral discharge smear.

The client will be scheduled for a follow-up phone conference about the laboratory results in 48 hours and a return visit in 7 days. The nurse conducts an information, education, and advice session before discharge from the clinic.

► *Complete Documentation*

The following is sample documentation for James Lewis.

SUBJECTIVE DATA: Seeking care for "pain in groin." Pain in groin bilateral. Denies trauma, heavy lifting, athletic activity, or "working out." Reports he is in "good health." Takes no medications except vitamins and non-Aspirin product for a headache. Denies nausea, vomiting, diarrhea, or fever. No pain in back or legs. Reports "okay" appetite. Reports fatigue. "Became a little worried about this problem and decided to come in

ASSESSMENT FORM	
Reason for Visit: *"Pain in groin"*	
History:	
Reproductive Disease:	*Gonorrhea 2 mos. ago*
Medications:	*Vitamins, non-ASA product for headache*
Sexual History:	*Multiple partners*
Condom Use:	*None*
HIV Testing:	*Unknown*
Erectile Function:	*Unknown*
Safety:	*Not inform partners of diagnosis*
Other:	*Burning on urination, cloudy urine, fatigue, okay appetite*
Physical Findings:	
External Genitalia:	*No lesions, no erythema*
Meatus:	*Milky discharge on compression of glans (specimen to labs)*
Inguinal Area:	*Lymphadenopathy (bilateral)*

for help." Achiness 1 week ago. Burning on urination, cloudy urine. Is sexually active with multiple partners, generally avoids condoms.

OBJECTIVE DATA: VS: B/P 128/86—P 96—RR 20—T 37°C. Colour pale, skin moist and warm. External genitalia intact, no lesions or erythema. Lymphadenopathy bilateral groin. Milky discharge on compression of glans. Culture to lab.

▶ Critical Thinking Questions

1. Describe the critical thinking process as applied by the nurse to direct the care of this client.
2. What additional data should the nurse seek when conducting the health assessment for this client?
3. What data informed the nurse of a need to provide education for the client?
4. What data will the nurse seek on the return visit with Mr. Lewis?

▶ Applying Nursing Diagnoses

1. *Ineffective sexuality patterns* is a nursing diagnosis in the NANDA-I taxonomy (see Appendix A ⬭). Do the data for Mr. Lewis support this diagnosis? If so, identify the data that support the diagnosis.

2. Identify additional diagnoses suggested in the data. Develop PES (problem, etiology, signs or symptoms) statements.

▶ Prepare Teaching Plan

LEARNING NEED: The data from the case study reveal that James Lewis is at an increased risk for contracting sexually transmitted infections. Education and counselling will be provided for this client.

The case study provides data that are representative of concerns about sexually transmitted infection of many individuals. Therefore, the following teaching plan is based on the need to provide information to members of any community about sexually transmitted infections.

GOAL: The participants in this learning program will have the knowledge to prevent contraction and transmission of sexually transmitted infections.

OBJECTIVES: At the completion of this learning session the participants will be able to do the following:

1. Describe sexually transmitted infections.
2. Identify symptoms of sexually transmitted infections.
3. Discuss treatment strategies.
4. Describe methods to prevent contraction and transmission of sexually transmitted infections.

Application of Objective 4: Describe methods to prevent contraction and transmission of sexually transmitted infections.		
Content	**Teaching Strategy**	**Evaluation**
• Avoid sexual contact with partners whose health status is unclear. • Use condoms correctly and consistently during sexual intercourse. • When infected, notify all sexual partners so they can be treated. Refrain from sexual contact for 1 week after treatment ends. Take all prescribed medications exactly as ordered.	• Lecture • Discussion • Audiovisual materials • Printed materials Lecture is appropriate when disseminating information to large groups. Discussion allows participants to bring up concerns and to raise questions. Audiovisual materials, such as illustrations of the genitals and reproductive structures, reinforce verbal presentation. Printed material, especially to be taken away with learners, allows review, reinforcement, and reading at the learner's pace.	• Written examination. May use short answer, fill-in, or multiple-choice items or a combination of items. If these are short and easy to evaluate, the learner receives immediate feedback.

HEALTH PROMOTION ASSESSMENT TOOL

Social Determinants of Health	Level of Action	Action Strategies
Social environments	Individual and community	**Develop personal skills** • Prevent the spread of the sexually transmitted infection by notifying the communicable disease and infection control within the local health region. • Explore barriers that could inhibit or factors that could facilitate Mr. Lewis's abstinence from sexual activity until he is told it is safe to have sex. • Assess his understanding of the complications of sexually transmitted infections and his understanding of the risks for his sexual partners, which include pelvic inflammatory disease or sterility, and if a sexual partner becomes pregnant her infant is at risk of contracting gonorrhea during delivery. • Collect information about all his sexual partners in the past three months. Provide information for Mr. Lewis to give to his sexual partners regarding their legal obligation to be tested for STIs, explaining that a public health official will contact them if they are not tested. • Highly recommend HIV screening and immunization for hepatitis B if Mr. Lewis has not already been vaccinated.
Gender	Individual	**Develop personal skills** • Explore Mr. Lewis's statement that he generally avoids condoms because "I've known these girls for a long time." • Examine his values and beliefs related to sexual relations and what it means to be the male partner in a relationship. What underlies his reluctance to use condoms? • Provide education as needed on the benefits of condom use related to the prevention of sexually transmitted infections (as Mr. Lewis may not be informed about the benefits of condoms beyond their usefulness for pregnancy prevention).

ABNORMAL FINDINGS

Abnormal findings of the male reproductive system include inguinal hernias, disorders of the penis, abnormalities of the scrotum, and problems in the perianal area. These are depicted in Figures 21.20 through 21.37.

Abnormalities of the Penis

Hypospadias

Hypospadias is congenital displacement of the meatus to the inferior surface of the penis (see Figure 21.20).

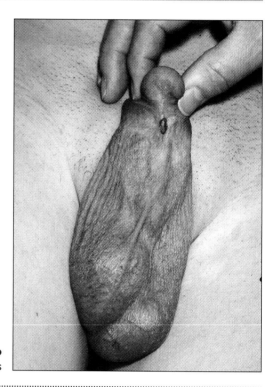

Figure 21.20 •
Hypospadias

Peyronie's Disease

In Peyronie's disease, hard plaques are found along the dorsum and are palpable under the skin. These plaques result in pain and bending of the penis during erection.

Carcinoma

Carcinoma of the penis usually occurs in the glans. It appears as a reddened nodule growth or ulcerlike lesion (see Figure 21.21).

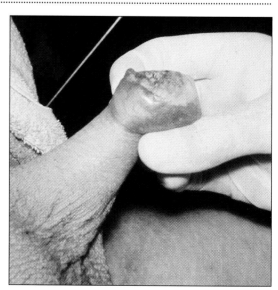

Figure 21.21 •
Carcinoma.

Genital Warts

Caused by human papillomavirus (HPV), genital warts are rapidly growing, papillar lesions (see Figure 21.22).

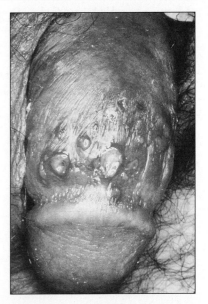

Figure 21.22 •
Genital warts.

Syphilitic Chancre

Syphilitic chancre are nontender lesions that appear as round or oval reddened ulcers (see Figure 21.23). Lymphadenopathy is present.

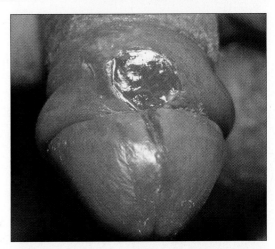

Figure 21.23 •
Syphilitic chancre.

Genital Herpes

Small vesicles appear in clusters on any part of the surface of the penis (see Figure 21.24) in genital herpes. These are painful, and the area around the vesicles is erythematous.

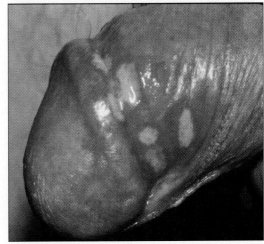

Figure 21.24 •
Genital herpes.

Abnormalities of the Scrotum

Hydrocele

A hydrocele is a fluid-filled mass that is nontender (see Figure 21.25). The mass occurs within the tunica vaginalis.

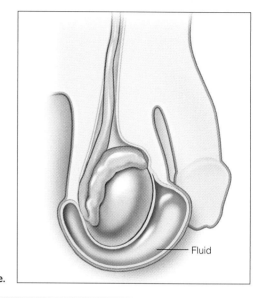

Fluid

Figure 21.25 ● Hydrocele.

Scrotal Hernia

A scrotal hernia is commonly an indirect inguinal hernia located within the scrotum (see Figure 21.26).

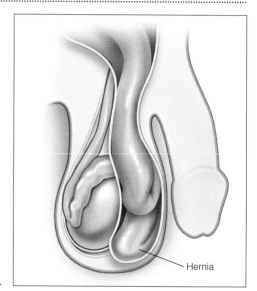

Hernia

Figure 21.26 ● Scrotal hernia.

Testicular Tumour

A testicular tumour is a painless nodule on the testes (see Figure 21.27). As it grows, the entire testicle seems to be overtaken.

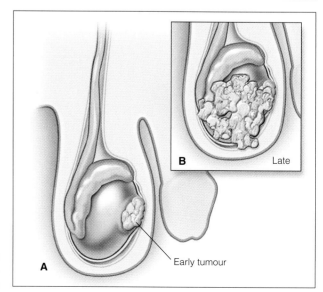

B   Late

A

Early tumour

Figure 21.27 ●
Testicular tumour.
A. Early. B. Late.

Orchitis

The inflammatory process of orchitis results in painful, tender, and swollen testes (see Figure 21.28).

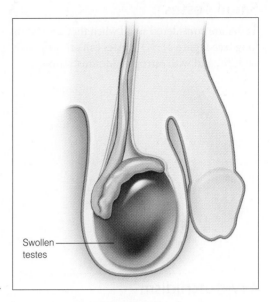

Swollen testes

Figure 21.28 ● Orchitis.

Epididymitis

Occurring in adults, epididymitis is often accompanied by urinary tract infection. The epididymis is inflamed and tender (see Figure 21.29).

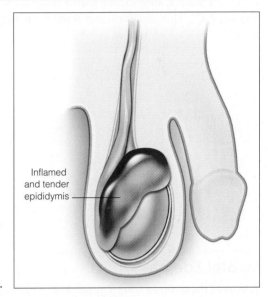

Inflamed and tender epididymis

Figure 21.29 ● Epididymitis.

Torsion of the Spermatic Cord

Torsion occurs with greatest frequency in adolescents. The twisting of the testicle or the spermatic cord creates edema and pain (see Figure 21.30). This condition requires immediate surgical intervention.

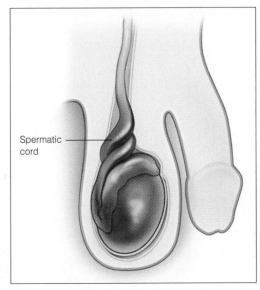

Spermatic cord

Figure 21.30 ●
Torsion of the spermatic cord.

Small Testes

Testes are considered small when they are less than 2 cm (1 in.) long (see Figure 21.31). Testes can atrophy in liver disease, in orchitis, and with estrogen administration.

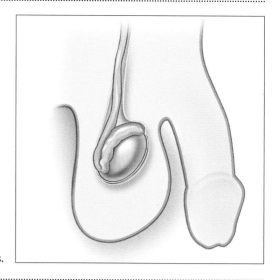

Figure 21.31 ● Small testes.

Cryptorchidism

Cryptorchidism is absence of a testicle in the scrotal sac (see Figure 21.32). This condition may result from undescended testicles.

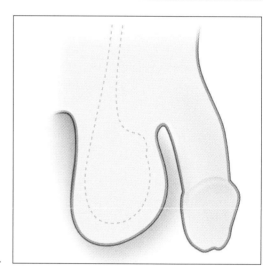

Figure 21.32 ● Cryptorchidism.

Scrotal Edema

Edema of the scrotum is seen in conditions causing edema of the lower body, including renal disease and heart failure (see Figure 21.33).

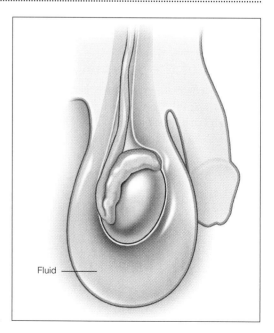

Fluid

Figure 21.33 ● Scrotal edema.

Abnormalities of the Perianal Area

Pilonidal Cyst

Pilonidal cysts are seen as dimpling in the sacrococcygeal area at the midline (see Figure 21.34). An opening is visible and may reveal a tuft of hair. Usually asymptomatic, these cysts can become acutely abscessed or drain chronically.

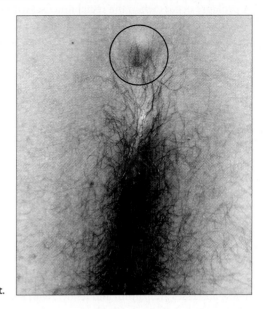

Figure 21.34 ● Pilonidal cyst.

Anal Fissure

Tears in the anal mucosa are known as fissures. These are usually seen in the posterior anal area. They are most frequently associated with passage of hard stools.

Hemorrhoids

Varicosities of the hemorrhoidal veins are called hemorrhoids or piles. These are considered normal findings in adults when they are asymptomatic.

Internal hemorrhoids occur in the venous plexus superior to the mucocutaneous junction of the anus (see Figure 21.35A). Internal hemorrhoids are rarely painful. They are identified by bright red bleeding unmixed with stool.

External hemorrhoids occur in the inferior venous plexus inferior to the mucocutaneous junction (see Figure 21.35B). External hemorrhoids rarely bleed. External hemorrhoids cause anal irritation and create difficulty with cleansing the area.

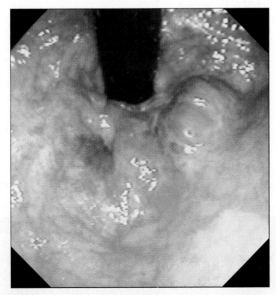

Figure 21.35A ● Hemorrhoids, internal.

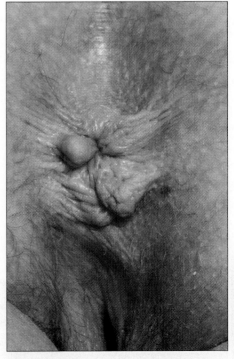

Figure 21.35B ● Hemorrhoids, external.

Prolapse of the Rectum

A prolapse occurs when the rectal mucosa, with or without the muscle, protrudes through the anus (see Figure 21.36). In mucosal prolapse, a round or oval pink protrusion is seen outside the anus. When the muscular wall is involved, a large red protrusion is visible.

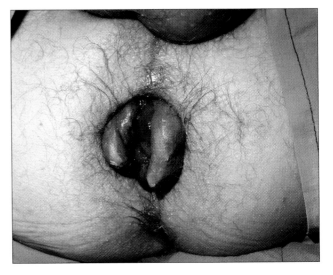

Figure 21.36 ●
Prolapse of the rectum.

Perianal Perirectal Abscess

These abscesses are painful and tender, with perianal erythema. They are generally caused by infection of an anal gland. Anal abscesses can lead to fistulas, which are openings between the anal canal and the outside skin (see Figure 21.37).

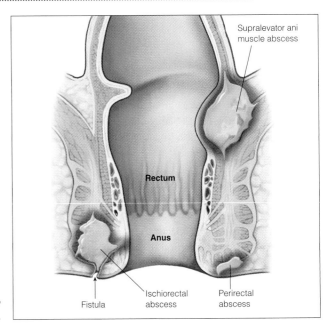

Figure 21.37 ●
Perianal perirectal abscess.

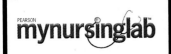

22

FEMALE REPRODUCTIVE SYSTEM

THE FEMALE REPRODUCTIVE SYSTEM PROVIDES FOR both human reproduction and sexual gratification. Many factors influence the female client's reproductive health on both physiological and psychological levels. Assessment of the client's psychosocial health, self-care habits, family, culture, and environment is an important part of the health history. The nurse must keep these findings in mind when conducting the physical assessment. The nurse also must have a thorough understanding of the constituents of a healthy reproductive system and be able to consider the relationship of other body systems to the reproductive system.

Throughout assessment of the female reproductive system, the nurse considers not only the function of the reproductive system but also the client's sexual fulfillment on both a physical and a psychological basis.

Nurses need to understand their own feelings and comfort about various aspects of sexuality to be efficient in gathering data. They must put aside personal beliefs and values about sexual practices and focus in a culturally competent and nonjudgmental manner on gathering data to determine the health status of the client.

It is essential to create an atmosphere that facilitates open communication and comfort for the client. Clients commonly experience anxiety, fear, and embarrassment when asked for information about a topic that, in most clients' minds, is very personal. These emotions may be expressed either verbally or nonverbally. The nurse should approach the client in as nonthreatening a manner as possible and assure the client that the information provided and the results of the physical examination will remain confidential.

ANATOMY AND PHYSIOLOGY REVIEW

The female reproductive system is unique in that it experiences cyclic changes in direct response to hormonal levels of estrogen and progesterone during the childbearing years. The uterus changes throughout the ovarian cycle, during which the ova (eggs) are prepared for fertilization with sperm. During the menstrual cycle, the uterine lining is prepared for the development of a fetus. The onset of menopause represents the end of the childbearing years.

Unlike the male reproductive system, the female reproductive tract is completely separate from the urinary tract. However, structures of the two tracts lie within close proximity.

The functions of the female reproductive system are the following:

- Manufacturing and protecting ova for fertilization
- Transporting the fertilized ovum for implantation and embryonic and fetal development
- Regulating hormonal production and secretion of several sex hormones
- Providing sexual stimulation and pleasure

External Genitalia

Female external genitalia include the mons pubis, labia, glands, clitoris, and perianal area. These will be described in the sections that follow.

Mons Pubis

The mons pubis is the mound of adipose tissue overlying the symphysis pubis (see Figure 22.1). In the mature female, it is thickly covered with hair and provides protection to the underlying reproductive structures.

Labia Majora and Labia Minora

The **labia** are a dual set of liplike structures lying on either side of the vagina (Figure 22.1). The exterior labia majora are two thick, elongated pads of tissue that become fuller toward the centre. An extension of the external skin surface, the labia majora are covered with coarse hair extending from the mons pubis. The enclosed labia minora are two thin,

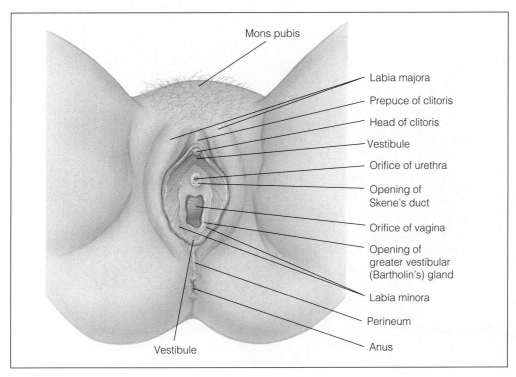

Figure 22.1 labels: Mons pubis, Labia majora, Prepuce of clitoris, Head of clitoris, Vestibule, Orifice of urethra, Opening of Skene's duct, Orifice of vagina, Opening of greater vestibular (Bartholin's) gland, Labia minora, Perineum, Anus, Vestibule

Figure 22.1 ● External female genitalia.

elongated pads of tissue that overlie the vaginal and urethral openings, as well as several glandular openings. Anteriorly, the labia minora join to form the prepuce, which covers the clitoris. Posteriorly, the labia join to form the *fourchette* (small fold of membrane). The labia minora border an almond-shaped area of tissue known as the *vestibule*. It extends from the clitoris to the fourchette. The urethral meatus, **introitus** (vaginal opening), Skene's glands, and Bartholin's glands lie within the vestibule. The major function of the labia is to protect the urethra and vagina, and ultimately other urinary and reproductive structures, from infection and physical injury.

Skene's and Bartholin's Glands

The Skene's glands, also called **paraurethral glands**, are located just posterior to the urethra (Figure 22.1). They open into the urethra and secrete a fluid that lubricates the vaginal vestibule during sexual intercourse. The **Bartholin's glands**, or greater vestibular glands, are located posteriorly at the base of the vestibule and produce mucus, which is released into the vestibule (Figure 22.1). This mucus actively promotes sperm motility and viability.

Clitoris

Located at the anterior of the vestibule is the **clitoris**, a small, elongated mound of erectile tissue (Figure 22.1). As the labia minora merge together anteriorly, a small hoodlike covering is formed that lies over the top of the clitoris. The clitoris is homologous with the penis. It is permeated with numerous nerve fibres that are responsive to touch. When stimulated, the clitoris becomes erect as its underlying corpus cavernosa become vasocongested. The major function of the clitoris is serving as the primary organ of sexual stimulation.

Perianal Area

The perianal area is bordered anteriorly by the top of the labial folds, laterally by the ischial tuberosities, and posteriorly by the anus (Figure 22.1). The anus is the terminal end of the gastrointestinal system. The anal canal opens onto the perineum at the midpoint of the gluteal folds. The external muscles of the anal canal are skeletal muscles, which form the part of the anal sphincter that voluntarily controls stool evacuation. The anal mucosa is smooth, moist, hairless, and darkly pigmented.

Internal Reproductive Organs

The internal female reproductive organs are the vagina, uterus, cervix, fallopian tubes, and ovaries. These organs will be described in the paragraphs that follow.

Vagina

The **vagina** is a long, tubular, muscular canal, approximately 9 to 15 cm (3.5 to 6 in.) long, that extends from the vestibule to the cervix at the inferior end of the uterus (see Figure 22.2A). The muscularity of the vaginal wall and its thick, transverse rugae (ridges) allow it to dilate widely to accommodate the erect penis and, during childbirth, the head of the fetus. At the point of juncture with the cervix, a continuous circular cleft called the *fornix* is formed. The major functions of the vagina are serving as the female organ of copulation, the birth canal, and the channel for the exit of menstrual flow.

Uterus

The **uterus** is a pear-shaped, hollow, muscular organ that is located centrally in the pelvis between the neck of the bladder and the rectal wall (Figure 22.2A). The body of the uterus is

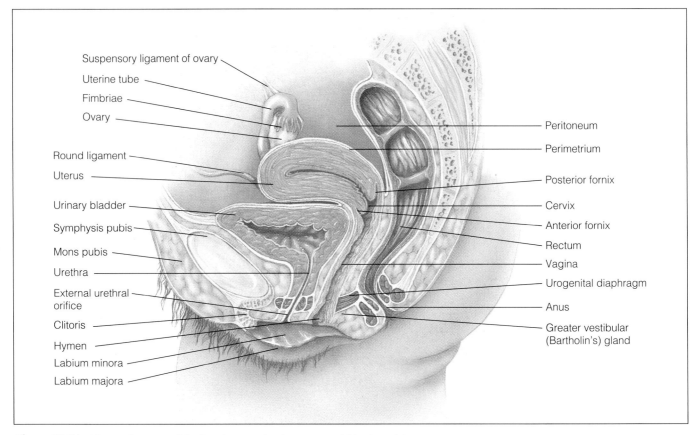

Figure 22.2A ● Internal organs of the female reproductive system within the pelvis.

about 4 cm (1.5 in.) wide and 6 to 8 cm (2.5 to 3 in.) long. Its walls are 2 to 2.5 cm (1 in.) thick and are composed of serosal, muscular, and mucosal layers. Anatomically, the uterus is divided into three segments: the fundus, the corpus, and the cervix. The **cervix** projects into the vagina about 2.5 cm (1 in.) and is about 2.5 cm (1 in.) round. A small central canal connects the vagina to the inside of the uterus. The external **cervical os**

is the inferior opening (the vaginal end of the canal), and the *internal cervical os* opens directly into the uterine chamber.

The uterus is easily moved within the pelvic cavity, but its basic position is secured with several ligaments that attach it to the pelvic floor. The ligaments also prevent the uterus from dropping into the vaginal canal. The major functions of the uterus are serving as the site of implantation of the fertilized

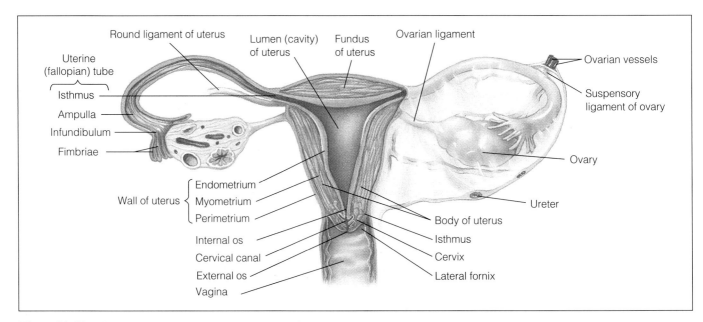

Figure 22.2B ● Cross-section of the anterior view of the female pelvis.

ovum and as a protective sac for the developing embryo and fetus.

Uterine Tubes

The **uterine tubes** (or fallopian tubes) are two ducts on either side of the fundus of the uterus (see Figure 22.2B). They are about 7 to 10 cm (3 to 4 in.) long and extend from the uterus almost to the ovaries. An ovum released by an ovary travels to the uterus within the uterine tubes. Normally, fertilization takes places within the uterine tubes. The major functions of the uterine tubes include serving as the site of fertilization and providing a passageway for unfertilized and fertilized ova to travel to the uterus.

Ovaries

Lying close to the distal end of either side of the uterine tubes are the **ovaries** (Figure 22.2B). These almond-shaped glandular structures produce ova, as well as estrogen and progesterone. They are about 3 cm (1.25 in.) long and 2 cm (1 in.) wide. The ovarian ligaments and suspensory ligaments hold the ovaries in place. The ovaries become fully developed after puberty and atrophy after menopause. The major functions of the ovaries are producing ova for fertilization by sperm and producing estrogen and progesterone.

SPECIAL CONSIDERATIONS

Throughout the assessment process, the nurse gathers subjective and objective data reflecting the client's state of health. By using critical thinking and the nursing process, the nurse identifies many factors to be considered when collecting the data. The subjective and objective data gathered throughout the assessment process inform the nurse about the client's state of health. A variety of factors, including age, developmental level, race, ethnicity, work history, living conditions, socioeconomics, and emotional well-being, influence health and must be considered during assessment. The impact of these factors is discussed in the sections that follow.

Developmental Considerations

Anatomy and physiology change with growth and development. The nurse must be aware of expected changes as data are gathered and findings are interpreted. The sections that follow describe specific variations in the female reproductive system across the age span.

Infants and Children

The female infant's labia majora will be enlarged at birth in response to maternal hormones. The labia majora should cover the labia minora. The urinary meatus and vaginal orifice should be visible. No inflammation should be present. Bloody and mucoid discharge (false menses) is commonly seen in newborns because of exposure to maternal hormones in utero.

The female child reaches puberty a few years before the male. Changes begin to occur at any time from 8 to 13 years of age; most commonly, breast changes begin at age 9 and

menstruation at age 12. Release of estrogen initiates the changes, which are first demonstrated in the development of breast buds and growth of pubic hair, followed several years later by menstruation. Table 22.1 describes Tanner's stages of maturation in girls.

TABLE 22.1	Maturation Stages in the Female
Stage 1	Preadolescent, no growth of pubic hair
Stage 2	Initial, scarcely pigmented straight hair, especially along medial border of the labia
Stage 3	Sparse, dark, visibly pigmented curly pubic hair on labia
Stage 4	Hair coarse and curly, abundant but less than in adults
Stage 5	Lateral spreading in triangle shape to medial surface of thighs
Stage 6	Further extension laterally and upward

The female child may experience a precocious puberty. These children develop the adult female sex characteristics of dense pubic and axillary hair, breasts, and menstrual bleeding before 8 years of age. Early maturation may be caused by hypothalamic tumour. Further, the early development of sexual characteristics allows for pregnancy before the child is intellectually or emotionally prepared for the experience. Early maturation can also lead to anemia related to menstrual bleeding and to psychosocial difficulties.

It is essential to assess for sexual molestation with female children. Some signs of sexual molestation are trauma, depression, eating disorders, and bruising, swelling, and inflammation in the vaginal, perineal, and anal areas. Additionally, the child may appear withdrawn. Often the child will deny the experience. Information about assessment in suspected child abuse is included in Chapter 25 of this text.

Adolescents often express interest in the changes related to puberty. The desire to explore sexual relationships and sexual contact, from kissing and fondling to intercourse, may be intense. Thus, adolescents need counselling on relationship issues, birth control, protection against sexually transmitted infections (STIs), and delaying sexual activity. A female adolescent may be concerned about or confused by an attraction to individuals of the same sex. Same-sex experimentation is developmentally normal in adolescents. It does not mean they are definitively lesbian or bisexual. The nurse should provide open communication so that the adolescent may ask questions and express her feelings and concerns.

The Pregnant Female

Pregnancy brings a multitude of changes to the female reproductive organs. The uterus, cervix, ovaries, and vagina undergo significant structural changes related to the pregnancy and the influence of hormones.

The uterus becomes hypertrophied and weighs about 1 kg (2 lb.) by the end of pregnancy. Its capacity increases to about 5 L (5 qt.). The growth of the uterus during pregnancy causes it to push up into the abdominal cavity and displace the liver and intestines from their normal positions. Contractions of the uterus occur. Throughout the pregnancy, the female may have irregular Braxton Hicks contractions, which are usually not painful. However, by the end of the pregnancy, these contractions may become more intense and cause pain.

During pregnancy, the vascularity of the cervix increases and contributes to the softening of the cervix. This softening is called **Goodell's sign**. The vascular congestion creates a blue-purple blemish or change in cervical colouration. This change is considered normal and is referred to as **Chadwick's sign**. Estrogen causes the glandular cervical tissue to produce thick mucus, which builds up and forms a mucus plug at the endocervical canal. The mucus plug prevents the introduction of any foreign matter into the uterus. At the initiation of labour, this plug is expelled. This expulsion is called the "bloody show."

The vagina undergoes changes similar to those of the uterus during pregnancy. Hypertrophy of the vaginal epithelium occurs. The vaginal wall softens and relaxes to accommodate the movement of the infant during birth. The vagina also displays Chadwick's sign. A thorough discussion of the pregnant female is found in Chapter 26.

The Older Adult

Reproductive ability in the female usually peaks in her late 20s. Over time, estrogen levels begin to decline. Between the ages of 46 and 55, menstrual periods become shorter and less frequent until they stop entirely. Menopause is said to have occurred when the female has not experienced a menstrual period in more than a year. Other symptoms of menopause can include mood changes and unpredictable episodes of sweating or hot flashes.

As the female progresses into older age, her sexual organs atrophy. Vaginal secretions are not as plentiful, and she may experience pain during intercourse. Intercourse may produce vaginal infections. The clitoris becomes smaller.

Even though older adults can achieve sexual gratification and participate in a satisfying sexual relationship, a decrease in sexual drive may contribute to the client's withdrawing from sexual experiences and relationships. Chronic or acute disease, medications, loss of a spouse or significant other, loss of privacy, depression, fatigue, stress, and use of alcohol and illicit drugs are factors known to influence sexual drive.

Psychosocial Considerations

Fatigue, depression, and stress can decrease sexual desire in a female client of any age. Grief over the loss of a relationship, whether because of separation, divorce, or death, can have long-term effects on a client's willingness to seek new relationships. Feelings of betrayal—for example, when a partner becomes intimate with another person—can have the same effect.

Past or recent trauma, as from childhood abuse, physical assault, and sexual assault, whether or not penetration occurred, may have a significant impact on a female client's ability to enjoy a sexual relationship. This may be true even if the trauma is unremembered.

Some females may fear sexual intimacy because of an altered body image related to their weight, body type, breast size, or other factors. Reproductive surgeries can affect a female client's self-image and sexual expression. For example, clients who have had a hysterectomy may feel free from the worry of unwanted pregnancy and experience an increase in sexual desire, or they may feel less feminine than before the surgery and withdraw from sexual relationships.

Social and Ethnocultural Considerations

Some cultures and religions have specific beliefs or encourage specific behaviours related to menstruation, female circumcision, and sexual practices. For example, many religions, such as Roman Catholicism, forbid premarital sex. When assessing clients, the nurse must never assume that they share all the beliefs or follow all the practices of their religious or cultural group.

Lack of privacy can inhibit the ability to engage in experiences that promote sexual gratification. Many adults today live with older parents or grandparents. As a result, the sexual experiences for all may be affected.

Sexual dysfunction can result from sexual, physical, or verbal abuse among family members. Negative family reactions to an individual's sexual orientation and lifestyle choices may affect the individual's ability to find a sexual partner and maintain a satisfying sexual relationship. Females may choose partners who do not meet their own needs or desires because of family pressures. This choice can have a negative emotional and physical impact, especially on female adolescents.

Several environmental and occupational exposures have been linked to birth defects, spontaneous abortions, low birth weight, and premature births. Oncology nurses exposed to antineoplastic drugs may have spontaneous abortions, fetal anomalies, change in the regularity of their menstrual cycles, or even cessation of their menstrual cycles. In assessing females in their reproductive stages, or those who express complaints about irregular menses, a thorough investigation of their workplace and occupational exposures should be conducted.

Maintaining the cleanliness of the female genitalia requires daily washing and changing of underclothes. Douching is not only unnecessary but may even be harmful. Douching has been shown to promote irritation, rashes, and infection in some females. The likelihood of rashes or infections can be reduced by keeping the genitals dry by changing sweaty underclothes after physical exercise, changing into dry clothes immediately after bathing or swimming, and changing an infant's diaper immediately after it is wet.

Although research has shown that infections can be transmitted sexually even when the partners are using a latex condom, its use significantly lowers the incidence of transmission. A history of human papillomavirus (HPV) and more than four sexual partners in a lifetime increases a female client's risk for cervical cancer. A history of STIs in children may indicate sexual abuse.

The risk for cervical cancer is increased in those females who participate in early (before age 18) and frequent sexual activity and have a history of many sexual partners. Obesity is a risk factor for uterine cancer.

Social and Ethnocultural Considerations

- Several environmental and occupational exposures have been linked to birth defects, spontaneous abortions, low birth weight, and premature births.
- Female circumcision or female genital mutilation (FGM) is a traditional or cultural practice in many countries and is becoming more commonly seen in Canada among some immigrant populations.

- In many cultures and religions, physical examination by a healthcare provider of the opposite sex is prohibited.
- Discussion of sexual activity and reproductive function is unacceptable in many cultural groups.

GATHERING THE DATA

Health assessment of the female reproductive system includes gathering subjective and objective data. Collection of subjective data occurs during the health history, before the physical assessment. The nurse uses a variety of communication techniques to elicit general and specific information about the health of the reproductive system. Health records and the results of laboratory and clinical examinations are important secondary sources to be reviewed and included in the data-gathering process. Physical assessment of the female reproductive system includes the techniques of inspection and palpation, as well as the use of equipment and techniques specific to the assessment of the female reproductive system.

HEALTH HISTORY

The health history of the female concerns data related to the structures and functions of the reproductive system. Subjective data related to that system are gathered during the health history. The nurse should be prepared to observe the client and listen for cues related to the function of this body system. Open-ended or closed questions are used to obtain information. Often, a number of follow-up questions or requests for descriptions are required to clarify data or gather missing information. Follow-up questions are aimed at identifying the source of problems, duration of difficulties, measures to alleviate problems, and clues about the client's knowledge of her own health.

Information about the genital areas, reproduction, and sexual activity is generally considered very private. The nurse must be sensitive to the client's need for privacy and carefully explain that all information is confidential. A conversational approach with the use of open-ended statements is often helpful in a situation that promotes anxiety and embarrassment. The client's terminology about body parts and functions should guide the nurse's questions.

The health history guides the physical assessment of the female reproductive system. The information is always considered in relation to normal parameters and expectations about the health of the system. Therefore, the nurse must consider age, gender, race, culture, environment, health practices, past and concurrent problems, and therapies when framing questions and using techniques to elicit information. To address all the factors when conducting a health history, specific questions related to the female reproductive status and function have been developed. These questions focus on the most common concerns or injuries associated with the female reproductive system; questions related to past health history; questions related to behaviours; questions that address environmental concerns; and those that are specific to clients according to age, including the pregnant female.

The nurse must consider the client's ability to participate in the health history and physical assessment of the reproductive system. If a client is experiencing pain or anxiety, attention must focus on relief of these symptoms. Because of the close proximity of some of the female reproductive structures to the urethra, data gathered during the health history will relate to the status of the urinary system as well. Questions related to the health and function of the female urinary system are discussed in Chapter 20. ⬡

Abnormal vaginal discharge, pelvic pain, inflammation, infection, and suspicion of contracting an STI are some of the more frequent problems that the female reports. Examination of the perianal area is included in assessment of the female reproductive system. Related problems include hemorrhoids, fissures, and infectious processes.

As the nurse gathers the data, she or he will shift the type of questions to direct questions that give the client room to explain or qualify. The mnemonic O-P-Q-R-S-T-U, which stands for onset (chronology), precipitating (or palliative), quality, region (or radiation), severity, timing, and understanding, will help the learner remember the dimensions of the symptoms. The nurse will keep in mind that not all these qualifiers will apply to each symptom.

HEALTH HISTORY QUESTIONS	RATIONALES

GATHERING THE DATA

The sections that follow provide sample questions and follow-up questions. Rationales for some questions are provided. The list of questions is not all-inclusive but rather represents the more common concern or injury questions required in a health history related to the female reproductive system. An example of using O-P-Q-R-S-T-U with pain is provided.

Questions Related to Common Concerns or Injuries

The most common concerns related to illness or injury of the female reproductive system are as follows:

- Abdominal or pelvic pain
- Abnormal vaginal bleeding
- Dysmenorrhea
- Infertility
- Vaginal discharge and itching
- Genital rashes
- Dyspareunia

1. **Abdominal or pelvic pain**
   - Are you having any pain at this time?

   ▶ Common causes of gynecological pain include infection, menstrual difficulties, endometriosis, ectopic pregnancy, threatened abortion, pelvic masses, uterine fibroids, and ovarian cancer.

   - When did you first notice the pain? How long does it last? *Onset (chronology)*
   - What makes the pain worse? better? *Precipitating (palliative)*
   - Can you describe the pain? Is it sharp? dull? burning? *Quality*
   - Does the pain radiate? Where? *Radiation*
   - How often do you experience the pain? How would you rate the pain on a scale of 1 to 10, with 10 being the worst pain? *Severity*
   - Is the pain associated with nausea? vomiting? abdominal distension? certain time of your cycle? *Timing*
   - What do you think is causing the pain? *Understanding*

   ▶ This question helps the nurse determine if the problem is current, experienced in the past only, or chronic.

   ▶ Some conditions, such as ovarian cysts or endometriosis, can be cyclical in nature.

HEALTH HISTORY QUESTIONS	RATIONALES

2. Abnormal vaginal bleeding
- Have you had any vaginal bleeding outside the time of your normal menstrual period?

▶ Abnormal bleeding may be related to hormonal influences and be easily corrected. Some conditions, such as uterine fibroids and several forms of cancer, can also cause abnormal bleeding patterns.

- How long have you noticed the vaginal bleeding?
- Do you experience this bleeding at particular times during your cycle?
- Are any clots present?
- How many pads or tampons do you use per day?
- Is the bleeding associated with headaches? breast tenderness? nausea?
- Describe your diet.

▶ Women with abnormally low percentages of body fat may have interruptions in their menses.

3. Dysmenorrhea
- How old were you when you had your first menstrual period?

▶ Onset of menses is influenced by a variety of factors, including percentage of body fat. Menarche (onset of menstruation) between the ages of 11 and 14 indicates normal development. Late onset is associated with endocrine problems.

- What was the first day of your last menstrual period?

▶ This establishes a pattern for the client and has significance for physical assessment in relation to physical changes that occur at points throughout the cycle (i.e., when to expect ovulation).

- How many days does your cycle usually last? Is this consistent?

▶ A cycle is defined as the first day of one period to the first day of the next.

- Describe your menstrual flow. How many tampons or pads do you use each day? Is this consistent?

▶ Clotting and excessive bleeding warrant additional follow-up.

- How do you usually feel just before your period? Has this gotten worse or better?
- Do you take any medications for cramps?

4. Infertility
- Do you have children? *If yes,* How many? *If no,* Have you tried to have children?

▶ The couple is not considered potentially infertile unless they have been unable to conceive for a year.

- How often to do you and your partner have intercourse?

▶ For couples attempting to become pregnant, it is important to engage in intercourse routinely, two to three times a week. Although nurses do not treat infertility, they may be involved in teaching the client about certain measures that may be helpful to determine the optimal time for intercourse. Concerns about infertility can produce great anxiety for many couples.

- Have you ever sought professional help for fertility problems? If so, describe this experience.

▶ This question may prompt the client to discuss any concerns about reproductive health.

- Has an inability to conceive placed a strain on your relationship with your partner? How are you feeling about this?

▶ Specific questions enable the client to affirm or deny relationship problems, to discuss changes in the relationship, and to discuss feelings about the partnership.

GATHERING THE DATA

HEALTH HISTORY QUESTIONS	RATIONALES

5. Vaginal discharge and itching
- Do you now have or have you ever had an illness or infection associated with the female reproductive system?

▶ If an infection or illness is identified, follow-up about the date, treatment, and outcomes is required. Common problems include dysmenorrhea (painful periods), uterine fibroids, cystitis, pelvic inflammatory disease, and uterine, ovarian, or vulvar cancer.

- Have you engaged in any sexual activities that would put you at risk of contracting a sexually transmitted infection?

▶ Many sexually transmitted infections can cause vaginal discharge and itchiness.

- Is there an odour associated with the discharge?

▶ Such conditions as vaginitis and *trichomoniasis* can produce a fishy odour.

- Have you experienced any itching in your labia or vaginal area?

▶ Crab lice, atrophic vaginitis, candidiasis (yeast infection), and contact dermatitis may cause intense itching.

6. Genital rashes
- Have you noticed any rashes, blisters, ulcers, sores, or warts on your genital area or surrounding areas?

▶ Rashes may occur with yeast infections, which are the most common female genital infections. Yeast infections generally produce redness, pruritus, and cheeselike discharge. Herpes infection causes small painful ulcerations, whereas syphilitic chancres are not painful. In the older client, a raised, reddened lesion may indicate carcinoma of the vulva. Reddened lesions that eventually weep and form crusts characterize contact dermatitis. Venereal warts are cauliflower shaped.

- Is there any itching or pain associated with the rash?

7. Dyspareunia
- Are you sexually active? If so, how would you describe your sexual relationship(s)?

▶ These questions may prompt the female client to discuss any concerns about reproductive health.

- Are there any obstacles to your ability to achieve sexual satisfaction?

▶ Causes of inability to achieve sexual satisfaction include fear of acquiring an STI, fear of being unable to satisfy the partner, fear of pregnancy, confusion regarding sexual orientation, unwillingness to participate in sexual activities enjoyed by the partner, job stress, financial considerations, crowded living conditions, loss of partner, or history of sexual trauma.

- Have you noticed a change in your sex drive recently? Can you associate the change with anything in particular?

▶ This may be indicative of some physical or psychological problems that need follow-up. Often clients can relate a decrease in sex drive with stress, illness, drug therapy, or some other factor.

Questions Related to Past Health History

1. Obstetrical history
- Have you ever been pregnant? If so, how many times?
- Did you have any problems during pregnancy, the delivery, or postpartum? If yes, describe the problem.
- Have you ever had a miscarriage? What was the cause? Was surgery required? How have you been emotionally since the miscarriage?

▶ Strong emotions often accompany the termination of a pregnancy by either spontaneous or surgical abortion. The nurse may want to follow up.

- Have you ever had an abortion? At how many weeks, and by what method? How have you been emotionally since the abortion?

GATHERING THE DATA

TECHNIQUES AND NORMAL FINDINGS	RATIONALES

2. **Have you ever been told that you had a sexually transmitted infection?**
   - If so, when did this occur?
   - Do you know the name of the infection?
   - Was it treated?
   - Was follow-up required?

Questions Related to Behaviours

Healthcare behaviours include both health practices and health patterns. Health practices consist of following recommendations for disease prevention, including screening for risks, screening for early detection of problems, and immunization. Health patterns are habits or acts that affect the client's health. Health behaviours may also include seeking healthcare from healthcare providers who use alternative methods to diagnose and treat illness. Clients should be questioned in a nonjudgmental way and areas for health teaching should be identified.

1. **For clients who are sexually active:**
   - What type of contraception do you use?

     ▶ This question helps determine the client's knowledge of the product being used and practices around contraception.

   - Would you like to know more about the use of contraceptives?

     ▶ This is a very important question to ask adolescents who shy away from talking about sexual practices but have said that they are sexually active.

2. **Do you check your genitals on a routine basis?**

   ▶ Self-examination of the genitals should be performed at least monthly for early detection of changes that need follow-up. Teaching may be indicated if the client is not performing self-examination.

3. **How do you protect yourself from sexually transmitted infections, including HIV?**

   ▶ Abstinence is the only 100% effective protection against STIs. Latex condoms offer significant protection, especially when treated with spermicide; however, they are not 100% effective.

4. **Do you drink alcohol? If so, how many drinks per week do you consume? Do you use recreational drugs? If so, what type and how much?**

   ▶ Drug and alcohol use may contribute to failure to use protection against STIs and unplanned pregnancy.

5. **Do you have routine Pap tests done?**
   - Have you ever had an abnormal Pap test? How long ago? What treatment did you receive? Did you have a follow-up Pap test? What were the results?

     ▶ A regular Pap test screens for cervical cancer and increases the likelihood of finding cervical cancer in the early stages. Once a female becomes sexually active, she should begin having regular Pap tests until 70 years of age. How frequently a Pap test is needed depends on a woman's history of negative results and can be anywhere from every 6 months to every 3 years.

Questions Related to the Environment

Environment refers to both internal and external environments. Questions related to the internal environment include all the previous questions and those associated with internal or physiological responses. Questions regarding the external environment include those related to home, work, or social environments.

HEALTH HISTORY QUESTIONS	RATIONALES

Internal Environment

1. Do you know if your mother received diethylstilbestrol (DES) treatment during pregnancy with you?

▶ Studies indicate that daughters of mothers who received DES during pregnancy have a significantly higher number of reproductive tract problems, including cervical cancer (Canadian Cancer Society, 2009), infertility, and ectopic pregnancy. This fact may have some bearing on the client's current problem. If the client answers yes to this question, the nurse should refer her to a physician.

2. Do you drink alcohol? How many drinks per week?

▶ Intake of alcoholic beverages can contribute to an individual taking chances, such as failing to ask her partner to use condoms.

3. Do you use illicit drugs? If so, what type and how much?

▶ Taken in sufficient amounts, some drugs, such as marijuana and opiates, may decrease libido. Drug use may also contribute to failure to use protection against STIs.

External Environment

The following questions deal with the physical environment of the client. That includes the indoor and outdoor environments of the home and the workplace, those encountered for social engagements, and any encountered during travel.

1. Do your family and friends support your relationship with your sexual partner?

▶ The client's family and friends can influence the client's sexual relationship in a variety of ways. The client may feel tension if the partner is not accepted.

2. Are you able to talk to your partner about your sexual needs?
   - Does your partner accept your needs and help you fulfill them?
   - Are you able to do the same for your partner?

▶ The ability to openly discuss sexual needs and preferences fosters strong and lasting relationships.

3. Some clients come to a healthcare provider to discuss sexual abuse.
   - Have you ever been forced to have sexual intercourse or other sexual contact against your will?
   - Have you ever been molested or sexually assaulted?
   - If the client answers yes: When was this?
   - Who abused you?
   - What was the experience?
   - What was done about the situation and for you?

Questions Related to Age

The health history must reflect the anatomical and physiological differences that exist along the age span.

Questions Regarding Infants and Children

1. Have you noticed any redness, swelling, or discharge that is discoloured or foul smelling in the child's genital areas?

▶ These symptoms may indicate inflammatory processes or infection.

2. Has the child complained of itching, burning, or swelling in the genital area?

▶ These symptoms may indicate the presence of pinworms, yeast infections and other infections, trauma, or sexual abuse.

The nurse should ask the preschool or school-age child the following questions:

1. Has anyone ever touched you where you didn't want him or her to? Where? (*The nurse may want to have the child point to a picture or doll.*)

2. Has anyone ever asked you to touch him or her where you didn't want to? (*If the child answers yes, the child may be sexually abused. The nurse should try to obtain additional information by asking the following questions but remember to be sensitive.*)

HEALTH HISTORY QUESTIONS	RATIONALES

3. Where did he or she ask you to touch him or her?

4. Who touched you? How many times did this happen? Who knows about this?

▶ The nurse must try to determine exactly what the person did to the child. Has there been more than touching? Has any other form of sexual contact occurred? The child may feel responsible for the situation and not want to discuss it. The abuser may be a parent or relative. The nurse should assure the child that she has not been bad and that it helps to talk to an adult about it. Referral should be made to a specialist immediately for sexual abuse assessment. Nurses also have the legal duty to report all suspected cases of child abuse to the local police or child welfare agency.

Questions Regarding Adolescents

Many of the questions nurses ask adolescents are similar to questions they ask adults. It is important to explore adolescents' feelings and concerns regarding their sexual development. The nurse can reassure the adolescent that these changes are normal. Some adolescents may be confused about their feelings of sexual attraction to the opposite or same sex. The nurse should ask open-ended questions and assure the adolescent that all such feelings are normal.

Whether or not an adolescent admits to being sexually active, it is important to offer information on teenage pregnancy, birth control, and protection against STIs. Some teenagers may be fearful that the nurse will relay this information to their parents. The nurse should reinforce that all information is confidential unless sexual abuse is reported.

1. Are you having sex with anyone now?

▶ Use of gender-neutral terms prevents value judgments about sexual orientation. This question allows clients to define what sex is to them. Many teens think anything that does not involve vaginal penetration is not sex. The nurse must stress that oral sex and other acts are indeed sexual activity.

Questions for the Pregnant Female

Questions for the pregnant female include menstrual, obstetrical, gynecological, family, and partner histories.

This information provides data about the client and her partner and identifies risk factors. Specific questions for the pregnant female are included in Chapter 26 of this text. ⫘

Questions for the Older Adult

The questions for aging female adults are the same as those for younger adults. In addition, the nurse should explore whether older clients perceive any changes in their sexuality related to advancing age. For example, an older female may notice a decrease in vaginal lubrication, even when she is fully aroused. The female older adult can be reassured that these changes are normal and do not indicate disease.

1. When did menopause begin for you?

▶ This information establishes a reference for the onset of physiological changes that accompany menopause.

2. Tell me about physical changes you have noticed since menopause.

▶ It is common for aging females to experience a variety of symptoms, including mood changes and hot flashes. Vaginal dryness causes dyspareunia (painful intercourse).

GATHERING THE DATA

HEALTH HISTORY QUESTIONS	RATIONALES
3. Have you had any vaginal bleeding since starting menopause?	▶ Some females assume that postmenopausal bleeding is normal and tend to ignore it. Postmenopausal bleeding may be suggestive of inadequate estrogen therapy and endometrial cancer. It could also be indicative of serious problems, such as genital tract cancer.

PHYSICAL ASSESSMENT

ASSESSMENT TECHNIQUES AND FINDINGS

Physical assessment of the female reproductive system includes the techniques of inspection and palpation. In addition, the speculum is used to visualize the vagina and cervix. During each procedure, the nurse is gathering data related to the health and function of the reproductive system. Knowledge of normal or expected findings is essential in determining the meaning of the data as the nurse conducts the physical assessment.

The adult female has pubic hair that is distributed in an even, inverted triangular pattern over the mons pubis. Hair distribution is less dense over the labia, perineum, and inner thighs. The labia majora are symmetrical, smooth, and without lesions. The labia minora are smooth, pink, and moist. The clitoris is smooth, midline, and about 1 cm (0.5 in.) long. The urethra is slitlike, midline, smooth, pink, and patent. The vaginal opening is pink and round. On bearing down, there should be no urine leakage at the meatus or protrusions from the vagina. The perineum is smooth and firm. The anus is intact, moist, darkly pigmented, and without lesions. On palpation the vaginal wall is rugated and soft; the Skene's glands and Bartholin's glands are nontender and without discharge. The examination with the speculum reveals a pink, moist, round, and centrally positioned cervix. The cervix is free of lesions, with clear, odourless secretions present. Palpation of the cervix reveals it as firm, smooth, and mobile, like the tip of the nose. The fornices are smooth and nontender. The uterus is palpated and found tilted upward above the bladder with the cervix tilted forward. Variations in uterine position may be anteverted, midline, or retroverted. When ovaries are palpable, they are smooth, firm, mobile, and almond shaped. They may be slightly tender. The uterine tubes are nonpalpable. The rectovaginal system is thin, smooth, and nontender.

Physical assessment of the female reproductive system follows an organized pattern. It begins with inspection of the external genitalia and perianal area, palpation of the vagina and glands, and speculum examination and specimen collection. This is followed by palpation of the cervix, fornices, uterus, uterine tubes, and ovaries. The assessment ends with the rectovaginal examination.

EQUIPMENT

examination gown and examination drape	Pap smear equipment
	speculum
clean, nonsterile examination gloves	hand-held mirror
	occult blood test
lubricant	

HELPFUL HINTS

- Provide a warm, private environment.
- Have the client void before the examination.
- Use appropriate draping to maintain the client's dignity.
- Determine if the client has had this kind of assessment before. If not, booklets with diagrams are helpful before proceeding.
- It is helpful to show the client pictures of equipment, slides, and the bimanual examination.
- Use an unhurried, deliberate manner and ask the client how she is doing as the examination proceeds.
- Explore and remedy cultural or language issues at the onset of the interaction.
- Use routine practices.

TECHNIQUES AND NORMAL FINDINGS	ABNORMAL FINDINGS AND SPECIAL CONSIDERATIONS

INSPECTION

1. Instruct the client.

- Explain to the client that you will be looking at and touching her external genital area. Tell her that it should not cause discomfort, but if pain occurs she should

TECHNIQUES AND NORMAL FINDINGS	ABNORMAL FINDINGS AND SPECIAL CONSIDERATIONS

tell you and you will stop. Explain that deep breathing is a good way to relax during the examination.

- Tell the client you will provide instructions and explanations at each point in the assessment.

2. Position the client.
   - Ask the client to lie down on the examination table.
   - Assist her into the lithotomy position (supine with knees and hips flexed so that feet rest flat on the examination table), and then have her slide her hips as close to the end of the table as possible.
   - Place her feet in the stirrups (see Figure 22.3).

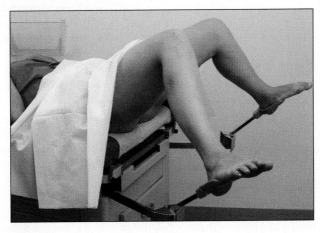

Figure 22.3 ●
Positioning the client.

3. Inspect the pubic hair.
   - Confirm that the hair grows in an inverted triangle and is scattered heavily over the mons pubis. It should become sparse over the labia majora, perineum, and inner thighs (see Figure 22.4).

▶ A sparse hair pattern may be indicative of delayed puberty. It is also a common and normal finding in Asian females. The older adult client's pubic hair will become sparse, scattered, and grey. Women may have different hair patterns because of waxing or other grooming practices. Confirm the use of these practices with the client. Table 22.1 depicts Tanner's stages of female development.

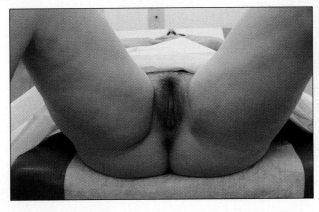

Figure 22.4 ●
Inspecting the pubic hair.

   - If the client has complained of itching in the pubic area, comb through the pubic hair with two or three fingers.
   - Confirm the absence of small, bluish-grey spots, or nits (eggs), at the base of the pubic hairs.

▶ These signs indicate pubic lice (crabs). Marks may be visible from persistent scratching to relieve the intense itching caused by the lice.

4. Inspect the labia majora.
   - Confirm that the labia majora are fuller and rounder in the centre of the structure and that the skin is smooth and intact.
   - Compare the right and left labia majora for symmetry.

▶ The labia majora of older females may be thinner and wrinkled.

PHYSICAL ASSESSMENT

TECHNIQUES AND NORMAL FINDINGS

ABNORMAL FINDINGS AND SPECIAL CONSIDERATIONS

- Observe for any lesions, warts, vesicles, rashes, or ulcerations. If you notice drainage, note the colour, distribution, location, and characteristics.

▶ These findings may signal a variety of conditions. *Contact dermatitis* appears as a red rash with associated lesions that are weepy and crusty. Scratch marks are often visible because of intense itching.

    Genital warts are raised, moist, cauliflower-shaped papules.

- Remember to change gloves as needed during the exam to prevent cross-contamination. Also remember to culture any abnormal discharge.
- Confirm the absence of any swelling or inflammation in the area of the labia majora.

▶ Red, painful vesicles accompanied by localized swelling are seen in *herpes infection.*

    Swelling over red, inflamed skin that is tender and warm to palpation may indicate an abscess in the Bartholin's gland. The abscess may be caused by gonorrhea.

5. **Inspect the labia minora.**
   - Confirm that the labia minora are smooth, pink, and moist.

▶ The older female may have drier, thinner labia minora.

   - Observe for any redness or swelling. Note any bruising or tearing of the skin.

▶ Redness and swelling indicate the presence of an infective or inflammatory process. Bruising or tearing of the skin may suggest forceful intercourse or sexual abuse, especially in the case of adolescents and children.

6. **Inspect the clitoris.**
   - Place your right or left hand over the labia majora and separate these structures with your thumb and index finger.
   - The clitoris should be midline, about 1 cm (0.5 in.) long, with more fullness in the centre. It should be smooth. (see Figure 22.5)

▶ An elongated clitoris may signal elevated levels of testosterone and warrants further investigation and referral to a physician.

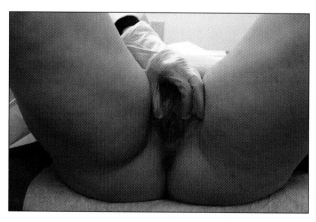

Figure 22.5 ●
Inspection of the clitoris.

   - Observe for any redness, lesions, or tears in the tissue.

7. **Inspect the urethral orifice.**
   - Confirm that the urethral opening is midline, pink, smooth, slitlike, and patent.

▶ Urine leakage indicates stress incontinence and weakening of the pelvic musculature.

   - Ask the client to cough. No urine should leak from the urethral opening.
   - Inspect for any redness, inflammation, or discharge.

▶ These symptoms indicate urinary tract infection.

8. **Inspect the vaginal opening, perineum, and anal area.**
   - Confirm that the vaginal opening or introitus is pink and round. It may be either smooth or irregular.

| TECHNIQUES AND NORMAL FINDINGS | ABNORMAL FINDINGS AND SPECIAL CONSIDERATIONS |

- Locate the **hymen**, which is a thin layer of skin within the vagina. It may be present in females who have never had sexual intercourse.
- Inspect for tears, bruising, or lacerations.

▶ Tears, bruising, or lacerations could be due to forceful, consensual sex or sexual assault. Additional follow-up is needed after examination. It is important not to ask any questions that the client may interpret as probing or threatening during the physical assessment.

- The **perineum**, the space between the vaginal opening and the anal area, should be smooth and firm.
- Scars from episiotomy procedures may be observed in parous females. These are normal.
- The anus should be intact, moist, and darkly pigmented. There should be no lesions.
- Have the client bear down.

▶ Thin, fragile perineal tissues indicate atrophy. Tears and fissures may indicate trauma.

- Inspect for any protrusions from the vagina.

▶ A **prolapsed uterus** may protrude right at the vaginal wall with straining, or it may hang outside the vaginal wall without any straining (see Figure 22.6).

A **cystocele** is a hernia that is formed when the urinary bladder is pushed into the anterior vaginal wall.

A **rectocele** is a hernia that is formed when the rectum pushes into the posterior vaginal wall.

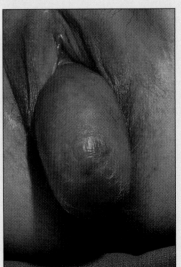

Figure 22.6 ● Prolapsed uterus.

PALPATION

1. Palpate the vaginal walls.
   - Explain to the client that you are going to palpate the vaginal walls. Tell her that she will feel you insert a finger into the vagina.
   - Place your left hand above the labia majora and spread the labia minora apart with your thumb and index finger.
   - With your right palm facing toward the ceiling, gently place your right index finger at the vaginal opening.
   - Insert your right index finger gently into the vagina.

PHYSICAL ASSESSMENT

TECHNIQUES AND NORMAL FINDINGS	ABNORMAL FINDINGS AND SPECIAL CONSIDERATIONS

- Gently rotate the right index finger counterclockwise. The vaginal wall should feel rugated, consistent in texture, and soft.
- Ask the client to bear down or cough.
- Note any bulging in this area.

▶ Bulging may occur with uterine prolapse, cystocele, or rectocele.

2. **Palpate the urethra and Skene's glands.**
   - Explain to the client that you are going to palpate her urethra. Tell her that she will again feel pressure against her vaginal wall.
   - Your left hand should still be above the labia majora and you should still be spreading the labia minora apart with your thumb and index finger.
   - Your right index finger should still be inserted in the client's vagina.
   - With your right index finger, apply very gentle pressure upward against the vaginal wall.
   - Milk the Skene's glands by stroking outward (see Figure 22.7).

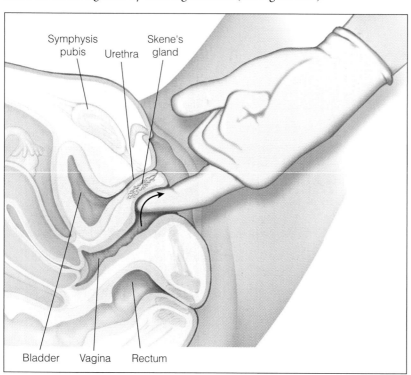

Figure 22.7 ● Palpating the Skene's glands.

- Now apply the same upward and outward pressure on both sides of the urethra.
- No pain or discharge should be elicited.

▶ Discharge from the urethra or Skene's glands may indicate an infection, such as gonorrhea. A culture must be obtained.

3. **Palpate the Bartholin's glands.**
   - With your right index finger still inserted in the client's vagina, gently squeeze the posterior region of the labia majora between your right index finger and right thumb (see Figure 22.8).
   - Perform this manoeuvre bilaterally, palpating both Bartholin's glands.
   - No lump or hardness should be felt. No pain response should be elicited. No discharge should be produced.

▶ Lumps, hardness, pain, or discharge suggest the presence of an abscess and infective process. Often the source is a gonorrheal infection. A culture should be obtained of any discharge.

TECHNIQUES AND NORMAL FINDINGS	ABNORMAL FINDINGS AND SPECIAL CONSIDERATIONS

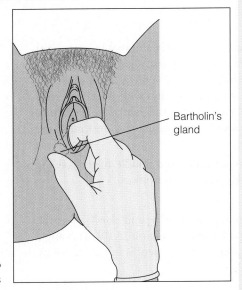

Bartholin's gland

Figure 22.8 ●
Palpating the Bartholin's glands.

INSPECTION WITH A SPECULUM

Be sure that the client has not douched or had sexual intercourse within 24 hours before obtaining cervical and vaginal specimens. Otherwise, the results of the test may be inaccurate.

1. **Select the speculum.**
   - Metal speculums and plastic disposable speculums are available. The following is a description of the proper use of a metal speculum.
   - Use a speculum that has been warmed with warm (not hot) water. Ensure that the majority of the water has been removed to avoid introducing water into the vagina. Do not use gel lubricant, as it may distort the cells in your specimen.
   - If you are using a plastic speculum, check the bills to ensure that there are no rough edges.

2. **Hold the speculum in your dominant hand.**
   - Place the index finger on top of the blades, the third finger on the bottom of the blades, and be sure to move the thumb just underneath the thumbscrew before inserting (see Figure 22.9).

▶ If the client has vaginitis, the speculum examination should be delayed until the problem has been treated, unless this is the client's chief complaint and the reason for her visit.

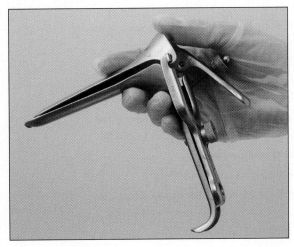

Figure 22.9 ●
Holding the speculum.

PHYSICAL ASSESSMENT

<table>
<tr><td>

TECHNIQUES AND NORMAL FINDINGS

</td><td>

</td></tr>
</table>

TECHNIQUES AND NORMAL FINDINGS

3. Insert the speculum.

- Tell the client that you are going to examine her cervix and that to do so, you are going to insert a speculum. If this is the client's first vaginal examination, show her the speculum, and briefly demonstrate how you will use it to visualize her cervix. Have a mirror available to share findings with the client. Also explain that she will feel pressure, first of your fingers, and then of the speculum. You may also want to show her a booklet with a picture demonstrating the technique.

- With your nondominant hand, place your index and middle fingers on the posterior vaginal opening and apply pressure gently downward.

- Turn the speculum blades obliquely.

- Place the blades over your fingers at the vaginal opening and *slowly* insert the closed speculum at a 45-degree downward angle (see Figure 22.10). This angle matches the downward slope of the vagina when the client is in the lithotomy position.

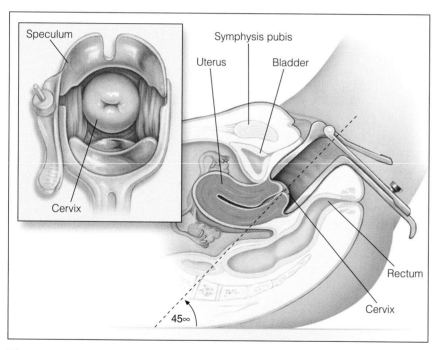

Figure 22.10 ● Speculum inserted into vagina.

- Once the speculum is inserted, withdraw your fingers and turn the speculum clockwise until the blades are in a horizontal plane.

- Advance the blades at a downward 45-degree angle until they are completely inserted.

- This manoeuvre should not cause the client pain.

- Avoid pinching the labia or pulling on the client's pubic hair. If insertion of the speculum causes the client pain, stop immediately and reevaluate your technique.

- To open the speculum blades, squeeze the speculum handle.

- Sweep the speculum blades upward until the cervix comes into view.

- Adjust the speculum blades as needed until the cervix is fully exposed between them.

- Tighten the thumbscrew to stabilize the spread of the blades.

PHYSICAL ASSESSMENT

TECHNIQUES AND NORMAL FINDINGS	ABNORMAL FINDINGS AND SPECIAL CONSIDERATIONS

TECHNIQUES AND NORMAL FINDINGS

4. Visualize the cervix.
   - Confirm that the cervix is pink, moist, round, and centrally positioned, and that it has a small opening in the centre called the os.
   - Note any bluish colouring.

   - Confirm that any secretions are clear or white and without odour.

   - Confirm that the cervix is free from erosions, ulcerations, lacerations, and polyps.

OBTAINING THE PAP SMEAR AND OTHER CULTURES

The Pap (Papanicolaou) smear screens for cervical cancer. The examiner should have the slides prelabelled with the client's identifying information and, if several slides are used, with the area that is sampled. Having spray fixative readily available is necessary as the slides must be fixed immediately to avoid drying of the cell samples.

There are several ways to prepare the cell samples for the Pap test. Some areas will use one slide for all samples, while others may require multiple slides. Some provinces and territories use a newer method of sampling called liquid-based cytology. The examiner must be familiar with the techniques used in her or his area of practice.

1. Perform an endocervical swab.
   - Carefully insert an endocervical brush into the vagina and into the cervical os.

   - Do not force insertion of the brush.

   - Rotate the brush in a complete circle (see Figure 22.11).

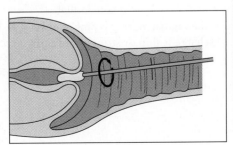

Figure 22.11 ●
The endocervical swab.

   - Roll a thin coat across the labelled slide.

   - If the slide will contain the cervical scrape as well, wait until this is complete before fixing the slide. If the slide is complete, spray fixative on the slide immediately.

ABNORMAL FINDINGS AND SPECIAL CONSIDERATIONS

▶ A bluish colouring is seen during the second month of pregnancy and is called *Chadwick's sign*. Otherwise, a bluish colour is indicative of cyanosis.

▶ Green discharge that has a foul smell is associated with gonorrhea. Thick discharge is seen in *candidiasis*. Frothy, yellow-green discharge is seen in *trichomoniasis*. A yellow discharge can also be seen in chlamydial infection. *Bacterial vaginosis* presents with a creamy-grey to white discharge that has a fishy odour.

▶ Erosions are associated with carcinoma or infections. Ulcerations can be due to carcinoma, syphilis, and tuberculosis. Yellow cysts or nodules are *nabothian cysts* (benign cysts that may appear after childbirth).

▶ The endocervical brush is contraindicated in pregnancy. A saline-moistened, cotton-tipped applicator is used in the pregnant client.

▶ If the brush cannot be slipped into the cervical os, a tumour may be blocking the opening.

▶ A thin coat is preferred because a thick coat may be difficult to assess under the microscope.

PHYSICAL ASSESSMENT

TECHNIQUES AND NORMAL FINDINGS

2. **Obtain a cervical scrape.**
   - Insert the longer end of a bifid or extended-tip spatula into the client's vagina.
   - Advance the fingerlike projection of the bifid or longer end gently into the cervical os.
   - Allow the shorter end to rest on the outer ridge of the cervix.
   - Rotate the applicator one full 360-degree turn clockwise to scrape cells from the cervix (see Figure 22.12).

▶ If the client has had a hysterectomy, obtain the scrape from the surgical stump.

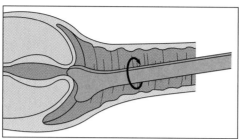

Figure 22.12 ●
The cervical scrape.

   - Do not rotate the applicator more than once or turn it in a counterclockwise manner.
   - Spread a thin smear across the slide from each side of the spatula.
   - Spray fixative on the slide immediately if no other samples are to be included on this slide.

3. **Obtain additional cultures.**
   - If indicated, the nurse may screen for STIs and obtain a gonorrhea or chlamydia culture.

▶ *Special consideration:* Nurses should check with the laboratory in their institution as techniques and protocols may differ. With some STI cultures, an endocervical sample is no longer required.

   - Insert a sterile cotton-tipped applicator into the os. Many manufacturers have applicators and transport medium prepackaged.
   - Leave the applicator in place for 20 seconds to allow full saturation of the cotton.
   - Place applicator in required transport medium tube.

4. **Remove the speculum.**
   - Gently loosen the thumbscrew on the speculum while holding the handles securely.
   - Slant the speculum from side to side as you slide it from the vaginal canal.
   - While you withdraw the speculum, note that the vaginal mucosa is pink, consistent in texture, rugated, and nontender. Discharge is thin or stringy, and clear or opaque.

▶ The infections that contribute to the development of discoloured or foul-smelling vaginal discharge are the same as those listed in the previous section on identifying cervical discharge.

   - Close the speculum blades before complete removal.

BIMANUAL PALPATION

Stand at the end of the examination table. The client remains in the lithotomy position.

1. **Palpate the cervix.**
   - Lubricate the index and middle fingers of your gloved dominant hand.
   - Inform the client that you are going to palpate her cervix.

PHYSICAL ASSESSMENT

Techniques and Normal Findings

- Place your nondominant hand against the client's thigh, then insert your lubricated index and middle fingers into her vaginal opening.
- Proceed downward at a 45-degree angle until you reach the cervix.
- Keep the other fingers of that hand rounded inward toward the palm and put the thumb against the mons pubis away from the clitoris (see Figure 22.13).

▶ Pressure on the clitoris may be painful for the client.

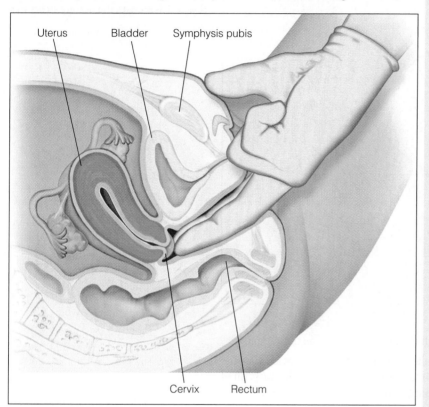

Figure 22.13 ● Palpating the cervix.

- Palpate the cervix. It should feel firm and smooth, somewhat like the tip of a nose.
- Gently try to move it. It should move easily about 1 to 2 cm (0.5 to 1 in.) in either direction.

▶ Nodules, hardness, or lack of mobility suggest a tumour.

▶ If the woman is pregnant, the cervix will be soft. This is a normal finding and is called Goodell's sign.

Pain on palpation or cervical excitation in the nulliparous woman can be indicative of inflammation.

2. **Palpate the fornices.**
   - Slip your fingers into the vaginal recess areas, called the fornices.
   - Palpate around the grooves.
   - Confirm that the mucosa of the vagina and cervix in these areas is smooth and nontender.
   - Leave your fingers in the anterior fornix when you have checked all sides.

3. **Palpate the uterus.**
   - Place the fingers of your nondominant hand on the client's abdomen.

▶ Note any tenderness, which could be indicative of inflammation.

TECHNIQUES AND NORMAL FINDINGS	ABNORMAL FINDINGS AND SPECIAL CONSIDERATIONS

- Invaginate the abdomen midway between the umbilicus and the symphysis pubis by pushing with your fingertips downward toward the cervix (see Figure 22.14).

▶ Note tenderness, masses, nodules, or bulging. These findings may indicate inflammation, infection, cysts, tumours, or wall prolapse. Note size, shape, consistency, and mobility of nodules and masses.

In the obese female, it may be difficult to clearly differentiate the uterine structures.

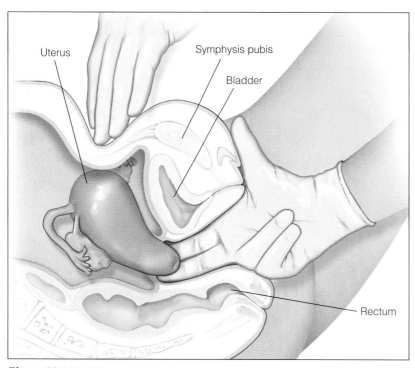

Figure 22.14 ● Palpating the uterus.

- Palpate the front wall of the uterus with the hand that is inside the vagina.
- As you palpate, note the position of the uterine body to determine that the uterus is in a normal position. When in a normal position, the uterus is tilted slightly upward above the bladder, and the cervix is tilted slightly forward.
- Normal variations of uterine position are as follows:
  - **Anteversion** (uterus tilted forward, cervix tilted downward; see Figure 22.15A)
  - **Midposition** (uterus lies parallel to tailbone, cervix pointed straight; see Figure 22.15B)
  - **Retroversion** (uterus tilted backward, cervix tilted upward; see Figure 22.15C)

▶ Abnormal variations of uterine position are as follows:
- **Anteflexion** (uterus folded forward at about a 90-degree angle, cervix tilted downward; see Figure 22.15D)
- **Retroflexion** (uterus folded backward at about a 90-degree angle, cervix tilted upward; see Figure 22.15E)

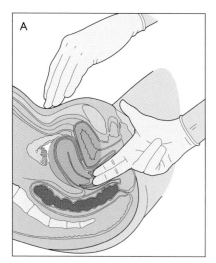
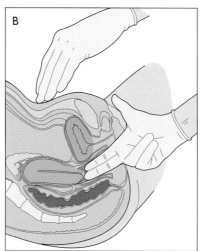
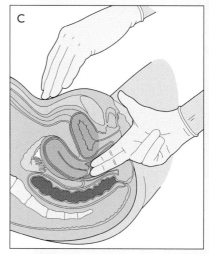

Figure 22.15 ● Variations in uterine position. A. Anteversion. B. Midposition. C. Retroversion.

TECHNIQUES AND NORMAL FINDINGS	ABNORMAL FINDINGS AND SPECIAL CONSIDERATIONS

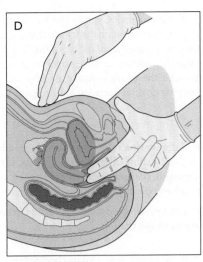 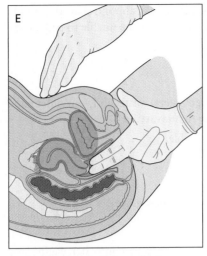

Figure 22.15 • Variations in uterine position. D. Anteflexion. E. Retroflexion.

- Move the inner fingers to the posterior fornix, and gently raise the cervix up toward your outer hand.
- Palpate the front and back walls of the uterus as it is sandwiched between the two hands.

4. **Palpate the ovaries.**
   - While positioning the outer hand on the left lower abdominal quadrant, slip the vaginal fingers into the left lateral fornix.

   - Push the opposing fingers and hand toward one another, and then use small circular motions to palpate the left ovary with your intravaginal fingers (see Figure 22.16).

▶ Masses, tenderness, nodules, or bulging require further evaluation.

▶ Extreme tenderness, nodularity, and masses are suggestive of inflammation, infection, cysts, malignancies, or tubal pregnancy.

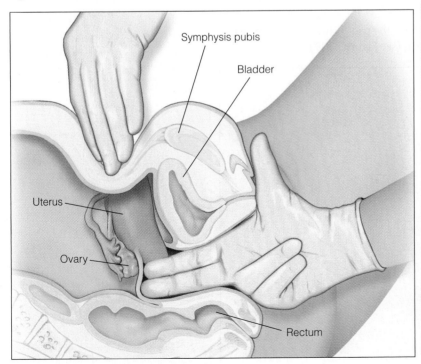

Symphysis pubis

Bladder

Uterus

Ovary

Rectum

Figure 22.16 • Palpating the ovaries.

Techniques and Normal Findings

- If you are able to palpate the ovary, it will feel mobile, almond shaped, smooth, firm, and nontender to slightly tender. Often you will be unable to palpate the ovaries, especially the right ovary.

- Slide your vaginal fingers around to the right lateral fornix and your outer hand to the lower right quadrant to palpate the right ovary.
- Confirm that the uterine tubes are not palpable.

- Remove your hand from the vagina and put on new gloves.

5. **Perform the rectovaginal exam.**
   - Tell the client that you are going to insert one finger into her vagina and one finger into her rectum to perform a rectovaginal exam. Tell her that this manoeuvre may make her feel as though she needs to have a bowel movement.
   - Lubricate the gloved index and middle fingers of the dominant hand.
   - Ask the client to bear down.
   - Touch the client's thigh with your nondominant hand to prepare her for the insertion.
   - Insert the index finger into the vagina (at a 45-degree downward slope) and the middle finger into the rectum.
   - Compress the rectovaginal septum between your index and middle fingers.
   - Confirm that it is thin, smooth, and nontender.
   - Place your nondominant hand on the client's abdomen.
   - While maintaining the position of your intravaginal hand, press your outer hand inward and downward on the abdomen over the symphysis pubis.
   - Palpate the posterior side of the uterus with the pad of the rectal finger while continuing to press down on the abdomen (see Figure 22.17).

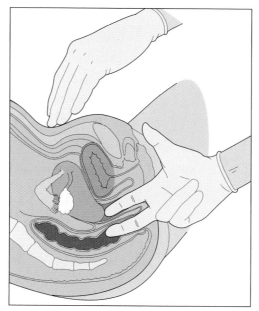

Figure 22.17 ●
Rectovaginal palpation.

ABNORMAL FINDINGS AND SPECIAL CONSIDERATIONS

▶ In obese females, it may not be possible to palpate the ovaries. In the female client who has been postmenopausal for more than 2.5 years, palpable ovaries are considered abnormal because the ovaries usually atrophy with the postmenopausal decrease in estrogen.

▶ If the uterine tubes are palpable, an inflammation or some other disease process, such as salpingitis (inflammation of the uterine tube) or an ectopic pregnancy, may be present.

▶ This prevents cross-contamination from the vagina to the rectum.

▶ Note tenderness, masses, nodules, bulging, and thickened areas.

TECHNIQUES AND NORMAL FINDINGS	ABNORMAL FINDINGS AND SPECIAL CONSIDERATIONS

- Confirm that the uterine wall is smooth and nontender.
- If the ovaries are palpable, note that they are normal in size and contour.
- Remove your fingers from the vagina and rectum slowly and gently.

▶ Tenderness, masses, nodules, bulging, or thickened areas require further evaluation.

6. **Examine the stool.**
   - Inspect feces remaining on the glove. Feces is normally brown and soft. Test feces for occult blood. Normally the test is negative.
   - Remove your gloves.

   - Wash your hands.
   - Assist the client into a comfortable position.
   - Give the client tissues to wipe the perineal area. Some clients may need a perineal pad.
   - Inform the client that she may have a small amount of spotting for a few hours after the speculum examination.

▶ Black, tarry stool indicates upper gastrointestinal tract bleeding.

▶ Rectal bleeding is suspected when bright red blood is on the surface of the stool. Feces mixed with blood signals bleeding above the rectum.

SAMPLE DOCUMENTATION

Subjective: 29-year-old female, G2P2, to clinic for annual gyne exam. No vaginal tenderness or redness noted. Menses regular, lasting 4 days. No additional vaginal discharge. Sexually active with no concerns. Uses oral contraceptives as birth control. No complaints of headaches or leg pain. Nonsmoker.

Objective: *External genitalia:* triangular hair distribution. No redness or lesions noted. No Bartholin's glands palpable. *Internal genitalia:* strong vaginal wall tone. Cervix pink, os visible. Pap swabs taken, no bleeding noted.

APPLICATION THROUGH CRITICAL THINKING

CASE STUDY

Jessica Krahn, a 24-year-old, arrives in the clinic with lower abdominal pain and nausea. She states, "I've had this throbbing pain for 3 days and it kept getting worse." She further states, "I haven't been able to eat. I feel awful. You have to do something for the pain."

The nurse explains that more information is needed so that the proper treatment can be initiated. In further interview the following information is obtained. Ms. Krahn's last menstrual period was 1 week ago and she had more crampiness than usual. She has had brownish, thick vaginal discharge on and off since then. She has had some itchiness in the vaginal area and burning when she voids. She states she has to go to the bathroom all the time: "All I did was pee little bits, until this pain got to me. I have hardly gone since last night."

When asked about the pain, Ms. Krahn says it is mostly 8 on a scale of 1 to 10 and getting pretty constant. "Nothing I do helps, except a little if I curl up and hold still."

Physical examination reveals a thin, pale female.

VS: B/P 108/64—P 92—RR 20—T 38.5°C (101°F).
Skin is hot, dry, decreased skin turgor with tenting
Mucous membranes dry.
Posture—abdominal guarding.
Abdomen BS × 4 tender in R & LLQ to palpation. Vulvar pruritus, thick purulent vaginal drainage, pain on cervical and uterine movement.

Cultures from vaginal secretions obtained	To lab
Blood drawn for CBC	To lab
Urine specimen obtained—clear, yellow	To lab

The client's clinic record reveals that she has been sexually active since age 16. She has had multiple partners and one abortion. She has been treated for sexually transmitted disease three times, most recently 2 months before this visit. The client is on birth control pills. She has no allergies to medications, and no family history of cardiovascular, abdominal, neurological, urological, endocrine, or reproductive disease.

Interpretation of the data suggests a diagnosis of pelvic inflammatory disease (PID). The options are outpatient treatment with antibiotics and education about limitations in activity and sexual practices, or inpatient treatment with intravenous fluids, antibiotics, analgesic, and bed rest.

Because Ms. Krahn is acutely ill, with pain and dehydration, she is admitted to the acute care facility with a diagnosis of PID.

▶ Complete Documentation

The following is sample documentation for Jessica Krahn.

SUBJECTIVE DATA: Throbbing abdominal pain for 3 days and getting worse. Rated 8 on scale of 1 to 10 with slight relief when "curled up and still." Nausea, unable to eat. LMP 1 week ago with increased crampiness. Brownish, thick vaginal discharge. Vaginal itchiness. Urgent, burning urination of small amounts until past 12 hours. Sexually active with history of multiple partners, recent STI. No family history of disease, no allergies to medication.

OBJECTIVE DATA: Thin, pale female. Dry mucous membranes, skin hot, dry, decreased skin turgor with tenting. Abdominal guarding, BS present × 4, tender RLQ, LLQ to light palpation. Vulvar pruritus, purulent vaginal discharge, adnexal tenderness with vaginal and bimanual examination.

ASSESSMENT FORM

Vital Signs

B/P: *108/64*

P: *92*

T: *38.5°C (101.4°F)*

Pain: Location: *R & L LQ*

Rating: *8*

Duration: *constant*

Relief: *curling up and being still*

Onset: *3 days*

Quality: *throbbing*

Skin

Colour: *pink*

Temperature: *hot*

Moisture: *dry*

Turgor: *poor*

Lesions: *none*

Respiratory

Respiratory rhythm: *regular*

Rate: *20*

Lung sounds: *clear all fields*

Abdomen

Contour: *round*

BS: *+ all Q*

Pain: *tender (R) (L) LQ*

Stool: *none*

Appetite: *poor—nausea*

Urinary

Frequency: *increased until past 12 hours*

Amount: *"a little at a time"*

Colour: *yellow*

Effort: *burning*

Endocrine

LMP: *1 week ago*

Blood sugar: *unknown*

Genitalia

Vulvar pruritus, purulent vaginal discharge

Adnexal tenderness with vaginal and bimanual examination

▶ Critical Thinking Questions

1. What clusters of information suggest the diagnosis of PID?
2. What additional information is required to develop a plan of care for Jessica Krahn?
3. What would discharge planning for Ms. Krahn include?

▶ Applying Nursing Diagnoses

1. *Ineffective sexuality patterns* is a diagnosis in the NANDA-I taxonomy (see Appendix A ⟳). Do the data in the case study support this diagnosis? Explain your response.
2. Use the data from the case study and the NANDA-I taxonomy (see Appendix A) to develop nursing diagnoses for Jessica Krahn.
3. Identify the data to support each diagnosis identified in the NANDA-I taxonomy.

▶ Prepare Teaching Plan

LEARNING NEED: Ms. Krahn initiated sexual activity at 16 years of age. She has had multiple partners and frequent episodes of STI. These data indicate a need to learn about PID and to discuss this infection with her partner.

GOAL: Ms. Krahn will decrease her risk for repeated episodes of PID.

OBJECTIVES: Jessica Krahn will be able to do the following:
1. Describe PID.
2. Relate personal practices to the occurrence of PID.
3. Describe treatment modalities for PID.

Application of Objective 2: Relate personal practices to the occurrence of PID (cognitive).

Content	Teaching Strategy	Evaluation
• Frequent douching: masks symptoms or pushes organisms internally • Sexual activity before age 25 • Multiple partners • Partner with multiple partners • Use of IUD • Not practising safe sex—use of condoms decreases risk • Untreated STI	• One-on-one discussion encourages learner participation, permits reinforcement of content, and is appropriate for sensitive subject matter.	• Learner relates personal practices to the occurrence of PID.

HEALTH PROMOTION ASSESSMENT TOOL

Social Determinants of Health	Level of Action	Action Strategies
Gender	Individual	**Reorient health services** (going beyond treating the illness to addressing the root causes of PID to prevent future reoccurrence) • Assess Ms. Krahn's sexual history (including circumstances related to her sexual initiation as a teen) and current activity. • Using a nonjudgmental approach, explore her lifestyle choices, how she views and values her body, and her possible use of sexuality to meet relational needs.
Social environments and health child development	Individual	**Reorient health services** • Explore Ms. Krahn's social environments, how they may have affected her understanding of what it means to be a woman, and how they are connected to her current sexual behaviour: • What did it mean to be a woman in her family of origin? • How were girls treated in her circle of friends, school environment, and other social environments? • Who were her female role models and what did she admire about them? • What did she learn about expressing her sexuality? • How were the women in her life treated by men and how did the women respond? • How has she been treated by men in her life (father, relatives, family friends, sexual partners)? • Explore her willingness and ability to communicate her personal needs and desires in relationships. *(continued)*

Health Promotion Assessment Tool

Social Determinants of Health	Level of Action	Action Strategies
Personal coping skills	Individual	**Develop personal skills** • Assess Ms. Krahn's knowledge and skill level for preventing STIs and PID, including her personal hygiene practices. • Assess her ability to negotiate the use of condoms with her sexual partners. • Teach Ms. Krahn about the use of barrier methods of preventing STIs, including male and female condoms. • Positively reinforce her use of oral contraceptive and assess the consistency of her use of birth control pills.

Abnormal Findings

Abnormal findings from assessment of the female reproductive system include but are not limited to problems with the external genitalia, perianal area, cervix, internal reproductive organs, and inflammatory processes. Problems in the perianal area are described in this chapter. Abnormal findings in the external genitalia are depicted and described in Figures 22.18 through 22.21. Abnormal findings of the cervix are illustrated and described in Figure 22.22. Abnormal findings of the internal reproductive organs, such as myomas or fibroids, ovarian cancer, and ovarian cysts, are illustrated and explained in Figures 22.23 through 22.25. Common inflammatory processes in the female reproductive system are depicted and described in Figures 22.26 through 22.29.

External Genitalia

Pediculosis Pubis

Nits are on and around roots of pubic hair and cause itching. The area is reddened and excoriated (scratched) (see Figure 22.18).

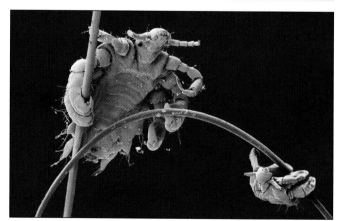

Figure 22.18 ●
Pediculosis pubis (crab lice).

Herpes Simplex

In herpes simplex, small vesicles appear on the genitalia and may spread to the inner thigh (see Figure 22.19). Ulcers are painful and erupt on rupture of vesicles. The virus may be dormant for long periods.

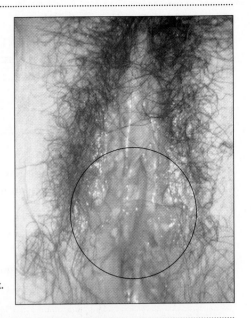

Figure 22.19 ● Herpes simplex.

Syphilitic Lesion

A syphilitic lesion is a nontender solitary papule that gradually changes to a draining ulcer (see Figure 22.20).

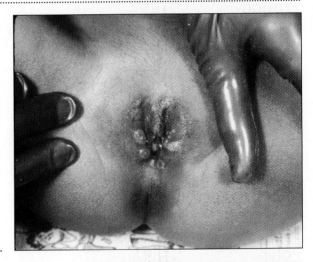

Figure 22.20 ● Syphilitic lesion.

Human Papillomavirus (HPV)

In HPV, wartlike, painless growths appear in clusters (see Figure 22.21). These are seen on the vulva, inner vagina, cervix, or anal area.

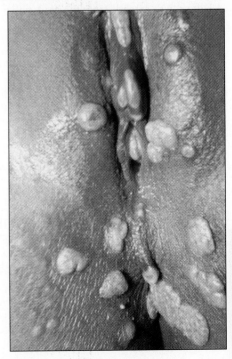

Figure 22.21 ●
Human papillomavirus
(genital warts).

Abscess of Bartholin's Gland

An abscess of the Bartholin's gland includes labial edema and erythema with a palpable mass. There is purulent drainage from the duct.

Cervix

Cyanosis

Cyanosis associated with hypoxic conditions, such as congestive heart failure, can cause this. Blue colouring of the cervix is normal in pregnancy.

Carcinoma

Ulcerations with vaginal discharge, postmenopausal bleeding or spotting, or bleeding between menstrual periods are characteristics of cervical carcinoma. Diagnosis is confirmed by Pap smear.

Erosion

Inflammation and erosion are visible on the surface of the cervix (see Figure 22.22). It is difficult to distinguish this from carcinoma without a biopsy.

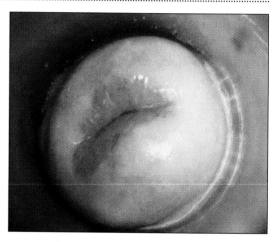

Figure 22.22 ● Erosion of the cervix.

Polyp

A soft growth extends from the os. A polyp is usually bright red and may bleed.

Diethylstilbestrol (DES) Syndrome

Abnormalities of the cervix arise in females who had prenatal exposure to DES. Epithelial abnormalities occur as granular patchiness extending from the cervix to the vaginal walls.

Internal Reproductive Organs

Myomas or Fibroids

Fibroids, also known as myomas and leiomyomas, are solid tumours located either inside the uterine cavity or on the muscle wall. They range in size from a few millimetres to several centimetres in diameter (see Figure 22.23).

Characteristics

• May be influenced by estrogen

Signs and Symptoms

- May be asymptomatic
- May cause excessive bleeding during menses
- Uterus may become enlarged
- May cause abdominal distension, pain, intestinal obstruction, frequent urination, and constipation

Treatment

- Depends on symptoms and whether the client is currently pregnant or wants to become pregnant
- Surgery

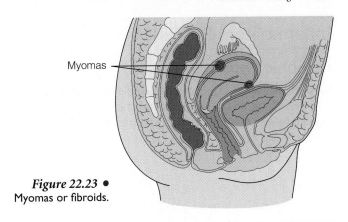

Figure 22.23 ●
Myomas or fibroids.

Ovarian Cancer

Ovarian cancer (see Figure 22.24) is a type of cancer that begins in the cells of the ovaries and includes the epithelial and germ cells.

Characteristics

- The Canadian Cancer Society (2009) reports 2500 new cases annually. It is known as the silent killer of women.
- The incidence is higher in females with a family history (first-degree relative), in women over 50 (with highest risk over age 60), in those who have not had children, in those who have had breast or colon cancer, and in those who have used fertility drugs, applied talc (talcum powder, baby powder) in the genital area, or used hormone replacement therapy (HRT).

Signs and Symptoms

- In early stages, it may be symptomatic. Some clients experience gastrointestinal disturbances (pressure, bloating, cramps, indigestion), pain in the calves of the legs, lower back pain, loss of appetite, weight gain or loss with no known reason, nausea, diarrhea, constipation, and frequent urination.

- Progression of the tumour leads to severe abdominal pressure and bloating, ascites, constipation, urinary frequency, abnormal bleeding from the vagina, and severe pain.

Treatment

- Depending on the stage and general health of the female, it may include surgery, chemotherapy, and radiation therapy.

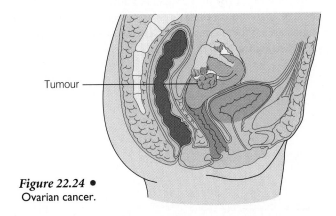

Figure 22.24 ●
Ovarian cancer.

Ovarian Cysts

Ovarian cysts are fluid-filled sacs within the ovary or on the surface of the ovary (see Figure 22.25).

Characteristics

- Nonmalignant cysts may develop during puberty and through menopause.

Signs and Symptoms

- Can be asymptomatic
- Some clients experience pelvic pain, abdominal distension, and lower back pain.

Treatment

- May be spontaneously resorbed within several months
- Surgery may be indicated

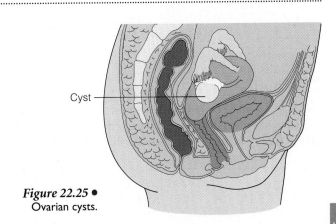

Figure 22.25 ●
Ovarian cysts.

Inflammatory Processes

Atrophic Vaginitis

Estrogen deficiency in postmenopausal females results in dryness, itching, and burning sensations in the vagina. The vaginal mucosa may appear pale, with mucusy discharge (see Figure 22.26).

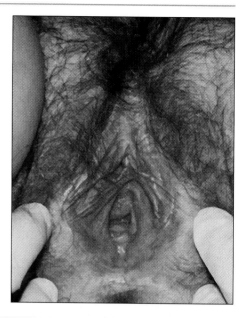

Figure 22.26 ●
Atrophic vaginitis.

Candidiasis

Alteration of the pH of the vagina or antibiotic use predispose the female to this candidiasis (yeast infection). The vulva and vagina are erythematous. Thick, cheesy, white discharge is seen (see Figure 22.27).

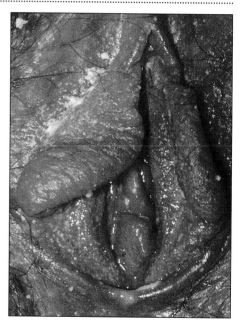

Figure 22.27 ●
Candidiasis (yeast infection).

Chlamydia

Chlamydia is an STI that is often asymptomatic. It is characterized by purulent discharge with tenderness on movement of the cervix. Chlamydia can cause sterility if untreated.

Gonorrhea

Gonorrhea is generally asymptomatic. It may produce vaginal discharge or bleeding of the cervix and abscesses in the Bartholin's or Skene's glands (see Figure 22.28).

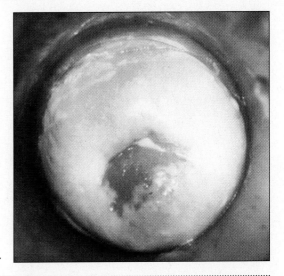

Figure 22.28 ● Gonorrhea.

Trichomoniasis

The female experiences painful urination, vulvular itching, and purulent vaginal discharge with this STI. The vagina and vulva are reddened and the discharge is yellow and foul smelling (see Figure 22.29).

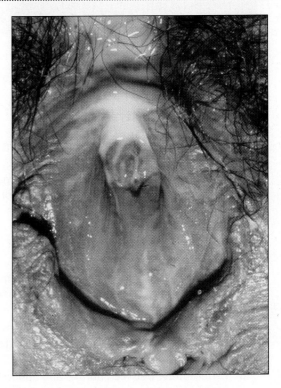

Figure 22.29 ● Trichomoniasis.

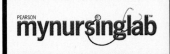

Visit the MyNursingLab website at **http://www.pearsoned.ca/mynursinglab**. This online homework and tutorial system puts you in control of your own learning with study and practice tools directly correlated to this chapter's content.

23

MUSCULOSKELETAL SYSTEM

THE PRIMARY FUNCTION OF THE MUSCULOSKELETAL SYSTEM is to provide structure and movement for the human body. The 206 bones of the musculoskeletal system and accompanying skeletal muscles allow the body to stand erect and move, and they support and protect body organs. This system produces red blood cells, stores fat and minerals, and generates body heat.

A thorough assessment of the musculoskeletal system provides data relevant to activity, exercise, nutrition, and metabolism. The physical assessment of the musculoskeletal system is extensive, requiring a head-to-toe approach because it extends throughout the body. Musculoskeletal assessment could be combined with assessment of other body systems to obtain data reflecting the client's total health status, because every other body system is affected by or affects this body system. For example, the nervous system innervates bone and joint capsules and helps stimulate and regulate muscle activity. Should the client have difficulty moving a specific part of the body, the nurse will need to determine the origin of the problem as being neurological or musculoskeletal. Red blood cells are formed in the bone marrow; therefore, if the cell count is low, the nurse will need to determine the source of the problem.

Bone density and curvatures vary widely among people of different cultural groups. Working conditions requiring heavy lifting, repetitive motions, or substantial physical activity present potential risks to this system. Participation in hobbies and athletic activities can contribute to wear and tear damage to joints and create risks for trauma to bones, muscles, and joints. Changes in bone density and injury to bone and muscle are factors in the goals for health promotion.

ANATOMY AND PHYSIOLOGY REVIEW

The musculoskeletal system consists of the body's bones, skeletal muscles, and joints. A thorough discussion of these anatomical structures is included in the following section.

Bones

The bones support and provide a framework for the soft tissues and organs of the body. They are classified according to shape and composition. Bone shapes include *long bones* (femur, humerus), *short bones* (carpals, tarsals), *flat bones* (the parietal bone of the skull, the sternum, ribs), and *irregular bones* (vertebrae, hip bones) as shown in Figure 23.1. Bones are composed of osseous tissue that is arranged in either a dense, smooth, compact structure or a cancellous, spongy structure with many small open spaces (see Figure 23.2). The bones of the human skeleton are illustrated in Figure 23.3.

The major functions of the bones include providing a framework for the body, protecting structures, acting as levers for movement, storing fat and minerals, and producing blood cells.

Skeletal Muscles

A skeletal muscle is composed of hundreds of thousands of elongated muscle cells or fibres arranged in striated bands that attach to skeletal bones (see Figure 23.4 on page 588). Although some skeletal muscles react by reflex, most skeletal muscles are voluntary and are under an individual's conscious control. Figure 23.5 on pages 589 and 590 illustrates the muscles of the human body. The major functions of the skeletal muscles include providing for movement, maintaining posture, and generating body heat.

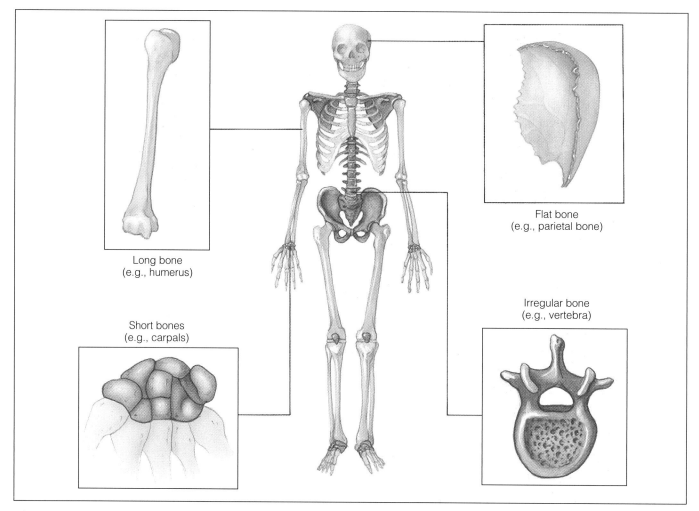

Figure 23.1 ● Classification of bones according to shape.

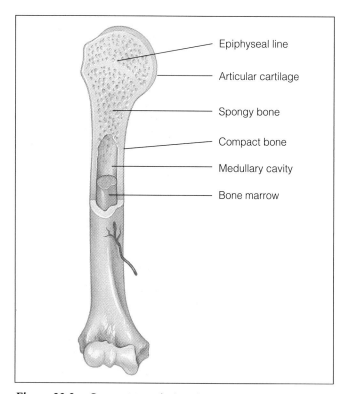

Epiphyseal line

Articular cartilage

Spongy bone

Compact bone

Medullary cavity

Bone marrow

Figure 23.2 ● Composition of a long bone.

Joints

A **joint** (or *articulation*) is the point at which two or more bones in the body meet. Joints can be classified structurally as fibrous, cartilaginous, or synovial. Bones joined by fibrous tissue, such as the sutures joining the bones of the skull, are called **fibrous joints**. Bones joined by cartilage, such as the vertebrae, are called **cartilaginous joints**. Bones separated by a fluid-filled joint cavity are called **synovial joints**. The structure of synovial joints allows tremendous freedom of movement, and all joints of the limbs are synovial joints. Most synovial joints are reinforced and strengthened by a system of *ligaments,* which are bands of flexible tissue that attach bone to bone. Some ligaments are protected from friction by small, synovial-fluid-filled sacs called **bursae**. **Tendons** are tough fibrous bands that attach muscle to bone, or muscle to muscle. Tendons, subjected to continuous friction, develop fluid-filled bursae called *tendon sheaths* to protect the joint from damage.

During the assessment of the musculoskeletal system, the nurse assesses the joint, its range of motion, and its surrounding structures of muscles, ligaments, tendons, and bursae. Table 23.1 on page 591 describes the classification of synovial joints, and Table 23.2 on page 592 describes the movements of the joints. A description of selected joints to be examined during the physical assessment of the musculoskeletal system follows.

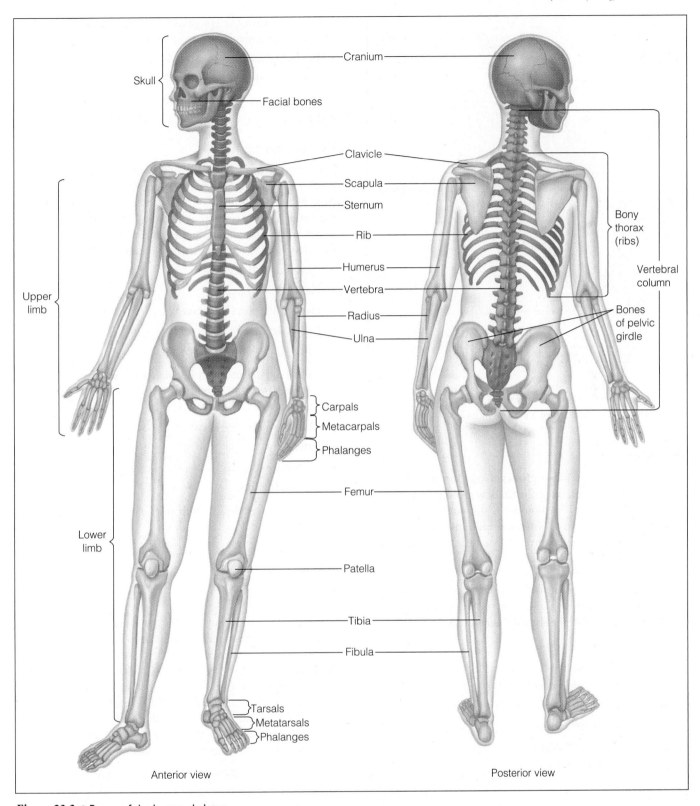

Figure 23.3 • Bones of the human skeleton.

Temporomandibular Joint

The temporomandibular joint (TMJ) permits articulation between the mandible and the temporal bone of the skull (see Figure 23.6 on page 594). Lying just anterior to the external auditory meatus, at the level of the tragus of the ear, the temporomandibular joint allows an individual to speak and chew. Temporomandibular movements include the following:

- Opening and closing of the lower jaw
- Protraction and retraction of the lower jaw
- Side-to-side movement of the lower jaw

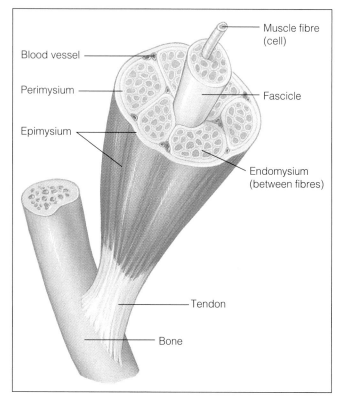

Muscle fibre (cell)

Blood vessel

Perimysium

Epimysium

Fascicle

Endomysium (between fibres)

Tendon

Bone

Figure 23.4 • Composition of a skeletal muscle.

Shoulder

The shoulder joint is a ball-and-socket joint in which the head of the humerus articulates in the shallow glenoid cavity of the scapula (Table 23.1). The shoulder is supported by the rotator cuff, a sturdy network of tendons and muscles, as well as a series of ligaments (see Figure 23.7 on page 594). The major landmarks of the shoulder include the scapula, the acromion process, the greater tubercle of the humerus, and the coracoid process. The subacromial bursa, which allows the arm to abduct smoothly and with ease, lies just below the acromion process. Movements of the shoulder include the following:

- Abduction (180 degrees)
- Adduction (50 degrees)
- Horizontal forward flexion (180 degrees)
- Horizontal backward extension (50 degrees)
- Circumduction (360 degrees)
- External rotation (90 degrees)
- Internal rotation (90 degrees)

Elbow

The elbow is a hinge joint that allows articulation between the humerus of the upper arm and the radius and ulna of the forearm (see Figure 23.8 on page 591). Landmarks include the lateral and medial epicondyles on either side of the distal end of the humerus and the olecranon process of the ulna. The olecranon bursa sits between the olecranon process and the skin. The ulnar nerve travels between the medial epicondyle and the olecranon process. When inflamed, the synovial membrane is palpable between the epicondyles and the olecranon process. Elbow movements include the following:

- Flexion of the forearm (160 degrees)
- Extension of the forearm (160 degrees)
- Supination of the forearm and hand (90 degrees)
- Pronation of the forearm and hand (90 degrees)

Wrist and Hand

The wrist (or *carpus*) consists of two rows of eight short carpal bones connected by ligaments as illustrated in Figure 23.9 on page 595. The distal row articulates with the metacarpals of the hand. The proximal row includes the scaphoid and lunate bones, which articulate with the distal end of the radius to form the wrist joint. Wrist movements include the following:

- Extension (70 degrees)
- Flexion (90 degrees)
- Hyperextension (30 degrees)
- Radial deviation (20 degrees)
- Ulnar deviation (55 degrees)

Each hand has metacarpophalangeal joints, and each finger has interphalangeal joints. Finger movements include the following:

- Abduction (20 degrees)
- Extension
- Flexion (90 degrees)
- Circumduction

Thumb movements include the following:

- Extension
- Flexion (80 degrees)
- Opposition

Hip

The hip joint is a ball-and-socket joint composed of the rounded head of the femur as it fits deep into the **acetabulum**, a rounded cavity on the right and left lateral sides of the pelvic bone (see Figure 23.10 on page 595). Although not as mobile as the shoulder, the hip is surrounded by a system of cartilage, ligaments, tendons, and muscles that contribute to its strength and stability. Landmarks include the iliac crest (not shown), the greater trochanter of the femur, and the anterior inferior iliac spine. Hip movements include the following:

- Extension (90 degrees)
- Hyperextension (15 degrees)
- Flexion with knee flexed (120 degrees)
- Flexion with knee extended (90 degrees)
- Internal rotation (40 degrees)
- External rotation (45 degrees)
- Abduction (45 degrees)
- Adduction (30 degrees)

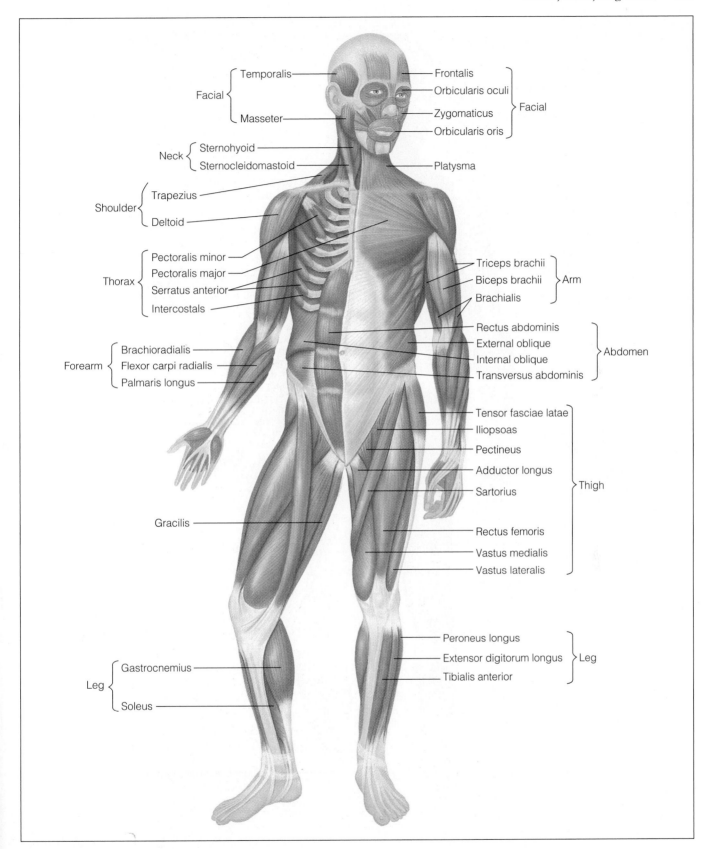

Figure 23.5A ● Anterior view of muscles of the human body.

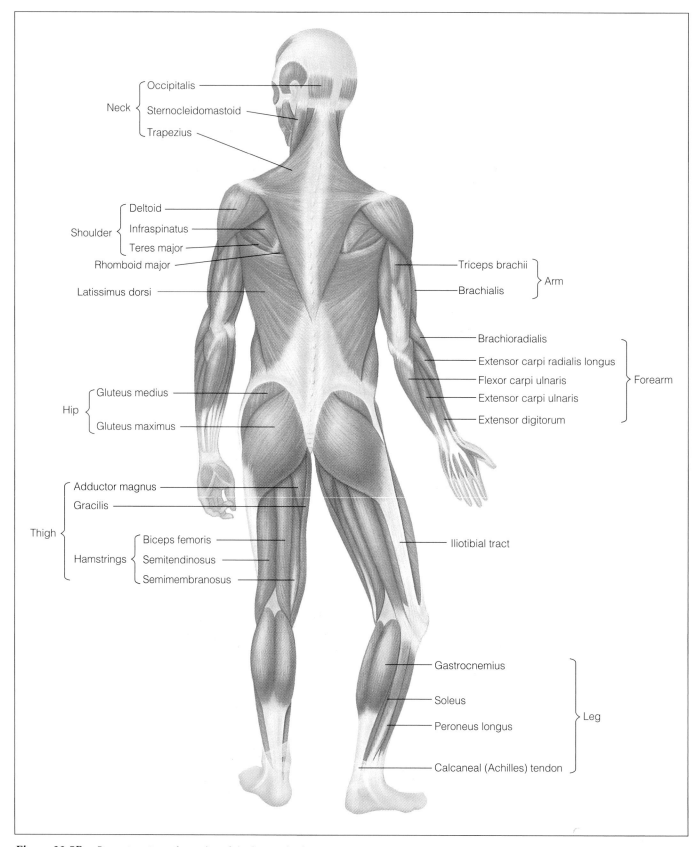

Figure 23.5B • Posterior view of muscles of the human body.

TABLE 23.1 | Classification of Synovial Joints

TYPE OF JOINT	DESCRIPTION
 A Plane joint	In *plane joints,* the articular surfaces are flat, allowing only slipping or gliding movements. Examples include the intercarpal and intertarsal joints, and the joints between the articular processes of the ribs.
 B Hinge joint	In *hinge joints,* a convex projection of one bone fits into a concave depression in another. Motion is similar to that of a mechanical hinge. These joints permit flexion and extension only. Examples include the elbow and knee joints.
 C Pivot joint	In *pivot joints,* the rounded end of one bone protrudes into a ring of bone (and possibly ligaments). The only movement allowed is rotation of the bone around its own long axis or against the other bone. An example is the joint between the atlas and axis of the neck.
 D Condyloid joint	In *condyloid joints,* the oval surfaces of two bones fit together. Movements allowed are flexion and extension, abduction, adduction, and circumduction. An example is the radiocarpal (wrist) joints.
 E Saddle joint	In *saddle joints,* each articulating bone has both concave and convex areas (resembling a saddle). The opposing surfaces fit together. The movements allowed are the same as for condyloid joints, but the freedom of motion is greater. The carpometacarpal joints of the thumbs are an example.

(continued)

TABLE 23.1	Classification of Synovial Joints *(continued)*

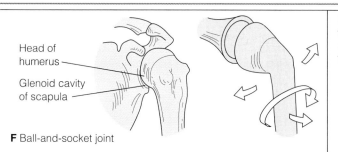

Head of humerus

Glenoid cavity of scapula

F Ball-and-socket joint

In *ball-and-socket joints,* the ball-shaped head of one bone fits into the concave socket of another. These joints allow movement in all axes and planes, including rotation. The shoulder and hip joints are the only examples in the body.

TABLE 23.2	Joint Movement

TYPE OF MOVEMENT	DESCRIPTION
	Gliding movements are the simplest type of joint movements. One flat bone surface glides or slips over another similar surface. The bones are merely displaced in relation to one another.
	Flexion is a bending movement that decreases the angle of the joint and brings the articulating bones closer together. **Extension** increases the angle between the articulating bones. **Hyperextension** is a bending of a joint beyond the neutral position or 180 degrees.
	Flexion of the ankle so that the superior aspect of the foot approaches the shin is called **dorsiflexion**. Extension of the ankle (pointing the toes) is called **plantar flexion.**
	Abduction is movement of a limb away from the midline or median plane of the body, along the frontal plane. When the term is used to describe movement of the fingers or toes, it means spreading them apart. **Adduction** is the movement of a limb toward the body midline. Bringing the fingers close together is adduction.
	Circumduction is the movement in which the limb describes a cone in space: while the distal end of the limb moves in a circle, the joint itself moves only slightly in the joint cavity.

(continued)

TABLE 23.2	Joint Movement *(continued)*

TYPE OF MOVEMENT	DESCRIPTION
	Rotation is the turning movement of a bone around its own long axis. Rotation may occur toward the body midline or away from it.
	The terms **supination** and **pronation** refer only to the movements of the radius around the ulna. Movement of the forearm so that the palm faces anteriorly or superiorly is called *supination*. In *pronation*, the palm moves to face posteriorly or inferiorly.
	The terms **inversion** and **eversion** refer to movements of the foot. In *inversion*, the sole of the foot is turned medially. In *eversion*, the sole faces laterally.
	Protraction is a nonangular anterior movement in a transverse plane. **Retraction** is a nonangular posterior movement in a transverse plane.
	Elevation is a lifting or moving superiorly along a frontal plane. When the elevated part is moved downward to its original position, the movement is called **depression**. Shrugging the shoulders and chewing are examples of alternating elevation and depression.
	Opposition *of the thumb* is only allowed at the saddle joint between metacarpal 1 and the carpals. It is the movement of touching the thumb to the tips of any of the other fingers of the same hand.

Knee

The knee is a complex joint consisting of the patella (knee cap), femur, and tibia (see Figure 23.11 on page 596). It is supported and stabilized by the cruciate and collateral ligaments, which have a stabilizing effect on the knee and prevent dislocation. The landmarks of the knee include the tibial tuberosity and the medial and lateral condyles of the tibia. Knee movements include the following:

- Extension (0 degree)
- Flexion (130 degrees)
- Hyperextension (15 degrees)

Ankle and Foot

The ankle is a hinge joint that accommodates articulation between the tibia, fibula, and *talus,* a large, posterior tarsal of the foot (see Figure 23.12 on page 596). The **calcaneus** (or heel bone) is just inferior to the talus. It is stabilized by a set of taut ligaments that are anchored from bony prominences at the distal ends of the tibia and fibula (the lateral and medial malleoli), and then extend and attach to the foot. Movements of the ankle and foot include the following:

- Dorsiflexion of ankle (20 degrees)
- Plantar flexion of ankle (45 degrees)

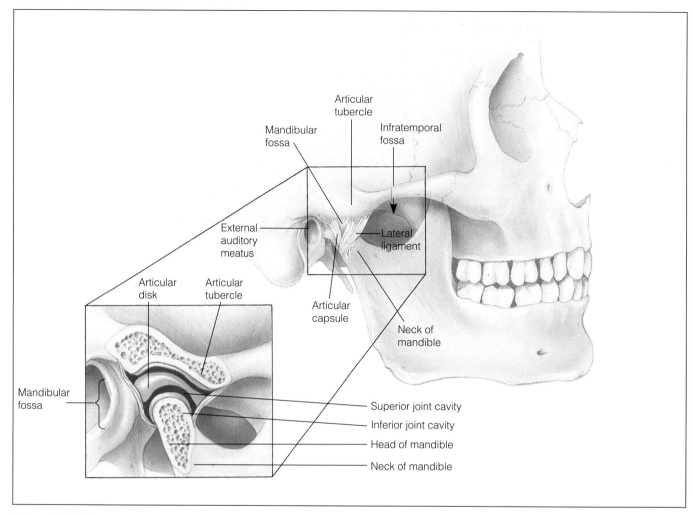

Figure 23.6 ● Temporomandibular joint. The enlargement shows a sagittal section through the joint.

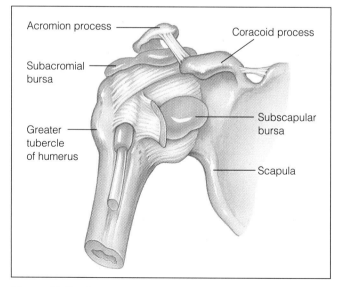

Figure 23.7 ● Shoulder joint.

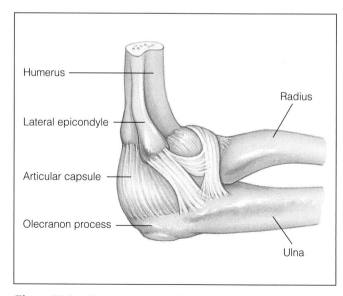

Figure 23.8 ● Elbow joint. Lateral view of the right elbow.

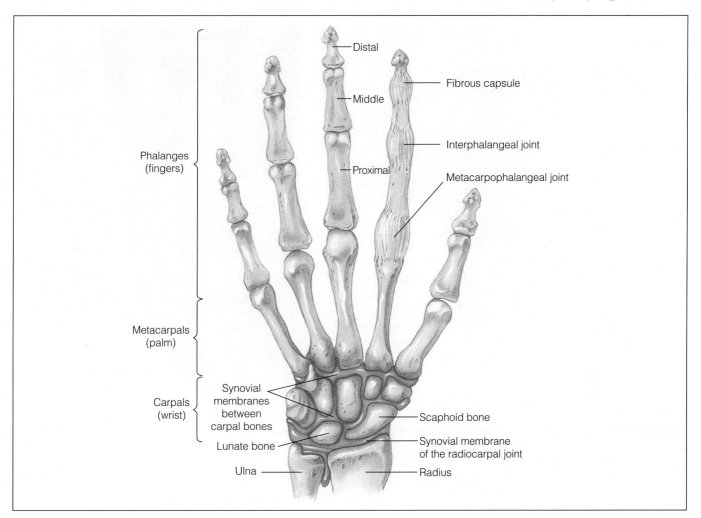

Figure 23.9 ● Bones of the wrist, hand, and phalanges.

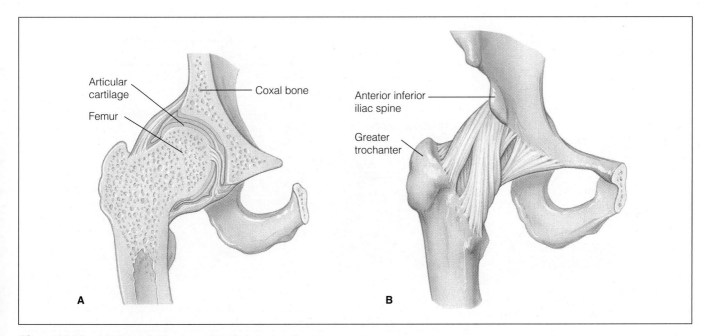

Figure 23.10 ● Hip joint. A. Cross section. B. Anterior view.

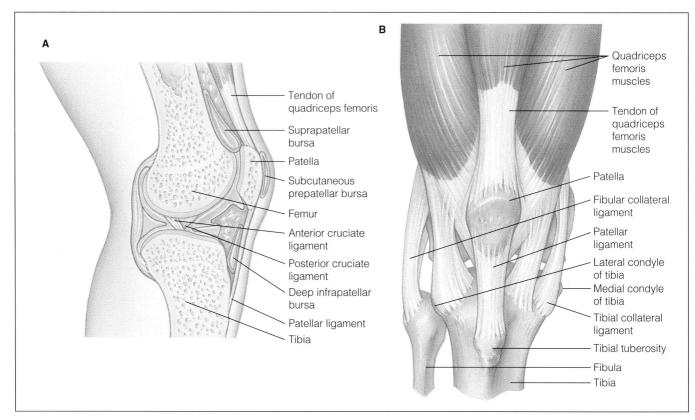

Figure 23.11 ● Knee joint. A. Sagittal section through the right knee. B. Anterior view.

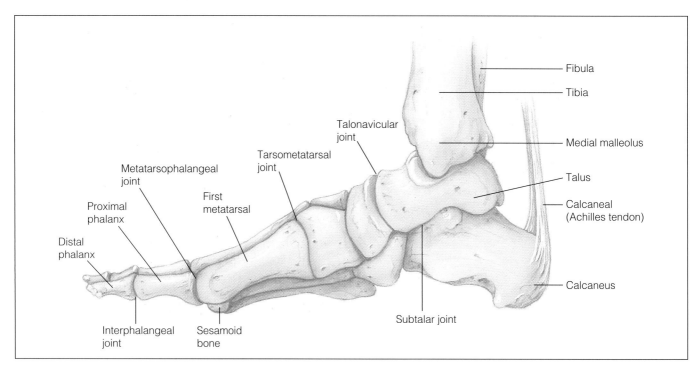

Figure 23.12 ● Medial view of joints of right ankle and foot.

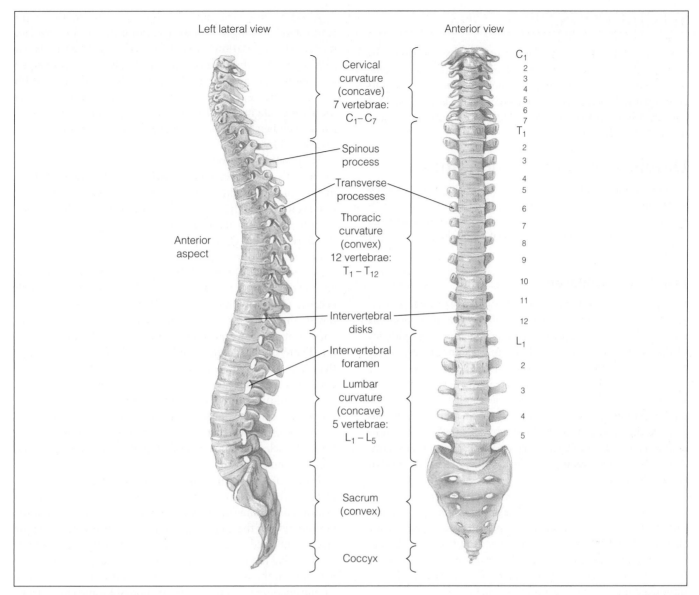

Left lateral view

Anterior view

Cervical curvature (concave) 7 vertebrae: C_1–C_7

Spinous process

Transverse processes

Thoracic curvature (convex) 12 vertebrae: T_1–T_{12}

Intervertebral disks

Intervertebral foramen

Lumbar curvature (concave) 5 vertebrae: L_1–L_5

Anterior aspect

Sacrum (convex)

Coccyx

C_1
2
3
4
5
6
7
T_1
2
3
4
5
6
7
8
9
10
11
12
L_1
2
3
4
5

Figure 23.13 ● The spine.

- Inversion of foot (30 degrees)
- Eversion of foot (20 degrees)

Movements of the toes include the following:

- Extension
- Flexion
- Abduction (10 degrees)
- Adduction (20 degrees)

Spine

The spine is composed of 26 irregular bones called vertebrae (see Figure 23.13). The seven *cervical vertebrae* support the base of the skull and the neck. All twelve *thoracic vertebrae* articulate with the ribs. The five *lumbar vertebrae* support the lower back. They are heavier and denser than the other vertebrae, reflecting their weight-bearing function. The *sacrum* shapes the posterior wall of the pelvis, offering strength and stability. The *coccyx* is a small, triangular tailbone at the base of the spine.

Viewed laterally, the spine has cervical and lumbar concavities and a thoracic convexity. As a person bends forward, the normal concavity should flatten, and there should be a single convex C-shaped curve. Figure 23.5B shows the main posterior muscles of the neck and the spine. Movements of the neck include the following:

- Flexion (45 degrees)
- Extension (55 degrees)
- Lateral flexion (bending) (40 degrees)
- Rotation (70 degrees)

Movements of the spine include the following:

- Lateral flexion (35 degrees)
- Extension (30 degrees)
- Flexion (90 degrees)
- Rotation (30 degrees)

SPECIAL CONSIDERATIONS

A variety of factors or special considerations contribute to health status, including age, developmental level, race, ethnicity, work history, living conditions, socioeconomics, and emotional well-being. The sections that follow describe special considerations for the nurse to include when gathering subjective and objective data.

Developmental Considerations

Accurate interpretation of findings requires knowledge of the variations in anatomy and physiology that occur with growth and development. Specific variations in the musculoskeletal system across the age span are described in the sections that follow.

Infants and Children

Fetal positioning and the delivery process may cause musculoskeletal anomalies in the infant. These include *tibial torsion,* a curving apart of the tibias, and *metatarsus adductus,* a tendency of the forefoot to turn inward. Many such anomalies correct themselves spontaneously as the child grows and walks.

Newborns normally have flat feet; arches develop gradually during the preschool years. Before learning to walk, infants tend to exhibit genu varum (bowlegs). Then, as the child begins to walk, this tendency gradually reverses. By the age of 4, most children tend to exhibit genu valgum (knock knees). This condition also resolves spontaneously, usually by late childhood or early adolescence.

The nurse should inspect the newborn's spine. Any tuft of hair, cyst, or mass may indicate spina bifida and requires further evaluation. The nurse also palpates the length of the clavicles at each office visit, noting any lumps or irregularities and observing the range of motion of the arms. The clavicle is frequently fractured during birth, and the fracture often goes unnoticed until a callus forms at the fracture site.

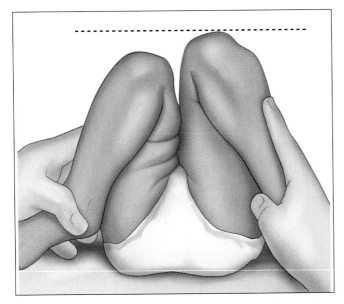

Figure 23.14 ● Allis' sign—demonstration of unequal knee height.

At every office visit, until the child is 1 year old, the infant is assessed for congenital hip dislocation using the Ortolani manoeuvre and Barlow's test, as described in Chapter 25, or Allis' sign. ◌ Allis' sign is used specifically to detect unequal leg length. The nurse is positioned at the child's feet. With the infant supine, the nurse flexes the infant's knees, keeping the femurs aligned, and compares the height of the knees. An uneven height indicates unequal leg length, as depicted in Figure 23.14.

While holding the infant, the nurse's hands should be beneath the infant's axillae. Shoulder muscle strength is present if the infant remains upright between the nurse's hands. Muscle weakness is indicated if the infant begins to slip through the hands.

Bone growth is rapid during infancy and continues at a steady rate during childhood until adolescence, at which time both girls and boys experience a growth spurt. Long bones increase in width because of the deposition of new bony tissue around the diaphysis (shaft). Long bones also increase in length because of a proliferation of cartilage at the growth plates at the epiphyses (ends) of the long bones. Longitudinal growth ends at about 21 years of age, when the epiphyses fuse with the diaphysis. Throughout childhood, ligaments are stronger than bones. Therefore, childhood injuries to the long bones and joints tend to result in **fractures** (partial or complete break in the continuity of the bone from trauma) instead of sprains. Individual muscle fibres grow throughout childhood, but growth is especially increased during the adolescent growth spurt. Muscles vary in size and strength because of genetics, exercise, and diet.

Much of the examination of the child and adolescent includes the same techniques of inspection, palpation, and assessment of range of motion and muscle strength used in the examination of the adult. However, children also have unique assessment needs. Children present wonderful opportunities for assessing range of motion and muscle strength as they play with toys in the waiting area or examination room. The nurse should encourage children to jump, hop, skip, and climb. Most children are eager to show off their abilities.

At each office visit, the nurse should ask children to demonstrate their favourite sitting position. If a child assumes the reverse tailor position (see Figure 23.15), common when watching television, the nurse should encourage the child to try other sitting positions. Parents should be told that the reverse tailor position stresses the hip, knee, and ankle joints of the growing child.

The nurse should ask the child to lie supine, then to rise to a standing position. Normally, the child rises without using the arms for support. Generalized muscle weakness may be indicated if the child places the hands on the knees and pushes the trunk up (Gowers' sign).

The child's spine is assessed for scoliosis at each office visit. It is also important to inspect the child's shoes for signs of abnormal wear, and assess the child's gait. Before age 3, the gait of the child is normally broad-based. After age 3, the child's gait narrows. At each visit, the nurse assesses the range of motion of each arm. **Subluxation** of the head of the radius occurs commonly when adults dangle children from their hands or remove their clothing forcibly.

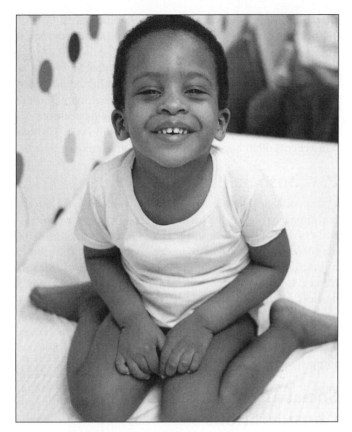

Figure 23.15 ● Reverse tailor position.

The nurse must obtain complete information on any sports activity the child or adolescent engages in, because participation in these can indicate the need for special assessments or preventive teaching, such as the use of helmets and other safety equipment.

The Pregnant Female

Estrogen and other hormones soften the cartilage in the pelvis and increase the mobility of the joints, especially the sacroiliac, sacrococcygeal, and symphysis pubis joints. As the pregnancy progresses, **lordosis** (exaggeration of the lumbar spinal curve) compensates for the enlarging fetus. The female's centre of gravity shifts forward, and she shifts her weight farther back on her lower extremities. This shift strains the lower spine, causing the lower back pain that is so common during late pregnancy (see Figure 23.16). As the pregnancy progresses, she may develop a waddling gait because of her enlarged abdomen and the relaxed mobility in her joints. Typically, a female resumes her normal posture and gait shortly after the pregnancy.

The Older Adult

As individuals age, physiological changes take place in the bones, muscles, connective tissue, and joints. These changes may affect the older client's mobility and endurance. Bone changes include decreased calcium absorption and reduced osteoblast production. If the older adult has a chronic illness, such as chronic obstructive lung disease or hyperthyroidism, or takes medications containing glucocorticoids, thyroid hormone preparation, or anticonvulsants, bone strength may be greatly compromised because of decrease in the bone density. Older adults who are housebound or immobile or whose dietary intake of calcium and vitamin D is low may also experience reduced bone mass and strength. During aging, bone resorption occurs more rapidly than new bone growth, resulting in the loss of bone density typical of osteoporosis. The entire skeleton is affected, but the vertebrae and long bones are especially vulnerable. Most aging adults develop some degree of osteoporosis, but it is more marked in females, especially those of European or Asian ancestry.

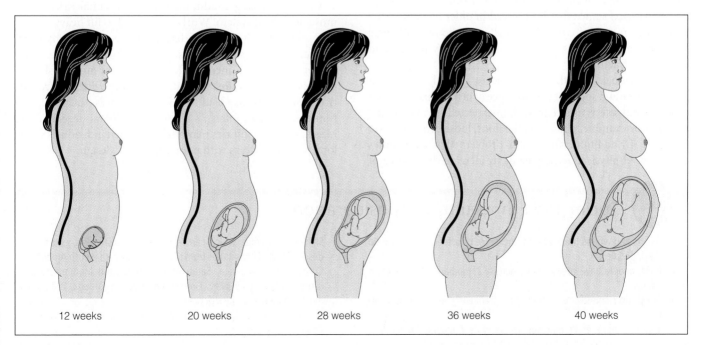

| 12 weeks | 20 weeks | 28 weeks | 36 weeks | 40 weeks |

Figure 23.16 ● Postural changes with pregnancy.

The decreased height of the aging adult occurs because of a shortening of the vertebral column. Thinning of the intervertebral discs during middle age and an erosion of individual vertebrae through osteoporosis contribute to this shortening. People experience an average decrease in height of 2.5 to 5 cm (1 to 2 in.) from the 20s through the 70s, and a further decrease in the 80s and 90s because of additional collapse of the vertebrae. **Kyphosis,** an exaggerated convexity of the thoracic region of the spine, is common. When the older adult is standing, the nurse may notice a slight flexion of the hips and knees. These changes in the vertebral column may cause a shift in the individual's centre of gravity, which in turn may put the older adult at an increased risk for falls.

The size and quantity of muscle fibres tend to decrease by as much as 30% by the 80th year of life. The amount of connective tissue in the muscles increases, and they become fibrous or stringy. Tendons become less elastic. As a result, the older client experiences a progressive decrease in reaction time, speed of movements, agility, and endurance.

Degeneration of the joints causes thickening and decreased viscosity of the synovial fluid, fragmentation of connective tissue, and scarring and calcification in the joint capsules. In addition, the cartilage becomes frayed, thin, and cracked, allowing the underlying bone to become eroded. Because of these changes, the joints of older people are less shock absorbent and have decreased range of motion and flexibility. These normal degenerative joint changes that occur from aging and use are referred to as *osteoarthrosis.* In some individuals, *Heberden's nodes*—hard, typically painless, bony enlargements associated with osteoarthritis—may occur in the distal interphalangeal joints.

The gait of an older client alters as the bones, muscles, and joints change with advancing age. Both males and females tend to walk slower, supporting themselves as they move. Older males tend to walk with the head and trunk in a flexed position, using short, high steps, a wide gait, and a smaller arm swing. The bowlegged stance that is observed in older females is due to reduced muscular control, thus altering the normal angle of the hip and leading to increased susceptibility to falls and subsequent fractures.

As individuals age, they experience a general decrease in reaction time and speed of performance of tasks. This can affect mobility and safety, especially with unexpected environmental stimuli (for example, objects on the floor, loose carpeting, wet surfaces). In addition, any health problem that contributes to decreased physical activity tends to increase the chance of alterations in the health of the musculoskeletal system. A well-balanced diet and regular exercise help to slow the progression of these musculoskeletal changes.

The physical assessment of the musculoskeletal system of the older person is similar to that of any other adult. When testing range of motion, the nurse must be careful not to cause pain, discomfort, or damage to the joint. The musculoskeletal exam is conducted at a slower pace when necessary because older clients often have health problems that affect endurance.

Psychosocial Considerations

Psychosocial problems, such as anxiety, depression, fear, altered body image, or a disturbance in self-esteem, may promote inactivity or isolation, which in turn may lead to musculoskeletal degeneration. Similarly, any health problem that contributes to inactivity may trigger or contribute to psychosocial disturbances. Impaired physical mobility may lead to stress, hopelessness, ineffective coping, social isolation, or other problems.

Physical abuse should be considered if a client has a history of frequent fractures, sprains, or other musculoskeletal trauma. The nurse must follow the provincial or territorial guidelines for referring the client to social or protective services.

Social and Ethnocultural Considerations

The bone density of Black people is significantly higher than that of white people. Asians typically have lower bone density than whites. The curvature of long bones varies widely among cultural groups and seems to be related to genetics and body weight. Thin people have less curvature than people of average weight; obese people display an increased curvature.

The number and distribution of vertebrae vary. Although 24 vertebrae is the average (present in about 85% to 90% of all people), 23 or 25 vertebrae are not uncommon.

Certain working conditions present potential risks to the musculoskeletal system. Workers required to lift heavy objects may strain and injure their back. Jobs requiring substantial physical activity, such as those of construction workers, fire fighters, or athletes, increase the likelihood of musculoskeletal injuries, such as sprains, strains, and fractures. Frequent repetitive movements may lead to misuse disorders, such as carpal tunnel syndrome, pitcher's elbow, or vertebral degeneration. Musculoskeletal injuries may also arise when individuals sit for long periods at desks with poor ergonomic design.

Social and Ethnocultural Considerations

- Asians and whites have a higher incidence of osteoporosis than do Black people.
- Black people have greater bone density compared with whites or Asians.
- Ankylosing spondylitis occurs more frequently in males than in females.
- Systemic lupus erythematosus occurs more frequently in females and with greater frequency and severity in Black people.

- Sickle-cell anemia, which can result in joint disruption, occurs in descendants of individuals from sub-Saharan Africa, South America, Cuba, Central America, Saudi Arabia, India, and Mediterranean countries, such as Turkey, Greece, and Italy. In Canada, it occurs most frequently in Black people.
- Paget's disease of bone occurs more frequently in whites than in other cultural groups.

GATHERING THE DATA

Health assessment of the musculoskeletal system includes gathering subjective and objective data. Subjective data collection occurs during the client interview, before the physical assessment. During the interview, various communication techniques are used to elicit general and specific information about the status of the client's musculoskeletal system and ability to function. Health records, the results of laboratory tests, X-rays, and imaging reports are important secondary sources to be included in the data-gathering process. During physical assessment of the musculoskeletal system, the techniques of inspection and palpation will be used to gather objective data.

HEALTH HISTORY

The health history for the musculoskeletal system concerns data related to the structures and functions of that system. Subjective data are gathered during the health history. The nurse must be prepared to observe the client and to listen for cues related to the function of the musculoskeletal system. The nurse may use open-ended or closed questions to obtain information. A number of follow-up questions or requests for descriptions may be required to clarify data or gather missing information. Follow-up questions are intended to identify the sources of problems, duration of difficulties, and measures used to alleviate or manage problems. They also provide clues about the client's knowledge of his or her own health.

The health history guides the physical assessment of the musculoskeletal system. The information is always considered in relation to norms and expectations about musculoskeletal function. Therefore, the nurse must consider age, gender, race, culture, environment, health practices, past and concurrent problems, and therapies when framing questions and using techniques to elicit information. To address all the factors when conducting a health history, specific questions related to musculoskeletal status and function have been developed. These questions focus on the most common concerns or injuries associated with the musculoskeletal system; questions related to past health history; questions related to behaviours; questions that address environmental concerns; and those that are specific to clients according to age, including the pregnant female.

The nurse must consider the client's ability to participate in the health history and physical assessment of the musculoskeletal system. Illness, discomfort, and disease may affect the ability to participate in the interview. Participation in the health history may be influenced by the ability to communicate in the same language. Language barriers interfere with the accuracy of data collection and cause anxiety in the client and examiner. A nurse may have to use a translator in conducting interviews and during the physical assessment. If the client is experiencing acute pain, recent injury, or anxiety, attention must be focused on relief of discomfort and relief of symptoms before proceeding with the in-depth interview.

As the nurse gathers the data, she or he will shift the type of questions to direct questions that give the client room to explain or qualify. The mnemonic O-P-Q-R-S-T-U, which stands for onset (chronology), precipitating (or palliative), quality, region (or radiation), severity, timing, and understanding, will help the learner remember the dimensions of the symptoms. The nurse will keep in mind that not all these qualifiers will apply to each symptom.

HEALTH HISTORY QUESTIONS | RATIONALES

The following sections provide sample questions and follow-up questions. Rationales for some questions are provided. The list of questions is not all-inclusive but rather represents the more common concern or injury questions required in a health history related to the musculoskeletal system. An example of using O-P-Q-R-S-T-U with pain is provided.

Questions Related to Common Concerns or Injuries

The most common concerns related to illness or injury of the musculoskeletal system are as follows:

- Pain
- Stiffness
- Swelling or heat
- Weakness
- Trauma

HEALTH HISTORY QUESTIONS	RATIONALES

1. **Pain**
   - Do you experience pain in your bones, joints, or muscles? *If yes:*
   - When did you first notice the pain? How long does it last? *Onset (chronology)*

   ► These questions help determine if the pain has a sudden or gradual onset.

   - What makes the pain worse? What makes the pain better? *Precipitating (palliative)*

   ► Certain activities, such as lifting heavy objects, can strain ligaments and vertebrae in the back, causing acute pain. Weight-bearing activities may increase the pain if the client has degenerative disease of hip, knee, and vertebrae.

   - Would you describe the pain as sharp? dull? burning? cramping? *Quality*

   ► Sensations of burning, tingling, or prickling (paresthesia) may accompany compression of nerves or blood vessels in that body region.

   - Where is the pain located? Does the pain radiate? *Region (radiation)*
   - How would you rate the pain on a scale of 1 to 10, with 10 being the worst pain? *Severity*
   - How often do you experience the pain? When does the pain occur, while walking, at rest, all day long? How long does it last? *Timing*
   - What do you think is causing the pain? *Understanding*

   ► The pain from hiatal hernia and from cardiac, gallbladder, and pleural conditions may be referred to the shoulder. Lumbosacral nerve root irritation may cause pain to be felt in the leg.

2. **Stiffness**
   - Do you have any stiffness in your joints? *If yes:*
   - When did you first notice the stiffness?

   ► Stiffness may be related to disorders of the musculoskeletal system, such as arthritis or trauma.

   - How long does it last?
   - What makes the stiffness worse? What makes the stiffness better?
   - How often do you experience stiffness? Does the pain affect your activities of daily living or other functions? How would you rate the stiffness on a scale of 1 to 10, with 10 being the most severe?
   - Is the stiffness associated with movement, time of day, weather?
   - What do you think is causing the stiffness?

3. **Swelling or heat**
   - Do you have any swelling or heat in your joints? *If yes:*

   ► Swelling or heat may be related to inflammation or disorders of the musculoskeletal system, such as arthritis or trauma.

   - When did you first notice the problem? How long does it last?
   - What makes the symptom worse? What makes the symptom better?
   - Does the swelling or heat affect your activities of daily living or other functions? How would you rate the problem on a scale of 1 to 10, with 10 being the most severe?
   - Where is the swelling or heat?
   - What do you think is causing the swelling or heat?

4. **Weakness**
   - Do you have any weakness in your muscle or joints? *If yes:*
   - When did you first notice the problem? How long does it last?
   - What makes the symptom worse? What makes the symptom better?
   - Does the weakness affect your activities of daily living or other functions? How would you rate the problem on a scale of 1 to 10, with 10 being the most severe?
   - Where is the weakness?
   - What do you think is causing the weakness?

5. **Trauma**
   - Have you had any fractures? *If yes:*
   - How many? How often do they occur?

HEALTH HISTORY QUESTIONS	RATIONALES

- Tell me about the causes, injuries, treatments, and present problems with daily activities.

▶ Older adults who have osteoporosis and osteomalacia (adult vitamin D deficiency) are prone to multiple bone fractures. Physical abuse should be considered when a client has a history of frequent fractures; however, disease or hereditary illness can predispose a person to fractures.

Questions Related to Past Health History

- Do you have any chronic diseases, such as diabetes mellitus, hypothyroidism, sickle-cell anemia, lupus, or rheumatoid arthritis?

▶ These conditions can predispose the client to musculoskeletal problems, such as osteomyelitis.

- Please describe any musculoskeletal problems of any family member.

▶ Some conditions, such as rheumatoid arthritis, are genetic or familial and recur in a family.

- Have you ever been diagnosed with a musculoskeletal illness? *If yes:*

▶ The client has an opportunity to provide information about a specific illness. If a diagnosed illness is identified, follow-up about the date of diagnosis, treatment, and outcomes is required. Data about each illness identified by the client are essential to an accurate health assessment. Illnesses can be classified as acute or chronic, and follow-up regarding each classification will differ.

- When were you diagnosed with the problem?
- Has the problem ever recurred? *(acute)*
- How are you managing the disease now? *(chronic)*
- Have you ever experienced any penetrating wounds (punctures from a nail or sharp object, stabbing, or gunshot)? *If yes:*
- Please describe the injuries.

▶ Penetrating wounds may be a causative factor for osteomyelitis.

Questions Related to Behaviours

Healthcare behaviours include both health practices and health patterns. Health practices consist of following recommendations for disease prevention, including screening for risks, screening for early detection of problems, and immunization. Health patterns are habits or acts that affect the client's health. Health behaviours may also include seeking healthcare from healthcare providers who use alternative methods to diagnose and treat illness. Clients should be questioned in a nonjudgmental way and areas for health teaching should be identified.

1. **Tell me about your exercise program.**

▶ A sedentary lifestyle leads to muscle weakness, contributes to poor coordination skills, and predisposes postmenopausal females to osteoporosis.

2. **Have you gained any recent weight?**

▶ Increased weight puts added stress on the musculoskeletal system.

Questions Related to the Environment

Environment refers to both internal and external environments. Questions related to the internal environment include all the previous questions and those associated with internal or physiological responses. Questions regarding the external environment include those related to home, work, or social environments.

Internal Environment

1. **Describe your typical daily diet.**
   - Do you have problems eating or drinking dairy products?

GATHERING THE DATA

HEALTH HISTORY QUESTIONS	RATIONALES

- If so, describe the problems you experience.

▶ Protein deficiency interferes with bone growth and muscle tone; calcium deficiency predisposes an individual to low bone density, resulting in osteoporosis; and vitamin C deficiency inhibits bone and tissue healing. Clients with intolerance to milk products frequently ingest low amounts of calcium, leading to musculoskeletal problems, such as osteoporosis.

2. **Are you currently taking any medications, such as steroids, estrogen, muscle relaxants, or any other drugs?**

▶ These drugs may cause a variety of symptoms, such as weakness, swelling, and increased muscle size, that could affect the musculoskeletal system.

External Environment

The following questions deal with the physical environment of the client. That includes the indoor and outdoor environments of the home and the workplace, those encountered for social engagements, and any encountered during travel.

1. **How much sunlight do you get each day?**

▶ Twenty minutes of sunshine each day helps the body manufacture vitamin D. Vitamin D deficiency can lead to osteomalacia.

2. **What kind of work do you do?**
   - Do you work on a computer?

▶ Frequent repetitive movements may lead to misuse syndromes, such as carpal tunnel syndrome, an inflammation of the tissues of the wrist that causes pressure on the median nerve. Work that requires heavy lifting or twisting may lead to lower back problems.

3. **Describe your hobbies or athletic activities.**

▶ Participation in athletic or sports activities can predispose the individual to trauma or wear and tear injuries. Sitting for long periods and repetitive motion, such as in sewing, crocheting, and woodworking, can cause musculoskeletal damage.

Questions Related to Age

The health history must reflect the anatomical and physiological differences that exist along the age span.

Questions Regarding Infants and Children

1. **Were you told about any trauma to the infant during labour and delivery?**
   - If so, describe the trauma.

▶ Traumatic births increase the risk for fractures, especially of the clavicle.

2. **Did the baby require resuscitation after delivery?**

▶ Periods of anoxia can result in increased muscle tone.

3. **Have you noticed any deformity of the child's spine or limbs, or any unusual shape of the child's feet and toes?**
   - If yes, please describe these deformities and any treatment the child has had.

▶ Some deformities correct themselves as the child grows. Others may require physical therapy or surgery.

4. **Please describe any dislocations or broken bones the child has had, including any treatment.**

▶ Dislocations or broken bones are more common in children with certain developmental disabilities or sensory or motor disorders, such as cerebral palsy or Down syndrome. They may also signal physical abuse. The latter will require further investigation.

HEALTH HISTORY QUESTIONS	RATIONALES

5. *For the school-age child:* **Do you play any sports at school or after school?**
- If so, describe the sports activities.

▶ Sports activities can cause musculoskeletal injuries, especially if played without adequate adult supervision or the use of protective equipment.

Questions for the Pregnant Female

1. Please describe any back pain you are experiencing.

- Tell me about the effects of the pain on your daily activities.

▶ Lordosis may occur in the last months of pregnancy, along with complaints of back pain.

Questions for the Older Adult

1. Have you noticed any muscle weakness over the past few months?
- If so, explain what effect this muscle weakness has on your daily activities.

▶ Muscle weakness is common as a person ages, especially in people with sedentary lifestyles.

2. Have you fallen in the past 6 months?
- If so, how many times?
- What prompted the fall(s)?
- Describe your injuries.
- What treatment did you receive?
- What effect did your injuries have on your daily activities?

▶ Older adults have an increased rate of falls because of a change in posture that can affect their balance. Loss of balance may also be caused by sensory or motor disorders, inner ear infections, the side effects of certain medications, and other factors.

3. Do you use any walking aids, such as a cane or walker, to help you get around?
- If so, please describe the aid or show it to me.

▶ These aids help the older adult ambulate, but they can also cause falls, especially if the client does not use the device properly.

4. *For postmenopausal females:* **Do you take calcium supplements?**

▶ Calcium supplementation may slow the development of some of the musculoskeletal changes associated with age, such as osteoporosis.

GATHERING THE DATA

PHYSICAL ASSESSMENT

ASSESSMENT TECHNIQUES AND FINDINGS

Physical assessment of the musculoskeletal system requires the use of inspection and palpation. During each of the procedures the nurse is gathering data related to the client's skeleton, joints, musculature, strength, and mobility. Knowledge of normal or expected findings is essential in determining the meaning of the data as the nurse conducts the physical assessment.

Adults have erect posture, an even gait, and symmetry in size and shape of muscles. A healthy adult is capable of active and complete range of motion in all joints. Joints are nonswollen and nontender. Muscle strength is equal bilaterally, and the movements against resistance are smooth and symmetrical. The spine is midline and cervical; thoracic and lumbar curves are present. The extremities are of equal length. The arm span

is equal to height, and the distance from head to pubis is equal to the distance from pubis to toes.

Physical assessment of the musculoskeletal system follows an organized pattern. It begins with a client survey and proceeds in a cephalocaudal direction to include inspection, palpation, assessment of range of motion of each joint, and assessment of muscle size, symmetry, and strength.

EQUIPMENT
examination gown
skin marking pen
clean, nonsterile examination gloves
goniometer
examination light
tape measure

HELPFUL HINTS

- Age and agility influence the client's ability to participate in the assessment.
- It is often more helpful to demonstrate the movements you expect of the client during this assessment than to use easily misunderstood verbal instructions. A "Simon Says" approach works well, especially with children.
- When assessing range of motion, do not push the joint beyond its normal range.
- Stop when the client expresses discomfort.
- Measure the joint angle with a goniometer when range of motion appears limited.
- Use an orderly approach: head to toe, proximal to distal, compare the sides of the body for symmetry.
- The musculoskeletal assessment may be exhausting for some clients. Provide rest periods or schedule two sessions.
- Use routine practices.

TECHNIQUES AND NORMAL FINDINGS	ABNORMAL FINDINGS AND SPECIAL CONSIDERATIONS

SURVEY

A quick survey of the client enables the nurse to identify any immediate problems and to determine the client's ability to participate in the assessment. Inspect the overall appearance, posture, and position of the client. Observe for deformities, inflammation, and immobility (see Figure 23.17).

▶ If a client is experiencing pain or inflammation, these issues must be addressed first. The complete assessment of the musculoskeletal system may have to be delayed until acute problems are attended to. Limited strength and mobility must be considered throughout the assessment.

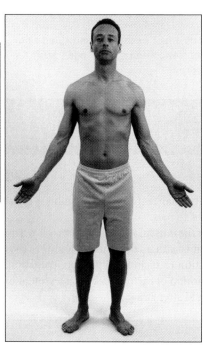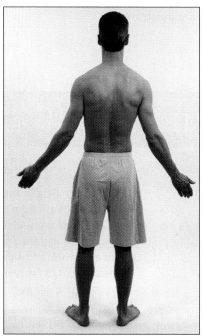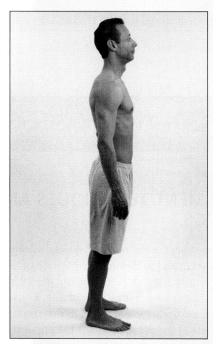

Figure 23.17 ● Survey and posture of client. A. Anterior view. B. Posterior view. C. Lateral view.

ASSESSMENT OF THE JOINTS

1. Position the client.

- The client should be in a sitting position with an examination gown on.

TECHNIQUES AND NORMAL FINDINGS	ABNORMAL FINDINGS AND SPECIAL CONSIDERATIONS

2. Instruct the client.

- Explain that you will be looking at all of the client's joints and muscles. Tell the client you will be touching bones, muscles, and joints and you will ask the client to move different parts of the body to determine the mobility of the joints. To assess muscle strength, the client will have to move against the resistance you provide. It is helpful to demonstrate or describe the movements expected of the client for one joint and to apply resistance as the client repeats the expected movement. Then explain that each joint will be assessed in a similar manner with the same amount of resistance and that you will provide direction with each examination. Explain that the assessment should not cause discomfort and tell the client to inform you of pain, discomfort, or difficulty with any assessment. Explain that you will provide assistance or support when necessary and can provide rest periods throughout the examination.

3. Inspect the temporomandibular joint on both sides.

- The joints should be symmetrical and not swollen or painful.

▶ An enlarged or swollen joint shows as a rounded protuberance.

4. Palpate the temporomandibular joints.

- Place the fingerpads of your index and middle fingers in front of the tragus of each ear. Ask the client to open and close the mouth while you palpate the temporomandibular joints (see Figure 23.18).

▶ Discomfort, swelling, crackling sounds, and limited movement of the jaw are unexpected findings that require further evaluation for dental or neurological problems or TMJ syndrome.

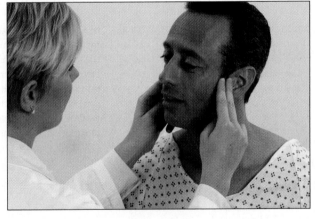

Figure 23.18 ●
Palpating the temporomandibular joints.

- As the client's mouth opens, your fingers should glide into a shallow depression of the joints. Confirm the smooth motion of the mandible.
- The joint may audibly and palpably click as the mouth opens. This is normal.

5. Palpate the muscles of the jaw.

- Instruct the client to clench the teeth as you palpate the masseter and temporalis muscles. Confirm that the muscles are symmetrical, firm, and nontender.

▶ Swelling and tenderness suggest arthritis and myofascial pain syndrome.

6. Test for range of motion of the temporomandibular joints.

- Ask the client to open the mouth as wide as possible. Confirm that the mouth opens with ease to as much as 3 to 6 cm (1.25 to 2.5 in.) between the upper and lower incisors.
- With the mouth slightly open, ask the client to push out the lower jaw and return the lower jaw to a neutral position. The jaw should protrude and retract with ease.
- Ask the client to move the lower jaw from side to side. Confirm that the jaw moves laterally from 1 to 2 cm (0.5 to 1 in.) without deviation or dislocation.
- Ask the client to close the mouth. The mouth should close completely without pain or discomfort.

▶ Temporomandibular joint dysfunction should be suspected if facial pain and limited jaw movement accompany clicking sounds as the jaw opens and closes.

PHYSICAL ASSESSMENT

TECHNIQUES AND NORMAL FINDINGS	ABNORMAL FINDINGS AND SPECIAL CONSIDERATIONS

7. Test for muscle strength and motor function of cranial nerve V.

- Instruct the client to repeat the movements in step 6 as you provide opposing force. The client should be able to perform the movements against your resistance. The strength of the muscles on both sides of the jaw should be equal.

- For more detailed testing of cranial nerve V, including sensory function, see Chapter 24. ⚭

THE SHOULDERS

1. With the client facing you, inspect both shoulders.

- Compare the shape and size of the shoulders, clavicles, and scapula. Confirm that they are symmetrical and similar in size both anteriorly and posteriorly.

▶ Swelling, deformity, atrophy, and misalignment, combined with limited motion, pain, and crepitus (a grating sound caused by bone fragments in joints), suggest degenerative joint disease, traumatized joints (strains, sprains), or inflammatory conditions (rheumatoid arthritis, bursitis, or tendinitis).

2. Palpate the shoulders and surrounding structures.

- Begin palpating at the sternoclavicular joint, and then move laterally along the clavicle to the acromioclavicular joint.

- Palpate downward into the subacromial area and the greater tubercle of the humerus.

- Confirm that these areas are firm and nontender, the shoulders symmetrical, and the scapulae level and symmetrical.

▶ Shoulder pain without palpation or movement may result from insufficient circulation to the myocardium. This cue, known as *referred pain,* can be a precursor to a myocardial infarction (heart attack). If the client exhibits other symptoms, such as chest pain, indigestion, and cardiovascular changes, medical assistance must be obtained immediately.

3. Test the range of motion of the shoulders.

- Instruct the client to use both arms for the following manoeuvres:
- Shrug the shoulders by flexing them forward and upward.
- With the elbows extended, raise the arms forward and upward in an arc. (The client should demonstrate a forward flexion of 180 degrees.)
- Return the arms to the sides. Keeping the elbows extended, move the arms backward as far as possible (see Figure 23.19). (The client should demonstrate an extension of as much as 50 degrees.)
- Place the back of the client's hands as close as possible to scapulae (internal rotation; see Figure 23.20).
- Ask the client to clasp his or her hands behind the head (external rotation; see Figure 23.21).

▶ If the client expresses discomfort, it is important to determine if the pain is referred. Conditions that increase intra-abdominal pressure, such as hiatal hernia and gastrointestinal disease, may cause pain in the shoulder area. When limitation or increase in range of motion (ROM) is assessed, the goniometer should be used to precisely measure the angle.

- With elbows extended, ask the client to swing the arms out to the sides in arcs, touching the palms together above the head. The client should demonstrate abduction of 180 degrees.

▶ In rotator cuff tears, the client is unable to perform abduction without lifting or shrugging the shoulder. This sign is accompanied by pain, tenderness, and muscle atrophy.

PHYSICAL ASSESSMENT

TECHNIQUES AND NORMAL FINDINGS

ABNORMAL FINDINGS AND SPECIAL CONSIDERATIONS

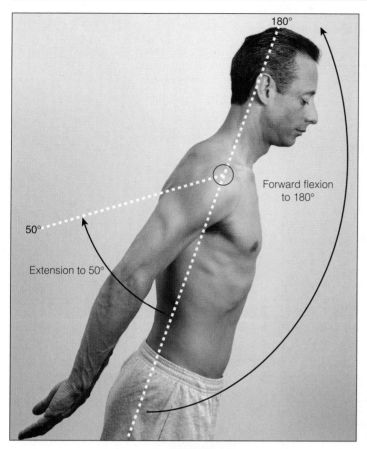

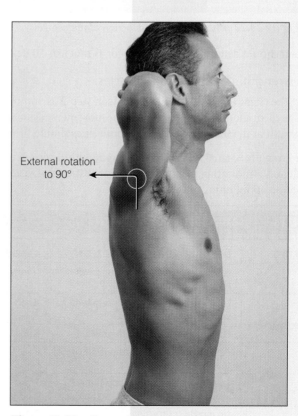

Figure 23.19 ● Flexion and extension of the shoulders.

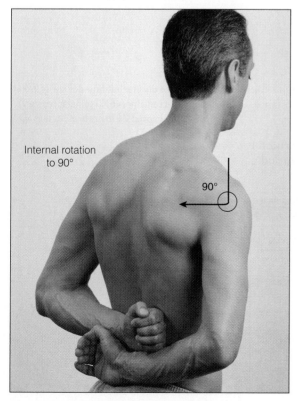

Figure 23.20 ● Internal rotation of the shoulders.

Figure 23.21 ● External rotation of the shoulders.

TECHNIQUES AND NORMAL FINDINGS	ABNORMAL FINDINGS AND SPECIAL CONSIDERATIONS

- With the elbows extended, ask the client to swing each arm toward the midline of the body (see Figure 23.22).

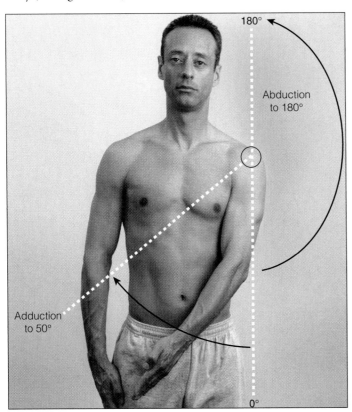

Figure 23.22 ● Abduction and adduction of the shoulder.

- The client should demonstrate adduction of as much as 50 degrees.

4. Test for strength of the shoulder muscles.

- Instruct the client to repeat the movements in step 3 as you provide opposing force. The client should be able to perform the movements against your resistance. The strength of the shoulder muscles on both sides should be equal.

- Muscle strength is rated on a scale of 0 to 5, with 0 representing absence of strength and 5 indicating maximum or normal strengths. Table 23.3 includes information about rating muscle strength.

▶ Full resistance during the shoulder shrug indicates adequate cranial nerve XI (spinal accessory) function. See Chapter 24 for more detail.

TABLE 23.3	Rating Muscle Strength	
RATING	**DESCRIPTION OF FUNCTION**	**CLASSIFICATION**
5	Full range of motion against gravity with full resistance	Normal
4	Full range of motion against gravity with moderate resistance	Good
3	Full range of motion with gravity	Fair
2	Full range of motion without gravity (passive motion)	Poor
1	Palpable muscle contraction but no movement	Trace
0	No muscle contraction	Zero

| TECHNIQUES AND NORMAL FINDINGS | ABNORMAL FINDINGS AND SPECIAL CONSIDERATIONS |

ELBOWS

1. Support the client's arm and inspect the lateral and medial aspects of the elbow.
   - The elbows should be symmetrical.

   ▶ Swelling, deformity, or misalignment requires further evaluation. If there is a subluxation (partial dislocation), the elbow looks deformed and the forearm is misaligned.

2. Palpate the lateral and medial aspects of the olecranon process.
   - Use your thumb and middle fingers to palpate the grooves on either side of the olecranon process.

   ▶ In the presence of inflammation, the grooves feel soft and spongy, and the surrounding tissue may be red, hot, and painful.

   - The joint should be free of pain, thickening, swelling, or tenderness.

   ▶ Inflammatory conditions of the elbow include arthritis, bursitis, and epicondylitis. *Rheumatoid arthritis* may result in nodules in the olecranon bursa or along the extensor surface of the ulna. Nodules are firm, nontender, and not attached to the overlying skin. *Lateral epicondylitis* (tennis elbow) results from constant, repetitive movements of the wrist or forearm. Pain occurs when the client attempts to extend the wrist against resistance. *Medial epicondylitis* (pitcher's or golfer's elbow) results from constant, repetitive flexion of the wrist. Pain occurs when the client attempts to flex the wrist against resistance.

3. Test the range of motion of each elbow.
   - Instruct the client to perform the following movements:
   - Bend the elbow by bringing the forearm forward and touching the fingers to the shoulder (see Figure 23.23). The elbow should flex to 160 degrees.

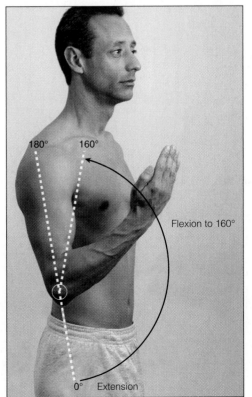

Figure 23.23 ●
Flexion and extension of the elbow.

TECHNIQUES AND NORMAL FINDINGS	ABNORMAL FINDINGS AND SPECIAL CONSIDERATIONS

- Straighten the elbow. The lower arm should form a straight line with the upper arm. The elbow in a neutral position is at 0 degree extension. The elbow should extend to 0 degree.

- Holding the arm straight out, turn the palm upward facing the ceiling, then downward facing the floor (see Figure 23.24). The elbow should supinate and pronate to 90 degrees.

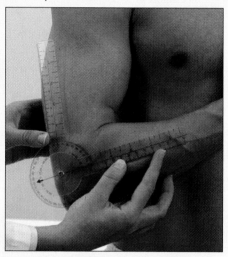

▶ To use the goniometer, begin with the joint in a neutral position and then flex the joint as far as possible. Measure the angle with the goniometer. Fully extend the joint and measure the angle with the goniometer. Compare the goniometer measurements to the expected degree of flexion and extension. See Figure 23.25 for an example.

Figure 23.25 ● Goniometer measure of joint range of motion.

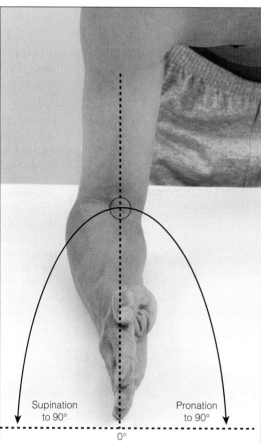

Supination to 90°   Pronation to 90°

0°

Figure 23.24 ●
Supination and pronation of the elbow.

- The client should be able to put each elbow through the normal range of motion without difficulty or discomfort.

4. **Test for muscle strength.**
   - Stabilize the client's elbow with your nondominant hand while holding the wrist with your dominant hand.
   - Instruct the client to flex the elbow while you apply opposing resistance (see Figure 23.26).
   - Instruct the client to extend the elbow against resistance.
   - The client should be able to perform these movements. The strength of the muscles associated with flexion and extension of each elbow should be equal. Muscle strength is measured by testing against the strength of the examiner as resistance is applied.

TECHNIQUES AND NORMAL FINDINGS	ABNORMAL FINDINGS AND SPECIAL CONSIDERATIONS

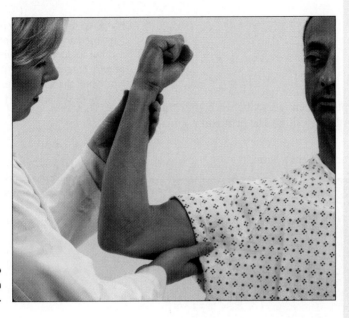

Figure 23.26 ●
Testing muscle strength by using opposing force.

WRISTS AND HANDS

1. **Inspect the wrists and dorsum of the hands for size, shape, symmetry, and colour.**
   - The wrists and hands should be symmetrical and free from swelling and deformity. The colour should be similar to that of the rest of the body. The ends of either the ulna or the radius may protrude further in some individuals.

▶ Redness, swelling, or deformity in the joints requires further evaluation. It is important to note any nodules on the hands or wrists, or atrophy of the surrounding muscles. In acute rheumatoid arthritis, the wrist, proximal interphalangeal, and metacarpophalangeal joints are likely to be swollen, tender, and stiff. As the disease progresses, the proximal interphalangeal joints deviate toward the ulnar side of the hand; the interosseous muscles atrophy, and rheumatoid nodules form, giving the rheumatic hand its characteristic appearance.

2. **Inspect the palms of the hands.**
   - There is a rounded protuberance over the thenar eminence (the area proximal to the thumb).

▶ Carpal tunnel syndrome is a nerve disorder in which an inflammation of tissues in the wrist causes pressure on the median nerve (which innervates the hand). Thenar atrophy is a common finding associated with carpal tunnel syndrome; however, some atrophy of the thenar eminence occurs with aging.

3. **Palpate the wrists and hands for temperature and texture.**
   - The temperature of the wrists and hands should be warm and similar to the rest of the body. The skin should be smooth and free of cuts. The skin around the interphalangeal joints may have a rougher texture.

4. **Palpate each joint of the wrists and hands.**
   - Move your thumbs from side to side gently but firmly over the dorsum, with your fingers resting beneath the area you are palpating (see Figures 23.27A and 23.27B). As you palpate, make sure you keep the client's wrist straight.

PHYSICAL ASSESSMENT

TECHNIQUES AND NORMAL FINDINGS

ABNORMAL FINDINGS AND SPECIAL CONSIDERATIONS

- Straighten the hand (extension).

► A ganglion is a typically painless, round, fluid-filled mass that arises from the tendon sheaths on the dorsum of the wrist and hand. It may require surgery. Ganglia that are more prevalent when the wrist is flexed do not interfere with range of motion or function.

- To palpate the interphalangeal joints, pinch them gently between your thumb and index finger (see Figure 23.27C). All joints should be firm and nontender, with no swelling.
- As you palpate, note the temperature of the client's hand.

► A cool temperature in the extremities may indicate compromised vascular function, which may in turn influence muscle strength.

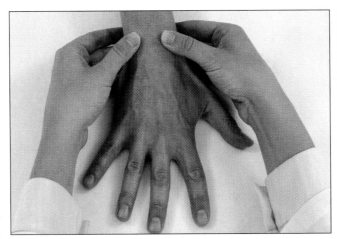

Figure 23.27A ●
Palpating the wrist.

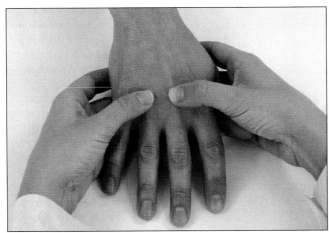

Figure 23.27B ●
Palpating the hand.

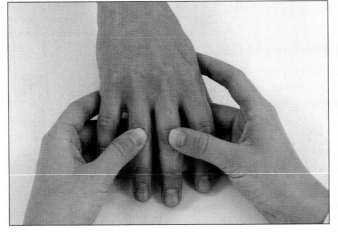

Figure 23.27C ●
Palpating the fingers.

TECHNIQUES AND NORMAL FINDINGS	ABNORMAL FINDINGS AND SPECIAL CONSIDERATIONS

5. **Test the range of motion of the wrist.**
   - Instruct the client to perform the following movements:
   - Using the wrist as a pivot point, bring the fingers backward as far as possible, and then bend the wrist downward (see Figure 23.28). The wrist should extend to 70 degrees and flex to 90 degrees.

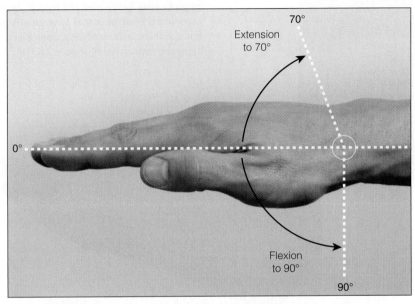

Figure 23.28 ● Hyperextension and flexion of the wrist.

   - Turn the palms down; move the hand laterally toward the fifth finger, then medially toward the thumb (see Figure 23.29). Be sure the movement is from the wrist and not the elbow. Ulnar deviation should reach as much as 55 degrees, and radial deviation should reach as much as 20 degrees.

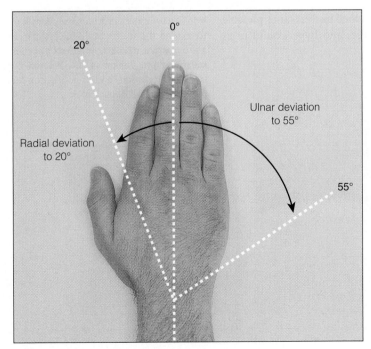

Figure 23.29 ● Ulnar and radial deviation of the wrist.

TECHNIQUES AND NORMAL FINDINGS

ABNORMAL FINDINGS AND SPECIAL CONSIDERATIONS

- Bend the wrists downward and press the backs of both hands together (*Phalen's test;* see Figure 23.30). This causes flexion of the wrists to 90 degrees. Normally clients experience no symptoms with this manoeuvre.

▶ When a Phalen's test is performed on individuals with carpal tunnel syndrome, **80%** experience pain, tingling, and numbness that radiates to the arm, shoulder, neck, or chest within 60 seconds. If carpal tunnel syndrome is suspected, it is important to check for Tinel's sign by percussing lightly over the median nerve in each wrist. If carpal tunnel syndrome is present, the client feels numbness, tingling, and pain along the median nerve (Figure 23.31).

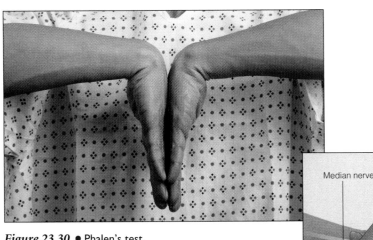

Figure 23.30 ● Phalen's test.

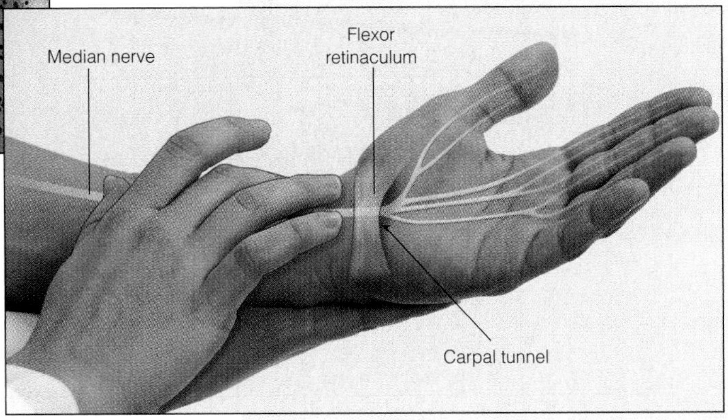

Figure 23.31 ●
Tinel's sign.

6. Test the range of motion of the hands and fingers. Instruct the client to perform the following movements:
   - Make a tight fist with each hand with the fingers folded into the palm and the thumb across the knuckles (thumb flexion).
   - Open the fist and stretch the fingers (extension).
   - Point the fingers downward toward the forearm and then back as far as possible (see Figure 23.32). Fingers should flex to 90 degrees and hyperextend to as much as 30 degrees.

▶ In *Dupuytren's contracture,* the client is unable to extend the fourth and fifth fingers. This is a progressive, painless, inherited disorder that causes severe flexion in the affected fingers, is usually bilateral, and is more common in middle-aged and older males.

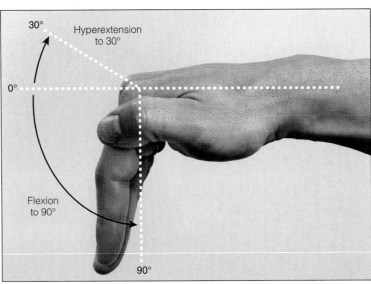

Figure 23.32 ● Flexion and extension of the fingers.

| **TECHNIQUES AND NORMAL FINDINGS** | **ABNORMAL FINDINGS AND SPECIAL CONSIDERATIONS** |

- Spread the fingers far apart and then push back together. Fingers should abduct to 20 degrees and should adduct fully (they should touch).
- Move the thumb toward the ulnar side of the hand and then away from the hand as far as possible.
- Touch the thumb to the tip of each of the fingers and to the base of the little finger.

7. **Test for muscle strength of the wrist.**
   - Place the client's arm on a table with his or her palm facing up.
   - Stabilize the client's forearm with one hand while holding the client's hand with your other hand.
   - Instruct the client to flex the wrist while you apply opposing resistance (see Figure 23.33). The client should be able to provide full resistance.

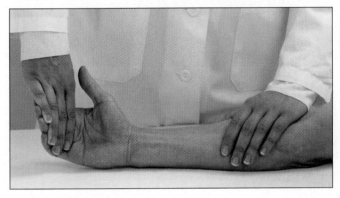

Figure 23.33 ● Testing the muscle strength of the wrist.

8. **Test for muscle strength of the fingers.**
   - Ask the client to spread his or her fingers, and then try to force the fingers together.
   - Ask the client to touch his or her little finger with the thumb while you place resistance on the thumb to prevent the movement.

▶ Clients with carpal tunnel syndrome manifest weakness when attempting opposition of the thumb.

HIPS

1. **Inspect the position of each hip and leg with the client in a supine position.**
   - The legs should be slightly apart and the toes should point toward the ceiling.

▶ External rotation of the lower leg and foot is a classic sign of a fractured femur.

2. **Palpate each hip joint and the upper thighs.**
   - The hip joints are firm, stable, and nontender.

3. **Test the range of motion of the hips.**

▶ Pain, tenderness, swelling, deformity, limited motion (especially limited internal rotation), and crepitus are diagnostic cues that signal inflammatory or degenerative joint diseases in the hip. A fractured femur should be suspected if the joint is unstable and deformed.

> **CLINICAL TIP**
> *Do not ask clients who have undergone hip replacement to perform these movements without the permission of the physician, because these motions can dislocate the prosthesis.*

- Instruct the client to perform the following movements:
- Raise each leg straight off the bed or table (see Figure 23.34). The other leg should remain flat on the bed. Hip flexion with straight knee should reach 90 degrees. Return the leg to its original position.

▶ This manoeuvre produces back and leg pain along the sciatic nerve in the client with a herniated disk.

TECHNIQUES AND NORMAL FINDINGS	ABNORMAL FINDINGS AND SPECIAL CONSIDERATIONS

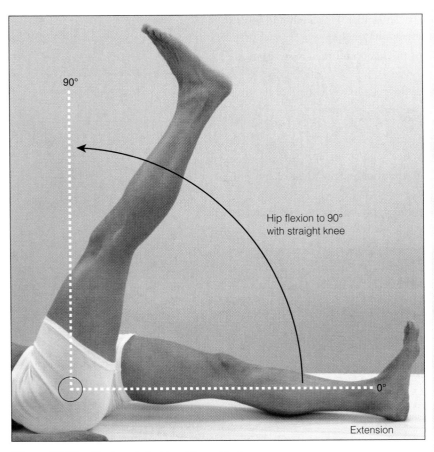

Figure 23.34 ● Flexion of the hip with straight knee.

● Raise the leg with the knee flexed toward the chest as far as it will go (see Figure 23.35). Hip flexion with flexed knee should reach 120 degrees. Return the leg to its original position.

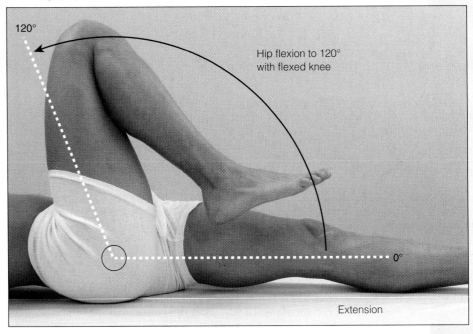

Figure 23.35 ● Flexion of the hip with flexed knee.

Techniques and Normal Findings	Abnormal Findings and Special Considerations

- Move the foot away from the midline as the knee moves toward the midline (see Figure 23.36). Internal hip rotation should reach 40 degrees.

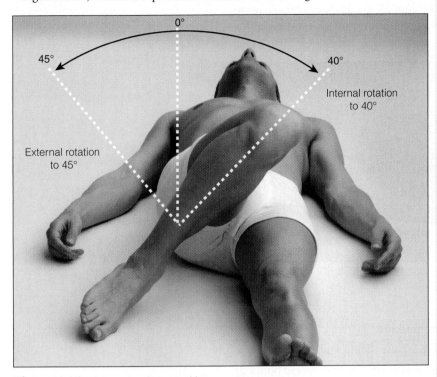

Figure 23.36 ● Internal and external hip rotation.

- Move the foot toward the midline as the knee moves away from the midline. External hip rotation should reach 45 degrees.

- Move the leg away from the midline (see Figure 23.37) and then as far as possible toward the midline. Abduction should reach 45 degrees. Adduction should reach 30 degrees.

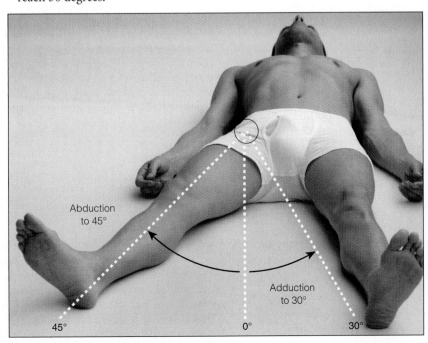

Figure 23.37 ● Abduction and adduction of the hip.

<table>
<tr><td>TECHNIQUES AND NORMAL FINDINGS</td><td>ABNORMAL FINDINGS AND SPECIAL CONSIDERATIONS</td></tr>
</table>

TECHNIQUES AND NORMAL FINDINGS

- Assist the client to turn onto his or her abdomen. An alternative position could be side lying. With the client's knee extended, ask the client to raise each leg backward and up as far as possible (see Figure 23.38). Hips should extend to 15 degrees. (You may also perform this test later, during assessment of the spine, with the client standing.)

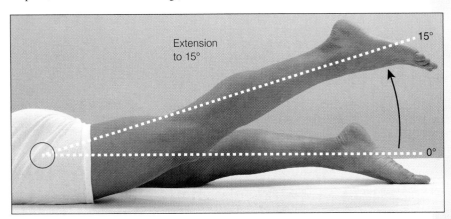

Figure 23.38 ● Hyperextension of the hip.

4. Test for muscle strength of the hips.
   - Assist the client in returning to the supine position.
   - Press your hands on the client's thighs and ask the client to raise his or her hip.
   - Place your hands outside the client's knees and ask the client to spread both legs against your resistance.
   - Place your hands between the client's knees, and ask the client to bring the legs together against your resistance.

KNEES

1. Inspect the knees.
   - With the client in the sitting position, inspect the knees.

   - The patella should be centrally located in each knee. The normal depressions along each side of the patella should be sharp and distinct. The skin colour should be similar to that of the surrounding areas.

2. Inspect the quadriceps muscle in the anterior thigh.
   - The muscles should be symmetrical.

3. Palpate the knee.
   - Using your thumb, index, and middle fingers begin palpating approximately 10 cm (4 in.) above the patella with your thumb, index, and middle fingers (see Figure 23.39). Palpate downward, evaluating each area.
   - The quadriceps muscle and surrounding soft tissue should be firm and non-tender. The suprapatellar bursa is usually not palpable.

ABNORMAL FINDINGS AND SPECIAL CONSIDERATIONS

▶ Swelling and signs of fluid in the knee and its surrounding structures require further evaluation. Fluid accumulates in the suprapatellar bursa, the prepatellar bursa, and other areas adjacent to the patella when there is inflammation, trauma, or degenerative joint disease.

▶ Atrophy in the quadriceps muscles occurs with disuse or chronic disorders.

▶ Any pain, swelling, thickening, or heat should be noted while palpating the knee. These diagnostic cues occur when the synovium is inflamed. Painless swelling frequently occurs in degenerative joint disease. A painful, localized area of swelling, heat, and redness in the knee is caused by the inflammation of the bursa (bursitis), such as *prepatellar bursitis*.

PHYSICAL ASSESSMENT

TECHNIQUES AND NORMAL FINDINGS	ABNORMAL FINDINGS AND SPECIAL CONSIDERATIONS

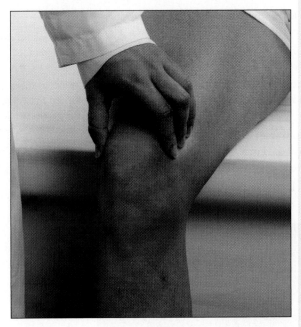

Figure 23.39 ●
Palpating the knee.

4. **Palpate the tibiofemoral joint.**
   - With the client's knee still in the flexed position, use your thumbs to palpate deeply along each side of the tibia toward the outer aspects of the knee.

   ▶ Signs of inflammation, including pain and tenderness, occur when the joint is inflamed or damaged and may indicate degenerative joint disease, synovitis, or a torn meniscus. Bony ridges or prominences in the outer aspects of the joint occur with osteoarthritis.

   - Then palpate along the lateral collateral ligament.
   - The joint should be firm and nontender.

5. **Test for the bulge sign.**
   - This procedure detects the presence of small amounts of fluid (4 to 8 mL or 0.1 to 0.3 fl.oz.) in the suprapatellar bursa.
   - With the client in the supine position, use firm pressure to stroke the medial aspect of the knee upward several times, displacing any fluid (see Figure 23.40).

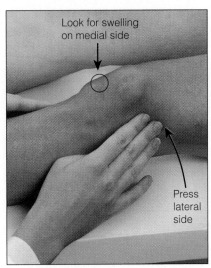

Look for swelling on medial side

Press lateral side

Figure 23.40 ●
Testing for the bulge sign.

TECHNIQUES AND NORMAL FINDINGS

ABNORMAL FINDINGS AND SPECIAL CONSIDERATIONS

- Apply pressure to the lateral side of the knee while observing the medial side.
- Normally no fluid is present.

▶ The medial side of the knee bulges if fluid is in the joint.

6. Perform ballottement.
   - **Ballottement** is a technique used to detect fluid, or to examine or detect floating body structures. The nurse displaces body fluid and then palpates the return impact on the body structure.
   - To detect large amounts of fluid in the suprapatellar bursa, use your thumb and fingers to firmly grasp the thigh just above the knee. This action causes any fluid in the suprapatellar bursa to move between the patella and the femur.
   - With the fingers of your left hand, quickly push the patella downward on the femur (see Figure 23.41).

▶ When there are abnormal fluid levels, fluid forced between the patella and femur causes the patella to "float" over the femur. A palpable click is felt when the patella is snapped back against the femur when fluid is present.

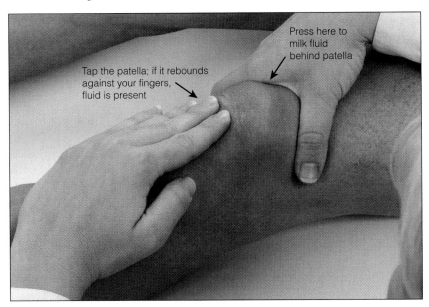

Figure 23.41 ● Testing for ballottement.

- Normally the patella sits firmly over the femur, allowing little or no movement when pressure is exerted over the patella.

7. Evaluate for tears in the meniscus of the knee.
   - The *McMurray test* is used to evaluate tears in the meniscus of the knee.
   - With the client supine, flex the knee.
   - With one hand on the medial aspect of the joint and the other on the palmar surface of the foot, rotate the leg externally and fully extend the knee. Normally the knee moves smoothly and is nonpainful.

If a palpable click is felt or the client experiences pain when the tibia rotated, it is a positive McMurray test. The meniscus should be investigated further for tears.

> **CLINICAL TIP**
> *The McMurray test is a basic screening test and further examination is required.*

8. Test the range of motion of each knee.
   - Instruct the client to bend each knee against the chest as far as possible (flexion; see Figure 23.42), and then return the knee to its extended position.

TECHNIQUES AND NORMAL FINDINGS	ABNORMAL FINDINGS AND SPECIAL CONSIDERATIONS

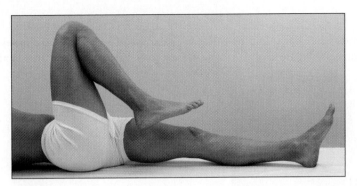

Figure 23.42 ● Flexion of the knee.

9. Test for muscle strength.
    * Instruct the client to flex each knee while you apply opposing force.
    * Now instruct the client to extend the knee again.
    * The client should be able to perform the movement against resistance.
    * The strength of the muscles in both knees is equal.

10. Inspect the knee while the client is standing.
    * Ask the client to stand erect. If the client is unsteady, allow the client to hold onto the back of a chair.

    ▶ Look for *genu varum* (bowlegs), *genu valgum* (knock knees), or *genu recurvatum* (excessive hyperextension of the knee with weight bearing caused by weakness of quadriceps muscles).

    * The knees should be in alignment with the thighs and ankles.
    * Ask the client to walk at a comfortable pace with a relaxed gait.

ANKLES AND FEET

1. Inspect the ankles and feet with the client sitting, standing, and walking.
    * The colour of the ankles and feet should be similar to that of the rest of the body. They should be symmetrical, and the skin should be unbroken. The feet and toes should be in alignment with the long axis of the lower leg. No swelling should be present, and the client's weight should fall on the middle of the foot.

    ▶ The following abnormalities require further evaluation:
    Gouty arthritis: The metatarsophalangeal joint of the great toe is swollen, hot, red, and extremely painful.
    Hallux valgus: The great toe deviates laterally from the midline, crowding the other toes.
    Bunion: Thickening and inflammation of the bursa of the joint of the great toe causes enlargement of the joint.
    Hammertoe: There is flexion of the proximal interphalangeal joint of a toe, while the distal metatarsophalangeal joint hyperextends. A callus or corn frequently occurs on the surface of the flexed joint from external pressure.
    Pes planus (flatfoot): The arch of the foot is flattened, sometimes coming in contact with the floor. The deformity may be noticeable only when an individual is standing and bearing weight on the foot.

PHYSICAL ASSESSMENT

Techniques and Normal Findings

ABNORMAL FINDINGS AND SPECIAL CONSIDERATIONS

2. Palpate the ankles.
   - Grasp the heel of the foot with the fingers of both hands while palpating the anterior and lateral aspects of the ankle with your thumbs (see Figure 23.43).

   ▶ Pain or discomfort on palpation and movement frequently indicate degenerative joint disease.

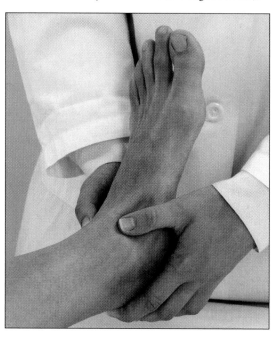

Figure 23.43 ●
Palpating the ankle.

   - The ankle joints should be firm, stable, and nontender.

3. Palpate the length of the calcaneal (Achilles) tendon at the posterior ankle.
   - The calcaneal tendon should be free of pain, tenderness, and nodules.

   ▶ Pain and tenderness along the tendon may indicate tendinitis or bursitis. Small nodules sometimes occur in clients with rheumatoid arthritis.

4. Palpate the metatarsophalangeal joints just below the ball of the foot.
   - The metatarsophalangeal joints should be nontender.

   ▶ Pain and discomfort with this manoeuvre suggest early involvement of rheumatoid arthritis. Acute inflammation of the first metatarsophalangeal joint suggests gout.

5. Deeply palpate each metatarsophalangeal joint.
   - The joints should be firm and nontender.

   ▶ Pain, swelling, or tenderness may be associated with inflammation or degenerative joint disease.

6. Test the range of motion of the ankles and feet.
   - Instruct the client to perform the following movements:

   ▶ Limited range of motion and painful movement of the foot and ankle without signs of inflammation suggest degenerative joint disease.

   - Point the foot toward the nose. Dorsiflexion should reach 20 degrees.
   - Point the foot toward the floor. Plantar flexion should reach 45 degrees.
   - Point the sole of the foot outward, then inward. The ankle should evert to 20 degrees and invert to 30 degrees (see Figure 23.44).
   - Curl the toes downward (flexion).
   - Spread the toes as far as possible (abduction), and then bring the toes together (adduction).

PHYSICAL ASSESSMENT

| TECHNIQUES AND NORMAL FINDINGS | ABNORMAL FINDINGS AND SPECIAL CONSIDERATIONS |

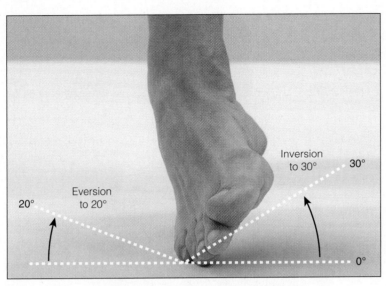

Figure 23.44 ● Eversion and inversion of the ankles.

7. **Test muscle strength of the ankle.**
   - Ask the client to perform dorsiflexion and plantar flexion against your resistance.

8. **Test muscle strength of the foot.**
   - Ask the client to flex and extend the toes against your resistance.

9. **Palpate each interphalangeal joint.**
   - As you did for the hand, note the temperature of the extremity. Confirm that it is similar to the temperature of the rest of the client's body.

▶ Pain, swelling, or tenderness may be associated with inflammation or degenerative joint disease.

A temperature in the lower extremities that is significantly cooler than the rest of the body may indicate vascular insufficiency, which in turn may lead to musculoskeletal abnormalities.

SPINE

1. **Inspect the spine.**
   - With the client in a standing position, move around the client's body to check the position and alignment of the spine from all sides. Confirm that the cervical and lumbar curves are concave and that the thoracic curve is convex (see Figure 23.45A).

▶ Lack of symmetry of the scapulae may indicate thoracic surgery. A scapula may appear higher if a lung has been removed on that side. In addition, the following abnormalities require further evaluation:

▶ *Kyphosis:* An exaggerated thoracic dorsal curve that causes asymmetry between the sides of the posterior thorax (see Figure 23.50 on page 633 in the Abnormal Findings section).

▶ *Lordosis:* An exaggerated lumbar curve that compensates for pregnancy, obesity, or other skeletal changes (see Figure 23.52 on page 634 in the Abnormal Findings section).

▶ *Flattened lumbar curve:* A flat lumbar curve frequently occurs when spasms affect the lumbar muscles.

▶ *List:* The spine leans to the left or right. A plumb line drawn from T_1 does not fall between the gluteal cleft. This condition may occur with spasms in the paravertebral muscles or a herniated disk.

Techniques and Normal Findings

Abnormal Findings and Special Considerations

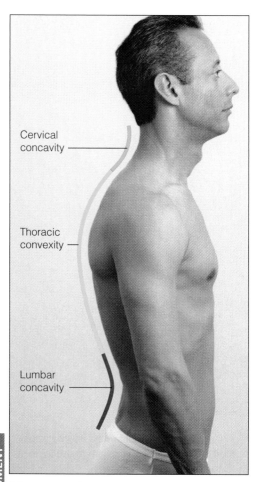

Figure 23.45A ● Lateral view of spine.

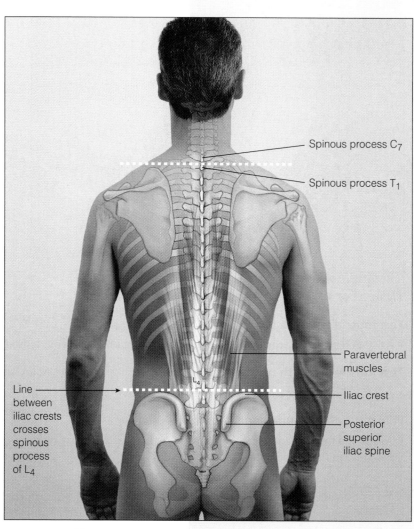

Figure 23.45B ●
Posterior view of spine.

▶ **Scoliosis:** The spine curves to the right or left, causing an exaggerated thoracic convexity on that side (see Figure 23.51 on page 634 in the Abnormal Findings section). The body compensates, and a plumb line dropped from T_1 falls between the gluteal cleft. Unequal leg length may contribute to scoliosis; therefore, if scoliosis is suspected, it is necessary to measure the client's leg length. With the client supine, measure the distance from the anterior superior iliac spine to the medial malleolus, crossing the tape measure at the medial side of the knee (see Figure 23.46).

- Imagine a vertical line falling from the level of T_1 to the gluteal cleft. Confirm that the spine is straight (see Figure 23.45B).
- Imagine a horizontal line across the top of the scapulae. Confirm that the scapulae are level and symmetrical (Figure 23.45B). Similarly, check that the heights

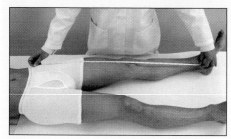

Figure 23.46 ●
Measuring leg length.

TECHNIQUES AND NORMAL FINDINGS	ABNORMAL FINDINGS AND SPECIAL CONSIDERATIONS

of the iliac crests and the gluteal folds are level (Figure 23.45B). Ask the client to bend forward, and assess the alignment of the vertebrae.

2. **Palpate each vertebral process with your thumb.**
   - The vertebral processes should be aligned, uniform in size, firm, stable, and nontender.

▶ A *compression fracture* should be considered if the client is older, complains of pain and tenderness in the back, and has restricted back movement. T_8 and L_3 are the most common sites for compression fractures.

3. **Palpate the muscles on both sides of the neck and back.**
   - The neck muscles should be fully developed and symmetrical, firm, smooth, and nontender.

▶ *Muscle spasms* feel like hardened or knot-like formations. When they occur, the client may complain of pain and restricted movement. Muscle spasms may be associated with temporomandibular joint dysfunction or with *spasmodic torticollis,* a disorder in which the spasms cause the head to be pulled to one side.

4. **Test the range of motion of the cervical spine.**
   - Instruct the client to perform the following movements.
   - Touch the chest with the chin (flexion).
   - Look up toward the ceiling (hyperextension).
   - Attempt to touch each shoulder with the ear on that side, keeping the shoulder level (lateral bending or flexion).
   - Turn the head to face each shoulder as far as possible (rotation).

5. **Test the range of motion of the thoracic and lumbar spine.**

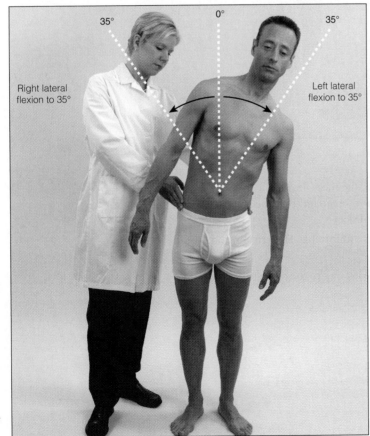

Figure 23.47 ●
Lateral flexion of the spine.

TECHNIQUES AND NORMAL FINDINGS	ABNORMAL FINDINGS AND SPECIAL CONSIDERATIONS

- Sit or stand behind the standing client. Stabilize the pelvis with your hands and ask the client to bend sideways to the right and to the left. Right and left lateral flexion should reach 35 degrees (see Figure 23.47).

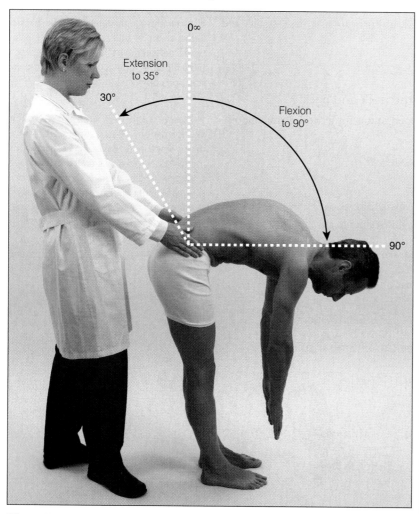

Figure 23.48 ● Forward flexion of the spine.

- Ask the client to bend forward and touch the toes (flexion). Confirm that the lumbar concavity disappears with this movement and that the back assumes a single C-shaped convexity (see Figure 23.48).
- Ask the client to bend backward as far as is comfortable. Hyperextension should reach 30 degrees.
- Ask the client to twist the shoulders to the left and to the right. Rotation should reach 30 degrees (see Figure 23.49).

▶ Limited range of motion, crepitation, or pain with movement in the joint requires further evaluation. If the client complains of sharp pain that begins in the lower back and radiates down the leg, perform the straight-leg-raising test: Keeping the knee extended, raise the client's leg until pain occurs, then dorsiflex the client's foot. Record the distribution and severity of the pain and the degree of leg elevation at the time the pain occurs. Also record whether dorsiflexion increases the pain. Pain with straight-leg raising may indicate a herniated disk.

TECHNIQUES AND NORMAL FINDINGS

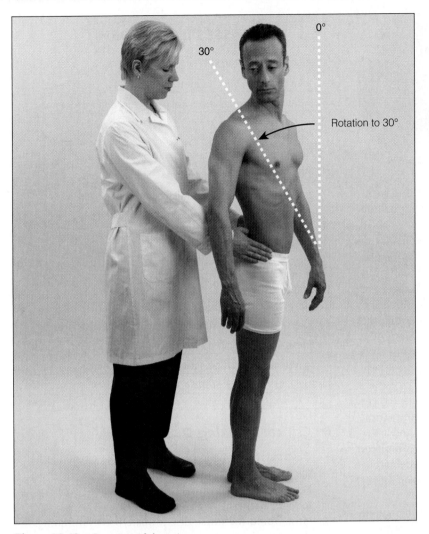

0°

30°

Rotation to 30°

Figure 23.49 ● Rotation of the spine.

SAMPLE DOCUMENTATION

Subjective: Client reports no history of pain, stiffness, swelling or heat, weakness, or trauma. No past personal or family history of musculoskeletal illness or injuries. On no medications, follows Canada's Food Guide, and exercises 4 to 5 times per week: low-impact aerobics. Patient does not spend long periods standing or sitting at work.

Objective: No masses, swelling, or deformities. Full ROM in all joints, no pain or crepitus noted with movement. Muscle strength equal to examiner's, rated as 5.

APPLICATION THROUGH CRITICAL THINKING

CASE STUDY

Mrs. Rhonda Barber is a 43-year-old teacher. She visits the clinic for assessment of swelling and stiffness all over, but especially in her hands.

The health history reveals that Mrs. Barber has had some stiffness in her joints when awakening from sleep and after long periods of physical activity "like housework" for several months. She became "alarmed" when her hands were "hot, red, and swollen" and that she "could hardly move them." She has had no recent illness but has "felt weak and tired" and has not had much of an appetite lately. She reports no family history of musculoskeletal disease. She reports that she has had regular physical examinations, including blood work, and that nothing has been abnormal. Her last exam was 6 months ago. She takes no prescribed medications but has been using Advil and Aleve for the stiffness with moderate relief. She states that she is concerned about her hands because she must write on the board and correct papers. She also fears that "if something is really wrong and I don't get relief, I won't be able to care for my family or myself for that matter."

Physical assessment reveals a well-developed female 160 cm (5′3″) tall, weighing 54 kg (120 lb.). Her skin is pale and warm. Her gait is steady. She has normal ROM in the upper and lower extremities. ROM of her wrists, hands, and fingers is limited. The joints of her fingers are erythematous, hot, and edematous bilaterally. Her joints are tender to touch and painful on movement. Pain is 6 to 7 on a scale of 1 to 10.

The nurse suspects that Mrs. Barber may have rheumatoid arthritis. The nurse will obtain laboratory tests and X-rays.

▶ Complete Documentation

The following is sample documentation from assessment of Rhonda Barber.

SUBJECTIVE DATA: Stiffness in joints when waking and after long periods of physical activity for several months. "Alarmed" when hands were hot, red, swollen, and could hardly move them. No recent illness. Weak, tired, and loss of appetite lately. No family history of musculoskeletal disease. Regular physical examinations with normal results and normal "blood work." Last examination 6 months ago. No prescribed medications. Advil and Aleve for stiffness—moderate relief. Concerned about ability to work as teacher and "if something is really wrong," about ability to care for family.

OBJECTIVE DATA: Well-developed 43-year-old female. 160 cm (5'3") tall, 54 kg (120 lb.). Skin pale, warm. Gait steady. Full ROM all extremities except hands and fingers. Joints of fingers erythematous, hot, edematous bilaterally, tender to touch and painful on movement. Pain 6 to 7 on a scale of 1 to 10.

ASSESSMENT FORM

REASON FOR VISIT

Joint stiffness , heat, redness, swelling of hands for several months Concerned about ability to work and care for family.

HISTORY

No history of recent illness. No family history of musculoskeletal disease. No prescribed medications. Advil and Aleve for stiffness—moderate relief. Regular physical examinations—no abnormalities. Last = 6 months.

FINDINGS

Skin pale, warm

160 cm 54 kg (5 3 ″120 lb.)

Gait steady

Joints—all within normal limits except hand and fingers

Bilateral hands/fingers—erythematous, hot, swollen, tender to touch, pain on movement

Pain 6 to 7 on scale of 1 to 10

▶ Critical Thinking Questions

1. Describe the thoughts and actions of the nurse that led to the suspicion of rheumatoid arthritis.
2. What information would help in developing a plan of care for Mrs. Barber?
3. How would the nurse discriminate between findings for rheumatoid arthritis and osteoarthritis?

▶ Applying Nursing Diagnoses

1. The NANDA-I taxonomy (see Appendix A ⚭) includes the nursing diagnosis of *impaired physical mobility*. Do the data for Mrs. Barber support this diagnosis? If so, identify the data required for the PES (problem, etiology, signs or symptoms) statement.
2. The NANDA-I taxonomy includes a diagnosis of *role conflict*. Do the data in the case study support this diagnosis? If so, identify the data.
3. Refer to the NANDA-I taxonomy to identify additional nursing diagnoses for Mrs. Barber.

▶ Prepare Teaching Plan

LEARNING NEED: The data in the case study revealed that Mrs. Barber may have rheumatoid arthritis. Her symptoms are typical for rheumatoid arthritis. She will undergo laboratory tests and X-rays to confirm the diagnosis.

The case study provides data that are representative of risks, symptoms, and behaviours of many individuals. Therefore, the following teaching plan is based on the need to provide information to members of any community about arthritis.

GOAL: The participants in this learning program will have increased awareness of risk factors and symptoms associated with arthritis.

OBJECTIVES: At the completion of this learning session, the participants will be able to do the following:

1. Describe arthritis.
2. Identify risk factors associated with arthritis.
3. List the symptoms of arthritis.
4. Discuss strategies in diagnosis and treatment of arthritis.

Application of Objective 2: Identify risk factors associated with arthritis.

Content	Teaching Strategy	Evaluation
• Age: Osteoarthritis risk increases after age 40. • Gender: Females have a higher incidence of arthritis. • Heredity: Family history and genetic factors increase risk for arthritis. • Obesity: Obesity increases risk for arthritis in weight-bearing joints. • Joint injury through sports or repeated stress in some occupations can increase the risk of osteoarthritis. • Joint misalignment or deformity can increase the risk for arthritis.	• Lecture • Discussion • Audiovisual materials • Printed materials Lecture is appropriate when disseminating information to large groups. Discussion allows participants to bring up concerns and to raise questions. Audiovisual materials, such as pictures and slides, reinforce verbal information. Printed material, especially to be taken away with the learner, allows review, reinforcement, and reading at the learner's pace.	• Written examination May use short answer, fill-in, or multiple-choice items or a combination of items. If these are short and easy to evaluate, the learner receives immediate feedback.

HEALTH PROMOTION ASSESSMENT TOOL

Social Determinants of Health	Level of Action	Action Strategies
Work and working conditions	Individual and community	**Building healthy public policy** • Assess how and when Mrs. Barber most often uses her hands at work (for example, when writing on the blackboard) and how the pain varies with time of day, type of activity, and length of time doing the activity. • Explore options within school policies (or provide support to lobby for changes to school policy) for teaching strategies that would enable Mrs. Barber to take intermittent breaks to minimize pain, weakness, and fatigue. Examples include recruiting students to write on the blackboard for her and exploring alternative ways of marking student assignments, such as giving oral instead of written feedback.
Social support networks	Individual	**Create supportive environments** • Assess Mrs. Barber's level of supports. • Assist her to access support networks through organizations such as Arthritis Canada, where she would have access to other professionals with similar limitations who have developed effective strategies within their own work settings and who can provide her with helpful hints and social support.

(continued)

HEALTH PROMOTION ASSESSMENT TOOL *(continued)*

Social Determinants of Health	Level of Action	Action Strategies
Personal coping skills	Individual and family	**Create supportive environments** • Assess Mrs. Barber's household routines and responsibilities with the goal of increasing her opportunities to get adequate rest and minimizing activities that induce pain. Strategies could include renegotiating divisions of household tasks with her husband or hiring a house cleaner. • Complete a nutritional assessment using a diet diary. Refer Mrs. Barber to a nutritionist to develop a diet that meets her nutritional needs and helps to stimulate her appetite while addressing dietary likes and dislikes.

ABNORMAL FINDINGS

Abnormal findings of the musculoskeletal system include rheumatic disease, abnormalities of the spine, joint disorders, and trauma-induced disorders. Common disorders of the musculoskeletal system are described and depicted in Figures 23.50 through 23.68. Table 23.4 lists and defines rheumatic diseases. Table 23.5 lists and provides definitions for trauma-induced disorders. Table 23.6 outlines the differences between rheumatoid arthritis and osteoarthritis.

TABLE 23.4	Rheumatic Diseases
DISEASE	**DESCRIPTION**
Osteoarthritis	In osteoarthritis the joint cartilage erodes, resulting in pain and stiffness. Disability is associated with osteoarthritic changes in the spine, knees, and hips.
Rheumatoid arthritis	Inflammation of the synovium of the joint occurs in rheumatoid arthritis. The inflammation leads to pain, swelling, damage to the joint, and loss of function. Rheumatoid arthritis affects the hands and feet symmetrically.
Juvenile rheumatoid arthritis	This form of arthritis can affect any body part. Inflammation causes pain, swelling, stiffness, and loss of function of joints. Symptoms may include fever and skin rash.
Systemic lupus erythematosus (SLE)	SLE is an autoimmune disease. The autoimmune response results in inflammation and damage to joints and other organs, including the kidneys, lungs, blood vessels, and heart.
Scleroderma	In scleroderma there is an overproduction of collagen in the skin or organs, which results in damage to skin, blood vessels, and joints.
Fibromyalgia	Fibromyalgia is a chronic disease that is characterized by pain in the muscles and soft tissues that support and surround joints. Pain is experienced in tender points of the neck, shoulders, ribs, elbows, gluteal area, hips, and knees.
Ankylosing spondylitis	Ankylosing spondylitis is a chronic inflammatory disease of the spine. It occurs more frequently in males than in females. Fusion of the spine results in stiffness and inflexibility. This disorder may also affect the hips.
Gout	Gout is a type of arthritis caused by uric acid crystal deposits in the joints. The deposits cause inflammation, pain, and swelling in the joint.
Infectious arthritis	Infectious arthritis refers to joint inflammatory processes that occur as a result of bacterial or viral infection. Infectious arthritis can occur as parvovirus arthritis, as gonococcal arthritis, or in Lyme disease.
Psoriatic arthritis	Psoriatic arthritis may occur in individuals with psoriasis. Joint inflammation occurs in the fingers and toes and occasionally in the spine.
Bursitis	Bursitis refers to inflammation of the bursae (fluid-filled sacs) that surround joints. The pain of bursitis may limit range of motion of the affected area.
Tendinitis	Overuse or inflammatory processes can result in tendinitis. The inflammation of the tendon results in pain and limitation in movement.
Polymyositis	Polymyositis refers to inflammation and weakness in skeletal muscles. This disease can affect the entire body and result in disability.
Osteomyelitis	Osteomyelitis is an inflammation of the bone caused by infection. The inflammation results in bone destruction, pain, and fever.

TABLE 23.5	Trauma-Induced Disorders
DISORDER	**DESCRIPTION**
Dislocation	A displacement of the bone from its usual anatomical location in the joint.
Muscle sprain	A stretching or tearing of the capsule or ligament of a joint due to forced movement beyond the joint's normal range.
Fracture	A partial or complete break in the continuity of the bone from trauma.
Muscle strain	A partial muscle tear resulting from overstretching or overuse of the muscle.

TABLE 23.6	Rheumatoid Arthritis and Osteoarthritis	
PARAMETERS	**RHEUMATOID ARTHRITIS (RA)**	**OSTEOARTHRITIS (OA)**
1. Disease and clinical manifestations	• A systemic inflammatory disease with exacerbations and remissions. • Cause: Unknown. • Manifestations may include fatigue, anorexia, generalized stiffness, inflamed joints symmetrically and bilaterally.	• A localized progressive noninflammatory, asymmetric degenerative joint disease (no organ involvement). • Cause: New joint tissue forms in response to cartilage destruction, which is due to constant friction of two surfaces. • Manifestations may include joint stiffness, pain, and enlarged joints.
2. Onset of disease	• Common in young to middle-aged adults.	• Cartilage destruction may begin as early as age 20.
3. Gender	• Females are at greater risk. After age 60, there is a decreased marked gender difference.	• The incidence of OA is more prevalent in women, usually after the age of 50.
4. Stiffness	• It may last from 1 hour to most of day. As the disease progresses, pain is present even during rest.	• It is common on arising and subsides after 30 minutes to 1 hour. Pain is worse at the end of the day or after periods of activity. As the disease progresses, pain is present even during rest.
5. Weight	• People may experience weight loss.	• Common in people who are overweight.
6. Complications	• Joint destruction indicated by flexion contractures, hand deformities, inflamed joints (Figures 23.54 and 23.55 on page 635), rheumatoid nodules (Figure 23.56 on page 636), and swan-neck and boutonnière deformities (Figure 23.60 on page 637).	• Complications range from mild discomfort to loss of function caused by joint pain. Heberden's nodes and Bouchard's nodes (Figure 23.61 on page 637) are common.

Abnormalities of the Spine

Kyphosis

Kyphosis is an exaggeration of the normal convex curve of the thoracic spine (see Figure 23.50). It may result from congenital abnormality, rheumatic conditions, compression fractures, or other disease processes, including syphilis, tuberculosis, and rickets.

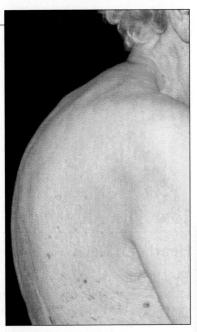

Figure 23.50 ●
Kyphosis (hunchback).

Scoliosis

Scoliosis is a lateral curvature of the spine (see Figure 23.51). Scoliosis may occur congenitally or as a result of disease or injury. In addition, scoliosis can occur from habitual improper posture, unequal leg length, weakening of musculature, and chronic head tilting in visual disorders. Functional scoliosis is flexible. It is visible when standing. Structural scoliosis is irreversible and visible when standing and bending.

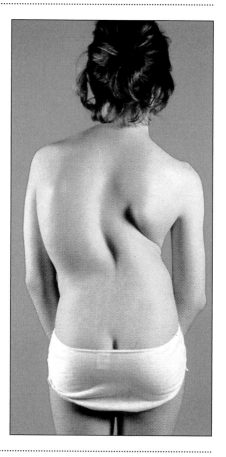

Figure 23.51 ● Scoliosis.

Lordosis

Lordosis is an exaggeration of the normal lumbar curve (see Figure 23.52). This occurs in pregnancy and in obesity to compensate for the protuberance of the abdomen.

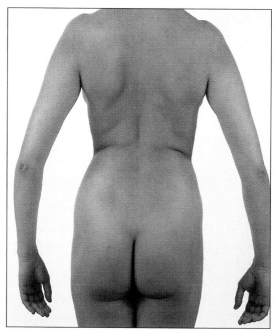

Figure 23.52 ● Lumbar lordosis.

Joint Disorders

Head and Neck

TMJ Syndrome

Inflammation or trauma can result in temporomandibular joint (TMJ) syndrome. Findings include swelling and crepitus or pain in the joint, especially on movement, such as opening and closing the mouth.

Shoulder

Rotator Cuff Tear

More common after the age of 40, rotator cuff tears arise from repeated impingement, injury, or falls. Findings include muscle atrophy of the infraspinatus and supraspinatus, tenderness, and pain. Impaired abduction of the glenohumeral joint occurs with a complete tear of the supraspinatus tendon. The appearance of shoulder shrugging occurs with attempts at abduction (see Figure 23.53).

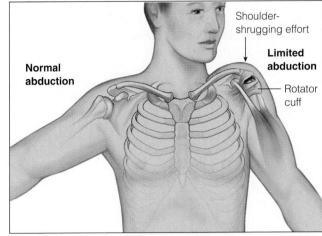

Figure 23.53 ●
Rotator cuff tear.

Elbow

Olecranon Bursitis

Trauma or inflammation from rheumatoid or gouty arthritis results in swelling of the olecranon bursa (see Figure 23.54).

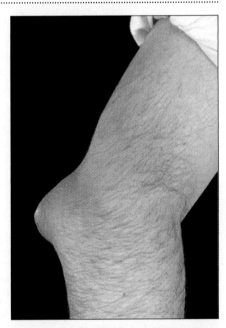

Figure 23.54 ●
Olecranon bursitis.

Wrist and Hand

Joint Effusion

Inflammatory joint disease results in fluid in the joint capsule (see Figure 23.55). The result is distension of the tissue seen.

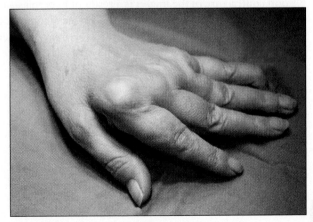

Figure 23.55 ●
Joint effusion of the hand.

Rheumatoid Nodules

Firm, nontender subcutaneous nodules occur along the extensor surface of the ulna (see Figure 23.56). They often are seen distal to the olecranon bursa in the hands and fingers.

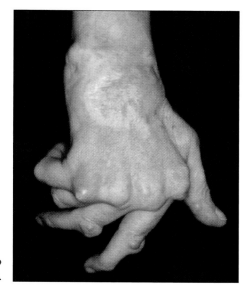

Figure 23.56 ●
Rheumatoid nodules.

Carpal Tunnel Syndrome

Chronic repetitive motion results in compression of the medial nerve, which lies inside the carpal tunnel. Decreased motor function leads to atrophy of the thenar eminence (see Figure 23.57). Findings include pain, numbness, and positive Phalen's test.

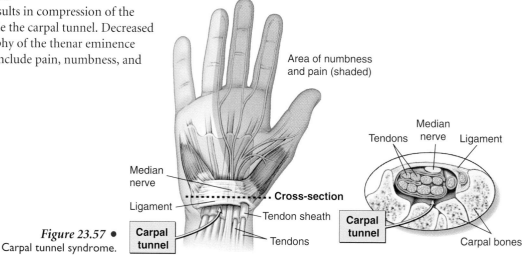

Area of numbness
and pain (shaded)

Median
nerve

Ligament

Cross-section

**Carpal
tunnel**

Tendon sheath

Tendons

Tendons

Median
nerve

Ligament

**Carpal
tunnel**

Carpal bones

Figure 23.57 ●
Carpal tunnel syndrome.

Dupuytren's Contracture

Flexion contracture of the fingers is a result of hyperplasia of the fascia of the palmar surface of the hand (see Figure 23.58). Range of motion is impaired. This contracture may be inherited or occur with diabetes or alcoholic cirrhosis.

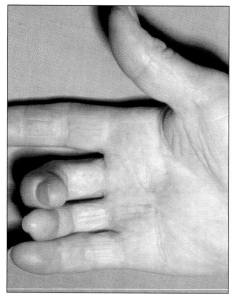

Figure 23.58 ●
Dupuytren's contracture.

Ulnar Deviation

In rheumatoid arthritis, the chronic inflammation of the metacarpophalangeal and interphalangeal joints leads to ulnar deviation (see Figure 23.59).

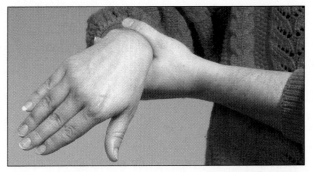

Figure 23.59 ●
Ulnar deviation.

Swan-Neck and Boutonnière Deformities

Flexion contractures associated with rheumatoid arthritis include (1) swan-neck contractures, in which the proximal interphalangeal joints are hyperextended while the distal interphalangeal joints are fixed in flexion; and (2) boutonnière deformities, in which the proximal interphalangeal joint is flexed in conjunction with distal interphalangeal joint hyperextension (see Figure 23.60).

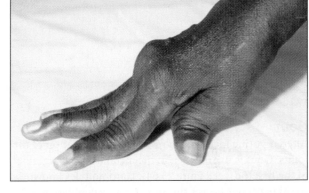

Figure 23.60 ●
Swan-neck and boutonnière
deformities.

Osteoarthritis

Bouchard's and Heberden's nodes occur in osteoarthritis (see Figure 23.61). These nodes are hard nodules over the proximal and distal interphalangeal joints. Osteoarthritis is a localized progressive degenerative disease. Wear and tear on the joints results in the formation of new tissue, which may result in mild to severe pain.

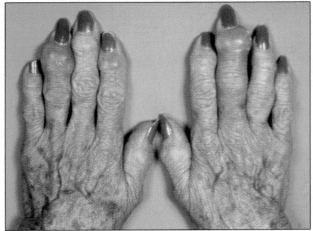

Figure 23.61 ●
Osteoarthritis.

© 1972–2004 American College of Rheumatology Clinical Slide
Collection. Used with permission.

Rheumatoid Arthritis

Rheumatoid arthritis results in symmetrical fusiform swelling in the soft tissue around the proximal interphalangeal joints (see Figure 23.62). It is a systemic inflammatory disease characterized by exacerbations and remissions. The cause is unknown and it affects people of all ages.

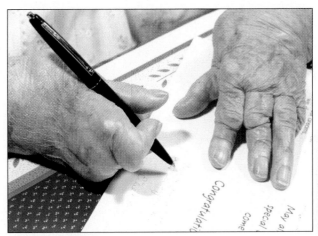

Figure 23.62 ●
Rheumatoid arthritis.

Synovitis

Effusion within the synovinum results in distension of the suprapatellar area and the lateral aspects of the knee (see Figure 23.63).

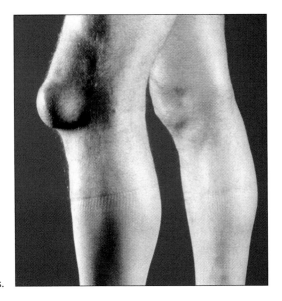

Figure 23.63 • Synovitis.

Foot

Gout

Altered purine metabolism results in inflammation of the joints. Gout is usually seen in the metatarsophalangeal joint of the first toe (see Figure 23.64). Hard nodules known as **tophi** may appear over the joint. Gout is manifested in erythema, pain, and edema.

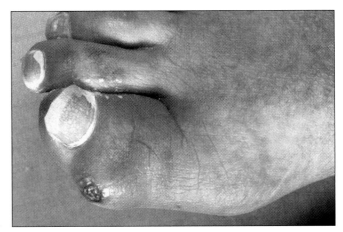

Figure 23.64 • Gout.

Bunion

Bunions are thickening and inflammation of the bursa of the joint of the great toe (see Figure 23.65). There is lateral displacement of the toe, with marked enlargement of the joint.

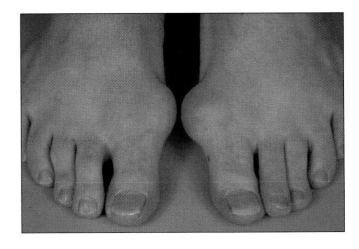

Figure 23.65 • Bunion.

Hallux Valgus

In hallux valgus the great toe is abnormally adducted at the metatarsophalangeal joint (see Figure 23.66).

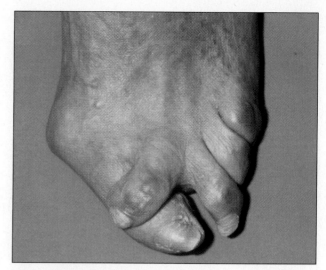

Figure 23.66 ● Hallux valgus.

Hammertoe

In hammertoe, the metatarsophalangeal joint of the toe hyperextends with flexion of the interphalangeal joint of the toe (see Figure 23.67).

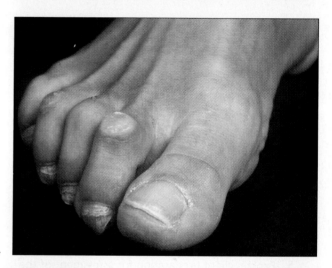

Figure 23.67 ● Hammertoe.

Osteomyelitis

In osteomyelitis, infections and inflammation cause bone destruction and skin breakdown (see Figure 23.68).

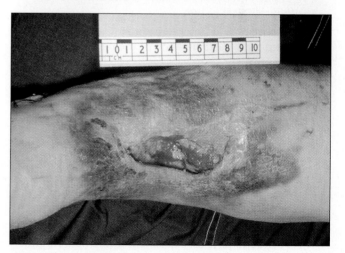

Figure 23.68 ● Osteomyelitis.

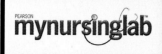

Visit the MyNursingLab website at **http://www.pearsoned.ca/mynursinglab**. This online homework and tutorial system puts you in control of your own learning with study and practice tools directly correlated to this chapter's content.

24

NEUROLOGICAL SYSTEM

The complex integration, coordination, and regulation of body systems, and ultimately all of body functions, are achieved through the mechanics of the nervous system. The intricate nature of the nervous system permits the individual to perform all physiological functions, perform all activities of daily living, function in society, and maintain a degree of independence. A threat to any aspect of neurological function is a threat to the whole person. A neurological deficit could alter self-concept, produce anxiety related to decreased function and loss of self-control, and restrict the client's mobility. Thus, it is essential to assess the psychosocial health status of a client experiencing a neurological deficit. Because such factors as diet, alcohol intake, smoking, and other healthcare practices can influence neurological health, the nurse must consider the client's self-care practices when assessing the client's neurological system. Factors relating to the client's occupation, environment, and genetic background also contribute to neurological health.

The nervous system is immature at birth. Many reflexes that are present in the newborn begin to disappear as the system matures. The older adult experiences a decrease in neurological function; the senses diminish, as do the reactions to stimuli. Degeneration of the nervous system may lead to a variety of psychosocial problems, such as social isolation, lowered self-esteem, stress, anxiety, and ineffective coping.

A healthy diet, exercise, and rest help ensure optimum neurological functions. Alcohol causes neurological impairments ranging from mild sedation to severe motor deficits. Caffeine is a mild stimulant that may cause restlessness, tremors, and insomnia.

A variety of home, work, and environmental factors may cause neurological impairments. For example, lead-based paint in older homes may cause lead poisoning and encephalopathy in children.

A thorough neurological assessment gives the nurse detailed data regarding the client's health status and self-care practices. It is imperative to develop and refine assessment skills regarding the wellness and normal parameters of the neurological functions in the body. The nurse needs to foster a keen discriminatory skill concerning the subtle changes that could be occurring in the client. Neurological assessment is an integral aspect of the client's health and must be carefully considered when conducting a thorough health assessment.

ANATOMY AND PHYSIOLOGY REVIEW

The neurological system, a highly integrated and complex system, is divided into two principal parts: the central nervous system (CNS) and the peripheral nervous system (PNS). The **central nervous system** consists of the brain and the spinal cord; the cranial nerves and the spinal nerves make up the **peripheral nervous system**. The two systems work together to receive an impulse, interpret it, and initiate a response, enabling the individual to maintain a high level of adaptation and homeostasis. The nervous system is responsible for control of cognitive function and both voluntary and involuntary activities.

The basic cell of the nervous system is the *neuron*. This highly specialized cell sends impulses throughout the body. Many of the nerve fibres that have a large diameter or are long are covered with a *myelin sheath*. This white, fatty coverage helps to protect the neuron while increasing the delivery of a nerve impulse, hence the term *white matter of the nervous system*.

Central Nervous System

The central nervous system includes the brain and spinal cord. These structures will be described in the sections that follow.

Brain

The brain is the largest portion of the central nervous system. It is covered and protected by the meninges, the cerebrospinal fluid, and the bony structure of the skull. The **meninges** are three connective tissue membranes that cover, protect, and nourish the central nervous system. The cerebrospinal fluid also helps to nourish the central nervous system; however, its primary function is to cushion the brain and prevent injury to the brain tissue. The brain is made up of the cerebrum, diencephalon, cerebellum, and brain stem (see Figure 24.1).

CEREBRUM. The **cerebrum** is the largest portion of the brain. The outermost layer of the cerebrum, the *cerebral cortex,* is composed of grey matter. Responsible for all conscious behaviour, the cerebral cortex enables the individual to perceive, remember, communicate, and initiate voluntary movements. The cerebrum consists of the frontal, parietal, and temporal lobes. The lobes of the cerebrum are illustrated in Figure 24.2.

The frontal lobe of the cerebrum helps control voluntary skeletal movement, speech, emotions, and intellectual activities. The prefrontal cortex of the frontal lobe controls intellect, complex learning abilities, judgment, reasoning, concern for others, and creation of abstract ideas.

The parietal lobe of the cerebrum is responsible for conscious awareness of sensation and somatosensory stimuli, including temperature, pain, shapes, and two-point discrimination—for example, the ability to sense a round versus square object placed in the hand or hot versus cold materials against the skin.

The visual cortex, located in the occipital lobe, receives stimuli from the retina and interprets the visual stimuli in relation to past experiences.

The temporal lobe of the cerebrum is responsible for interpreting auditory stimuli. Impulses from the cochlea are transmitted to the temporal lobe and are interpreted regarding pitch, rhythm, loudness, and perception of what the individual hears. The olfactory cortex is also in the temporal lobe and transmits impulses related to smell.

DIENCEPHALON. The diencephalon is composed of the thalamus, hypothalamus, and epithalamus. The **thalamus** is the gateway to the cerebral cortex. All input channelled to the cerebral cortex is processed by the thalamus.

The hypothalamus, an autonomic control centre, influences such activities as blood pressure, heart rate, force of heart contraction, digestive motility, respiratory rate and depth, and perception of pain, pleasure, and fear. Regulation of body temperature, food intake, water balance, and sleep cycles are also regulated by the hypothalamus.

The epithalamus helps control moods and sleep cycles. It contains the choroid plexus, where the cerebrospinal fluid is formed.

CEREBELLUM. The **cerebellum** is located below the cerebrum and behind the brain stem. It coordinates stimuli from the cerebral cortex to provide precise timing for skeletal muscle coordination and smooth movements. The cerebellum also assists with maintaining equilibrium and muscle tone.

BRAIN STEM. The **brain stem** contains the midbrain, pons, and medulla oblongata. Located between the cerebrum and spinal cord, the brain stem connects pathways between the higher and lower structures. Ten of the 12 pairs of cranial nerves originate in the brain stem. As an autonomic control centre, the brain stem influences blood pressure by controlling vasoconstriction. It also regulates respiratory rate, depth, and rhythm, as well as vomiting, hiccupping, swallowing, coughing, and sneezing.

Spinal Cord

The **spinal cord** is a continuation of the medulla oblongata. About 42 cm (17 in.) long, it passes through the skull at the

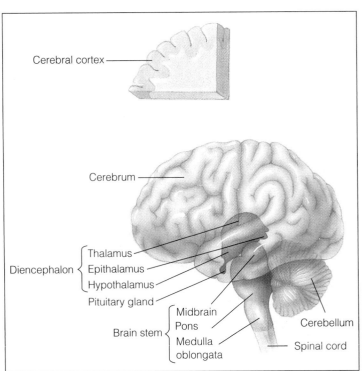

Figure 24.1 ● Regions of the brain.

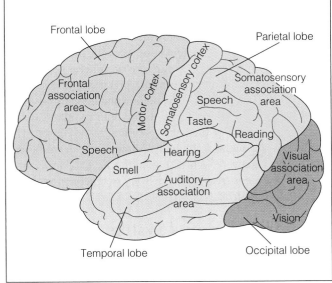

Figure 24.2 ● Lobes of the cerebrum.

foramen magnum and continues through the vertebral column to the first lumbar vertebra. The meninges, cerebrospinal fluid, and bony vertebrae protect the spinal cord. The spinal cord has the ability to transmit impulses to and from the brain via the ascending and descending pathways. Some reflex activity takes place within the spinal cord; however, for this activity to be useful, the brain must interpret it.

Reflexes

Reflexes are stimulus-response activities of the body. They are fast, predictable, unlearned, innate, and involuntary reactions to stimuli. The individual is aware of the results of the reflex activity and not the activity itself. The reflex activity may be simple and take place at the level of the spinal cord, with interpretation at the cerebral level. For example, if the tendon of the knee is sharply stimulated with a reflex hammer, the impulse follows the afferent nerve fibres. A synapse occurs in the spinal cord, and the impulse is transmitted to the efferent nerve fibres, leading to an additional synapse and stimulation of muscle fibres. As the muscle fibres contract, the lower leg moves, causing the knee-jerk reaction. The individual is aware of the reflex after the lower leg moves and the brain has interpreted the activity. Figure 24.3 illustrates two simple reflex arcs.

Peripheral Nervous System

The peripheral nervous system includes the 12 pairs of cranial nerves and the paired spinal nerves. They will be described in the paragraphs that follow.

Cranial Nerves

The 12 pairs of cranial nerves originate in the brain and serve various parts of the head and neck (see Figure 24.4). The first 2 pairs originate in the anterior brain, and the remaining 10 pairs originate in the brain stem. The vagus nerve is the only cranial nerve to serve a muscle and body region below the neck. The cranial nerves are numbered by using roman numerals and many times are discussed by number rather than name. Composition of the cranial nerve fibres varies, producing sensory nerves, motor nerves, and mixed nerves. A summary of the name, number, function, and activity of the cranial nerves is presented in Table 24.1.

Spinal Nerves

The spinal cord supplies the body with 31 pairs of spinal nerves that are named according to the vertebral level of origin as shown in Figure 24.5.

There are eight pairs of cervical nerves, twelve pairs of thoracic nerves, five pairs of lumbar nerves, five pairs of sacral nerves, and one pair of coccygeal nerves. At the cervical level, the nerves exit superior to the vertebra except for the eighth cervical nerve. This nerve exits inferior to the seventh cervical vertebra. All remaining descending nerves exit the spinal cord and vertebral column inferior to the same-numbered vertebrae. Spinal nerves are all classified as mixed nerves because they contain motor and sensory pathways that produce motor and sensory activities. Each pair of nerves is responsible for a par-

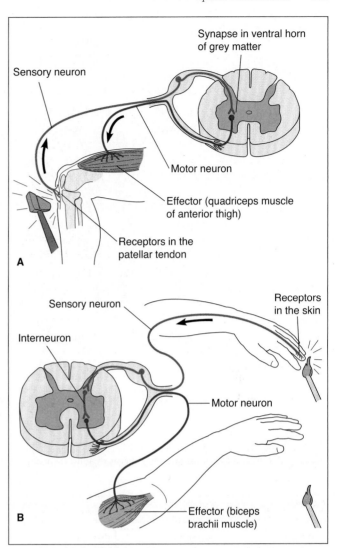

Figure 24.3 • Two simple reflex arcs. A. In the two-neuron reflex arc, the stimulus is transferred from the sensory neuron directly to the motor neuron at the point of synapse in the spinal cord. B. In the three-neuron reflex arc, the stimulus travels from the sensory neuron to an interneuron in the spinal cord, and then to the motor neuron. (Sensory nerves are shown in blue; motor nerves, in red.)

ticular area of the body. The nerves provide some overlap of the body segments they serve. This overlap is more complete on the trunk than on the extremities.

A **dermatome** is an area of skin innervated by the cutaneous branch of one spinal nerve. All spinal nerves except the first cervical (C_1) serve a cutaneous region. The anterior and posterior views of the dermatomes of the body are shown in Figure 24.6.

SPECIAL CONSIDERATIONS

Throughout the assessment process, the nurse gathers subjective and objective data about the client's state of health. By using critical thinking and the nursing process, the nurse identifies many factors to be considered when collecting the data, including age, developmental level, race, ethnicity, work history, living conditions, and socioeconomics. Physical and emotional wellness are also among the many factors or special

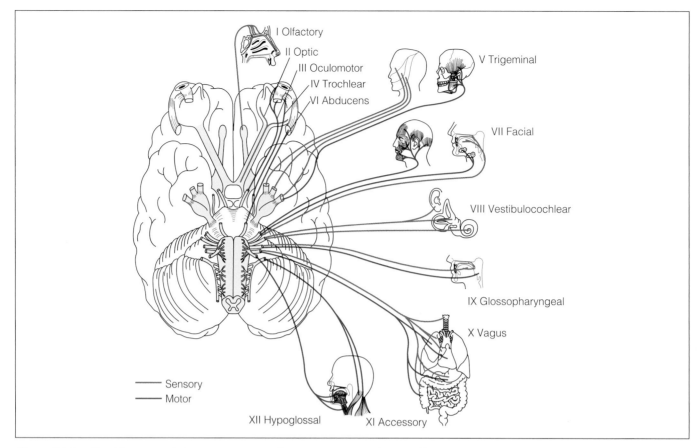

Figure 24.4 • Cranial nerves and their target regions. (Sensory nerves are shown in blue; motor nerves, in red.)

TABLE 24.1	Cranial Nerves		
NAME	**NUMBER**	**FUNCTION**	**ACTIVITY**
Olfactory	I	Sensory	Sense of smell.
Optic	II	Sensory	Vision.
Oculomotor	III	Motor	Pupillary reflex, extrinsic muscle movement of eye.
Trochlear	IV	Motor	Eye-muscle movement.
Trigeminal	V	Mixed	*Ophthalmic branch:* Sensory impulses from scalp, upper eyelid, nose, cornea, and lacrimal gland.
			Maxillary branch: Sensory impulses from lower eyelid, nasal cavity, upper teeth, upper lip, palate. *Mandibular branch:* Sensory impulses from tongue, lower teeth, skin of chin, and lower lip. Motor action includes teeth clenching, movement of mandible.
Abducens	VI	Mixed	Extrinsic muscle movement of eye.
Facial	VII	Mixed	Taste (anterior two thirds of tongue). Facial movements such as smiling, closing of eyes, frowning. Production of tears and salivary stimulation.
Vestibulocochlear	VIII	Sensory	*Vestibular branch:* Sense of balance or equilibrium. *Cochlear branch:* Sense of hearing.
Glossopharyngeal	IX	Mixed	Produces the gag and swallowing reflexes. Taste (posterior third of the tongue).
Vagus	**X**	Mixed	Innervates muscles of throat and mouth for swallowing and talking. Other branches responsible for pressoreceptors and chemoreceptor activity.
Accessory	XI	Motor	Movement of the trapezius and sternocleidomastoid muscles. Some movement of larynx, pharynx, and soft palate.
Hypoglossal	XII	Motor	Movement of tongue for swallowing, movement of food during chewing, and speech.

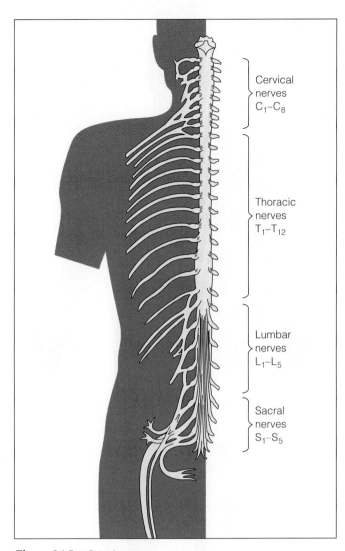

Figure 24.5 ● Spinal nerves.

Cervical
nerves
C_1–C_8

Thoracic
nerves
T_1–T_{12}

Lumbar
nerves
L_1–L_5

Sacral
nerves
S_1–S_5

considerations that affect a client's health status. The sections that follow describe the ways in which neurological health is affected by these special considerations.

Developmental Considerations

Growth and development are dynamic processes that describe change over time. The following discussion presents specific variations for different age groups across the life span. The structures and functions of the neurological system undergo change as a result of normal growth and development. Accurate interpretation of subjective and objective data from assessment of the neurological system is dependent upon knowledge of expected variations. The discussion of age-related variations is presented in the sections that follow.

Infants and Children

The growth of the nervous system is very rapid during the fetal period. This rate of growth does not continue during infancy. Some research indicates that no neurons are formed after the third trimester of fetal life. It is believed that during infancy the neurons mature, allowing for more complete actions to

take place. The cerebral cortex thickens, brain size increases, and myelinization occurs. The maturational advances in the nervous system are responsible for the cephalocaudal and proximal-to-distal refinement of development, control, and movement.

The neonate has several primitive reflexes at birth. These include but are not limited to sucking, stepping, startle (Moro), and the Babinski reflex, in which stimulation of the sole of the foot from the heel toward the toes results in dorsiflexion of the great toe and fanning of other toes. The Babinski reflex and the tonic neck reflex are normal until around 2 years of age. (See Table 25.3, Primitive Reflexes of Early Childhood.) By about 1 month of age, the reflexes begin to disappear, and the child takes on more controlled and complex activity.

The cry of the newborn helps place the infant on the health-illness continuum. *Strong* and *lusty* are terms used to describe the cry of a healthy newborn. An absent, weak, or "catlike" or shrill cry usually indicates cerebral disease.

Throughout infancy and the early childhood years, it is important to assess the fine and gross motor skills, language, and personal-social skills of the child. The nurse identifies benchmarks or milestones related to the age and level of functioning of the child and compares the child's actual functioning with an anticipated level of functioning. Developmental delays or learning disabilities may be related to neurological conditions, such as fetal alcohol syndrome, autism, and attention deficit disorder.

The Pregnant Female

As the uterus grows to accommodate the fetus, pressure may be placed on nerves in the pelvic cavity, thus producing neurological changes in the legs. As the pressure is relieved in the pelvis, the changes in the lower extremities are resolved. As the fetus grows, the centre of gravity of the female shifts, and the lumbar curvature of the spine is accentuated. This change in posture can place pressure on roots of nerves, causing sensory changes in the lower extremities. These sensory changes are reversible following relief of pressure and postural changes. Hyperactive reflexes may indicate pregnancy-induced hypertension (PIH).

The Older Adult

As the individual ages, many neurological changes occur. Some of these changes are readily visible, whereas others are internal and are not easily detected. The internal changes could be primary in nature, or secondary to other changes, and contribute to the aging process. In general, the aging process causes a subtle, slow, but steady decrease in neurological function. These changes can be more pronounced and more troublesome for the individual when they are accompanied by a chronic illness, such as heart disease, diabetes, or arthritis. Impulse transmission decreases, as does reaction to stimuli. Reflexes are diminished or disappear, and coordination is not as strong as it once was. Deep tendon reflexes are not as brisk. Coordination and movement may be slower than and not as smooth as they were at one time.

The senses—hearing, vision, smell, taste, and touch—are not as acute as they once were. Taste is not as strong; therefore,

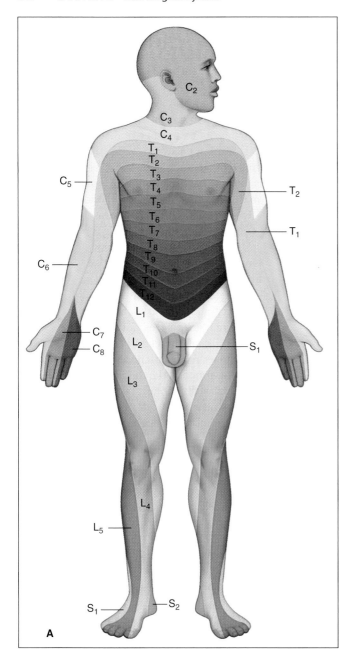

Figure 24.6A ● Dermatomes of body, anterior view.

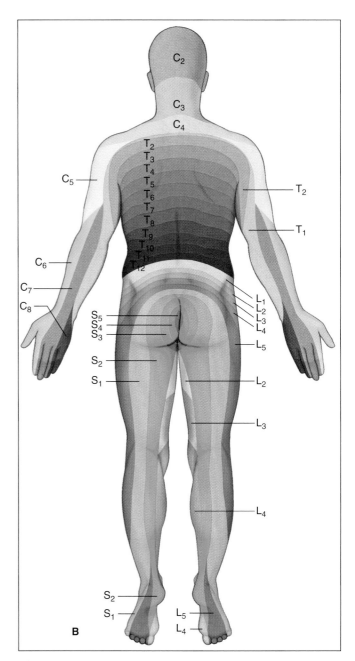

Figure 24.6B ● Dermatomes of body, posterior view.

the older adult tends to use more seasonings on food. Visual acuity and hearing also begin to diminish as the individual ages.

As muscle mass decreases, the older individual moves and reacts more slowly than during youth. The client's gait may now include short, shuffling, uncertain, and perhaps unsteady steps. The posture of the older adult demonstrates more flexion than in earlier years.

Assessment techniques used with the older adult are the same as those used for the younger or middle-aged adult. However, because the older adult tires more easily, the nurse may need more than one visit to complete the total assessment. The nurse should allow more time than usual when performing the neurological assessment of the older adult. It is also imperative to obtain a detailed history, because chronic health problems can influence the findings.

Psychosocial Considerations

Changes in nervous system functioning may alter an individual's ability to control body movements, speech, and elimination patterns, and to engage in activities of daily living. Inevitably, these changes will affect the individual's psychosocial health. Clients' self-esteem may suffer as they suddenly or progressively become unable to carry out the roles they previously assumed in their family and society. Another common psychosocial problem associated with neurological disorders is social isolation. For example, an individual in the first stage of Alzheimer's disease will decline invitations to social functions because the individual feels anxious and confused in unfamiliar surroundings. Such problems indicate a need for improved coping strategies and increased support systems.

As stresses accumulate, an individual becomes increasingly susceptible to neurological problems, such as forgetfulness, confusion, inability to concentrate, sleeplessness, and tremors. For example, a fourth-year university student who is studying for examinations, writing applications for graduate school, and has just broken up with his or her significant other might experience one or all of these symptoms. Chronic stress may also contribute to clinical depression in some clients.

Social and Ethnocultural Considerations

Huntington's disease is a genetically transferred neurological disorder. However, the genetic link to most other degenerative neurological disorders, such as Alzheimer's disease, multiple sclerosis, myasthenia gravis, and others, is unclear.

Research is inconclusive on the effects of environmental toxins, most notably aluminum, on the development of degenerative neurological disorders like Alzheimer's disease. Other research indicates that toxins, such as carbon monoxide, manganese, and mercury, may cause some cases of Parkinson's disease. Peripheral neuropathy, damage to the peripheral nerves, occurs more often among farm workers exposed to the organophosphates in many insecticides.

Lead poisoning also causes peripheral neuropathy and encephalopathy. Although not as common as in the past, the risk for lead poisoning still remains high among preschool children who live in old apartments or houses in which walls are painted with lead-based paints. Lead poisoning is not limited to those who live in low-cost, inner-city dwellings and may also occur in wealthy families living in restored older homes.

Social and Ethnocultural Considerations

- Very low-birth-weight babies are at risk for neurological problems, including intraventricular hemorrhage.
- Women have higher rates of Alzheimer's disease than do men.

- High blood pressure increases the risk of brain attack (stroke).
- Cleft lip and palate occur with greatest frequency in Asians and least often in Black people.

GATHERING THE DATA

Health assessment of the neurological system includes gathering subjective and objective data. Subjective data are collected during the client interview, before the physical assessment. During the interview, various communication techniques are used to elicit general and specific information about the status of the client's neurological system and ability to function. Health records, results of laboratory tests, X-rays, and imaging reports are important secondary sources to be included in the data-gathering process. During the physical assessment, the techniques of inspection and palpation, as well as techniques and methods specific to neurological function, will be used.

HEALTH HISTORY

The health history for the neurological system concerns data related to the functions of this body system. Subjective data are collected during the health history. The nurse must be prepared to observe the client and to listen for cues related to the function of the neurological system. The nurse may use open-ended or closed questions to obtain information. A number of follow-up questions or requests for descriptions can be required to clarify data or gather missing information. Follow-up questions are intended to identify the sources of problems, duration of difficulties, measures to alleviate or manage problems, and clues about the client's knowledge of his or her own health.

The health history guides the physical assessment of the neurological system. The information is always considered in relation to norms and expectations of neurological function. Therefore, the nurse must consider age, gender, race, culture, environment, health practices, past and concurrent problems, and therapies when framing questions and using techniques to elicit information. To address all the factors when conducting a health history, specific questions related to disorders of the neurological system and function have been developed. These questions focus on the most common symptoms or injury associated with the neurological system; questions related to past health history; questions related to behaviours; questions that address environmental concerns; and those that are specific to clients according to age, including the pregnant female.

The nurse must consider the client's ability to participate in the health history interview and physical assessment of the neurological system. Participation in the health history is influenced by the ability to communicate in the same language. Language barriers interfere with the accuracy of the data and cause anxiety in the client. The nurse may have to use a translator in conducting an interview and in the physical assessment. If the client is experiencing pain, recent injury, or anxiety, attention must focus on relief of symptoms or discomfort before proceeding with an in-depth interview.

As the nurse gathers the data, she or he will shift the type of questions to direct questions that give the client room to explain or qualify. The mnemonic O-P-Q-R-S-T-U, which stands for onset (chronology), precipitating (or palliative), quality, region (or radiation), severity, timing, and understanding, will help the learner remember the dimensions of the symptoms. The nurse will keep in mind that not all these qualifiers will apply to each symptom.

GATHERING THE DATA

HEALTH HISTORY QUESTIONS	RATIONALES

The sections that follow provide sample questions and follow-up questions. Rationales for some questions are provided. The list of questions is not all-inclusive but rather represents the more common concern or injury questions required in a health history related to the neurological system. An example of using O-P-Q-R-S-T-U with a headache is provided.

Questions Related to Common Concerns or Injuries

The most common symptoms related to illness or injury of the neurological system are as follows:

- Headache
- Head injury
- Seizures
- Numbness or tingling
- Dizziness or vertigo
- Change in senses
- Difficulty swallowing
- Difficulty speaking

1. **Headache**
   - Do you have a headache? *If yes:*

   ▶ The nurse is developing the database to determine if the headaches are migraines, tension headaches, cluster headaches, unilateral headaches, bilateral headaches, or headaches associated with other disease. (Refer to the section on the types of headaches in Chapter 12. ⊙)

   - When did you first notice the pain? How long does it last? *Onset (chronology)*
   - What makes the pain worse? What makes the pain better? *Precipitating (palliative)*
   - Would you describe the pain as throbbing? sharp? dull? burning? *Quality*
   - Where is the pain located? Does the pain radiate? *Region (radiation)*
   - How would you rate the pain on a scale of 1 to 10, with 10 being the worst pain? *Severity*
   - How often do you experience the pain? When does the pain occur? How long does it last? *Timing*
   - What do you think is causing the pain? *Understanding*

2. **Head injury**
   - Have you ever injured your head or back?

   ▶ The database being developed relates to past incidents and residual deficits.

3. **Seizures**
   - Do you experience fainting spells or have a history of seizures or convulsions?

   ▶ The client should be encouraged to identify the type of seizures: partial, complex, or mixed. The questions focus on an aura, a muscular activity, a postictal period, and the use of medications. Lifestyle changes are important, because individuals with these disorders need to be cautioned regarding driving and the use of dangerous equipment. (Epilepsy is described later in this chapter.)

HEALTH HISTORY QUESTIONS	RATIONALES

4. Tingling or numbness
- Do you have numbness or tingling in any part of your body?

▶ Numbness or tingling may result from neurological changes alone or as a result of systemic or circulatory disease.

5. Dizziness or vertigo
- Do you have any difficulty maintaining your balance?

▶ Balance is regulated by the cerebellum and disease or injury to the area may cause some incoordination or loss of balance.

6. Change in senses
- Have you experienced any change in your hearing, vision, sense of smell, or sense of taste?

▶ Changes in hearing and ringing in the ears may indicate a problem with cranial nerve VIII or auditory function.

Changes in vision may indicate problems with cranial nerve II, III, IV, or VI, a brain tumour, increased intracranial pressure, or ocular disease.

Changes in the ability to smell may be related to symptoms of the common cold, smoking, hereditary, caused by a zinc deficiency, or indicate a problem with cranial nerve I.

Change in the sense of taste may indicate damage to cranial nerves VII or IX or both.

7. Difficulty swallowing
- Do you have any difficulty swallowing?

▶ Dysphagia (difficulty swallowing), may be due to a neurological problem (damage to cranial nerves IX or X or both) or a gastrointestinal problem, or it may be related to ill-fitting dentures or malocclusion. Achalasia, a chronic difficulty in swallowing caused by constriction of the esophagus, may be related to anxiety or stress. Finally, painful or difficulty swallowing could be related to cancer of the throat or esophagus.

8. Difficulty speaking
- Do you have any difficulty speaking?

▶ Vocal changes could be indicative of lesions, paralysis, or other conditions.

Questions Related to Past Health History

1. Do have any chronic diseases, such as diabetes or hypertension?

▶ Chronic diseases, such as diabetes and hypertension, can predispose clients to neurological problems.

2. Do you or any member of your family have any neurological illness, such as stroke, paresis, epilepsy, multiple sclerosis, and myasthenia gravis, or infections, such as meningitis, encephalitis, or poliomyelitis? *If yes:*
- When were you diagnosed with the problem?
- Has the problem ever recurred? *(acute)*
- How are you managing the disease now? *(chronic)*

▶ This is a comprehensive and easy way to elicit information about all neurological diagnoses and gives the client the opportunity to provide information about a specific illness. If a diagnosed illness is identified, follow-up about the date of diagnosis, treatment, and outcomes is required. Data about each illness identified by the client are essential to an accurate health assessment. Illnesses can be classified as acute or chronic, and follow-up regarding each classification will differ. It is important to ask about the client's family, as some neurological conditions are familial.

Questions Related to Behaviours

Healthcare behaviours include both health practices and health patterns. Health practices consist of following recommendations for disease prevention, including screening for risks, screening for early detection of problems, and immunization. Health patterns are habits or acts that affect the client's health. Health behaviours may also include seeking healthcare from healthcare providers who use alternative methods to diagnose and treat illness. Clients should be questioned in a nonjudgmental way and areas for health teaching should be identified.

GATHERING THE DATA

HEALTH HISTORY QUESTIONS	RATIONALES

1. **Do you now use or have you ever used recreational drugs or alcohol?** *If yes:*
   - What drugs do you use?
   - How often?

▶ *Recreational drugs* is a common term used to describe illegal substances. This category includes heroin, cocaine, marijuana, ketamine, oxycodone, and other substances. Use of social drugs and alcohol can create risk for neurological symptoms or disorders that may be temporary or have long-term consequences.

2. **Do you have any problems with your memory?** *If yes:*
   - Do you need to make a list or write things down so you won't forget?
   - Do you lose things easily?

▶ Memory loss is indicative of the aging process and neurological or psychiatric diseases, such as Alzheimer's disease, depression, or stroke. This question helps to develop a baseline regarding the client's memory and the ability to recall recent and distant events.

Questions Related to the Environment

Environment refers to both internal and external environments. Questions related to the internal environment include all the previous questions and those associated with internal or physiological responses. Questions regarding the external environment include those related to home, work, or social environments.

Internal Environment

1. **Describe your daily diet.**
   - Do you have problems eating or drinking certain products?

▶ The diet provides nutrients and electrolytes responsible for neuromuscular activity and electrical activity in the nervous system.

2. **Are you currently taking any medications?**
   - What are the medications?
   - Do you use prescribed, over-the-counter, herbal, or culturally derived medications?
   - Do you use home remedies?

▶ Medications can cause neurological side effects. The interaction of medications, herbs, or other products may alter or affect the absorption or effects of prescribed medications.

External Environment

The following questions deal with the physical environment of the client. That includes the indoor and outdoor environments of the home and the workplace, those encountered for social engagements, and any encountered during travel.

1. **Are you now or have you ever been exposed to environmental hazards, such as insecticides, organic solvents, lead, toxic wastes, or other pollutants?** *If yes:*
   - Which one, when, and for how long were you exposed?
   - What treatment did you seek?
   - Do you have any problems because of the exposure?

▶ Such exposure could contribute to neurological deficits and neoplastic activity in the body.

Questions Related to Age

The health history must reflect the anatomical and physiological differences that exist along the age span.

HEALTH HISTORY QUESTIONS	RATIONALES

Questions Regarding Infants and Children

1. **Describe, if you can, the pregnancy with this child, including any health problems, medications taken, or alcohol or drugs used.**
   - Was the child premature, at term, or late?
   - Describe the birth of the child, including any complications occurring during or shortly after the birth.

▶ Health problems during the antepartal period and the use of medications, alcohol, or drugs may affect the neurological health of the child. Similarly, complications during or shortly after birth may have residual effects on the infant. For example, research indicates that some cases of epilepsy, a seizure disorder, may be due to prenatal or birth trauma.

2. **Has the child ever had a seizure?** *If yes:*
   - How often has this happened?
   - Describe what happens when the child has a seizure.
   - Has the child had a high fever when the seizures occurred?

▶ Seizures in feverish infants and toddlers are not uncommon. Seizures without accompanying fever may indicate a seizure disorder, such as epilepsy.

3. **Have you noticed any clumsiness in the child's activities? For example, does the child frequently drop things, have difficulty manipulating toys, bump into things, have problems walking or climbing stairs, or fall frequently?**

▶ These signs may indicate neurological disease.

4. **Are you aware of any surfaces in the home that are painted with lead-based paint?**
   - Have you ever seen the child eating paint chips?

▶ Lead poisoning may lead to developmental delays, peripheral nerve damage, or brain damage.

5. **How is the child doing in school?**
   - Does the child seem to be able to concentrate on homework assignments and complete them on time?
   - Have you ever been told that the child has a learning disability?
   - Have you ever been told that the child is hyperactive?
   - Do you agree with these assessments? Why or why not?
   - Have any medications or therapies been prescribed for the hyperactivity?
   - If so, please provide details.

Questions for the Pregnant Female

1. **Do you have a history of seizures?**
   - Have you had any seizures during this pregnancy or previous pregnancies?
   - If so, how often?
   - Please describe the seizures.

2. **Are you taking any vitamins or other nutritional supplements?**
   - Please describe these.

▶ Prenatal supplements are important to provide for the neurological health of the growing fetus. For example, vitamin A is required for nerve myelinization, and folic acid has been shown to reduce the incidence of neural tube defects.

Questions for the Older Adult

1. **Do you require more time to perform tasks today than perhaps 2 years ago? 5 years ago? Explain.**

▶ Endurance decreases with aging; therefore, more time is required for all activities.

2. **When you stand up, do you have trouble starting to walk?**

▶ Trouble initiating movement may indicate Parkinson's disease, which is more common in older adults.

3. **Do you notice any tremors?**

▶ Tremors may indicate motor nerve disease, or they may be attributable to certain medications or excessive consumption of caffeine.

4. **What safety features have you added to your home?**

▶ Safety precautions are essential to prevent neurological trauma from falls and other accidents.

GATHERING THE DATA

PHYSICAL ASSESSMENT

ASSESSMENT TECHNIQUES AND FINDINGS

Physical assessment of the neurological system requires the use of inspection, palpation, auscultation, and special equipment and procedures to test the functions of the system. During each part of the assessment, the nurse is gathering objective data related to the functioning of the client's central and peripheral nervous systems. The examination begins with assessment of the client's mental status and includes cranial nerves, motor and sensory function, balance, and reflexes. Knowledge of normal or expected findings is essential in the interpretation of the data.

Adults have erect posture and a smooth gait. Facial expressions correspond to the content and topic of discussion. The speech is clear and vocabulary and word choice are appropriate to age and experience. Adults are well groomed, clean, and attired appropriately for the season and setting. The adult is oriented to person, place, and time and can respond to questions and directions. The adult demonstrates intact short- and long-term memory, is capable of abstract thinking, and can perform calculations. The cranial nerves are intact. Motor function is intact, and movements are coordinated and smooth. Sensory function is demonstrated in the ability to identify touch, pain, heat, and cold; to sense vibrations; to identify objects; and to discriminate between place and points of touch on the body. The response to testing of reflexes is 2+ on a scale of 0 to 4+. Carotid arteries are without bruits.

Physical assessment of the neurological system follows an organized pattern. It begins with assessment of the client's mental status and proceeds to assessment of cranial nerves, motor and sensory function, reflexes, and auscultation of carotid arteries. Assessment proceeds in a cephalocaudal manner. The nurse tests distal to proximal and moves from gross function to fine function, always comparing corresponding body parts. More than one technique can be used to assess one function.

> **EQUIPMENT**
>
> | | |
> |---|---|
> | examination gown | penlight |
> | applicators | substances to smell, such as vanilla, mint, and coffee |
> | clean, nonsterile exam gloves | |
> | hot and cold water in test tubes | ophthalmoscope |
> | percussion hammer | substances to taste, such as sugar, salt, lemon, and grape |
> | gauze pads | |
> | tuning fork | stethoscope |
> | tongue blade | visual acuity charts (Snellen or E for distance vision, Rosenbaum for near vision) |
> | sterile cotton balls | |
> | objects to touch, such as coins, paper clips, or safety pins | sterile safety pins |

> **HELPFUL HINTS**
>
> - Data gathering begins with the initial nurse-client interaction. As nurses meet clients, they make assessments regarding their general appearance, personal hygiene, and ability to walk and sit down. These activities are related to cerebral function.
> - Physical assessment of the neurological system proceeds in a cepahalocaudal and distal to proximal pattern, and includes comparison of corresponding body parts.
> - Several assessments may occur at one time. For example, asking the client to smile tests cranial nerve VII, hearing, and the functions of the cerebral cortex, indicated by the ability to follow directions and initiate voluntary movements.
> - Provide specific information about what is expected of the client. Demonstrate movements.
> - Explain and demonstrate the purposes and uses of the equipment.
> - Use routine practices.

TECHNIQUES AND NORMAL FINDINGS	ABNORMAL FINDINGS AND SPECIAL CONSIDERATIONS

MENTAL STATUS

The nurse assesses the mental status of the client when meeting the client for the first time. This process begins with taking the health history and continues with each client contact.

A variety of tools are available to conduct mental status assessment. These tools are described in Table 24.2.

| TECHNIQUES AND NORMAL FINDINGS | ABNORMAL FINDINGS AND SPECIAL CONSIDERATIONS |

Table 24.2	Tools for Assessment of Mental Status

TOOL	ASSESSMENT
Mini-Mental State Examination (MMSE)	Cognitive status; conducted via interview
Addenbrooke's Cognitive Examination	Detects early dementia
Confusion Assessment Method (CAM)	Tests for delirium
Telephone Interview for Cognitive Status (TICS)	Similar to MMSE; cognitive function assessed via telephone interview
Cornell Scale for Depression in Dementia	Assessment of behavioural problems
Dementia Signs and Symptoms Scale	Assessment of behavioural problems
Psychogeriatric Dependency Rating Scale	Assessment of behavioural problems
Hopkins Competency Assessment Test	Assessment of ability to make decisions about healthcare
General Health Questionnaire	Assessment of psychosocial disturbance in those with normal cognitive ability
Hamilton Depression Rating Scale	Assessment of depression in clients with impaired cognition
Short Portable Mental Status Questionnaire (SPMSQ)	Assessment of organic brain deficit

1. **Instruct the client.**
   * Explain to the client that you will be conducting a variety of tests. Tell the client that you will provide instructions before beginning each examination. Explain that moving about and changing position during the examination will be required. Provide reassurance that the tests will not cause discomfort; however, the client must inform you of problems if they arise during any part of the assessment. Identify the types of equipment you will use and describe the purpose in relation to neurological function. Tell the client that you will begin the assessment with some general questions about the present and past. Then you will ask the client to respond to number and word questions.

2. **Position the client.**
   * The client should be sitting on the examination table wearing an examination gown (see Figure 24.7).

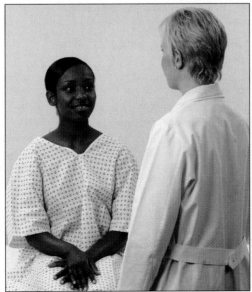

Figure 24.7 ●
Positioning the client.

TECHNIQUES AND NORMAL FINDINGS	ABNORMAL FINDINGS AND SPECIAL CONSIDERATIONS

3. Observe the client.
   - Look at the client and note hygiene, grooming, posture, body language, facial expressions, speech, and ability to follow directions.

▶ Changes could be indicative of depression, schizophrenia, organic brain syndrome, or obsessive-compulsive disorder.

4. Note the client's speech and language abilities.
   - Throughout the assessment, note the client's rate of speech, ability to pronounce words, tone of voice, loudness or softness (volume) of voice, and ability to speak smoothly and clearly.
   - Assess the client's choice of words, ability to respond to questions, and ease with which a response is made.

▶ Changes in speech could reflect anxiety, Parkinson's disease, depression, or various forms of aphasia.

5. Assess the client's sensorium.
   - Determine the client's orientation to date, time, place, and reason for being here. Grade the level of alertness on a scale from full alertness to coma.

▶ Neurological disease can produce a sliding or changing degree of alertness. Change in the level of consciousness may be related to cortical or brain stem disease. A stroke, a seizure, or hypoglycemia could also contribute to a change in the level of consciousness.

6. Assess the client's memory.
   - Ask for the client's date of birth, social insurance number, names and ages of any children or grandchildren, educational history with dates and events, work history with dates, and job descriptions. Ask questions for which the response can be verified.

▶ Loss of long-term memory may indicate cerebral cortex damage, which occurs in Alzheimer's disease.

7. Assess the client's ability to calculate problems.
   - Start with a simple problem, such as $4 + 3$, $8 \div 2$, or $15 - 4$.

▶ Inability to calculate simple problems may indicate the presence of organic brain disease, or it may simply indicate lack of exposure to mathematical concepts, nervousness, or an incomplete understanding of the examiner's language. In an otherwise unremarkable assessment, a poor response to calculations should not be considered an abnormal finding.

   - Progress to more difficult problems, such as $(10 \times 4) - 8$, or ask the client to start with 100 and subtract 7 ($100 - 7 = 93$, $93 - 7 = 86$, $86 - 7 = 79$, and so on).
   - Remember to use problems that are appropriate for the developmental, educational, and intellectual level of the client.
   - Asking the client to calculate change from one dollar for the purchase of items costing 25, 39, and 89 cents is a quick test of calculation.

8. Assess the client's ability to think abstractly.
   - Ask the client to identify similarities and differences between two objects or topics, such as wood and coal, king and president, orange and apple, and pear and celery. Quote a proverb and ask the client to explain its meaning. For example:
   - "A stitch in time saves nine."
   - "The empty barrel makes the most noise."
   - "Don't put all your eggs in one basket."
   - Be aware that age and culture influence the ability to explain North American proverbs and slang terms.

▶ Responses made by the client may reflect lack of education, developmental disabilities, or dementia. Clients with personality disorders, such as schizophrenia or depression, may make bizarre responses.

TECHNIQUES AND NORMAL FINDINGS	ABNORMAL FINDINGS AND SPECIAL CONSIDERATIONS

9. **Assess the client's mood and emotional state.**
   - Observe the client's body language, facial expressions, and communication technique. The facial expression and tone of voice should be congruent with the content and context of the communication.

   ▶ Lack of congruence of facial expression and tone of voice with the content and context of communication may occur with neurological problems, psychosocial disturbance, or a psychogenic disorder, such as schizophrenia or depression.

   - Ask if the client generally feels this way or if he or she has experienced a change and if so over what period.
   - Ask the client if it is possible to identify an event or incident that fostered the change in mood or emotional state.
   - The client's mood and emotions should reflect the current situation or response to events that trigger mood change or call for an emotional response (e.g., a change in health status, a loss, or a stressful event).

   ▶ Lack of emotional response, lack of change in facial expression, and flat voice tones can indicate problems with mood or emotional responses. Other abnormal findings in relation to mood and emotional state include anxiety, depression, fear, anger, overconfidence, ambivalence, euphoria, impatience, and irritability. Mood disorders are associated with bipolar disorder, anxiety disorders, and major depression.

10. **Assess perceptions and thought processes.**
    - Listen to the client's statements. Statements should be logical and relevant. The client should complete his or her thoughts.
    - Determining the client's awareness of reality assesses perception.

    ▶ Disturbed thought processes can indicate neurological dysfunction or mental disorder.

    ▶ Disturbances in sense of reality can include hallucination and illusion. These are associated with mental disturbances as seen in schizophrenia.

11. **Assess the client's ability to make judgments.**
    - Determine if the client is able to evaluate situations and to choose a realistic course of action. For example, ask the client about future plans related to employment.
    - The plans should reflect the reality of the client's health, psychological stability, and family situation and obligations. The client's responses should reflect an ability to think abstractly.

    ▶ Impaired judgment can occur in emotional disturbances, schizophrenia, and neurological dysfunction.

CRANIAL NERVES

1. **Instruct the client.**
   - Tell the client you will be testing special nerves and the senses of smell, vision, taste, and hearing. Explain that several of the tests will require the client to close both eyes. You will be asking the client to make changes in facial expression. Occasionally, you will touch the client with your hands while using different types of equipment during each test.

2. **Test the olfactory nerve (cranial nerve I).**
   - If you suspect the client's nares are obstructed with mucus, ask the client to blow the nose.
   - Ask the client to close both eyes and to close one naris. Place a familiar odour under the open naris (see Figure 24.8).
   - Ask the client to sniff and identify the odour. Use coffee, vanilla, perfume, cloves, and so on. Repeat with the other naris.

   ▶ **Anosmia**, the absence of the sense of smell, may be due to cranial nerve dysfunction, a cold, rhinitis, or zinc deficiency, or it may be genetic. A unilateral change in this sense may be indicative of a brain tumour.

TECHNIQUES AND NORMAL FINDINGS

ABNORMAL FINDINGS AND SPECIAL CONSIDERATIONS

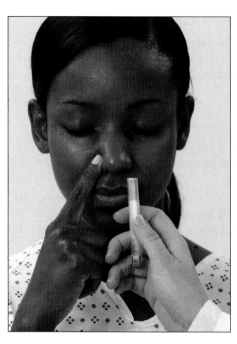

Figure 24.8 ●
Olfactory nerve assessment.

3. Test the optic nerve (cranial nerve II).

- Test near vision by asking the client to read from a magazine, newspaper, or the Rosenbaum card. Observe closeness or distance of page to client's eyes (35.5 cm or 14 in. is normal vision acuity). Also note the position of the head.

- Use the Snellen chart to test distance vision (see Figure 13.7).

▶ Pathological conditions of the optic nerve include retrobulbar neuritis, papilledema, and optic atrophy. **Retrobulbar neuritis** is an inflammatory process of the optic nerve behind the eyeball. Multiple sclerosis is the most common cause.

- Use the ophthalmoscope to inspect the fundus of the eye. Locate the optic disc and describe the colour and shape.

▶ **Papilledema** (or *choked disc*) is a swelling of the optic nerve as it enters the retina. A symptom of increased intracranial pressure, papilledema can be indicative of brain tumours or intracranial hemorrhage.

Immediate medical attention is required if intracranial hemorrhage is suspected.

Optic atrophy produces a change in the colour of the optic disc and decreased visual acuity. It can be a symptom of multiple sclerosis or brain tumour.

- See Chapter 13 for a detailed description of the technique for all of these activities. ⬭

4. Test the oculomotor, trochlear, and abducens nerves (cranial nerves III, IV, and VI).

- Test the six cardinal points of gaze.

▶ Pathological conditions include nystagmus, strabismus, diplopia, or ptosis of the upper lid. **Nystagmus** is the constant involuntary movement of the eyeball. A lack of muscular coordination, *strabismus*, causes deviation of one or both eyes. **Diplopia** is double vision. A dropped lid, or *ptosis* of the lid, is usually related to weakness of the muscles.

TECHNIQUES AND NORMAL FINDINGS	ABNORMAL FINDINGS AND SPECIAL CONSIDERATIONS

- Test direct and consensual pupillary reaction to light (cranial nerve III).
- Test convergence and accommodation of the eyes.
- These three tests are described in detail in Chapter 13. ⚭

5. **Explain the procedure for testing sensation.**
   - Show the client the cotton wisp. Touch the arm with the wisp and explain that the wisp will feel like that when a body part is touched. Ask the client to close both eyes.
   - Touch the arm with the wisp. Ask the client to say "now" when the wisp is felt. Explain that further tests with the wisp will be carried out with the eyes closed, and "now" is to be stated when the wisp is felt.
   - Show the client the opened sterile safety pin. Explain while you touch the arm with the rounded end that the sensation is dull and with the point that the sensation is sharp.
   - Tell the client that both eyes must be closed during several tests with the pin.
   - The client is expected to identify each touch or sensation as sharp or dull.

6. **Test the trigeminal nerve (cranial nerve V).**
   - Test the sensory function.
   - Ask the client to close both eyes.
   - Touch the face with a wisp of cotton (see Figure 24.9).

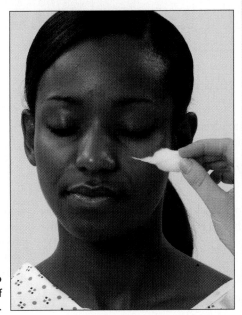

Figure 24.9 ●
Testing sensory function of
the trigeminal nerve.

- Direct the client to say "now" every time the cotton is felt. Repeat the test by using sharp and dull stimuli.
- Be random with the stimulation. Do *not* establish a pattern when testing. Be sure all three branches of the nerve are assessed.
- Test the corneal reflex.
- Ask the client to look straight ahead.
- Use a wisp of cotton to touch the cornea from the side.
- Anticipate a blink.

▶ Document any loss of sensation, pain, or noted fasciculations (fine rapid muscle movements).

TECHNIQUES AND NORMAL FINDINGS	ABNORMAL FINDINGS AND SPECIAL CONSIDERATIONS

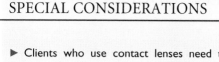

- Details for this procedure are presented in Chapter 13. ⚭

▶ Clients who use contact lenses need to remove them before testing. Most likely these clients will have a decreased or absent reflex because the corneal reflex has diminished in response to long-term contact lens use.

- Test the motor function of the nerve. Ask the client to clench the teeth tightly. Bilaterally palpate the masseter and temporalis muscles, noting muscle strength (see Figure 24.10).

▶ Muscle pain, spasms, and deviation of the mandible with movement can indicate myofascial pain dysfunction.

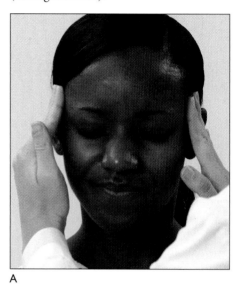

A

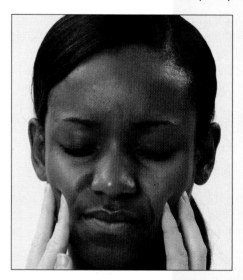

B

Figure 24.10 ● Testing muscle strength. A. Masseter muscles. B. Temporalis muscles.

- Ask the client to open and close the mouth several times. Observe for symmetry of movement of the mandible without deviation from midline.

7. Test the facial nerve (cranial nerve VII).
   - Test the motor activity of the nerve.
   - Ask the client to perform several functions, such as the following: smile, show your teeth, close both eyes, puff your cheeks, frown, and raise your eyebrows (see Figure 24.11).

▶ Asymmetry or muscle weakness may indicate nerve damage. Muscle weakness includes drooping of the eyelid and changes in the nasolabial folds.

   - Look for symmetry of facial movements.
   - Test the muscle strength of the upper face.
   - Ask the client to close both eyes tightly and keep them closed.

▶ Inability to perform motor tasks could be the results of a lower or upper motor neuron disease.

Techniques and Normal Findings

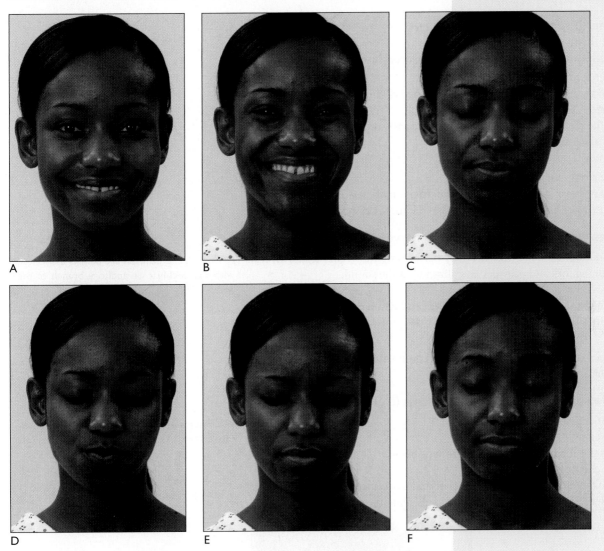

Figure 24.11 ● Testing motor function of cranial nerve VII. A. Smile. B. Show teeth. C. Close both eyes. D. Puff cheeks. E. Frown. F. Raise eyebrows.

- Try to open the eyes by retracting the upper and lower lids simultaneously and bilaterally (see Figure 24.12).

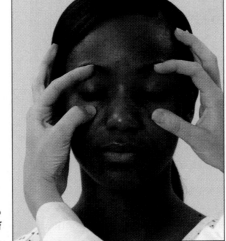

Figure 24.12 ●
Testing the strength of
the facial muscles.

TECHNIQUES AND NORMAL FINDINGS	ABNORMAL FINDINGS AND SPECIAL CONSIDERATIONS

- Test the muscle strength of the lower face.
  - Ask the client to puff the cheeks.
  - Apply pressure to the cheeks, attempting to force the air out of the lips.
- Test the sense of taste.
  - Moisten three applicators and dab one in each of the samples of sugar, salt, and lemon.
  - Touch the client's tongue with one applicator at a time and ask the client to identify the taste.
  - Water may be needed to rinse the mouth between tests.
- Test the corneal reflex.
  - This may have been tested with the trigeminal nerve assessment (see Figure 13.14). Cranial nerve VII regulates the motor response of this reflex.

8. **Test the vestibulocochlear nerve (cranial nerve VIII).**
   - Test the auditory branch of the nerve by performing the Weber test. This test uses the tuning fork and provides lateralization of the sound.

     ▶ Tinnitus and deafness are deficits associated with the cochlear or auditory branch of the nerve.

   - Perform the Rinne test. This compares bone conduction of sound with air conduction. Both the Weber and Rinne tests are described in detail in Chapter 14. ⚭
   - The Romberg test assesses coordination and equilibrium. It is discussed later in this chapter.

9. **Test the glossopharyngeal and vagus nerves (cranial nerves IX and X).**
   - Test motor activity.
     - Ask the client to open the mouth.
     - Depress the client's tongue with the tongue blade.
     - Ask the client to say "ah."
     - Observe the movement of the soft palate and uvula (see Figure 24.13).
     - Normally, the soft palate rises and the uvula remains in the midline.

     ▶ Unilateral palate and uvula movement indicate disease of the nerve on the opposite side.

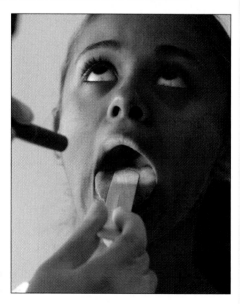

Figure 24.13 ●
Testing cranial nerves IX and X.

- Test the gag reflex. This tests the sensory aspect of cranial nerve IX and the motor activity of cranial nerve X.
- Inform the client that you are going to place an applicator in the mouth and lightly touch the throat.

  ▶ Clients with a diminished or absent gag reflex have an increased potential for aspiration and need medical evaluation.

TECHNIQUES AND NORMAL FINDINGS

- Touch the posterior wall of the pharynx with the applicator.
- Observe pharyngeal movement.
- Test the motor activity of the pharynx.
  - Ask the client to drink a small amount of water and note the ease or difficulty of swallowing.
  - Note the quality of the voice or hoarseness when speaking.

▶ **Dysphagia**, difficulty swallowing, could be related to cranial nerve disease.

▶ Vocal changes could be indicative of lesions, paralysis, or other conditions.

10. Test the accessory nerve (cranial nerve XI).
- Test the trapezius muscle.
- Ask the client to shrug the shoulders.
- Observe the equality of the shoulders, symmetry of action, and lack of fasciculations (see Figure 24.14).

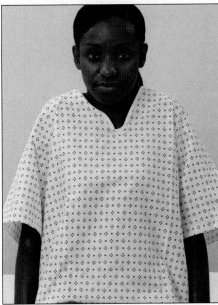

Figure 24.14 ●
Trapezius muscle movement.

- Test the sternocleidomastoid muscle.
  - Ask the client to turn the head to the right and then to the left.
  - Ask the client to try to touch the right ear to the right shoulder without raising the shoulder (see Figure 24.15).

▶ Abnormal findings include muscle weakness, muscle atrophy, fasciculations, uneven shoulders, and the inability to raise the chin following flexion.

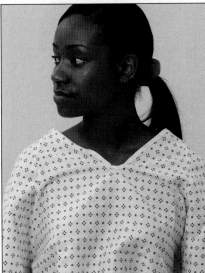

Figure 24.15 ●
Sternocleidomastoid muscle
movement.

TECHNIQUES AND NORMAL FINDINGS	ABNORMAL FINDINGS AND SPECIAL CONSIDERATIONS

- Repeat with the left shoulder.
- Observe ease of movement and degree of range of motion.
- Test trapezius muscle strength.
  - Have the client shrug the shoulders while you resist with your hands (see Figure 24.16).

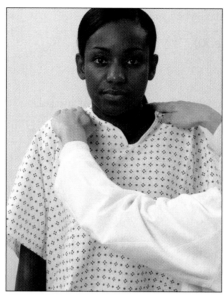

Figure 24.16 ●
Testing the strength of the trapezius muscle against resistance.

- Test sternocleidomastoid muscle strength.
  - Ask the client to turn the head to the left to meet your hand.
  - Attempt to return the client's head to midline position (see Figure 24.17).
  - Repeat the preceding steps with the client turning to the right side.

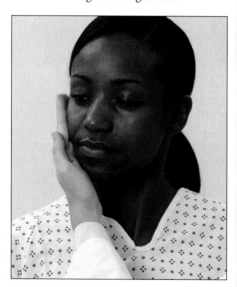

Figure 24.17 ●
Testing the strength of the sternocleidomastoid muscle against resistance.

11. Test the hypoglossal nerve (cranial nerve XII).

- Test the movement of the tongue.
  - Ask the client to protrude the tongue.
  - Ask the client to retract the tongue.
  - Ask the client to protrude the tongue and move it to the right and then to the left.
  - Note ease of movement and equality of movement (see Figure 24.18).

▶ Note atrophy, tremors, and paralysis. An ipsilateral paralysis will demonstrate deviation and atrophy of the involved side.

TECHNIQUES AND NORMAL FINDINGS	ABNORMAL FINDINGS AND SPECIAL CONSIDERATIONS

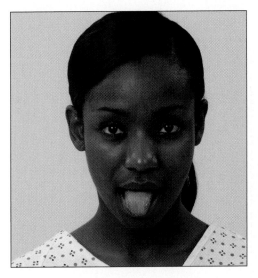

Figure 24.18A ● Protruding movement of tongue.

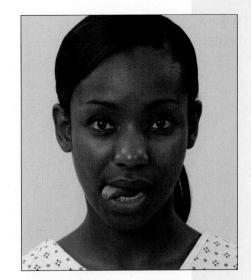

Figure 24.18B ● Lateralization of tongue.

- Test the strength of the tongue.
  - Ask the client to push against the inside of the cheek with the tip of the tongue.
  - Provide resistance by pressing one or two fingers against the client's outer cheek (see Figure 24.19).
  - Repeat on the other side.

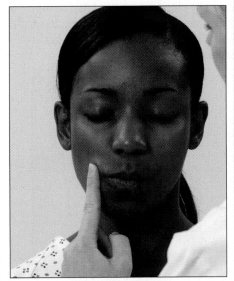

Figure 24.19 ●
Testing the strength of
the tongue.

MOTOR FUNCTION

Motor function requires the integrated efforts of the musculoskeletal and the neurological systems. Assessment of the musculoskeletal system is discussed in detail in Chapter 23. ⚭ The neurological aspect of motor function is directly related to activities of the cerebellum, which is responsible for coordination and smoothness of movement, and equilibrium. All of the following tests focus on activities of the cerebellum.

CLINICAL TIP
Be ready to support and protect the client to prevent an accident, an injury, or a fall.

TECHNIQUES AND NORMAL FINDINGS	ABNORMAL FINDINGS AND SPECIAL CONSIDERATIONS

1. Assess the client's gait and balance.

- Ask the client to walk across the room and return (see Figure 24.20).

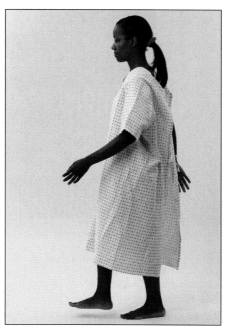

Figure 24.20 ●
Evaluation of gait.

- Ask the client to walk heel to toe (or tandem) by placing the heel of the left foot in front of the toes of the right foot, and then the heel of the right foot in front of the toes of the left foot. Be sure the client is looking straight ahead and not at the floor. Continue this pattern for several metres (see Figure 24.21).

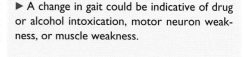

▶ A change in gait could be indicative of drug or alcohol intoxication, motor neuron weakness, or muscle weakness.

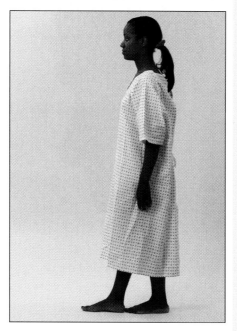

Figure 24.21 ●
Heel-to-toe walk.

- Ask the client to walk on his or her toes.
- Ask the client to walk on the heels. Observe the client's posture. Does the posture demonstrate stiffness or relaxation? Note the equality of steps taken, the pace of walking, the position and coordination of the arms when walking, and the ability to maintain balance during all these activities.

TECHNIQUES AND NORMAL FINDINGS	ABNORMAL FINDINGS AND SPECIAL CONSIDERATIONS

2. Perform the Romberg test.

- The **Romberg test** assesses coordination and equilibrium (cranial nerve VIII).

- Ask the client to stand with feet together and arms at the sides. The client's eyes are open.

- Stand next to the client to prevent falls. Observe for swaying.

- Ask the client to close both eyes without changing position.

- Observe for swaying with the eyes closed. Swaying normally increases slightly when the eyes are closed (see Figure 24.22).

▶ If swaying greatly increases or the client falls, suspect disease of the posterior columns of the spinal cord.

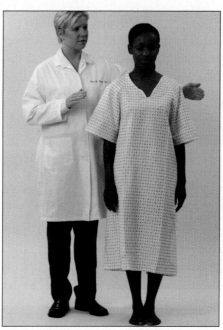

Figure 24.22 •
The Romberg test for balance.

3. Perform the finger-to-nose test.

- The finger-to-nose test also assesses coordination and equilibrium. It is sometimes called the pass-point test.

- Ask the client to resume a sitting position.

- Ask the client to extend both arms from the sides of the body.

- Ask the client to keep both eyes open.

- Ask the client to touch the tip of the nose with the right index finger, and then return the right arm to an extended position.

- Ask the client to touch the tip of the nose with the left index finger, and then return the left arm to an extended position.

- Repeat the procedure several times.

- Ask the client to close both eyes and repeat the alternating movements (see Figure 24.23).

- Observe the movement of the arms, the smoothness of the movement, and the point of contact of the finger. Does the finger touch the nose, or is another part of the face touched?

▶ With the eyes closed, the client with cerebellar disease will reach beyond the tip of the nose, because the sense of position is affected.

TECHNIQUES AND NORMAL FINDINGS	ABNORMAL FINDINGS AND SPECIAL CONSIDERATIONS

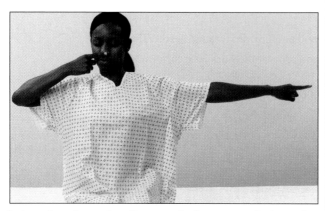

Figure 24.23 ● Finger-to-nose test.

- An alternative technique is to have the client touch the nose with the index finger and then touch that finger to the finger of the nurse (see Figure 24.24).

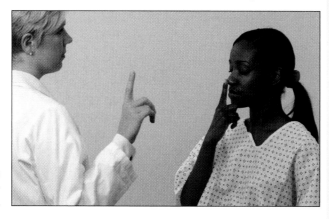

Figure 24.24 ● Alternative for pass-point test.

4. Assess the client's ability to perform a rapid alternating action.

- Ask the client to sit with the hands placed palms down on the thighs (see Figure 24.25A).
- Ask the client to turn the hands palms up (see Figure 24.25B).

▶ Inability to perform this task could indicate upper motor neuron weakness.

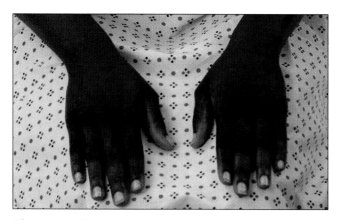

Figure 24.25A ● Testing rapid alternating movement, palms down.

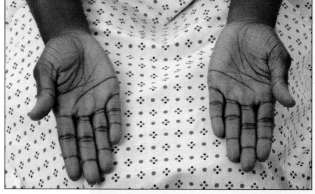

Figure 24.25B ● Testing rapid alternating movement, palms up.

- Ask the client to return the hands to a palms-down position.
- Ask the client to alternate the movements at a faster pace. If you suspect any deficit, test one side at a time.
- Observe the rhythm, rate, and smoothness of the movements.

| TECHNIQUES AND NORMAL FINDINGS | ABNORMAL FINDINGS AND SPECIAL CONSIDERATIONS |

- Figure 24.26 demonstrates the finger-to-finger test, which is an alternative method to assess coordination.

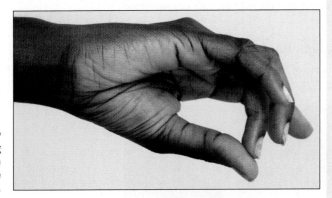

Figure 24.26 ● Testing coordination by using the finger-to-finger test.

- Ask the client to touch the thumb to each finger in sequence with increasing pace.

5. **Ask the client to perform the heel-to-shin test.**

- Assist the client to a supine position.
- Ask the client to place the heel of the right foot below the left knee.
- Ask the client to slide the right heel along the shinbone to the ankle (see Figure 24.27).

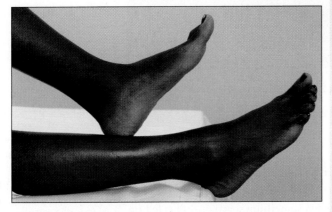

Figure 24.27 ● Heel-to-shin test.

- Ask the client to repeat the procedure, reversing the legs.
- Observe the smoothness of the action. The client should be able to move the heel in a straight line so that it does not fall off the lower leg.

▶ Inability to perform this test could indicate disease of the posterior spinal tract.

SENSORY FUNCTION

This part of the physical assessment evaluates the client's response to a variety of stimuli. This assessment tests the peripheral nerves, the sensory tracts, and the cortical level of discrimination. A variety of stimuli are used, including light touch, hot and cold, sharp and dull, and vibration. Stereognosis, graphesthesia, and two-point discrimination are also assessed. Each assessment is described in the sections that follow.

CLINICAL TIP

The client may tire during these procedures. If this happens, stop the assessment and continue at a later time. Be sure to test corresponding body parts. Take a distal-to-proximal approach along the extremities. When the client describes sensations accurately at a distal point, it is usually not necessary to proceed to a more proximal point. If a deficit is detected at a distal point, then it becomes imperative to proceed to proximal points while attempting to map that specific area of the deficit. Repeat testing to determine accuracy in areas of deficits.

TECHNIQUES AND NORMAL FINDINGS	ABNORMAL FINDINGS AND SPECIAL CONSIDERATIONS

Remember, always ask the client to describe the stimulus and the location. Do not suggest the type of stimulus or location. Tell the client to keep both eyes closed during testing. To promote full client understanding, you may have to demonstrate what you will do.

1. Assess the client's ability to identify light touch.
   - Use a wisp of cotton to touch various parts of the body, including feet, hands, arms, legs, abdomen, and face (see Figure 24.28).

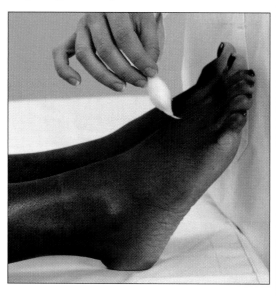

Figure 24.28 ●
Evaluation of light touch.

   - Touch at random locations and use random time intervals.
   - Ask the client to say "yes" or "now" when the stimulus is perceived. Be sure to test corresponding dermatomes.

▶ **Anaesthesia** is the inability to perceive the sense of touch. **Hyperesthesia** is an increased sensation, whereas *hypoesthesia* is a decreased but not absent sensation.

2. Assess the client's ability to distinguish the difference between sharp and dull.
   - Ask the client to say "sharp" or "dull" when something sharp or dull is felt on the skin.
   - Touch the client with the tip of a sterile safety pin (see Figure 24.29A).
   - Now touch the client with the blunt end of the pin (see Figure 24.29B).

▶ The absence of pain sensation is called **analgesia**. Decreased pain sensation is called **hypalgesia**. These conditions may result from neurological disease or circulatory problems such as peripheral vascular disease.

   - Alternate between sharp and dull stimulation.
   - Touch the client by using random locations, random time intervals, and alternating patterns.
   - Be sure to test corresponding body parts.
   - Discard the pin.

TECHNIQUES AND NORMAL FINDINGS

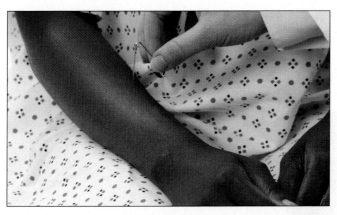

Figure 24.29A • Testing client's ability to identify sharp sensations.

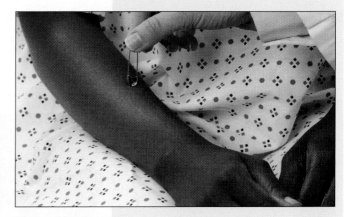

Figure 24.29B • Testing client's ability to identify dull sensations.

3. **Assess the client's ability to distinguish temperature.**
   - Perform this test only if the client demonstrates an absence or decrease in pain sensation.
   - Randomly touch the client with a test tube containing warm water and one containing cold water.
   - Ask the client to describe the temperature.
   - Be sure to test corresponding body parts.

4. **Assess the client's ability to feel vibrations.**
   - Set a tuning fork in motion and place it on bony parts of the body, such as the toes, ankle, knee, iliac crest, spinal process, fingers, sternum, wrists, or elbows (see Figure 24.30).

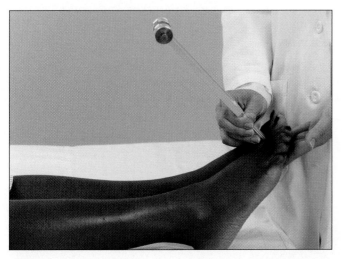

Figure 24.30A • Testing the client's ability to feel vibrations, the toe.

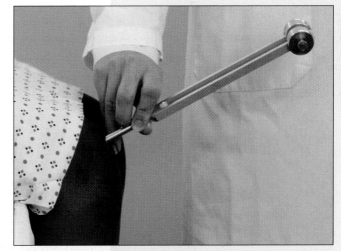

Figure 24.30B • Testing the client's ability to feel vibrations, the knee.

- Ask the client to say "now" when the vibration is perceived and "stop" when it is no longer felt.
- If the client's perception is accurate when you test the most distal aspects (toes, ankles, fingers, and wrist), end the test at this time.
- Proceed to proximal points if distal perception is diminished.

▶ The inability to perceive vibration may indicate neuropathy. This may be associated with aging, diabetes, intoxication, or posterior column disease.

PHYSICAL ASSESSMENT

TECHNIQUES AND NORMAL FINDINGS	ABNORMAL FINDINGS AND SPECIAL CONSIDERATIONS

5. Test stereognosis, the ability to identify an object without seeing it.
   * Direct the client to close both eyes. Place a safety pin in the client's right hand and ask the client to identify it.
   * Place a different object in the left hand and ask the client to identify it.
   * Place a coin in the right hand and ask the client to identify it (see Figure 24.31).

▶ Inability to identify a familiar object could indicate cortical disease.

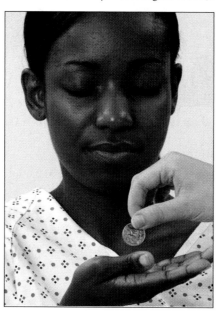

Figure 24.31 ●
Testing stereognosis by using a coin.

   * Place a different coin in the left hand and ask the client to identify it.
   * The objects you use must be familiar and safe to hold (no sharp objects).
   * Test each object independently.

6. Test graphesthesia, the ability to perceive writing on the skin.
   * Direct the client to keep both eyes closed.
   * Use the noncotton end of an applicator or the base of a pen to scribe a number, such as 3, into the palm of the client's right hand (see Figure 24.32).

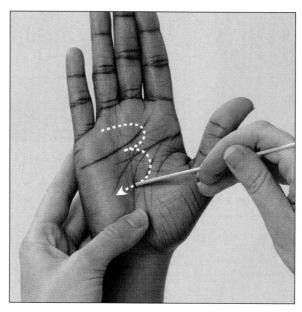

Figure 24.32 ●
Testing graphesthesia.

| TECHNIQUES AND NORMAL FINDINGS | ABNORMAL FINDINGS AND SPECIAL CONSIDERATIONS |

- Be sure the number faces the client.
- Ask the client to identify the number.
- Repeat in the left hand by using a different number, such as 5 or 2.
- Ask the client to identify the number.

▶ Inability to perceive a number on the skin may indicate cortical disease.

7. **Assess the client's ability to discriminate between two points.**
   - Simultaneously touch the client with two stimuli over a given area (see Figure 24.33).

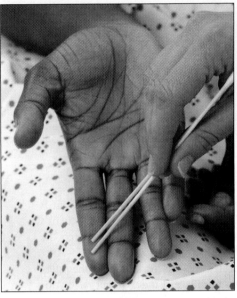

Figure 24.33 ●
Two-point discrimination.

- Use the unpadded end of two applicators.
- Vary the distance between the two points according to the body region being stimulated. The more distal the location, the more sensitive the discrimination.
- Normally, the client is able to perceive two discrete points at the following distances and locations:

Fingertips	0.3 to 0.6 cm (0.1 to 0.2 in.)
Hands and feet	1.5 to 2 cm (0.75 to 1 in.)
Lower leg	4 cm (1.5 in)

- Ask the client to say "now" when the two discrete points of stimulus are first perceived.

▶ An inability to perceive two separate points within normal distances may indicate cortical disease.

- Note the smallest distance between the points at which the client can perceive two distinct stimuli.
- Discard the applicators.

8. **Assess topognosis, the ability of the client to identify an area of the body that has been touched.**
   - This need not be a separate test. Include it in any of the previous steps by asking the client to identify what part of the body was involved. Also ask the client to point to the area you touched.

▶ Inability of the client to identify a touched area demonstrates sensory or cortical disease.

9. **Assess position sense of joint movement.**
   - Ask the client to close both eyes. Grasp the great toe. Move the joint into dorsiflexion, plantar flexion, and abduction.

Techniques and Normal Findings	Abnormal Findings and Special Considerations

- Ask the client to identify the movement (see Figure 24.34).

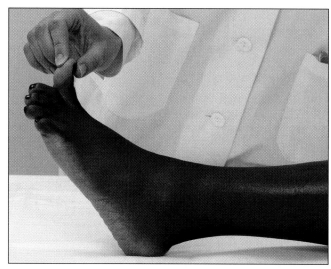

Figure 24.34 ●
Position sense of joint
movement.

REFLEXES

Reflex testing is typically the last part of the neurological assessment. The client is usually in a sitting position; however, you can use a supine position if the client's physical condition so requires. Position the client's limbs properly to stretch the muscle partially.

Proper use of the reflex hammer requires practice. Hold the handle of the reflex hammer in your dominant hand between your thumb and index finger. Use your wrist, not your hand or arm, to generate the striking motion. Proper wrist action will provide a brisk, direct, smooth arc for stimulation with the flat or pointed end of the hammer. Stimulate the reflex arc with a brisk tap to the tendon, not the muscle. Through continued practice and experience, you will learn the amount of force to use. Strong force will cause pain, and too little force will not stimulate the arc. After striking the tendon, remove the reflex hammer immediately.

Evaluate the response on a scale from 0 to 4+:

0	no response
1+	diminished
2+	normal
3+	brisk, above normal
4+	hyperactive

Before concluding that a reflex is absent or diminished, repeat the test. Encourage the client to relax. It may be necessary to distract the client to achieve relaxation of the muscle before striking the tendon. Distraction techniques include clenching the teeth, counting ceiling blocks, or humming.

1. **Assess the biceps reflex (C₅, C₆).**

   - Support the client's lower arm with your nondominant hand and arm. The arm needs to be slightly flexed at the elbow with palm up.

   - Place the thumb of your nondominant hand over the biceps tendon.

   - Use the pointed side of a reflex hammer to briskly tap your thumb (see Figure 24.35).

   - Look for contraction of the biceps muscle and slight flexion of the forearm.

▶ Neuromuscular disease, spinal cord injury, or lower motor neuron disease may cause absent or diminished (hypoactive) reflexes. Hyperactive reflexes may indicate upper motor neuron disease. **Clonus**, rhythmically alternating flexion and extension, confirms upper motor neuron disease.

TECHNIQUES AND NORMAL FINDINGS	ABNORMAL FINDINGS AND SPECIAL CONSIDERATIONS

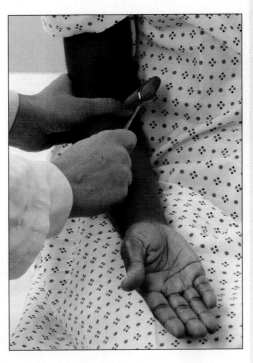

Figure 24.35 ●
Testing the biceps reflex.

2. Assess the triceps reflex (C_6, C_7).

    - Support the client's elbow with your nondominant hand.
    - Sharply percuss the tendon just above the olecranon process with the flat end of the reflex hammer (see Figure 24.36).
    - Observe contraction of the triceps muscle with extension of the lower arm.

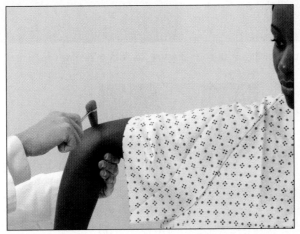

Figure 24.36 ●
Testing the triceps reflex.

3. Assess the brachioradialis reflex (C_5, C_6).

    - Position the client's arm so the elbow is flexed and the hand is resting on the client's lap with the palm down (pronation).
    - Use the flat end of the reflex hammer to briskly strike the tendon toward the radius about 5 to 7 cm (2 to 3 in.) above the wrist (see Figure 24.37).
    - Observe flexion of the lower arm and supination of the hand.

PHYSICAL ASSESSMENT

TECHNIQUES AND NORMAL FINDINGS

ABNORMAL FINDINGS AND SPECIAL CONSIDERATIONS

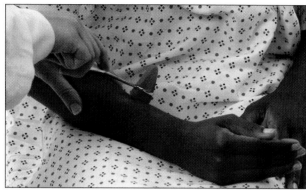

Figure 24.37 ● Testing the brachioradialis reflex.

4. Assess the patellar (knee) reflex (L$_2$, L$_3$, L$_4$).

   • Palpate the patella to locate the patellar tendon inferior to the patella.

   • Briskly strike the tendon with the flat end of the reflex hammer (see Figure 24.38).

   • Note extension of lower leg and contraction of the quadriceps muscle.

▶ Flex the leg at the knee. Occasionally, the response is not obtained. Distraction, such as that depicted in Figure 24.39, may be required.

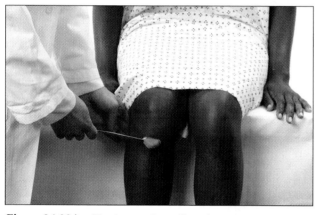

Figure 24.38A ● Testing patellar reflex, client in a sitting position.

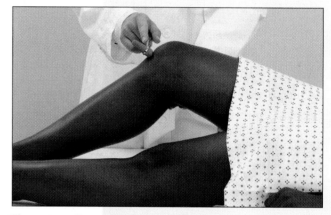

Figure 24.38B ● Testing patellar reflex, client in a supine position.

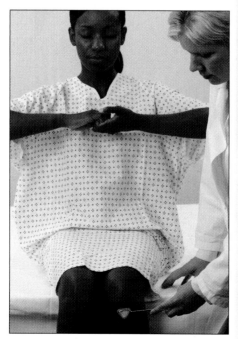

Figure 24.39 ● Testing patellar reflex with distraction.

| TECHNIQUES AND NORMAL FINDINGS | ABNORMAL FINDINGS AND SPECIAL CONSIDERATIONS |

TECHNIQUES AND NORMAL FINDINGS

5. Assess the Achilles tendon (ankle) reflex (S_1).
   - Flex the leg at the knee.
   - Dorsiflex the foot of the leg being examined.
   - Hold the foot lightly in the nondominant hand.
   - Strike the Achilles tendon with the flat end of the reflex hammer (see Figure 24.40).
   - Observe plantar flexion of the foot; the heel will "jump" from your hand.

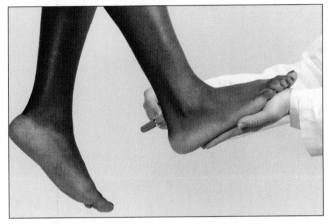

Figure 24.40A ● Testing the Achilles tendon reflex with client in a sitting position.

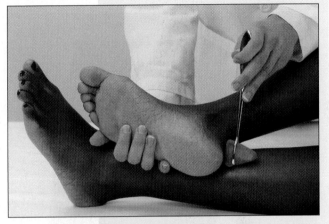

Figure 24.40B ● Testing the Achilles tendon reflex with client in a supine position.

6. Assess the plantar reflex (L_5, S_1).
   - Position the leg with a slight degree of external rotation at the hip.
   - Stimulate the sole of the foot from the heel to the ball of the foot on the lateral aspect. Continue the stimulation across the ball of the foot to the big toe.
   - Observe for plantar flexion, in which the toes curl toward the sole of the foot (see Figure 24.41). It may be necessary to hold the client's ankle to prevent movement.

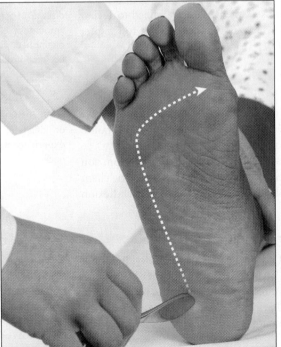

Figure 24.41 ●
Testing the plantar reflex.

ABNORMAL FINDINGS AND SPECIAL CONSIDERATIONS

▶ A **Babinski response** is the fanning of the toes with the great toe pointing toward the dorsum of the foot (see Figure 24.42). This is called dorsiflexion of the toe and is considered an abnormal response in the adult. It may indicate upper motor neuron disease.

A positive Babinski response is considered a normal response in the child until about 2 years of age.

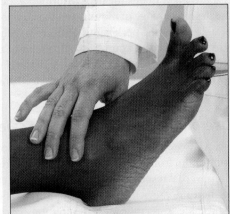

Figure 24.42 ● Babinski response.

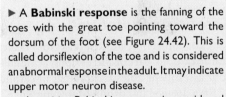

PHYSICAL ASSESSMENT

TECHNIQUES AND NORMAL FINDINGS	ABNORMAL FINDINGS AND SPECIAL CONSIDERATIONS

7. Assess the abdominal reflexes (T_8, T_9, T_{10} for upper and T_{10}, T_{11}, T_{12} for lower).

- Use an applicator or a tongue blade to briskly stroke the abdomen from the lateral aspect toward the umbilicus (see Figure 24.43).

- Observe muscular contraction and movement of the umbilicus toward the stimulus.

▶ Obesity and upper and lower motor neuron pathology can decrease or diminish the response.

- Repeat this procedure in the other three quadrants of the abdomen.

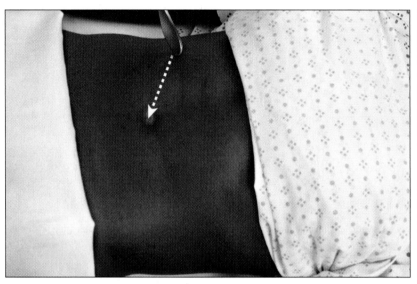

Figure 24.43 • Abdominal reflex testing pattern.

ADDITIONAL ASSESSMENT TECHNIQUES

Carotid Auscultation

Auscultation of the carotid arteries may be performed with the assessment of the head and neck or as part of the peripheral vascular assessment. You may need to review your assessment notes for findings of carotid artery auscultation. (Refer to Chapter 17 for a detailed discussion of this content. ⊂⊃)

▶ A bruit may be indicative of an obstructive disease process, such as atherosclerosis. The amount of blood flow to the brain may be diminished. This decrease in oxygen could be responsible for subtle changes in client responses.

Meningeal Assessment

Ask the client to flex the neck by bringing the chin down to touch the chest. Observe the degree of range of motion and the absence or presence of pain. The client should be able to flex the neck about 45 degrees without pain.

When the client complains of pain and has a decrease in the flexion motion, you will observe for *Brudzinski's sign.* With the client in a supine position, assist the client with neck flexion. Observe the legs. Brudzinski's sign is positive when neck flexion causes flexion of the legs and thighs.

▶ When the meningeal membranes are irritated or inflamed, as in meningitis, the client will experience **nuchal rigidity** or stiffness of the neck.

Use of the Glasgow Coma Scale

The *Glasgow Coma Scale* assesses the level of consciousness of the individual on a continuum from alertness to coma (see Figure 24.44). The scale tests three body functions: verbal response, motor response, and eye response. A maximum total score of 15 indicates the person is alert, responsive, and oriented. A total score of 3, the lowest achievable score, indicates a nonresponsive comatose individual.

▶ **Syncope** is a brief loss of consciousness and is usually sudden. **Coma** is a prolonged state of unconsciousness with possible altered responses to verbal and neuromuscular stimuli and pupillary reaction to light. A client experiencing any loss of consciousness needs immediate medical interventions.

PHYSICAL ASSESSMENT

TECHNIQUES AND NORMAL FINDINGS

ABNORMAL FINDINGS AND SPECIAL CONSIDERATIONS

GLASGOW COMA SCALE

BEST EYE-OPENING RESPONSE
4 = Spontaneously
3 = To speech
2 = To pain
1 = No response
(Record "C" if eyes closed by swelling)

BEST MOTOR RESPONSE to painful stimuli
6 = Obeys verbal command
5 = Localizes pain
4 = Flexion—withdrawal
3 = Flexion—abnormal
2 = Extension—abnormal
1 = No response
(Record best upper limb response)

BEST VERBAL RESPONSE
5 = Oriented × 3
4 = Conversation—confused
3 = Speech—inappropriate
2 = Sounds—incomprehensible
1 = No response
(Record "E" if endotracheal tube in place, "T" if tracheostomy tube in place)

Figure 24.44 ●
Glasgow Coma Scale.

▶ The Glasgow Coma Scale has limitations. For example, a client with an endotracheal tube or tracheostomy cannot communicate. As a result, the score is carried out according to each individual component of the scale. The verbal response score would then indicate intubation or tracheostomy. In addition, the motor response scale is invalid in a client with a spinal cord injury, and eye opening may be impossible to assess in those individuals with severe orbital injury.

SAMPLE DOCUMENTATION

Subjective: No history of headache, head injury, seizures, muscle weakness, change in senses, numbness or tingling, dizziness or vertigo, difficulty swallowing or difficulty speaking. No past history of neurological disease, hypertension, or diabetes. Nonsmoker, nondrinker, and has never used prescription or nonprescription drugs. Wears protective gear while participating in contact sports. No change in memory. Healthful diet.

Objective: Mental status:

Appropriate appearance, affect, mood, and responses to questions related to calculating problems, thinking abstractly and making judgments, oriented 3, long- and short-term memory intact.

Cranial nerves: I: No alteration in sense of smell

II: Snellen 20/20 both eyes. Rosenbaum 14/14 both eyes. Peripheral vision equal by confrontation

III, IV, and VI: EOM intact by six cardinal fields and symmetric corneal light reflex, PERRLA

V: TMJ: Full ROM, no pain or crepitus noted with movement. Muscle strength 5, sensation intact, corneal reflex present

VII: Full ROM with facial movement. No alteration in sense of taste

VIII: Weber, no lateralization, Rinne, AC > BC, whisper test, client able to correctly repeat spoken words

IX and XI: Gag reflex intact, uvula midline, no difficulty swallowing

X: Full ROM and strength in muscles

XII: Tongue midline, no tremors

Sensorimotor: Motor: No muscular atrophy and full strength against resistance. Smooth coordinated gait and no involuntary movements. Romberg negative, smooth movement with RAM.

Sensation: Sense of touch intact: light, sharp, and dull. Intact vibration, two-point discrimination and point location.

Stereognosis: Identified key and graphesthesia identified number.

Reflexes: Deep tendon reflexes 2+ and equal bilaterally, negative Babinski, contraction of abdominal muscle to stimuli.

PHYSICAL ASSESSMENT

APPLICATION THROUGH CRITICAL THINKING

CASE STUDY

Mr. John Phelps, age 65, is a Black male who comes to the community health clinic. He and his wife, Helen, recently celebrated their 40th wedding anniversary. He has a 35-year-old daughter, a 32-year-old son, and three grandchildren. Mr. Phelps retired 4 months ago from a busy accounting firm where he worked as a CPA for 25 years. He and his wife have been planning their retirement and are looking forward to travelling across the country to visit family.

Mr. Phelps's chief complaint is tremors that seem to be getting worse over the past few months. He noticed the tremors about 6 months ago and thought they were related to fatigue, since the office was very busy and he was working long hours. He anticipated that the tremors would stop after he retired and became rested. Mrs. Phelps indicates her husband's handwriting has become small and almost illegible and that she had to write several cheques for him last week. She also comments that her husband seems depressed about his recent retirement, since he has a "blank look" on his face and his speech is slow. Mari Chung, RN, conducts a health history and then proceeds with the physical assessment. She gathers the following objective and subjective data:

- Mood swings
- Tremors, movement of thumb and index finger in a circular fashion
- Shuffling gait, falls easily
- Constipation
- Fatigue
- Loss of 4.5 kg (10 lb.)
- Drooling
- Speaks in a monotone; voice slow, weak, and soft
- Rigidity during passive ROM
- Jerky movements
- Muscle pain and soreness
- Decrease in corneal response
- Posture not erect, forward flexion
- Unable to perform finger-to-nose test and rapid alternating movement
- Difficulty standing from sitting position without assistance

Ms. Chung consults with the clinic physician. After further evaluation, Mr. Phelps is admitted to the neurological unit of the community hospital with a diagnosis of Parkinson's disease.

▶ Complete Documentation

The following is sample documentation from health assessment of John Phelps.

SUBJECTIVE DATA: Complains of tremors, getting worse over 6 months. He has had "some mood changes, has lost weight, and is constipated frequently." He has occasional drooling. Experiences muscle pain and soreness. Requires assistance to get up from a chair and falls easily. Wife states writing increasingly illegible. She reports he has become depressed, has a "blank" look, and has slow speech.

OBJECTIVE DATA: Posture not erect—forward flexion, shuffling gait, jerky movements. Voice monotone, slow, weak, soft. Decreased corneal response. Rigidity during passive range of motion (ROM). Unable to perform finger-to-nose and rapid alternating movement tests. Drooling. Weight loss 4.5 kg (10 lb.) since last exam.

▶ Critical Thinking Questions

1. What data were considered in the medical diagnosis of Parkinson's disease?
2. What additional data would be required to confirm a diagnosis of Parkinson's disease?
3. What are the nursing considerations for Mr. Phelps?

▶ Applying Nursing Diagnoses

1. Use the NANDA-I taxonomy (see Appendix A ⬭) to develop two nursing diagnoses from the data provided.
2. *Falls, risk for* and *self-esteem, risk for situational loss* are included as nursing diagnoses in the NANDA-I taxonomy. Do the data in the case study support these nursing diagnoses? Explain your answer.

▶ Prepare Teaching Plan

LEARNING NEED: The data in the case study revealed that Mr. Phelps has symptoms of Parkinson's disease. His symptoms include tremors, weight loss, fatigue, constipation, falling, and others. He was admitted to the hospital and will begin treatment for his problem. He and his wife will require education about the disease and his care on discharge.

The case study provides data that are representative of risks, symptoms, and behaviours of many individuals. Therefore, the following teaching plan is based on the need to provide information to members of any community about Parkinson's disease.

GOAL: The participants in this learning program will have increased knowledge about Parkinson's disease and its management.

OBJECTIVES: At the completion of this learning session, the participants will be able to do the following:

1. Describe Parkinson's disease.
2. Identify risk factors associated with Parkinson's disease.
3. List the symptoms of Parkinson's disease.
4. Discuss strategies in management of Parkinson's disease.

ASSESSMENT FORM

History:		No	Yes	Describe
	Tremors		X	*6 mos. worsening*
	Mood change		X	*"Depression"*
	Pain		X	*Muscle pain*
	Stiffness		X	*Extremities*
	Speech (change)		X	*Slow, weak*
Describe:	Facial Expression	*"Blank"*		
	ADL	*"Needs assistance to get up from chair"*		
Other:	Constipation			
	Weight loss			
	Falls easily			
Physical Findings:		Yes	No	Describe
	Posture (erect)		X	*Forward flexion*
	Gait (smooth)		X	*Shuffling*
	Movement (smooth/coordinated)		X	*Jerky—finger-nose, rapid alt. movement*
	CN (intact)		X	*Decreased corneal reflex*

Application of Objective 4: Discuss strategies in management of Parkinson's disease.

Content

- Medication is used to manage problems with tremor and movement.
- Surgery may improve movement.
- Deep brain stimulation refers to implantation of a device to reduce trembling.
- Self-care includes a healthful diet. Fibre reduces problems with constipation. Including folate in the diet or as a supplement may protect against Parkinson's disease. Eating and swallowing carefully reduces risk of choking.
- Regular exercise improves mobility, balance, range of motion, and emotional well-being.
- Reduce the risk of injury from falls by making the home environment safe (no throw rugs; install handrails and grab bars).
- Seek assistance from physical and occupational therapists for guidelines to improve ease of ambulation and carrying out daily tasks.
- Communication requires speaking louder than believed necessary. Practise reading aloud. Seek assistance from a speech pathologist.

Teaching Strategy and Rationale

- Lecture
- Discussion
- Audiovisual materials
- Printed materials

Lecture is appropriate when disseminating information to large groups.

Discussion allows participants to bring up concerns and to raise questions.

Audiovisual materials, such as illustrations, reinforce verbal presentation.

Printed materials, especially to be taken away with learners, allow review, reinforcement, and reading at the learner's pace.

Evaluation

- Written examination.

May use short answer, fill-in, or multiple-choice items, or a combination of items.

If these are short and easy to evaluate, the learner receives immediate feedback.

Health Promotion Assessment Tool

Social Determinants of Action	Level of Action	Action Strategies
Social support networks	Individual and family	**Create supportive environments** • Assess the personal support networks for both Mr. and Mrs. Phelps. Work with them to determine how to mobilize their supports in an optimal way. Examples include sharing the diagnosis with family and significant others; discussing their upcoming travel plans to see family and suggesting alternate options such as having their family travel to see them instead. What were their retirement plans, and how could these be modified to retain as much that is meaningful to the couple as possible? • In this situation, the wife is the primary support for her husband so it is important to assess her knowledge of Parkinson's disease, including the signs and symptoms, illness trajectory, prognosis, and her capacity to support and care for her husband. It is just as important to anticipate that Mrs. Phelps may need breaks from caregiving; engage in a discussion with her about possibilities for respite care to give her breaks. • Assess the couple's knowledge of community supports; educate them on support available; assist in making the necessary referrals to services such as home care or caregiver support groups and Parkinson Society Canada (http://www.parkinson.ca).
Personal coping skills and physical environment	Individual	**Create supportive environments** • Develop a safe and accommodating environment that supports Mr. Phelps's mobility and independence. • Assess for feasible environmental changes that would allow him to continue to participate in society in a meaningful way and to remain engaged with family, friends, and his life interests. • Plan an occupational therapy and falls prevention assessment through a home care referral. Falls prevention interventions could include the installation of railings in the home, grab bars in the shower, an elevated toilet seat, and the removal of hazards like area rugs.

Abnormal Findings

Problems commonly associated with the neurological system include changes in motor function, including gait and movement, seizures, spinal cord injury, infections, degenerative disorders, and cranial nerve dysfunction. These conditions are described below and in Tables 24.3 and 24.4.

TABLE 24.3	Problems with Motor Function
GAIT	**MOVEMENT**
Ataxic gait: A walk characterized by a wide base, uneven steps, feet slapping, and a tendency to sway. This type of walk is associated with posterior column disease or decreased proprioception regarding extremities. Seen in multiple sclerosis and drug or alcohol intoxication.	*Fasciculation:* Commonly called a twitch, this is an involuntary, local, visible muscular contraction. It is not significant when it occurs in tired muscles. It can be associated with motor neuron disease.
Scissors gait: A walk characterized by spastic lower limbs and movement in a stiff, jerky manner. The knees come together; the legs cross in front of one another; and the legs are abducted as the individual takes short, progressive, slow steps. This is seen in individuals with multiple sclerosis.	*Tic:* Commonly called a *habit,* a tic is usually psychogenic in nature. The involuntary spasmodic movement of the muscle is seen in a muscle under voluntary control, usually in the face, neck, or shoulders.
Steppage gait: Sometimes called the "foot drop" walk. The individual flexes and raises the knee to a higher-than-usual level yielding a flopping of the foot when walking. This usually is indicative of lower motor neuron disease. Seen in individuals with alcoholic neuritis and progressive muscular atrophy.	*Tremor:* A rhythmic or alternating involuntary movement from the contraction of opposing muscle groups. Tremors vary in degree and are seen in Parkinson's disease, multiple sclerosis, uremia (a form of kidney failure), and alcohol intoxication.
Festination gait: Referred to as the "Parkinson's walk." The individual has stooped posture, takes short steps, and turns stiffly. There is a slow start to the walk and frequent, accelerated steps. This gait is associated with basal ganglia disease.	*Athetoid movement:* A continuous, involuntary, repetitive, slow, "wormlike," arrhythmic muscular movement. The muscles are in a state of hypotoxicity, producing a distortion to the limb. This movement is seen in cerebral palsy.
Dystonia: Similar to athetoid movements, dystonia involves larger muscle groups. The twisting movements yield a tortuous change in the individual's posture. Torticollis, or wryneck, is an example of dystonia.	*Myoclonus:* A continual, rapid, short spasm involving a muscle, part of a muscle, or even a group of muscles. Frequently occurs in an extremity as the individual is falling asleep. Myoclonus is also seen in seizure disorders.

TABLE 24.4	Problems Associated with Dysfunction of Cranial Nerves
CRANIAL NERVE	**DYSFUNCTION**
I Olfactory	Unilateral or bilateral anosmia
II Optic	Optic atrophy, papilledema, amblyopia, field defects
III Oculomotor	Diplopia, ptosis of lid, dilated pupil, inability to focus on close objects
IV Trochlear	Convergent strabismus, diplopia
V Trigeminal	Tic douloureux, loss of facial sensation, decreased ability to chew, loss of corneal reflex, decreased blinking
VI Abducens	Diplopia, strabismus
VII Facial	Bell's palsy, decreased ability to distinguish tastes
VIII Vestibulocochlear	Tinnitus, vertigo, deafness
IX Glossopharyngeal	Loss of gag reflex, loss of taste, difficulty swallowing
X Vagus	Loss of voice, impaired voice, difficulty swallowing
XI Accessory	Difficulty with shrugging of shoulders, inability to turn head to left and right
XII Hypoglossal	Difficulty with speech and swallowing, inability to protrude tongue

Seizures

Seizures are sudden, rapid, and excessive discharges of electrical energy in the brain. They are usually centred in the cerebral cortex. Some seizure disorders stem from neurological problems that occur before or during birth, or they can develop secondary to childhood fevers. In children and adults, seizures can result from a variety of factors including trauma, infections, cerebrovascular disease, environmental toxins, drug overdose, and withdrawal from alcohol, sedatives, or antidepressants. *Epilepsy* is a chronic seizure disorder.

Spinal Cord Injuries

The spinal cord extends from the medulla oblongata of the brain stem. As it continues down the back, the cervical, thoracic, and lumbar vertebrae protect it. Spinal cord injuries result from trauma to the vertebrae, which causes dislocation fractures that in turn compress or transect the spinal cord. The most common causes of this type of trauma are automobile and motorcycle accidents; sports accidents, such as football and diving accidents; and penetrating injuries, such as stab wounds and gunshots. Generally, the higher level of the injury, the greater the loss of neurological function. Injuries to the cervical region are the most common and the most devastating.

Infections of the Neurological System

Infections of the neurological system include meningitis, myelitis, brain abscess, and Lyme disease. Each will be described in the sections that follow.

Meningitis

Meningitis is caused by a virus or bacteria that infects the coverings, or meninges, of the brain or spinal cord. Meningitis may result from a penetrating wound, fractured skull, or upper respiratory infection, or it may occur secondary to facial or cranial surgery.

In some cases, meningitis may spread to the underlying brain tissues, causing encephalitis. *Encephalitis* is defined as an inflammation of the tissue of the brain. It usually results from a virus, which may be transmitted by ticks or mosquitoes, or it may result from a childhood illness, such as chickenpox or the measles.

Myelitis

Myelitis is an inflammation of the spinal cord. Poliomyelitis and herpes zoster infection are two common causes. It may develop after an infection, such as measles or gonorrhea, or it may follow vaccination for rabies.

Brain Abscess

A *brain abscess* is usually the result of a systemic infection. It is marked by an accumulation of pus in the brain cells. Most brain abscesses develop secondary to a primary infection. Others result from skull fractures or penetrating injuries, such as a gunshot wound.

Lyme Disease

Lyme disease is an infection caused by a spirochete transmitted by a bite from an infected tick that lives on deer. Its major symptoms are arthritis, a flulike syndrome, and a rash. If untreated, Lyme disease may cause severe neurological disorders.

Degenerative Neurological Disorders

Degenerative neurological disorders include Alzheimer's disease, amyotrophic lateral sclerosis, Huntington's disease, multiple sclerosis, myasthenia gravis, and Parkinson's disease. These will be discussed in the paragraphs that follow.

Alzheimer's Disease

Alzheimer's disease is a progressive degenerative disease of the brain that leads to dementia. Although it is more common in people over age 65, its onset may occur as early as middle adulthood. Symptoms include a loss of memory, particularly of recent events, shortened attention span, confusion, and disorientation. Eventually, the client with Alzheimer's disease may experience paranoid fantasies and hallucinations.

Amyotrophic Lateral Sclerosis

Amyotrophic lateral sclerosis, commonly known as Lou Gehrig's disease, is a chronic degenerative disease involving the cerebral cortex and the motor neurons in the spinal cord. The result is a progressive wasting of skeletal muscles that eventually leads to death. Although the cause is unknown, research has implicated viral infection.

Huntington's Disease

Huntington's disease is an inherited disorder characterized by uncontrollable jerking movements, called *chorea,* which literally means "dance." It typically progresses to mental deterioration and ultimately death. Symptoms usually first appear in early middle age; thus, those with Huntington's disease often have had children before they know they have the disorder.

ABNORMAL FINDINGS

Multiple Sclerosis

Multiple sclerosis is the deterioration of the protective sheaths, composed of myelin, of the nerve tracts in the brain and spinal cord. The first attack usually occurs between the ages of 20 and 40. Early symptoms include temporary tingling, numbness, or weakness that may affect only one limb or one side of the body. Other symptoms include unsteadiness, blurred vision, slurred speech, and difficulty in urinating. Some individuals experience repeated attacks that progress in severity. In these individuals, permanent disability with progressive neuromuscular deficits develops.

Myasthenia Gravis

Myasthenia gravis is a chronic neuromuscular disorder involving increasing weakness of voluntary muscles with activity, and some abatement of symptoms with rest. Onset is gradual and usually occurs in adolescence or young adulthood. The precise etiology is unknown, but it is believed that myasthenia gravis is an *autoimmune* disorder, that is, the individual's immune system attacks the individual's own normal cells rather than foreign pathogens. Some of the most common symptoms include ptosis (drooping eyelids), diplopia (double vision), a flat affect, and a weak, monotone voice.

Parkinson's Disease

Parkinson's disease is a degeneration of the basal nuclei of the brain, which are collections of nerve cell bodies deep within the white matter of the cerebrum. These nuclei are responsible for initiating and stopping voluntary movement. Parkinson's disease is characterized by slow movements, continuous "pill-rolling" tremor of the forefinger and thumb, rhythmic shaking of the hands, bobbing of the head, and difficulty in initiating movement. The individual may have a masklike facial expression, difficulty in speaking clearly, and difficulty maintaining balance while walking. Although the precise etiology is unknown, research indicates that environmental toxins, such as carbon monoxide or certain metals, may cause some cases of Parkinson's disease. It may also result from previous encephalitis.

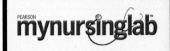

ABNORMAL FINDINGS

25

ASSESSMENT OF INFANTS, CHILDREN, AND ADOLESCENTS

Canadian Contributor: Deborah Askin, University of Manitoba

CHAPTER OBJECTIVES

On completion of this chapter, you will be able to

1. Relate knowledge of anatomy and physiology to the physical examination of infants, children, and adolescents.

2. Identify anatomical differences between children and adults, and identify landmarks that guide assessment of infants and children.

3. Explain client preparation for assessment of infants, children, and adolescents.

4. Perform an age-appropriate and comprehensive health history and physical assessment of a child.

5. Relate knowledge of the principles of communication to the health history interview.

6. Differentiate between normal and abnormal findings in pediatric physical assessment.

7. Incorporate the physical, cognitive, and emotional development of children into comprehensive health and physical assessment.

8. Apply critical thinking in selected situations related to pediatric physical assessment.

9. Document findings of the pediatric physical assessment by using appropriate terminology.

CHAPTER OUTLINE

THE PREVIOUS CHAPTERS IN THIS BOOK INCLUDE TECHNIQUES USED to elicit health histories and perform physical assessment of adult clients. Much of the information from previous chapters is appropriate for pediatric clients. However, children are not little adults, and significant differences exist between infants, children, adolescents, and adults. These differences include variations in physiology, development, and cognition that must be incorporated into the nursing assessment. This chapter uses the word *parent* to represent parents, caregivers, or guardians.

The head-to-toe approach to physical assessment is useful in many situations and with different types of clients, but it may not work with young children. Adults and adolescents will usually sit on an examination table, wear a paper gown, and follow the nurse's instructions. However, infants and toddlers often refuse to sit still or cooperate.

Young children do not have the cognitive or verbal ability to describe symptoms or comply with complex instructions. Nurses must possess strong assessment skills to overcome the communication and situational challenges involved in pediatric physical assessment. This chapter focuses on the health history questions, physical assessment and examination techniques, and developmental information necessary to obtain an accurate and comprehensive health status assessment of infants, children, and adolescents.

CHILDHOOD DEVELOPMENTAL STAGES

Babies are not born with the ability to walk, talk, and independently care for themselves. Just as the brain is not fully mature at birth, all the major organ systems are immature and develop throughout childhood. The most dramatic development changes occur primarily in infancy and adolescence, although each stage of childhood is marked by unique changes. Knowledge of the normal physical, psychological, and cognitive development of children is essential. It may be helpful to review the material in Chapter 3. ⚭

Newborns are children between birth and 1 month of age. **Infants** are children between 1 and 12 months of age. Infancy is characterized by dramatic changes in height and weight, and the development of gross physical and social skills. Young children have **cephalocaudal** physical growth. That is, their development progresses in a head-to-toe fashion. Development and growth begin proximally before developing distally. For example, fine motor skills follow gross motor skills, and the ability to grasp precedes the ability to stand or walk. **Toddlers** are children who are at least 1 year old but who have not yet reached 3 years of age. Toddlerhood is marked by slower, steadier growth, fine motor skill improvement, and language development. **Preschoolers** are children between 3 and 5 years of age. The preschool years are characterized by motor and language skill refinement and beginning social skill development. **School-age** children are between 6 and 10 years old. The major developmental tasks of school-age children involve cognitive and social growth. **Adolescence** is characterized by periods of rapid growth, sexual maturation, and cognitive refinement. Adolescence is the period between 11 and 21 years of age.

NUTRITIONAL ASSESSMENT

Nutrition is an important factor contributing to the health and well-being of children. A thorough nutritional assessment is important to identify those infants and children at risk for malnutrition and obesity, as well as those at risk from potentially harmful feeding practices. When assessing children, it may be helpful to conduct the nutrition history portion before the physical assessment to establish rapport and make the child more comfortable with the process. Rapport is essential, especially when assessing an adolescent. Infants and younger children need a parent present to assist with the assessment and to answer questions. Adolescents may be more comfortable having privacy during the assessment. It is best to discuss the assessment arrangement with the adolescent and parent separately to allow the adolescent to give an unpressured answer. A caregiver can be interviewed separately if appropriate. When there are known existing nutritional issues, such as disordered eating or obesity, the nurse should be sensitive to the needs of the child and parent. Both must feel their respective needs to provide information are met.

Nutritional History

A diet recall, food frequency, and food diary can all remain appropriate tools when assessing dietary intake in children. School-age children and children in daycare should be assessed for food habits on at-home days and on days away from home. Differences in intake may also exist for weekend days for the child who is not in school or daycare full-time. Children who participate in many outside activities may have varying nutritional habits throughout the week with missed meals, meals on the run, or frequent take-out meals contrasting with more regular eating patterns on other days. The nurse should inquire about the child's schedule and activities to determine the extent of variation and need for additional data. Box 25.1 outlines specific data to gather for infants, children, and adolescents during the nutritional history and health history.

Physical Assessment

The parameters of the physical assessment in children primarily are the same anthropometric measurements and clinical observations as in the adult, with references and standards that are unique to age. Growth rate during the first year of life is most rapid compared with later childhood and adolescence. Developmental milestones have important nutrition implications throughout childhood and should become part of a complete assessment.

Anthropometric Measurements

Assessing the growth of an infant or a child is the most useful measure of nutritional status and of health, yet it is an area that is often overlooked or done improperly. Anthropometric measurements in children should be obtained by using equipment appropriate for the pediatric population. Recumbent length and weight measurements are needed in the infant and young child. Weight should be measured wearing only a clean, dry diaper. Older children can have standing height and weight measured as described. Children with musculoskeletal

---

BOX 25.1	Nutritional History Data for Assessment of Infants, Children, and Adolescents

The nurse should gather the following data for infants, children, and adolescents during the nutritional history and health history:

Breastfed baby
- Number and lengths of feedings
- Number of wet diapers
- Supplemental vitamin D at hospital discharge and additional vitamin D for infants from Northern Canada
- Iron source by 6 months
- Vitamin C source concomitant with iron for improved absorption
- Vegan mother: assess for her vitamin B_{12} source

Bottle-fed baby
- Type and amount of formula
- Iron source by 6 months (formula or fortified cereal)
- Vitamin C source concomitant with iron for improved absorption

Assess for intake of solids at age 4 to 6 months and thereafter. Note type, amount, intolerances, or allergies.

Assess for effect of any medical condition on diet: feeding difficulties, therapeutic diet, food or nutrient as medication interactions, altered nutrient needs.

Assess nutrition knowledge and beliefs of the parent, including religious and cultural influences.

Assess whether feeding skills are appropriate to the child's developmental stage. Note delays. Note whether food texture is appropriate for development (chewing and swallowing abilities, self-feeding, sitting upright).

Assess for feeding practices that are not recommended:
- Sleeping with a bottle (assess for baby-bottle tooth decay)
- Solids before age 4 to 6 months or not after 7 to 9 months
- Solids added to formula in a bottle
- Cow's milk before age 1
- Honey before age 1 (botulism risk)
- Fat restriction
- Inappropriately textured foods for developmental stage
- Foods likely to cause choking: hot dogs, grapes, nuts, whole raw vegetables (e.g., carrots), gum, hard candy, chunks of unpeeled fruit
- Supplements not prescribed by healthcare provider

- Use of food for punishment or reward
- Self-prescribed diet or restrictive eating habits (especially in adolescents)

CLINICAL TIP

It is recommended that children limit intake of unsweetened juice to 125 mL (4 fl.oz.) per day. Excess intake of juice is associated with obesity.

Assess for appropriate feeding practices:
- All meals and snacks: portion, preparation method
- Meal and snack pattern: frequency, number, missed meals
- Liquid intake: volume, type, presence of caffeine or alcohol intake, sugary drinks
- Food intolerances or allergies
- Therapeutic diet
- Use of supplements: type, dose, frequency

CLINICAL TIP

Adolescents may choose to follow a vegetarian diet for a number of reasons. Ask about this. Although religious, ethical, and health beliefs are often cited, many adolescents choose a vegetarian diet to mask attempts at weight loss or disordered eating.

- Family, child, and caregiver beliefs and knowledge about food, including cultural or religious influences
- Body satisfaction (older children and adolescents). Ask: "What do you think about your body or body weight? Have you ever tried to gain or lose weight? Tell me what you tried."
- Activity level. Note amount and type. Assess adequacy of intake for active children. Include assessment of daily "screen time" (time spent watching television, playing computer games, using the computer).

CLINICAL TIP

Increased screen time is associated with incidence of overweight and obesity in children.

disorders and contractures can have knee height measured. Skinfold measurements should be done by using calipers calibrated to 1 mm since small changes in measurement can cause changes in assessment classification. The World Health Organization (WHO) recommends weight for height as the standard in measuring children since skinfold and circumference measurements are prone to errors that could result in misclassification of nutritional health.

Head circumference is a measurement unique to assessing growth in children at or under 2 years of age. Beyond age 2, head circumference is not a valid tool to assess growth and nutritional status. Body mass index (BMI) for age should be used to screen all children over the age of 2 years to identify children at risk for obesity.

Anthropometric measurements have age-specific references and a number of organizations have published pediatric growth charts. Canada does not have a national system for collecting pediatric growth data. The Dietitians of Canada, Canadian Paediatric Society, College of Family Physicians of Canada, and Community Health Nurses Association of Canada (2010) have jointly recommended that Canadian healthcare providers use the World Health Organization's 2006 Child Growth Standards (birth to 5 years) and the 2007 WHO Growth Reference (5 to 19 years) to assess the growth of children. In children under 20 years of age, references are described by using charts with age-specific percentiles for height, weight, BMI, and, for children under 36 months, head circumference. **Percentiles** are used to assess growth rate and health of weight for height. Percentile charts are derived from the distribution of data from population studies and are age- and gender-specific descriptions of anthropometric measurements. Newer infant growth charts are more representative of the population-matched prevalence of breastfed infants compared with charts published before 2000. Breastfed infants normally grow at a slightly slower rate than formula-fed babies do. Infants, children, and adolescents can be compared with their age-matched peers to determine their individual percentile within the population. A best use of percentile charts is in monitoring individual growth over time. Normally, children will remain within a narrow percentile range for each measurement over the course of childhood. For example, a child assessed sequentially in the 25th percentile for height (length) for age may have a small frame and parents with small stature and may not be at risk for poor nutritional health. A child sequentially in the 50th percentile for height for age who drops to the 25th percentile may be at risk for undernutrition. A significant drop or increase in percentile category is cause for further investigation to assess for undernutrition or overnutrition. Overweight and obesity in children are defined as BMI for age greater than the 85th percentile and the 95th percentile, respectively. Undernutrition is defined as BMI for age less than the 5th percentile. Separate growth references are used for children with some chronic diseases and for knee-height estimates of stature.

Clinical Examination

Clinical signs of possible poor nutritional health include those in Table 9.5, as well as some unique findings. Certain diseases and conditions, such as HIV infection, congenital heart disease, or premature birth, can predispose children to nutritional risk. During the clinical exam, the nurse should be mindful of the potential negative influences of existing medical issues on nutritional health. Undernutrition can occur because of insufficient intake, increased nutrient losses, or increased nutritional needs that are not met. Insufficient intake can occur for a variety of reasons. Feeding difficulties, as with cleft palate, food intolerances, and food insecurity, are among the many contributors to poor intake. Nutrient losses can occur with malabsorptive conditions and drug-nutrient interactions. Unmatched increased nutritional needs, such as with chronic fever, fracture, or wound healing, will lead to undernutrition.

Bottle-fed children should be assessed for signs of baby-bottle tooth decay (see Figure 25.1). Caries can result from the inappropriate practice of putting children to sleep with a bottle containing milk or juice.

Insufficient vitamin D status from lack of intake or little exposure to sunlight can lead to changes in bone formation that affect a growing child. Rickets, rachitic rosary, pigeon-breast formation of the rib cage, and widened bone epiphyses can occur. Breastfed infants require daily supplemental vitamin D until their diet provides adequate amounts of vitamin D or until 1 year of age (Canadian Paediatric Society, 2005). Because of the climate, infants living in Northern Canada are at particular risk of developing vitamin D deficiency. Additional supplementation is recommended for this population. Signs and symptoms consistent with disordered eating should also be included in the assessment of older children and adolescents. Box 25.2 outlines clinical findings of disordered eating.

An assessment of development in younger children and pubertal status in older children can be included in a nutritional assessment. Poor nutritional health can negatively affect sexual maturation, growth, and muscle development in the adolescent. A determination of sexual maturity can be included in the assessment, as discussed on page 694.

Feeding skills coincide with developmental skills and determine the type of foods a young child can handle. Foods included in the diet should be developmentally appropriate. Introduction of solid foods into the diet should not occur until age 4 to 6 months, when an infant can sit with support

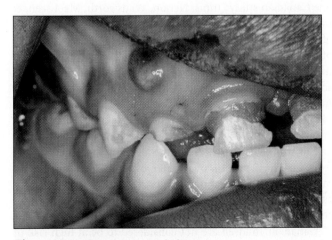

Figure 25.1 ● Baby-bottle tooth decay.

BOX 25.2	Clinical Findings Consistent with Eating Disorders

The following signs and symptoms are associated with disordered eating.

Bulimia or Binge-Purge Behaviour
- Bloodshot eyes
- Broken blood vessels on the face
- Swollen parotid glands or "chipmunk cheeks"
- Dental erosion
- Hoarse voice
- Scarring on the dorsal surface of the hand from teeth during purge attempts
- Poor or lacking gag reflex
- Weight fluctuations

Anorexia or Restrictive Eating Behaviour
- Cold intolerance
- Lanugo, soft white hair growth on body
- Pedal edema
- Dry skin
- Alopecia
- Bradycardia
- Hypotension
- Amenorrhea in nonpregnant postmenarcheal females
- Loss of strength and muscle tone

General Eating Disorder Findings
- Body dissatisfaction. Ask: "How do you feel about your weight?" followed by "Have you ever tried to gain or lose weight? Tell me what you did."
- Constipation
- Bloating
- Fatigue

and transfer food to the rear of the mouth for swallowing. As the ability to chew improves around age 9 to 12 months, more texture-appropriate foods can be introduced. Solids introduced too soon can result in aspiration. Delays in development may affect nutritional health if diet is not carefully monitored. Developmental milestones that affect nutritional health are discussed on page 697.

Laboratory Measurements

The nutritional components of a laboratory assessment in children are the same as described for the general population. In one Canadian study (Innis, Nelson, Wadsworth, MacLaren, & Lwanga, 1997), iron deficiency anemia was found in up to 7% of otherwise healthy 9-month-old infants. Decreased intake of iron-rich foods and increased needs during growth contribute to the prevalence of anemia. Adolescent males require additional iron as muscle mass and blood volume increase. Adolescent females require additional iron to compensate for menstrual losses. Infants living in First Nations communities are at increased risk of iron deficiency anemia. Routine screening for iron deficiency is recommended for Aboriginal infants from age 6 to 12 months of age. Hemoglobin screening in other infants should be based on an assessment of risk factors, such as premature birth, chronic illness, excessive consumption of cow's milk, or inadequate dietary intake of iron.

Canadian children are not considered to be at high risk of developing lead poisoning; however, screening for lead should be considered in children with a history of exposure to lead-based paint (used before 1978), lead solder (used in water pipes before 1986), or pottery from countries that use lead-based glazes or paints. Infants exposed to low levels of lead are usually asymptomatic but can develop brain damage. Signs of severe lead poisoning include abdominal pain, headaches, vomiting, confusion, muscle weakness, and seizures.

Immunization History

National immunization recommendations are set forth by the Public Health Agency of Canada (2007) (see Chapter 3 for the full immunization schedules ⬭) but jurisdictional variations exist. Provincial and territorial immunization schedules are published by the Department of Health in each province and territory. Routine childhood immunizations are strongly recommended but, in most provinces and territories, they are not required. It is therefore important to determine the immunization status of each child. Parents may report that their child's immunizations are up-to-date, but the parents may not be aware of all the potential vaccinations available. A thorough immunization history will confirm whether or not the child has received all of the recommended immunizations.

Vital Signs

Accurate heart rates and respiratory rates must be taken for 1 minute. The nurse takes an apical pulse for children under 1 year of age. Infants have irregular breathing patterns characterized by frequent, brief rate accelerations or decelerations. This is a normal variant that disappears during the first few months of life. Blood pressure accuracy depends on the selection of an appropriate sized cuff. Blood pressure cuffs must be wide enough to cover at least 80% of the upper arm (from the acromion process to the olecranon process). The length of the blood pressure cuff should be large enough so that half of the circumference of the arm does not exceed 40% of the cuff's length, as shown in Figure 25.2. If the cuff is too narrow, the reading will be falsely high. If the cuff is too wide, it will be falsely low. Blood pressure readings should be done with the child's arm supported at the heart level. The diastolic pressure is recorded as the point when the Korotkoff sounds disappear. See Table 25.1 for a listing of the normal childhood vital signs.

PHYSICAL VARIANTS IN CHILDHOOD

Children are physically different from adults. The following sections include discussion of common physical variants in childhood.

Integument

The skin is one of the last systems to develop in utero. Infants have less developed corneum stratum and a thinner epidermis than older children and adults. As a result, infants and newborns are more prone to heat and water loss from skin evaporation, and cold stress from radiant heat loss. The

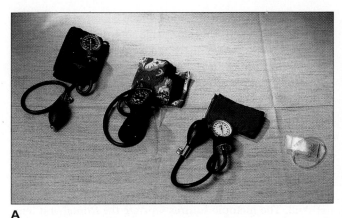

A

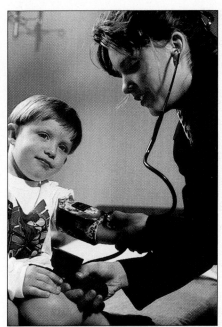

B

Figure 25.2 ● A. Blood pressure cuffs are available in various types and sizes for infants and children. B. Measuring blood pressure with an aneroid manometer.

TABLE 25.1	Normal Childhood Vital Signs		
AGE	**HEART RATE (BEATS PER MIN)**	**RESPIRATORY RATE (BREATHS PER MIN)**	**BLOOD PRESSURE RANGE (95TH PERCENTILE)**
Newborn	90–160	30–50	(60–90)/(40–60)
1–11 months	85–170	24–45	(94–104)/(50–60)
1–2 years	70–150	22–38	(98–109)/(56–63)
3–5 years	72–140	21–30	(100–115)/(59–71)
6–10 years	68–130	18–24	(105–123)/(67–80)
11–14 years	65–120	14–20	(110–131)/(64–84)
15+ years	55–100	14–20	(113–130)/(50–84)

thinner epidermis allows for increased transdermal absorption of substances and medications placed on the skin. It is essential to use special caution with topical medications and preparations in infants under 6 months of age because of the potential for systemic absorption. The sebaceous glands do not begin to function until around the first birthday, causing infants to be at greater risk for heat intolerance. The apocrine sweat glands and sebaceous glands do not fully function until puberty.

Milia are tiny (less than 0.5 mm), smooth, white cysts of the hair follicle, as depicted in Figure 11.3. They are often present at birth and are common on the forehead and nose. Milia on the palate are called Epstein's pearls. Milia are normal infant variations. **Lanugo** is a covering of fine hair in newborns that is most prominent on the upper chest, shoulders, and back. Lanugo disappears within the first few weeks of life. Premature infants generally have more lanugo than full-term infants. **Salmon patches,** also known as stork bites, are small macules and patches caused by visible intradermal capillaries. This normal variant occurs in 30% to 50% of newborns. The most common locations for salmon patches are the forehead, the eyelids, the upper lip, the nasal bridge, and the nape of the neck. Anything that causes the skin to flush, such as fever or crying, will cause these lesions to be more noticeable.

Salmon patches spontaneously resolve during infancy in all but a few children. **Mongolian spots** are areas of dark-bluish pigmentation that are common in Aboriginal, Black, Asian, and Hispanic children (refer to Figure 11.4). These benign patches are caused by increased concentrations of melanocytes and can be found anywhere on the body, but are most common at the base of the spine. Mongolian spots are darkest in the newborn period, and they fade during the first 2 years of life. **Acrocyanosis** is a commonly seen, normal finding in newborns and infants. During times of stress, especially exposure to cold environments, the hands and feet appear cyanotic; it is often accompanied by increased mottling of the distal arms and legs. Nurses must distinguish this benign condition from true cyanosis that is accompanied by a bluing of the tongue and oral mucous membranes. **Vernix caseosa** is a cheeselike white substance that coats the skin surfaces at birth. Vernix consists of a combination of epithelium cells and sebum. It is generally more pronounced in term and postterm infants. The integumentary assessment of older children and adolescents is similar to that of adults.

Morbilliform, or "measleslike," rashes consist of erythematous, confluent macules and papules. Morbilliform rashes are caused by viruses and occur most often in toddlers and pre-

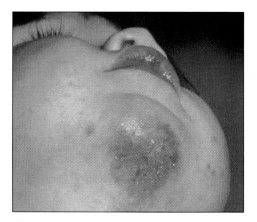

Figure 25.3 • Chronic eczema.

schoolers. Atopic dermatitis, also know as **eczema,** is a chronic skin disorder characterized by intense itching, patches, erythema, and papules that typically begins in the first year of life, as depicted in Figure 25.3. Infantile eczema is common on the face, the neck, the popliteal space, and the antecubital space. By the school-age years, eczema presents with the same distribution noted in adults. The hair should be examined for texture and distribution. Some syndromes, such as Cornelia de Lange, are associated with abnormal hair distribution and such findings as one continuous eyebrow. The nails are examined for texture and strength. Brittle or striated nails may be a sign of nutritional deficiencies, infections, or diseases, such as psoriasis.

Head and Neck

The bones of the cranium are not fused at birth. The infant's skull has openings, called fontanelles and sutures, which protect the brain during birth and allow for skull and brain growth during infancy. The **posterior fontanelle** is located in the superior occiput and may not be palpable at birth. It is usually 1 to 2 cm (0.5 to 1 in.) in diameter and closes by 2 months of age. The **anterior fontanelle** is a 2 to 4 cm (1 to 1.5 in.) diamond-shaped opening, also known as a "soft spot," located at the top of the skull.

The skin covering the anterior fontanelle should be even with the skull surface. The anterior fontanelle normally closes between 9 and 18 months of age. Children with premature or delayed fontanelle closure require further evaluation and assessment.

The **cranial sutures** are palpable gaps between the bones of the skull. The **metopic sutures** separate the frontal and temporal bones. The **lambdoidal sutures** separate the temporal and occipital bones. The **sagittal suture** lies in the middle of the skull and crosses the anterior and posterior fontanelles, as illustrated in Figure 25.4. **Craniosynostosis** is a condition that results in cranial deformity caused by premature fusion of the cranial bones. In craniosynostosis, the skull appears flattened as a body ridge develops along the suture lines (see Figure 12.17). If untreated, this disorder results in impaired brain growth and cognitive impairment. The nurse should promptly refer any child with suspected craniosynostosis for further evaluation and treatment.

The head is the largest body surface area in infants. Heat loss and cold stress can result from leaving a newborn's head uncovered in cool environments. The head remains disproportionately large in comparison to the body until approximately 5 years of age. As a result, young children are top heavy and prone to minor head injury from falls.

Newborns who are large for gestational age, those born vaginally, and those with birth histories of cephalopelvic disproportion or prolonged or difficult labours often have misshapen skulls from trauma or compression during labour and

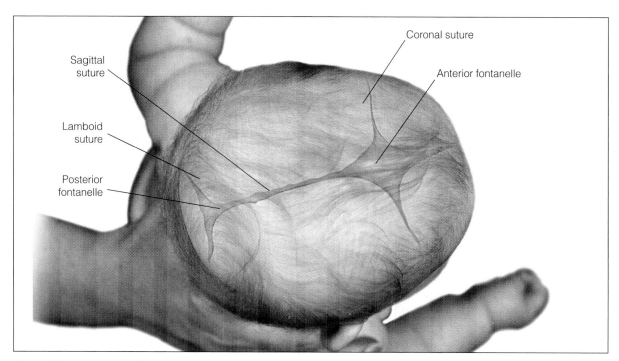

Figure 25.4 • Sutures and fontanelles of the skull.

delivery. **Caput succedaneum** is characterized by edema that results from a collection of fluid in the tissue at the top of the skull. The swelling associated with caput succedaneum crosses the cranial suture lines. **Cephalohematomas** are blood collections inside of the skull's periosteum and do not cross suture lines. Children with cephalohematomas are at increased risk of developing jaundice during the first week of life.

The lymph nodes are present at birth, but differentiation and growth of lymphatic tissue occurs primarily between ages 4 and 8 years. As such, preschoolers and school-age children often have "shotty" lymph nodes. Shotty nodes are noninfected, nontender, slightly enlarged lymph nodes that move when palpated and feel firmer than normal. Most children under 6 to 7 years have palpable, shotty femoral or cervical lymph nodes. Newborns and infants with a history of internal fetal monitoring during labour often have palpable occipital lymph nodes. Enlarged, noninfected tonsils are common in children ages 4 to 8. The presence of supraclavicular or cervical nodes should prompt the examiner to consider diseases, such as Hodgkin's lymphoma, that may present in adolescents between 10 and 14 years of age.

The maxillary and ethmoid sinuses are present at birth, but they are proportionately smaller than in adults. The sphenoid sinuses develop before age 5 and the frontal sinuses by age 10. Children rarely have infections of the ethmoid sinuses. The frontal sinuses cause infection only in older school-age children and adolescents. Children under the age of 5 years often have yellow-green nasal discharge during upper respiratory infections because they cannot efficiently clear their nasal passages.

The external auditory canals of children are smaller and less straight than those of adults. The nurse should pull the earlobe of children under the age of 4 years down and back when examining the tympanic membrane with the otoscope,

as illustrated in Figure 25.5. The eustachian tubes of infants, toddlers, and preschoolers are shorter, straighter, and more level than those in older children and adults. This normal variant, in combination with increased frequency of colds and respiratory infections, results in an increased incidence of **otitis media,** or middle ear infections, in children under the age of 4. The occurrence of otitis media peaks between 6 and 18 months of age. Children with middle ear infections typically present with fever, decreased appetite, irritability, and the inability to sleep lying down. The tympanic membrane appears opaque, bulging, and yellow-orange or red during otitis media episodes (see Figure 14.31). The tympanic membrane is a vascular tissue that appears red with infection, fever, or any condition that results in skin flushing. Children with red tympanic membranes and no purulent discharge in the middle ear space do not have bacterial otitis media.

Universal hearing screening before hospital discharge is a standard of practice in some Canadian provinces. In other jurisdictions, hearing screening may be carried out in at-risk infants, such as those born prematurely or those requiring medications, such as aminoglycosides, that are associated with hearing loss. Any infant or child demonstrating signs of hearing loss, such as failure to turn toward a noise or failure to meet normal language milestones, and children with recurrent episodes of otitis media should also be referred for hearing screening.

Teeth first erupt between 4 and 6 months of age. Normally, children lose their primary teeth, also known as baby teeth, in the order they erupt. No medical significance is associated with the order of tooth eruption. As long as a child cuts the first tooth by 15 months of age, no further evaluation is necessary. Most children lose their first primary tooth by 7 years of age. Figure 25.6 shows a typical sequence of tooth eruption for both deciduous and permanent teeth.

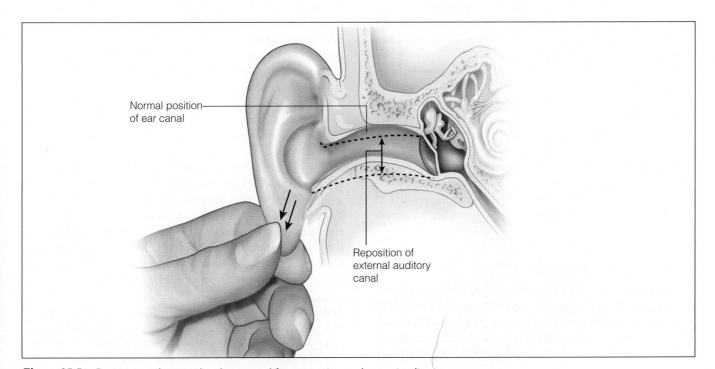

Normal position of ear canal

Reposition of external auditory canal

Figure 25.5 ● Positioning of external auditory canal for tympanic membrane visualization.

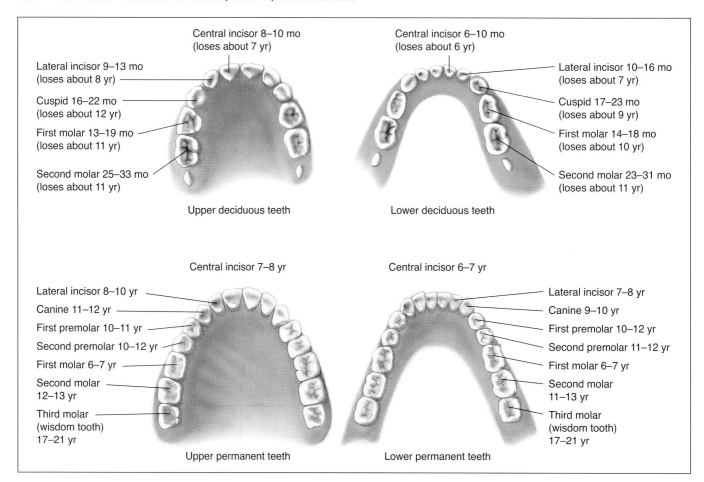

Figure 25.6 • Typical sequence of tooth eruption for both deciduous and permanent teeth. Notice that bottom teeth come in first for each kind of tooth, incisors, cuspids, and molars.

Infants have shorter necks than older children and adults. The neck should be assessed for the presence of redundant skin or webbing, which may be associated with syndromes, such as Turner syndrome. The thyroid gland cannot be palpated until adolescence. Infants do not develop good head control until approximately 4 months of age.

Babies can see at birth, but the visual acuity of newborns is not as sharp as adults. Children typically have 20/20 vision by the age of 7 years. Uncoordinated eye gaze is normal until 4 months of age.

An infant who cannot focus on objects at birth needs further evaluation. A whitened red reflex occurs with congenital cataracts. Infants and preschool children with the cancer retinoblastoma often present a history of a diminished red reflex or a "white glow" in the pupil. Almond-shaped eyes and up-turned epicanthal folds in white infants may be a marker for Down syndrome.

Respiratory System

Lung development is complete in healthy full-term newborns; however, significant differences exist between child and adult respiratory tracts. Infants have thinner, less muscular chest walls with a more noticeable xiphoid process. Breath sounds are louder and harsher. Referred sounds from the upper airways are common. The anterior-posterior chest diameter is approximately equal in infants, and the ribs appear more horizontal. Infants are obligate nose breathers until 6 months of age; they cannot breathe through their mouths. The nurse should carefully assess children under the age of 6 months with nasal congestion for signs of respiratory distress. Abdominal breathing is common until age 6 years. Thoracic breathing begins in the school-age years.

Children have smaller, more pliant airways until early adolescence. Until that time, children are more prone to airway collapse and blockage. Infants and young children should be assessed for the presence of such symptoms as nasal flaring, the use of accessory muscles for breathing, or the presence of intercostal or subcostal retractions. Oxygen needs are higher in small children because their increased metabolic rates result in higher oxygen consumption. It is important to carefully assess and manage children who show signs of dyspnea and respiratory distress. The risk of respiratory failure is greatest in infants, toddlers, and preschoolers, but children of all ages experience respiratory failure much more quickly than adults.

CLINICAL TIP

Children are much more likely to die from respiratory failure than from cardiovascular collapse. Any child with altered sensorium should be immediately evaluated for respiratory compromise.

Choanal atresia is a relatively rare congenital defect that results from a membranous or bony obstruction of the nasal passages. If undetected or untreated, severe respiratory distress results. All newborns should be carefully assessed for nasal patency. **Laryngomalacia** or **tracheomalacia** are congenital defects of the cartilage in the larynx and trachea, respectively. Infants with laryngomalacia or tracheomalacia have airways that easily collapse. Parents frequently describe children with laryngomalacia or tracheomalacia as "noisy breathers." Continuous inspiratory and expiratory stridor that improves during the first year of life characterizes these abnormalities.

Cardiovascular System

Prenatally, the blood shunts away from the heart and liver through the **ductus venosus,** the **ductus arteriosus,** and the **foramen ovale.** When the umbilical cord is clamped and newborns take their first breath, a combination of increased thoracic pressure, increased blood oxygen levels, and changes in intracardiac pressures close these shunts. However, both the ductus venosus and the ductus arteriosus may remain open for 12 to 72 hours after birth. **Sinus arrhythmia,** also known as heart period variability, presents with heart rate increases during inspiration and decreases during expiration. This normal variant is common until early adulthood and results from parasympathetic enervation of the heart. Cardiac output is more dependent on heart rate than stroke volume in children. Therefore, bradycardia results in rapid decompensation and should be considered life threatening. Children in shock experience hypotension later than adults because the elasticity of a child's blood vessels is greater.

The thinner chest wall of children causes heart sounds to seem louder. Infants have a point of maximal impulse (PMI) that is difficult to assess and is located approximately one intercostal space higher than in adults. An S_2 split with inspiration may be detected in children under the age of 6. The physiological S_2 split disappears with expiration. Any S_2 split that persists throughout the cardiac cycle merits further evaluation. Preadolescents may have a physiological S_3 gallop that results from vibrations during rapid ventricular filling.

Seventy percent of children will have a detectable innocent, or functional, murmur sometime during childhood. Any condition that increases metabolism, like fever or anemia, will make innocent murmurs more pronounced. By definition, innocent murmurs arise from increased blood flow across normal heart structures. All innocent murmurs have the following characteristics: they are grade I to II or VI in intensity, are systolic (with the exception of the venous hum), and are not associated with thrills or other cardiac symptoms. See Table 25.2 for a description of the most common innocent murmurs.

A number of congenital cardiac defects occur in the newborn period. **Coarctation of the aorta** results in the narrowing of the aorta with decreased femoral pulses and bounding upper extremity pulses. Also noticeable are discrepancies in blood pressure and oxygen saturation between the upper and lower extremities. The nurse should carefully assess all infants and newborns for cardiac murmurs, altered pulse intensity, and cyanosis. It is important to promptly refer any child with suspected congenital heart disease.

CLINICAL TIP

Congestive heart failure (CHF) in infants may be the first sign of an acyanotic congenital heart defect. Common symptoms of CHF include sweating and fatigue while feeding, and frequent respiratory tract congestion.

Breasts

Inverted nipples are evident at birth and common until adolescence. Because of circulating maternal estrogen and prolactin, male and female infants may have a milky white discharge from their nipples that is commonly called "witches' milk." This condition will resolve within 1 to 2 weeks after birth when maternal hormone levels decrease.

Thelarche, or breast budding, is usually the first pubertal sign in females. Breast development follows a clear pattern described by the Tanner stages as illustrated in Figure 25.7. **Gynecomastia** is the benign development of breast tissue in males and results in a tender, mobile knot under the areola in as many as one third of adolescent males (see Figure 16.28). This condition is more common in overweight males and in teens who use performance-enhancing steroids.

Abdomen

Typically, the umbilical cord will dry and fall off within 3 weeks of birth. When the cord stump is still present, it should be assessed for the presence of bleeding, redness around the base, discharge, or odour. The liver edge may be palpable at the right

TABLE 25.2	Common Innocent Heart Murmurs		
NAME	**LOCATION**	**TIMING**	**CHARACTERISTICS**
Venous hum	Upper left or right sternal borders near the clavicles	Continuous	Loudest in sitting position—disappears when child is supine. May also disappear with light pressure on jugular vein or when child turns his or her head to the side.
Still's murmur	Apex or left lower sternal border	Systolic ejection	Most common innocent murmur. May change with position changes.
Pulmonary flow	Pulmonic area or upper left sternal border	Systolic	Usually heard in newborns. Disappears with Valsalva's manoeuvre.

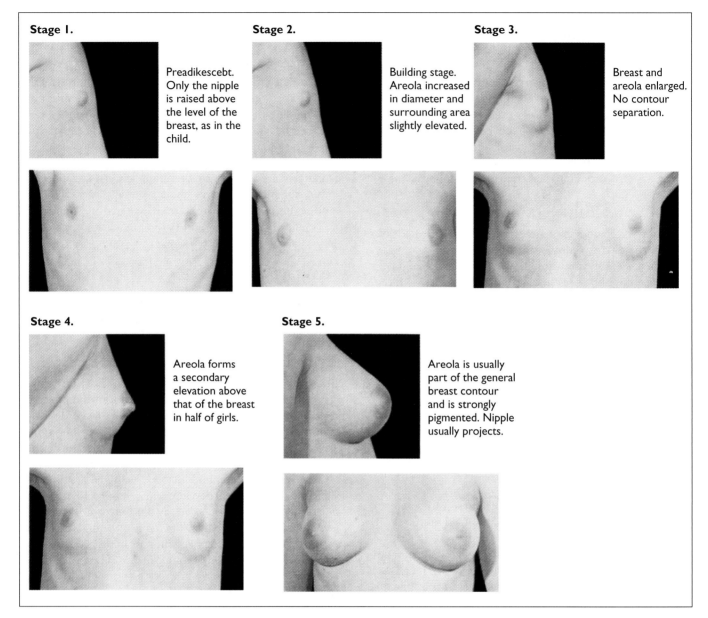

Stage 1.
Preadikescebt.
Only the nipple
is raised above
the level of the
breast, as in the
child.

Stage 2.
Building stage.
Areola increased
in diameter and
surrounding area
slightly elevated.

Stage 3.
Breast and
areola enlarged.
No contour
separation.

Stage 4.
Areola forms
a secondary
elevation above
that of the breast
in half of girls.

Stage 5.
Areola is usually
part of the general
breast contour
and is strongly
pigmented. Nipple
usually projects.

Figure 25.7 ● Tanner stages of breast development.

lower costal margin because the thoracic cage of young children is smaller. Any liver edge palpable more than 2 cm below the costal margin indicates hepatomegaly and should be evaluated. **Umbilical hernias** cause a protrusion at the umbilicus and are visible at birth (see Figure 19.29). Umbilical hernias are common in Black children and in those with Mediterranean heritage. More than 95% resolve spontaneously before 6 years of age. Umbilical hernias require no medical intervention since they do not incarcerate. Toddlers and infants have prominent abdomens that result in a potbelly appearance (see Figure 19.7). This variance diminishes by age 5 years. Infectious mononucleosis is most common in school-age children. Splenomegaly results in up to 25% of acute mononucleosis cases. Enlarged spleens are vulnerable to trauma because they no longer fit completely behind the thoracic cage. Careful abdominal assessment is indicated in any child with suspected mononucleosis.

Genitourinary and Reproductive Systems

Children do not have adult bladder capacities (around 500 mL or 17 fl.oz.) until adolescence. A quick way to estimate a child's bladder capacity is to use the following formula: the child's age (in years) times 30 plus or minus 60 mL (2 fl.oz.). For example, a 4-year-old child has a bladder capacity of 60 to 180 mL (2 to 6 fl.oz.).

On average, children attain bladder sphincter control at approximately 3 years for females and age 3.5 for males. Bladder training requires bladder sphincter control. Normal urine output for children is at least 2 mL/kg/h.

Minimal genital growth occurs before puberty. The onset of genital development is expected by age 11 in females and 13 in males. Refer to the Tanner stages, Table 21.2 for males and Table 22.1 for females.

Uncircumcised males have unretractile foreskins until 2 to 3 years of age. **Cryptorchidism** is the failure of one or both testicles to descend through the inguinal canal during the final stages of fetal development. This condition is more common in premature infants and is detectable at birth. Males with undescended testicles should be referred for surgical evaluation by 6 months of age because there is an increased risk of testicular cancer in retained testicles, and spontaneous descent is rare after this age.

Infant females may have a bloody vaginal discharge during the first 2 weeks of life. This "false menses" is the result of exposure to maternal estrogen and progesterone. **Labial adhesions** occur when the labia minora fuse together. They are common in preadolescent females because decreased estrogen levels result in labial and genital atrophy. When present, labial adhesions extend from the posterior fourchette and look like a skin covering all or part of the introitus. They are of medical concern if there is blockage of urinary flow or if they result in recurrent urinary tract infections.

Musculoskeletal System

The human skeleton does not fully ossify until 18 years of age. As a result, most children's skeletons are more cartilaginous and structurally weaker than adults' skeletons. During trauma, preadolescent children are more likely to fracture a bone than to injure a ligament, muscle, or tendon. Bone growth occurs at the epiphyseal plates located in the ends of the bones. Fractures of the **epiphyseal plates** can result in bone growth failure and limb length discrepancy. Muscular development increases with age and completes after puberty.

Genu varum, or bowlegs, is common until 1 or 2 years of age. Preschoolers and school-age children less than 7 years of age are often knock kneed, also known as **genu valgum.** Both genu varum and genu valgum are normal findings in children from the age groups previously listed. Because of well-developed fat pads, children under the age of 2 years appear flatfooted.

Scoliosis is a lateral curvature of the lumbar or thoracic spine that is more common in children with neuromuscular deficits. Screening for scoliosis should begin by age 5 years and continue annually until after puberty because increases in height may worsen the spinal curvature. Figure 25.8 on page 697 depicts a teenage girl with mild scoliosis.

Developmental dysplasia of the hip is a congenital disorder that results from inadequate development of the hip socket. This disorder often manifests in the early newborn period, but it may be noted anytime before 2 years of age.

Muscular dystrophy is an X-linked genetic disorder that results in progressive loss of muscle function. Males are affected four times as often as females. Both smooth and skeletal muscles are affected. The first signs of muscular dystrophy are often noted around age 3, when a child shows muscle weakness and impaired gait.

Neurological System

Myelin is a fatty substance that covers the neurons of the brain and spinal cord. Myelin speeds nerve impulse conduction. The myelin sheath grows until 2 to 3 years of age. Infants have a number of primitive reflexes that gradually disappear as the brain matures (see Table 25.3). Developmental milestones are related to brain development. As a general rule, children acquire and refine gross motor skills before fine motor skills. Table 25.4 on page 697 lists the major developmental milestones of childhood. Children require more sleep than adults. Table 25.5 on page 697 lists the normal sleep requirements for infants and children.

SPECIAL CONSIDERATIONS

The nurse must consider the psychosocial and cultural factors that affect the health of infants, children, and adolescents. These are described in the sections on page 698.

TABLE 25.3	Primitive Reflexes of Early Childhood		
REFLEX	**HOW TO ELICIT**	**AGE WHEN DISAPPEARS**	**EXAMPLE**
Tonic neck	Turn the infant's head to one side while the infant is supine. The infant will extend the arm and leg on the side the head is turned to while flexing the opposite arm and leg.	2 to 6 months	Tonic neck

(continued)

| TABLE 25.3 | Primitive Reflexes of Early Childhood *(continued)* |

REFLEX	HOW TO ELICIT	AGE WHEN DISAPPEARS	EXAMPLE
Palmar grasp	The infant will grasp fingers or objects placed in the palm of the hand.	3 to 4 months	Palmar grasp
Plantar grasp	The infant will curl the toes when the base of the toes is touched.	6 to 8 months	Plantar grasp
Rooting	Lightly stroke the infant's cheek. The infant will turn the head with the mouth open toward the stroked side.	3 to 4 months	
Moro (startle)	The infant will extend the arms with the fingers spread and flex the legs while making loud sounds or if the infant's body drops suddenly.	4 to 6 months	Moro
Stepping	The infant will flex the leg and take steps when the infant is upright with the feet touching a surface.	4 to 5 months	Stepping

(continued)

TABLE 25.3	Primitive Reflexes of Early Childhood		
REFLEX	**HOW TO ELICIT**	**AGE WHEN DISAPPEARS**	**EXAMPLE**
Babinski	Gently stroke the plantar surface of the foot from heel to toe. The infant will extend and fan the toes and flex the foot.	18 to 24 months	Babinski

TABLE 25.4	Major Developmental Milestones of Childhood
MILESTONE	**AGE ATTAINED**
Smiles socially	2 months
Places objects in mouth	3 to 4 months
Babbles and coos	4 months
Extends forearms to support upper body when prone	4 to 5 months
Rolls from front to back	4 to 5 months
Rolls from back to front	5 to 6 months
Sits with support	6 to 7 months
Transfers objects from one hand to another	6 to 7 months
Sits without support	7 to 8 months
Supports weight when stands	7 to 8 months
Pulls self to standing position	8 months
Creeps or crawls	8 to 9 months
Attains pincer grasp	9 months
Cruises (walks holding on to furniture or objects)	9 to 10 months
Plays peekaboo and patty cake	10 months
Says one word	11 months
Walks independently	12 to 15 months
Runs or climbs	14 to 18 months
Goes up and down stairs two feet per step	2 years
Goes up and down stairs alternating feet	3 years
Pedals tricycle	3 years
Copies circle	3 years
Prints name	5 years

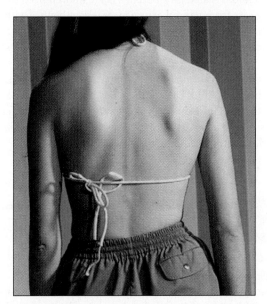

Figure 25.8 ● A child may have varying degrees of scoliosis. For mild forms, treatment will focus on strengthening and stretching. Moderate forms will require bracing. Severe forms may need surgery and fusion. Clothes that fit at an angle, such as this teenage girl's shorts, and anatomical asymmetry of the back provide clues for early detection.

TABLE 25.5	Sleep Requirements for Children and Adolescents
AGE	**AVERAGE HOURS OF SLEEP PER 24 HOURS**
Newborn	16
3 months	15
12 months	13.5
2 years	11.5
6 years	9.5
12 years	11.5

Psychosocial Considerations

Children and adults have different understandings of health and illness. It is common for children to believe they are ill because of bad thoughts or behaviours. The belief that illness is a punishment for wrongdoing is common. Young children cannot identify or modify health risks. Children do not have the cognitive ability to understand cause and effect relationships until late school age or early adolescence. Parents function as proxies for their children in most healthcare decisions.

Nurses should use a caring, supportive, yet firm approach with children. Whenever possible, play should be incorporated into nursing procedures. It is helpful to allow children to touch and manipulate equipment. Adhesive bandages or empty syringes can be provided for playacting with dolls. The nurse should encourage children to express their fears and concerns. Depending on the child's age, it may be appropriate to encourage the child to express his or her feelings through drawings or puppet play. Painful procedures should not be performed while a child is seated on a parent's lap. Children need to know they are safe from painful experiences when they are with their parents.

When a child is ill, parents suffer from increased stress that results from interrupted sleep, concern for the child's well-being, and frustration at the inability to fix what is hurting or bothering their child. Each of these factors may affect a parent's ability to recall information or to follow complex instructions. Nurses should consider parental stress levels when conducting the health history and developing care plans.

Social and Ethnocultural Considerations

Most of the world's cultures value children. However, significant variation exists among cultures with respect to what constitutes acceptable child behaviour and expectations for health or caregiving. Nurses must be aware of the cultural influences on children and families. For example, European cultures encourage independence at an early age, whereas other groups, such as Asians, Hispanics, and Arabs, stress a strong commitment to family. Commonly, children from these cultural groups are taught to respect elder family members and to place the needs of the family before their personal needs. Hispanics and First Nation parents tend to be more permissive with their children, especially with male children.

All the dominant North American cultures view mothers as the primary child caregivers. Overall, females are viewed as nurturers who are responsible for guiding and caring for children. It is common for mothers to make the decisions regarding home care of child illness and complaints. However, many groups, including East Indian and Arab Canadians, have patriarchal hierarchies where the father must be consulted before any professional healthcare decisions are made.

Many cultures have taboos against physical assessment of postpubertal children by healthcare providers of different genders. The nurse must identify and respect privacy, modesty, and cultural issues of the individual.

Social and Ethnocultural Considerations

Aboriginal

- Direct eye contact may be avoided.
- Mongolian spots are commonly located over the lower back and buttocks; they will begin to fade by age 2 or 3.
- Most newborns have dark grey-brown eyes that will not change much as they get older.
- Hypertension and insulin-resistant diabetes are more common in Aboriginal youth.

Asian

- As a sign of respect, many Asian parents may be reluctant to disagree with or displease a healthcare provider.
- Direct eye contact may be viewed as impolite.
- Mongolian spots are common.
- Most infants have dark-grey eye colour at birth.
- Vietnamese families believe the head is sacred. The nurse should avoid touching the head of the mother and baby without first asking permission.
- Chinese families practise cupping, where a heated cup is placed over the skin to draw out illness. Vietnamese families use coin rubbing, where a coin is rubbed on the trunk. Neither practice should be considered abuse.

- Many Asian families use the concept of hot and cold illnesses. Certain illnesses are considered to be hot or cold, and treatments should counter the effect of the illness. Therefore, hot illnesses should be treated with cold medicines and foods, whereas cold illnesses should be treated with hot medicines and foods.

Middle Eastern

- Direct eye contact may be viewed as impolite or improper, especially with members of the opposite sex.
- Physical examination by individuals of different gender is taboo after adolescence.
- Thalassemias are more common in children of Middle Eastern heritage than in children of European descent.
- Modesty may be important and should be respected.
- Females may defer to the male head of the family for healthcare decisions.

All Races and Cultures

- Babies within all races and cultures are born with lighter, pinker skin. The true skin colour will develop over the first year.
- All cultures and ethnic groups have folk beliefs that centre on childbirth and child rearing. The nurse should assess for positive folk practices and incorporate them into nursing care.

GATHERING THE DATA

The basic components of a health history are the same whether the nurse works with children or adults. However, a number of variations must be incorporated into the pediatric health history. This section focuses on the unique issues involved in taking the history of a child.

It is essential that the nurse determine the relationship between the child who seeks healthcare and the adult who presents with the child. The nurse must never assume legal or family ties between children and adults who accompany them. Nannies, babysitters, friends, siblings, and stepparents often transport children to healthcare appointments. Provincial and territorial law determines which individuals can legally consent to medical treatment of a minor child. Privacy laws limit access to protected health information. Directly asking about relationships is the easiest way to ensure compliance with the legal and ethical concerns regarding the medical treatment of children.

HEALTH HISTORY

Many children are nonverbal or possess limited language ability; therefore, nurses depend on parents for health history information. This can limit the specificity of the history information. However, it is important to ask preschoolers and older children about their chief complaint and symptoms even though the information they provide may not be as detailed as the information provided by their parents. This chapter uses the word *parent* to represent parents, caregivers, or guardians.

The nurse should determine if the parent is stressed or distracted before the health interview. Many parents of ill children are sleep deprived because of their child's altered sleep patterns. Sleep deprivation can result in altered recall, limited ability to follow complex questions, and diminished ability to remember verbal instructions. The presence of other children can be distracting, especially if the children are loud, active, or irritable. Nurses can distract energetic or fussy children with books, crayons, or toys.

The nurse should listen carefully to the parent and use open-ended questions to elicit health information. Parents know their children better than anyone else does. They are able to detect subtle differences in their child's behaviour. It is essential to pay special attention to the chief complaints that parents provide. A thorough physical assessment is based on the issues and concerns raised in the health history.

The nurse should call the child by his or her name and use words that the child understands. For example, most pre-adolescents are not familiar with the word *abdomen,* but most children use the word *tummy* or *belly* from infancy. Instead of asking "Does your head hurt?" the nurse should ask the child to touch the head where it hurts. It is necessary to be patient. Children often pause between words or repeat phrases when they are excited or nervous.

Children who are at least 10 years old should be given the option of being examined without their parents present. The child is the client, not the parent. The nurse's legal and ethical responsibility is to the child first. The nurse must respect the confidentiality of the information provided by older children and be aware of federal and provincial or territorial laws regarding parental notification. The parent and the child should be told what the nurse can and cannot keep confidential. For example, statements like "What you and I talk about will be between the two of us, unless you tell me that you are thinking about harming yourself or someone else, or if you tell me that someone is hurting you" help establish rapport and boundaries to the nurse-child and nurse-parent relationship. If a nurse is required to report health interview information to others (e.g., public health departments or child protection agencies), the nurse should always inform the child of the need to share the information with others before actually doing so. Failure to do so can jeopardize the rapport between nurse and child.

HEALTH HISTORY QUESTIONS

RATIONALES

The following sections provide sample questions and follow-up questions. Rationales for some questions are provided. The list of questions is not all-inclusive but rather represents the more common concern or injury questions required in a health history related to a pediatric assessment.

Questions About the Birth History

All children under 6 years of age, children with congenital defects, and children who have developmental or neurological delays require a documented birth history. The birth history includes the following questions:

HEALTH HISTORY QUESTIONS	RATIONALES
1. For the mother of the child: • Did you have prenatal care? • How much weight did you gain during the pregnancy? • Were there any complications during the pregnancy? • Were you ill during the pregnancy? • Did you use any medications, alcohol, drugs, or herbal or complementary medicines during pregnancy?	▶ Poor or absent prenatal care is associated with an increased risk of developmental delay and neurological conditions. Exposure to **teratogens** (substances known to cause birth defects) is associated with genetic defects, congenital abnormalities, and physical and mental syndromes, especially when the exposure occurs during the first trimester of pregnancy. Most of the organ systems develop during the third to eighth week of pregnancy. Exposure to teratogens is especially worrisome when it occurs during this gestational period. Maternal illness can affect embryonic or fetal development during any gestational age. The nurse should note infectious diseases and illnesses that cause high fevers or alter placental blood flow.
2. How was your labour and delivery? What was your child's due date?	▶ Premature and postmature infants have an increased risk of hypoglycemia. Pregnancies that last at least 37 weeks are considered full term. The nurse should determine the child's birth weight and Apgar scores. Very low birth weight is correlated with negative health outcomes of prematurity, such as significant respiratory complications and neurological deficits. It is important to note the type of delivery (vaginal versus caesarean section). If the child was born by caesarean section, the nurse should ask why the caesarean was performed. The nurse should also ask if the child was admitted to the regular nursery, the special care nursery, or the intensive care unit. Cerebral palsy and other developmental disorders occur more often in children with traumatic birth histories.
3. How did your child do after the birth? • How are you doing with the changes since the baby was born? • How did your husband or partner, parents, siblings, or family members adapt to the new baby?	▶ The nurse should determine if the child needed medical care to assist with feeding, breathing, and so on. The nurse also asks about hearing and vision problems. Did the child receive medications associated with ototoxicity (such as vancomycin or gentamicin)? Untreated or complicated neonatal jaundice can result in neurological damage. Separation, illness (maternal or infant), or stress often affect early parent-child attachment. Pediatric nurses and physicians often notice postpartum depression.
4. Is there anything else about the pregnancy, labour, or delivery that you think I should know?	▶ This question allows parents to add information they feel is pertinent but that they perceived was not covered by the preceding questions.

Questions Related to Illness or Infection

1. What brings you here today? • How long has the child been ill? • What symptoms does the child have and how have they changed since the beginning of the illness?	▶ These questions establish the chief complaint and the history of the present illness.

GATHERING THE DATA

HEALTH HISTORY QUESTIONS	RATIONALES

- Follow-up questions should include timing of the symptoms (day vs. night, at rest vs. when playing), activity levels, effect on the child's appetite and temperament, and whether symptoms disrupt the child's sleep. The nurse should ask verbal children why they are there.
- Do the child's symptoms happen during the day, at night, or both?
- What is the child's activity level like?
- How well is the child eating?
- How much is the child drinking?
- Does the child seem more irritable than usual?
- Is the child having a hard time sleeping because of the symptoms?

▶ Commonly, small children will complain of a "tummy ache" or "my throat hurts" while parents may be concerned about fussiness or altered sleep patterns. Postnasal drip causes a cough that worsens with activity, when arising from bed, or when supine. Preadolescent children will complain of stomach pain when they are gassy, if they are nauseated, or if they actually feel abdominal pain. Children with sore throats often present with a history of normal fluid intake but decreased solid food intake. Anxious or frightened preschool and school-age children may complain of headache or stomach ache.

2. **Has the child been exposed to other people with the same symptoms?**

▶ The nurse should determine if the child attends daycare or group babysitting and the number of hours per week. This helps to identify the origin of infectious diseases.

3. **Have you given your child any medicines?**
   - If so, what medicines, what doses, and what frequency?
   - Do you use herbal or complementary medicine?

▶ Many parents do not think it is important to inform nurses about over-the-counter and herbal preparations since they are readily available. Therefore, it is important for the nurse to ask specific questions regarding these preparations. The data on the safety of herbal and complementary medicine in children are limited.

Questions Related to Well Children and Health Promotion

1. **How is the child doing?**
   - Do you have concerns about the child's hearing, vision, physical development, or speech?

▶ These questions help to identify parental concerns and expectations. Parents often compare their child's abilities with those of other children. They may have unrealistic expectations related to inappropriate age comparisons or incorrect understanding of normal child development. Parents may notice subtle developmental differences that are difficult to assess in clinical settings.

2. **How does the child do in school?**
   - Does the child seem to make friends and get along with other children?

▶ This is an easy way to get an overall sense of social and cognitive functioning in an older child.

3. **Does the child play sports?**
   - What types of activities does the child like to do? Does the child like to eat foods from all the food groups (dairy, fruits, vegetables, meats, and grains)?
   - How much juice, milk, pop, and tea does the child drink every day?

▶ These items help identify children at risk for nutritional deficiencies and health problems related to inactivity.

HEALTH HISTORY QUESTIONS	RATIONALES

- How often does the child eat fast food?
- What types of beverages does the child drink?

4. **For adolescent children, the nurse should ask about sexual activity (including age of first activity and risky sexual behaviour), and tobacco, drug, and alcohol use.**

▶ Adolescence is a time of experimentation and limit testing. Initial drug, alcohol, and substance use often occurs before age 21. Many adolescents are sexually active, have multiple sexual partners, or do not consistently use birth control or protection against sexually transmitted disease. Most adolescents will not disclose information regarding these topics unless they are specifically questioned about these behaviours.

PHYSICAL ASSESSMENT

The skills and equipment needed to assess a child are the same as those needed for adult physical assessment. This section focuses on physical assessment techniques that are unique to pediatric clients. Refer to the previous text chapters for greater system-specific details.

ASSESSMENT TECHNIQUES AND FINDINGS

The nurse can do many things to make the examination fun. Children should be allowed to touch equipment. For example, the nurse can ask a young child to put the otoscope's "hat" (i.e., speculum) on the light. Before examining the tympanic membrane, the nurse can ask toddlers and preschoolers if they have elephants or cartoon characters in their ears. Young children can be encouraged to take deep breaths by having them blow bubbles or blow out the light on the otoscope. Toys can be used to distract children. Examples include finger puppets, small animals placed on the stethoscope, and whistles or small music boxes. It is important to keep toys with small pieces out of the reach of infants, toddlers, and preschoolers.

EQUIPMENT

examination gown and drape	otoscope with pneumatic bulb
clean, nonsterile examination gloves	appropriately sized specula
stethoscope	measuring tape
ophthalmoscope	tongue depressor
appropriately sized sphygmomanometer	

HELPFUL HINTS

- Children have the same needs as adults to protect their modesty and privacy.
- Explain procedures and techniques in words that children can understand.
- Young children are more comfortable and compliant when they sit on their parents' laps.
- Establish rapport with the parent and child before initiating any physical examination.
- A flexible approach to assessment is essential. Begin with the least threatening examinations.
- Keep painful or invasive procedures at the end of the assessment.
- Auscultate the thorax of the sleeping child.
- Use routine practices.

TECHNIQUES AND NORMAL FINDINGS	ABNORMAL FINDINGS AND SPECIAL CONSIDERATIONS

GENERAL SURVEY

Observe the child's interaction with the adults present. How does the child react to them? If the child is ill, is he or she consolable? How comfortably do the adults interact with the child? Does the child's development match the chronological age? Assess the child's vital signs.

▶ Poor eye contact between child and adult may indicate impaired attachment. Seriously ill and septic children are often irritable and inconsolable.

| TECHNIQUES AND NORMAL FINDINGS | ABNORMAL FINDINGS AND SPECIAL CONSIDERATIONS |

GROWTH AND DEVELOPMENT

1. Obtain accurate height and weight.

    - Measure the recumbent length of children under 2 years old. Have the child lie supine on the examination table. Hold the child's leg straight with the hips and knees extended. Mark and measure the distance between the heel and the top of the head as shown in Figure 25.9. Make sure the child is flat during the measurement. Plot recumbent length on the growth charts for children between birth and 36 months of age.

    ▶ Assess for height and weight discrepancies. Height and weight should be within one standard deviation of each other. For example, a child whose height is at the 50th percentile should weigh between the 25th and 75th percentile. Reduced height velocity may indicate endocrine deficiencies or chronic renal disease. Poor weight gain may indicate nutritional deficiency, impaired parent-infant interaction, or chronic congestive heart disease. Overweight and obese children have increased risk of developing type 2 diabetes and acquired cardiovascular disease.

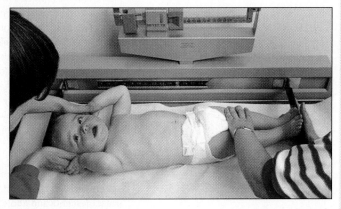

Figure 25.9 ●
Nurse measuring the recumbent height of a toddler.

    - Obtain a standing height for children older than 2 years. (Note: Some children between 24 and 36 months of age will not be able to stand still long enough to get an accurate reading. Recumbent height is better in this situation.) Make sure the child's heels are flat against the wall. Use a stadiometer for the highest accuracy. Plot standing heights on growth charts for children between 2 and 18 years of age.

    - Use an infant scale to weigh children under 2 years. Infants and toddlers should be naked except for a clean, dry diaper. Use a robe for preschoolers, school-age children, and adolescents. Note: A single height or weight measurement cannot be used to determine insufficient growth patterns. Children with a body mass index (BMI) less than the 5th percentile for their age are underweight. Children with a BMI greater than the 95th percentile for their age are overweight.

2. Measure head circumference for children under 3 years old.

    - Hold the measuring tape taut against the child's skull from the forehead (just above the eyebrows) across the parietal region, and over the occipital prominence, as shown in Figure 25.10. Plot the measurement on the growth chart.

    ▶ Any child whose head circumference is below the 5th percentile has **microcephaly**. Microcephaly may be caused by genetic disorders or intrauterine exposure to cocaine or alcohol. Any child whose head circumference is above the 95th percentile has macrocephaly. **Macrocephaly** is associated with hydrocephalus, brain tumour, and increased intracranial pressure. Any child with microcephaly, with macrocephaly, or who has greater than 1 standard deviation change in head circumference percentile should be referred for medical evaluation.

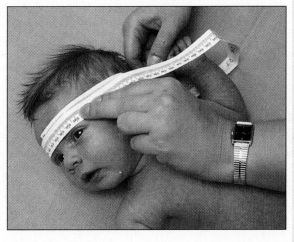

Figure 25.10 ●
Head circumference landmarks.

PHYSICAL ASSESSMENT

TECHNIQUES AND NORMAL FINDINGS	ABNORMAL FINDINGS AND SPECIAL CONSIDERATIONS

SKIN, HAIR, AND NAILS

1. Inspect the skin for colour and the presence of lesions, birthmarks, or discolourations.
   - Use a measuring tape to determine the exact size of lesions and birthmarks. Carefully document the appearance, distribution, and characteristics of all skin lesions. Cyanosis is best detected by inspecting the mucous membranes. Detect jaundice by inspecting the sclera or by noting a yellow undertone after skin blanching.

▶ Contact diaper rashes occur on the skin surfaces that touch the diaper and typically do not involve the skinfolds. Diaper rashes caused by *Candida albicans* (yeast) are characterized by beefy erythema that concentrates in the intertriginous folds and have small, red satellite lesions along the rash margins.

▶ Strawberry hemangiomas initially present during the first few weeks after birth as red macules that blanch with pressure and grow into spongy, vascular nodules. Strawberry hemangiomas grow until approximately 1 year of age and spontaneously resolve by age 9.

▶ Mongolian spots are blue-black patches that are most common at the base of the spine in Aboriginal, Black, Hispanic, and Asian infants (refer to Figure 11.4).

▶ Acne vulgaris appears on the face, neck, upper back, upper chest, and upper arms of preadolescents and adolescents.

▶ Newborn jaundice that appears within 24 hours of birth, appears in children with maternal ABO/Rh incompatibility, or persists more than 2 to 3 weeks after birth must be carefully evaluated because of the increased risk of significant complications and underlying disease.

▶ The presence of more than five café au lait lesions may indicate neurofibromatosis. Viral exanthems are morbilliform rashes common in preschool children.

▶ The classic viral exanthem is a nonpruritic, erythematous, macular rash that worsens with skin flushing, coalesces to give a lacy appearance, begins on the trunk and spreads to the extremities, and blanches with light pressure.

2. Inspect the hair and nails for texture, distribution, and moisture.
   - Infants who cannot sit upright independently may have areas of friction alopecia on the occiput caused by rubbing and friction. Newborns have thin, brittle nails.

▶ Nail clubbing indicates chronic hypoxemia. Growth of pubic hair, facial hair, and axillary hair in a prepubescent child indicates endocrinological disease. Areas of alopecia with hair follicle breakage at the skin level characterize tinea capitis, also known as scalp ringworm.

HEAD AND NECK

1. Inspect and palpate the skull for the presence of deformity.
   - The scalp should be intact, round, smooth, and free of lesions. Fontanelles and sutures, if present, should be smooth and flat.

▶ Premature closure of the cranial sutures causes craniosynostosis, a condition characterized by abnormal skull flattening and altered brain growth (see Figure 12.17). Birth trauma may result in cephalohematoma or caput succedaneum.

PHYSICAL ASSESSMENT

TECHNIQUES AND NORMAL FINDINGS	ABNORMAL FINDINGS AND SPECIAL CONSIDERATIONS

2. **Palpate the lymph nodes of the head and neck.**

- Assess the lymph nodes of the head and neck in the same order as in the adult. Before the exam, ask young children if they have "tickles" in their neck. Shotty lymph nodes are a normal variant in preschoolers and school-age children. Shotty nodes are noninfected, nontender, slightly enlarged lymph nodes that move when palpated and feel firmer than normal. Most children under 6 to 7 years old have palpable, shotty femoral or cervical lymph nodes. Enlarged, noninfected tonsils are common in 4- to 8-year-old children.

▶ Anterior cervical and tonsillar lymphadenopathies are common in children with upper respiratory tract infection. Newborns and infants with a history of internal fetal monitoring during labour often have palpable occipital lymph nodes. Mononucleosis causes lymphadenitis of the anterior and posterior cervical chains.

EYES AND VISION

1. **Inspect the eyes for symmetry, position, and movement.**

- Note the position of the eyes in relation to the upper margin of the external ear. Normally, the outer canthus of the eye will be even with or slightly higher than the upper margin of the ear. Both eyes should be approximately the same size and shape. Note the presence of discharge, lesions, or edema.

- Nonconvergent strabismus is normal in children under 2 months of age. Assess for esotropia (inward gaze) and exotropia (outward gaze) with the corneal light reflection test and the cover-uncover test. Figure 25.11 illustrates normal and abnormal corneal light refraction. Elicit the corneal light reflection by standing about 0.75 m (2 ft.) in front of the child; ask the child to look at you while you shine the light from the otoscope in his or her eye. The light reflection should be in the same position, slightly medial to the centre of the pupil, in both eyes. Asymmetry of the light reflexes indicates eye deviation. To perform the cover-uncover test, have the child stare at an object approximately 1 m (3 ft.) in front of him or her. Cover one eye with your hand for at least 10 seconds. Remove your hand and determine the presence of eye movement (Canadian Paediatric Society, 2009).

▶ Low-set ears are associated with various genetic disorders, including Down syndrome. Dacryostenosis is the congenital blockage of the tear ducts and is a normal variant until 9 months of age. Children older than 9 months who have symptoms of dacryostenosis should be referred to ophthalmology for evaluation. It presents with unilateral increased tearing and nonpurulent crusting. Refer children older than 3 months with strabismus for ophthalmological evaluation. Esotropia causes the covered eye to move inward (medially), and exotropia causes the covered eye to move outward (laterally) during the cover-uncover test. Periorbital cellulitis is a fast-progressing, serious bacterial infection of the periorbital tissues. Carefully assess all children with edema and erythema of the eye for fever, altered ocular movement, and lymphadenitis.

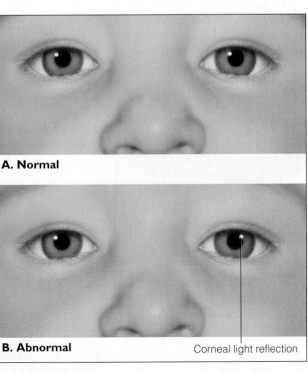

A. Normal

B. Abnormal   Corneal light reflection

Figure 25.11 ● Normal and abnormal corneal light reflection test.

PHYSICAL ASSESSMENT

TECHNIQUES AND NORMAL FINDINGS	ABNORMAL FINDINGS AND SPECIAL CONSIDERATIONS

2. Assess the inner eye structures.

- Assess the red reflex. Inspect the cornea for translucency. The pupils should be equally round and reactive to light accommodation. The red reflex should be symmetrical.

▶ An absent or "white glow" red reflex may indicate the presence of a retinoblastoma. Congenital cataracts cause the cornea to appear hazy.

3. Assess vision.

- Use modified Snellen charts to assess the vision of children older than 3 to 4 years. Assess the ability to track objects with a blinking light made by rapidly moving your finger in front of the otoscope light. Normal newborns visually track moving objects. Chapter 13 of this text provides a thorough discussion of the eye. ∞

EARS AND HEARING

1. Assess the outer ear.

- Inspect and palpate the auricle. Note the presence of lesions and nodules. Assess ear position. Determine patency of the external auditory canal.

▶ Small, abnormally shaped and low-set ears occur with many genetic syndromes and renal malformations. Mastoiditis, an acute infection of the mastoid bone, causes the external ear to protrude forward. Preschoolers frequently insert foreign objects, such as beads or rocks, in the external auditory canal.

2. Inspect the auditory canal and tympanic membrane.

- Restrain young or uncooperative children (see Figure 25.12). Young children have narrower auditory canals that angle downward. To assess the tympanic membrane of children under the age of 4 years, pull the tragus of the external ear down and back. Carefully insert the speculum of the otoscope into the ear, following the curve of the auditory canal. Assess the tympanic membrane for colour, opacity, mobility, position, and the presence of fluid or other abnormal findings. Use a speculum that fits tightly into the ear canal and gently press the bulb insufflator to assess tympanic membrane mobility. Look for dimpling, or inward movement, of the tympanic membrane lateral to the umbo. Normal tympanic membranes are pearly-grey, transparent, mobile, and neutrally positioned. The tympanic membrane is a vascular organ; it will redden with conditions that cause flushing (fever, crying, etc.).

▶ Reddening of the tympanic membrane, in the absence of purulent discharge, does not indicate the presence of middle ear infection. Otitis media causes full, orange-yellow coloured tympanic membranes with decreased motility. Otitis media with effusion, or serous otitis media, is the presence of nonpurulent fluid in the middle ear space caused by edema of eustachian tubes. Otitis media with effusion results in tympanic membranes that are amber-coloured, immobile, and in neutral to full positions. Figure 14.31 depicts otitis media. Otitis externa, or "swimmer's ear," results in pain with pinna manipulation and erythematous, edematous ear canals with or without purulent discharge. Figure 14.30 shows otitis externa.

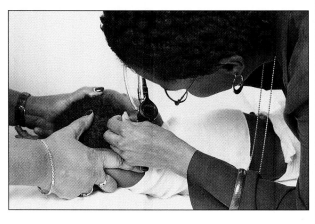

Figure 25.12 ●
Parent restraint of
a young child during
examination of
the ear.

3. Assess hearing.

- Use standardized hearing tests for children older than 4 years. Assess infants for the startle reflex or blinking with loud noises. To assess hearing in preschoolers, stand approximately 1.25 m (4 ft.) behind the child and whisper simple commands or ask simple questions.

▶ Refer any abnormalities or parental concerns about hearing for further evaluation.

PHYSICAL ASSESSMENT

| TECHNIQUES AND NORMAL FINDINGS | ABNORMAL FINDINGS AND SPECIAL CONSIDERATIONS |

NOSE AND SINUSES

1. **Assess the nose for nasal patency and septal deviation.**

   - Children under 6 months of age are obligate nose breathers. They will develop respiratory distress with blocked nasal passages. Determine and document the presence, colour, and consistency of any nasal discharge.

   ▶ Unilateral nasal discharge may indicate septal deviation, foreign body, or nasal polyps. Pale, boggy nasal turbinates occur with nasal allergies. Infection typically results in erythematous, edematous nasal turbinates, and mucosa. Purulent nasal discharge commonly occurs at the end of viral upper respiratory infection and is caused by ineffective clearing of the nasal passages.

2. **Assess the sinuses.**

   - The maxillary and ethmoid sinuses are present at birth, but they are proportionately smaller than in adults. The sphenoid sinuses develop before age 5 and the frontal sinuses by age 10. Children rarely have infections of the ethmoid sinuses. The frontal sinuses cause infection only in older school-age and adolescent children. Transillumination of the sinuses is not recommended because of poor sensitivity and specificity.

   ▶ Sinus pressure and tenderness of greater than 10 days' duration indicates sinusitis.

MOUTH AND THROAT

1. **Assess the mouth and teeth.**

   - Inspect and palpate the palate of newborns. Determine the location and order of the teeth. Document the presence of lesions and discharge. Movement of the uvula, tongue, and lips should be symmetrical.

   ▶ *Macroglossia* occurs with congenital hypothyroidism and Down syndrome. White plaques on the gums and buccal mucosa characterize oral thrush, caused by *Candida albicans* infection.

2. **Assess the pharynx and tonsils.**

   - Ask the child to open the mouth, and demonstrate what you want the child to do. Orient young children to the oropharyngeal exam by examining the mouth of a parent or a doll. Preschool and younger children are frightened by the oral exam; therefore, always assess the oropharynx last. Determine the presence and characteristics of postnasal drainage on the posterior pharynx. Children between 3 and 8 years of age often have enlarged, noninfected tonsils.

   ▶ Strep throat infection, caused by group A beta-hemolytic *Streptococcus pyogenes,* may cause yellow tonsillar exudates, erythematous and edematous pharynx, red tongue with prominent taste buds (strawberry tongue), and petechial hemorrhages on the soft palate near the uvula. Epiglottitis is an acute life-threatening infection caused by infection with Haemophilus influenzae type B that results in infection and edema of the epiglottis. Symptoms include high fever, marked stridor, drooling, forward sitting, and respiratory distress.

CLINICAL TIP

Never assess the oropharynx of a preschool child with suspected epiglottis because coughing, crying, or gagging precedes acute respiratory failure.

CHEST AND LUNGS

1. **Inspect the chest.**

   - Young children under the age of 6 years have round chests with prominent xiphoid processes. Abdominal breathing is common until age 6. Thoracic breathing begins in the school-age years. Infants have irregular breathing patterns that increase and decrease often. Pay special attention to respiratory effort and the presence of accessory muscle use. Note the presence of supernumerary nipples (if more than two).

   ▶ *Apnea* is the cessation of breathing for greater than 20 seconds. Funnel chest (pectus excavatum) causes a depression of the lower part of the sternum. Pigeon chest (pectus carinatum) causes bowing of the sternum. Illustrations of pigeon chest and funnel chest can be found in Box 15.3. Wide spacing of the nipples occurs with genetic syndromes, such as Turner syndrome.

PHYSICAL ASSESSMENT

| TECHNIQUES AND NORMAL FINDINGS | ABNORMAL FINDINGS AND SPECIAL CONSIDERATIONS |

2. Auscultate the chest.

- Lung sounds are louder in children because of their thinner chest wall. Listen carefully in all lung fields, including the apex of the lungs. Children can be encouraged to take deep breaths by blowing bubbles or blowing out the otoscope light.

▶ Referred sounds from upper airway congestion are common and are often described as "chest rattling." To distinguish upper airway congestion from lower airway congestion, listen at the trachea and near the mouth. Lung sounds are always loudest at the point of origin.

CARDIOVASCULAR

1. Assess the child for cyanosis and chest pulsations, and determine the PMI.

- Central cyanosis is more pronounced in the mucous membranes. Apical pulsation is normal in young children. The PMI of children under 4 years of age is difficult to assess and is located approximately one intercostal space higher than in adults.

▶ Pericardial heaves are always abnormal findings. Children with heaves should be referred to cardiology for evaluation.

2. Palpate pulses for symmetry, rate, and rhythm.

- Evaluate the symmetry and amplitude of the femoral pulses in newborns, infants, and toddlers.

▶ Coarctation of the aorta causes a narrowing of the descending aorta and results in diminished femoral pulses and bounding radial pulses.

3. Auscultate heart sounds.

- Sinus arrhythmia presents with heart rate increases during inspiration and decreases during expiration. An S_2 split with inspiration may be detected in children under the age of 6. The physiological S_2 split disappears with expiration. Any S_2 split that persists throughout the cardiac cycle merits further evaluation. Preadolescents may have a physiological S_3 gallop that results from vibrations during rapid ventricular filling. Refer to Table 25.2 for the common innocent heart murmurs. Pathological heart murmurs are described in Table 25.6.

TABLE 25.6	Common Pathological Heart Murmurs	
NAME	**LOCATION**	**TIMING OR ASSOCIATED CHARACTERISTICS**
Pulmonary valve stenosis	Upper left sternal border	Ejection click in early systole
Aortic valve stenosis	Midsternum and upper right sternal border	Early systolic ejection click. Growth failure with congestive heart failure.
Tetralogy of Fallot	Mid- to upper left sterna border	Continuous murmur. Cyanosis and poor weight gain.
Ventricular septal defect	Lower left sternal border	Pansystolic murmur. Signs of congestive heart failure and poor growth if large.
Atrial septal defect	Upper left sternal border	Systolic ejection murmur.
Patent ductus arteriosus	Upper left sternal border	Continuous murmur. Bounding pulses.

ABDOMEN

1. Inspect abdominal contour and movement.

- Infants and toddlers have prominent abdomens that result in a potbelly appearance. Umbilical hernias cause a protrusion at the umbilicus and are visible at birth.

▶ Umbilical hernias are common in Black children and in those of Mediterranean descent.

PHYSICAL ASSESSMENT

| TECHNIQUES AND NORMAL FINDINGS | ABNORMAL FINDINGS AND SPECIAL CONSIDERATIONS |

2. Ausculate the abdomen.

- Use deeper pressure for children with ticklish abdomens. Bowel sounds are present in all quadrants.

▶ Absence of bowel sounds requires further evaluation.

3. Palpate the abdomen.

- The lower liver edge is palpable 1 to 2 cm (0.5 to 1 in.) below the costal margin in most infants. Detect the presence of tenderness or masses.

▶ Constipation may result in a palpable cigar-shaped mass in the left lower quadrant. Wilms' tumour is a malignancy of the kidney commonly diagnosed in infants and toddlers. The most common presentation of Wilms' tumour is parental history of an abdominal mass felt during bathing or diaper changes. Refer children with suspected Wilms' tumour for immediate evaluation.

GENITALIA

1. Inspect the external genitalia.

- Genital maturation follows distinct patterns described by the Tanner stages, as illustrated in Table 21.2 and Table 22.1. Examination of the female internal genitalia is rare in children who are not sexually active. Refer to Chapter 22 for detailed information about the female pelvic examination. ⊂⊃ Examine the genitalia with the child in the supine position.

- Males: Determine the location of the urethral meatus. The normal urethra is centred at the tip of the glans penis. The scrotum should be symmetrical and should have a uniform colour.

▶ Males: Chordee is a fixed downward curving of the penile shaft. Hypospadias presents with an abnormal positioning of the urethral opening along the ventral glans or shaft of the penis as illustrated in Figure 25.13. Scrotal swelling may be caused by hydrocele or inguinal hernia.

CLINICAL TIP

The foreskin of uncircumcised males will not retract until the child is between 2 and 3 years old. Do not forcefully retract the foreskin of infants and toddlers. In older children with retractile foreskins, always return the foreskin to the natural position after urethral or glans examination.

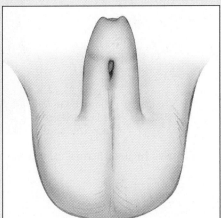

Figure 25.13 ● In hypospadias, the urethral canal is open on the ventral surface of the penis.

- Females: Facilitate inspection of the perineal area by placing the child supine with knees and hips flexed and externally rotated. This position is also referred to as the frog-leg position. To visualize the perivaginal area, grasp the labia majora between your thumb and forefinger and gently pull the labia majora up and out. Inspect the vaginal opening and the urethral meatus. Determine hymen patency. Newborns may present with a clear mucoid or blood-tinged vaginal discharge. Exposure to maternal hormones in utero causes "false menses."

▶ Females: Foreign bodies commonly cause malodorous, blood-tinged vaginal discharge. Vaginal foreign bodies, with the exception of those caused by retained toilet paper, are suspicious for sexual abuse. Box 25.3 lists signs of sexual abuse in children.

TECHNIQUES AND NORMAL FINDINGS

ABNORMAL FINDINGS AND SPECIAL CONSIDERATIONS

BOX 25.3	Signs of Sexual Abuse in Children

- Presence of vaginal foreign body (exception: retained toilet paper)
- Presence of condyloma acuminata (warts spread by sexual contact)
- Genital bruises, lacerations, or abrasions without plausible history of trauma
- Absence of hymenal tissue between the 3-o'clock and 9-o'clock positions
- Presence of perianal lacerations that extend to the anal sphincter
- Presence of purulent genital discharge (may indicate the presence of a sexually transmitted infection)

2. Palpate the external genitalia.
   - Males: Verify testicular positioning in the scrotum (see Figure 25.14). Foreskin retraction is impossible at birth. Normal foreskin retraction occurs between 2 and 3 years of age.

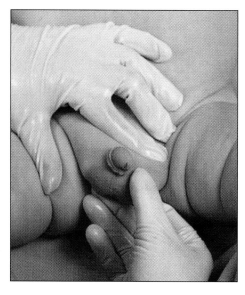

Figure 25.14 •
Palpating the scrotum for descended testicles and spermatic cords.

▶ Males: Hydrocele causes a painless, nonreducible, serous fluid accumulation in the scrotum. No treatment is necessary unless the hydrocele persists after the child's first birthday. Inguinal hernias cause a mass at the external inguinal ring. Incarcerated, or nonreducible, inguinal hernias are surgical emergencies that merit immediate surgical evaluation. Refer children with reducible inguinal hernias for surgical evaluation within 1 to 2 weeks. Cryptorchidism, or undescended testicle, is more common in preterm infants. Refer children with undescended testicles between 6 and 12 months of age for medical evaluation.

   - Females: Inguinal hernias cause a painful swelling of the labia majora in females.

▶ Females: Decreased estrogen production and genital atrophy cause labial adhesions. Labial adhesions present as a fused labia majora that obscures all or most of the perivaginal area. Refer any child with labial adhesions that impair urinary outflow for further evaluation and treatment.

TECHNIQUES AND NORMAL FINDINGS	ABNORMAL FINDINGS AND SPECIAL CONSIDERATIONS

MUSCULOSKELETAL

1. **Observe the child's gait and movements.**

   - Movements should be coordinated and equal. Ask preschoolers and older children to duck walk. The duck walk involves squatting and moving forward while flapping the upper arms. Any child who can duck walk has normal range of motion of the major joints, and normal muscle strength and coordination.

2. **Assess the upper extremities and neck.**

   - Notice symmetry and coordination of hand grip. Assess range of motion. Bilaterally inspect muscle symmetry and note the presence of weakness, masses, and swelling. Determine shoulder strength by having the child push, pull, and shrug the shoulders against resistance.

▶ *Polydactyly* is the presence of an extra finger or toe (see Figure 25.15). *Syndactyly* is webbed fingers or toes (see Figure 25.16). Birth trauma may result in a brachial plexus injury. One type of brachial plexus injury is Erb's palsy, a transient condition that results in paralysis of the shoulder and upper arm. Infants with Erb's palsy present with an intact palmar grasp and the inability to move the upper arm. Entire brachial plexus palsy results in no movement of the shoulder, arm, and hand. Unfortunately, this type of brachial plexus injury has a poor prognosis.

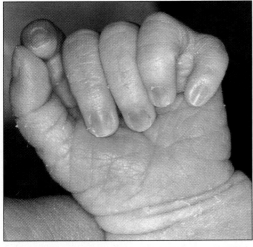

Figure 25.15 ● Polydactyly.

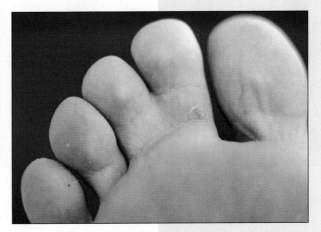

Figure 25.16 ● Syndactyly.

3. **Assess the lower extremities.**

   - Assess range of motion. Bilaterally inspect muscle symmetry and note the presence of weakness, masses, and swelling. Determine hip strength by having the child push and pull against resistance with the knees and hips flexed. Check for pelvic girdle weakness by assessing for Gowers' sign. Gowers' sign is the inability to get up from a seated or squatting position without pushing up with the arms (see Figure 25.17). Children under 2 years of age appear flatfooted. Genu varum, or bowlegs, is common until 1 to 2 years of age. Preschoolers and school-age children under 7 years old are often knock kneed, also known as genu valgum.

▶ Metatarsus adductus results in a C-shaped appearance of the foot that is caused by adduction of the forefoot. *Osgood-Schlatter disease* is a disorder of older children and adolescents caused by repetitive strain at the insertion of the quadriceps ligament at the tibial tubercle. It is more common in active children, especially those who participate in activities that require running, jumping, and squatting. Children with Osgood-Schlatter disease present with knee pain and tenderness over the tibial tubercle.

TECHNIQUES AND NORMAL FINDINGS	ABNORMAL FINDINGS AND SPECIAL CONSIDERATIONS

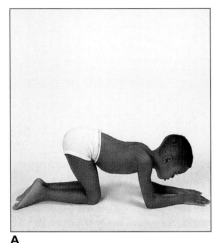

A

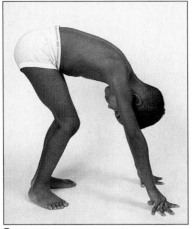

B

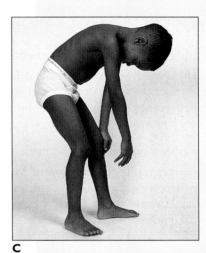

C

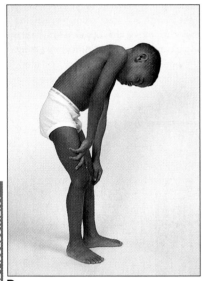

D

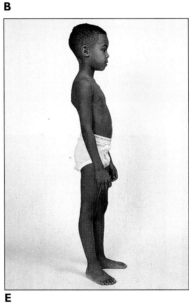

E

Figure 25.17 ● Gowers' manoeuvre. Since the leg muscles of children with muscular dystrophy are weak, these children must perform the Gowers' manoeuvre to raise themselves to a standing position. A and B. The child first manoeuvres to a position supported by arms and legs. C. The child next pushes off the floor and rests one hand on the knee. D and E. The child then pushes himself upright.

4. Assess the hips.

   ● Careful hip assessment is critical in children under 2 years of age. Abnormal development of the acetabulum causes developmental dysplasia of the hip. Determine symmetry of the fat folds of the gluteus and upper thighs. Place infants in a supine position with their legs extending toward you. To perform Ortolani's manoeuvre, flex the hips and knees at a 90-degree angle and abduct the hips while placing your thumb over the greater trochanter and your forefinger over the lesser trochanter. To perform Barlow's manoeuvre, keep your fingers in the same position and adduct the hip while gently lifting the thigh and placing pressure on the trochanter (see Figure 25.18).

CLINICAL TIP

Assess the hip of any child with a complaint of anterior thigh or knee pain.

▶ None of the following signs indicate definitive diagnosis of hip dysplasia. Refer any child with these findings for further evaluation and treatment. Unequal fat folds occur with improper acetabular placement as shown in Figure 25.19. A manual or audible clunk is positive for Ortolani's sign and Barlow's sign. Place the infant supine and bend both knees with the feet together. Positive Galeazzi's and Allis' signs present with unequal knee heights. Legg-Calvé-Perthes disease results from an avascular necrosis of the femoral head in children between 7 and 12 years of age. This disorder presents with refusal to bear weight on the affected side, altered gait, and pain with internal rotation and flexion of the hip. Slipped capital femoral epiphysis is the most common hip disorder of adolescents. It is more common in obese children and results in a limp or complete refusal to bear weight on the affected side and pain with internal rotation and flexion

PHYSICAL ASSESSMENT

TECHNIQUES AND NORMAL FINDINGS	ABNORMAL FINDINGS AND SPECIAL CONSIDERATIONS

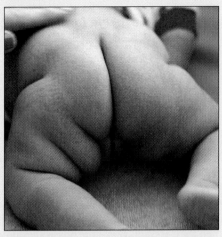

of the hip. Children with these disorders often present with a complaint of anterior thigh or knee pain.

Figure 25.19 ● The asymmetry of the gluteal and thigh fat folds is easy to see in this child with developmental dysplasia of the hip.

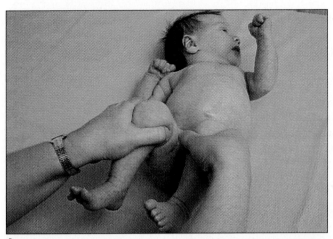

A

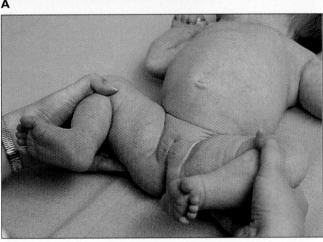

B

Figure 25.18 ● Ortolani-Barlow manoeuvre. A. Place the infant on his or her back and flex the hips and knees at a 90-degree angle. Place a hand over each knee with the thumb over the inner thigh, and the first two fingers over the upper margin of the femur. Move the infant's knees together until they touch, and then put downward pressure on one femur at a time to see if the hips easily slip out of their joints or dislocate. B. Slowly abduct the hips, moving each knee toward the examining table. Any resistance to abduction or a clunk felt on palpation can be an indication of a congenital hip dislocation.

5. Assess the spine.
   - Have the child stand with feet together and assess for symmetry of the trunk, spine, hips, and scapula. Stand in front of the child and ask him or her to bend forward with the arms extended until the fingers touch the floor. Carefully inspect the back, hips, and scapula for asymmetry.

▶ Scoliosis is a lateral curvature of the spine that usually presents during adolescence. Children with scoliosis present with uneven shoulders, hips, or scapula.

NEUROLOGICAL

1. Assess the child's mental status.
   - Determine the orientation of younger children by asking, "Is it time for breakfast, lunch, or dinner?" or "Who is your friend?" Note the child's energy level and ability to follow instructions. Normal preschoolers are active and alert and able to follow simple commands.

▶ Any change in the mental status, reflexes, cranial nerve function, and sensation and movement require further evaluation.

TECHNIQUES AND NORMAL FINDINGS	ABNORMAL FINDINGS AND SPECIAL CONSIDERATIONS

2. **Assess the child's development and determine the presence of infant reflexes.**

- Table 25.3 depicts and describes primitive reflexes in early childhood.

3. **Assess cranial nerve functioning and deep tendon reflexes.**

- Examine the cranial nerves and deep tendon reflexes with the same techniques discussed in Chapter 24 of this text. ⬭ Deep tendon reflexes are difficult to assess in young children because of their tendency to tense their muscles during the procedure. Tell preschoolers that you can make their legs "dance" before assessing the patellar reflex.

4. **Assess for coordination, sensation, and movement.**

- Ask if the child feels "tickles" during light stimulation. Ask children older than 3 years to draw a circle.

Many of the techniques provided in previous chapters are used during the pediatric health assessment. Remain flexible and take opportunities to assess specific systems when they present. Make the physical examination fun. Children will be less anxious and more cooperative if they view the nurse in a positive light.

APPLICATION THROUGH CRITICAL THINKING

CASE STUDY

Leon is a healthy 18-month-old who presents to the outpatient clinic for his well-child examination. His mother reports that Leon was born at 40 weeks' gestation after an uncomplicated pregnancy and vaginal delivery. Leon has met each developmental milestone at the normal age. Leon's mother tells the nurse that Leon is "a bundle of energy."
He sleeps approximately 10 hours each night and takes a 2- to 3-hour nap in the afternoon. He began walking at 13 months of age, and he now runs and climbs. His mother reports that Leon is "very picky" and will not eat "anything that is good for him." She reports that "Leon is healthy as a horse" and that he has never been ill "except for two ear infections last winter and colds every 2 months or so." Leon lives at home with his mother, his father (his parents are not married), and his older sister Martha (4 years old). The mother denies family problems.

▶ Complete Documentation

The following is a sample of the documentation from Leon's visit.

SUBJECTIVE DATA: Child presents for 18-month well-child examination. Birth history and past medical history negative for significant findings. 24-hour diet recall is as follows: breakfast—1 blueberry waffle, 1/2 banana, 250 mL (8 fl.oz.) whole milk; morning snack—170 g (6 fl.oz.) "fish" crackers and water; lunch—1 serving macaroni and cheese, 1/2 cup fruit cocktail (in fruit juice, not heavy syrup), and 250 mL (8 fl.oz.) whole milk; afternoon snack—1 apple and 175 mL (6 fl.oz.) apple juice; dinner—1/2 boneless, skinless chicken breast, 1 serving green beans, tossed salad, 1 dinner roll, 250 mL (8 fl.oz.) whole milk. He uses a sippy cup and a pacifier. Sleeps 12 to 13 hours per 24 hours. Mother denies concerns with Leon's health or development but is concerned about the adequacy of his dietary intake. Has soft, formed bowel movements daily. Wets at least 8 diapers every 24 hours.

OBJECTIVE DATA: Weight 13 kg (28 lb.), 70th percentile; height 85 cm (33.5 in.), 80th percentile.

▶ Critical Thinking Questions

1. Is Leon's growth and development normal?
2. Describe the nursing actions needed for Leon's heart murmur. Include discussion of management and evaluation parameters.
3. Document the above information using the SOAP format.

ASSESSMENT FORM

Vital Signs: *P 92—RR 24.*

Head: *Anterior fontanelle nonpalpable.*

Eyes: *Bilateral red reflux extra ocular movement intact (EOMI).*

Nose: *Patent. No discharge noted.*

Mouth: *16 teeth, large second molar bulges. Tonsils 21,*
pharynx pink and moist.

Ears: *TMs pearly grey in a neutral position with normal*
movement. No fluid noted.

Lymphatic: *Shotty anterior cervical nodes.*

Lungs: *Breath sounds clear.*

Heart: *Regular rate and rhythm. Clear S_1, S_2. II/VI systolic*
ejection murmur heard along left lower sternal border
when child supine. Murmur disappears when upright.
Femoral pulses equal bilaterally, 21 intensity.

Abdomen: *Soft, nondistended with potbelly appearance.*
No palpable tenderness or masses.

Spine: *Negative for asymmetry, tenderness, or masses.*

Genitalia: *Tanner 1 male with descended testes bilaterally.*

Musculoskeletal: *Full range of motion in all extremities.*
Normal muscle mass. Coordinated gait.
Genu varum present.

Neurological: *Speech 70% understandable. Uses one- to*
two-word sentences. Runs and climbs. Follows
one-step commands. Patellar, bicep, tricep
deep tendon reflexes. Cranial nerves I–XII intact.

▶ Applying Nursing Diagnoses

1. Use the NANDA-I taxonomy (see Appendix A ⚭) to identify one wellness diagnosis and one problem-oriented nursing diagnosis from the data provided in this case study.
2. From the data provided in this case, is the nursing diagnosis *alteration in cardiovascular function* (as stated in the NANDA-I taxonomy) a legitimate diagnosis? Explain your answer.
3. Through a subjective interaction with the mother, the nurse learns that the child has never been sick except for two ear infections in the last 2 months and "he seems to constantly have a runny nose." From this information, use the NANDA-I taxonomy to formulate at least two nursing diagnoses that would be appropriate for this child's illness episodes.

▶ Prepare Teaching Plan

LEARNING NEED: From the information obtained from the health history, the child has had two episodes of ear infections in 2 months and "seems to constantly have a runny nose."

GOAL: The child will experience a decrease in the number of ear infections and colds.

OBJECTIVES: At the completion of the session, the mother of the child will be able to do the following:

1. Identify risk factors for upper respiratory and ear infection.
2. Identify ways to reduce the spread of infection between family members.

Application of Objective 1: **Identify risk factors for upper respiratory and ear infection.**

Content	Teaching Strategy	Evaluation
• Children under the age of 2 have smaller eustachian tubes and more frequent upper respiratory infections because of their immature immune systems. Review the causes of upper respiratory infections in children. Review how a child of 18 months is not able to expectorate and effectively clear the nasal passages. • Children of this age group frequently place objects in the mouth, thus making them more susceptible to viral illness transmission. Bottle and pacifier use after the age of 6 months increases the risk of ear infection. Other risk factors include daycare attendance, exposure to cigarette smoke, allergies, and cleft lip or cleft palate.	• One-on-one discussion with the mother. • Provide printed materials. • Provide pamphlets about proper hand-washing. • The mother states she will return home and disinfect or clean Leon's toys.	• The mother states she will keep track of the number of colds and ear infections that both of her children have. • The mother identifies Leon's risk factors for upper respiratory infection and ear infection. • The mother identifies strategies that she can use to modify these risk factors.

(continued)

Application of Objective 1: Identify risk factors for upper respiratory and ear infection.		
Content	**Content (continued)**	
• Children often spread infection to other children. Leon has a sister who is 4 years old. Review the mechanism of transmission of microorganisms between individuals. • A few simple things can be done to help reduce the number of colds and ear infections that Leon is having. Everyone should use good hand-washing techniques after using the bathroom, after blowing the nose, after coughing, and anytime the hands are obviously soiled.	• If the daughter has a cold, it is best to keep her away from Leon and his toys. This might be difficult, but it will help Leon. • Leon needs plenty of fluids to keep his secretions thin. This will help clear them out of his nose and sinuses and could reduce the buildup that is leading to ear infections. • Noncompliance with therapy for otitis media increases the risk of subsequent resistant infection. Teach parents to give prescribed medicines as ordered and to follow up with the care provider as recommended.	

HEALTH PROMOTION ASSESSMENT TOOL

Social Determinants of Action	Level of Action	Action Strategies
Healthy child development	Family	**Develop personal skills** • Review Leon's 24 hour diet recall with his mother • Discuss her concerns about his dietary intake and "picky" eating habits. • Educate Leon's mother regarding normal child growth and development. Include the normalcy of variations in appetite, expected quantities of food an 18-month-old will ingest at each meal, and types of healthy food toddlers prefer. • Engage his mother in comparing Leon's intake to Canada Food Guide guidelines, together identifying healthy areas of his diet for improvement. • Provide Leon's mother with public health educational resources for review and for additional information. Include recipe ideas, normal child development, and food safety materials.
Physical environment	Family	**Create supportive environments** • Leon is running and climbing, therefore safety is an issue. Review the family's current safety precautions, such as playpen use, locked cabinets for storing medications and dangerous household chemicals and items, and removal of furniture close to windows to prevent Leon from accessing window blind cords (strangulation hazard) or from falling out windows. Additional precautions include placing childproof locks on cupboards and protective covers on electrical outlets.

Abnormal Findings

A number of abnormalities occur commonly during childhood. The following discussion includes descriptions of the typical assessment findings of some of the more common childhood abnormalities. Refer to pediatric nursing textbooks for more detailed and comprehensive information.

Otitis Media

Otitis media, or middle ear infections, results from bacterial or viral infection and is the leading cause of community-based nursing visits (see Figure 14.31). Acute otitis media (AOM) is a frequent complication of allergic rhinitis and upper respiratory infection whose peak incidence occurs between 6 and 18 months of age. Eustachian tubes connect the middle ear to the posterior pharynx and are shorter, straighter, and more level in young children than those in older children and adults. AOM results from the accumulation of middle ear fluid that contains viruses or bacteria. Children with middle ear infections typically present with pain, fever, decreased appetite, irritability, and altered sleep patterns. The tympanic membrane appears opaque, bulging, and yellow-orange or red during otitis media episodes. The tympanic membrane is a vascular tissue that appears red with infection, fever, or any condition that results in skin flushing. Children with red tympanic membranes and no purulent discharge in the middle ear space do not have bacterial otitis media. Risk factors for AOM include the following: bottle or pacifier use after 6 months of age, daycare attendance, exposure to cigarette smoke, personal history of Down syndrome, cleft lip, or cleft palate. Most cases of AOM result in antibiotic therapy, although recent clinical guidelines allow for watchful waiting for low-risk children.

Allergic Rhinitis

Allergic rhinitis is an immune hypersensitivity disorder that results from exposure to an allergen. Immune complex response results in the release of histamine, which causes increased mucus production, nasal congestion, lacrimation, and sneezing. Allergic rhinitis occurs in children from infancy through adolescence. Common clinical findings include darkening of the periorbital tissue under the eyes (also known as "allergic shiners"), periorbital edema, erythematous conjunctiva, clear nasal discharge, edematous and pale, often blue-tinged, nasal turbinates, and a cobblestone appearance of the posterior pharynx. Important findings include child or family history of atopic disease (asthma, allergy, eczema, hives) and history of recent exposure to pollen, animal dander, insect bites, or new goods. Parents of children with allergies often report sneezing "fits" where the child sneezes multiple times in succession, mouth breathing, and halitosis. The cornerstone therapy for allergic rhinitis is removal of the offending substances. Toddlers and older children may be treated with antihistamines, nasal corticosteroids, and leukotriene modifiers.

Asthma

Asthma is one of the most common chronic illnesses in childhood. Asthma is characterized by airway hypersensitivity, bronchospasm, and airway inflammation (see Figure 15.23). Initial asthma episodes may present from infancy through adolescence. Common asthma triggers include allergens (foods, pollens, danders, mould, grasses, weeds, and cockroaches), smoke, and viruses. Children with acute asthma episodes present with expiratory wheezes, dyspnea (retractions, nasal flaring, and grunting), tachypnea, and prolonged expiratory phases. Risk factors for asthma include infection with respiratory syncytial virus (RSV) and personal or family history of atopy. Asthma therapy is tailored to the severity and frequency of symptoms and includes inhaled bronchodilators, inhaled corticosteroids, leukotriene modifiers, and trigger avoidance.

Acne Vulgaris

Bacterial infections with *Propionibacterium acnes* and sebaceous gland occlusion cause acne vulgaris. Acne typically occurs on the face, upper chest, upper back, neck, and upper arms of adolescents. Acne is common during adolescence because of the influence of androgens on sebaceous gland secretion. Acne lesions may be open comedones (blackheads), closed comedones (whiteheads), and cysts (see Figure 25.20). Common acne treatments include cleansing with mild soap, keratolytics such as benzoyl peroxide, and topical antibiotic therapy.

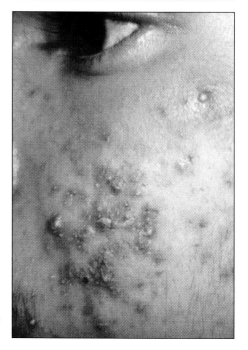

Figure 25.20 ●
Open and closed comedones of acne.

Scalp Ringworm (Tinea Capitis)

Tinea capitis is a superficial fungal infection of the scalp hair follicles that results in areas of alopecia characterized by hair follicle breakage at the skin surface (see Figure 11.77). The peak incidence occurs during school age. Epidermal scaling may occur inside the bald spots. Treatment of this disorder includes oral antifungals, such as griseofulvin, and selenium sulphide shampoo.

Acute Gastroenteritis

Acute gastroenteritis (AGE) is an acute, common diarrhea disease that may or may not be accompanied by vomiting. Nine percent of hospital admissions during childhood result from episodes of AGE. Additional symptoms include abdominal pain, cramping, and fever. Pertinent history findings include frequency and amount of diarrhea, vomiting, magnitude and duration of fever, and presence and location of abdominal pain. Exposure to infectious substances (salmonella, shigella, etc.) and people with similar symptoms, as well as questions regarding hydration status, are important parts of the history. Abdominal examination may reveal hyperactive bowel sounds. Assessment of hydration status is essential and should include documentation of level of consciousness, presence of thirst, time and amount of last urination, vital signs (heart rate and blood pressure), skin turgor, and capillary perfusion of less than 2 seconds.

CLINICAL TIP

Level of consciousness is the most accurate indicator of dehydration. Vital signs, skin turgor, and capillary perfusion will be present only with moderate to severe dehydration and indicate risk of cardiovascular collapse.

Nursing management of gastroenteritis focuses on the correction of electrolyte imbalances with oral rehydration therapy, intravenous fluid resuscitation, and administration of an age-appropriate diet in a nondehydrated child.

ABNORMAL FINDINGS

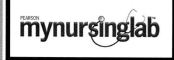

Visit the MyNursingLab website at **http://www.pearsoned.ca/mynursinglab**. This online homework and tutorial system puts you in control of your own learning with study and practice tools directly correlated to this chapter's content.

26

THE PREGNANT FEMALE

CHAPTER OBJECTIVES

On completion of this chapter, you will be able to

1. Relate knowledge of anatomy and physiology to the physical examination of the pregnant and postpartum client.
2. Identify landmarks that guide assessment of the pregnant female.
3. Relate knowledge of the principles of communication to the health history interview.
4. Conduct a health history interview that represents a comprehensive account of the client's physical and psychosocial health status in relation to her pregnancy.
5. Explain client preparation for assessment of the pregnant female.
6. Describe the different assessment techniques required for examination of the pregnant female.
7. Perform a physical examination of a pregnant client by using appropriate equipment and assessment techniques.
8. Differentiate between normal and abnormal findings in assessment of the pregnant female.
9. Describe developmental, psychosocial, ethnocultural, and environmental variations in assessment techniques and findings in relation to the pregnant female.
10. Apply critical thinking in selected situations related to assessment of the pregnant female.
11. Document findings of the examination of the pregnant female by using appropriate terminology.

CHAPTER OUTLINE

Pregnancy and the postpartum period offer a unique opportunity for health promotion, disease prevention, and changes in lifestyle behaviours through the actions of the nurse. For the vast majority of childbearing females, pregnancy and postpartum are normal processes that can be enhanced through education, healthcare, and supportive intervention. Changes in personal lifestyle behaviours and healthcare can influence not only the course of the pregnancy and the health of mother and child but also the health behaviours of the entire family in the future. Knowledge of variations in body systems during the three trimesters of pregnancy and postpartum periods will enable the nurse to differentiate normal from abnormal changes. The risk for and development of many pathological conditions in pregnancy and postpartum can be ascertained and prevented by a careful, thorough interview. Past medical, obstetric, gynecological, family, genetic, and social history will influence the focus of the physical assessment examination and teaching. Knowledge of lifestyle and health practices, nutrition and exercise history, environmental exposures, and current symptoms will also guide assessment and teaching. The physical assessment also provides an opportunity for client education and clarification of misperceptions. Cultural, familial, and personal beliefs can be discussed, as appropriate, during the history and examination. Whether the nurse is perceived as kind, personable, knowledgeable, and helpful, or cold, bureaucratic, ill informed, and ineffective will influence the client's willingness and ability to implement health recommendations. This life transition is also an opportunity for sharing much joy and excitement with childbearing families. The nurse can influence a whole generation through caring, accurate, and appropriate assessment and intervention (see Figure 26.1).

NUTRITIONAL ASSESSMENT

A comprehensive nutritional history is important when assessing the nutritional health of a pregnant female. Diet recall and food frequency questionnaires remain important tools to use to assess intake. Assessment of preconception diet should also be obtained in general detail as it provides the foundation for nutritional health in early pregnancy and beyond. Lactation needs are also addressed. Box 26.1 outlines specific data to be assessed when conducting a nutritional history of a pregnant female.

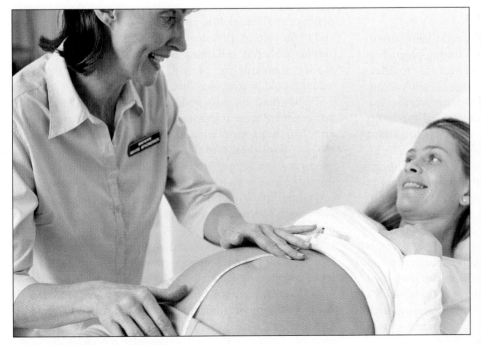

Figure 26.1 ● Nurse with pregnant client and family.

BOX 26.1	Nutritional History Data for Gestation and Lactation

Specific data must be gathered when conducting a nutritional history of a pregnant female:

Assess for Specific Foods and Nutrients

- Folic acid: fortified flour and cereals, orange juice, green leafy vegetables, legumes
- Calcium and vitamin D: dairy, fortified juices, fortified soy products
- Iron: meats, poultry, shellfish, fortified cereals and grains, legumes, dried fruit
- Vitamin B_{12}: if vegan, must be synthetic as plant sources are not bioavailable
- Fluids: include alcohol
- Caffeine: coffee, tea, cola and other soft drinks, cocoa, chocolate, OTC medications
- Mercury: recommendation is to limit large cold or fresh water fish to 340 g (12 oz.) per week

Assess for Eating Patterns and Behaviours

- Weight gain with any prior pregnancies
- Restrictive eating, missed meals, dieting attempts
- Cultural beliefs related to food and pregnancy
- Food aversions
- Pica (eating of nonfood items)
- Gastrointestinal complaints and any resultant alterations in diet

Assess for Supplement Use

- Prenatal vitamin compliance
- Iron supplement compliance
- Other vitamins: high intake of vitamin A is teratogenic
- Herbs: most untested in pregnant or lactating females
- Remedies for any pregnancy symptoms

TABLE 26.1	Guidelines for Gestational Weight Gain Ranges	
BMI CATEGORY	**RECOMMENDED TOTAL GAIN**	
	(KILOGRAMS)	**(POUNDS)**
BMI < 18.5	12.5–18.0	28–40
BMI 18.5–24.9	11.5–16	25–35
BMI 25.0–29.9	7.0–11.5	15–15
BMI ≥ 30ᵃ	5.0–9.0	11–20

Source: Health Canada. (2010). Canadian gestational weight gain recommendations. Retrieved from http://www.hc-sc.gc.ca/fn-an/nutrition/prenatal/qa-gest-gros-qr-eng.php
Note: These guidelines do not apply to women carrying multiple fetuses.
ᵃ A narrower range of weight gain may be advised for women with a prepregnancy BMI of 35 or greater. Individualized advice is recommended for these women.

Physical Assessment

The clinical examination of a pregnant female should include parameters to assess the nutritional health of the client and weight gain patterns necessary to support a healthy pregnancy.

Anthropometric Measurements

Weight, weight history, and gestational weight gain pattern and amount are important considerations during pregnancy. Preconception weight, height, and BMI are necessary to determine gestational weight gain goals. In pregnant adolescents, **gynecological age** should be determined to assess whether linear growth may still be occurring. Gynecological age is the difference between current age and age at menarche. Young women with a gynecological age of 3 years or less are considered to still be completing linear growth and will have competing nutritional needs between their own growth and that of the fetus. Weight gain guidelines are outlined in Table 26.1. Adolescents females are encouraged to strive for the upper limits of weight gain for their BMI because of the incidence of low-birth-weight babies in that population. Adolescents should gain weight early and continuously. Shorter women (less than 157 cm or 62 in.) are encouraged to gain weight at the lower end of their BMI range. Weight gain guidelines for specific racial and ethnic groups have had insufficient research to establish a consensus. For each client, the nurse should develop individual weight gain guidelines.

During the physical assessment the nurse can screen for factors for low weight gain patterns. Smoking, alcohol consumption, drug use, lack of social support, and depression have all been associated with low weight gain. An adolescent trying to hide a pregnancy may be at risk for low weight gain.

The nurse can also ask questions about the presence of physical symptoms that may be affecting nutritional status. Gastrointestinal discomfort, nausea and vomiting, constipation, and heartburn occur during pregnancy and can alter dietary intake and food tolerance. Follow-up questions should seek information on remedies used to relieve symptoms. A pregnant female with a history of an eating disorder and hyperemesis gravidarum (persistent and severe pregnancy-related vomiting) should be screened for current signs of an eating disorder. Box 26.2 outlines physical findings with an eating disorder.

Laboratory Measurements

Laboratory assessment of the pregnant female should routinely include screening for iron-deficiency anemia. The increased iron needs during pregnancy put many females at risk for iron deficiency. Hemoglobin and hematocrit decrease until the end of the second trimester because of the expansion of blood volume and red cell mass during pregnancy. Pregnancy-specific standards for normal hemoglobin and hematocrit values should be used (see Table 26.2).

Fasting plasma glucose and, if found to be above 7.0 mmol/L, subsequent glucose tolerance is performed between weeks 24 and 28 of the pregnancy to assess for gestational diabetes. Both the nutritional health of the mother and the outcome of the pregnancy can be negatively affected if diet changes are not instituted in females found to have gestational diabetes.

Plasma lipid levels increase during pregnancy as normal physiology and may be unrelated to nutrition, requiring no intervention.

Special consideration should be given to screen for plasma lead in females who report **pica**, the eating of nonfood items or ice, as consumption of earth or clay can be a source of environmental contamination. Females following a **vegan** diet, with no consumption of animal products, are at risk for vitamin B_{12} deficiency unless the diet is fortified or supplemented. Plant sources of vitamin B_{12} are not considered biologically avail-

BOX 26.2	Clinical Findings Consistent with Eating Disorders

The following are signs and symptoms of an eating disorder:

Bulimia or Binge-Purge Behaviour

- Bloodshot eyes
- Broken blood vessels on the face
- Swollen parotid glands or "chipmunk cheeks"
- Dental erosion
- Hoarse voice
- Scarring on the dorsal surface of the hand from teeth during purge attempts
- Poor or lacking gag reflex
- Weight fluctuations

Anorexia or Restrictive Eating Behaviour

- Cold intolerance
- Lanugo: soft, white hair growth on body
- Pedal edema
- Dry skin
- Alopecia
- Bradycardia
- Hypotension
- Amenorrhea in nonpregnant postmenarcheal females
- Loss of strength and muscle tone

General Eating Disorder Findings

- Body dissatisfaction. Ask: "How do you feel about your weight?" followed by "Have you ever tried to gain or lose weight? Tell me what you did."
- Constipation
- Bloating
- Fatigue

Table 26.2	Gestational Hemoglobin and Hematocrit References for Anemia

	FIRST AND THIRD TRIMESTERS	SECOND TRIMESTER
Hemoglobin (g/L)	<110	<105
Hematocrit (%)	<0.33	<0.32

Source: Compiled by author based on information from Public Health Agency of Canada. (2006). The Canadian guide to clinical preventive health care: Prenatal and perinatal preventive care. Retrieved from http://origin.phac-aspc.gc.ca/publicat/clinic-clinique/sec1-eng.php

able. Women without added synthetic vitamin B_{12} should be assessed for vitamin B_{12} status. Pregnant females with a history of phenylketonuria should have a plasma assay for phenylalanine to screen for elevated levels. Elevated phenylalanine levels are harmful to fetal brain development.

ANATOMY AND PHYSIOLOGY REVIEW

To implement programs of prenatal care to promote health, the nurse must understand the adaptations that occur in the female body during pregnancy and postpartum. The anatomical and physiological changes during the 40 weeks of pregnancy serve three important functions:

- Maintaining normal maternal physiological function
- Meeting maternal metabolic needs as the woman adapts to the pregnancy
- Meeting the growth and development needs of the fetus

An examination of the changes in each body system during pregnancy and postpartum will enable the nurse to interpret findings in the interview and assessment.

The Placenta

The physiological and anatomical changes in pregnancy are due to the hormones secreted by the fetus and placenta and the mechanical effects of the growing fetus. The human placenta is a unique organ that promotes and provides for fetal growth and development. Its functions include metabolism, transport of gases and nutrients, and secretion of hormones. It develops from the fertilized ovum, but generally also includes the maternal uterine lining at the site of implantation. The **placenta** is an ovoid organ that weighs approximately one sixth of the fetus and covers one third of the inner surface area of the uterus at term. Implantation of the fertilized egg, called a *blastocyst*, in the endometrium or lining of the uterus begins 6 days after fertilization. The umbilical blood vessels and placenta develop. Two arteries and a vein exit the fetus at the umbilicus, forming the umbilical cord, and insert in the centre of the placenta (see Figure 26.2). The fetal vessels branch out into treelike chorionic villi, where the fetal capillaries are the sites of exchange between the maternal and fetal circulations. The fetal and maternal circulations are kept essentially separate by the placental membrane covering the villi. The exchange of nutrients from the maternal to the fetal circulation takes place here, as well as passage of waste products, such as carbon dioxide and uric acid, from the fetal to maternal circulation. The placenta, in conjunction with the fetus and maternal uterine lining, also produces hormones, such as human chorionic gonadotropin (hCG), estrogen, progesterone, relaxin, prolactin, and other hormones.

Fetal Development

Pregnancy is divided into three trimesters, each lasting approximately 13 weeks (3 months in lay terms). The age of the fetus can be referred to in weeks beyond fertilization, used in discussion of fetal development, or **gestational age**, the age in weeks from the last normal menstrual period, more commonly used in prenatal care.

The first 2 weeks after fertilization are the early embryo stage, and disruptions in development, such as from environmental agents, usually cause death, or miscarriage. From 2 to 8 weeks after fertilization, the **embryo** is in the stage of *organogenesis*. During this period a **teratogen,** an agent, such as a virus, a drug, a chemical, or radiation, that causes malformation of an embryo or fetus, may induce major congenital anomalies. The fetal stage is from 8 weeks until birth (see Figure 26.3).

By the end of the first trimester, all major systems have formed. **Viability,** the point at which the fetus can survive outside the uterus, may occur as early as 22 weeks or at the weight

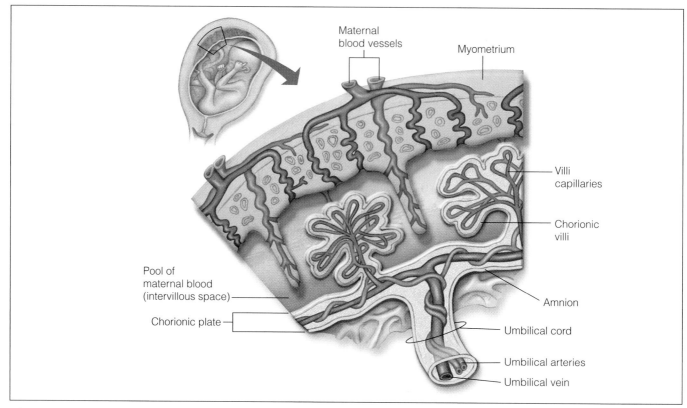

Figure 26.2 • Cross section of the placenta.

of 500 g (1 lb.). During the fetal period, the body grows, and differentiation of tissues, organs, and systems occurs.

Although fetal movement can be detected as early as 7 weeks through diagnostic techniques, **quickening,** the fluttery initial sensations of fetal movement perceived by the mother, usually occurs at approximately 18 weeks, possibly earlier in females who have given birth before.

The fetal heart begins beating at 22 days. During assessment, the fetal heartbeat can be heard via Doppler starting between 7 and 12 weeks of pregnancy. The uterine souffle, the sound of the uterine arteries, which is synchronous with the maternal pulse, may be heard, as well as the funic souffle, the sound of the umbilical vessels that is synchronous with the fetal heartbeat.

Fetal circulation before birth has three shunts that enable the fetus to maximize oxygenation from the maternal circulation since the lungs are not yet functional for oxygen exchange. Oxygenated blood from the placenta is carried via the umbilical vein to the fetus, entering at the umbilicus. The fetal liver is partially bypassed by the **ductus venosus,** so that highly oxygenated blood continues on to the heart. More highly oxygenated blood flows into the second shunt, the **foramen ovale,** which connects the fetal right atrium to the fetal left atrium. The other half of the blood continues to the right ventricle. The more highly oxygenated blood from the umbilical vein continues to the left ventricle and is shunted across the **ductus arteriosus** into the descending aorta. In this way, only a small part of the blood flow enters the pulmonary bed. The oxygenated blood then perfuses the rest of the fetal body and returns to the placenta via the umbilical arteries (see Figure 26.4).

Reproductive System Changes

In addition to the fetus and placenta, extensive changes occur in the reproductive organs. The uterus, cervix, fallopian tubes, and vagina undergo massive changes in size and function.

Uterus

The uterus is profoundly transformed in pregnancy. The crisscross muscle fibres of the body of the uterus increase in size and number because of the effects of progesterone and estrogen. The uterus increases in size from 70 to 1000 g (2.5 oz. to 2 lb.), and from 7.5 cm (3 in.) long, 5 cm (2 in.) wide, and 2.5 cm (1 in.) deep to 25 cm (10 in.) long, 20 cm (8 in.) wide, and 22.5 cm (9 in.) deep, and its capacity increases from 10 to 5000 mL (0.5 to 170 fl.oz.). During the second and third trimesters, the growing fetus also mechanically expands the uterus.

Early in pregnancy, the uterus retains its nonpregnant pear shape but becomes more globular by 12 weeks. Bimanual palpation is used to assess the size of the uterus during the early weeks. The early sizes can be compared to fruits: 6 weeks, lemon; 8 weeks, small orange; 10 weeks, large orange; 12 weeks, grapefruit. The growing uterus can be palpated abdominally by about 10 to 12 weeks, at which time the top of the uterus or **fundus** is slightly above the symphysis pubis. The female begins to "show" externally at approximately 14 to 16 weeks, later for a **primigravida,** a female pregnant for the first time, and earlier for a **multigravida,** a female who has been pregnant before. At 16 weeks, the fundus is halfway between the symphysis and umbilicus. Between 20 and 22 weeks, the fundus reaches the umbilicus. Fundal height increases until 38 weeks. The distance

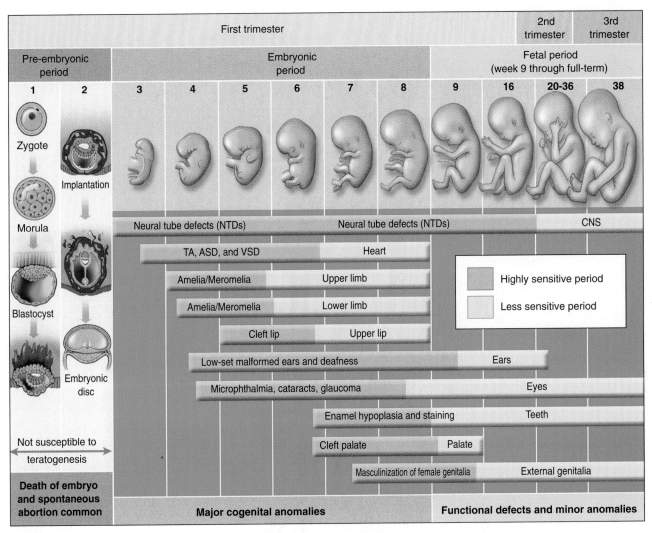

First trimester | 2nd trimester | 3rd trimester

Pre-embryonic period | Embryonic period | Fetal period (week 9 through full-term)

Zygote | Implantation | Morula | Blastocyst | Embryonic disc

Not susceptible to teratogenesis

Death of embryo and spontaneous abortion common

Neural tube defects (NTDs) | Neural tube defects (NTDs) | CNS

TA, ASD, and VSD | Heart

Amelia/Meromelia | Upper limb

Amelia/Meromelia | Lower limb

Cleft lip | Upper lip

Low-set malformed ears and deafness | Ears

Microphthalmia, cataracts, glaucoma | Eyes

Enamel hypoplasia and staining | Teeth

Cleft palate | Palate

Masculinization of female genitalia | External genitalia

Highly sensitive period | Less sensitive period

Major cogenital anomalies | **Functional defects and minor anomalies**

Figure 26.3 ● Fetal development.

from the symphysis pubis to the fundus is measured with a measuring tape to assess fetal growth and dating in pregnancy. **McDonald's rule** for estimating fetal growth states that after 20 weeks in pregnancy, the weeks of gestation approximately equal the **fundal height** in centimetres (see Figure 26.5). Between 38 and 40 weeks, **lightening**, or the descent of the fetal head into the pelvis, occurs, and the fundal height drops slightly.

Throughout pregnancy the uterus softens, as does the region that connects the body of the uterus and cervix, referred to as **Hegar's sign**. **Piskacek's sign** is the irregular shape of the uterus caused by the implantation of the ovum. The decidua or lining of the uterus becomes four times as thick during pregnancy. Amenorrhea, or the absence of menstruation, one of the first signs of pregnancy, occurs. The contractility of the uterus increases because of the action of estrogen. **Braxton Hicks contractions,** painless and unpredictable contractions of the uterus that do not dilate the cervix, start in the first trimester, are palpable to the nurse by the second trimester, and are felt by the mother usually starting in the third trimester. **Ballottement,** a technique of palpation, in which the examiner's hand is used to push against the uterus and detect the presence or position of a fetus by its return impact, can be elic-

ited after about 20 weeks, because the **amniotic fluid,** a clear, slightly yellowish liquid that surrounds the fetus, is greater in comparison with the still small fetus.

Cervix and Vagina

The cervix, or opening of the uterus, develops a protective **mucus plug** during pregnancy, through the action of progesterone, which also causes **leukorrhea,** a profuse, nonodorous, nonpainful vaginal discharge that protects against infection. Increased glycogen in vaginal cells predisposes the mother to yeast infections in pregnancy. **Goodell's sign** is the softening of the cervix starting at about 6 weeks. At the same time, increased vascularity causes the cervix and vagina to appear bluish (**Chadwick's sign**). Because of these changes the cervix is more friable and may bleed slightly with sexual intercourse or vaginal examination. Near the end of pregnancy, cervical **ripening,** or softening, and **effacement,** or thinning, occurs in preparation for labour. Progressive **dilation,** or opening of the cervix, does not usually occur until the onset of active labour. Externally, the labia majora, labia minora, clitoris, and vaginal introitus enlarge because of hypertrophy and increased vascularity.

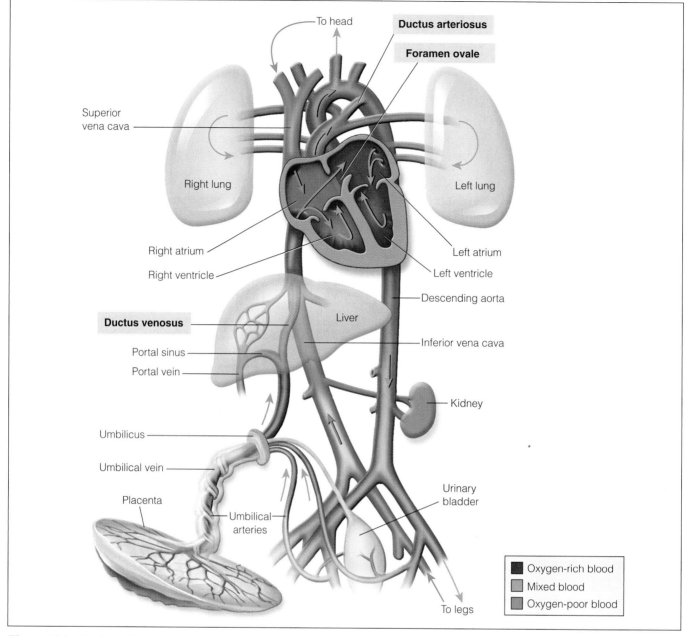

Figure 26.4 • Fetal circulation.

Changes in Breasts

One of the first symptoms in pregnancy is breast tenderness, enlargement, and tingling, which is noticeable at 4 to 6 weeks' gestation. These changes are caused by the growth of the alveoli and ductal system and the deposition of fat in the breasts under the influence of estrogen and progesterone. The nipple and the **areola,** the pink circle around the nipple, darken in colour in pregnancy, and the sebaceous glands on the areola, **Montgomery's glands** (or Montgomery's tubercles), enlarge and produce a secretion that protects and lubricates the nipples. With the doubling of the blood flow to the breasts, the vascular network above the breasts enlarges and becomes more visible. **Colostrum,** a yellowish specialized form of early breast milk, is produced starting in the second trimester and is replaced by

mature milk during the early days of lactation after labour (see Figure 26.6).

Respiratory System Changes

Mechanical and biochemical changes during pregnancy allow the respiratory needs of both mother and fetus to be met. The enlarging uterus lifts the diaphragm up 4 cm (1.5 in.), the transverse diameter of the chest increases, the ribs flare, and the subcostal angle increases. The increasing hormonal levels of progesterone and relaxin allow these changes in the thorax.

The respiratory-stimulating properties of progesterone contribute to the following:

- A slight increase in respiratory rate of about 2 breaths per minute

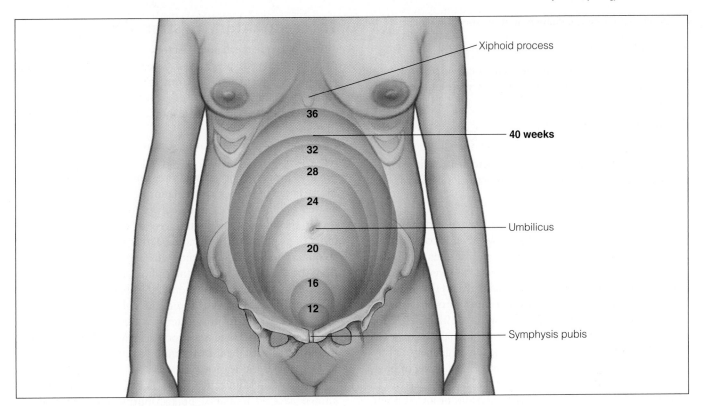

Figure 26.5 ● Fundal height in pregnancy.

- A lowered threshold for carbon dioxide, contributing to a sense of dyspnea by the pregnant female
- Decreased airway resistance
- Increased tidal volume and inspiratory capacity
- Decreased expiratory volume

The vital capacity is unchanged, but oxygen consumption is increased 20% to 60%. The pregnant female may report great fatigue, particularly in the first trimester, because of these changes. Hyperventilation may occur, and rales in the base of the lung may be heard as a result of compression by the growing uterus.

Cardiovascular and Hematological System Changes

The most significant hematological change is an increase in blood and plasma volume of 30% to 50%, and even greater in multiple pregnancies, beginning at 6 to 8 weeks. This change is facilitated by three factors:

- The increased progesterone leads to decreased venous tone.
- The increased progesterone combined with increased estrogen results in increased sodium retention and an increase in total body water.
- The shunt of blood to uteroplacental circulation provides physical space for increased plasma volume.

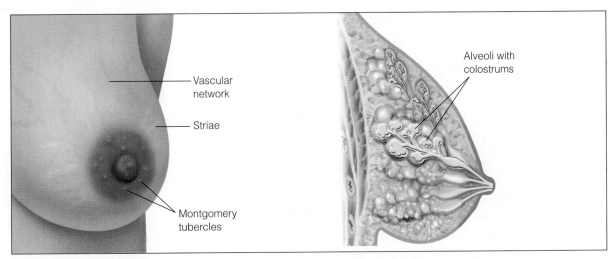

Figure 26.6 ● Breast changes in pregnancy.

Other hematological changes include the following:

- A 25% to 33% increase in red blood cells (RBCs)
- A decrease in hemoglobin and hematocrit or **physiological anemia** caused by plasma volume increase outpacing the increase in RBCs
- A gradual increase in reticulocytes
- An increase in white blood cells (WBCs)
- A hypercoagulable state caused by increased activity of most coagulation factors and decreased activities of factors that inhibit coagulation

Physical changes in the cardiac system include cardiac enlargement caused by the increased blood volume and accompanying increase in cardiac output. The upward displacement of the diaphragm by the growing uterus shifts the heart upward and to the left. Most pregnant females will have an S_1 sound that is louder. Systolic murmurs are usually heard. A murmur over the mammary vessels, the **mammary souffle,** caused by increased blood flow, is occasionally heard. The heart rate gradually increases by 10 to 20 beats per minute (bpm) during the pregnancy.

Blood pressure remains the same at the beginning of pregnancy. The decrease in vascular resistance leads to a decrease in diastolic blood pressure that reaches its nadir, or lowest point, during the second trimester and gradually returns to baseline by the time of delivery.

The changes in hemodynamics can cause orthostatic stress when the female changes position from sitting to standing or lying to sitting. **Supine hypotension syndrome,** also known as the vena cava syndrome, occurs when pressure from the pregnant uterus compresses the aorta and the inferior vena cava when the female is in the supine position (see Figure 26.7). She may experience dizziness, syncope, and a significant drop in heart rate and blood pressure.

Decreased peripheral resistance leads to increased filling in the legs, but the pressure of the growing uterus on the femoral veins restricts venous return, leading to increased dependent edema, and varicosities in the legs, vulva, and rectum (hemorrhoids).

Integumentary System Changes

Hormonal and mechanical factors cause the integumentary changes seen with pregnancy. Categories of change include alterations in pigmentation, connective tissue, vascular system, secretory glands, skin, hair, and pruritus. The changes are not usually pathological but are a source of concern to expectant mothers.

Alterations in pigmentation, the most common integumentary changes in pregnancy, are caused by the increase in estrogen and progesterone early in pregnancy and by the increase in placental hormones and melanocyte-stimulating hormone, as well as others, later in pregnancy. Any areas of pigmentation in the body, including the areolae, axillae, perineum, and inner thighs, will usually become darker for females of all skin colours. The *linea alba,* a tendinous line that extends midline from the symphysis pubis to the xiphoid, darkens with the progression of the fundus up through the abdomen and becomes the **linea nigra.** *Melasma,* also called chloasma or the "mask of pregnancy," occurs in a butterfly pattern over the forehead, nose, and cheeks. There is a strong genetic predisposition, and it is also seen with the use of combined oral contraceptive pills. Freckles, nevi, and scars may also darken in pregnancy.

A change in connective tissue is **striae gravidarum,** also known as stretch marks, pinkish-purplish streaks that are depressions in the skin. Caused by the stretching of the collagen in skin, they develop in the second half of pregnancy and fade to silver in the postpartum; unlike most integumentary changes, they do not resolve completely after pregnancy. They may develop in the lower abdomen, breasts, thighs, and buttocks.

Vascular alterations that affect the integumentary system are spider angiomas or nevi, and palmar erythema. Spider angiomas or nevi are arterioles dilated at the centre, with branches radiating outward, appearing on the face, neck, and arms. They fade after pregnancy, but do not usually disappear. They often occur with palmar erythema, a reddening or mottling of the palms or fleshy side of the fingers, which occurs after the first trimester, has a genetic predisposition, and regresses by the first week after birth.

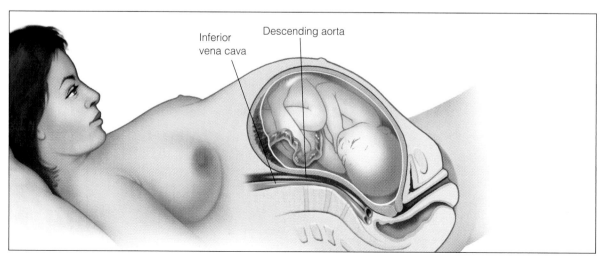

Figure 26.7 ● Supine hypotension in pregnancy. The weight of the uterus compresses the vena cava, trapping blood in the lower extremities.

Alterations in secretory glands in pregnancy include a decrease in apocrine sweat gland activity in the axillae, abdomen, and genitalia. The eccrine sweat glands in the palms, soles, and forehead increase in activity because of increases in thyroid and metabolic activity, allowing for dissipation of increased heat. Some females experience a "glow" in their skin during pregnancy, while some experience an increase in acne caused by increased sebaceous gland activity.

A skin change that sometimes occurs in the second half of pregnancy is the development of soft, pedunculated, flesh-coloured or pigmented skin tags. They occur on the sides of the face and neck, on the upper axillae, between and under the breasts, and in the groin.

Because of the hormonal influence of estrogen in pregnancy, more hairs enter the growth phase. Some females experience mild hirsutism and report thicker hair. Consequently, more than the usual number of hairs reach maturity and fall out in the postpartum period during months 1 to 5. Usually all hair regrows by 6 to 15 months postpartum. Occasionally nails become soft or more brittle.

Pruritus (itching) is common in the abdomen in the third trimester. If it is severe, it must be distinguished from rare dermatological disorders in pregnancy, such as cholestasis of pregnancy, pruritic urticarial papules and plaques of pregnancy (PUPPP), herpes gestationis, and prurigo of pregnancy. Figure 26.8 depicts integumentary changes in pregnancy.

Changes in the Ear, Nose, Throat, and Mouth

An increase in estrogen increases vascularity throughout the body in pregnancy. Increased vascularity of the middle ear may cause a feeling of fullness or earaches. Increased blood flow (hyperemia) to the sinuses can cause rhinitis and epistaxis. The sense of smell is heightened in pregnancy. Edema of the vocal cords may cause hoarseness or deepening of the voice. Hyperemia of the throat can lead to an increase in snoring. In the mouth, small blood vessels and connective tissue increase. Gingivitis or inflammation of the gums occurs in many females. This leads to bleeding and discomfort with brushing and eating.

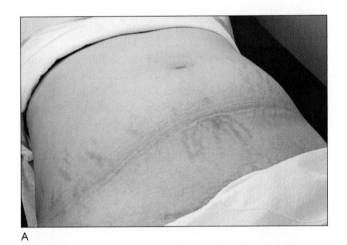

A

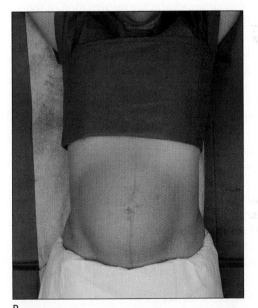

B

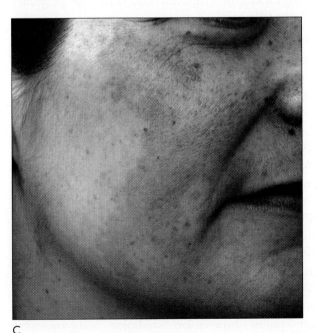

C

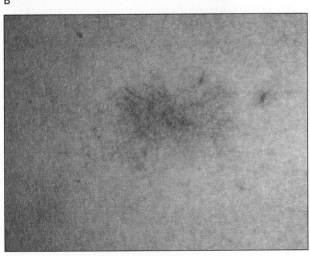

D

Figure 26.8 ● Integumentary changes in pregnancy. A. Striae. B. Linea nigra. C. Melasma. D. Spider angioma.

Occasionally a hyperplasic overgrowth forms a mass on the gums called epulis, which bleeds easily and recedes after birth.

Gastrointestinal System Changes

Nausea and vomiting are common beginning at 4 to 6 weeks and usually resolve by 12 weeks' gestation. The exact cause is unknown, although hormonal and psychological factors have been implicated. Other gastrointestinal changes occur during the second and third trimesters. *Ptyalism,* an increase in saliva production, may occasionally occur with nausea and vomiting. The pregnant female may also report pica, an abnormal craving for and ingestion of nonnutritive substances such as starch, dirt, or ice. Mechanical pressure from the growing uterus contributes to displacement of the small intestine and reduces motility. The increased secretion of progesterone further reduces motility because of decreased gastric tone and increased smooth muscle relaxation; thus, the emptying time of the stomach and bowel is prolonged, and constipation is common. Progesterone's relaxing effect on smooth muscle also accounts for the prolonged emptying time of the gallbladder, and gallstone formation may result. *Pyrosis,* or heartburn, the regurgitation of the acidic contents of the stomach into the esophagus, is related to the enlarging uterus displacing the stomach upward and to the relaxation of the esophageal sphincter. Hemorrhoids are another common finding in the third trimester, resulting from the increasing size of the uterus creating pressure on the pelvic veins. If the mother is constipated, the pressure on the venous structures from straining to move the bowels can also lead to hemorrhoids.

Nutritional demands of the pregnancy and fetus increase the maternal requirements. Each day, the mother requires an increased intake of 300 calories, and 15 g (0.5 oz.) or more of protein. Most nutrient requirements increase from 20% to 100%. The recommended weight gain for females of average weight is 11.5 to 16 kg (25 to 35 lb.), 12.5 to 18 kg (28 to 40 lb.) if underweight, 7.0 to 11.5 kg (15 to 25 lb.) if overweight, and 5.0 to 9.0 kg (11 to 20 lb.) if obese.

Urinary System Changes

The growing uterus causes displacement of the ureters and kidneys, especially on the right side. A slower flow of urine through the ureters causes physiological hydronephrosis (stretching) and hydroureter (distension of the ureter). Estrogen causes increased bladder vascularity, predisposing the mucosa to bleed more easily. Urinary frequency occurs in the first trimester as the uterus grows and puts pressure on the bladder. Relief from frequency occurs after the uterus moves out of the pelvis, only to return in the third trimester when the enlarged uterus again presses on the bladder.

The functional changes in the urinary system include the following:

- Increased renal blood flow of 35% to 60%
- Increased glomerular filtration rate by as much as 50% above prepregnancy levels
- Decreased reabsorption of filtered glucose in the renal tubules, contributing to glycosuria

- Increased tubular reabsorption of sodium, promoting necessary retention of fluid
- Decreased bladder tone because of the effects of progesterone on smooth muscle, and increased capacity
- Dilation of ureters leading to increased risk of urinary tract infection
- Nocturia (increased urination at night) caused by dependent edema resolving while recumbent

Musculoskeletal Changes

Anatomical changes in the musculoskeletal system result from the influence of hormones, growth of the fetus, and maternal weight gain. Round ligaments, which attach to the uterus just under the fallopian tubes and insert in the groin, may cause sharp, shooting lower abdominal and groin pain in early pregnancy as the uterus enlarges. As pregnancy advances, the growing uterus tilts the pelvis forward, increasing the lumbosacral curve and creating a gradual lordosis, and the stretching of the broad ligament attaching the uterus to the sacrum may cause back pain (see Figure 26.9). The enlarging breasts pull the shoulders forward, and the client may assume a stoop-shouldered stance. The pelvic joints and ligaments are relaxed by progesterone and relaxin. The rectus abdominis muscles that run vertically down the midline of the abdomen may separate during the third trimester. This is called **diastasis recti abdominis** and may allow the abdominal contents to protrude (see Figure 26.10). The weight of the uterus and breasts, along with the relaxation of the pelvic joints, changes the client's centre of gravity, stance, and gait. Muscle cramps and ligament injury are more frequent in pregnancy. Shoe size, especially width, may increase permanently.

Neurological System Changes

Neurological changes frequently associated with pregnancy include the following:

- Increase in frequency of vascular headaches
- Entrapment neuropathies caused by mechanical pressures in the peripheral nervous system
- Sciatica (pain, numbness, or tingling) in the thigh, caused by pressure of the growing uterus on the sciatic nerve
- Carpal tunnel syndrome: pressure on the median nerve beneath the carpal ligament of the wrist, causing burning, tingling, and pain in the hand
- Change in corneal curvature, increased corneal thickness or edema, or change in the tear production, causing changes in optical prescription
- Increased total sleep time and insomnia in first and third trimesters
- Leg cramps, which may be caused by inadequate intake of calcium
- Dizziness and light-headedness, which may be associated with supine hypotension syndrome and vasomotor instability

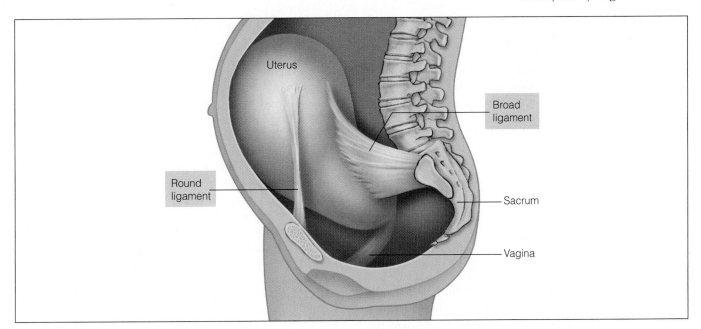

Figure 26.9 ● Round and broad ligaments.

Endocrine System Changes

Changes in the endocrine system facilitate the metabolic functions that maintain maternal and fetal health throughout the pregnancy. Human chorionic gonadotropin (hCG), the hormone that is detected by pregnancy tests, is secreted by tissue surrounding the embryo soon after implantation. It serves as a messenger to the corpus luteum to maintain progesterone and estrogen production until the placenta starts to produce these hormones at approximately 5 weeks. It also may be involved in the suppression of maternal immunological rejection of the fetal tissue.

The fetus and placenta become additional sites for synthesis and metabolism of hormones. The pituitary, thyroid, parathyroid, and adrenal glands enlarge because of estrogen stimulation and increased vascularity. Increases in the production of thyroid hormones, particularly T_3 and T_4, increase the basal metabolic rate (BMR), cardiac output, vasodilation, heart rate, and heat intolerance. The BMR may increase eightfold.

Changes also occur in the metabolism of protein, glucose, and fats because of the increasing production of human placental lactogen (hPL) by the placenta. Throughout pregnancy, protein is metabolized more efficiently to meet fetal needs. In the second trimester, insulin production increases in response to the rising glucose levels, and falls to prepregnancy levels at the end of pregnancy. In addition, the mother's body tissues develop a decreased sensitivity to insulin, sometimes referred to as the diabetogenic state of pregnancy. This ensures an adequate supply of glucose, which the fetus requires in large amounts. A disruption in this delicate homeostatic balance results in gestational diabetes mellitus (GDM). A form of glucose-sparing called accelerated starvation causes the metabolism of fats stored in pregnancy, which makes more glucose available to the fetus but puts the pregnant female at greater risk of ketosis;

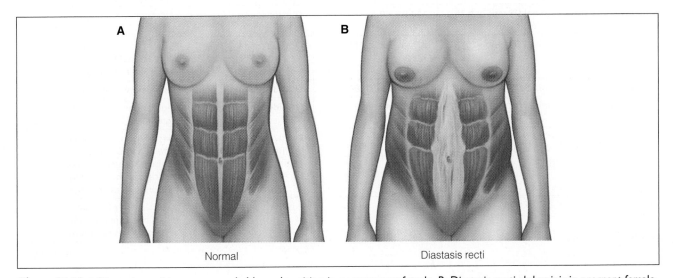

Figure 26.10 ● Diastasis recti in pregnancy. A. Normal position in nonpregnant female. B. Diastasis recti abdominis in pregnant female.

ketones are harmful to the fetal brain. Pregnant females are at increased risk of lipolysis during pregnancy secondary to hypoglycemia or prolonged fasting.

After birth, *oxytocin,* secreted by the posterior pituitary, stimulates uterine contractions and causes milk ejection in the mammary glands. Prolactin, secreted by the anterior pituitary, increases production of breast milk after delivery.

SOCIAL AND ETHNOCULTURAL VARIATIONS

At the time of pregnancy and birth, women of various cultures will have unique perspectives and practices regarding delivery. Culturally safe nurses will know or seek information about cultural practices of specific groups; however, they will not stereotype clients and assume that the clients ascribe to specific cultural practices. With the diverse cultural population in Canada, nurses need to be aware that many different beliefs about pregnancy, childbirth, the postpartum period, and the newborn exist.

In 2001, the Society of Obstetricians and Gynaecologists of Canada (SOGC) created a clinical practice guideline titled *A Guide for Health Professionals Working with Aboriginal Peoples* and in 2003 published a policy statement on diversity to make a visible commitment to the advancement of Aboriginal women's health and well-being. The SOGC is also working toward the removal or reduction of systemic barriers that have prevented the participation of minorities as consumers of healthcare.

Some ethnic backgrounds are at greater risk for carrying particular genetic disorders. For example, the Ashkenazi Jewish population is routinely screened for a variety of conditions, such as Tay-Sachs disease, that tend to have an increased incidence of occurring in that population. Although population-based screening is not currently recommended for the French-Canadian population, Tay-Sachs disease is also common in that group, and a thorough familial history must be obtained for all pregnant women.

The best tool for providing a healthy start for a child is to ensure that the mother's determinants of health are met. Working with mothers at risk for poor child health outcomes is a key program strategy for public health worldwide and a priority in the World Health Organization's millennium goals. Access to prenatal care, early childhood development, and the reduction of risky health behaviours significantly affect the health of the mother and, ultimately, the fetus.

LABORATORY TESTS IN PREGNANCY

Several types of laboratory tests are performed during pregnancy. Table 26.3 provides information about the tests, when they should be performed during pregnancy, the normal and abnormal values, and any client education that is needed as follow-up.

TABLE 26.3	Tests in Pregnancy			
NAME OF TEST	**TIMING OF TEST IN PREGNANCY**	**NORMAL VALUE**	**ABNORMAL VALUES**	**SPECIAL TEACHING**
Blood type, Rh factor, and antibody screen	Initial OB visit and 26 weeks for Rh-negative females	A, B, AB, O, Rh+ or Rh–; no irregular antibodies	Irregular antibodies found	If not her first pregnancy, inquire about previous Rh immune globulin WinRho administration if Rh⁻.
Hematocrit	Initial OB visit and 36 weeks	0.33 to 0.44 (33% to 44%)	Outside range	Eat iron-rich foods. Report any bleeding.
Hemoglobin	Initial OB visit and 36 weeks	110 to 140 g/L	Outside range	Effects of pregnancy on iron needs.
CBC	RBC	Initial OB visit	3.8 to 5.2 1012/L	Outside range	Red cell indices will also be examined to R/O hemoglobinopathies.
	WBC	Initial OB visit	4.5 to 11.8 109/L	Outside range	Report signs of infection.
	Platelets	Initial OB visit	140 to 440 109/L	Outside range	Report abnormal bleeding from gums, bruising.
HIV		Offered at initial OB visit and prn	Negative	Positive Confirmed by further testing: Western blot	Specific informed consent obtained prior to testing. Advise of dramatic decrease in vertical (mother to child) transmission with medication.
Hepatitis B		Initial OB visit	Negative	Positive	Inform client of sexual transmissibility. Explain importance of prophylaxis for infant.

(continued)

TABLE 26.3 | Tests in Pregnacy *(continued)*

Gonorrhea	Initial OB visit; third trimester if high risk	Negative	Positive	Educate client about infection. Empathetic listening if +. Stress importance of compliance and partner treatment.
Chlamydia	Initial OB visit; third trimester if high risk	Negative	Positive	Address STI prevention.
Rubella titre	Initial OB visit	Immune	Nonimmune	Recommend maternal immunization after birth. Stress the avoidance of pregnancy for 3 months after immunization. Avoid first-trimester exposure to infection because of risk of congenital rubella syndrome.
Tuberculin skin testing	Initial OB visit if high risk	Negative	Positive induration > 10 mm in nonimmuno-compromised client	Educate mother about infection. Teach respiratory precautions. Encourage smoking cessation.
Urinalysis	Initial OB visit	Negative	Presence of protein, glucose, ketones, RBCs, WBCs	
Urine culture	Initial OB visit	Negative	Positive bacteria > 100 000 col	Wipe from front to back during toileting. Report urgency, flank pain, frequency, burning on urination.
Papanicolaou smear	Initial OB visit (if not done in previous 6–12 months)	Negative	Epithelial cell abnormalities or neoplasms present	Refrain from intercourse or douching 2 to 3 days before test (for accuracy). Discuss individualized schedule of testing.
VDRL (syphilis)	Initial OB visit; third trimester	Nonreactive	Reactive FTA-ABS reports a ratio	Educate about infection stages and treatment; advise compliance and abstinence during treatment; reinforce importance of follow-up.
Maternal serum triple screen	15 to 20 weeks' gestation; first trimester	No increased risk	Elevated risk	Discuss conditions screened for and limitations of test. Emphasize need for diagnostic testing if screen is positive.
50 g glucose challenge test	24 to 28 weeks; may be done at initial prenatal visit for clients with increased risk of GDM	< 7.8 mmol/L	> 7.8 mmol/L	Not fasting; blood drawn exactly 1 hour after glucose is drunk.
Oral glucose tolerance test (OGTT)	Follow-up to elevated 1 hour screen	Fasting ≥ 5.3 mmol/L 1 h plasma glucose (PG) ≥ 10.6 mmol/L 2 h PG ≥ 8.9 mmol/L	Two or more values met or exceeded	Three days of unrestricted carbohydrates and physical activity; fasting before test; no smoking or caffeine before and during test; inform re: schedule of blood draws.
Group B streptococcus	Third trimester/35 to 37 weeks	Positive	Negative	IV antibiotics will be given in active labour to decrease risk of transmission to infant.
Ultrasound	Optional, frequently at 16 to 20 weeks, dependent on rationale	Normal	Abnormal	Client can decide whether she wants to know the sex of the child; some ultrasound studies require vaginal probe; nuchal translucency test at 11 weeks is to screen for chromosomal abnormalities.

THE POSTPARTUM FEMALE

The critical role of the nurse in assisting clients through the maternity cycle continues after the birth with postpartum assessment.

Anatomy and Physiology Review

During the postpartum period, the reproductive organs return to the nonpregnant state through the process of involution. Immediately after the delivery of the placenta, the uterine fundus is located midway between the symphysis pubis and the umbilicus. The fundus rises to the umbilicus by 12 hours later, and decreases approximately 1 cm (0.5 in.) or a fingerbreadth per day until it is nonpalpable externally by 10 days. The contracted uterus is firm, preventing postpartum hemorrhage through ligation of the uterine arteries by the contraction. The uterus is longer and wider in mothers who have a caesarean section and shorter in mothers who breastfeed.

The uterine lining or endometrium returns to the nonpregnant state through the process of a postpartum vaginal discharge called lochia. The initial *lochia rubra* contains blood from the placental site, amniotic membrane, cells from the decidua basalis, vernix and lanugo from the infant's skin, and meconium. It is dark red and has a fleshy odour, and lasts anywhere from 2 days to 18 days. Next the discharge becomes pinkish and is called *lochia serosa*. It is composed of blood, placental site exudates, erythrocytes, leukocytes, cervical mucus, microorganisms, and decidua, and lasts approximately a week. Finally, the discharge becomes whitish-yellow, *lochia alba,* and is composed of leukocytes, mucus, bacteria, epithelial cells, and decidua. Most females will have vaginal discharge from 10 days to 5 or 6 weeks.

The cervix closes over the next 2 weeks, and the vagina regains the folds or rugae. Decreased lubrication and lacerations or surgical incisions to the perineum cause discomfort. Hemorrhoids caused by pelvic pressure during pregnancy or pushing during childbirth may occur. Gastric motility slows during labour and resumes afterward. Bowel movements usually restart after 2 to 3 days postpartum. The urethra may be bruised, swollen, or damaged by childbirth or episiotomy.

After birth, the breasts become engorged or full from the swelling of the lymphatic tissue and initial milk production. At days 2 to 4, the mature milk starts to be produced by the alveoli, with a lower protein and immunoglobulin content and higher fat content than the initial colostrum, and engorgement occurs.

The hormones estrogen and progesterone, secreted by the placenta, decrease rapidly after birth. Prolactin, which controls milk production, increases after birth. Oxytocin acts on the smooth muscle of the uterus and muscle cells surrounding the breast alveoli. In nonbreastfeeding mothers, menses return at 6 to 10 weeks postpartum. In lactating mothers, menses usually does not return for 12 or more weeks; with exclusive breast-feeding and introduction of solid foods after 6 months, amenorrhea may last a year or more. Eighty percent of first menses in lactating mothers are preceded by anovulatory cycles caused by the action of prolactin. These hormonal swings, combined with role changes and exhaustion, can contribute to the development of postpartum depression.

In the circulatory system, it may take up to 6 weeks for slowed blood velocity and relaxed veins to return to the nonpregnant state, so a risk of thromboembolism remains during the postpartum period. In the renal system, diuresis occurs days 2 to 5, and decreased bladder tone and urinary retention can be worsened by birth trauma.

The BUBBLESHE Head-to-Toe Postpartum Assessment

With all the physiological changes occurring in the postpartum period, a thorough postpartum assessment plays an important role in healthcare. The mnemonic BUBBLESHE can be used to remember the steps in assessing a postpartum client.

B	Breast
U	Uterus
B	Bowel
B	Bladder
L	Lochia
E	Episiotomy and perineum
S	Support system
H	Homans' sign and extremities
E	Emotional state

In preparation for the postpartum assessment, the nurse gathers the following supplies: lab coat, stethoscope, black ink pen, and penlight. Before entering the room, it is important to review the data needed to fill out the assessment flow sheet (data on pain, urinary tract infection [UTI] symptoms, voiding, stooling, flatus, bleeding, support system, bonding, etc.) as well as to complete the physical assessment. Establishing a good rapport with the client is important while conducting the physical exam. The nurse should project caring and confidence, and use eye contact.

Throughout all aspects of the assessment the nurse must be sure to maintain the client's privacy and dignity.

Assess the vital signs, and auscultate the lungs, the heart, and the abdomen. Inspect the IV saline lock site. Examine the client's breasts, palpate for costovertebral angle tenderness, and palpate the fundus.

Inspect the lower extremities for vascular changes, and assess for edema. Some facilities may still use the Homans' test to assess for deep vein thrombosis (DVT); however, this test has been found to have low sensitivity in predicting the presence of a clot. Look for colour changes, warmth, and increase in calf circumference as other means to assess for DVTs. Place the client in a lateral position to inspect the perineum and rectum.

Gathering the Data

The role of the nurse in assessment of the pregnant female includes collecting subjective data from the health history. Objective data are obtained from the physical assessment. Objective data are also obtained from secondary sources, such as health records, the results of laboratory tests, and radiological and ultrasound studies. Preparation includes gathering equipment, positioning, and informing the client about the physical examination.

HEALTH HISTORY

At the first prenatal visit, a very thorough history is conducted. Important information that may dramatically affect the health of the fetus and mother can be obtained; the quality of the relationship with the client for the entire pregnancy is begun. The environment for the interview should be comfortable, quiet, private, and relaxing.

Health History Questions	Rationales

The following sections provide sample questions for the pregnant female. Rationales for most questions are provided. The list of questions is not comprehensive but represents the type of questions required in a comprehensive prenatal health history.

Confirmation of Pregnancy

Before the provision of a prenatal history and physical assessment, the nurse must be sure that the client is indeed pregnant. Pregnancy can be determined through urine and serum pregnancy tests, as well as signs and symptoms of pregnancy.

Urine pregnancy tests test for the beta subunit of hCG and can be accurate 7 days after implantation or can indicate pregnancy before the missed menstrual period. These tests produce results in 1 to 5 minutes and are 99% accurate. Serum pregnancy tests may indicate pregnancy as soon as 7 to 9 days after ovulation or just after implantation. This test can be qualitative, with a value of positive or negative, or quantitative, with a level of hCG reported. Serum progesterone can also be obtained if necessary; nonviable pregnancies have lower levels than normal pregnancies.

Presumptive signs of pregnancy are symptoms the client reports that may have multiple causes other than pregnancy. These presumptive signs include amenorrhea, breast tenderness, nausea and vomiting, frequent urination, quickening or the client's perception of fetal movement, skin changes, and fatigue. Probable signs are elicited by the nurse and have few causes other than pregnancy. Probable signs include positive pregnancy test, abdominal enlargement, Piskacek's sign, Hegar's sign, Goodell's sign, Chadwick's sign, and Braxton Hicks contractions. Positive signs of pregnancy have no possible explanation other than pregnancy. These include hearing the fetal heart with Doppler, or ultrasound, fetal movements verified by the examiner, and visualization of the fetus via ultrasound or radiology.

Demographics

For the purposes of identification, statistics, and record keeping, the following information must be collected for each pregnant client.

1. **What is your complete name and nickname?**

   ▶ Knowing the client's nickname is important during stressful situations, such as labour.

2. **What is your address?**

3. **What is your date of birth?**

   ▶ This also screens for age-related complications.

4. **What is your race or ethnic background?**

   ▶ See Chapter 4 for more detail regarding questions about race and ethnic identity. ⚭ This question also screens for race- or ethnicity-related genetic disorders.

HEALTH HISTORY QUESTIONS	RATIONALES

5. **Do you work outside the home? How many hours per week do you work? Describe your activities at work.**

▶ This also screens for occupational hazards to the mother and fetus.

6. **Are you married, single, divorced, or widowed, or do you have a partner?**

7. **What is your baby's father's name?**

8. **What is your partner's name, if that is a different person?**

9. **Who is your emergency contact, and what is his or her phone number?**

10. **Who lives with you?**

▶ Questions 6 to 10 provide information about the client's support system.

11. **What is your religion?**

▶ This provides information that may relate to maternity care, such as attitudes toward blood products.

12. **How many years of school have you completed?**

▶ This information will assist in the development of the teaching plan.

Menstrual History

1. **When was the date of your last menstrual period?**

▶ The estimated date of birth (EDB), also known as the estimated date of delivery (EDD), estimated date of confinement (EDC), or due date, is usually calculated by using the first day of the last menstrual period (LMP), which may also be useful in estimating gestational age.

2. **Were you using any methods of contraception at the time you conceived?**

▶ Although oral contraceptive pills have not shown any adverse effects on pregnancy, their use does affect the timing of ovulation. An IUD in place at the time of conception can cause complications in the pregnancy.

3. **Describe your usual menstrual cycle.**

▶ The typical menstrual cycle is 28 days. Prolonged, shortened, or irregular menstrual cycles affect the EDB. If the LMP was not normal for the client, it may have been implantation bleeding or a menstrual dysfunction. Some prenatal charts ask for last normal menstrual period (LNMP) to assist in dating the pregnancy.

4. **Have you had any cramping, bleeding, or spotting since your LMP?**

▶ Cramping, bleeding, or spotting may indicate a problem with hormonal support of the endometrium and may lead to a spontaneous abortion.

5. **How old were you when you got your first menstrual period?**

▶ The number of years since **menarche**, or age of first menstrual period, helps determine physical maturity of the client.

Calculating Estimated Date of Birth and Gestational Weeks

A pregnancy lasts approximately 266 days from conception, or 280 days from the LMP, based on a 28-day cycle. **Naegele's rule** can be used to compute the EDB based on the LMP (see Box 26.3). To use this approximate guide to determine the due date, 7 days are added to the day of the month of the first day of the LMP, 3 is subtracted from the number of the month (12 is added to the month number if the LMP occurs in January, February, or March), and the year of the due date is the year of the LMP, plus one year if January 1 is passed during the pregnancy.

HEALTH HISTORY QUESTIONS	RATIONALES

BOX 26.3	Using Naegele's Rule to Compute an Estimated Date of Birth (EDB)

EXAMPLE: LMP = January 29, 2012

Rule = first day of LMP + 7, number of month – (year of LMP + 1 if January 1 is passed during pregnancy)

Jan 29

30	Day 1	Month Dec = 12th month
31	2	Jan = 13 (if LMP is in January, February, or March)
Feb 1	3	Feb = 14 (add 12 to month to prevent negative number) 14 – 3 = 11 = November
2	4	
3	5	
4	6	
5	7	

Due date = November 5, 2012

A gestational wheel is a two-layer, round, computational device, usually made of laminated paper, which can also be used to compute the EDB and weeks of gestation. Each day of the month in the year has a line on the outer wheel, and each day of the week of the pregnancy has a line on the inner wheel. Zero weeks and days indicates the LMP, and 40 weeks indicates the EDB on the inner wheel. If the zero or LMP line on the inner wheel is aligned with the date of the LMP on the outer wheel, the EDB can be found by determining which date lines up with 40 weeks. If the LMP or EDB is correctly lined up with its date on the outer wheel, the current date on the outer wheel will line up with the gestational age (e.g., 36 weeks and 4 days, often recorded as 36.4 or 36-4/7, based on a 7-day week).

The third way that the EDB can be determined is through the use of ultrasound in the first half of pregnancy. The EDB should be shared with the client as soon as it is determined, along with its degree of certainty. The fact that a due date actually is the middle day of a month straddling the due date by 2 weeks on each side should be emphasized.

Obstetrical and Gynecological History

1. **Have you experienced any discomfort or unusual occurrences since your LMP?**

▶ The client's response allows the nurse to evaluate whether the symptoms reported are expected or if they suggest development of a complication. The client will most likely report subjective signs of pregnancy, such as absence of menstrual periods, nausea, vomiting, breast tenderness, fatigue, abdominal enlargement, or urinary frequency. Client teaching and other nursing interventions can also be identified.

Reaction to Pregnancy

1. **Was this pregnancy planned?**

▶ Confirmation of pregnancy usually causes ambivalent feelings whether or not the pregnancy was planned. If the pregnancy was unplanned, the nurse needs to assess the mother's desire to maintain the pregnancy and explain available options.

2. **How do you feel about this pregnancy? How does your family (if applicable) and partner (if applicable) feel about the pregnancy?**

▶ This discussion can strengthen the relationship between the nurse and the client and provide important cues to the client's home environment.

HEALTH HISTORY QUESTIONS	RATIONALES

Past Obstetrical History

1. **Have you been pregnant before? If so, how many times?**

▶ Multiparity, especially if there have been more than four previous pregnancies, increases the maternal risks of antepartal and postpartal hemorrhage and fetal or neonatal anemia. Teaching needs are also affected by the client's previous experiences.

2. **Have you had any spontaneous or induced abortions?**
   - If so, how far along in weeks were you?
   - Did you have any follow-up, such as a D&C (dilation and curettage) procedure?

▶ Previous history of persistent spontaneous abortion (miscarriage or stillbirth) places the client at higher risk for subsequent spontaneous abortions. Induced abortions may cause trauma to the cervix and may interfere with cervical dilation and effacement during labour.

3. **Describe any previous pregnancies, including the length of the pregnancy, the length of labour, problems during pregnancy, medications taken during pregnancy, prenatal care received, type of birth, and your perception of the experience.**

▶ Discussion of the client's previous pregnancies helps the nurse anticipate needs and complications of the current pregnancy.

4. **Describe your birth experience, including labour or delivery complications, the infant's condition at birth, the infant's weight, and whether the infant required additional treatment or special care after birth.**

▶ Reviewing the client's previous birth experience(s) helps to anticipate needs and complications of the current pregnancy and to assess the client's current knowledge base and the success with which the client integrated the previous birth experience into her life experiences. An example of a previous complication that would affect the current pregnancy is group B streptococcus (GBS) colonization. If a client has a history of GBS colonization of the vagina in a previous pregnancy, her baby has a risk for early-onset infection that has serious morbidity and mortality, so she will need to be treated in labour with antibiotics.

5. **Do you attend or plan to attend prenatal education classes?**

▶ Assessment of prenatal education provides information on the client's current knowledge base and attitude toward education for self-care.

6. **What are your expectations for this pregnancy?**

▶ Identification of the client's desires helps the nurse provide guidance in formulating the birth plan in the present pregnancy.

Past Gynecological History

1. **When was your most recent Pap smear and what was the result?**

▶ Abnormal Pap smears must be followed up during pregnancy the same way as at any time.

2. **What methods of birth control have you used in the past? How satisfied were you with each method?**

▶ This will influence teaching on this topic later in the pregnancy.

3. **Have you previously been tested for STIs? If so, when and what was the result?**

▶ This addresses risk for sexually transmitted infections (STIs).

4. **Have you ever had a sexually transmitted infection?**
   - What was the treatment?
   - Were your partners treated and notified?

▶ Untreated STIs can cause complications in pregnancy.

5. **Have you had any problems with or surgeries on your breasts, vagina, fallopian tubes, ovaries, or urinary tract?**

▶ Problems in the genitourinary system may affect pregnancy. Fibroids will affect the measurement of fundal height during pregnancy. Some types of vaginitis can cause preterm labour.

GATHERING THE DATA

Health History Questions

Rationales

6. **Have you ever been sexually assaulted? Did you receive any care afterward?**

▶ A history of sexual abuse is linked to complications in pregnancy and may influence a client's psychological adaptation to pregnancy.

7. **Do you have a history of infertility?**

▶ Many causes of previous infertility can affect the current pregnancy. For example, pelvic inflammatory disease increases a client's risk of an ectopic pregnancy.

Past Medical History and Family History

1. **Have you or any members of your family or your partner's family had any of the following conditions?**
   - Hypertension
   - Heart disease
   - Asthma
   - Kidney or gallbladder problems
   - Diabetes mellitus
   - Blood or bleeding disorders
   - Hepatitis
   - Cancer
   - Infectious diseases, such as HIV, tuberculosis, and chickenpox
   - Allergies

▶ The nurse needs to assess the family medical history to identify and investigate risk factors thoroughly. Preexisting maternal conditions may increase maternal and fetal risk.

▶ *Hypertension:* Mild to moderate hypertension poses the risk of intrauterine growth restriction (IUGR) and fetal death. When combined with smoking, there is an increased risk of placental abruption, when the placenta shears off the uterus, which is highly dangerous to mother and child.

▶ *Heart disease:* Mitral valve prolapse complicated by regurgitation requires antibiotic prophylaxis to prevent bacteremia (bacterial infection of the blood).

▶ *Asthma:* The nurse should ask if asthma is well controlled, how stable medication levels have been, and which medications are currently being used. Asthma can cause fetal growth restriction and may necessitate serial ultrasounds to follow growth in the intrapartum period. Meperdine and morphine for pain relief, and prostaglandin F2a to control postpartum hemorrhage, are not recommended for use by clients with asthma.

▶ *Kidney and gallbladder disease:* Previous occurrences of urinary tract infection may increase risk for asymptomatic bacteriuria, the presence of bacteria in the urine without the usual symptoms of cystitis of urinary frequency, burning on urination, and flank pain. Asymptomatic bacteriuria may lead to pyelonephritis (kidney infection). Urinary tract infections in pregnancy are associated with preterm labour and birth, low birth weight, anemia, amnionitis (infection of the membrane inside the uterus), hypertension, and preeclampsia. Gallbladder problems may be exacerbated in pregnancy.

▶ *Diabetes:* Pregestational diabetes (diabetes that was present before the pregnancy) is associated with fetal anomalies and pregnancy loss.

▶ *Blood and bleeding disorders:* Blood disorders, such as anemia, are associated with urinary tract infections, preterm delivery, low birth weight, preeclampsia, and perinatal mortality, if the anemia occurs before the third trimester. Females with sickle-cell anemia and thalassemia have an increase in maternal and perinatal mortality and morbidity. If the client has sickle-cell trait, she may have an increase in UTIs and iron- and folate-deficiency anemia.

Health History Questions

Rationales

Female clients with thalassemia minor should be monitored for anemia.

▶ *Hepatitis:* If a pregnant client has a past history of hepatitis B and is part of the 6% to 10% that go on to become carriers, there is a risk of transmission to the newborn, as well as to her sexual partners. The infant should receive hepatitis B immunoglobulin as well as the HBV vaccine.

▶ *Cancer:* If cancer of the cervix was treated with cone biopsy, the client is at risk for pre-term labour.

▶ *Infectious diseases:* HIV transmission to the newborn can be dramatically reduced by treat-ment in pregnancy. Tuberculosis treatment in pregnancy decreases neonatal mortality and morbidity. If the client does not report a history of varicella (chicken-pox) and is not immune by blood test, she is susceptible to infection during pregnancy, which can be very harmful to the fetus or newborn. Varicella-zoster immune globulin can be given to exposed mothers and infants.

▶ *Allergies:* Allergies are identified in the prenatal period in case medications are rec-ommended during the perinatal period. The nurse should note the type of reaction.

2. **What medications have you taken since your last menstrual period?**

▶ This will help identify any teratogenic exposures as well as medications for illnesses and symptoms. Drugs in pregnacy are rated in risk categories A, B, C, D, and X (see Box 26.4).

BOX 26.4	Drugs in Pregnancy: Risk Categories

A: Adequate and well-controlled studies in pregnant women have not shown an increased risk of fetal abnormalities.

B: Animal studies have revealed no evidence of harm to the fetus; however, there are no adequate and well-controlled studies in preg-nant women, or animal studies have shown an adverse effect, but adequate and well-controlled studies in pregnant women have failed to demonstrate a risk to the fetus.

C: Animal studies have shown an adverse effect and there are no adequate and well-controlled studies in pregnant women, or no animal studies have been conducted and there are no adequate and well-controlled studies in pregnant women.

D: Adequate well-controlled or observational studies in pregnant women have demon-strated a risk to the fetus. However, the ben-efits of therapy may outweigh the potential risk.

X: Adequate well-controlled or observational studies in animals or pregnant women have demonstrated positive evidence of fetal abnormalities. The use of the product is con-traindicated in women who are or who may become pregnant.

HEALTH HISTORY QUESTIONS	RATIONALES

3. **Have you ever had a blood transfusion?**

▶ This will help identify increased risk for abnormal antibody reactions, or blood-borne pathogens.

4. **What infections and immunizations have you had?**
   - Did you have chickenpox as a child?

▶ Some infections, such as rubella, can cause birth defects. If the client has hepatitis B, her newborn may need hepatitis B immunoglobulin and vaccine after birth. Prior immunizations and exposures affect the client's risk for contracting certain infections during pregnancy. Chickenpox, or varicella, can cause abnormalities in the fetus if contracted between 8 and 20 weeks in pregnancy.

5. **Review of systems questions: For each body system the nurse should discuss benign and worrisome changes in pregnancy. For example, "Describe any changes you have experienced regarding your skin, digestion, bowel function, muscles and joints, or vision."**

▶ This discussion will ensure that the pregnant client recalls each system, and it provides an important teaching opportunity.

Genetic Information

To obtain information to determine genetic risk factors, the nurse will ask the client about three generations of her family. This is called a medical family tree or genetic pedigree. These questions refer to the client's brothers and sisters, her mother and father, her aunts and uncles on both sides, her grandparents and their siblings, all her children, and all her cousins on both sides. This information is also needed for the baby's father's family.

1. **Please tell me the date of birth and, if applicable, death, as well as any health problems or diseases for each of these individuals. For those who have died, tell me what the cause was, and date of death.**

▶ Three generations of medical history are needed to determine recessive and dominant genetic diseases.

2. **Do you or the baby's father, or anybody in your families, have any of the following conditions?**
   - Sickle-cell anemia or trait
   - Thalassemia
   - Down syndrome
   - Cystic fibrosis
   - Huntington's disease
   - Muscular dystrophy
   - Tay-Sachs
   - Hemophilia
   - Any other blood or genetic disorders

▶ Sometimes charting the medical family tree will not jog the memory of the client, but a specific mention of the condition will.

3. **What is your ethnic background?**

▶ Tay-Sachs occurs more frequently in Ashkenazi Jews and French Canadians in Eastern Quebec. Cystic fibrosis trait occurs in 1 in 29 northern Europeans (see Table 26.4).

TABLE 26.4	Genetic Disorders and Traits with Increased Frequency by Ethnicity
ETHNIC GROUP OR GEOGRAPHIC LOCATION	**GENETIC DISORDERS AND TRAITS WITH INCREASED FREQUENCY**
Africans and Descendants	Sickle-cell anemia Alpha- and beta-thalassemia Glucose-6-phosphate dehydrogenase (G6PD) Fy (Duffy) antigen Rh positive Arcus cornea Café au lait spots Clubbing of digits Polydactyly Vitiligo Abnormal separation of sutures Earlobe absent Keloid Hereditary hypertrophic osteoarthropathy Scaphocephaly Alpha-antitrypsin deficiency

(continued)

TECHNIQUES AND NORMAL FINDINGS

RATIONALES

TABLE 26.4	Genetic Disorders and Traits with Increased Frequency by Ethnicity *(continued)*
ETHNIC GROUP OR GEOGRAPHIC LOCATION	**GENETIC DISORDERS AND TRAITS WITH INCREASED FREQUENCY**
Europeans and Descendants	Cystic fibrosis Neural tube defects Congenital spherocytic anemia Phenylthiocarbamide (PTC) taster Red-green colour vision defect Alpha1-antitrypsin deficiency Baldness Cleft lip and palate Hemophilia A Congenital dislocation of the hip Hereditary spherocytosis Phenylketonuria XYY syndrome
Ashkenazi Jews	Tay-Sachs disease Niemann-Pick disease Gaucher's disease Canavan's disease Torsion dystonia Familial dysautonomia Nonclassical 21-hydroxylase deficiency Bloom's syndrome Hereditary breast cancer
Sephardic and Oriental Jews	G6PD Familial Mediterranean fever Gaucher's disease Beta-thalassemia Laron-type dwarfism
Puerto Rican	Sickle-cell anemia
Mediterranean	Sickle-cell anemia Alpha-thalassemia
Southeast Asian	Alpha-thalassemia Beta-thalassemia
Italian	Beta-thalassemia
Greek	Beta-thalassemia
Middle Eastern	Sickle-cell anemia
French Canadian	Tay-Sachs disease Familial hypercholesterolemia
Lebanese	Familial hypercholesterolemia
Denmark	Alpha1-antitrypsin deficiency
Hispanic	Sickle-cell anemia
Scotland	Phenylketonuria
Finland	Phenylketonuria Gyrate atrophy
Japan	Phenylketonuria

Sources: Mahowald, M. B., McKusick, V. A., Scheuerle, A. S., & Aspinwall, T. J. (2001). *Genetics in the clinic: Clinical, ethical, and social implications for primary care.* St. Louis, MO: Mosby; Lea, D. H., Jenkins, J. F., & Francomano, C. A. (1998). *Genetics in clinical practice: New directions for nursing and health care.* Boston, MA: Jones & Bartlett; Nussbaum, R. L., McInnes, R. R., & Willard, H. F. (2001). *Thompson & Thompson genetics in medicine.* Philadelphia, PA: W. B. Saunders.

GATHERING THE DATA

HEALTH HISTORY QUESTIONS	RATIONALES

Lifestyle and Social Health Practices

1. **How much do you smoke per day? Does anyone in your household smoke?**

   ▶ Smoking doubles the risk of a low-birth-weight baby and increases the risk of ectopic pregnancy or placental complications. It also increases the infant's risk of sudden infant death syndrome (SIDS), asthma, and autism after birth. Second-hand smoke exposure also may contribute to low birth weight.

2. **Since the start of pregnancy, how many alcoholic drinks have you consumed each day?**

   ▶ Any amount of alcohol consumption during pregnancy can cause fetal alcohol syndrome and related disorders, composed of physical, neurological, and behavioural defects in the infant.

3. **What recreational drugs have you used since your last menstrual period? This includes marijuana, cocaine, heroin, prescription painkillers, methadone, and so on.**

   ▶ Cocaine and other drugs have been shown to cause miscarriage and multiple fetal defects.

4. **Have you ever been emotionally or physically abused by your partner or someone important to you?**
   - Within the last year, have you been pushed, shoved, slapped, hit, kicked, or otherwise physically hurt by someone?
   - If yes, by whom?
   - Within the last year, have you been forced to have sex?
   - If yes, by whom?
   - Are you afraid of your partner or anyone else?

   ▶ All female clients should be screened during each trimester for abuse. At least 4% to 8% of females report abuse during pregnancy (Public Health Agency of Canada, 2004), which makes abuse more common than most complications screened for in pregnancy, such as diabetes and hypertension. Abuse can cause miscarriage, fetal trauma, maternal stress, smoking, and drug abuse. Risk factors for abuse in pregnancy include unintended pregnancy, unhappiness with pregnancy, young maternal age, single maternal status, higher parity, late or absent entry to care, and substance abuse. The nurse should notify the physician or midwife of any positive findings and work together to develop a plan of care.

Nutrition and Exercise History

1. **What kind of exercise do you currently engage in? How many days per week for how many minutes do you do it?**

   ▶ Current recommendations state all pregnant clients should be screened for risk factors, such as heart disease, lung disease, a cervix that dilates prematurely, preterm labour, multiple births, frequent vaginal bleeding, placenta previa, or hypertension. If no high-risk conditions exist, all normal pregnant clients should be counselled to engage in an accumulated 30 minutes of moderate exercise on most if not all days each week. Exercise in pregnancy can prevent complications, such as gestational diabetes, and build stamina for labour. Sports that are not safe in pregnancy include soccer, vigorous racquet sports, gymnastics, basketball, ice hockey, horseback riding, kickboxing, downhill skiing, and scuba diving. Females should not perform any exercises that require lying on the back after the first trimester.

CLINICAL TIP

If a pregnant female experiences any of the following conditions during exercise, she should stop exercising and call her healthcare provider:

- *Bleeding from the vagina*
- *Difficulty or laboured breathing before she exercises*
- *Dizziness, headache, or chest pain*
- *Muscle weakness, calf pain, or swelling*
- *Preterm labour symptoms*
- *Decreased movement of the fetus*
- *Leakage of fluid from the vagina*

HEALTH HISTORY QUESTIONS

RATIONALES

2. **Describe everything you have consumed for the past 24 hours. Include water, vitamins, and supplements.**

TABLE 26.5	Recommended Dietary Allowances for Select Nutrients, Women 19 to 50 Years	
ALLOWANCE	**PREGNANT**	**BREASTFEEDING**
Folate (mcg/day)	600	500
Iron (mg/day)	27	9
Vitamin A (mcg retinol activity equivalent/day)	770	1300
Vitamin C (mg/day)	85	120
Vitamin D (mcg/day)	5	5
Calcium (mg/day)	1000	1000
Zinc (mg/day)	11	12
Vitamin B_6 (mg/day)	1.9	2.0
Magnesium (mg/day)	350 (19–30 y) 360 (31–50 y)	310 (19–30 y) 320 (31–50 y)
Vitamin B_{12} (mcg/day)	2.6	2.8

Source: Health Canada. (2009). *Prenatal nutrition guidelines for health professionals: Background on Canada's Food Guide.* Retrieved from http://www.hc-sc.gc.ca/fn-an/pubs/nutrition/guide-prenatal-eng.php

Note: Nutrient amounts in bold indicate an Adequate Intake.

▶ During pregnancy, females should include the following in their diet: four or more servings of fruits and vegetables for vitamins and minerals; four or more servings of whole-grain or enriched bread and cereal for energy; four or more servings of milk and milk products for calcium; three or more servings of meat, poultry, fish, eggs, nuts, dried beans, and peas for protein (see Table 26.5 for recommended dietary allowances in pregnancy and while breastfeeding). Clients often need education on portion size: one serving equals 1 slice of bread, 1 potato the size of a computer mouse, 3/4 cup of juice, 1 cup milk, 60 to 90 g (2 to 3 oz.) of meat or poultry, 1/2 cup beans, or 1/2 cup vegetables, for example.

Caffeine is a stimulant found in coffee, tea, chocolate, and many medications. In large quantities it may cause miscarriage or low-birth-weight babies and dehydration for the mother, and should be avoided. Calcium needs increase 40% in pregnancy. Dairy foods are an excellent source of calcium; other excellent sources include collard greens, sesame seed meal, blackstrap molasses, bok choy and other greens, soybeans, and tortillas. It is important that females consume eight glasses of water each day. Sodium is a required nutrient in pregnancy, 2000 to 8000 mg; pregnant females should salt foods to taste and not consume overly processed highly salted foods.

Females should avoid consuming non-food items such as clay, cornstarch, laundry starch, dry milk of magnesia, paraffin, coffee grounds, or ice. Pregnant females should also avoid these foods: swordfish, shark, king mackerel, and tilefish due to potentially risky levels of mercury; more than 180 g (6 oz.) of albacore ("white") tuna per week; game fish unless first checking its safety with the local health department; raw fish, especially shellfish (oysters, clams); undercooked meat, poultry, or seafood; hot dogs and deli meats (such as ham, salami, and bologna); soft-scrambled eggs and all foods made with raw or lightly cooked eggs; soft cheeses, such as Brie, feta, Camembert, Roquefort, and Mexican-style, unless they are labelled as made with pasteurized milk; unpasteurized milk and any foods made from it; unpasteurized juices; and raw sprouts, especially alfalfa sprouts, if there is a danger of salmonellosis and E. coli infections. Everyone, but especially pregnant females, should practise safe food handling, including hand washing, keeping refrigerator temperature below 5°C (40°F), cleaning the refrigerator regularly, refrigerating

HEALTH HISTORY QUESTIONS	RATIONALES

and freezing food promptly, and avoiding cross-contamination between cooked and uncooked foods, to avoid listeriosis and other food-borne infections.

Some herbal supplements and vitamin supplements can be a problem during pregnancy. As research in herbs in pregnancy is continuing, it is recommended that females check with their healthcare provider before consuming herbal teas and supplements. A partial list of common herbs known to be harmful in pregnancy includes aloe vera, black cohosh, blue cohosh, comfrey, dong quai, goldenseal, mugwort, pennyroyal, and wild yam. Although most healthcare providers recommend that pregnant clients consume a prenatal vitamin during pregnancy, some vitamin supplements (such as vitamin A) can cause harm if consumed beyond the recommended daily allowance.

Environmental Exposure

1. What kind of chemicals are you exposed to in your home and workplace?

▶ To prevent birth defects and miscarriage, pregnant females should avoid cigarette smoke, lead (in water and paint), carbon monoxide, mercury, pesticides, insect repellents, some oven cleaners, solvents, such as alcohol and degreasers, paint, paint thinners, benzene, and formaldehyde. If the pregnant female must be around these substances, she should minimize her exposure by ensuring good ventilation; wearing protective gear, such as facemask and gloves; and checking with the water or health department about the quality of the drinking water. For X-rays, 5 rads is the level of exposure believed to be necessary to cause birth defects; dental, chest, or mammogram X-rays are less than 0.02 rads of exposure. Federal guidelines prohibit exposure in the workplace to more than 0.5 rads accumulated during pregnancy, if the pregnant female has notified her employer of her pregnancy (see Figure 26.11).

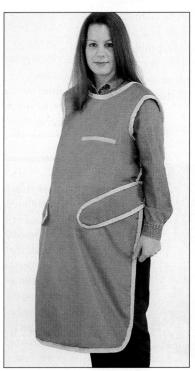

Figure 26.11 ●
Pregnant woman wearing a lead apron.

PHYSICAL ASSESSMENT

The room should be warm and private. For prenatal blood tests, a variety of collection tubes and collection equipment will be required and differs for each site.

The nurse should ask the client to empty her bladder and explain how to collect a clean-catch urine specimen. If this is the client's first gynecological exam, the nurse should explain the components and general purposes of the physical exam to the client, using pictures and the equipment as necessary, and ask the client if she has any special needs or questions about the exam. It is important to provide privacy while the client puts on the gown with the opening in back and lays a drape across her lap.

For the initial parts of the physical exam the client can be sitting and later be assisted to a semi-Fowler's position on the examination table. During the pelvic part of the exam, the client should be assisted to the lithotomy position. Some clients may need to have this exam in the side-lying position with top knee bent. The nurse assists the client in placing her feet in the stirrups, which should be padded if possible. The legs should be symmetrically and comfortably positioned. The client can then be instructed to move her buttocks down to the end of the table. For the initial part of the pelvic exam, it is helpful to tell the client what she will feel before the nurse touches her ("You will feel me touching your leg, you will feel me touching your labia," etc.). Some clients will be more relaxed if they assist in the insertion of the speculum (see Figure 26.12).

Remember to use routine practices throughout the assessment.

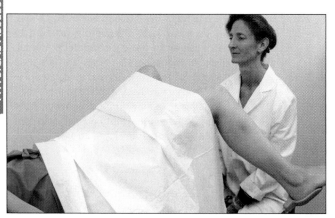

Figure 26.12 ● Pregnant female in lithotomy position.

EQUIPMENT

examination gown and drape
sphygmomanometer
adjustable light source
high-performance stethoscope
centimetre tape measure
reflex hammer
fetal Doppler and ultrasonic gel
urine collection containers
urine testing strips
perineal cleansing wipes
otoscope and specula
tongue depressor

For the pelvic exam, the nurse will need the following materials:

clean, nonsterile examination gloves
labelled slides and fixative or labelled containers for cytology
slide for vaginitis check
saline drops
plastic or metal speculum
spatula
cytology brush or cervical broom
tissues
hand mirror (optional, per client preference)
water-soluble lubricant
cervical culture swabs

HELPFUL HINTS

- Ask the client to empty her bladder before the examination.
- Explain the purposes and processes of each part of the examination. Use pictures or diagrams as needed.
- Assist the client to the sitting, lying, and lithotomy positions.
- Explain what the client will feel before touching her.
- The nurse must be sure to maintain the client's dignity throughout the examination.
- The side-lying position may be used to examine the perineum and rectum of the postpartum client.
- Use routine practices.

PHYSICAL ASSESSMENT

TECHNIQUES AND NORMAL FINDINGS	ABNORMAL FINDINGS AND SPECIAL CONSIDERATIONS

GENERAL SURVEY

1. Measure the client's height and weight.

   - At the initial exam, take these measurements to establish a baseline. In the first trimester, the client should gain 2 to 3 kg (4 to 6 lb.). The client should gain 0.5 kg (1 lb.) per week in both the second and the third trimesters, for a total weight gain of about 11.5 to 16.0 kg (25 to 35 lb.), if she is of normal weight when she conceives.

   ▶ A gain of 3 kg (6.5 lb.) or more per month may be associated with a large-for-gestational-age baby or the development of preeclampsia. A gain of less than 1 kg (2 lb.) per month may cause preterm birth, small-for-gestational-age infant, or IUGR.

2. Assess the client's general appearance and mental status.

   - Tiredness and ambivalence are normal in early pregnancy. Most females express well-being and energy during the second trimester. During the third trimester, most report increased fatigue and concern regarding upcoming birth.

   ▶ It is important to watch for signs of depression, such as decreased appetite, persistent feelings of sadness, guilt or worry, and suicidal thoughts.

3. Take the client's vital signs.

   - The respiratory rate may increase slightly during pregnancy, the heart rate increases, and the blood pressure may drop to below prepregnancy baseline during the second trimester.

   ▶ Blood pressure should not be greater than 140/90. Higher blood pressure could be a sign of gestational hypertension or, if accompanied by significant proteinuria, preeclampsia.

CLINICAL TIP

As preeclampsia worsens, multiple systems of the body are affected, producing such symptoms as (from head to toe) the following:

- *Headache unrelieved by acetaminophen*
- *Blurred vision, dizziness, or vision changes*
- *Dyspnea or difficulty breathing*
- *Epigastric (upper abdominal) pain*
- *Nausea, vomiting, or malaise ("I don't feel right")*
- *Sudden weight gain or sudden, severe edema of face, hands, and legs*

Signs noted by healthcare providers include hypertension greater than 140/90, proteinuria ≥+1, oliguria (decreased urine output), hyperreflexia, and abnormal laboratory values, such as elevated liver enzymes and uric acid.

---

4. Test the client's urine for glucose and protein.

   - Occasional mild glycosuria or trace protein can be normal findings in pregnancy.

   ▶ Persistent glycosuria may indicate gestational diabetes and necessitates follow-up. Greater than trace protein may indicate preeclampsia. If the client has lost weight, it is important to check the urine for ketones, indicating ketoacidosis, which is harmful to the fetus.

5. Observe the client's posture.

   - Increasing lordosis is a normal adaptation to pregnancy.

6. Assist the client to a sitting position.

SKIN, HAIR, AND NAILS

1. Observe the skin, hair, and nails for changes associated with pregnancy.

   - These include linea nigra, striae, melasma, spider nevi, palmar erythema, and darkened areola and perineum. Softening and thinning of nails is common. Hair may become thicker in pregnancy.

   ▶ Bruises may indicate physical abuse. Lesions may indicate infection. Scars along veins may indicate intravenous drug abuse.

PHYSICAL ASSESSMENT

TECHNIQUES AND NORMAL FINDINGS	ABNORMAL FINDINGS AND SPECIAL CONSIDERATIONS

HEAD AND NECK

1. Inspect and palpate the neck.
   - Slight thyroid gland enlargement is normal in pregnancy.

▶ Enlarged or tender lymph nodes may indicate infection or cancer. Marked thyroid gland enlargement may indicate hyperthyroidism.

EYES, EARS, NOSE, MOUTH, AND THROAT

1. Inspect the eyes and ears.
   - There are no visible changes associated with pregnancy.

▶ Redness or discharge may indicate infection.

2. Inspect the nose.
   - Increased swelling of nasal mucosa and redness may accompany the increased estrogen of pregnancy.

▶ Epistaxis may occur if the vascular increase is extreme.

3. Inspect the mouth.
   - Hypertrophy of gum tissue is normal.

▶ Epulis nodules or poor condition of teeth warrant referral to a dentist. Pale gums may indicate anemia. Redness or exudates may indicate infection.

4. Inspect the throat.
   - The throat should appear pink and smooth.

THORAX AND LUNGS

1. Inspect, palpate, percuss, and auscultate the chest.
   - Note diaphragmatic expansion and character of respirations. Later in pregnancy, pressure from the growing uterus produces a change from abdominal to thoracic breathing.

   - Observe for symmetrical expansion with no retraction or bulging of the intercostal spaces. Confirm that the lungs are clear in all fields.

▶ Unequal expansion or intercostal retractions are signs of respiratory distress. Rales, crackles, wheezes, rubs, and absent or unequal sounds may indicate pulmonary disease.

THE HEART

1. Auscultate the heart.
   - Confirm that the rhythm is regular and that the rate is from 70 to 90 bpm. The heart rate in pregnancy increases 10 to 20 bpm above the baseline. Short systolic murmurs are due to increased blood volume and displacement of the heart.

▶ Irregular rhythm, dyspnea, or markedly decreased activity tolerance may indicate cardiac disease.

2. Position the client.
   - Assist the client into a semi-Fowler's position, and pull out the bottom of the table extension so the client can lie backward on the slightly elevated headrest.

BREASTS AND AXILLAE

1. Inspect the breasts.
   - Normal changes include enlargement, increased venous pattern, enlarged Montgomery's glands, presence of colostrum after 12 weeks, striae, and darkening of nipple and areola (see Figure 26.6).

▶ Flat or inverted nipples can be treated with breast shells in the last month of pregnancy.

▶ Bloody discharge or fixed, unchanging masses or skin retraction could indicate breast cancer.

PHYSICAL ASSESSMENT

TECHNIQUES AND NORMAL FINDINGS	ABNORMAL FINDINGS AND SPECIAL CONSIDERATIONS

2. Palpate the breasts and axillae.

- Breasts are more tender to touch and more nodular during pregnancy.

EXTREMITIES

1. Inspect and palpate the extremities.

- Varicose veins in the lower extremities are normal with pregnancy. Mild dependent edema of the hands and ankles is common in pregnancy. Inspect and palpate the extremities for raised or tender veins. Palpate for ankle or lower leg edema.

▶ Raised, hard, tender, warm, painful, or reddened veins may indicate thrombophlebitis (inflammation of the veins). Marked edema may indicate preeclampsia.

NEUROLOGICAL SYSTEM

1. Percuss the deep tendon reflexes.

- Reflexes should be +1/+2 and bilaterally equal.
- Refer to Chapter 24 for more detail.

▶ Hyperreflexia and clonus are signs of preeclampsia.

ABDOMEN AND FETAL ASSESSMENT

1. Inspect and palpate the abdomen.

- The uterus becomes an abdominal organ after 12 weeks in pregnancy. Uterine contractions are palpable after the first trimester. Palpate uterine contractions by laying both hands on the abdomen. The *frequency* of contractions is determined by measuring the interval from the beginning of one contraction to the beginning of the next contraction. Indent the uterus with a finger to measure *intensity* or strength of contractions. The strength can be classified as mild, moderate, or strong. These distinctions can be described by comparing the rigidity of the uterus to the firmness of certain other body features. Mild contractions are comparable to the firmness of the nose, moderate contractions feel like the chin, and strong contractions are as hard and unyielding as the forehead. The *duration* of contractions is measured from the beginning to the end of the contraction.

▶ Liver enlargement is abnormal.
▶ Hyperreflexia and clonus are signs of preeclampsia.
▶ More than five contractions per hour may indicate preterm labour.

2. Assess fetal growth through fundal height assessment.

- Before 20 weeks, fundal height is measured by indicating the number of fingerbreadths or centimetres above the symphysis pubis or below the umbilicus. Once the uterus rises above the umbilicus, a tape measure is used.
- The 0 line of the measuring tape is placed at the superior edge of the symphysis pubis.
- The other hand is placed at the xiphoid with the ulnar surface against the abdomen. When the superior edge of the uterus is encountered by the descending hand, the top of the uterus has been located.
- The measuring tape is stretched from the top of the symphysis pubis to the fundus. The superior aspect of the tape is held between the middle fingers of the hand that is resting perpendicular to the fundus. The fundal height in centimetres is noted and compared with the weeks of pregnancy. Uterine size in centimetres is approximately equal to the weeks of pregnancy. The uterus should measure within 2 units of the weeks of pregnancy (see Figure 26.13).

▶ If the uterus is more than 2 cm (1 in.) larger or smaller than the weeks of pregnancy, a growth disorder, such as IUGR or macrosomia (large-for-gestational-age baby), multiple gestation, amniotic fluid disorders, incorrect dating, fetal malpresentation, or anomalies may be occurring.

PHYSICAL ASSESSMENT

Techniques and Normal Findings

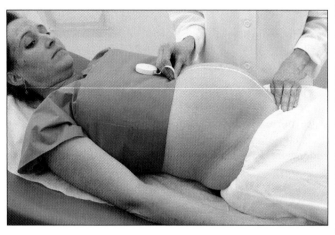

Figure 26.13 ●
Fundal height
measurement.

3. Assess fetal activity.

- After 24 weeks, fetal movement is palpable by the examiner. Maternal perception of movement occurs between 16 and 18 weeks in pregnancy.

4. Assess fetal lie, presentation, and position.

- **Leopold's manoeuvres** use a specialized palpation of the abdomen sequence to answer a series of questions to determine the position of the fetus in the abdomen and pelvis after 28 weeks' gestation.

  - *First Leopold's manoeuvre: What is in the fundus?* With the client in a supine position, stand facing her head. Place the ulnar surface of both hands on the fundus, with the fingertips pointing toward the midline. Palpate the shape and firmness of the contents of the upper uterus. A longitudinal lie will find the head or breech in the fundus. A round, firm mass is the fetal head. A soft, irregular mass is the fetal breech (see Figure 26.14). Nothing in the fundus indicates a transverse lie. The fetus can also be oblique, at an oblique angle to the midline.

▶ A woman should feel four fetal movements within one hour. If four movements are not felt within one hour, the woman should monitor movement for a second hour. If, after two hours, four movements have not been felt, the fetus should be assessed. However, routine daily counting, followed by appropriate action when movements are reduced, does not reduce fetal or neonatal mortality over informal inquiry about movements during standard antenatal assessments and selective use of formal counting in high-risk cases.

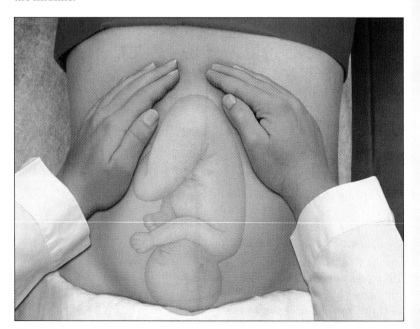

Figure 26.14 ● First Leopold's manoeuvre.

| TECHNIQUES AND NORMAL FINDINGS | ABNORMAL FINDINGS AND SPECIAL CONSIDERATIONS |

- *Second Leopold's manoeuvre: Where is the fetal back?* Move the hands down the sides of the abdomen along the uterine contour. A smooth, long, firm, continuous outline is found on the side with the fetal back (see Figure 26.15). Irregular, lumpy, moving parts are found on the side with the fetal small parts, or feet and hands. Note whether the back is found on the client's left or right side; if an indentation about the size of a dinner plate is seen at the midline and movements are at the centre of the abdomen, the fetal back may be against the mother's spine (posterior position).

- *Third Leopold's manoeuvre: What part of the fetus is presenting at the pelvis?* Next, slide your hands down to the area above the symphysis pubis to determine the "presenting" part of the fetus, the part of the fetus entering the pelvic inlet. Palpate the shape and firmness of the presenting part. Use the thumb and third finger of one hand to grasp the presenting part. This may require pressing into the area above the symphysis pubis with some pressure. Try to move the presenting part with one hand and see if the part of the fetus in the fundus moves with it by using the other hand. If the breech is presenting, the whole mass of the fetus will move when the presenting part is moved, and it will feel irregular and soft above the symphysis pubis. If a hard, round, independently movable mass is palpated in the pelvis, it is the head (see Figure 26.16).

- *Fourth Leopold's manoeuvre: How deep in the pelvis is the presenting part?* Now, face the client's feet. Place the ulnar surface of your two hands on each side of the client's abdomen. Follow the uterine or fetal contour to the pelvic brim. If the fingers come together above the superior edge of the symphysis pubis, the presenting part is floating above the pelvic inlet. If the fingers snap over the brim of the pelvis before coming together, the presenting part has descended into the pelvis. A prominent part on one side is the *cephalic prominence* if the presenting part is the fetal head; this indicates a face presentation if felt on the same side as the back. If a prominence is felt on both sides, the forehead is presenting. If no prominence is felt or the prominence is felt on

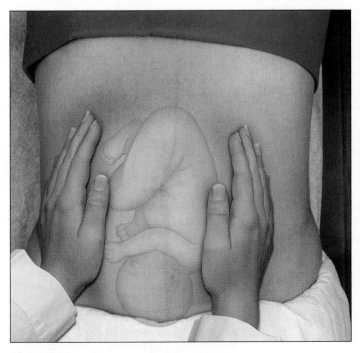

Figure 26.15 ● Second Leopold's manoeuvre.

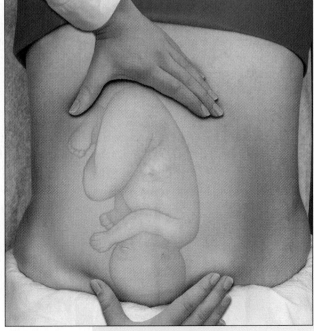

Figure 26.16 ● Third Leopold's manoeuvre.

TECHNIQUES AND NORMAL FINDINGS

ABNORMAL FINDINGS AND SPECIAL CONSIDERATIONS

the same side as the small parts, the fetus is well flexed, with the chin on the chest (flexion) (see Figure 26.17).

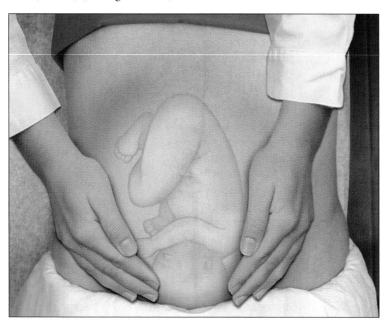

Figure 26.17 • Fourth Leopold's manoeuvre.

- *Fetal position.* The position of the fetus is the relationship of the presenting part to the four quadrants of the maternal pelvis. The fetus can be in the left or right half of the maternal pelvis, and in the anterior, posterior, or transverse portion of the pelvis. Three notations are used to designate the fetal position. The first notation is L or R for left or right, indicating in which half of the maternal pelvis the presenting part is found. The second notation is a letter abbreviating the part of the fetus that is presenting at the top of the pelvis. The most common notations for presenting part are O, indicating occiput, or the back of the head in a flexed position; S, indicating sacrum for a breech presentation; Sc, indicating scapula in a transverse lie; and M, indicating mentum or face presentation. The third notation indicates if the presenting part is in the anterior, posterior, or transverse portion of the pelvis. For example, a position of LOA indicates that the presenting part is the occiput, and it is in the left half of the anterior part of the pelvis.

5. Auscultate fetal heart rate.
   - Once the position of the fetus has been determined, the fetal heart tones (FHTs) can be located. They are usually heard loudest over the left scapula of the fetus, so this is the area that should be auscultated (see Figure 26.18).
   - Place the fetal Doppler in the location where the FHTs are most likely to be heard given the findings of Leopold's manoeuvres. Place ultrasonic gel, warmed if possible, on the Doppler before placement on the abdomen.

   - Auscultate the FHT for 1 minute.

▶ If the fetal heartbeat is not found by 12 weeks with a fetal Doppler, ultrasound evaluation of the fetal viability may be indicated. Other causes could be incorrect dating of pregnancy or retroverted uterus.

▶ Irregular heartbeats, tachycardia (heart rate above 160 bpm), bradycardia (heart rate below 120 bpm, or 110 bpm in postterm fetuses), or decelerations in fetal heart rate below the baseline should be followed up with electronic fetal monitoring.

| TECHNIQUES AND NORMAL FINDINGS | ABNORMAL FINDINGS AND SPECIAL CONSIDERATIONS |

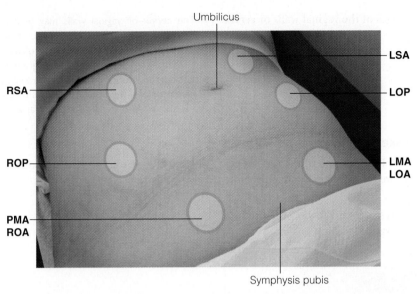

Figure 26.18 ● Location of fetal heart tones for various fetal positions.

6. Assist the client into the lithotomy position for the next portion of the assessment.

EXTERNAL GENITALIA

1. Inspect the external genitalia.
    * Normal findings include enlargement of the clitoris and labia, gaping vaginal introitus for multiparas (clients who have given birth before), scars on perineum from previous births, small hemorrhoids, and darkened pigmentation (see Figure 26.19).

▶ Varicosities can occur in the labia and upper thighs. Lesions may indicate sexually transmitted infection. Redness may indicate vaginitis.

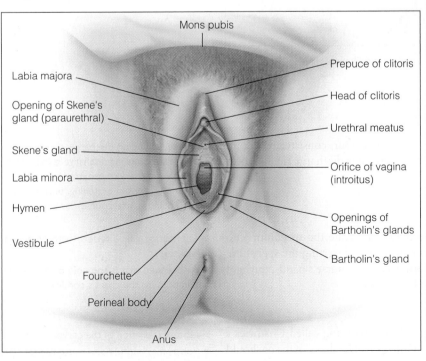

Figure 26.19 ● External female genitalia.

PHYSICAL ASSESSMENT

TECHNIQUES AND NORMAL FINDINGS	ABNORMAL FINDINGS AND SPECIAL CONSIDERATIONS

- Ask the client to bear down, and note any bulges of the vaginal walls or cervix outside the vagina.

► The cervix or vaginal walls may protrude from the vagina in cases of uterine, bladder (cystocele), or rectal (rectocele) prolapse. If the cervix is at the introitus, it is graded as a first-degree uterine prolapse. In a second-degree prolapse, the uterus descends through the introitus. In a third-degree prolapse, the entire uterus is outside the vagina.

2. Palpate Bartholin's gland, urethra, and Skene's glands.

- Insert a gloved index finger into the vagina. Press thumb and index finger together at the 5-o'clock and 7-o'clock positions at the vaginal introitus. Note any masses or discharge (see Figure 26.20).
- Insert the index finger into the vagina and press upward toward the urethra. Milk the urethra and Skene's glands for discharge or swelling.

► Note any masses or discharge that may indicate infection.

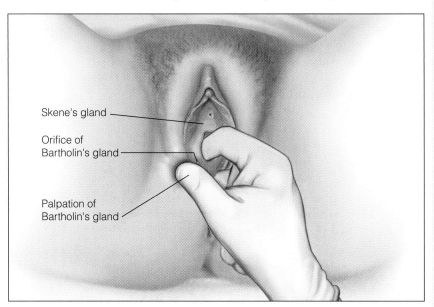

Skene's gland

Orifice of
Bartholin's gland

Palpation of
Bartholin's gland

Figure 26.20 ● Palpation of Bartholin's gland, urethra, and Skene's glands.

INSPECTION OF VAGINA AND CERVIX

1. Observe the vagina.

- The vagina may be bluish in pregnancy. Note the colour, consistency, odour, and amount of discharge. Increased whitish, odourless discharge (leukorrhea) is normal in pregnancy.

► White, clumping discharge or grey, green, bubbly, fishy-smelling discharge is indication of vaginitis or sexually transmitted infections. The client may complain of itching, burning, dyspareunia (pain on intercourse), or pelvic pain.

2. Visualize the cervix.

- Select the appropriate speculum for the client. Lubricate the speculum with water only. (See Chapter 22 for more instructions on inserting the speculum. ⊙⊙) The speculum can be warmed by warm water, the nurse's hands, the light source, or a heating pad kept in the speculum drawer.

► Lubricating gels interfere with some cytological tests.
► A speculum that is too cold or too warm is detrimental to the client's comfort.

3. Inspect the cervix.

- Expected changes in pregnancy include a bluish colouring called Chadwick's sign, or a slitlike cervical opening (os) for multiparas. The shape of the os should match the obstetric history. The os will usually be round and about the size of a

► Note any dilation of the cervix.
► Polyps may rupture and cause vaginal bleeding during pregnancy.

PHYSICAL ASSESSMENT

Techniques and Normal Findings	Abnormal Findings and Special Considerations

TECHNIQUES AND NORMAL FINDINGS

ABNORMAL FINDINGS AND SPECIAL CONSIDERATIONS

pencil tip for a primigravida. The os is usually slitlike in multigravidas. Note any lacerations, ulcerations, erosions, polyps, or other masses on the cervix.

- Note the colour and texture of the cervix, and note character and amount of any discharge from the os.

▶ A rough, reddened texture may represent the growth of cells from the internal cervical canal to the outside of the os (ectopy). It is seen in multiparas, and females who use oral contraceptives. If the speculum is pushed too deeply into the fornices or corners of the vagina, the internal canal may also appear; this eversion should be eliminated by pulling the speculum back slightly.

- If the cervix is covered with secretions, and you will be obtaining a Papanicolaou (Pap) smear, use a gauze pad on a sponge stick or a large swab to blot the cervix.
- Note the size, position, shape, and any friability (bleeding) of the cervix. The cervix should be 2 to 3 cm (1 in.) in diameter.

▶ Increased friability is common in pregnancy.

4. Obtain the Pap smear and cervical cultures.
   - See Chapter 22 for guidelines. ⚭

▶ Because of the risks of sexually transmitted infections to the fetus during pregnancy, cervical cultures are frequently obtained. The cervical brush is the best method for collection of endocervical cells during pregnancy. Cotton swabs interfere with the growth of chlamydia.

5. Proceed to pelvic assessment.
   - Unlock and remove speculum.

▶ If the speculum is not closed before removal, there is uncomfortable stretching for the client.

PALPATION OF PELVIS

Some nurses with advanced training assess the size and shape of the pelvis to screen for problems during birth.

1. Assess the angle of the pubic arch.
   - Place the thumbs at the midline of the lower border of the symphysis pubis (see Figure 26.21). Follow the edge of the pubic bone down to the ischial tuberosity. Estimate the angle of the pubic arch. A pubic arch greater than 90 degrees is best for vaginal birth.

▶ An angle less than 90 degrees may be more difficult for a fetus to navigate in labour.

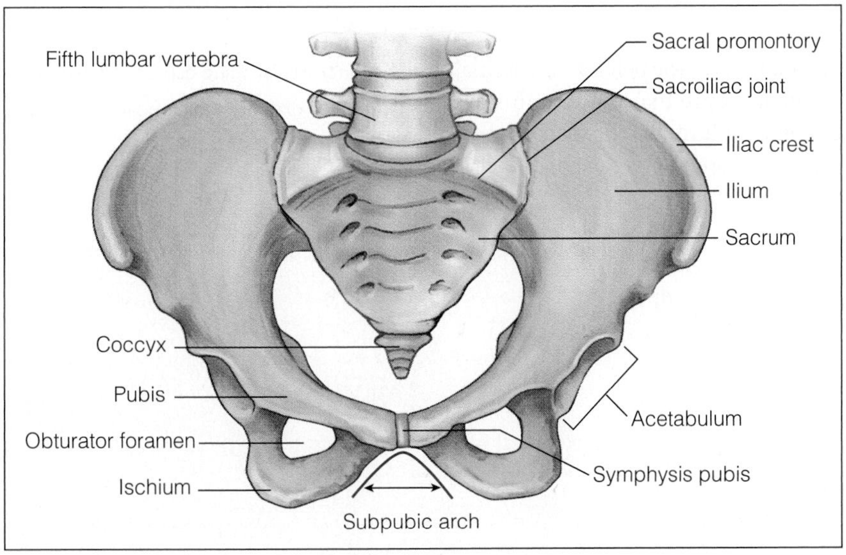

Figure 26.21 ● Internal structures of the female pelvis for landmarks.

TECHNIQUES AND NORMAL FINDINGS	ABNORMAL FINDINGS AND SPECIAL CONSIDERATIONS

2. **Lubricate the gloved fingers.**

   • Apply a teaspoon or more of lubricating jelly to the index and middle fingers.

3. **Estimate the angle of the subpubic arch.**

   • Insert the index and middle fingers slightly into the vagina, palmar side up. Keep the fingers separated slightly to prevent pressure on the urethra. Palpate the inner surface of the symphysis pubis. Using both thumbs, externally trace the descending sides of the pubis down to the tuberosities. The symphysis pubis should be at least two fingerbreadths wide, and parallel to the sacrum, without any abnormal thickening (see Figure 26.22).

   ▶ An anterior or a posterior tilting, or width less than two fingerbreadths, is abnormal.

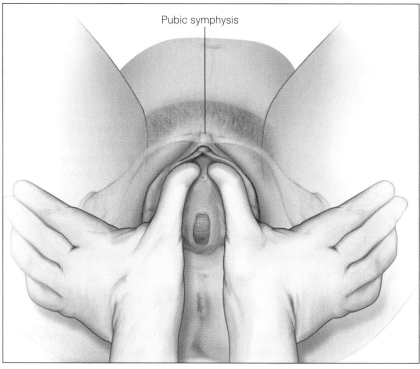

Pubic symphysis

Figure 26.22 • Estimation of angle of subpubic arch.

4. **Assess the interspinous diameter.**

   • Turn the fingers to the side and follow the lateral walls of the pelvis to the ischial spine. (As the fingers go deeper into the vagina, ensure that the thumb stays away from the perineum.) Determine if the spine is blunt, flat, or sharp. Sweep your fingers across the pelvis to the opposite ischial spine. Average diameter is approximately 10.5 cm (4 in.) (see Figure 26.23).

   ▶ A pointy ischial spine can impede labour.

   ▶ A smaller diameter may mean a contracted pelvis.

TECHNIQUES AND NORMAL FINDINGS	ABNORMAL FINDINGS AND SPECIAL CONSIDERATIONS

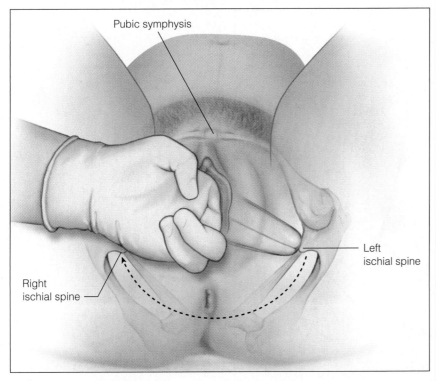

Figure 26.23 ● Assessing the interspinous diameter.

5. **Assess the curvature of the sacrum.**
    - Sweep your fingers upward as far as you can reach. Determine if the sacrum is concave, flat, or convex. Note if the coccyx at the posterior end of the sacrum is movable or fixed by pressing down on it.

6. **Measure the diagonal conjugate.**
    - Next, position the fingers in the back of the vagina next to the cervix. Drop your wrist so your fingers are at an upward angle of 45 degrees.
    - Reach as far toward the sacrum as you can, and raise your wrist until your hand touches the symphysis pubis. If your fingers reach the sacral promontory, note the distance from the tip of your middle finger touching the sacral promontory to the symphysis pubis. If you cannot reach the sacral promontory, the diagonal conjugate is greater than the length of your examining fingers. The diagonal conjugate is an approximation of the pelvic inlet and should be greater than 11.5 cm (4.5 in.) (see Figure 26.24).

▶ A hollow sacrum provides more room for the fetus moving through the pelvis.

▶ A diagonal conjugate of less than 11.5 cm (4.5 in.) may prevent a vaginal birth.

PHYSICAL ASSESSMENT

TECHNIQUES AND NORMAL FINDINGS	ABNORMAL FINDINGS AND SPECIAL CONSIDERATIONS

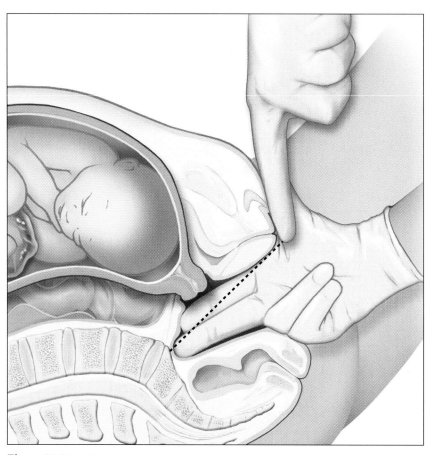

Figure 26.24 • Measuring the diagonal conjugate.

PALPATION OF CERVIX, UTERUS, ADNEXA, AND VAGINA

1. **Assess the cervix.**

   • Run your fingers around the cervix, and feel the length, width, consistency, and opening. The cervix is usually 1.5 to 2 cm (0.75 to 1 in.) long and 2 to 3 cm (1 to 1.25 in.) wide. In multiparas, the outside of the os may be open up to 2 to 3 cm (1 to 1.25 in.).

   ▶ The cervix is softer during pregnancy (Goodell's sign). It becomes even softer and jellylike as the client approaches labour. The outer opening of the cervix may be open but the internal os should be closed before term, 37 weeks of pregnancy or more. A shortened cervix is also a symptom or predictor of possible preterm labour.

   • Assess the texture and position of the cervix. It should be smooth.

   ▶ Note the roughness of ectopy or any nodules or masses. Nabothian cysts may become infected or be a sign of cervicitis. Normal variations include a retroverted uterus, which will have an anterior cervix, and an anteverted uterus, which will have a posterior cervix.

   • Move the cervix from side to side with your fingers.

   ▶ Cervical motion tenderness (CMT) is a sign of pelvic inflammatory disease and other abnormalities.

TECHNIQUES AND NORMAL FINDINGS	ABNORMAL FINDINGS AND SPECIAL CONSIDERATIONS

2. Perform bimanual palpation of the uterus.

- Place the nondominant hand on the abdomen, halfway between the umbilicus and the symphysis pubis. Press the palmar surface of the fingers toward the fingers in the vagina.

- Insert the fingers of the dominant hand into the vagina. Move the fingers to the sides of the cervix, palmar surfaces upward, and press upward toward the abdomen.

- Estimate the size, consistency, and shape of the uterus captured between your hands. The uterus softens in pregnancy, and the isthmus, the area between the cervix and the upper body of the uterus, is compressible (Hegar's sign).

- The uterus will feel about the size of an orange at 10 weeks' gestation and a grapefruit at 12 weeks' gestation. If the gestation is beyond the first trimester, abdominal fundal height measurement is used (see Figure 26.25).

▶ If the uterine size is not consistent with what is expected for the gestation, then incorrect dating, multiple gestation, or fibroids should be suspected.

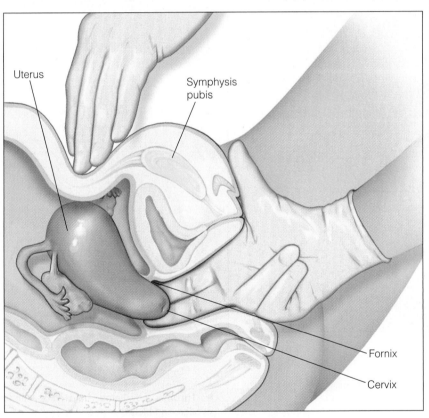

Figure 26.25 ● Bimanual palpation of the uterus.

Labels: Uterus, Symphysis pubis, Fornix, Cervix

3. Palpate the adnexa.

- The fallopian tubes and ovaries, or adnexa, sometimes cannot be palpated, especially after the uterus enters the abdominal cavity as pregnancy progresses.

▶ Any adnexal masses are abnormal and require referral. Bilateral pain is a symptom of pelvic inflammatory disease. During pregnancy an enlarged fallopian tube could indicate ectopic or tubal pregnancy and must be referred to a physician.

4. Assess vaginal tone.

- Withdraw your fingers to just below the cervix, and ask the client to squeeze her muscles around your fingers as hard and long as she can. Normal strength is demonstrated by a snug squeeze lasting a few seconds and with an upward movement. This provides an opportunity to teach the client about pelvic floor strengthening exercises.

TECHNIQUES AND NORMAL FINDINGS	ABNORMAL FINDINGS AND SPECIAL CONSIDERATIONS

ANUS AND RECTUM

1. Perform the rectovaginal exam.
   - The exam is sometimes deferred, but it enables the nurse to evaluate internal structures more deeply and is especially important if any fistulas are noted in the vagina, or if an early pregnancy is in a retroflexed or retroverted uterus.

2. Measure the intertuberous diameter of the pelvic outlet.
   - This part of the pelvic assessment is done at the end of the internal exam. As you gently withdraw your hand, make a fist with your thumb on the downward side, and press it in between the ischial tuberosities. A diameter of 11 cm (4.25 in.) is average, and 8.5 cm (3.25 in.) or greater usually is adequate. You must know the diameter of your fist to make this determination (see Figure 26.26).

▶ A diameter smaller than 8.5 cm (3.25 in.) may inhibit fetal descent during expulsion.

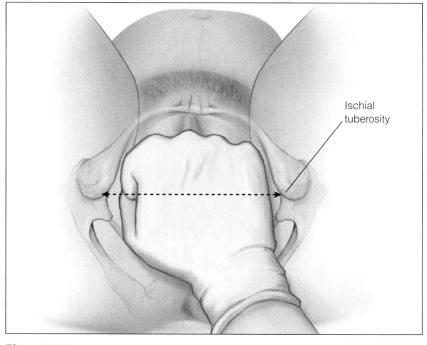

Ischial tuberosity

Figure 26.26 ● Assessing the pelvic outlet.

3. Inspect the rectum.
   - Hemorrhoids are common in pregnancy.

▶ Thrombosed hemorrhoids are tender, swollen, and bluish.

4. Conclude the exam.
   - Use the tissue to wipe the client's perineum, or offer tissues to her to do so. Dispose of speculum, swabs, and gloves in a biohazard container. Offer your hand to assist her to the sitting position, and leave the room so she can dress in privacy. Share your findings with her.

PHYSICAL ASSESSMENT

APPLICATION THROUGH CRITICAL THINKING

CASE STUDY

Susan Li, gravida 1, para 1, age 22, is married to a 23-year-old sales clerk who is required to work as much as possible because of family financial problems. She has 2 years of college education and was working as a server before this pregnancy. She speaks very good English. Her only local family member is her sister, who also works full time. The rest of her family is in China. She gave birth to a 3400 g (7 lb. 4 oz.) female infant 24 hours ago. Ms. Li's blood loss at birth was 400 cc (13.5 fl.oz.), and her placenta delivered intact. A first-degree laceration occurred during birth and was repaired, and a small cluster hemorrhoid developed during the pushing stage of labour. She had an unmedicated birth. She breastfed her baby girl in the delivery room and twice since for approximately 5 minutes each time. No family members have been to see her since the birth.

▶ Complete Documentation

The case study information is documented on page 762.

▶ Critical Thinking Questions

1. What should the nurse's priority assessments for Ms. Li be during this postpartum assessment exam at 24 hours after birth?
2. Ms. Li complains that her stitches and hemorrhoids are painful at the level of 7 on a 10-point pain scale. Describe the recommended nursing assessment and relief measures.
3. At 5 weeks postpartum, Ms. Li's sister brings her to the clinic nurse. Ms. Li tells the nurse she feels hopeless and overwhelmed and has been irritable and anxious for the past 3 weeks. What should the nurse's action be?

▶ Applying Nursing Diagnoses

1. *Ineffective breast-feeding* is a NANDA-I nursing diagnosis that applies to this client. Provide the related factors and defining characteristics for this diagnosis statement.

2. List one additional physical and one psychosocial diagnosis for this client based on the case study.
3. Rank these three nursing diagnoses in order of importance:
   a. *Pain, acute related to episiotomy, and hemorrhoids*
   b. *Ineffective breast-feeding*
   c. *Interrupted family processes*

▶ Prepare Teaching Plan

LEARNING NEED: Ms. Li has just delivered her first child. She is physically stable but is experiencing severe perineal pain. She has a small hemorrhoid that may be contributing to her pain. She has begun breastfeeding but has not established it yet. She is receiving no support from her family at this time. Like most new mothers, she has pain, self-care, and knowledge deficit, and social support and breastfeeding needs that must be addressed by the nurse. The following teaching plan is focused on individual care and education for Ms. Li.

GOAL: The new mother will demonstrate safe care of herself and her newborn, and the family will experience a successful transition to parenthood.

OBJECTIVES: On completion of this educational session, the participant will be able to do the following:

1. Identify two pharmacological and two nonpharmacological measures for perineal pain relief.
2. Describe the components of a good latch in breastfeeding, the recommended feeding frequency during the first week of life, and indicators of adequate breastfeeding.
3. List three ways in which family members, friends, and community nurses can provide social support to the new mother and family.
4. Demonstrate the use of a sitz bath and other measures for hemorrhoidal pain relief.
5. Explain the difference between baby blues, postpartum depression, and postpartum psychosis, and list two resources for additional help.

Postpartum Flow Sheet	Client Label *Li, Susan*

Maternal Data		Allergy _____ *PCN* _____

Age ___ *22* _____   GI T0 PI A0 L0

Del _*8/ 15/ 12*_ Time _*08: 14*_   SVD

Incision Type Abd Intact ①②③④ Provider *Jones*

Blood Type A ⓑ O +   Rub Imm Ⓝⓞⓝ

Newborn M Ⓕ Ⓝⓢⓨ NICU BR Ⓕⓞⓡ MD: __ *Night* ___

Problems Identified:

1. ___ ⤴*Social Support* _____
2. _____
3. _____
4. _____
5. _____

Year 2012	Date/Time	*8/15 8 am*		
Vital Signs	Temp/Pulse/Resp	*36.8/76/16*		
	Blood pressure	*98/62*		
Pain Assessment	1–10 scale	*6/10*		
	Location	*perineal*		
	Management 1=Pharm 2=Heat/Cold 3=Touch/Massage 4=Position/Movement	*1, 2*		
Activity	1=Complete bedrest 2=Partial bedrest 3=Out of bed	*3*		
	ADL 1=Self 2=Assist	*2*		
Gastrointestinal	Nutrition	*Reg*		
	Fluid intake	*750 mL*		
Breasts	Milk tension	*Filling*		
	Nipple condition	*Intact*		
Reproductive	Fundus (consistency, height, position)	*FF@U-1*		
	Lochia (type, amount)	*Rubra* *small*		
	Incision Redness Ecchymosis Edema Discharge Approximation Dressing	*NA* — + — — + *NA*		
Elimination	UTI Sx	*None*		
	Voiding	*200cc*		
	Bowel: (sounds, flatus, stool)	*+ + −*		
	Hemorrhoids	*small*		
Extremities	Edema	*slight pedal*		
	Homans'	—		
Psychosocial	Rest/sleep	*Adequate*		
	Bonding	*+*		
	Adaptation Taking in, Taking hold	*Taking In*		
	Social work consult Y/N	*Y*		
Signature		*E. Crownheart, RN*		

Application of Objective 1: Identify two pharmacological and two nonpharmacological measures for perineal pain relief.		
Content	**Teaching Strategy**	**Evaluation**
• Sutures are reabsorbed by the body and do not need to be removed. • Ibuprofen or acetaminophen can be used safely by breastfeeding mothers for perineal pain relief. Witch hazel pads assist with drying, and anaesthetic sprays may provide topical relief. • Cold packs, a peribottle filled with warm water and squirted on the perineum, and sitz baths are also used to decrease perineal pain. • Do not sit cross-legged (tailor-sit) or place undue stress on stitches until they have healed. • Pain should stay the same or get better each day. • Increased perineal pain should be reported to the healthcare provider. • Good hand-washing technique and frequency should be maintained.	• Discussion • Audiovisual materials • Printed materials • Group instruction • Individual discussion allows the client to verbalize specific concerns as well as fears. • Videos on the postpartum unit can allow clients to schedule the timing of the teaching and provide visual instructions for those with limited English. • Printed materials can reinforce teaching performed by the nurse and provide a reference for the client later. • Small teaching groups provide support and can be more time efficient to ensure that all the basic components of postpartum care are taught to all clients. Large lecture classes are not appropriate for new mother-infant dyads.	• The client verbalizes understanding. For example, client states, "I should call the physician or midwife if my stitches start hurting more." • The client provides counter-demonstration. For example, the client sets up sitz bath unassisted in the nurse's presence. • The nurse observes client. For example, the nurse observes the client put the infant to the breast and obtain a good latch unassisted.

HEALTH PROMOTION ASSESSMENT TOOL

Social Determinants of Health	**Level of Action**	**Action Strategies**
Income and social status	Individual and family	**Create supportive environments** • Assess the family's current financial status. • Explore whether Ms. Li has applied for Employment Insurance for financial support during her maternity leave. • Assess the couple's plans to meet their financial needs with the addition of a new family member. • Refer Ms. Li to additional local community resources, including city social services.

Social support networks and culture	Family and community	**Create supportive environments**
		• Explore Ms. Li's plans or resources for childcare breaks, adult companionship, and emotional support with this significant lifestyle change.
		  • What emotional and physical support can her husband and sister provide?
		  • What supports does she have outside of her family in Canada and has she made any plans to access their support or assistance?
		• Refer Ms. Li to additional local community resources, including (as appropriate) her cultural or faith community, community association, or other social services.

ABNORMAL FINDINGS

Disease processes can result in abnormal assessment findings or abnormal laboratory results. Cultural variations may lead to unexpected psychosocial adaptation and behaviours if the nurse is not familiar with cultural groups and sources of variation.

Common Complications in Pregnancy

During pregnancy the role of the nurse is to educate the client to prevent complications of pregnancy and to assist in the screening process to detect complications, identify risk factors, and effectively implement treatment if complications develop. Table 26.6 describes the common complications of pregnancy.

TABLE 26.6	Common Complications in Pregnancy	
COMPLICATION	**DESCRIPTION**	**ASSESSMENT FINDINGS**
First Trimester		
Spontaneous abortion	Loss of pregnancy; lay term is miscarriage.	Vaginal bleeding accompanied by cramping and loss of fetus, placenta, and membranes through dilated cervix. No heart tones heard when expected. Fundal height less than expected.
Ectopic pregnancy	Implantation of fertilized ovum in fallopian tube or other abnormal location.	Client complains of pelvic pain, vaginal bleeding; bimanual exam reveals tenderness in adnexa; mass palpated near uterus; may reveal gestational sac smaller than expected size for gestational age.
Anemia	Deficiency in iron, folate, or B_{12}.	Abnormal iron values in CBC; tachycardia; client reports fatigue, light-headedness, pica, cold intolerance.
Substance abuse	Use of illicit drugs, alcohol.	Positive screening questionnaire; inappropriate affect; irregular prenatal care; possibly preterm labour.
Molar pregnancy or gestational trophoblastic disease	Abnormal growth of placental trophoblast.	Vaginal bleeding; fundal height large for dates; fetal heart tones not heard at appropriate time.
Mood disorders	Depression	Symptoms present: depressed mood, diminished interest in activities, sleep disorders, weight changes, fatigue, decreased concentration, suicidal ideation.
Second and Third Trimester		
Premature dilation of the cervix	Passive, painless dilation of cervix during second trimester.	History of second-trimester loss; short cervix; abnormal cervical ultrasound findings.
Preeclampsia	Multisystem reaction to vasospasm.	Elevated blood pressure above 140/90 after 20 weeks; proteinuria >1 dipstick; pathological edema of face, hands, and abdomen unresponsive to bed rest.
Gestational diabetes	Glucose intolerance during pregnancy.	Abnormal screen; positive history; glycosuria.
Preterm labour	Uterine contractions at 20 to 37 weeks that cause cervical change.	Uterine contractions more frequent than every 10 minutes; change in cervical or vaginal discharge; progressive cervical change: effacement > 80%, dilation > 2 cm (1 in.); short cervix; positive fetal fibronectin or salivary estriol test.
Intrauterine growth restriction	Fetal growth below norms.	Fundal height less than expected; weight gain less than recommended.
Placental abnormalities	Abnormal placental implantation, including placenta previa (placenta is implanted over the cervix) and abruptio placenta (placenta detaches from uterus).	Vaginal bleeding; abdominal pain; nonreassuring fetal heart rate pattern; abnormal ultrasound.

Common Complications in the Postpartum Period

Several, common complications are found during the postpartum period. These complications are discussed in Table 26.7.

TABLE 26.7	Common Complications in the Postpartum Period
COMPLICATION	**ASSESSMENT FINDINGS**
Postpartum hemorrhage	Estimated blood loss (EBL) reported to be greater than 500 cc (17 fl.oz.) at birth for vaginal delivery or greater than 1000 cc (34 fl.oz.) after caesarean birth; a 10% decrease in hematocrit between admission and postpartum; vaginal bleeding that saturates more than one menstrual pad per hour is considered excessive bleeding; uterine fundus may be relaxed or "boggy," even after circular massage if caused by uterine atony; if caused by lacerations of genital tract, fundus may be firm but bleeding continues.
Preeclampsia	Elevated blood pressure; excessive edema in hands or face; proteinuria greater than +1; headaches, blurred vision, abdominal pain, dyspnea.
Subinvolution of the uterus	Uterine fundus is above expected level; at 6 weeks postpartum, uterus has not returned to nonpregnant size.
Disseminated intravascular coagulation (DIC)	Bleeding from IV site, gums, or nose; petechiae; tachycardia, diaphoresis; decreased platelets and abnormal clotting factor values.
Endometriosis	Fever, tachycardia, chills; extreme pelvic pain when fundus assessed; increased or foul-smelling lochia.
Deep vein thrombophlebitis	Unilateral pain in lower extremity; warmth, redness, swelling over vein; vein feels cordlike; Homans' sign may be positive (see Figure 26.27). Homans' sign has a low sensitivity in predicting the presence of blood clots. Other changes (i.e., colour, temperature, circumference) should be assessed.

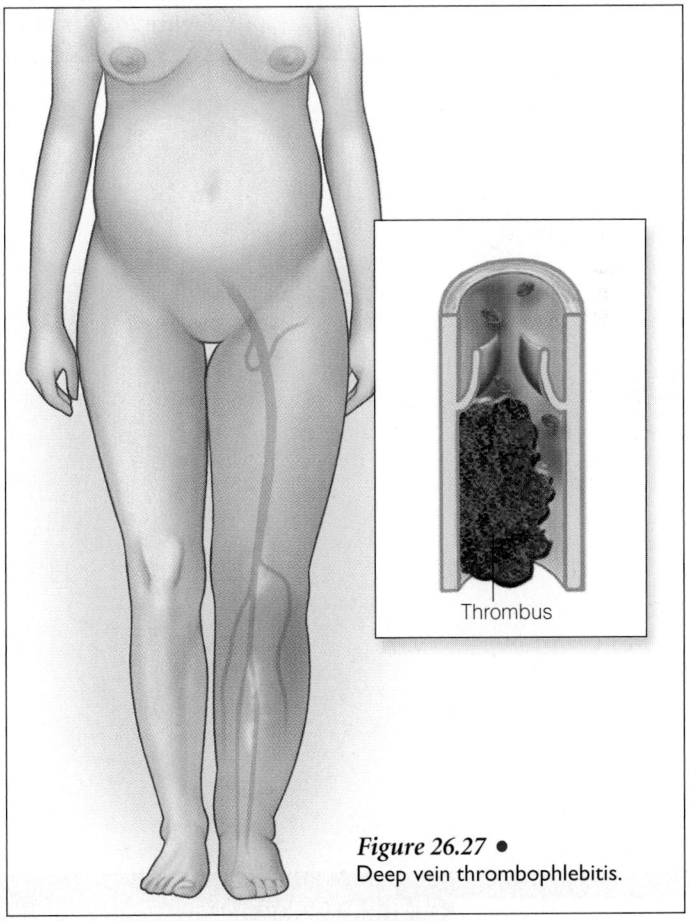

Figure 26.27 ●
Deep vein thrombophlebitis.

(continued)

TABLE 26.7 Common Complications in the Postpartum Period *(continued)*

COMPLICATION	ASSESSMENT FINDINGS
Hematoma	Bulging, bluish, painful area in perineum.
Mastitis	Unilateral red streaks on breast; flulike symptoms, fever; mastalgia (breast pain) (see Figure 26.28). 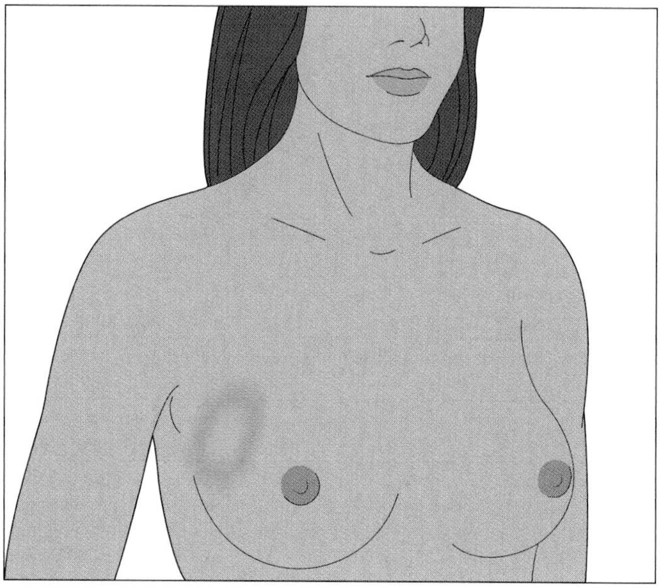 *Figure 26.28* ● Mastitis.

Visit the MyNursingLab website at **http://www.pearsoned.ca/mynursinglab**. This online homework and tutorial system puts you in control of your own learning with study and practice tools directly correlated to this chapter's content.

ASSESSING THE OLDER ADULT

In 2005, an estimated 4.2 million Canadians were 65 years of age or older, more than two thirds more than reported in 1981. As the baby boomers (individuals born between 1946 and 1966) age, "the number of seniors in Canada is projected to increase from 4.2 million to 9.8 million between 2005 and 2036, which is nearly one in four Canadians" (Statistics Canada, 2006a, p. 12). The number of Canadians 85 years or older is growing rapidly: in 2001, more than 430 000 Canadians were at least 85, close to three times as many as in 1981, and more than 20 times as many as in 1921 (Statistics Canada, 2006a).

As the population shifts with this increasing proportion of older adults, the process of aging is no longer being viewed as a disease. It is a normal growth and developmental stage, one that is often filled with happiness and fulfillment (see Figure 27.1). Some of the conditions once tolerated as expected age changes are now being aggressively treated as diseases. Such conditions as incontinence, tooth loss, and some mental confusion can be treated and cured.

THEORIES OF AGING

Theories of aging include those related to environmental influences and to cellular changes caused by wear and tear, chemical alteration, and genetic influences. In the wear-and-tear theory, the body is likened to a machine (Miller, 2004). Over time, cells wear out and cannot be replaced. This eventually leads to death of the entire organism. Within this theory, healthy behaviours have a positive effect because they protect cell wear and tear and may allow cells to repair themselves. When the wear and tear of aging affects the immune system, some believe a greater incidence of cancer, infections, and autoimmune diseases occurs.

In some newer theories, the wear and tear on the cells is expressed by a buildup of detritus, or abnormal collection of malformed or inappropriate molecules within the cells. In the cross-linkage theory, strands of DNA that should remain separate are linked together damaging the DNA and leading to decreased cell function and cell death. In the free radical theory, highly reactive molecules that can be created by irradiation, pollut-

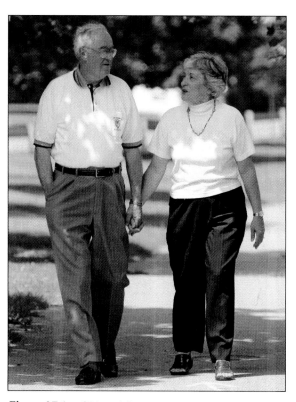

Figure 27.1 ● Older adults.

ants, or normal metabolism interact with and damage cellular components. Although these free radicals can be removed by antioxidants, including beta-carotene and vitamins C and E, over time the damage that is caused interrupts cellular function enough so that death occurs.

The genetic theories of aging focus on chromosomal differences between people and chromosomal effects on cellular makeup, function, and longevity. One estimate is that genes have up to 33% influence on longevity and healthy aging, with the remaining influence being composed of environment and other health-related factors (Perls, Kunkel, & Puca, 2002). Genetic theories serve to explain why some families produce people with longer lifespans than others.

The apoptosis theory seeks to explain why the process of apoptosis, the regulation of cells through death or growth restriction, appears to get out of control in aging. This theory is thought by some to possibly explain the increased incidence of cancer, autoimmune disease, cardiovascular disease, and neurodegenerative diseases seen in aging people (Joaquin & Gollapudi, 2001).

Miller (2004, p. 49) concluded the following about biological aging: (1) It affects all living organisms. (2) It is natural, inevitable, irreversible, and progressive. (3) The course of aging varies from individual to individual. (4) The rate of aging for different organs and tissues varies within individuals. (5) Biological aging is influenced by nonbiological factors. (6) The processes are different from pathological processes. (7) Biological aging increases a person's vulnerability to disease. For these reasons,

health assessment of the older adult can be among the most complex and the most fulfilling of nursing care.

Social and Ethnocultural Considerations

Older adults in Canada come from very diverse ethnocultural backgrounds. For example, 13% of seniors mainly speak a language at home other than English or French (Statistics Canada, 2006b). Many seniors may be isolated because they do not speak English or French, or because they have a different ethnocultural background from others in their community. In addition, in 2006, the estimated 56 465 Aboriginal seniors represented 4.8% of the total Aboriginal population (Statistics Canada, 2010), a heterogeneous population with varied histories, languages, beliefs, values, and practices. For example, many Aboriginal seniors were negatively affected by residential school experiences.

When conducting a health assessment with an older adult, the nurse needs to consider many factors, such as a person's ethnocultural history, gender, ability, language, literacy, education level, employment background, and health beliefs and practices, including beliefs regarding what constitutes health and well-being and general attitudes about age and aging, family, and so on. All these factors can influence how the nurse conducts an assessment and inform decisions, such as whether an interpreter is needed or whether a family member or friend may need to be present during the assessment.

Social and Ethnocultural Considerations

- From a dominant cultural perspective, aging is sometimes seen as a disadvantage, but in many other cultures aging is a sign of strength and wisdom. Nurses need to be aware of the assumptions that they have about the abilities of older persons.
- For many Aboriginal peoples, an *elder* is a person with strength and wisdom. The title is not necessarily related to age and is a status generally conferred by others.

- Older persons tend to be considered a homogeneous group. Older persons need and have the right to expect individualized treatment and to be considered a key member of the healthcare team.

ANATOMY AND PHYSIOLOGY REVIEW WITH CHANGES OF AGING

Aging has an impact on all the organs and systems of the body. The sections that follow describe age-related changes in each of the body systems.

Integumentary System

Skin-related changes are affected by lifestyle and environmental changes, as well as by normal aging. Exposure to the sun and other radiation, to chemicals, and to the effects of nicotine and alcohol on circulatory function all serve to speed aging skin effects. Over time, corneocytes, which make up 85% of the epidermal cells, become larger and more variable. This change alters skin appearance, making it coarser and

rougher. Melanocytes, which protect the skin from radiation and are located in the basal layer of epidermal tissue, progressively decline in number, thus increasing the risk of radiation changes. The melanocytes tend to clump irregularly, leading to patchy pale spots of pigment loss or to denser spots of colour, commonly called liver spots, also known as **lentigo senilis**. These skin discolourations caused by melanocyte clumping are relatively small. The white "freckles" should not be confused with vitiligo, which may affect large areas of the skin (see Figure 11.16). With age, the rate of epidermal turnover decreases, and the skin becomes thinner and drier.

Wrinkles appear on the face, especially at the corners of the eyes and mouth. Wrinkles are caused by loss of skin elasticity, as well as loss of underlying subcutaneous tissue. These signs of aging are disliked by many, but some people see them as marks of experience and wisdom. The face may have bony prominences along the cheeks and jaws, and the eyes may appear sunken because of loss of fat pads around these structures. Eyelids may droop because of loss of skin elasticity or may bulge along the lower lids due to herniation of fat tissue. The nose droops lower. Ears may appear larger than they did when the person was younger because of loss of facial fat deposits, balding, and stretched, pendulous earlobes.

Partial or complete baldness is common, especially in men, and often to a partial extent in women with male pattern baldness genes. Men's beards may remain full, and women may experience increased coarse facial hair growth, especially on the chin. The hair loses its colour and becomes white or grey because of a decrease in melanin production. Hair thins all over the body.

The number and functional ability of sweat glands also decrease with aging. This loss reduces an older person's ability for thermoregulation. Sebaceous glands, which help to lubricate the skin, prevent loss of water, and stop the entry of microorganisms, begin to decrease their sebum production. This change contributes to the dryness of the older adult's skin and opens portals for infection because skin dryness and scaliness can cause pruritus and scratching.

Mouth, Nose, and Throat

The senses of smell and taste diminish with age because of a decrease in olfactory fibres, taste buds, and saliva production. In some older persons, however, saliva increases, causing the **cheilitis** (angular stomatitis) at the corners of the mouth. Partial or complete loss of teeth may also occur, especially in the oldest adults who lived half of their lives before the use of prophylactic fluoride and other modern dental care. Poor dental health is decreasing, however, now that dental care is improving for people of all ages, and the current generation of older adults has lived most of their lives drinking fluoridated water and observing modern dental hygiene.

Edentulism (being toothless) can give the mouth a pursed or sunken look. Persons both with and without teeth should be examined for gingivitis and signs of periodontal disease. This pathology must be differentiated from normal gums that may recede to an extent, making teeth appear longer.

Eyes

Several alterations are associated with normal aging and are not related to vision or eye problems. **Xanthelasma** are soft, yellow plaques on the lids at the inner canthus. These plaques are sometimes associated with high cholesterolemia but usually have no pathological significance as they appear on persons with normal cholesterol counts. **Pingueculae** are yellowish nodules on the sclera that are thickened areas of the bulbar conjunctiva caused by prolonged exposure to sun, wind, and dust. They may occur on either side of the pupil and cause no problems. However, they must be differentiated from **pterygium**, an opacity of the bulbar conjunctiva that can grow over the cornea and block vision. **Arcus senilis** is a light-grey or white ring surrounding the iris at the corneal margin caused by the deposition of lipids. This is a common finding that does not affect vision.

A **cataract** is clouding of the lens, which can significantly alter vision in terms of both light perception and clarity of sight. This condition is now easily correctable by outpatient surgery that replaces the lens in a 20- to 30-minute procedure. The lens also loses the ability to accommodate, and many older people cannot focus well on near objects, such as print. **Presbyopia** is the name for this vision change, and it is treated with reading glasses or bifocals.

Ears

The tympanic membrane may appear more opaque than in a younger person. The client may have difficulty hearing whispered words. This change is due to **presbycusis**, the hearing loss that occurs over time and that causes high-frequency sounds not to be heard. Older clients may complain that they do not hear consonants well when listening to normal conversation. This problem is due to the loss of hair cells in the organ of Corti in the inner ear. However, conductive sound loss can often occur through an accumulation of earwax that is drier and becomes more impacted than in a younger person. Any older persons complaining of difficulty hearing should be checked for outer ear canal blockage and have their ears cleaned before any further testing is performed.

Respiratory System

The stiffening and inelasticity in all the soft tissue that occurs with aging also affects the lungs. The chest wall does not expand as well, and breaths are therefore shallower. Sagging of nasal and upper airway structures further impedes airflow. Mucus lining the respiratory passages becomes drier. The older person uses more accessory muscles and therefore must work harder and use more energy to take in air.

The number of capillaries in the pulmonary tissue decreases, and less blood flow is available for gas exchange. Normal alveoli enlarge and their walls become thinner. Since they are less elastic, it becomes more difficult to maintain positive pressure and keep the small airways open. Gas exchange becomes compromised, especially in the bases of the lungs.

It is important for the older adult to be vaccinated against influenza and pneumonia. These two diseases have a significant impact on morbidity and mortality in the older adult. Each year a new influenza vaccine is formulated based on the best prediction of that year's dominant flu strains. The Public Health Agency of Canada (2006) recommends that the influenza vaccine be administered once a year in the fall to adults 65 and older. The immunization is effective for most older people but only for those organisms covered in that vaccine. The older person is therefore not protected against other respiratory infections. The pneumococcal vaccine is recommended for all persons 65 years of age and older. It protects against 23 types of infections that cause 85% to 90% of all cases of pneumonia.

Cardiovascular System

With aging, the heart must pump against a stiffening aorta. Blood pressure gradually rises and pulse pressure gradually widens throughout adulthood, with mean systolic values for healthy persons peaking between ages 70 and 75 years at a high of 158, followed by a slow decline to the 140s by age 100. Diastolic pressure stays relatively constant at a little above 80, declining slightly in the advanced years. Hypertension is usually defined as blood pressure consistently above 140/90. The incidence of hypertension in older adults is high, and diagnosing it in older people who may have an increasing high systolic pressure can be important. It is a major risk factor in coronary artery disease, congestive heart failure, renal disease, retinopathy, ruptured aortic aneurysm, and stroke. This fact should be considered in the diagnosis or treatment of the disease in the client. It has been estimated that one in five adult Canadians has hypertension. The Canadian Hypertension Education Program (2009) predicts that the lifetime risk of developing hypertension for adults between the ages of 55 and 65 increases to nine out of ten. Blood Pressure Canada has established a public education program for individuals of all ages aimed at the prevention and control of hypertension and at ultimately reducing the incidence of cardiovascular disease in Canada.

Gastrointestinal System

The intensity of the propulsive esophageal wave decreases in aging. However, it is thought that this does not seriously affect swallowing and digestion. A pathological cause should be sought if an older person is experiencing esophageal dysfunction.

Gastric emptying times are significantly slowed with aging, which can cause feelings of premature fullness and contribute to gastritis and peptic ulcers caused by *Helicobacter pylori* infections. Although it was formerly thought that diminished secretion of gastric acid occurred in older people, thereby decreasing the rate of digestion, recent studies indicate that this is not a normal aging finding and that a pathological cause for the condition should be determined if it occurs (Jensen, McGee, & Binkley, 2001).

Once food leaves the stomach and reaches the small intestine, absorption of some nutrients is slowed in the older person because of atrophy of muscle fibres and mucosal surfaces. Lymphatic and vascular circulation in the villi is reduced, and the villi become flatter and less effective.

In the large intestine, water and electrolytes are absorbed. The walls of the colon become weaker and more flaccid with age. There is less mucus production, and older persons may experience more constipation, especially if they have had a lifetime of poor bowel habits, insufficient fibre intake, and overdependence on laxative use. Continuous overdistension of the bowel and straining to pass stools may result in **diverticula** (outpouchings in the wall of the colon) formation and **hemorrhoids** (varicosities of the hemorrhoidal veins), or even **rectal prolapse**.

Nutrition

Many older adults are just as interested in the latest nutritional information as are many younger adults. They may be very knowledgeable about reading food labels and as informed about nutritional recommendations for healthy lifestyles as many younger people (see Figure 27.2). But as with younger

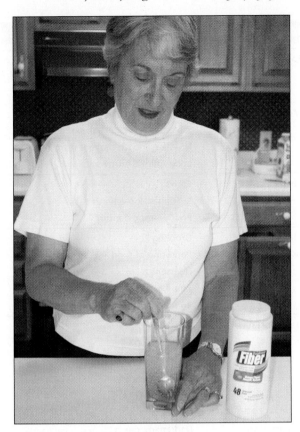

Figure 27.2 ● Adding fibre to the diet.

adults, they may not always follow the recommendations, and fad diets may have more serious side effects on less robust older adults or those with chronic diseases.

Eating Well with Canada's Food Guide (Health Canada, 2007) recommends a balanced lifestyle by eating a variety of foods, choosing more grain products and low-fat options, and maintaining a healthy body weight by participating in physical activity on a regular basis.

Nutritional Assessment

A diet recall, food frequency questionnaire, or more in-depth health history can provide complementary information to the laboratory assessment and physical assessment. A careful diet history can uncover risk factors for poor nutritional health. Sensitivity is essential when gathering nutritional history data, as an older adult may be reluctant or embarrassed to divulge personal information. Insufficient funds for food, decline in functional status leading to food preparation challenges, or sadness and depression have all been reported as contributors to malnutrition in older adults, but the clients may not volunteer whether they are affected by these factors. Table 27.1 outlines important nutritional history data to obtain when assessing the older adult.

Other older clients may have underlying or serious nutritional deficiencies caused by lack of knowledge; disease processes that affect digestion and absorption of nutrients; lack of ability to obtain food because of economic, psychological, or mobility problems; edentulism or the pain of periodontal and tooth disease; or alcoholism.

TABLE 27.1	Nutritional Risk Factors on Physical Assessment and Nutritional History in Older Adults		
Face	Sunken eyes Temporal wasting Note any changes from Table 9.4		Impaired vision Loss of hearing Impaired taste and smell
Mouth	Changes in taste perception (and smell) Xerostomia (lack of saliva production) Note any mouth changes from Table 9.4 Long tongue furrows		**CLINICAL TIP** *Taste and smell losses are often related to medications and not aging.*
Teeth	Caries Missing or loose teeth Poorly fitting dentures	Nervous system	Note any changes that impair food shopping, preparation, or self-feeding: • Tremors • Altered gait • Neuropathy • Impaired cognition Confusion, headache, lethargy
Chewing and swallowing mechanics	Drooling Pocketing of food Hoarseness Coughing with swallow Complaint of lump in throat	Functional capacity (activities of daily living, instrumental activities of daily living)	Note any changes that impair food shopping, preparation, or self-feeding: • Altered mobility or flexibility • Pain • Vision • Strength • Energy level/fatigue
Gastrointestinal	Anorexia Nausea Vomiting Diarrhea Constipation Heartburn	Psychosocial	Depressive symptoms Bereavement Social isolation Dependency Food insecurity
Genitourinary	Darkened urine Low-volume urine	Medical condition	Acute or chronic disease Multiple medications
Skin	Decubitus ulcer (pressure sore) Poorly healing wounds Note any rashes listed in Table 9.4 Dry mucous membranes Dry axillae **CLINICAL TIP** *Tenting is not an accurate assessment of dehydration in older adults because of altered skin elasticity.*	Diet	Restrictive therapeutic diet **CLINICAL TIP** *Most older adults do not need to be on strict therapeutic diets. Each person should be individually evaluated for the appropriateness of restrictions, and diet should be liberalized unless contraindicated.* Missed meals—assess reason Alcohol Lack of access to culturally familiar foods
Skeleton/trunk	Loss of subcutaneous fat Muscle wasting Note any skeletal changes from Table 9.4 Sensory		

The nutritional assessment starts with calculation of body mass index (BMI). This calculation requires the measurement of height and weight, which is usually done during the assessment or during the registration process at the beginning of the assessment time. The weight in kilograms divided by the height in metres squared equals the BMI. An older person may be considered underweight if he or she has a BMI of less than 23. A client is considered to be obese if he or she has a BMI of 30 or more. Persons with BMIs of more than 28 are at significantly higher risk for morbidity and mortality. Because body shape has also been correlated with certain diseases, attention should be given to that if the BMI is elevated. A waist-hip ratio greater than 0.95 puts older adults at high risk for health prob-

lems, especially coronary disease (Grodner, Long, & DeYoung, 2004).

Although body weight increases with aging up to the sixth decade of life, it usually decreases in the seventh decade and above. Lean body mass lessens as muscles atrophy, and bone density decreases. Height shrinks because of thinning of the vertebrae and vertebral disks, and increasing curvatures of the spine. The distribution of fat also changes, with more deposited on the hips and abdomen and less on the face and periphery.

Skinfold thickness and limb measurements are used with mixed results in assessing older adults. Changes in skin integrity and connective tissue, as well as loss of muscle tone and fat redistribution, can make accurate measurements a challenge.

Reference values are available from national survey data and include age, gender, and racial subgroup information. As with younger populations, skinfold and limb measurements are best used to monitor progress or changes in an individual.

LABORATORY MEASUREMENTS. Laboratory measurements for plasma proteins, anemia screening, or nitrogen balance may be included when assessing the older adult client. In particular, any macrocytosis should be evaluated for folic acid and vitamin B_{12} status. Absorption of vitamin B_{12} diminishes with age because of a decreased acid environment in the stomach and decreased production of the intrinsic factor needed for absorption. Iron absorption also requires an acid medium in the stomach. Medications may further alter gastric acid by buffering the contents or decreasing production.

Fluid Intake

Fluid intake should be assessed along with nutritional intake. Older people may consciously or unconsciously decrease fluid intake because they do not feel thirsty when it is appropriate to drink, because they fear incontinence or nocturia, or because they lack the mobility to have easy access to beverages. Dehydration may lead to confusion, digestion problems, constipation, and bladder infections.

Genitourinary System

By age 75 to 80, a loss of 50% of nephrons has occurred; thus, glomerular filtering is decreased. This loss has major implications for drug toxicity in older adults. Atherosclerosis of renal arteries can decrease renal blood flow and may lead to atrophy of the kidneys. Tubular function also diminishes, and urine is not as effectively concentrated as at a younger age; maximum specific gravity may be only 1.024.

Urinary incontinence can cause embarrassment and lead to social isolation, infection, and skin breakdown. It is the leading cause of institutionalization into long-term care facilities. It is related to diminished bladder elasticity, bladder capacity, and sphincter control, as well as to cognitive impairment. Stretching of perineal muscles through childbirth and obesity further contributes to stress incontinence in females. Prostatic enlargement, which occurs in 95% of all males by age 85, results in problems of urinary retention with frequent overflow voiding, especially during the night.

Endocrine changes, described in the next section, affect size, lubrication, and function of genital structures in both men and women. Decreased hormone production affects both libido and performance.

Endocrine System

Areas of concern regarding function of the endocrine system in the older adult include sleep, fatigue, and sexual function.

Sleep

One of the myths of aging is that older people need less sleep than younger ones. This is not necessarily true, although the pattern and quality of sleep do change. Often, older adults will either have trouble getting to sleep or wake up in the middle of the night and not be able to get back to sleep. Many older people take one or more naps. This makes their total sleep time equal that of a younger person. However, if they are not able to nap during the day because of the scheduling of jobs and activities, and if they continue to have trouble with sleep patterns at night, they may become sleep deprived. Clients should be questioned about their sleep patterns and whether they feel they are getting enough satisfying sleep. Hypnotic medication may be useful for short-term treatment. However, lifestyle changes may be necessary, such as change of bedtimes, change of environment, and inclusion of some sort of formal exercise. Naps of 1 hour or less should be used judiciously. Nutritional intake should be examined and large, heavy meals omitted near bedtime. A small protein and carbohydrate snack, to increase serotonin levels, can be helpful before going to sleep.

Normal age changes cause a decreased amount of growth hormone to be produced during sleep. Further endocrine changes cause a decrease in dopamine, an increased release of somatostatin, a lessening of the feedback inhibition of adrenocorticotropic hormone (ACTH) by glucocorticoids, a decrease in estrogen production, a diminished availability of testosterone, a decrease in sperm production, and an increase in follicle-stimulating hormone (FSH) (Terry & Halter, 1994). Women become menopausal, with greater vaginal dryness and more rapid loss of vaginal vasoconstriction. Men usually have decreased sperm production, decreased volume of seminal fluid, and less testosterone. Changes in collagen and the vascular endothelium may impair erection stiffness or frequency. Both men and women may experience body image changes secondary to illness, surgery, or psychosocial factors.

Fatigue

Whenever an older person complains of feeling tired, weak, or unwell, the thyroid should be screened for malfunction. Some symptoms that many people expect with aging, such as weight loss, slowed mental functioning, slowed physical movement, and feeling unwell, may be signs of thyroid malfunction. Although it was once thought to affect mainly younger adults, the rate of hyperthyroidism is actually higher in older people than in younger ones (Burke & Walsh, 1997).

Sexual Function

Nurses must recognize that if individuals maintain overall health, normal aging may not compromise sexual functioning. The results of a global study of sexual attitudes and behaviours indicated that 73% of Canadians between the ages of 40 and 80 were sexually active (Pfizer Inc., 2002). Additionally, 94% expressed emotional satisfaction and 91% expressed physical satisfaction with their relationships (Pfizer Inc., 2002). Quality of life and overall health were associated with emotional and sexual satisfaction.

Once the assessment interview has become comfortable for both the client and the nurse, the older client should be asked about sexual health. The nurse should consider the culture of the client and try to determine the level of interest that the client has in sexual activities. Some clients may not want to pursue such activities because of the loss of a long-time partner. Others may be very interested but too shy to bring up the subject. Much too often, this area of health is omitted from assessment. Sometimes this omission is due to embarrassment, not only on the part of the client but also largely on the part of the nurse, who may feel that this is not a proper topic to discuss with an older person.

Some causes of sexual dysfunction, such as medication use, can be easily changed. More is known about the effect of medications on male sexual dysfunction than on female dysfunction. It is thought that medications may diminish female lubrication, decrease libido, or interfere with achieving orgasm (Miller, 2004). Medications that may cause erectile dysfunction include antidepressants, such as serotonin reuptake inhibitors, monoamine oxidase inhibitors, and tricyclic antidepressants; tranquilizers; anticholinergics; phenothiazines; and antihypertensives, such as beta-adrenergic blockers. Cimetidine (for gastroesophageal reflux disease) may cause erectile dysfunction as well as gynecomastia. Imipramine (a tricyclic antidepressant) may reduce libido; methyldopa (an antihypertensive) may inhibit erection by reducing pelvic blood flow (Doerfler, 1999).

Musculoskeletal System

By the age of 80, about 30% of muscle mass is lost. Coupled with structural loss is loss of neurons that control muscle function. Thus, both strength and agility decline.

Bone loss also increases because of increased resorption, diminished calcium absorption, impaired osteoblast activity, and decreased numbers of bone marrow cells. Decreased estrogen production in women and decreased testosterone production in men speed this bone loss. Bone fractures can occur with minimal force. The vertebrae and intervertebral discs dry and flatten, providing less support and resulting in a shortening of several centimetres of height after age 65.

Weight-bearing joints suffer from the wear and tear of repeated use, especially if subjected to heavy weights. The viscosity of synovial fluid decreases, and degeneration of supporting collagen and elastin cells occurs. All this contributes to inflexibility and the aches and pains of osteoarthritis. Gait can become unsteady, and falls become a safety issue.

Neurological System

The conduction of neurological impulses slows with aging, decreasing reaction time, slowing learning, and decreasing short-term memory. However, the idea that all older persons lose mental capacity is wrong and causes much harm. Any decrease in mental acuity should be investigated to determine its pathological cause. Too often older people and their families suffer needlessly with conditions that can be treated and relieved. Often the fear of mental incapacity alone decreases quality of life for the older person. Many older persons contribute significantly to their own happiness and to that of their families and society by continuing to share the intelligence and experience that they have gained over their lifetimes, even if they provide it at a somewhat slower rate.

Aging does bring a series of losses, however, and that can lead to depression. These losses can include loss of spouse and friends through death or illness, loss of occupation or living arrangement through functional disability, loss of body image, loss of favoured recreation, and loss of independence. Of all persons 65 years of age or older, 2.5% report having experienced serious **psychological distress** within the last 30 days, with women more likely affected than men (Ni, Coriaty-Nelson, Schiller, Cohen, & Barnes, 2004). Clients should be asked whether they have had such distress and whether they have been medically treated for it.

The interview should give the nurse opportunity to form some opinion of the mental processes of the client. The client's mood and affect should be assessed, along with the ability to concentrate on the questions being asked, to reason competently, and to recall both recent and remote memories.

Clients in early stages of memory loss and even dementia, however, may be able to convey adequate mental ability, especially to people doing the assessment who may not have known them over time. Changes in mental status may be missed unless a formal instrument is used to compare against norms and to use as a baseline measure for future trend comparisons. This type of testing should not be done at the very outset of the interview, even though it is described at this point in this chapter. Likewise, mental screening should not be done at the very end of the assessment when the client may be tired. The screening should be done toward the end of the verbal part of the interview, when the client has learned to feel comfortable with the nurse and a rapport has developed. Many older clients, whether experiencing signs of mental decline or not, are very fearful of such a condition. If they believe that they actually have symptoms, they may be even more reticent to participate in formal testing.

The **Mini-Mental State Examination (MMSE)** (Folstein, Folstein, & McHugh, 1975) is one screening instrument of cognitive reasoning that has been used extensively for 30 years. It is familiar to most practitioners and rates well as a reliable and valid tool for detecting dementia and delirium relating to organic disease. It is easy to use. It takes less than 10 minutes to administer and requires no special testing materials other than paper and pencil.

One problem with the MMSE is that it is so widely used that clients may become irritated when they find themselves taking the test over and over. It also becomes easy for anyone, young or old, with dementia or not, to become confused between the answers on one test and the next when they are given too close together. Were the words to be remembered *ball*, *bat*, and *chair*, or was that from the test given yesterday?

Older clients who take the test on a periodic basis begin to learn the scoring system and keep track of their scores. They may become fearful of this progression of numbers and resist giving an opportunity for comparison if they feel it will show decline.

GATHERING THE DATA

Comprehensive health assessment of the older adult includes the interview and physical assessment. Subjective data are gathered during the health history, in which the client's own words and perceptions are recorded. Objective data are collected during physical assessment, from client records, results from laboratory, and other diagnostic studies.

GUIDELINES FOR INTERVIEWING OLDER ADULTS

It is important to respect the older client's worth and individuality (see Figure 27.3). He or she should initially be interviewed alone and considered to be mentally competent unless mental status is previously known. If caregivers or family members remain in the room for the interview, the client may not feel comfortable telling the "whole truth." When the client is very frail, the nurse may tend to address the spouse or adult child of the client rather than the client. This may happen unconsciously when the client is slow to answer or does not interact as quickly as the nurse would like. Frailness does not necessarily mean an inability to respond appropriately, however, and ignoring the client at the beginning of the interview is not a way to gain trust and gather information. If it is established in the initial, private interview that the client is unable to communicate sufficiently to supply the nurse with all the needed information, then it is appropriate to meet later with family or other caregivers. The nurse should consider cultural differences when asking about state of health and functional abilities, and save sensitive subjects, like sexual and cognitive function, until rapport has been established.

The temperature of the room should be in a comfortable range, with the client dressed appropriately for that temperature. A robe, blanket, or slippers may be necessary if the patient is not wearing street clothes. Thin paper or cotton examining gowns often make the older client feel uncomfortably chilly and less able to attend to the health history questions.

To facilitate clients' abilities to see and hear clearly, the nurse should make sure clients are wearing their glasses and that hearing aids are turned on. The nurse should minimize background noise, turn off background music, and shut the door or screen the area. Once both participants are seated, the client should have his or her back to the window or strong light source. Thus, glare is reduced, and the light falls on the face of the examiner. If the older person is known to have a vision impairment, additional lighting may be needed. Eye contact should be maintained at eye level. The interviewer should sit if the client is sitting or lying and be sure that the client has a back support.

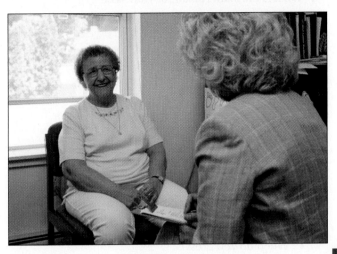

Figure 27.3 ● Establishing rapport with the older adult.

The nurse should address the client by his or her last name. It is also appropriate for the nurse doing the assessment to introduce herself or himself by using a last name. It often puts the older person more at ease and builds trust when the client knows that the person doing the assessment is approaching it in a professional manner. As rapport is established, a more informal approach can develop.

Once the comforts of seating, lighting, and environmental distractions are cared for, it is important to know whether the client is in pain and whether pharmaceutical or alternative pain therapies should be considered before conducting the interview. It is also important to consider sleepiness and the effects of any recent medication.

The interview precedes the physical assessment; this allows the client and nurse time to become comfortable with each other. After the initial questions and fact-finding are done, and rapport is established, the physical assessment can be started. It often prompts information if questions about function are asked while that body system is being physically assessed.

Asking clients how they assess their own health may yield insight into functionality problems or lack thereof. Often older people are more satisfied with their health than might be apparent.

HEALTH HISTORY

Subjective data are collected during the health history. The nurse organizes the questions for the client, family members, and caregivers. The following is a sample of questions to be used during the health history.

HEALTH HISTORY QUESTIONS	RATIONALES

Questions for the Client

1. What is the main reason for your visit?

▶ This question will elicit information in an open-ended manner, although it is important to remember that fear or embarrassment may cause clients' deep concerns to be withheld until trust and comfort increase. Starting with only one concern allows time to establish rapport before going on to further issues.

2. Can you tell me more about that?

▶ The nurse should ask follow-up questions to each point that the client raises. Not only are data lost without these, but a lack of real concern is also conveyed to the client if the nurse does not follow up, and information sharing begins to lessen.

3. Tell me about what you do during a typical day.
- When do you wake up?
- When do you get up?
- When do you dress?
- When and what do you eat?
- When do you start daily activities? Tell me what they are.

▶ These questions need to be broken into specific sections to find out information not only about physical health habits, such as sleep, diet, mobility, and other basic activities of daily living, but also about psychological health, energy, and interaction and socialization with other people.

4. How long do you usually sleep each night?
- Are you satisfied with your night's sleep?
- Do you rate your sleep as sufficient in terms of both quality and quantity?
- Do you nap during the day, if so how often and for how long?

▶ Many older people awaken early but may get up for a cup of coffee and read the newspaper and then return to bed and sleep, not really starting their day until several hours later. So only asking what time they wake up in the morning might elicit an answer of 5 a.m. but not give an accurate picture of their sleep-wake cycle. Poor sleep quality can be rated on a scale of 0 to 10, similar to pain rating. Zero represents totally adequate sleep with no sleep quality problems. Ten represents totally inadequate sleep quality, usually related to severe insomnia.

5. How much exercise, planned or informal, do you do during the day?

▶ For many older adults, a decline in physical activity is due to onset of some disability or limitation. According to Statistics Canada (2006a) men are more physically active than women. Individuals who live in warmer areas, such as British Columbia, are more physically active and participate in outdoor activities more often than people who live in colder climates.

6. Do you experience any dizziness or difficulties when you try to walk or exercise? *If yes:*
- Do you have any of these symptoms when you are at rest?
- Do you feel energetic or tired most of the time?
- If you are tired, can you relate it to any specific cause?

▶ The answers to these questions can lead to the need for laboratory or other diagnostic testing to determine a physical cause but may also relate to psychological and social interaction difficulties that must be addressed.

7. Have you ever fallen as a result of feeling dizzy?

▶ Approximately one in three older adults living outside of institutions fall every year and half of those individuals fall more than once. If the nurse suspects that the client is at high risk, the nurse assesses the client's physical health and the conditions in and around the client's home (Public Health Agency of Canada, 2002).

GATHERING THE DATA

HEALTH HISTORY QUESTIONS	RATIONALES
8. Where do you live? With whom do you live? What is your place in the household?	▶ The nurse should follow up any responses that might indicate a housing problem, whether or not the client lives alone, or those that hint at elder or spousal abuse.
9. Are you responsible for your own care needs and personal business, or do you depend on someone else?	▶ The number of individuals requiring help during their activities of daily living increases as they get older. A complete assessment will assist in identifying individuals who require help with their personal care.
10. Do you have a job, either within or outside the home? *If yes:* • Are you happy doing it? Do you receive compensation for the job? • Does the workplace environment and work situation seem safe?	▶ These questions provide information about activity and socioeconomic status, as well as safety. They also give insight into personal satisfaction and sense of worth.
11. Do you smoke, drink alcohol, or use recreational drugs? *If yes:* • How much and for how long? • Have you ever tried to quit? • Have you ever done any of these things in the past? • If so, when did you stop?	▶ Seventy-five percent of men age 75 and over have smoked versus 40% of women (Statistics Canada, 2006a). Almost half of all seniors consume an alcoholic drink each month, and approximately 12% of men and 3% of women age 65 to 74 were considered heavy drinkers. Heavy drinking is defined as the consumption of five or more drinks on one occasion (Statistics Canada, 2006a).
12. What prescribed and over-the-counter medications do you take routinely or occasionally?	▶ When discussing prescribed medications, the nurse must determine whether the client actually takes them as ordered. Inconvenient scheduling, confusion, ignorance, and thrift are all reasons why older adults may not be taking prescribed medications. Such medications can be extremely expensive, and the prescriptions may never have been filled, or the client may cut pills in half or take them on a delayed schedule. If possible, the client should bring all of his or her pill bottles to the interview. Not only will the names and amounts of the prescribed medications be more accurately known, but attention can also be paid to the dates on which the prescriptions were filled and whether the amount of medication in the bottle matches what should be there at the time of the interview. The nurse should make sure the client understands what each medication is for and assess whether any special instructions for taking them are being followed. The nurse should also record the list of over-the-counter medications, vitamins, and any herbal remedies that the client may be taking.
13. Do you have any problem holding your urine? How many times a night do you get up to urinate?	▶ This is a concern that often causes embarrassment. The question should be asked late in the interview once rapport has been established. Urinary incontinence may have a significant impact on quality of life and functional ability. Negative answers to earlier functionality questions may give hints of this problem that should be followed up.

GATHERING THE DATA

HEALTH HISTORY QUESTIONS	RATIONALES

14. **Do you have any problems with constipation or moving your bowels? What is your normal bowel pattern?**

▶ Asking whether the client feels he or she has constipation problems yields information about elimination expectations as well as actual problems. Here is an opportunity for the nurse to teach about the variations of normality and ways that regular elimination can be established. Answers to these questions may also hint at laxative abuse.

15. **Do you experience any pain or discomfort in any particular part of your body?**
If yes:
- When did you first notice the pain? How long does it last? *Onset (chronology)*
- What makes the pain worse? What makes the pain better? *Precipitating (palliative)*
- Would you describe the pain as sharp? dull? burning? cramping? *Quality*
- Where is the pain located? Does the pain radiate? *Region (radiation)*
- How would you rate the pain on a scale of 1 to 10, with 10 being the worst pain? *Severity*
- How often do you experience the pain? When does the pain occur, while walking, at rest, all day long? How long does it last? *Timing*
- What do you think is causing the pain? *Understanding*

▶ It is especially important to consider cultural differences when clients are talking about their pain and to determine exactly where the pain is and when it occurs.

16. **Do you have times that you feel especially sad or lonely? (Depending on the answer to this question, the nurse should follow up with questions about what clients do to relieve the feeling. Do they have social support? Do they ever consider ending their lives?)**

▶ Following up may lead to the opportunity to ask whether the client has ever thought of taking his or her own life. Depression and suicide are major concerns with older adults, especially those who have debilitating illnesses or those who have lost a significant person. The nurse can use the Yesavage/Brink Geriatric Depression Scale to assess further if this seems warranted (see Figure 27.4).

1. Are you basically satisfied with your life? (no)
2. Have you dropped many of your activities and interests? (yes)
3. Do you feel that your life is empty? (yes)
4. Do you often get bored? (yes)
5. Are you hopeful about the future? (no)
6. Are you bothered by thoughts that you just cannot get out of your head? (yes)
7. Are you in good spirits most of the time? (no)
8. Are you afraid that something bad is going to happen to you? (yes)
9. Do you feel happy most of the time? (no)
10. Do you often feel helpless? (yes)
11. Do you often get restless and fidgety? (yes)
12. Do you prefer to stay home at night, rather than go out and do new things? (yes)
13. Do you frequently worry about the future? (yes)
14. Do you feel that you have more problems with memory than most? (yes)
15. Do you think it is wonderful to be alive now? (no)
16. Do you often feel downhearted and blue? (yes)
17. Do you feel pretty worthless the way you are now? (yes)
18. Do you worry a lot about the past? (yes)
19. Do you find life very exciting? (no)
20. Is it hard for you to get started on new projects? (yes)
21. Do you feel full of energy? (no)
22. Do you feel that your situation is hopeless? (yes)
23. Do you think that most persons are better off than you are? (yes)
24. Do you frequently get upset over little things? (yes)
25. Do you frequently feel like crying? (yes)
26. Do you have trouble concentrating? (yes)
27. Do you enjoy getting up in the morning? (no)
28. Do you prefer to avoid social gatherings? (yes)
29. Is it easy for you to make decisions? (no)
30. Is your mind as clear as it used to be? (no)

Figure 27.4 ● Geriatric depression scale.

Source: Adapted with permission from Yesavage, J. A., & Brink, T. L. (1983). Development and validation of a geriatric depression screening scale: A preliminary report. *Journal of Psychiatric Research, 17*:41. Copyright © 1983. Pergamon Journals Ltd.

HEALTH HISTORY QUESTIONS	RATIONALES

17. Do you have any concern about your memory or thinking process?

▶ This is a very sensitive question for many older people. Almost all will answer that they have such concerns. The interview up to this point will yield information from which the nurse can make conclusions about this topic. If the client does voice concerns, it is important to ask for specific examples to determine whether the client suffers from actual mental impairment or simply self-ageism and fear of possible mental decline. The MMSE can be used as a quick screening tool.

Questions for Family Members and Caregivers

These questions will need to be tailored according to the competence and functionality exhibited by the client in the client interview. Independent older people who are cognitively intact can be expected to give their own accurate interview answers. However, questions that go unanswered during the interview, or that seem to elicit confused or inaccurate answers, need to be followed up. This follow-up should be done privately with the family caregivers while the older person waits in another room. Examples of additional questions to caregivers are:

1. **Have you noticed any forgetfulness or changes in the way (the client) normally does things?** *If yes:*
   - Has (the client) stopped doing any of his or her normal activities?
   - Have you noticed any unusual behaviours?

▶ Responses can help the nurse identify changes in mental status or deterioration of function, which might put the client at risk for injury.

2. **Do you have any concerns about (the client) that you want to tell me but do not want to discuss in front of him or her?**

▶ This gives family members permission to share fears or to ask questions that they are reluctant to mention for fear of worrying the older person.

GATHERING THE DATA

PHYSICAL ASSESSMENT

ASSESSMENT TECHNIQUES AND FINDINGS

Before beginning the physical assessment, the nurse should wash his or her hands in warm water, warm the stethoscope, ask whether the client needs to void before the examination, and ask whether the client is warm enough and comfortable.

EQUIPMENT	
examination gown	vision screener
sphygmomanometer	stethoscope
drape	tuning fork
centimetre measuring device	ophthalmoscope
examination gloves	reflex hammer
tongue blade	otoscope
examination light	sharp and dull objects
cotton	substances to taste and smell
penlight	

HELPFUL HINTS

- To prevent discomfort caused by temperature sensitivity, the nurse should provide gowns and wraps of sufficient warmth. Older adults may remain clothed and remove only what is necessary for a particular examination.
- Lying or sitting on a hard examining table is difficult for many older adults. A bed that can be elevated or a table with a padded mattress can be used.
- The client's energy should be conserved by organizing the assessment so activities are grouped for a minimum of position changes.
- Many older adults are uncomfortable with a much younger examiner, especially if the examiner is of the opposite sex. The nurse should maintain a mature and professional attitude while demonstrating care and concern.
- A great deal of information about the client's functional abilities can be obtained by observation of movements, the ability to carry out requests, and communication and interaction with the examiner. These also provide information about the ability to hear and understand requests.
- Explain each step of the procedure and ask questions about the findings. Older adults are often more at ease when asked to explain a scar or physical alteration.
- Consider the client's need or desire to have a family member present for the assessment.
- Use routine practices.

TECHNIQUES AND NORMAL FINDINGS	ABNORMAL FINDINGS AND SPECIAL CONSIDERATIONS

GENERAL SURVEY

1. **Position the client.**
   - The client should be in a comfortable sitting position with some back support. Lighting must be adequate to detect skin colour changes, discharge, and lesions.

2. **Observe the client.**
   - Note signs of distress, quality of dress and hygiene, and posture or any physical abnormalities.

   ▶ Facial grimacing, rocking, rigid posture, pallor, or perspiration could indicate pain. Inappropriate dress, body odour, and inadequate hygiene may indicate cognitive or functional problems. Obvious poor care and poor interaction may indicate elder abuse issues, although this should not be assumed. Culture must also be considered. Physical abnormalities may indicate pathological conditions. Breath and body odours may also give clues to illness, such as infection or diabetes mellitus, or to excess alcohol intake.

   - Note any breath or body odour.
   - Note the client's interactions with family members or caregivers.

3. **Evaluate the client's nutritional status.**
   - Observe for a wasted or apathetic appearance.

   ▶ Muscle and fat are normally lost with aging, and facial features may sag, but extreme loss may indicate decreased nutrition or be a symptom of disease, such as cancer.

   - Measure height and weight and ask about usual values and whether there has been any recent change.
   - Calculate BMI.

   ▶ Determine classification of BMI. Underweight, overweight, and obesity all indicate risk conditions.

PHYSICAL ASSESSMENT

TECHNIQUES AND NORMAL FINDINGS	ABNORMAL FINDINGS AND SPECIAL CONSIDERATIONS

- Measure the waist at the smallest circumference and hips at the largest circumference, and calculate waist-hip ratio.
- Assess hydration by looking at skin for dryness, flakiness, or scaling, as well as tenting when skin is pinched up. Check oral mucous membranes for dryness.

▶ Increased waist-hip ratio has been found to correlate with cardiovascular risk.

▶ Dehydration is a common problem in older adults, who may not experience thirst appropriately or who may withhold fluids due to nocturia or urinary incontinence. It may also be a sign of problems with caregiving. Dehydration can lead to cognitive problems. Alcohol intake may decrease other food and fluid intake and lead to dehydration through diuresis.

CLINICAL TIP

Tenting is not an accurate assessment of dehydration in older adults because of altered skin elasticity.

4. Measure vital signs.
- Take the blood pressure in both arms with the client reclining, sitting, and standing. Allow a minute or two between each measurement.
- Use an appropriately sized cuff. A child's cuff can be used for very thin persons; a thigh cuff can be used for extremely fatty upper arms.

▶ Orthostatic hypotension (a drop of 20 mm Hg or more when standing) may occur in older adults as a result of medications or vascular impairment.

CLINICAL TIP

It is important to assist the client to a sitting or standing position before retaking the blood pressure and to be cautious that the client does not fall.

- Take the pulse both apically and radially and compare, checking for pulse deficit. Note regularity and strength of beats at both sites.

▶ Weak beats and arrhythmias may not be conducted to the radial pulse. Consider the effect that any of the client's medications may have on pulse rate. For example, beta blockers or digoxin may slow the pulse, whereas adrenergics may increase the rate.

- Take an oral temperature, being sure that the client's mouth is closed around the device.

▶ In the absence of illness, body temperature in older adults is lower than at a younger age. The mean is 36.2°C (97.2°F). Because temperature regulation is not as effective in older adults, however, attention should be paid to whether the client has just come in from the cold or is overly bundled on a warm day.

- Count respirations for a full minute at a time other than when the thermometer is in the client's mouth. It is best to count the respirations after listening to the last beat of the apical pulse.

▶ It may be difficult for the client to hold an electronic thermometer or even keep his or her mouth closed tightly around a lighter one and still breathe normally. Be sure that clients do not think you want them to take deep breaths when you are listening to their apical pulse.

- Ask the client to rate his or her current pain on a scale of 0 to 10, with 0 being no pain at all and 10 being the most pain imaginable.

▶ Pain is an important vital sign to measure with all clients. It is especially important in older persons who may experience acute as well as chronic conditions and who may not report the pain because they believe it is a normal part of aging.

INTEGUMENTARY SYSTEM

1. Inspect the skin for colour.
- Note any overall redness, cyanosis, jaundice, pallor, or transparency.

PHYSICAL ASSESSMENT

TECHNIQUES AND NORMAL FINDINGS

ABNORMAL FINDINGS AND SPECIAL CONSIDERATIONS

- Check for erythema on bony prominences and in moist areas, such as the groin and under the breasts.

▶ Skin in older adults is normally paler and more transparent, but pallor can indicate anemia, malnutrition, or edema. Redness can indicate inflammation, skin infection, or a beginning decubitus ulcer. Differentiate visible veins, especially on lower extremities, from cyanosis or ecchymosis.

CLINICAL TIP

Although it is insulting to wear gloves for casual, upper body inspection, gloves should be worn when examining areas that cannot be easily visualized and that might contain open wounds or body fluids, such as scalp, under the breasts, and between the toes.

2. Palpate the skin.
   - Note moisture or dryness, scaliness, texture, and thinness.

▶ Skin dryness and scaliness may indicate dehydration, malnutrition, or such conditions as eczema or psoriasis.

   - Note overall temperature as well as that in individual areas, especially on the periphery. Compare bilaterally.

▶ Overall skin temperature is usually cooler than in younger adults. However, cold spots, especially on the periphery, may indicate circulatory disease.

CLINICAL TIP

Skin can be extremely thin and fragile, especially in very old people. This is especially true in persons taking corticosteroids over a long term. Care must be taken to avoid tearing and bruising.

3. Measure and describe all skin lesions.
   - Look for lesions that are common and nonsignificant in aging skin: cherry angiomas, senile lentigines, seborrheic keratoses, and acrochordons. (See Chapter 11. ⬤) Describe and measure these so that new lesions or changes can be identified later. Inspect precancerous actinic keratoses for cancerous lesions, such as melanoma or basal or squamous cell carcinomas. Identify any areas of trauma, decubitus, or vascular ulcers.

▶ Herpes zoster is more common in older adults. Look for painful, red vesicular or pustular lesions that may be in a line or in patches on the thorax, front or back. Ecchymoses, petechiae, or purpura may indicate a bleeding disorder. Excessive bruising or burns may be signs of abuse, falling, or cognitive problems.

4. Inspect the hair.
   - Observe the amount, distribution, and colour of hair.
   - Note excessive or total loss of hair; abnormal location of hair, especially gender related; and dry, brittle, or coarse hair.

▶ Hair usually becomes grey or white because of the loss of melanocytes. Be sure to check the colour at the roots if it is dyed. Balding of hair in men and thinning of head hair in women is common. However, hairiness increases in the nose and ears. Women may experience an increase of facial hair, especially on the chin. Excessive hair changes may indicate hormonal disorders, use of gonadotropic hormones for cancer chemotherapy, or excessive use of corticosteroids. Dry, brittle hair may indicate malnutrition. Dull, coarse hair could indicate hypothyroidism. Dishevelled hair may indicate lack of care or mental impairment.

TECHNIQUES AND NORMAL FINDINGS	ABNORMAL FINDINGS AND SPECIAL CONSIDERATIONS

5. Inspect the nails and nail beds.
   - Note the condition, hygiene, nail-bed angle, and blanching.

▶ Nails become thicker and may be more brittle. However, extreme brittleness and tearing may indicate a protein deficiency. Very thick nails are seen in vascular insufficiency and diabetes. Long, dirty nails are signs of caregiver or self-care neglect. Increased nail-bed angle (clubbing) is related to chronic lung or cardiac diseases.

HEAD AND NECK

1. Observe the face.
   - Aging changes result in more wrinkles and a softer, more jowly appearance.

▶ Excessive sagging and drooping, especially when it is unilateral, may indicate a stroke or other neurological damage.

2. Inspect the nose and nares.
   - Note colour, size, and any excessive dryness.

▶ Dryness is a sign of senile rhinitis, and redness in the nares may indicate chronic allergy. The nose tends to get larger with age, but a swollen papular, red nose indicates rhinophyma, a severe rosacea of the lower half of the nose. Usually seen in males, rhinophyma is characterized by lobulated overgrowth of sebaceous glands and epithelial connective tissue.

3. Evaluate the client's sense of smell.
   - Use identifiable substances, such as coffee, mint, or lemon.

▶ Smell and taste diminish with age, but perceiving unusual odours may be a sign of temporal lobe epilepsy. An inability to distinguish pungent, common odours could be related to neurological dysfunction, such as stroke.

4. Inspect the oral mucous membranes, gums, throat, and tongue.
   - Note colour, exudate, swelling, and lesions.
   - Have the client say "ah" as you depress the tongue with a tongue blade. Check for symmetrical elevation of the soft palate.

▶ Pale mucous membranes can indicate malnutrition or anemia; white patches could be precancerous leukoplakia. If the client's own teeth are present, redness and spongy swelling with recession of the gum from the neck of the tooth indicate periodontal disease. If the client is wearing dentures, redness and leukoplakia are signs of poorly fitting, irritating dentures. A bright red tongue could indicate thiamine (B_1) or vitamin C deficiency; a dark red, swollen tongue with white or yellow adherent patches is a sign of fungal infection, which older people taking antibiotics commonly experience. A dry and red tongue with longitudinal furrows indicates dehydration, especially in people taking diuretics or having elevated blood sugar levels. Unequal elevation or loss of elevation of the soft palate occurs with impairment of cranial nerves IX and X, seen with cerebral vascular accident. In this case, the person is at risk for choking and aspiration.

PHYSICAL ASSESSMENT

TECHNIQUES AND NORMAL FINDINGS	ABNORMAL FINDINGS AND SPECIAL CONSIDERATIONS

5. Palpate and auscultate the carotid arteries.
   - Proceed gently, palpating one artery at a time.
   - Auscultate with the bell of the stethoscope.

   ▶ Bruits are signs of carotid stenosis and impending cerebral vascular accident. If you hear bruits, check the aortic and pulmonic valve areas of the chest for murmurs, which may be radiating into the neck.

   - Note any bruits.

6. Inspect and palpate the neck veins.
   - Assess the veins first with the client lying flat and then with the client elevated above a 45-degree angle.

   ▶ All vessels enlarge with age and are more visible because of decreased subcutaneous tissue, but they are normally soft and compressible. If the veins are flat when the client is supine, suspect dehydration. If the neck veins are visible, firm to the touch, or tortuous when the client is elevated 45 degrees, suspect increased venous pressure and right-sided heart failure.

   - Note any firmness and distension.

7. Evaluate the range of motion of the neck.
   - Do not overextend the neck.

   ▶ Limited range of motion in the neck is often related to cervical arthritis, degenerative disc disease, or muscle spasm. Overextension may be painful. It may also decrease blood flow to basal arteries if any are stenosed. If kyphosis is present, hyperextension of the neck is difficult. Dizziness may also occur with motion if there are any existing inner ear pathologies.

EYE

1. Inspect the eyelids, cornea, and iris.
   - Note the position of the lid on the iris, identifying any tumours or cloudiness of the cornea, rings over the limbus, irregularities of the iris, and inturning or drooping of lids.

   ▶ The eyelids cover more of the iris in the aging eye because of decreased muscle tone, but frank ptosis in which the upper lid covers a considerable portion of the pupil, especially if unilateral, is a sign of dysfunction of cranial nerves III and IV, possibly because of cerebral vascular accident (brain attack). Bilateral ptosis may be due to ocular myasthenia gravis. Pterygium is not significant, nor is arcus senilis. Cloudiness over the iris and pupil could be due to beginning cataracts. Irregularities of the iris may be genetic in origin but more likely caused by previous surgery for glaucoma. Entropion and ectropion are the result of loss of muscle tone.

2. Check the pupils for size, equality, and reactivity.
   - Note both consensual and direct response to light. Ensure that the room is dimly lighted and that the client is facing away from sources of outside light.

   ▶ Pupils decrease in size with age, and because of their smallness it may be difficult to elicit pupillary constriction. Lack of consensual response or inequality of size may indicate damage to cranial nerve III. Unusually small pupils (smaller than 2 mm) may be due to ophthalmic miotic medications for glaucoma.

PHYSICAL ASSESSMENT

TECHNIQUES AND NORMAL FINDINGS	ABNORMAL FINDINGS AND SPECIAL CONSIDERATIONS

3. **Measure visual acuity.**
   - Be sure that the light is now comfortably bright.

▶ Loss of accommodation and power (holding the screener more than 35 cm [14 in.] away from the eyes and requiring bright light to read by), called presbyopia, is a normal finding. However, the client should be asked when he or she last had a full vision screening and reading glasses prescription update. Loss of central vision indicates macular degeneration. Blurring or cloudiness could be related to glaucoma, diabetic retinopathy, or cataracts.

   - Use a hand-held Rosenbaum card, testing each eye separately while the client has glasses on. Then test both eyes together.

4. **Check peripheral fields of vision.**
   - Especially note any losses of either left or right fields of vision.

▶ A right or left hemispheric stroke can result in a loss in the contralateral visual field. Bilateral loss of peripheral vision may indicate cataracts or glaucoma.

5. **Inspect the fundus of the eye with an ophthalmoscope.**
   - Note any dark areas in the red reflex, changes in the optic disc, and the appearance of the blood vessels.

▶ Tiny pupils make funduscopic inspection difficult. Changes of aging include narrower and straighter vessels. Black spots in the red reflex are signs of opacities as may be seen in cataracts. "Cupping" of the disc is a sign of glaucoma, and a "fuzzy disc" indicates cerebral edema. Narrowing and tapering of the arterioles are seen in hypertensive disease, and small red spots or creamy round lesions are punctate hemorrhages and exudate seen in diabetic retinopathy.

6. **Gently palpate the eyeball.**
   - Ask the client to close his or her eyes. Note tension or firmness.

▶ Very soft or boggy eyeballs indicate dehydration, whereas rock-hard orbits could mean glaucoma.

EAR

1. **Inspect the outer ear, ear canal, and tympanic membrane.**
   - Use an otoscope to inspect the ear canal and tympanic membrane.

▶ Excessive cerumen may cause a conductive hearing loss. Cerumen tends to be drier in older adults and may not be easy to remove. Improper ear-cleaning habits (e.g., use of cotton swabs) can pack cerumen tightly in the canal, interfering with hearing and obscuring visualization of the tympanic membrane. Scarring and sclerosis of the tympanic membrane from repeated inflammation or infection give a darkened appearance or dark lines.

   - Note any excessive cerumen or changes in the tympanic membrane.

PHYSICAL ASSESSMENT

TECHNIQUES AND NORMAL FINDINGS

ABNORMAL FINDINGS AND SPECIAL CONSIDERATIONS

2. Evaluate the client's hearing.
   - Use the whisper, Rinne, and Weber tests.

▶ Hearing loss with aging begins with diminished perception of high-frequency sounds. Subtle changes are found when using higher-frequency tuning forks. Sensorineural losses are more common than conductive losses in older adults because of loss of hair cells in the organ of Corti. This loss is called presbycusis. In sensorineural hearing loss, the Rinne test is normal (AC > BC), but the Weber test shows the sound lateralizing to the good ear or equal in both if hearing is diminished bilaterally.

RESPIRATORY SYSTEM

1. Inspect the shape of the thorax.
   - Look for increased anterior to posterior diameter and spinal curvature abnormalities that may affect respiration.

▶ Loss of bone density and weakened thoracic musculature result in an increased anteroposterior diameter. Severe barrel chest is a sign of chronic obstructive pulmonary disease. Also, kyphosis and scoliosis may decrease lung expansion. (See Chapter 15. ⬭)

2. Assess the chest wall and ribs.
   - Assess pain or tenderness to touch, crepitus, or bruising.
   - Palpate for tactile fremitus.

▶ Pain on palpation of the ribs is a sign of pathological fractures of the ribs, which can occur without any major trauma in the client with osteoporosis. Also look for bruising in conjunction with rib pain, which could be due to falls or physical abuse.

Increased fremitus, especially in the periphery, indicates fluid accumulation or tissue consolidation.

3. Percuss the lung fields.
   - Check for hyperresonance or dullness.

▶ Anticipate hyperresonance in the older adult with chronic obstructive pulmonary disease. Dullness indicates fluid accumulation from pulmonary edema or retained secretions. Dullness could also indicate tissue consolidation from a tumour or mass.

4. Auscultate the lung fields.
   - Auscultate all lung fields and note characteristics of sounds.

▶ Scattered rales in the bases are quite common in healthy older adults. Rales that extend upward and do not temporarily clear with cough suggest pulmonary edema. Scattered or discrete rales can be due to alveolar or small airway exudate. Coarse, loud rales may be signs of pulmonary fibrosis seen in people with long-standing lung disease. Because lung expansion decreases with age, breath sounds are not heard as far down as in younger adults. If the person has increased trapped air from emphysema, which is present to some degree in the very old as a normal finding, breath sounds and vocal resonance will be diminished. Difficulty hearing any breath sounds, harsh

TECHNIQUES AND NORMAL FINDINGS

ABNORMAL FINDINGS AND SPECIAL CONSIDERATIONS

rhonchi, or bronchovesicular breath sounds in the periphery are indicative of advanced chronic lung disease.

CLINICAL TIP
When listening to breath sounds, care should be taken to allow the older adult to intersperse the necessary deep breaths with shallower ones so that the client does not hyperventilate and become dizzy. Care should also be taken to keep the client warm and not overly exposed.

BREASTS

1. Assess the female and male breasts.
   - Note changes in symmetry, lumps or thickening of tissue, lesions or sores, inflammation, changes in the nipples, or drainage from open lesions or from the nipples. (See Chapter 16. ⚭)

▶ Hormonal changes can increase breast tissue in males and put them at risk for breast cancer. In Canada, less than 1% of breast cancers occur in men, more commonly in those over 60 years old (Canadian Cancer Society, 2009).

Females on postmenopausal hormone therapy are at increased risk for breast cancer, especially if female relatives have had it. Decreased fat in the female breast may make masses easier to feel. Risk for all cancers increases with age, and early identification of tumours is vital.

CARDIOVASCULAR SYSTEM

1. Auscultate the precordium.
   - Auscultate at five points on the precordium. Listen for S_1 and S_2.
   - Check for murmurs, clicks, and S_3 or S_4 gallops.
   - Use the bell of the stethoscope to listen for low-pitched murmurs during S_3 and S_4.
   - Use the diaphragm to listen for high-pitched murmurs, clicks, and snaps.
   - If you hear a murmur, move the stethoscope away from the site in several directions to check for radiation. Describe murmurs by using specified criteria. (See Chapter 17. ⚭)

▶ Murmurs, usually holosystolic and grade 3 without radiation, and S_3 are common in older people because of decreased cardiac muscle tone. Loud murmurs grade 4 or greater and with thrills or radiation suggest a failing heart, valvular stenosis, or incompetency. Murmurs that radiate from the apex to the anterior axillary area are usually of mitral origin. Murmurs that radiate from the base near the sternal border, right or left, up into the neck are usually related to aortic or pulmonic valve disease. Clicks and snaps are opening sounds and point to aortic or mitral calcifications. A fixed splitting of the second heart sound (not heard just on inspiration but throughout the respiratory cycle) is noted in pulmonary hypertension or chronic obstructive pulmonary disease.

PHYSICAL ASSESSMENT

TECHNIQUES AND NORMAL FINDINGS

ABNORMAL FINDINGS AND SPECIAL CONSIDERATIONS

2. Take the apical pulse.
   - Note rate and rhythm.

▶ Arrhythmias are quite common in healthy seniors. Abnormally slow rates could indicate heart block or sinus arrest, especially if accompanied by syncope. Fast or grossly irregular rhythms point to potentially serious tachyarrhythmias, especially if accompanied by chest pain or dizziness. After periods of immobilization, increased heart rate can indicate decompensation.

ABDOMEN

1. Inspect the abdomen.
   - Observe for shape, symmetry, and pulsations.

▶ Flaccid or "potbelly" abdomen is common because of loss of collagen and muscle, and deposition of fat. A scaphoid and flaccid abdomen is seen in the very old with additional fat loss but may also be a sign of rapid weight loss accompanying malnutrition or cancer. A distended abdomen is seen with ascites (fluid in the peritoneal cavity) or excessive gas. Asymmetry may indicate tumours, hernia, constipation, or bowel obstruction. Although the slight up-and-down pulsation from a normal aorta is more readily seen in clients with thin abdominal walls, lateral pulsations or soft, pulsatile masses indicate an aortic aneurysm. Visible tortuous veins on the abdominal wall near the umbilicus, in conjunction with a firm and distended abdomen, indicate portal hypertension with ascites.

2. Auscultate the abdomen.
   - Note the number and quality of bowel sounds.
   - Check for vascular bruits over the aorta, in flank areas for the renal arteries, and over the groin for the femoral and iliac arteries.

▶ Bowel sounds may be hypoactive. Borborygmi may be due to bleeding or inflammatory bowel disease. High-pitched hyperactive bowel sounds accompanied by colicky pain and distension are signs of small bowel obstruction, which occurs more often in older males. Bruits heard over any of the arteries are signs of stenosis or aneurysms.

3. Percuss the abdomen.
   - Percuss the four quadrants of the abdomen and note tympany and dullness over most of the abdomen.

▶ Because of the normally thinner abdominal wall, tympany may be more noticeable but should still be within normal ranges. Areas of dullness in the lower left quadrant and sigmoid area are probably related to stool, but it is essential to rule out tumours.

   Shifting dullness, especially when accompanied by firm dullness, suggests ascites.

   Dullness above the symphysis pubis could indicate a full bladder.

4. Palpate the abdomen.
   - Use light and then deep palpation and note tenderness, firmness, rigidity, and masses.

TECHNIQUES AND NORMAL FINDINGS	ABNORMAL FINDINGS AND SPECIAL CONSIDERATIONS

- Palpate the costal margin at the right midclavicular line and midsternal line for liver enlargement.

▶ Tenderness with moderate distension could be due to flatus but could also indicate irritation of the stomach or bowel. The thinner abdominal wall of the older adult makes it easier to feel the underlying bowel. A soft mass or small firm masses felt in the left lower quadrant may be stool, especially because constipation is common. Firmness is associated with fluid or excessive gas, but rigidity is a sign of peritoneal inflammation. Distension just above the symphysis pubis may be caused by bladder distension because of prostatic hypertrophy or incomplete emptying. If the liver can be palpated below the costal margins, the liver is probably enlarged. Enlargement may reflect passive congestion from congestive heart failure or liver disease, especially if the liver feels nodular.

GENITOURINARY SYSTEM

Female

1. **Check the underclothing for staining.**
   - If present, note the colour, amount, and odour.

   ▶ Staining indicates urinary or bowel incontinence or vaginal discharge.

2. **Inspect the external genitals.**
   - Note changes in colour, appearance, and odour in the external genitalia. Atrophy of the labia is usual.

   ▶ Redness, swelling, or odour can indicate incontinence, yeast infections, inadequate self-care, or caretaker neglect. Fecal-like odour could signal a urinary fistula.

3. **Perform a pelvic examination.**
   - Assist the client into the left lateral position.

   ▶ Bulging of tissue or muscle into the vagina or rectum indicates cystocele, rectocele, or uterine prolapse. Vaginal atrophy and dryness may make examination painful. Malodorous vaginal discharge could be a sign of cancer or infection.

4. **Examine the rectum.**
   - Note sphincter control.
   - Check for hemorrhoids.
   - Take a stool sample and check for occult blood.

   ▶ Sphincter control decreases with age, resulting in incontinence. Rectal cancer is more common in older adults; occult blood in the stool is an early sign of cancer.

Male

1. **Check the underclothing for staining.**
   - Note colour and odour of stains.

   ▶ Staining indicates incontinence. Small amounts of dried blood could indicate intermittently bleeding hemorrhoids.

2. **Examine the external genitals.**
   - Observe for swelling, redness, or odour.

   ▶ Testicular and penile atrophy is normal, but swelling could be a sign of infection or prostatic hypertrophy. Swelling, redness, and odour can be a sign of infection, incontinence, poor self-care, or caretaker neglect.

PHYSICAL ASSESSMENT

TECHNIQUES AND NORMAL FINDINGS	ABNORMAL FINDINGS AND SPECIAL CONSIDERATIONS

PHYSICAL ASSESSMENT

3. Perform a rectal examination.

- Note sphincter control.
- Check for prostate enlargement and any rectal abnormalities, such as hemorrhoids.
- Take a stool sample and check for occult blood.

▶ Prostatic hypertrophy can be benign or malignant; encourage the client to have a prostate-specific antigen (PSA) test. Elevated levels usually indicate carcinoma of the prostate. The occult blood test can detect colon cancer, which increases in incidence in men over age 40. Hemorrhoids can cause bright red bleeding, as well as a red stain on the stool. A mass in the rectum could be rectal cancer.

MUSCULOSKELETAL SYSTEM

1. Position the client.

- Help the client to a comfortable sitting position while maintaining safety.

2. Assess the spinal column.

- Note abnormal curvatures, deformities, pain or tenderness with palpation of vertebrae, and bruising or other signs of trauma.

▶ Shortening of the spine through flattening of the discs is very common. Loss of bone matrix and decreased muscle mass and tone can result in increased curvatures, such as kyphosis, lordosis, or scoliosis. Arthritis and degenerative disc disease can cause spinal deformities. Pain on palpation of the vertebrae and generalized back pain indicate pathological fractures from osteoporosis. Bruising or unusual lesions on the back could indicate falls or physical abuse.

3. Assess all joints.

- Assess for pain, heat, redness, swelling, deformity, and range of motion.

▶ Heat, redness, swelling, and pain on movement of joints indicate bursitis or gouty or septic arthritis. Rheumatoid arthritis also produces these symptoms but is more likely to be seen in younger adults. Osteoarthritis causes swelling and joint deformity with early morning stiffness and pain. Hands and weight-bearing joints, such as hips and knees, are most often affected.

4. Assess the muscles.

- Inspect the muscles for size, comparing one side with the other.
- Palpate muscles for tone.

▶ Loss of innervation to specific muscle groups or paralysis from cerebral vascular accident or other neurological diseases results in atrophy and loss of or increased tone.

5. Assess the feet.

- Note colour, skin integrity, any deformities, and signs of inflammation, infection, or ulcerations.
- Palpate pedal pulses.

▶ Bunions and corns are common. If home remedies have been used to treat corns, inflammation and ulceration may result. Pedal pulses may diminish with aging, but the inability to palpate pulses, especially if the feet are red or dusky in colour, indicates arterial insufficiency. Pitting edema of feet and legs because of venous incompetency or right-sided heart failure may be present.

TECHNIQUES AND NORMAL FINDINGS	ABNORMAL FINDINGS AND SPECIAL CONSIDERATIONS

NEUROLOGICAL SYSTEM

1. Evaluate mental status.

- Do this at the end of the examination when rapport has been well established with the client, as long as the client is not overly tired. If at any point the client seems to be tiring, dividing the examination into two sessions should be considered, and the mental status assessment should be done when the client is rested.
- Use a tool designed for older people, such as the MMSE.
- Screen for depression, if indicated.

▶ These tools can identify subtle changes in memory and mental functioning that the client could disguise in ordinary conversation by confabulation. The results are especially valuable when compared over successive evaluations. However, clients can get very apprehensive over the possibility of poor performance, and the tools must be used with empathy and understanding.

2. Assess cranial nerves.

- Assess cranial nerves as described in Chapter 24. ⟳

▶ Tests are performed by using the same techniques. Findings may include slowed or diminished responses.

3. Evaluate balance and coordination.

- Assess the client's ability to walk heel to toe forward and backward.
- Ask the client to perform the Romberg test first with the eyes opened and then with the eyes closed.
- Look for swaying and loss of balance.
- Stand close to the client with arms outspread, ready to prevent fall or injury.

▶ The heel-to-toe walk is often impaired and is not indicative of any specific disease, but it can place the person at risk for falls. Older people have a tendency to fall sideways. Falling forward and a propulsive gait are indicative of Parkinson's disease. If the person can correct balance with the eyes open, the defect is probably proprioceptive rather than of basal ganglion or cerebellar origin.

CLINICAL TIP
Any time that clients are asked to close their eyes, special care should be taken to protect them from falling.

4. Inspect for tremors of the head, face, and extremities.

- Note the kind of tremor and whether it is present at rest or primarily with movement.

▶ Gross tremor of the head (head bobbing), jaw, and tongue is called a senile tremor and is not treatable. A resting tremor, which diminishes with willed movement, and a pill-rolling tremor of the hands is seen in Parkinson's disease. People taking bronchodilator drugs have a fine tremor that increases with activity.

5. Evaluate motor strength.

- Assess the client's arm drift. Have the client stand with his or her feet comfortably apart and the arms held straight out at shoulder level. Check arm drift first with the client's eyes closed and then with them open.
- Assess the client's grip and extremity strength against resistance.

▶ Subtle hemiparesis is indicated by slow downward drift and pronation of hand on affected side when the eyes are closed; if the client is able to correct the drift when the eyes are opened, suspect proprioceptive dysfunction (sensory-position sense). Unilateral diminished grip and loss of strength against resistance can indicate a stroke.

6. Evaluate sensation.

- Assist the client to a sitting position.
- Ask the client to close his or her eyes for all sensory evaluation.
- Check various sites for sensitivity to touch (use sharp and dull objects) and vibration (use a tuning fork on joints). Ask the client to identify where the sensation is felt by pointing or verbally identifying the location.

▶ Sensation and discrimination normally decrease in older people, as does vibratory sense in the toes. Suspect neurological disease, such as cerebrovascular accident, if sensation is absent in any area, especially unilaterally. Diminished or absent sensation symmetrically in lower extremities is a sign of diabetic peripheral neuropathy.

PHYSICAL ASSESSMENT

TECHNIQUES AND NORMAL FINDINGS	ABNORMAL FINDINGS AND SPECIAL CONSIDERATIONS

- Assess stereognosis by asking the client to close the eyes and identify a key or other familiar object placed in the client's hand.
- Assess graphesthesia by asking the client to identify numbers you write with your finger on each of the client's hands.
- Evaluate proprioception by having the client identify the position to which you move a toe or finger.

7. Evaluate reflexes with a reflex hammer.

- Note diminished or increased reflexes.

▶ Reflexes normally diminish with aging. If they are absent, suspect upper motor neuron disease; if they are hyperactive, especially with clonus, suspect lower motor neuron disease.

APPLICATION THROUGH CRITICAL THINKING

CASE STUDY

Mary Sutton is an 83-year-old grandmother of five who lives alone in a seniors' high-rise apartment in downtown Toronto. Her husband died 15 years ago. She has two daughters who live in Montreal and St. John's. They visit her every month or so, and she talks to them on the phone weekly. Mrs. Sutton has always been proud of her independence and has stated firmly that although she loves her family, she would never want to move in with either of her daughters and lose this independence.

She retired from her position as an executive secretary to a bank president when she was 67 years old, and she had been busy until recently volunteering in several community projects, visiting friends, and caring for her own daily needs. She has come to the clinic for a routine physical examination. Everyone in the clinic looks forward to her visits, because she frequently brings homemade cookies and is always smiling and friendly.

Mrs. Sutton's health has been fairly good up until now, although she has experienced angina and arthritis pain in the past. She is being treated for hypertension with atenolol 25 mg (beta blocker) and nifedipine 10 mg (calcium channel blocker) each day, as well as furosemide 40 mg (loop diuretic). Her blood pressure is usually 140/80. She takes allopurinol 200 mg (antihyperuricemic) to control symptoms of gout, and simvastatin 40 mg for hyperlipidemia. She also takes a daily low-dose enteric-coated Aspirin, has nitroglycerine tablets, and takes ibuprofen as needed for pain. She is on a low-fat, low-salt diet.

Today Mrs. Sutton seems quieter and smiles less than normal. She apologizes when she comes in that she was unable to bring any homemade goodies as she did not have a chance to go out to buy sugar and eggs. When asked how she has been feeling, she answers, "Okay." But when asked about some of her volunteer activities, she states that she has not been able to get involved as much as before. She is dressed nicely, although in quiet colours, and does not appear ill. Her hair is combed neatly, although she mentions that she did not get a chance to get her monthly permanent wave at the beauty parlour. She has no specific complaints.

When Mrs. Sutton weighs in, the nurse finds that she has lost 4.5 kg (10 lb.) since her last visit 3 months ago. Her vital signs are as follows: B/P 152/85—P 74—RR 18—T 37.6°C (99.8°F)—Pain 4. All of these values are elevated since her last visit. Her muscle strength is somewhat diminished but adequate. Her gait is slow, steady, and balanced.

Examination of her head, neck, and throat reveals no abnormalities or signs of inflammation or illness, although her skin is dry and she appears to have more wrinkles than the nurse remembers her having. Her hearing is unchanged, as is her vision. She is wearing bifocals that were updated 6 months ago. Her teeth appear to be in good condition and she does not exhibit any bad mouth odour. However, her mucous membranes are somewhat pale and dry. Her lung fields are clear and her respirations are not laboured. Her breasts are soft and without palpable masses. When listening to her heart, the nurse hears the systolic murmur that has been present for some time. It does not seem to have changed from the previous visit. Her abdomen is soft and not distended. No bruits or abnormal sounds are auscultated, although bowel sounds are somewhat hypoactive. No tenderness, firmness, rigidity, or masses are palpated.

Although Mrs. Sutton was asked to remove her clothing and put on an examination gown before the physical assessment, she chose to keep on her underpants. When asked to slide these down so that her genitourinary system could be assessed, she became somewhat flustered and anxious, but did so. The nurse sees that Mrs. Sutton has a wad of damp tissue inside her pants. There is no obvious stain on the tissue, but there is a strong odour of urine. The skin of her perineum and thighs is inflamed with a red, papular rash. When asked how long she has had the rash, Mrs. Sutton states that it has been getting worse for the last 2 months and that nothing she has tried has helped it. When asked what she has tried she answers, "Cornstarch or talcum powder, witch hazel, and soap."

The nurse asks why she is using the tissues. Mrs. Sutton answers that it is just a way to stay clean. The nurse then asks if she has any trouble holding her urine, and Mrs. Sutton says, "Of course. I'm 83, aren't I?" The nurse asks whether there is anything else that Mrs. Sutton does to help this, and she says that she puts pads on all the chairs she sits on and on her bed at night. She also says that she does not allow herself to drink water after 3 p.m. On further questioning Mrs. Sutton starts to wipe tears from her eyes and says that she cannot go out anymore and visit her friends because she is afraid of ruining their furniture. She admits that this is why she has given up her volunteer activities and why she does not get out to the store or the hairdresser anymore. She does not have her friends come to her apartment because she is embarrassed to have them see the pads on the furniture, and sometimes she is afraid that there is a bad odour. She ends by saying, "It's not fun to be old and have to be like this."

As the nurse questions Mrs. Sutton about the specifics of her urinary incontinence, the nurse learns that this problem has been increasing since shortly after the last clinic visit. Mrs. Sutton states she loses urine every time that she laughs, sneezes, coughs, carries heavy bundles, or even stands up quickly. This happens more when she is tired and when her bladder is full. Some days she skips taking her furosemide pill because it makes the problem worse. The rash is very annoying; it itches and stings at times. Lately her urine has started to burn her when she voids. Because of these symptoms, Mrs. Sutton has curtailed all social activity.

The rest of the physical assessment is normal. Mrs. Sutton's cognitive ability has not changed and she does not score highly on the depression screening scale. However, her affect is sad, and her enthusiasm for life is missing.

▶ Complete Documentation

The following is sample documentation for Mary Sutton.

SUBJECTIVE DATA: 83-year-old female seen for routine physical assessment. States urinary incontinence and rash for 3 months that is unrelieved by talcum powder, witch hazel, or soap. States incontinence episodes occur with laughing, sneezing, coughing, carrying heavy bundles, or standing up quickly. Reports that she restricts fluid intake after 3 p.m., sometimes withholds furosemide, and has withdrawn from community involvement and confined herself to her home for fear of embarrassment from wetness and odour. Sees the reason for this as "old age." Also states she has recently felt pain on voiding.

OBJECTIVE DATA: Vital signs slightly elevated since last visit 3 months ago. Mucous membranes are pale and dry. All other systems are within normal limits for client except for a red, papular rash on perineum and upper, inner thighs, and strong urine odour on wadded tissues in underpants. No concerns

regarding client's cognitive ability and her depression screening is normal. Her affect is sad and her personality more listless than normal for her. Her hair is not "permed" as usual, and her clothes are less colourful than is normal for her. A urinalysis yielded the following abnormal information: hazy, amber urine with a specific gravity of 1.035 that tested positive for bacteria. Other urine values were normal.

▶ Critical Thinking Questions

Clustering the objective and subjective data obtained from the interview will lead to several nursing diagnoses. However, Mrs. Sutton has also given some hints that may require follow-up to obtain additional information.

1. What additional information would help the nurse to plan care for this client?
2. How should information be clustered to guide decision making?
3. What recommendations would you provide for this client?

▶ Applying Nursing Diagnoses

1. *Stress urinary incontinence* is a nursing diagnosis in the NANDA-I taxonomy. Do the data for Mary Sutton support this diagnosis? If so, identify the data.
2. Another NANDA-I diagnosis is *impaired social interaction*. Do the data for Mrs. Sutton support this diagnosis? If so, identify the data.
3. Another NANDA-I diagnosis is *impaired skin integrity*. Do the data for Mrs. Sutton support this diagnosis? If so, identify the data.
4. Use the NANDA-I taxonomy in Appendix A to develop additional diagnoses for Mrs. Sutton. ∞
5. Identify the data required for the PES (problem, etiology, signs or symptoms) statement.

▶ Prepare Teaching Plan

LEARNING NEED: Mary Sutton came to the clinic for a routine physical assessment. She was experiencing stress incontinence, which had caused her embarrassment, fear, sorrow, inflammation, dehydration, possible infection, and social isolation. Mrs. Sutton saw this incontinence as a normal part of aging, causing her to adopt a hopeless attitude and not to seek treatment. Although she initially denied any health problems, her significant problems were found on genitourinary examination and follow-up questioning. In addition to the incontinence and rash, the issue of Mary's self-ageism must be addressed so that she can learn how to control her stress incontinence, clear up her rash, and once again enjoy her vibrant, outgoing lifestyle.

The case study presents a problem that is all too common among older clients. It is frequently underreported and undertreated because of ageism on the part of both the client and the healthcare provider. The following teaching plan on managing stress incontinence can be used for all clients experiencing this problem, but it is directed toward an older woman.

GOAL: The participant will be able to control incontinence.

OBJECTIVES: On completion of this educational session, the participant will be able to do the following:

1. State normal voiding patterns for older adults.
2. Identify causes of stress incontinence.
3. Describe measures to manage stress incontinence.
4. Describe measures to protect skin from incontinence episodes.

Application of Objective 1: State normal voiding patterns for older adults.

Content	Teaching Strategy	Evaluation
<ul><li>Incontinence is not "normal" in older people.</li><li>The amount of urine that an older person can store comfortably in the bladder is between 200 and 300 mL (7 to 10 fl.oz.).</li><li>This is less than the 350 to 450 mL (12 to 16 fl.oz.) held comfortably by younger adults, because of thickening of the bladder wall with age, which makes distension more difficult.</li><li>The presence of urine in the bladder triggers the neurological control to void.</li><li>Given normal kidney function, the amount of urine produced each hour depends on the amount of fluid taken in. This alters the times between voidings.</li><li>Some fluid is lost through sweat, respiration, and bowel movements, so the intake does not exactly match the output.</li><li>Medications, such as diuretics, increase the amount of urine produced.</li><li>Drinks that contain caffeine or alcohol also increase urine production.</li></ul>	<ul><li>Lecture</li><li>Discussion</li><li>Audiovisual materials</li><li>Printed materials</li><li>Samples of equipment</li></ul>Lecture is appropriate when disseminating information to large groups. Discussion allows participants to bring up concerns and to raise questions. Audiovisual materials, such as illustrations of the structures of the urinary system, reinforce verbal presentation. Printed materials, especially to be taken away with learners, allows review, reinforcement, and reading at the learner's own pace.	<ul><li>Having learners state orally the various points that they have learned is the best way to test their knowledge. This eliminates any problems with reading, writing, or the anxiety caused by a formal test situation.</li><li>Some learners in the early stages may not feel comfortable using the vocabulary or discussing out loud a topic area that they still find embarrassing or shameful. For them, written questions may be best.</li></ul>

Health Promotion Assessment Tool

Social Determinants of Action	Level of Action	Action Strategies
Social environments	Individual	**Develop personal skills** (to regain independence and a balanced lifestyle) • Assess Mrs. Sutton's physical limitations and comfort level and create a plan with her to facilitate ongoing social support. Components of the plan may include • shorter outings • outings when well rested • alternate means to keep social contact when she can't go out due to health reasons, for example, contact by telephone or email
Social support networks	Individual and community	**Create supportive environments** • Refer Mrs. Sutton to a nonjudgmental support group for seniors experiencing isolation due to health concerns. • Address ageist beliefs with Mrs. Sutton and explore the potential value to be gained from sharing challenges and solutions with other older adults.
Income and social status	Individual	**Develop personal skills** • Explore the meaning of Mrs. Sutton's statement "It's not fun to be old and have to be like this," and gently challenge her beliefs and attitudes related to being an older adult in relation to • changes in body image and acceptability of her body • independence • social status • value and contribution to society • Develop a plan with Mrs. Sutton to create an improved sense of social acceptability and her intrinsic self worth as an older adult. Start with identifying her contributions to others, including the clinic staff (homemade cookies and her friendly personality).

ABNORMAL FINDINGS

Abnormal findings common in older adults include skin lesions, insulin resistance syndrome, diabetes mellitus, and drug and alcohol abuse.

Skin Lesions

The aging skin is subject to a variety of lesions. (See Chapter 11. ⟳) The cause is unknown but may be related to altered DNA causing a change in cell types. Xanthelasma is a tiny, tumourlike fatty deposit on the eyelid that may be related to hyperlipidemia. **Acrochordons**, or skin tags, are pedunculated, flesh-coloured lesions of collagen and subcutaneous tissue that occur on the neck, back, axillary area, and eyelids. **Actinic keratoses** are normal aging growths, especially in fair–skinned people, but are considered precancerous. They appear as calluslike red, yellow, or flesh-coloured plaques on exposed areas, such as the ears, cheeks, lips, nose, upper extremities, or a balding scalp. **Seborrheic keratoses** are benign, greasy, wartlike lesions that are yellow-brown in colour. They can appear anywhere on the body but are seen most frequently on the neck, chest, and back. Vascular lesions can include **cherry angiomas**, which are nonsignificant tiny red spots, either macules or papules, rarely larger than 3 to 4 mm (0.12 to 0.16 in.), seen usually on the trunk. Another more serious vascular lesion is **senile purpura**, which can occur spontaneously or in response to minimal trauma in the very old client with fragile blood vessels. It is a coalescence of petechiae that begins as tiny individual red-to-purple spots caused by rupture of small capillaries. The petechiae converge from large purple to brown patches.

Cheilitis (angular stomatitis) is seen in persons who have poorly fitting dentures or who are not swallowing saliva well because of stroke or muscular weakness. This condition is marked by sore, reddened, cracked skin at either side of the mouth caused by excess salivation and *Candid0a* (yeast) infection.

Insulin Resistance Syndrome

Insulin resistance syndrome is a disorder in which is a whole complex of symptoms come together, including obesity, heart disease, hypertension, gout, polycystic ovaries, and type 2 diabetes. Insulin resistance syndrome is difficult to understand and to treat. It involves more than just transient hyperglycemia. The hyperinsulinemia resulting from the increased blood sugar levels causes hypoglycemia if meals are delayed. This may cause excess production of adrenal hormones (Lerman-Garber et al., 2000), which increases the heart rate and causes physical tremors.

The enzyme lipoprotein lipase, which helps break down triglycerides, is also altered in the presence of hyperinsulinemia. Thus, elevated triglyceride levels are found in persons experiencing the condition, especially in those who have central obesity. Such persons also show higher than usual incidence of atherosclerosis and gout. Each of these conditions is associated with increased risk for heart disease. In the case of atherosclerosis, this is due to stenosis caused by plaque buildup. In gout, it is due to the role of uric acid in thrombotic tendency (Longo-Mbenza, Luila, Mbete, & Vita, 1999).

Polycystic ovary syndrome is also related to hyperinsulinemia. In the presence of excess insulin levels, androgens are formed, leading to male pattern hair loss, excessive body hair, and ovarian cysts. There is an increased potential for endometrial hyperplasia and malignancy. Even though the older woman may have undergone menopause, taking a good menstrual history, with attention to irregular menstrual cycles and infertility, may identify possible polycystic ovary syndrome in an older, obese, hypertensive, hyperinsulinemic woman who may be experiencing insulin resistance syndrome.

Diabetes Mellitus

The chance of becoming diabetic doubles with every decade of life. A very small percentage of older clients have type 1 diabetes, and approximately 90% of all Canadians age 65 and older with diabetes have type 2 diabetes (Public Health Agency of Canada, 2008). In most populations, the incidence is higher in men than in women and non-whites are about 20% more likely to develop the disease (Ni et al., 2004).

The Public Health Agency of Canada (2008) believes that the chance of developing type 1 diabetes is increased for people who are genetically related to someone with diabetes or who have been exposed to a virus. Risk factors that influence the development of type 2 diabetes include age, obesity, a high-fat diet, a family history, physical inactivity, hypertension, and hypercholesterolemia.

The most reliable method to diagnose diabetes is a simple blood test followed by at least one confirmatory test. A fasting plasma glucose of 7.0 mmol/L, a casual (without consideration to the last meal) plasma glucose of 11.0 mmol/L, or a plasma glucose 2 hours after a meal of 11.0 mmol/L is indicative of nongestational diabetes (Canadian Diabetes Association, 2008). Examination of the glycated hemoglobin A (A1C) value shows the amount of blood glucose that is attached to the hemoglobin and indicates the average blood glucose level for the previous 120 days. The A1C is a useful test for monitoring the efficacy of glycemic control and checking for the effectiveness of health maintenance activities.

Drug and Alcohol Abuse

Some 12% of men and 3% of women ages 65 to 74 report having had more than five drinks of alcohol in one day at least once in the last year (Statistics Canada, 2006a). Alcohol intake must be considered when performing a nutritional assessment. The client should be asked the amount and type of alcoholic beverages he or she drinks. Although intake of one glass of wine or beer is associated with increased well-being, excessive alcohol intake may lead to malnutrition and to serious complications, such as pancreatitis or liver disease. If the client reports a high daily alcohol intake, the **CAGE** questionnaire (Ewing, 1984), which has been extensively validated against psychiatric criteria for alcoholism and alcohol abuse, may be used. The designer of the questionnaire recommends that even one "yes" identifies the need for further workup: **(C)** Have you ever had to *cut back* on your drinking? **(A)** Have people *annoyed you* with criticism about your drinking? **(G)** Have you ever felt *guilty* about your drinking? **(E)** Have you ever needed to start the day with a drink (an *eye-opener*)?

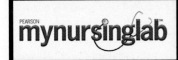

DOMAIN 1: HEALTH PROMOTION

Ineffective Health Maintenance
Ineffective Self Health Management
Impaired Home Maintenance
Enhanced Immunization Status, Readiness for
Self Neglect
Enhanced Nutrition, Readiness for
Ineffective Family Therapeutic Regimen Management
Enhanced Self Health Management, Readiness for

DOMAIN 2: NUTRITION

Ineffective Infant Feeding Pattern
Imbalanced Nutrition: Less Than Body Requirements
Imbalanced Nutrition: More Than Body Requirements
Imbalanced Nutrition: More Than Body Requirements,
    Risk for
Impaired Swallowing
Unstable Blood Glucose Level, Risk for
Neonatal Jaundice
Impaired Liver Function, Risk for
Electrolyte Imbalance, Risk for
Enhanced Fluid Balance, Readiness for
Deficient Fluid Volume
Excess Fluid Volume
Deficient Fluid Volume, Risk for
Imbalanced Fluid Volume, Risk for

DOMAIN 3: ELIMINATION AND EXCHANGE

Functional Urinary Incontinence
Overflow Urinary Incontinence
Reflex Urinary Incontinence
Stress Urinary Incontinence
Urge Urinary Incontinence
Urge Urinary Incontinence, Risk for
Impaired Urinary Elimination
Enhanced Urinary Elimination, Readiness for
Urinary Retention
Bowel Incontinence
Constipation
Perceived Constipation
Constipation, Risk for
Diarrhea
Dysfunctional Gastrointestinal Motility
Dysfunctional Gastrointestinal Motility, Risk for
Impaired Gas Exchange

DOMAIN 4: ACTIVITY/REST

Insomnia
Disturbed Sleep Pattern
Sleep Deprivation
Enhanced Sleep, Readiness for
Risk for Disuse Syndrome
Deficient Diversional Activity
Sedentary Lifestyle
Impaired Bed Mobility
Impaired Physical Mobility
Impaired Wheelchair Mobility
Delayed Surgical Recovery
Impaired Transfer Ability
Impaired Walking
Disturbed Energy Field
Fatigue
Activity Intolerance
Activity Intolerance, Risk for
Bleeding, Risk for
Ineffective Breathing Pattern
Decreased Cardiac Output
Ineffective Peripheral Tissue Perfusion
Decreased Cardiac Tissue Perfusion, Risk for
Ineffective Cerebral Tissue Perfusion, Risk for
Ineffective Gastrointestinal Perfusion, Risk for
Ineffective Renal Perfusion, Risk for
Shock, Risk for
Impaired Spontaneous Ventilation
Dysfunctional Ventilatory Weaning Response
Enhanced Self-care, Readiness for
Bathing Self-care Deficit
Dressing Self-care Deficit
Feeding Self-care Deficit
Toileting Self-care Deficit

DOMAIN 5: PERCEPTION/ COGNITION

Unilateral Neglect
Impaired Environmental Interpretation Syndrome
Wandering
Disturbed Sensory Perception (Specify: Visual, Auditory,
    Kinesthetic, Gustatory, Tactile, Olfactory)
Acute Confusion
Chronic Confusion
Risk for Acute Confusion

Deficient Knowledge
Enhanced Knowledge, Readiness for
Impaired Memory
Ineffective Activity Planning
Impaired Verbal Communication
Enhanced Decision Making, Readiness for
Enhanced Communication, Readiness for

DOMAIN 6: SELF-PERCEPTION

Compromised Human Dignity, Risk for
Hopelessness
Disturbed Personal Identity
Loneliness, Risk for
Readiness for Enhanced Power
Powerlessness
Powerlessness, Risk for
Enhanced Self-Concept, Readiness for
Situational Low Self-Esteem
Chronic Low Self-Esteem
Situational Low Self-Esteem, Risk for
Disturbed Body Image

DOMAIN 7: ROLE RELATIONSHIPS

Caregiver Role Strain
Caregiver Role Strain, Risk for
Impaired Parenting
Enhanced Parenting, Readiness for
Impaired Parenting, Risk for
Impaired Attachment, Risk for
Dysfunctional Family Processes
Interrupted Family Processes
Enhanced Family Processes, Readiness for
Effective Breastfeeding
Ineffective Breastfeeding
Interrupted Breastfeeding
Parental Role Conflict
Enhanced Relationship, Readiness for
Ineffective Role Performance
Impaired Social Interaction

DOMAIN 8: SEXUALITY

Sexual Dysfunction
Ineffective Sexuality Pattern
Enhanced Childbearing Process, Readiness for
Disturbed Maternal/Fetal Dyad, Risk for

DOMAIN 9: COPING/STRESS TOLERANCE

Post-Trauma Syndrome
Post-Trauma Syndrome, Risk for
Rape-Trauma Syndrome
Relocation Stress Syndrome
Relocation Stress Syndrome, Risk for
Anxiety
Death Anxiety
Risk-Prone Health Behavior
Compromised Family Coping
Defensive Coping
Disabled Family Coping
Ineffective Coping
Ineffective Community Coping
Enhanced Coping, Readiness for
Enhanced Community Coping, Readiness for
Enhanced Family Coping, Readiness for
Ineffective Denial
Fear
Grieving
Complicated Grieving
Complicated Grieving, Risk for
Impaired Individual Resilience
Enhanced Resilience, Readiness for
Compromised Resilience
Chronic Sorrow, Risk for
Stress Overload
Autonomic Dysreflexia
Autonomic Dysreflexia, Risk for
Disorganized Infant Behavior
Disorganized Infant Behavior, Risk for
Enhanced Organized Infant Behavior, Readiness for
Decreased Intracranial Adaptive Capacity

DOMAIN 10: LIFE PRINCIPLES

Enhanced Hope, Readiness for
Enhanced Spiritual Well-Being, Readiness for
Decisional Conflict
Moral Distress
Noncompliance
Impaired Religiosity
Impaired Religiosity, Risk for
Enhanced Religiosity, Readiness for
Spiritual Distress
Spiritual Distress, Risk for

DOMAIN 11: SAFETY/PROTECTION

Infection, Risk for
Ineffective Airway Clearance
Aspiration, Risk for
Sudden Infant Death Syndrome, Risk for
Impaired Dentition
Falls, Risk for
Injury, Risk for
Perioperative-Positioning Injury, Risk for
Impaired Oral Mucous Membrane
Peripheral Neurovascular Dysfunction, Risk for
Ineffective Protection
Impaired Skin Integrity
Impaired Skin Integrity, Risk for
Suffocation, Risk for
Impaired Tissue Integrity
Trauma, Risk for
Vascular Trauma, Risk for
Self-Mutilation
Self-Mutilation, Risk for
Suicide, Risk for
Other-Directed Violence, Risk for
Self-Directed Violence, Risk for
Contamination
Contamination, Risk for
Poisoning, Risk for

Latex Allergy Response
Latex Allergy Response, Risk for
Imbalanced Body Temperature, Risk for
Hyperthermia
Hypothermia
Ineffective Thermoregulation
Enhanced Immunization Status, Readiness for

DOMAIN 12: COMFORT

Enhanced Comfort, Readiness for
Impaired Comfort
Nausea
Acute Pain
Chronic Pain
Social Isolation

DOMAIN 13: GROWTH/ DEVELOPMENT

Adult Failure to Thrive
Delayed Growth and Development
Disproportionate Growth, Risk for
Delayed Development, Risk for

In order to make safe and effective judgments using NANDA-I nursing diagnoses it is essential that nurses refer to the definitions and defining characteristics of the diagnoses listed in this work.

Source: Nursing Diagnoses—Definitions and Classification 2009–2011 © 2009, 2007, 2005, 2003, 2001, 1998, 1996, 1994 NANDA International. Used by arrangement with Wiley-Blackwell Publishing, a company of John Wiley & Sons, Inc.

MODES OF TRANSMISSION

Transmission of infectious agents requires three elements: a source (or reservoir) of infectious agents, a susceptible host with a portal of entry receptive to the agent, and a mode of transmission. Historically, in hospital epidemiology the routes of transmission have been classified as airborne, contact, and droplet.

Airborne transmission: Airborne transmission occurs by dissemination of either airborne droplet nuclei or small particles in the respirable size range containing infectious agents that remain infective over time and distance. These microorganisms are widely dispersed by air currents and can be inhaled by susceptible hosts who may be some distance away from the infected source. Control of airborne transmission is the most difficult as it requires control of air flow through special ventilation systems.

Contact transmission: The most common mode of transmission is contact and it is subdivided into two categories: direct and indirect contact.

- **Direct contact transmission:** Direct transmission occurs when microorganisms are transferred from one infected person to another person. Examples include:

  - Blood or other blood-containing body fluids from a person directly enters another person's body through contact with a mucous membrane or cut in the skin

  - Mites from a scabies-infected person are transferred to the skin of another person while he or she has direct skin-to-skin contact

- **Indirect contact transmission:** Indirect transmission involves the transfer of an infectious agent through a contaminated intermediate object or person. Examples include:

  - Contaminated hands of care providers may transmit pathogens after touching an infected wound on one person and providing care to another person without performing hand hygiene

  - Equipment, such as glucose monitoring devices, may transmit pathogens if used while contaminated with blood from another person

  - Instruments that are inadequately cleaned after use may transmit pathogens

Droplet transmission: Refers to large droplets, greater than or equal to 5 mL in diameter, generated from the respiratory tract of the source (infected individual) during coughing or sneezing, or during procedures such as suctioning or bronchoscopy. These droplets are propelled a distance of less than 1–2 metres through the air and are deposited on the nasal or oral mucosa of the new host (susceptible individual) or in the immediate environment. Since these large droplets do not remain suspended in the air special ventilation is not required.

PERSONAL PROTECTIVE EQUIPMENT

Personal protective equipment (PPE) is any type of specialized clothing, barrier product, or breathing (respiratory) device used to protect workers from serious injuries or illnesses while doing their jobs. Personal protective equipment acts as a barrier between infectious materials and the skin, mouth, nose, or eyes (mucous membranes). In healthcare PPE includes gloves, gowns, and face protection: masks, goggles, and face shields. The CDC has a PowerPoint presentation on the procedures for donning and removing PPE available at http://www.cdc.gov/ncidod/dhqp/ppe.html

Gloves: Wear gloves when contact is anticipated with blood or other potentially infectious materials, mucous membranes, nonintact skin, or potentially contaminated intact skin.

- Wear gloves with fit and durability appropriate to the task
- Use gloves as an additional measure, not as a substitute for hand hygiene
- Change gloves during direct care if the hands move from a contaminated body site to a clean body site
- Remove gloves after providing care or after contact with contaminated medical equipment or potentially contaminated environmental surfaces
- Do not wear the same pair of gloves for the care of more than one person

- Do not wash gloves for the purpose of reuse
- Wash hands immediately after removing gloves

Gowns: Wear a gown, appropriate to the task, to protect skin and prevent soiling or contamination of clothing during procedures and direct care activities when contact with blood, body fluids, secretions, or excretions is anticipated.

- The routine use of a gown is not recommended
- Wear a gown for direct contact activities if the person has uncontained secretions or excretions
- Do not reuse gowns, even for repeated contacts with the same person

Mouth, nose, eye protection: PPE should be worn where appropriate to protect the mucous membranes of the eyes, nose and mouth during procedures and patient care activities likely to generate splashes or sprays of blood, body fluids, secretions, or excretions.

- Select masks, goggles, face shields, and combinations of each according to the need anticipated by the task performed
- During aerosol-generating procedures (e.g., bronchoscopy, endotracheal intubation) wear one of the following: a face shield that fully covers the front and sides of the face, a mask with attached shield, or a mask and goggles.

HAND HYGIENE

Hand hygiene is the single most important way to prevent the transmission of infection.

- Educate personnel regarding the types of healthcare activities that can result in hand contamination and the advantages and disadvantages of various methods used to clean their hands
- Monitor healthcare workers' adherence with recommended hand hygiene practices and provide personnel with information regarding their performance
- Alcohol-based hand rubs should be 60–90% concentration ethyl or isopropyl alcohol
- An interactive computer assisted hand hygiene education program is available at the following website: http://www.health.gov.on.ca/english/providers/program/pubhealth/handwashing/hw-pilot.html
- Wash hands with soap and water when hands are visibly dirty
- Use an alcohol-based hand rub to decontaminate the hands if hands are not visibly soiled

- Wash hands with soap and water if contact with spores (e.g., *Clostridium difficile*) is likely to have occurred
- The physical action of washing and rinsing hands under such circumstances is recommended because alcohols, chlorhexidine, iodophors, and other antiseptic agents have poor activity against spores
- Do not wear artificial fingernails or extenders if duties include direct care with persons at high risk for infection and adverse outcomes

Perform hand hygiene:

- Before and after providing direct care
- After contact with blood, body fluids or excretions, mucous membranes, nonintact skin, or wound dressings
- If hands will be moving from a contaminated body site to a clean body site during direct care
- After contact with potentially contaminated inanimate objects in the environment
- After removing gloves

NESTLÉ NUTRITION SERVICES

Nestlé

Mini Nutritional Assessment
MNA®

Last name:	First name:	Sex:	Date:

Age:	Weight, kg:	Height, cm:	I.D. Number:

Complete the screen by filling in the boxes with the appropriate numbers.
Add the numbers for the screen. If score is 11 or less, continue with the assessment to gain a Malnutrition Indicator Score.

Screening

A Has food intake declined over the past 3 months due to loss of appetite, digestive problems, chewing or swallowing difficulties?
0 = severe loss of appetite
1 = moderate loss of appetite
2 = no loss of appetite ☐

B Weight loss during the last 3 months
0 = weight loss greater than 3 kg (6.6 lbs)
1 = does not know
2 = weight loss between 1 and 3 kg (2.2 and 6.6 lbs)
3 = no weight loss ☐

C Mobility
0 = bed or chair bound
1 = able to get out of bed/chair but does not go out
2 = goes out ☐

D Has suffered psychological stress or acute disease in the past 3 months
0 = yes   2 = no ☐

E Neuropsychological problems
0 = severe dementia or depression
1 = mild dementia
2 = no psychological problems ☐

F Body Mass Index (BMI) (weight in kg) / (height in m)²
0 = BMI less than 19
1 = BMI 19 to less than 21
2 = BMI 21 to less than 23
3 = BMI 23 or greater ☐

Screening score (subtotal max. 14 points) ☐ ☐
12 points or greater   Normal – not at risk – no need to complete assessment
11 points or below   Possible malnutrition – continue assessment

Assessment

G Lives independently (not in a nursing home or hospital)
0 = no   1 = yes ☐

H Takes more than 3 prescription drugs per day
0 = yes   1 = no ☐

I Pressure sores or skin ulcers
0 = yes   1 = no ☐

Ref.: Guigoz Y, Vellas B and Garry PJ. 1994. Mini Nutritional Assessment: A practical assessment tool for grading the nutritional state of elderly patients. *Facts and Research in Gerontology.* Supplement #2:15-59.
Rubenstein LZ, Harker J, Guigoz Y and Vellas B. Comprehensive Geriatric Assessment (CGA) and the MNA: An Overview of CGA, Nutritional Assessment, and Development of a Shortened Version of the MNA. In: "Mini Nutritional Assessment (MNA): Research and Practice in the Elderly". Vellas B, Garry PJ and Guigoz Y, editors. Nestlé Nutrition Workshop Series. Clinical & Performance Programme, **vol.** 1. Karger, Bâle, in press.

J How many full meals does the patient eat daily?
0 = 1 meal
1 = 2 meals
2 = 3 meals ☐

K Selected consumption markers for protein intake
• At least one serving of dairy products (milk, cheese, yogurt) per day?   yes ☐   no ☐
• Two or more servings of legumes or eggs per week?   yes ☐   no ☐
• Meat, fish or poultry every day   yes ☐   no ☐
0.0 = if 0 or 1 yes
0.5 = if 2 yes
1.0 = if 3 yes ☐ . ☐

L Consumes two or more servings of fruits or vegetables per day?
0 = no   1 = yes ☐

M How much fluid (water, juice, coffee, tea, milk…) is consumed per day?
0.0 = less than 3 cups
0.5 = 3 to 5 cups
1.0 = more than 5 cups ☐ . ☐

N Mode of feeding
0 = unable to eat without assistance
1 = self-fed with some difficulty
2 = self-fed without any problem ☐

O Self view of nutritional status
0 = views self as being malnourished
1 = is uncertain of nutritional state
2 = views self as having no nutritional problem ☐

P In comparison with other people of the same age, how does the patient consider his/her health status?
0.0 = not as good
0.5 = does not know
1.0 = as good
2.0 = better ☐ . ☐

Q Mid-arm circumference (MAC) in cm
0.0 = MAC less than 21
0.5 = MAC 21 to 22
1.0 = MAC 22 or greater ☐ . ☐

R Calf circumference (CC) in cm
0 = CC less than 31   1 = CC 31 or greater ☐

Assessment (max. 16 points) ☐ ☐ . ☐

Screening score ☐ ☐

Total Assessment (max. 30 points) ☐ ☐ . ☐

Malnutrition Indicator Score
17 to 23.5 points   at risk of malnutrition ☐
Less than 17 points   malnourished ☐

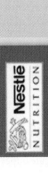

Nestlé
NUTRITION

MNA Home Page
► Introduction

▼ Clinical practice
User Guide
MNA Forms
MNA Score
Feedback

▲ Research & validation
▲ News
▲ References
▲ Links

Interpreting the MNA® score

The MNA was specifically designed to identify elderly people at risk of malnutrition and guide nutritional intervention in order to improve nutritional status.

MNA score > 23.5	MNA score 17-23.5	MNA score < 17
Satisfactory nutritional status. (see 1)	Malnutrition risk with good prognosis given early intervention. (see 2)	Protein energy malnutrition. (see 3)

1

Repeat MNA every 3 months. Provide guidelines for a balanced diet.

back to top

2

Analyse the MNA results to identify the reasons for the low score.

Perform a detailed diet history / interview.

▲ Does their medication interfere with their food intake?
▲ Do they have difficulty preparing or obtaining their meals?
▲ Does their mental status interfere with their oral intake?
▲ Is their diet unbalanced?
▲ Do they have shin lesions?
▲ Discuss these issues with their physician and / or provide the patient with the appropriate resources or educational information.
▲ Follow up with a repeat MNA in 3 months.

back to top

3

Analyse the score as described above. Perform a dietary interview. Investigate for other causes of malnutrition, e.g. disease states, increased metabolic needs, nutritional intervention must be initiated immediately. Consider use of nutritional supplements to enhance oral diet and or initiation of enteral tube feeding.

back to top

805

Glossary

abdomen The largest cavity of the body that contains organs and structures belonging to various systems of the body

abduction A movement of a limb away from the midline or median plane of the body, along the frontal plane

Aboriginal peoples In Canada, the First Nations, Metis, and Inuit

accessory digestive organs The structures connected to the alimentary canal by ducts—the liver, gallbladder, and pancreas—that contribute to the digestive process of foods

accommodation The ability of the eye to automatically adjust vision from far to near or a variety of distances

acetabulum A rounded cavity on the right and left lateral sides of the pelvic bone

acini cells Glandular tissue in each breast that produce milk

acrochordons Pedunculated, flesh-coloured lesions of collagen and subcutaneous tissue that occur on the neck, back, axillary area, and eyelids; also called skin tags

acrocyanosis A normal finding in newborns and infants in which during times of stress, especially exposure to cold environments, the hands and feet appear cyanotic; often accompanied by increased mottling of the distal arms and legs

acromegaly A disorder caused by overproduction of growth hormone by the pituitary gland, causing enlargement of the skull and cranial bones, enlargement of the lower jaw, and enlargement of the lips, tongue, hands, and feet

actinic keratoses Normal aging growths, especially in fair-skinned people, that are considered precancerous; they appear as calluslike red, yellow, or flesh-coloured plaques on exposed areas, such as the ears, cheeks, lips, nose, upper extremities, or a balding scalp

acute pain Pain that lasts only through the expected recovery period from illness, injury, or surgery, whether it has a sudden or slow onset and regardless of the intensity

adduction The movement of a limb toward the body midline

adolescence The period between 12 and 21 years of age; the transition period from childhood to adulthood

adventitious sounds Added sounds heard during auscultation of the chest that are superimposed on normal breath sounds and may indicate an underlying airway problems or diseases

advocacy and activism in nursing Engaging in activities to support and garner resources for an individual, a community, or a cause, or creating awareness of a health issue, fostering social acceptance or acquiring resources, and engaging in policy and organizational change to achieve a health goal; direct action taken to support health goals

air conduction The transmission of sound through the tympanic membrane to the cochlea and auditory nerve

alimentary canal A continuous, hollow, muscular tube that begins at the mouth and terminates at the anus

Allen test A test used to determine patency of the radial and ulnar arteries

alopecia areata Sudden patchy or complete loss of body hair for unknown cause; occurs most often on scalp but may occur over the entire body

amniotic fluid A clear, slightly yellowish liquid that surrounds the fetus during pregnancy

anaesthesia The inability to perceive the sense of touch

analgesia The absence of pain sensation

angle of Louis A horizontal ridge formed at the point at which the manubrium joins the body of the sternum; also called the sternal angle

angular stomatitis A clinical finding of poor nutrition; cracks at the corner of the mouth

anorexia nervosa A complex psychosocial and physiological problem characterized by a severely restricted intake of nutrients and a low body weight

anosmia The absence of the sense of smell, which may be due to cranial nerve dysfunction, colds, rhinitis, or zinc deficiency, or it may be genetic

anteflexion An abnormal variation of uterine position in which the uterus is folded forward at about a 90-degree angle, and the cervix is tilted downward

anterior fontanelle A small diamond-shaped open area located at the top of an infant's skull where the bones of the skull have not as yet closed; protects the brain during birth and allows for skull and brain growth during infancy; also called a soft spot

anterior triangle A landmark area of the anterior neck bordered by the mandible, the midline of the neck, and the anterior aspect of the sternocleidomastoid muscles

anteversion The normal uterine position in which the uterus is tilted forward and the cervix is tilted downward

anthropometric Any scientific measurement of the body

anus The terminal end of the large intestine, where it exits the body

apocrine glands Glands in the axillary and anogenital regions that are dormant until the onset of puberty, and produce a secretion made up of water, salts, fatty acids, and proteins, which is released into hair follicles

aqueous humour A clear, fluidlike substance found in the anterior segment of the eye that helps maintain ocular pressure

arcus senilis A light-grey ring around the outer pupil caused by the deposition of lipids

areola A circular, pigmented field of wrinkled skin on the breast that contains the nipple

arterial aneurysm A bulging or dilation in the wall of an artery caused by a weakness in the wall

arterial insufficiency Inadequate arterial circulation, usually because of the buildup of fatty plaque or calcification of the arterial wall

arteries Tubular elastic-walled vessels that carry oxygenated blood throughout the body

ascites An abnormal collection of fluid in the peritoneal cavity

assessment The first step of the nursing process, which includes the collection, organization, and validation of subjective and objective data

astigmatism A condition in which the refraction of light is spread over a wide area rather than on a distinct point on the retina

atlas The first cervical vertebra, which carries the skull

atrioventricular (AV) node A node located in the wall of the right atrium in the heart that works with the bundle of His to receive the current that has finished spreading throughout the atria, slowing the impulse before it passes onto the bundle branches; capable of initiating electrical impulses in the event of SA node failure

atrioventricular (AV) valves Heart valves that separate the atria from the ventricles

atrophic papillae A clinical finding of poor nutritional health in which the small bumps on the tongue shrink or vanish entirely

attending Giving full-time attention to verbal and nonverbal messages

auricle The external portion of the ear

auscultation The use of a stethoscope to listen to the sounds produced by the body

axillary tail Breast tissue that extends superiolaterally into the axilla; also called the tail of Spence

axis The second cervical vertebra (C_2), which supports the movement of the head

Babinski response During a plantar flexion text, the toes fan out, with the great toe pointing toward the dorsum of the foot; considered an abnormal response in the adult that may indicate upper motor neuron disease

ballottement A palpation technique used to detect fluid or examine floating body structures by using the hand to push against the body

Bartholin's glands Glands located posteriorly at the base of the vestibule of the vulva that produce mucus, which is released into the vestibule and actively promotes sperm motility and viability; also called greater vestibular glands

Bell's palsy A temporary disorder affecting cranial nerve VII and producing a unilateral facial paralysis

blepharitis The inflammation of the eyelids

blood pressure Pressure caused by waves of blood as it ebbs and flows within the systemic arteries

Blumberg's sign The experience of sharp stabbing pain as the compressed area returns to a noncompressed state

body mass index (BMI) A formula for assessing appropriate weight for height: BMI = weight (kg)/height^2 (metres)

bone conduction The transmission of sound through the bones of the skull to the cochlea and auditory nerve

brain stem The part of the brain located between the cerebrum and spinal cord; contains the midbrain, pons, and medulla oblongata and connects pathways between the higher and lower structures

Braxton Hicks contractions Painless and unpredictable contractions of the uterus that do not dilate the cervix

bronchial sounds Loud, high-pitched sounds heard in the upper airways and region of the trachea; expiration is longer than inspiration

bronchophony Auscultation of voice sounds; client says, "ninety-nine," and normal lung sound will be muffled

bronchovesicular sounds Sounds that are medium in loudness and pitch and heard as auscultation moves from the large central airways toward the periphery of the lungs; inspiration and expiration are equal in duration

bruit A loud blowing heart sound; an abnormal finding, most often associated with a narrowing or stricture of the carotid artery usually associated with atherosclerotic plaque

bulbourethral glands Small, round glands located below the prostate within the urethral sphincter; just before ejaculation, they secrete clear mucus into the urethra that lubricates the urethra and increases its alkaline environment; also called Cowper's glands

bundle branches Expressways of conducting fibres in the heart that spread the electrical current through the ventricular myocardial tissue; capable of initiating electrical charges in case both the SA node and AV node fail

bundle of His A part of the wall of the right atrium in the heart that works with the atrioventricular node to receive the current that has finished spreading throughout the atria, slowing the impulse before it passes onto the bundle branches

bursae Small, synovial-fluid-filled sacs that protect ligaments from friction

calcaneus A tarsal bone of the foot; also called the heel bone

calculi Stones that block the urinary tract, usually composed of calcium, struvite, or a combination of magnesium, ammonium, phosphate, and uric acid content in water

capillaries The smallest vessels of the circulatory system; exchange gases and nutrients between the arterial and venous systems

caput succedaneum A condition that is characterized by edema that results from a collection of fluid in the tissue at the top of the skull

cardiac conduction system The heart's conduction system, which can initiate an electrical charge and transmit that charge via cardiac muscle fibres throughout the myocardial tissue

cardiac cycle The events of one complete heartbeat: the contraction and relaxation of the atria and ventricles

cardiac output The amount of blood ejected from the left ventricle in 1 minute

cartilaginous joint Bones joined by cartilage

cataract A condition in which the lens of the eye thickens and yellows, forming a dense area that reduces lens clarity and results in a loss of central vision

central nervous system The nervous system of the body that consists of the brain and the spinal cord

cephalocaudal Head to toe direction

cephalohematomas Blood collections inside of the skull's periosteum that do not cross suture lines

cerebellum The part of the brain located below the cerebrum and behind the brainstem, it coordinates stimuli from the cerebral cortex to provide precise timing for skeletal muscle coordination and smooth movements; assists with maintaining equilibrium and muscle tone

cerebrum The largest portion of the brain, responsible for all conscious behaviour

cerumen Yellow-brown wax secreted by glands in the external auditory canal

cervical os The inferior opening at the vaginal end of the canal between the vagina and uterus

cervix Round part of the uterus that projects 2.5 cm (1 in.) into the vagina

Chadwick's sign Vascular congestion that creates a blue-purple blemish or change in cervical colour

cheilitis Inflammation of the lip; also called angular stomatitis

cheilosis An abnormal condition of the lips characterized by scaling of the surface and by the formation of fissures in the corners of the mouth

cherry angiomas Vascular lesions; nonsignificant tiny red spots, either macules or papules, rarely larger than 3 to 4 mm, seen usually on the trunk

chloasma A skin condition that develops during pregnancy resulting in hyperpigmented patches on the face; also called melasma, gravidum, or "the mask of pregnancy"

choanal atresia A congenital defect that results in a thin membrane that obstructs the nasal passages

choroid The middle layer; the vascular, pigmented layer of the eye

chronic pain Pain that is prolonged, usually recurring or persisting over 6 months or longer, and interferes with functioning

circumduction The movement in which the limb describes a cone in space: while the distal end of the limb moves in a circle, the joint itself moves only slightly in the joint cavity

client record A legal document used to plan care, to communicate information among healthcare providers, and to monitor quality of care

clitoris The primary organ of sexual stimulation; a small, elongated mound of erectile tissue located at the anterior of the vestibule of the vulva

clonus Rhythmically alternating flexion and extension of a reflex; confirms upper motor neuron disease

clubbing Flattening of the angle of the nail and enlargement of the tips of the fingers; a sign of oxygen deprivation in the extremities

coarctation of the aorta A congenital cardiac defect in the newborn that results in the narrowing of the aorta with decreased femoral pulses and bounding upper extremity pulses; causes discrepancies in blood pressure and oxygen saturation between the upper and lower extremities

cochlea A spiral chamber in the inner ear that contains the receptors for hearing

cognitive theory How people learn to think, reason, and use language

cold sores Lesions or blisters that occur on the lip or corner of the mouth, caused by a herpes simplex virus; also called fever blisters

colostrum Thick, yellow discharge that may leak from a pregnant woman's breasts in the month before she gives birth, in preparation for lactation

coma A prolonged state of unconsciousness, with pronounced and persistent changes

communication Exchange of information, feelings, thoughts, and ideas

concreteness Speaking to the client in specific terms rather than in vague generalities

confidentiality Protecting information, sharing only with those directly involved in client care

consensual constriction The simultaneous response of one pupil to the stimuli applied to the other

convergence Turning inward of the eyes so that an image falls at corresponding points in both retinas

cornea The clear, transparent part of the sclera that forms the anterior part of the eye, considered to be the window of the eye

cortex The outer portion of each kidney composed of more than 1 million nephrons, which form urine

costovertebral angle (CVA) The area on the lower back formed by the vertebral column and the downward curve of the last posterior rib

cranial sutures Palpable gaps between the bones of the skull

craniosynostosis A condition that results in cranial deformity caused by premature fusion of the cranial bones

cremasteric reflex A reflexive action that may cause the testicles to migrate upward temporarily; cold hands, a cold room, or the stimulus of touch could cause this response

critical thinking A process of purposeful and creative thinking about resolutions for problems or the development of ways to manage situations

cryptorchidism The failure of one or both testicles to descend through the inguinal canal during the final stages of fetal development

cues Bits of information that hint at the possibility of a health problem

cultural competence The capacity of nurses or health service delivery systems to effectively understand and plan for the needs of culturally diverse clients

cultural safety A method to avoid stereotypes by considering the uniqueness of each client and addressing historical, social, political, and economic inequalities of certain groups within society—those persons often most marginalized by social and structural inequity

cultural sensitivity The practice of being sensitive to the values, beliefs, and practices of all people

culture The nonphysical traits, such as values, beliefs, attitudes, and customs, that are shared by a group of people and passed from one generation to the next

Cushing's syndrome Increased adrenal hormone production that leads to a rounded "moon" face, ruddy cheeks, prominent jowls, and excess facial hair

cutaneous pain Pain that originates in the skin or subcutaneous tissue

cuticle A fold of epidermal skin along the base of the nail that protects the root and sides of each nail

cystocele A hernia that is formed when the female urinary bladder is pushed into the anterior vaginal wall

dandruff White or grey dead, scaly flakes of epidermal cells (skin)

database An electronic storage unit that contains subjective and objective data gathered about a client's medical history and physical examination findings

deep somatic pain Pain that is diffuse and arises from ligaments, tendons, bones, blood vessels, and nerves, which tends to last longer than cutaneous pain

depression For the musculoskeletal system, the movement in which the elevated part is moved downward to its original position

dermatome An area of skin innervated by the cutaneous branch of one spinal nerve

dermis A layer of connective tissue that lies just below the epidermis

development An orderly, progressive increase in the complexity of the total person; involves the continual, irreversible, complex evolution of intelligence, personality, creativity, sociability, and morality

developmental dysplasia of the hip A congenital disorder that results from inadequate development of the hip socket

diaphoresis Profuse perspiration or sweating that may occur during exertion, fever, pain, and emotional stress and in the presence of some metabolic disorders, such as hyperthyroidism

diastasis recti abdominis A separation of the rectus abdominis muscles that run vertically down the midline of the abdomen, which may allow the abdominal contents to protrude; can occur during the third trimester of pregnancy

diastole The phase of ventricular heart relaxation; the ventricles relax and are filled as the atria contract; also the bottom number of a blood pressure reading

diastolic pressure The lowest arterial blood pressure of the cardiac cycle occurring when the heart is at rest

diet recall A remembrance of all food, beverages, and nutritional supplements or products consumed in a set time, such as 24 hours

dilation Progressive opening of the cervix

diplopia Double vision

diverticula Outpouchings in the walls of the colon caused by continual overdistension of the bowel and straining to pass stools

dorsiflexion Flexion of the ankle so that the superior aspect of the foot moves upward, toward the shin

downstream approaches Interventions focused on treatment and cures

Down syndrome A chromosomal defect that causes varying degrees of mental retardation; people with it typically have slanted eyes, a flat nasal bridge, a flat nose, a protruding tongue, and a short neck

ductus arteriosus A shunt in fetal circulation that shunts blood into the descending aorta

ductus venosus A shunt in fetal circulation that enables the fetus to maximize oxygenation from the maternal circulation

dullness A flat percussion tone that is soft and of short duration

dysphagia Difficulty swallowing

dyspnea Shortness of breath or difficulty taking a breath

dysreflexia Bladder distension that causes a sympathetic response that can trigger a potentially life-threatening hypertensive crisis in clients with spinal cord injuries at level T_7 or higher

ecchymosis Bruising resulting from the escape of blood from a ruptured blood vessel into the tissues

eccrine glands Glands that produce a clear perspiration made up mostly of water and salts, which they release into funnel-shaped pores at the skin surface

ectropion The eversion of the lower eyelid caused by muscle weakness

eczema A chronic skin disorder characterized by intense itching, patches, erythema, and papules that typically begins in the first year of life; also called atopic dermatitis

edema An increased accumulation of fluid in the intercellular spaces of a dependent body part

effacement Thinning of the cervix occurring near the end of pregnancy in preparation for labour

egophony Auscultation of voice sounds; when client says "E," normal lungs sound like "eeeeee"

electrocardiogram (ECG) Electrical representations of the cardiac cycle documented by deflections on recording paper

elevation Lifting or moving superiorly along a frontal plane such as occurs in chewing

embryo A child during any development stage of pregnancy before birth

emmetropia The normal refractive condition of the eye

empathy Understanding, being aware of, and being sensitive to the feelings, thoughts, and experiences of another person

encoding The process of formulating a message for transmission to another person

endocardium The innermost layer of the heart, a smooth layer that provides an inner lining for the chambers of the heart

entropion The inversion of the lid and lashes caused by muscle spasm of the eyelid

enuresis Involuntary urination that occurs after 4 years of age

epicardium The outer layer of the heart wall; also called the visceral pericardium

epidermis The outer layer of skin on the body

epididymis A comma- or crescent-shaped system of ductules emerging posteriorly from the testis that holds the sperm during maturation

epididymitis A common infection in males characterized by a dull, aching pain

epiphyseal plates Plates located in the ends of the bones

epispadias A condition in which the urethral meatus is located on the superior aspect of the glans

epitrochlear node Node located on the medial surface of the arm above the elbow that drains the ulnar surface of the forearm and the third, fourth, and fifth digits

esophagitis Inflammatory process of the esophagus, caused by a variety of irritants

esophoria Inward turning of the eye toward the nose

ethnic group A group that shares heritage, culture, language, or religion

ethnicity Notions of blood, kinship, a common sense of belonging, and often a common geographic or national origin

eupnea The regular, even-depth, rhythmic pattern of inspiration and expiration; normal breathing

eustachian tube The bony and cartilaginous auditory tube that connects the middle ear with the nasopharynx and helps to equalize the air pressure on both sides of the tympanic membrane

eversion A movement in which the sole of the foot is turned laterally

exophoria Outward turning of the eye

extension A bending movement around a joint that increases the angle between the bones of the limb at the joint

false reassurance The client is assured of a positive outcome with no basis for believing in it

fever blisters Lesions or blisters on the lips may be caused by the herpes simplex virus; also called cold sores

fibrous joint Bones joined by fibrous tissue

flag sign Dyspigmentation of the mouth or a part of the mouth

flatness A dull percussion tone that is soft and has a short duration

flexion A bending movement that decreases the angle of the joint and brings the articulating bones closer together

food frequency questionnaire A questionnaire that assesses intake of a variety of food groups on a daily, weekly, or longer basis

foramen ovale A shunt in fetal circulation before birth that connects the fetal right atrium to the fetal left atrium

formal teaching Organized information sharing that occurs in response to an identified learning need of an individual, a group, or a community

fracture A partial or complete break in the continuity of the bone from trauma

fremitus The palpable vibration on the chest wall when the client speaks

friction rub A rough, grating sound caused by the rubbing together of organs or an organ rubbing on the peritoneum

functional assessment An observation to gather data while the client is performing common or routine activities

fundal height Size of the fundus; after 20 weeks' pregnancy, the weeks of gestation is equal to the fundal height in centimetres

fundus (eye) The inner back surface of the eye

fundus (uterine) The top portion of the uterus, or the part farthest from the cervix

galactorrhea Lactation not associated with childbearing or breastfeeding

general survey Impressions based on what is seen, heard, or smelled during the initial phase of assessment

genital warts Raised, moist, cauliflower-shaped papules

genogram A pictorial representation of family relationships and medical history

genu valgum A condition of the musculoskeletal system in which the knees touch each other but the ankles do not; also called knock knees

genu varum A condition of the musculoskeletal system where the ankles touch each other but the knees do not; also called bowlegs

genuineness The ability to present yourself honestly and spontaneously

gestational age The age of the fetus, which can be referred to in weeks from the last normal menstrual period

gliding The simplest type of joint movements: one flat bone surface glides or slips over another similar surface; bones are merely displaced in relation to one another

glomeruli Tufts of capillaries in the kidneys that filter more than 1 L (1 qt.) of fluid each minute

glossitis An inflammation or redness of the tongue often seen in malnutrition

goitre Enlargement of the thyroid gland that is commonly visible as swelling of the anterior neck; often caused by lack of iodine intake

Goodell's sign An increase in cervical vascularity that contributes to the softening of the cervix during pregnancy

growth Measurable physical change and increase in size; indicators of growth include height, weight, bone size, and dentition

gynecological age The difference between a woman's current age and her age at menarche

gynecomastia Benign temporary breast enlargement in one or both breasts in males

hair A thin, flexible, elongated fibre composed of dead, keratinized cells that grow out in a columnar fashion

hallux valgus The great toe is abnormally adducted at the metatarsophalangeal joint

hard palate The anterior portion of the roof of the mouth formed by bones

health A state of physical, mental, and social well-being

health assessment A systematic method of collecting data about a client to determine the client's current and ongoing health status, predict risks to health, and identify health-promoting activities

health equity The ideal in which all persons are entitled equally to health protection, basic income levels, and opportunities to be healthy

health history Information about the client's health in his or her own words and based on the client's own perceptions as part of gathering subjective data; includes biographical data, perceptions about health, past and present history of illness and injury, family history, a review of systems, and health patterns and practices

health inequality A term used to designate differences, variations, and disparities in the health status of individuals and groups

health pattern A set of related traits, habits, or acts that affect a client's health

health promotion The process of enabling people to increase control over and to improve their health

health promotion across nursing settings The process of using health promotion in the places or social groups in which people interact

heart An intricately designed pump composed of a meticulous network of synchronized structures; responsible for receiving unoxygenated blood from the body and returning oxygenated blood to the body

heart murmurs Atypical sounds of the heart that often indicate a functional or structural abnormality

Hegar's sign The softening of the uterus and the region that connects the body of the uterus and cervix that occurs throughout pregnancy

helix The external large rim of the auricle of the ear

hematuria Blood in the urine

hemorrhoids A mass of dilated veins in swollen tissue caused by continuous overdistension of the bowel and straining to pass stools

hepatitis An inflammatory process of the liver caused by viruses, bacteria, chemicals, or drugs

hernia A protrusion of an organ or structure through an abnormal opening or weakened area in a body wall

holism Considering more than the physiological health status of a client and including all factors that affect the client's physical and emotional well-being

Homans' sign A diagnostic manoeuvre in which pain occurring with sharp dorsiflexion of the foot may indicate a blood clot in the leg

hydrocephalus The enlargement of the head caused by inadequate drainage of cerebrospinal fluid, resulting in abnormal growth of the skull

hymen A thin layer of skin within the vagina

hyoid A bone that is suspended in the neck approximately 2 cm (1 in.) above the larynx

hypalgesia Decreased pain sensation

hyperalgesia Excessive sensitivity to pain

hyperesthesia An increased sensation

hyperextension A bending of a joint beyond 180 degrees

hyperopia Farsightedness: a condition in which the light rays focus behind the retina

hyperresonance Abnormally loud auscultatory tone that is low and of long duration

hyperthermia Body temperature that is greater than expected; it may be caused by an infection, trauma, surgery, or a malignancy; also called a fever

hyperthyroidism The excessive production of thyroid hormones, resulting in enlargement of the gland, exophthalmos (bulging eyes), fine hair, weight loss, diarrhea, and other alterations

hypodermis A cellular layer of subcutaneous tissue consisting of loose connective tissue; stores approximately half of the body's fat cells, cushions the body against trauma, insulates the body from heat loss, and stores fat for energy

hypospadias A condition in which the urethral meatus is located on the underside of the glans

hypothermia Body temperature that is lower than expected; usually a response to prolonged exposure to cold

hypothyroidism A metabolic disorder causing enlarged thyroid as a result of an autoimmune response or iodine deficiency

immunization The process of protecting people from communicable diseases through injected or oral vaccines that contain a minute quantity of the disease that is either very weak or dead and cannot cause illness

incontinence The inability to retain urine; classified as functional, reflex, stress, urge, or total

infant A child from birth to 1 year of age

inffective endocarditis A condition caused by bacterial infiltration of the lining of the heart's chambers

informal teaching Teaching that occurs as a natural part of a client encounter, with the nurse providing instructions, explaining a question or procedure, or reducing anxiety

inguinal hernia When a separation of the abdominal muscle exists, the weak points of these canals afford an area for the protrusion of the intestine into the groin region

innocent murmurs Heart sounds that arise from increased blood flow across normal heart structures, are graded I to II or VI in intensity, are systolic (with the exception of the venous hum), and are not associated with thrills or other cardiac symptoms

inspection The skill of observing the client in a deliberate, systematic manner

interactional skills Actions that are used during the encoding and decoding process to obtain and disseminate information, develop relationships, and promote understanding of the self and others

interdependent relationship A relationship in which an individual establishes a bond with someone based on some single factor, such as trust or a common goal

interpretation of findings Determinations made about all the data collected in the health assessment process

intractable pain Pain that is highly resistant to relief

introitus Vaginal opening

inversion A movement in which the sole of the foot is turned medially or inward

iris The circular, coloured muscular aspect of the eye's middle layer located in the anterior portion of the eye

iritis A serious eye disorder characterized by redness around the iris and cornea; the pupil is often irregular, vision is decreased, and the client experiences deep, aching pain.

joint The point where two or more bones in the body meet; also called articulation

keratin A fibrous protein that gives the epidermis its tough, protective qualities

kidneys Bean-shaped organs located in the retroperitoneal space on either side of the vertebral column

koilonychia A clinical finding of poor nutrition; spoon-shaped nails

kyphosis An exaggerated thoracic dorsal curve that causes asymmetry between the sides of the posterior thorax

labia A dual set of liplike structures lying on either side of the vagina

labial adhesion A condition common in preadolescent females that occurs when the labia minora fuse together

lambdoidal sutures Palpable gaps between the bones of the skull that separate the temporal and occipital bones

landmarks Thoracic reference points and specific anatomical structures used to help provide an exact location for the assessment findings and an accurate orientation for documentation of findings

lanugo A fine, downy hair in newborns that is most prominent on the upper chest, shoulders, and back

laryngomalacia Congenital defect of the cartilage in the larynx

left atrium The heart chamber that receives oxygenated blood from the pulmonary system

left ventricle The most powerful heart chamber; pumps the oxygenated blood outward through the aorta to the periphery of the body

lens Situated directly behind the pupil, a biconvex (convex on both surfaces), transparent, flexible structure that separates the anterior and posterior segments of the eye

lentigo senilis Relatively small darker spots of colour on the skin caused by melanocyte clumping; also called liver spots

Leopold's manoeuvres A special palpation sequence of the abdomen used to determine the position of the fetus after 28 weeks' gestation

leukorrhea A profuse, nonodourous, nonpainful vaginal discharge that protects against infection

lightening The descent of the fetal head into the pelvis

linea nigra A dark line running from the umbilicus to the pubic area

listening Paying undivided attention to what the client says and does

lobe A small flap of flesh at the inferior end of the auricle of the ear

lordosis An exaggerated lumbar curve of the spine that compensates for pregnancy, obesity, or other skeletal changes

lunula A moon-shaped crescent that appears on the nail body over the thickened nail matrix

lymph Clear fluid that passes from the intercellular spaces of the body tissue into the lymphatic system

lymph nodes Rounded lymphoid tissues that are surrounded by connective tissue; located along the lymphatic vessels in the body

lymphadenopathy The enlargement of lymph nodes, which is often caused by infection, allergies, or a tumour

lymphatic vessels Vessels that extend from the capillaries and collect lymph in organs and tissues

macrocephaly A child's head circumference above the 95th percentile; the condition is associated with hydrocephalus, brain tumour, and increased intracranial pressure

macula A hyperpigmented spot on the temporal aspect of the retina that is responsible for central vision

malnutrition An imbalance, whether a deficit or an excess, of the required nutrients of a balanced diet

mammary ridge Part of the breast tissue that extends from each axilla to the groin; also called the milk line

mammary souffle A murmur over the mammary vessel caused by increased blood flow and occasionally heard during pregnancy

manual compression test A manoeuvre to determine the length of varicose veins

manubrium The superior or upper portion of the sternum

mapping The process of dividing the abdomen into quadrants or regions for the purpose of examination

Marfan's syndrome A degenerative disease of the connective tissue, which over time may cause the ascending aorta of the heart to either dilate or dissect, leading to abrupt death

mastoiditis Inflammation of the mastoid that can occur secondary to a middle ear or a throat infection

McDonald's rule A method for estimating fetal growth that states that after 20 weeks in pregnancy, the weeks of gestation approximately equal the fundal height in centimetres

mediastinal space The area in which the heart sits obliquely within the thoracic cavity, between the lungs and above the diaphragm

mediastinum Part of the thorax, or thoracic cavity, that contains the heart, trachea, esophagus, and major blood vessels of the body

medulla The inner portion of the kidney composed of structures called pyramids and calyces

melanin Skin pigment produced in the melanocytes in the stratum basale

menarche Age of first menstrual period

meninges Three connective tissue membranes that cover, protect, and nourish the central nervous system

metopic sutures Palpable gaps between the bones of the skull that separate the frontal and temporal bones

microcephaly A child's head circumferences below the 5th percentile; may be caused by genetic disorders or intrauterine exposure to cocaine or alcohol

middle adulthood The period of a person's life between 40 and 65 years of age

midposition A normal variation of uterine position in which the uterus lies parallel to the tailbone, with the cervix pointed straight

milia Harmless skin markings on newborns; areas of tiny white facial papules caused by sebum that collects in the openings of hair follicles

Mini-Mental State Examination (MMSE) A screening instrument of cognitive reasoning for detecting dementia and delirium relating to organic disease

miosis Constriction of the pupil of the eye in response to light

Mongolian spots Grey, blue, or purple spots in the sacral and buttocks areas of newborns, which fade during the first year of life

Montgomery's glands Sebaceous glands on the areola that enlarge and produce a secretion that protects and lubricates the nipples; also called Montgomery's tubercles

morbilliform "Measleslike" rashes

mucus plug A protective covering of the cervix that develops during pregnancy because of progesterone

multigravida A female who has been pregnant two or more times

muscular dystrophy An X-linked genetic disorder that results in progressive loss of muscle function

mydriasis Excessive or prolonged dilation of the pupil of the eye

myocardium The second, thick, muscular layer of the heart, made up of bundles of cardiac muscle fibres reinforced by a branching network of connective tissue fibres called the fibrous skeleton of the heart

myopia Nearsightedness: a condition in which the light rays focus in front of the retina

Naegele's rule A formula that can be used to compute the fetus' expected date of birth (EDB) based on the mother's last menstrual period (LMP)

nails Thin plates of keratinized epidermal cells that shield the distal ends of the fingers and toes

nasal polyps Smooth, pale, benign growths found along the turbinates of the nose

neuropathic pain Pain resulting from current or past damage to the peripheral or central nervous system rather than a particular stimulus

newborn A child between birth and 1 month of age

nociception The physiological processes related to pain perception

nociceptors The receptors that transmit pain sensation

nocturia Nighttime urination

nuchal rigidity Stiffness of the neck as experienced when the meningeal membranes are irritated or inflamed

nursing diagnosis The second step of the nursing process in which the nurse uses critical thinking and applies knowledge from the sciences and other disciplines to analyze and synthesize the data

nursing process A systematic, rational, dynamic, and cyclic process used by the nurse for planning and providing care for the client

nutritional health The physical result of the balance between nutrient intake and nutritional requirements

nystagmus Rapid fluttering or constant involuntary movement of the eyeball

obesity A body mass index of 30.0 or more

objective data Data observed or measured by the nurse, also known as *overt data* or *signs* since they are detected by the nurse; these data can be seen, felt, heard, or measured

older adulthood The period of a person's life after 65 years of age

oliguria Diminished volume of urine

onycholysis The separation of the nail plate from the nail bed; may be caused by trauma, infection, or skin lesions

opposition The movement of touching the thumb to the tips of any of the other fingers of the same hand

optic atrophy Degeneration of the optic nerve, resulting in a change in the colour of the optic disc and decreased visual acuity

optic disc The creamy-yellow area on the retina of the eye where the optic nerve leaves the eye

orchitis Inflammation of the testicles

ossicles Bones of the middle ear: the malleus, the incus, and the stapes

otitis externa Infection of the outer ear or ear canal; also called swimmer's ear

otitis media Middle ear infection

Ottawa Charter for Health Promotion A document defining health promotion and outlining the components of health promotion actions, produced by the World Health Organization, Health and Welfare Canada, and the Canadian Public Health Association following the first International Conference on Health Promotion that was held in Ottawa in 1986

ovaries Almond-shaped glandular structures that produce ova, estrogen, and progesterone

overnutrition Excessive intake or storage of essential nutrients

overweight A body mass index of 25.0 to 29.9

oxygen saturation The percentage of oxygen in the blood

pain A highly unpleasant sensation that affects a person's physical health, emotional health, and well-being

pain rating scale A standardized measurement tool to assess the intensity of pain; may be numbers, words, or pictures, and provides the client the opportunity to describe the degree of discomfort

pain reaction Responses to pain, including the autonomic nervous system and behavioural responses to pain

pain sensation The acknowledgement of pain, often known as pain threshold

pain threshold The point at which the sensation of pain is perceived

pain tolerance The maximum amount and duration of pain that an individual is able to endure without relief

palpation The skill of assessing the client through the sense of touch to determine specific characteristics of the body

palpebrae The eyelid

palpebral fissure The opening between the upper and lower eyelids

papilledema Swelling and protrusion of the blind spot of the eye, caused by edema

paranasal sinuses Mucous-membrane-lined, air-filled cavities that surround the nasal cavity and perform the same air-processing functions of filtration, moistening, and warming

paraphrasing Restating the client's basic message to test whether it was understood

paraurethral glands Glands located just posterior to the female urethra that open into the urethra and secrete a fluid that lubricates the vaginal vestibule during sexual intercourse; also called Skene's glands

paronychia An inflammation of the cuticle, sometimes caused by infection

peau d'orange An "orange peel" appearance of the skin of the breast caused by edema from blocked lymphatic drainage in advanced cancer

pediculosis capitis Small parasitic insects that live on the scalp and neck; often called head lice

penis The male organ used for both elimination of urine and ejaculation of sperm during reproduction

percentiles Comparisons of various measurement values used to assess growth rate and healthy weights versus height

percussion "Striking through" a body part with an object, finger, or a reflex hammer, ultimately producing a measurable sound

pericardium A thin sac composed of a fibroserous material that surrounds the heart

perineum The space between the vaginal opening and anal area in a female; the space between the scrotum and anus in a male

periorbital edema Swelling of the soft tissue in the periorbital area; the swelling is often found in the dependent tissue space

peripheral nervous system The nervous system of the body that consists of the cranial nerves and spinal nerves

peripheral vascular system The blood vessels of the body that, together with the heart and the lymphatic vessels, make up the body's circulatory system

peritoneum A thin, double layer of serous membrane in the abdominal cavity

peritonitis A local or generalized inflammatory process of the peritoneal membrane of the abdomen

Peyronie's disease A disease that causes the shaft of the penis to be crooked during an erection

phantom pain Painful sensation experienced in a missing body part (amputation) or paralyzed area

phimosis A condition in which the foreskin of a penis cannot be fully retracted

physical assessment Hands-on examination of the client; components are the survey and examination of systems

physiological anemia A decrease in hemoglobin and hematocrit caused by plasma volume increase outpacing the increase in red blood cells (RBCs)

pica Abnormal craving for or eating of nonfood items, such as chalk or dirt

pingueculae Yellowish nodules on the sclera of the eye that are thickened areas of the bulbar conjunctiva caused by prolonged exposure to sun, wind, and dust; may occur on either side of the pupil and cause no problems

pinna The external portion of the ear

Piscacek's sign The irregular shape of the uterus caused by the implantation of the ovum

placenta A vascular organ that connects the fetus to the mother before birth and mediates the exchange of nutrients between the mother and fetus; covers one third of the inner surface area of the uterus at term

plantar flexion Extension of the ankle (pointing the toes) away from the body

pleximeter The device that accepts the tap or blow from a hammer

plexor A hammer or tapping finger used to strike an object

Population Health Promotion (PHP) model A model that explains the relationship between population health and health promotion and shows how a population health approach can be implemented through action on the full range of health determinants by means of multiple health promotion strategies as outlined in the Ottawa Charter for Health Promotion

positive regard The ability to appreciate and respect another person's worth and dignity with a nonjudgmental attitude

posterior fontanelle A small diamond-shaped open area located on the infant's skull in the superior occiput, where the bones of the skull have not as yet closed; protects the brain during birth and allows for skull and brain growth during infancy; also called a soft spot

posterior triangle A landmark area of the posterior neck bordered by the trapezius muscle, the sternocleidomastoid muscle, and the clavicle

preinteraction The period before first meeting with the client in which the nurse reviews information and prepares for the initial interview

presbycusis High-frequency hearing loss that occurs over time and is associated with aging

presbyopia Decreased ability of the eye lens to change shape to accommodate for near vision

preschooler A child between 3 and 5 years of age

primary healthcare An approach adopted by the World Health Organization in 1978 as the conceptual basis for effective, affordable healthcare delivery, which includes the concepts of accessibility, public participation, health promotion, appropriate technology, and intersectoral cooperation

primary lesion The initial lesion of a disease

primary prevention Strategies designed to prevent or reduce the risk of disease occurring by improving or maintaining general health, boosting the immune system, or preventing injury

primary source The client; the best source because he or she can describe personal symptoms, experiences, and factors leading to the current concerns

primigravida A female pregnant for the first time

prolapsed uterus A condition in which the uterus may protrude right at the vaginal wall with straining, or it may hang outside of the vaginal wall without any straining

pronation Movement of the forearm so that the palm faces down, posteriorly or inferiorly

prostate gland Organ that borders the urethra near the lower part of the bladder, it lies just anterior to the rectum and is composed of glandular structures that continuously secrete a milky, alkaline solution

protein-calorie malnutrition A nutrient deficiency resulting from undernutrition

protraction A nonangular anterior joint movement in a transverse plane, such as moving the jaw forward

pruritus Itching, usually caused by dry skin, that may increase with age

psychoanalytic theory Defines the structure of personality as consisting of three parts: the id, the ego, and the superego

psychological distress A mental condition that can be brought on by many factors, including loss of spouse and friends through death or illness, loss of occupation or living arrangement through functional disability, loss of body image, loss of favoured recreation, or loss of any other item of significance

psychosocial functioning The way a person thinks, feels, acts, and relates to self and others, the ability to cope and tolerate stress, and the capacity for developing a value and belief system

psychosocial health Being mentally, emotionally, socially, and spiritually well

psychosocial theory States that culture and society influence development across the entire lifespan

pterygium Opacity of the bulbar conjunctiva that can grow over the cornea and block vision

ptosis Drooping in one eyelid

pulse Wave of pressure felt at various points in the body cause by the force of the blood against the walls of the arteries

Purkinje fibres Fibres in the heart that fan out and penetrate into the myocardial tissue to spread the current into the tissues themselves

quickening The fluttery initial sensations of fetal movement perceived by the mother

race The socially constructed identification of an individual or a group by shared genetic heritage and biological or physical characteristics

racialization An assumption that the construct of race is a neutral way to categorize people and that the people in these categories have consistent behavioural characteristics

radiating pain Pain perceived at one location that then extends to nearby tissues

rales Discontinuous sounds that are intermittent, nonmusical, and brief; also called crackles

Raynaud's disease A condition in which the arterioles in the fingers develop spasms, causing intermittent skin pallor or cyanosis and then rubor (red colour)

rectal prolapse A condition caused by continuous overdistension of the bowel and straining to pass stools, whereby the lower rectal tissue may be forced out of the body through the anus

rectocele A hernia that is formed when the female rectum pushes into the posterior vaginal wall

red reflex A glowing red colour that fills the pupil as light from the ophthalmoscope reflects off the retina

referred pain Pain felt in a part of the body that is considerably removed or distant from the area actually causing the pain

reflecting A communication technique used in letting the client know that the nurse empathizes with the thoughts, feelings, or experiences expressed

reflexes Automatic stimulus-responses that involve a nerve impulse passing from a peripheral nerve receptor to the spinal cord and then moving outward to an effector muscle without passing through the brain; muscles typically contract following stimulation of the nerve receptors

resonance A long, low-pitched, hollow sound elicited with percussion over the lungs

respiratory cycle Consists of an inspiratory and expiratory phase of breathing

respiratory rate The number of times the individual inhales and exhales during 1 minute

retina The third and innermost membrane of the eye; the sensory portion of the eye; a direct extension of the optic nerve

retraction A nonangular posterior joint movement in a transverse plane, such as pulling the jaw backward after protraction

retrobulbar neuritis An inflammatory process of the optic nerve behind the eyeball

retroflexion An abnormal variation of uterine position in which the uterus is folded backward at about a 90-degree angle, and the cervix is tilted upward

retroversion A normal variation of uterine position in which the uterus is tilted backward, and the cervix is tilted upward

rhonchi A range of whistling or snoring sounds heard during auscultation when there is some type of airway obstruction; types of rhonchi include sibilant wheezes, sonorous rhonchi, and stridor; also called sonorous wheezes

rickets A clinical finding associated with poor nutritional health that results in bowed legs

right atrium A thin-walled chamber located above and slightly to the right of the right ventricle that forms the right border of the heart; receives unoxygenated blood from the periphery of the body

right ventricle Triangle-shaped part of the heart that makes up much of the anterior or sternocostal surface of the heart; pushes unoxygenated blood out to the pulmonary vessels, where oxygenation occurs

ripening Softening of the cervix near the end of pregnancy in anticipation of birth

role development The individual's capacity to identify and fulfill the social expectations related to the variety of roles assumed in a lifetime

Romberg test A test that assesses coordination and equilibrium

root cause of a health issue The identified reason for the presence of that health issue—the origin of the existing problem

rotation The turning movement of a bone around its own long axis

S₁ The first heart sound (*lub*) heard when the AV valves close; closure of these valves occurs when the ventricles are filled

S₂ The second heart sound (*dub*) heard when the aortic and pulmonic valves close; valves close when the ventricles have emptied their blood into the aorta and pulmonary arteries when the ventricles have emptied their blood into the aorta and pulmonary arteries

S₃ A third heart sound heard when the AV valves open and blood flows into the ventricles, causing vibrations during diastole that may be heard after S₂ in children, in young adults, or in pregnant females in their third trimester; may also be associated with pathological conditions, such as myocardial infarction (MI) or heart failure; also called a ventricular gallop

S₄ A fourth heart sound caused by atrial contraction and ejection of blood into the ventricles in late diastole that may be heard in children, well-conditioned athletes, and even healthy older adults without cardiac disease; may also be associated with pathological conditions, such as myocardial infarction (MI) or heart failure; also called an atrial gallop

sagittal suture Palpable gap between the bones of the skull that lies in the middle of the skull and crosses the anterior and posterior fontanelles

salmon patches Small macules and patches caused by visible intradermal capillaries; also called stork bites

school age A child between 6 and 12 years old

sclera The outermost layer of the eye; an extremely dense, hard, fibrous membrane that helps to maintain the shape of the eye

scoliosis A lateral curvature of the lumbar or thoracic spine that is more common in children with neuromuscular deficits

scrotum A loosely hanging, pliable, pear-shaped pouch of darkly pigmented skin located behind the penis that houses the testes, which produce sperm

sebaceous glands Oil glands that secrete sebum, an oily secretion, which generally is released into hair follicles

seborrheic keratoses Benign, greasy, wartlike lesions that are yellow-brown in colour; they can appear anywhere on the body but are seen most frequently on the neck, chest, and back

secondary lesion Skin condition or change to the skin that occurs following a primary lesion

secondary prevention Measures that focus on early detection of disease or conditions in a particular population, with the goal of either achieving a cure or minimizing the severity of the disease

secondary source A person or record beyond the client that provides additional information about the client

seizures Sudden and rapid physical manifestations (as convulsions or loss of consciousness), resulting from excessive discharges of electrical energy in the brain

self-concept The beliefs and feelings a person holds about himself or herself

self-observation The part of critical reflection that involves attending to and reflecting on thoughts, emotions, and bodily responses in the moment to enhance the opportunity to respond with intention, that is, in a way that is supportive of the individual or family

semilunar valves Heart valves that separate the ventricles from the vascular system

seminal vesicles A pair of saclike glands, located between the bladder and rectum, that are the source of 60% of the semen produced

senile purpura A vascular lesion that can occur spontaneously or in response to minimal trauma in the very old client with fragile blood vessels

sinoatrial (SA) node The part of the heart located at the junction of the superior vena cava and right atrium that initiates the electrical impulse

sinus arrhythmia A heart rate that increases during inspiration and decreases during expiration; also called heart period variability

smegma A white, cheeselike sebaceous matter that collects between the glans of the penis and the foreskin

social determinants of health The economic and social conditions that influence the health of individuals and their communities

social justice The fair distribution of society's benefits, responsibilities, and consequences

soft palate The posterior and somewhat mobile aspect of the roof of the mouth formed by muscle; moves with swallowing, breathing, and phonation

somatic protein Another term for muscle mass or skeletal muscle

spermatic cord A cord composed of fibrous connective tissue; its purpose is to form a protective sheath around the nerves, blood vessels, lymphatic structures, and muscle fibres associated with the scrotum

spermatocele A cyst located in the epididymis

sphygmomanometer An instrument used to measure arterial blood pressure

spinal cord A continuation of the medulla oblongata that has the ability to transmit impulses to and from the brain via the ascending and descending pathways

spirituality That dimension of the self that is most often associated with the search for meaning

sternum The flat, narrow centre bone of the upper anterior chest

strabismus A condition in which the axes of the eyes cannot be directed at the same object

stress Perceived or physical response to environmental factors; the body's response to thoughts and feelings that may result in a behavioural or physiological response

striae A change in connective tissue resulting in silvery, shiny, irregular markings on the skin, often seen in obesity, pregnancy, and ascites; also called stretch marks

striae gravidarum Pinkish-purplish skin depressions in connective tissue that develop in the second half of pregnancy; also called stretch marks

stroke volume The amount of blood that is ejected with every heartbeat

subjective data Information that the client experiences and communicates to the nurse, known as *covert data* or *symptoms*

subluxation A partial dislocation of the bones in a joint, such as the head of the radius, which may occur when a child is dangled by his or her hands

summarizing Tying together the various messages that the client has communicated throughout the interview

supination Movement of the forearm so that the palm faces up, anteriorly or superiorly

supine hypotension syndrome Pressure from the pregnant uterus compresses the aorta and the inferior vena cava when the female is in the supine position, causing dizziness, fainting, and a drop in heart rate and blood pressure; also called vena cava syndrome

suspensory ligaments Ligaments that extend from the connective tissue layer through the breast and attach to the fascia underlying the breast; also called Cooper's ligaments

sutures Nonmovable joints that connect two bones

syncope A brief, usually sudden, loss of consciousness

synovial joint Bones separated by a fluid-filled joint cavity

systole The phase of ventricular heart contraction; the filled ventricles contract to expel blood into the aorta and pulmonary arteries; also the top number of a blood pressure reading

systolic pressure The highest arterial blood pressure during the height of a ventricular contraction; the first number in a blood pressure reading

temperature The degree of hotness or coldness within the body as measured by a thermometer

tendons Tough fibrous bands that attach muscle to bone, or muscle to muscle

teratogen An agent that causes birth defects, such as a virus, a drug, a chemical, or radiation

terminal hair Dark, coarse, long hair that appears on the eyebrows, scalp, axillae, pubic region, and legs of both sexes, and on the face and chest of most males

tertiary prevention Strategies that occur later in a disease process and focus on reducing loss of function, maximizing health, and minimizing disability

testes Two firm, rubbery, olive-shaped structures that manufacture sperm and are thus the primary male sex organs

thalamus The largest subdivision of the diencephalon, which is the gateway to the cerebral cortex; the location in which all input channelled to the cerebral cortex is processed

thelarche Breast budding; often the first pubertal sign in females

thrill A soft vibratory sensation assessed by palpation with either the fingertips or palm flattened to the chest

thyroid gland The largest gland of the endocrine system; is butterfly shaped and located in the anterior portion of the neck

toddler A child between 1 and 3 years old

tophi Gout-related hard nodules that appear over the joint

torticollis A spasm of the sternocleidomastoid muscle on one side of the body, which often results from birth trauma

tracheal sounds Harsh, high-pitched sounds heard over the trachea when the client inhales and exhales

tracheomalacia Congenital defect of the cartilage in the trachea

tragus A small projection on the external ear that is positioned in front of the external auditory canal

tympanic membrane Membrane separating the external ear and middle ear that vibrates in response to sound waves entering the auditory canal and striking it; also called the eardrum

tympany A loud, high-pitched, drumlike tone of medium duration characteristic of an organ that is filled with air

umbilical hernias Protrusion at the umbilicus visible at birth

undernutrition Insufficient intake or storage of essential nutrients; also called malnutrition

upstream approaches Primary and secondary health prevention and promotion efforts

ureters Mucous-membrane-lined narrow tubes approximately 25 to 30 cm (10 to 12 in.) in length and 6 to 12 mm (0.25 to 0.5 in.) in diameter, whose major function is transporting urine from the kidney to the urinary bladder

urethra A mucous-membrane-lined tube that transports urine from the urinary bladder to the exterior

urethral stricture Condition indicated by pinpoint appearance to the urinary meatus

urinary retention A chronic state in which the client cannot empty his or her bladder

uterine tubes Ducts on either side of the fundus of the uterus; also called fallopian tubes

uterus A pear-shaped, hollow, muscular organ that is located centrally in the pelvis between the neck of the bladder and the rectal wall

uvula A fleshy pendulum that hangs from the edge of the soft palate in the back of the mouth; it moves with swallowing, breathing, and phonation

vagina A long, tubular, muscular canal that extends from the vestibule to the cervix at the inferior end of the uterus; major function is serving as the female organ of copulation, the birth canal, and the channel for the exit of menstrual flow

varicocele A varicose enlargement of the veins of the spermatic cord that causes a soft compressible mass in the scrotum; may lead to infertility

varicosities Distended and dilated veins that have a diminished blood flow and an increased intravenous pressure

vegan A dietary choice in which no animal products are consumed

veins Tubular walled vessels that carry deoxygenated blood from the body periphery back to the heart

vellus hair Pale, fine, short hair that appears over the entire body except for the lips, nipples, palms of hands, soles of feet, and parts of external genitals

venous insufficiency Inadequate circulation in the venous system usually because of incompetent valves in deep veins or a blood clot in the veins

verbal communication Spoken language to share information and ideas

vernix caseosa A cheeselike white substance that coats the skin surfaces at birth

vesicular sounds Soft and low-pitched breath sounds heard over the periphery; inspiration is longer than expiration

viability The point at which the fetus can survive outside the uterus

visceral layer of pericardium The inner layer that lines the surface of the heart

visceral pain Pain that results from stimulation of pain receptors deep within the body, such as the abdominal cavity, cranium, or the thorax

visual field Refers to the total area of vision in which objects can be seen while the eye remains focused on a central point

vital signs The systematic measurement of temperature, pulse, respirations, blood pressure, and pain status

vitiligo A skin condition identified by patchy depigmented skin over various areas of the body

vitreous humour A refractory medium; a clear gel within the eye that helps maintain the intraocular pressure and the shape of the eye, and transmits light rays through the eye

waist circumference The measurement around the waist at the top of the ilium, at the midaxillary point; measurement should be less than 88 cm (35 in.) in women and 102 cm (40 in.) in men

wheezes High-pitched squeaky or sibilant breath sounds, heard on expiration

whispered pectoriloquy Auscultation of voice sounds; as patient whispers, "one, two, three," normal lung sounds will be faint, almost indistinguishable

xanthelasma Soft, yellow plaques on the lids at the inner canthus, which are sometimes associated with high cholesterolemia

xerophthalmia A clinical finding of poor nutrition, dry mucosa

young adult A person between 21 and 40 years of age

References

Chapter 1

Alfaro-LeFevre, R. (2003). *Critical thinking and clinical judgment: A practical approach.* Philadelphia, PA: Saunders.

Canadian Nurses Association. (2010). *Vision and mission.* Retrieved from http://www.cna-nurses.ca/CNA/about/mission/default_e.aspx

Health Canada. (2009). *About Health Canada.* Retrieved from http://www.hc-sc.gc.ca/ahc-asc/index-eng.php

Leavell, H. R., & Clark, E. G. (1965). Preventive medicine for the doctor in the community. New York, NY: McGraw-Hill.

Leininger, M. M. (Ed.). (1991). *Culture care diversity and universality: A theory of nursing.* New York, NY: National League for Nursing Press.

NANDA International. (2009). Nursing diagnoses: Definitions and classification, 2009–2011. Oxford, UK: Wiley-Blackwell.

Neuman, B., & Fawcett, J. (2002). *The Neuman systems model* (4th ed.). Upper Saddle River, NJ: Prentice Hall.

Nightingale, F. (1969). *Notes on nursing: What it is and what it is not.* New York, NY: Dover Books. (Original work published 1860)

Orem, D. E. (1971). *Nursing: Concepts of practice.* Hightstown, NJ: McGraw-Hill.

Pender, N. J., Murdaugh, C. L., & Parsons, M. J. (2002). *Health promotion in nursing practice* (4th ed.). Upper Saddle River, NJ: Prentice Hall.

Public Health Agency of Canada. (2001). *What determines health?* Retrieved from http://www.phac-aspc.gc.ca/ph-sp/determinants/index-eng.php

Roy, C., & Andrews, H. (1999). *The Roy adaptation model* (2nd ed.). Stamford, CT: Appleton & Lange.

World Health Organization. (1947). *Constitution of the World Health Organization.* Geneva, Switzerland: Author.

Chapter 2

Bensaude De Castro Freire, S., Manoncourt, E., & Mukhopadhyay, A. (2009). IUHPE and social determinants of health: Setting an action agenda. *Global Health Promotion, Suppl. 1,* 89–92.

Best Start. (2007). *Reflecting on the trend: Pregnancy after age 35.* Retrieved from http://www.beststart.org/resources/rep_health/pdf/bs_pregnancy_age35.pdf

Canadian Broadcasting Corporation. (2010). *TB rate 185 times higher for Inuit than others.* Retrieved from http://www.cbc.ca/health/story/2010/03/10/tuberculosis-inuit.html

Canadian Federation for Sexual Health. (2007). *Sexual health in Canada baseline 2007.* Retrieved from http://www.cfsh.ca/files/publications/sexual_health_in_canada_baseline_2007_final.pdf

Canadian Nurses Association. (2006). *Social justice . . . a means to an end, an end in itself.* Ottawa, ON: Author.

Canadian Nurses Association. (2007). *Framework for the practice of registered nurses in Canada.* Ottawa, ON: Author.

Canadian Nurses Association. (2009). *Determinants of health* (Draft revised position statement—November 2009). Ottawa, ON: Author.

Canadian Public Health Association. (2010). *Public health—community health nursing practice in Canada: Roles and activities* (4th ed.). Ottawa, ON: Author.

Chen, Y., Jiang, Y., & Mao, Y. (2009). Association between obesity and depression in Canadians. *Journal of Women's Health, 18*(10), 1687–1692.

College of Family Physicians of Canada. (2004). *Infant feeding policy statement.* Retrieved from http://www.cfpc.ca/local/files/Communications/Health%20Policy/Final_04Infant_Feeding_Policy_Statement.pdf

Community Health Nurses Association of Canada. (2008). *Canadian community health nursing standards of practice* (Rev. ed.). Toronto, ON: Author.

Darroch, J. E., Singh, S., & Frost, J. J. (2001). Differences in teenage pregnancy rates among five developed countries: The roles of sexual activity and contraception use. *Family Planning Perspectives, 33*(6), 244–250, 281.

DiFranza, J. F., & Lew, R. A. (1995). Effect of maternal cigarette smoking on pregnancy complication and sudden infant death syndrome. *Journal of Family Practitioners, 40*(4), 385–394.

Edgington, E. M., Pimlott, J. F., & Cobban, S. J. (2009). Societal conditions driving the need for advocacy education in dental hygiene. *Canadian Journal of Dental Hygiene, 43*(6), 267–274.

Emrich, R. E., & Mazier, P. (2009). Impact of nutritional education on university students' fat consumption. *Canadian Journal of Dietetic Practice and Research, 70*(4), 187–192.

Epp, J. (1986). *Achieving health for all: A framework for health promotion.* Ottawa, ON: Minister of Supply and Services Canada.

Federal, Provincial, and Territorial Advisory Committee on Population Health. (1999). *Towards a healthy future: Second report on the health of Canadians.* Charlottetown, PE: Author.

Flynn, L. (1999). *Population health promotion model. Revised from original model developed by N. Hamilton and T. Bhatti, Health Promotion Development Division, Health Canada, 1996.* Winnipeg, MB: Health Canada, Manitoba/Saskatchewan Region.

Halton Suicide Prevention Coalition. (2009). *If you or anyone you know is feeling suicidal, CALL 911.* Retrieved from http://www.suicidepreventionhalton.ca/index.html

Hampton, M., Fahlman, S., Goertzen, J. R., & Jeffery, B. L. (2005). A process evaluation of the youth education about health (YEAH) program: A peer-designed and peer-led sexual health education program. *SEICCAN Newsletter, 40*(2), 129–140.

Health Canada. (2004). *Trends in workplace injuries, illnesses and policies in healthcare across Canada.* Retrieved from http://www.hc-sc.gc.ca/hcs-sss/pubs/hhrhs/2004-hwi-ipsmt/2004-hwi-ipsmt-eng.php

Health Canada. (2006a). *Youth and tobacco.* Retrieved from http://www.hc-sc.gc.ca/hc-ps/pubs/tobac-tabac/youth-jeunes/programs-eng.php

Health Canada. (2006b) *Obesity.* Retrieved from http://www.hc-sc.gc.ca/hl-vs/iyh-vsv/life-vie/obes-eng.php

Health Canada. (2007). *Eating well with Canada's Food Guide.* Retrieved from http://www.hc-sc.gc.ca/fn-an/food-guide-aliment/index-eng.php

Health Canada. (2008a). *Healthy pregnancy.* Retrieved from http://www.phac-aspc.gc.ca/hp-gs/know-savoir/smoke-fumer-eng.php

Health Canada. (2008b). *Mental health—coping with stress.* Retrieved from http://www.hc-sc.gc.ca/hl-vs/iyh-vsv/life-vie/stress-eng.php

Health Canada. (2010). *First Nations, Inuit and Aboriginal health: Diabetes.* Retrieved from http://www.hc-sc.gc.ca/fniah-spnia/diseases-maladies/diabete/index-eng.php#adi-ida

Human Resources and Skills Development Canada. (2010). *Health and safety.* Retrieved from http://www.rhdcc-hrsdc.gc.ca/eng/labour/health_safety/index.shtml

Hyman, Z, (2006). Brief interventions for high-risk drinkers. *Issues in Clinical Nursing, 15,* 1383–1396.

International Union for Health Promotion and Education & Canadian Consortium for Health Promotion Research. (2007). *Shaping the future of health promotion: Priorities for action.* Ottawa, ON: Public Health Agency of Canada.

Lalonde, M. (1974). *A new perspective on the health of Canadians: A working document.* Ottawa, ON: Government of Canada.

Layne, D. M., Rogers, B., & Randolf, S A. (2009). Health and gender comparisons in the long-haul trucking industry. *American Association of Occupational Health Nurses Journal, 57*(10), 405–413.

Martin, J. A., Hamilton, B. E., Sutton, P. D., Ventura, S. J., Menacker, F., & Munson, M. L. (2003). *Births: Final data for 2002* (National statistics report 52). Hyattsville, MD: Center for Health Statistics.

McKinlay, J. (1994). *An annotated bibliography of works held in the library of Australasia.* Adelaide, Australia: Royal Geographical Society of Australasia, South Australian Branch.

National Institute for Health and Clinical Excellence. (2007). *The social determinants of health: Developing an evidence base for political action.* Final report to World Health Organization Commission on the Social Determinants of Health. Retrieved from http://www.who.int/social_determinants/resources/mekn_final_report_102007.pdf

Nutbeam, D. (1998). Evaluating health promotion—progress, problems and solutions. *Health Promotion International, 13,* 27–44.

Polivy, J., & Herman, C. P. (2005). Mental health and eating behaviours. *Canadian Journal of Public Health, 96*(Suppl. 3), S43–S46.

Public Health Agency of Canada. (2001). *Population health promotion: An integrated model of population health and health promotion.* Retrieved from http://www.phac-aspc.gc.ca/ph-sp/php-psp/php3-eng.php

Public Health Agency of Canada. (2002). *Joint statement on shaken baby syndrome.* Retrieved from http://www.phac-aspc.gc.ca/dca-dea/publications/jointstatement_web-eng.php

Public Health Agency of Canada. (2003). *Get active your way every day—for life.* Retrieved from http://www.phac-aspc.gc.ca/hp-ps/hl-mvs/pag-gap/start-commence-eng.php

Public Health Agency of Canada. (2008). *What kinds of programs and services are available for people with diabetes?* Retrieved from http://www.phac-aspc.gc.ca/cd-mc/diabetes-diabete/diabetes_services-diabete_services-eng.php

Public Health Agency of Canada. (2009a). *Public health guidance for the prevention and management of influenza-like-illness (ILI), including the pandemic (HIN1) 2009 influenza virus, related to mass gatherings.* Retrieved from http://www.phac-aspc.gc.ca/alert-alerte/h1n1/phg-ldp-eng.php

Public Health Agency of Canada. (2009b). *Injury prevention.* Retrieved from http://www.phac-aspc.gc.ca/seniors-aines/publications/pro/injury-blessure/index-eng.php

Public Health Agency of Canada. (2009c). *Vaccines prevent disease.* Retrieved from http://www.phac-aspc.gc.ca/im/iyc-vve/prevention-eng.php#diseases

Public Health Agency of Canada. (2009d). *The FACTS on the safety and effectiveness of HPV vaccine.* Retrieved from http://www.phac-aspc.gc.ca/std-mts/hpv-vph/fact-faits-vacc-eng.php

Public Health Agency of Canada. (2010). *A-Z infectious diseases.* Retrieved from http://www.phac-aspc.gc.ca/id-mi/az-index-eng.php#measles

Raeburn, J., & Rootman, I. (1998). *People-centred health promotion.* Chichester, England: John Wiley & Sons.

Raine, K. D. (2005). Determinants of healthy eating in Canada: An overview and synthesis. *Canadian Journal of Public Health, 96*(Suppl. 3), S8–S14.

Raphael, D. (2002). Social justice is good for our hearts: Why societal factors—not lifestyles— are major causes of heart disease in Canada and elsewhere. Toronto, ON: CSJ Foundation for Research and Education.

Raphael, D. (2004). *Social determinants of health: Canadian perspectives.* Toronto, ON: Canadian Scholars' Press.

Raphael, D. (2006). Social determinants of health: Present status, unanswered questions, and future directions. *International Journal of Health Services, 36*(4), 651–677.

Search Institute (2010). *What are developmental assets?* Retrieved from http://www.search-institute.org/content/what-are-developmental-assets

Sex Information and Education Council of Canada. (2009). *Sexual health education in the schools: Questions & answers* (3rd ed.). Retrieved from http://www.sieccan.org/pdf/SHES_QA.pdf

Stamler, L. L., & Yiu, L. (2008). *Community health nursing: A Canadian perspective* (2nd ed.). Toronto, ON: Pearson Prentice Hall.

Statistics Canada. (2007). *Canadian community health survey—Cycle 1.1.* Retrieved from http://www.statcan.gc.ca/concepts/health-sante/index-eng.htm

United Nations General Assembly. (2002). *Resolution adopted by the general assembly: A world fit for children* (Report No. S-27/2). Retrieved from http://www.unicef.org/specialsession/docs_new/documents/A-RES-S27-2E.pdf

U.S. Department of Health and Human Services, Centers for Disease Control and Prevention, & National Center for Chronic Disease Prevention and Health Promotion. (2004). *The health consequences of smoking: A report of the surgeon general.* Atlanta, GA: Office on Smoking and Health.

Vollman, A. R. (2008). Population health promotion: Essentials and essence of practice. In A. R. Vollman, E. T. Anderson, & J. McFarlane (Eds.), *Canadian community as partner* (2nd ed., pp. 2–25). Philadelphia, PA: Lippincott Williams & Wilkins.

Wallerstein, N. (2002). Empowerment to reduce health disparities. *Scandinavian Journal of Public Health, 30*(Suppl. 59), 72–77.

World Health Organization. (1978). *Declaration of Alma-Ata on primary health care.* Geneva, Switzerland: Author.

World Health Organization. (2008). *Closing the gap in a generation: Health equity through action on the social determinants of health* (Commission on social determinants of health final report/executive summary). Geneva, Switzerland: WHO Press.

World Health Organization. (2010a). *The five elements of DOTS.* Retrieved from http://www.who.int/tb/dots/whatisdots/en/index.html

World Health Organization. (2010b). *Obesity and overweight.* Retrieved from http://www.who.int/mediacentre/factsheets/fs311/en/index.html

World Health Organization, Health and Welfare Canada, & Canadian Public Health Association. (1986). *Ottawa charter for health promotion.* Geneva, Switzerland: WHO.

Chapter 4

Aboriginal Nurses Association of Canada. (2009). *Cultural competence and cultural safety in nursing education: A framework for First Nations, Inuit and Metis nursing.* Ottawa, ON: Author.

Ahmad, W. I. U. (1993). Making black people sick: "Race," ideology and health research. In W. I. U. Ahmad (Ed.), *"Race" and health in contemporary Britain* (pp. 11–33). Buckingham, UK: Open University Press.

Anderson, J. M., & Reimer Kirkham, S. (1998). Constructing nation: The gendering and racializing of the Canadian health care system. In V. Strong-Boag, S. Grace, A. Eisenberg, & J. Anderson (Eds.), *Painting the maple: Essays on race, gender, and the construction of Canada* (pp. 242–261). Vancouver, BC: UBC Press.

Anderson, J. M., & Reimer Kirkham, S. (1999). Discourses on health: A critical perspective. In H. Coward & P. Ratanakul (Eds.), *A cross-cultural dialogue on health care ethics* (pp. 47–67). Waterloo, ON: Wilfred Laurier University Press.

Anderson, J. M., Perry, J., Blue, C., Browne, A. J., Henderson, A., Lynam, J.,..., & Smye, V. (2003). "Re-writing" cultural safety within the postcolonial and postnationalist feminist project: Toward new epistemologies of healing. *Advances in Nursing Science, 26*(3), 196–214.

Anderson, J. M., Reimer Kirkham, S., Waxler-Morrison, N., Herbert, C. Murphy, M., & Richardson, E. (2005). Conclusion: Delivering culturally responsive health care. In N. Waxler-Morisson, J. M. Anderson, E. Richardson, & N. Chambers (Eds.), *Cross-cultural caring: A handbook for health professionals* (2nd ed., pp. 323–352). Vancouver, BC: UBC Press.

Assembly of First Nations. (2005). *International reports highlight Canada's lack of progress in addressing First Nations poverty: UNICEF ranks Canada 19th out of 26 countries in child poverty.* Retrieved from http://www.afn.ca/article.asp?id=200

British Columbia Provincial Health Services Authority. (2009). *On-line cultural competency training program.* Retrieved from http://www.phsa.ca/AgenciesAndServices/Services/Provincial-Language-Service/TrainingServices/default.htm

Browne, A. J. (2005). Discourse influencing nurse's perceptions of First Nations patients. *Canadian Journal of Nursing Research, 37*(4), 62–87.

Browne, A. J. (2007). Clinical encounters between nurses and First Nations women in a Western Canadian hospital. *Social Science and Medicine, 64*(10), 2165–2176.

Browne, A. J., & Fiske, J. (2001). First Nations women's encounters with mainstream health care services. *Western Journal of Nursing Research, 23*(2), 126–147.

Browne, A. J., & Smye, V. (2002). A postcolonial analysis of health care discourses addressing Aboriginal women. *Nurse Researcher, 9*(3), 28–41.

Browne, A. J., & Varcoe, C. (2006).Critical cultural perspectives and health care involving Aboriginal peoples. *Contemporary Nurse, 22*(2), 155–167.

Browne, A. J., & Varcoe, C. (2009). Cultural and social considerations in health assessment. In C. Jarvis, A. J. Browne, J. MacDonald-Jenkins, & M. Luctkar-Flude (Eds.), *Physical examination and health assessment* (1st Cdn ed., pp. 35–50). Toronto, ON: Elsevier.

Browne, A. J., Fiske, J., & Thomas, G. (2000). *First Nations women's encounters with mainstream health care services and systems.* Vancouver, BC: British Columbia Centre of Excellence for Women's Health.

Browne, A. J., Smye, V., & Varcoe, C. (2005). The relevance of postcolonial theoretical perspectives to research in Aboriginal health. *Canadian Journal of Nursing Research, 37*(4), 16–37.

Browne, A. J., Varcoe, C., Smye, V., Reimer Kirkham, S., Lynam, M. J., & Wong, S. (2009). Cultural safety and the challenges of translating critically oriented knowledge in practice. *Nursing Philosophy, 10*(3), 167–179.

Cairns, A. C. (2000). Citizens plus: Aboriginal peoples and the Canadian state. Vancouver, BC: UBC Press.

Canadian Nurses Association. (2004). *Position statement: Cultural competence.*Retrieved from http://www.cna-nurses.ca/CNA/documents/pdf/publications/PS73_Promoting_Culturally_Competent_Care_March_2004_e.pdf

College of Registered Nurses of Nova Scotia. (2006). *Position Statement: Promoting culturally competent care.* Retrieved from http://www.crnns.ca/documents/PositionStatementCultural06.pdf

Culley, L. (1996). A critique of multiculturalism in health care: The challenge for nurse education. *Journal of Advanced Nursing, 23*, 564–570.

Dei, G. J. S. (1996). *Anti-racism education: Theory and practice.* Halifax, NS: Fernwood Publishers.

Doane, G. H. & Varcoe, C. (2005). *Family nursing as relational inquiry: Developing health promoting practice.* Philadelphia, PA: Lippincott, Williams and Wilkins.

Drevdahl, D. J., Philips, D. A., & Taylor, J. Y. (2006). Uncontested categories: the use of race and ethnicity variables in nursing research. *Nursing Inquiry, 13*(1), 52–63.

Gilroy, P. (2000). *Against race: Imagining political culture beyond the color line.* Cambridge, MA: Harvard University Press.

Gilroy, P. (2001). The end of antiracism. In P. Essed & D. T. Goldberg (Eds.), *Race critical theories: Text and context*(pp. 249–264). Malden, MA: Wiley-Blackwell.

Guruge, S., & Gastaldo, D. (2008). Violencia en la pareja e inmigración: ?Cómo ser parte de la solución? [Violence in couples and immigration: How to be part of the solution?] (Editorial). *Presencia,* n.8.

Gustafson, D. (2007). White on whiteness: Being radicalized about race. *Nursing Inquiry, 14*(2), 153–161.

Health Canada. (2001). *The health determinants: Population health promotion model.* Retrieved from http://www.phac-aspc.gc.ca/ph-sp/determinants/index-eng.php#key_determinants

Health Canada. (2009). *Non-insured health benefits.* Retrieved from http://www.hc-sc.gc.ca/fniah-spnia/pubs/nihb-ssna/index-eng.php

Henry, F., Tator, C., Mattis, W., & Rees, R. (2005). *The colour of democracy: Racism in Canadian society* (3rd ed.). Toronto, ON: Nelson.

Hyman, I., Guruge, S., & Mason, R. (2008). The impact of post-migration changes on marital relationships: A study of Ethiopian immigrant couples in Toronto. *Journal of Comparative Family Studies, 39*(2), 149–164.

Indian Residential Schools Adjudication Secretariat. (2008). *Frequently asked questions.* Retrieved from http://www.irsad-sapi.gc.ca/ab-ap-eng.asp?action=faq-1

Kawachi, I., Subramanian, S. V. & Almeida-Filho, N. (2002). A glossary for health inequalities. *Journal of Epidemiology and Community Health, 56*(9), 647–652.

Kelm, M. (1998). *Colonizing bodies: Aboriginal health and healing in British Columbia 1900–50.* Vancouver, BC: UBC Press.

Kendall, J., & Hatton, D. (2002). Racism as a source of health disparity in families with children with attention deficit hyperactivity disorder. *Advances in Nursing Science, 25*, 22–39.

Kleinman, A. (1980). *Patients and healers in the context of culture.* Berkeley, CA: University of California Press.

Kleinman, A., & Benson, P. (2006). Anthropology in the clinic: The problem of cultural competency and how to fix it. *PloSMedicine—A Peer-Reviewed Open-Access Journal, 3*(1), 1673–1676.

Lipp, A. (2007). Developing the reflexive dimension of reflection: A framework for debate. *International Journal of Multiple Research Approaches,1*(1), 18–26.

Lock, M. (1990). On being ethnic: The politics of identity breaking and making in Canada, or, Nevra on Sunday. *Culture, Medicine and Psychiatry, 14*, 237–252.

McConaghy, C. (2000). *Rethinking indigenous education: Culturalism, colonialism and the politics of knowing.* Brisbane, AU: Post Pressed.

Mental Health Commission of Canada. (2009). *First Nations, Inuit and Metis.* Retrieved from http://www.mentalhealthcommission.ca/English/Pages/FirstNationsInuitandMetis.aspx

Narayan, U. (2000). Essence of culture and a sense of history: A feminist critique of cultural essentialism. In U. Narayan & S. Harding (Eds.), *Decentering the center: Philosophy for a multicultural, postcolonial, and feminist world* (pp. 80–100). Bloomington, IN: University Press.

National Aboriginal Health Organization. (2008). *Cultural competency and safety: A guide for health care administrators, providers and educators.* Retrieved from http://www.naho.ca/publications/culturalCompetency.pdf

Native Mental Health Association of Canada. (2009). *Charting the future of Native mental health in Canada: The NMHAC's ten-year strategic plan.* Retrieved http://www.heretohelp.bc.ca/publications/aboriginal-people/bck/4

O'Neil, J. D., Lemchuk-Favel, L., Allard, Y., & Postl, B. (1999). Community healing and aboriginal self-government: Is the circle closing? In J. Hylton (Ed.), *Aboriginal self-government in Canada: Current trends and issues* (2nd ed., pp. 67–89). Saskatoon, SK: Purich Publishing.

Omi, M., & Winant, H. (2002). Racial formation. In P. Essed & D. T. Goldberg (Eds.) *Race critical theories: Text and context* (pp. 123–145). Malden, MA: Wiley-Blackwell.

Pederson, A., & Raphael, D. (2006). Gender, race and health inequities. In D. Raphael, T. Bryant, & M. Rioux (Eds.), *Staying alive: Critical perspectives on health, illness and health care* (pp. 159–191). Toronto, ON: Canadian Scholars' Press.

Pesut, B., Fowler, M., Johnston Taylor, Reimer Kirkham, S., & Sawatzky, R. (2008). Conceptualizing spirituality and religion for healthcare. *Journal of Clinical Nursing, 17*(21), 2803–2810.

Polaschek, N. R. (1998). Cultural safety: A new concept in nursing peoples of different ethnicities. *Journal of Advanced Nursing, 27*(3), 452–457.

Ramsden, I. (2000). Cultural safety/Kawa whakaruruhau ten years on: A personal overview. *Nursing Praxis in New Zealand, 15*(1), 4–12.

Raphael, D. (2006). Addressing health inequalities in Canada: Little attention, inadequate action, limited success. In M. O'Neill, A. Pederson, S. Dupere & I. Rootman (Eds.), *Health promotion in Canada: Critical perspectives* (2nd ed., pp. 106–122).

Raphael, D. (2007). *Poverty and policy in Canada: Implications for health and quality of life.* Toronto, ON: Canadian Scholars' Press.

Reid, C. (2007). Women's health and the politics of policy and exclusion. In M. Morrow, O. Hankivsky, & C. Varcoe (Eds.), *Women's health in Canada: Critical theory, policy and practice* (pp. 199–220). Toronto, ON: University of Toronto Press.

Reimer Kirkham, S., & Anderson, J. M. (2002). Postcolonial nursing scholarship: From epistemology to method. *Advances in Nursing Science, 25*(1), 1–17.

Reimer Kirkham, S., Pesut, B. Meyerhoff, H., & Sawatzky, R. (2004). Spiritual caregiving at the juncture of religion, culture, and state. *Canadian Journal of Nursing Research, 36*(4), 148–169.

Reimer Kirkham, S., Smye, V., Tang, S., Anderson, J., Browne, A. J., Coles, R.,..., & Shapero, L. (2002). Rethinking cultural safety while waiting to do fieldwork: Methodological implications for nursing research. *Research in Nursing and Health, 25*, 222–232.

Smye, V. (2007, July). *Integrating Culture into Practice: Developing a Peer Review Framework for Nurses.* Victoria, BC: Intertribal Health, University of Victoria & Vancouver Island Health Authority, Aboriginal Programs. Funded by the Nursing Directorate, B.C. Ministry of Health.

Smye, V., & Browne A. J. (2002). "Cultural safety" and the analysis of health policy affecting Aboriginal people. *Nurse Researcher, 9*(3), 42–56.

Smye, V., Browne, A., & Varcoe, C. (under review). Harm reduction and methadone maintenance treatment: Intersections of gender, class, race and ability. *Social Science and Medicine.*

Spector, R. E. (2004). *Cultural diversity in health and illness*(2nd ed.). Upper Saddle River, NJ: Prentice Hall.

Srivastava, R. H. (2007). *The health professional's guide to clinical cultural competence.* Toronto, ON: Elsevier.

Statistics Canada. (2007a). *Immigration in Canada: A portrait of the foreign-born population, 2006 census.* Retrieved from http://www.statcan.gc.ca/bsolc/olc-cel/olc-cel?catno=97-557-X2006001&lang=eng

Statistics Canada. (2007b). *Portrait of the Canadian population by age and sex.* Retrieved from http://www.statcan.ca/english/census06/analysis/agesex/index.cfm

Statistics Canada. (2007c). 2006 census: Immigration, citizenship, language, mobility and migration. *The Daily,* December 4. Retrieved from http://www.statcan.ca/Daily/English/071204/d071204a.htm

Statistics Canada. (2008a). 2006 census: Ethnic origin, visible minorities, place of work and mode of transportation. *The Daily,* April 2. Retrieved from http://www.statcan.gc.ca/daily-quotidien/080402/dq080402a-eng.htm

Statistics Canada. (2008b). *Annual demographic estimates: Canada, provinces and territories.* Retrieved from http://www.statcan.gc.ca/bsolc/olc-cel/olc-cel?catno=91-215-XIE&lang=eng

Statistics Canada. (2008c). Aboriginal peoples in Canada in 2006: Inuit, Metis and First Nations. *The Daily,* January 15. Retrieved from http://www.statcan.gc.ca/daily-quotidien/080115/dq080115a-eng.htm

Statistics Canada. (2009). *2006 census: Portrait of the Canadian population in 2006: Subprovincial population dynamics.* Retrieved from http://www12.statcan.ca/census-recensement/2006/as-sa/97-550/p17-eng.cfm

Tang, S. (1999). Interpreter services in healthcare: Policy recommendations for healthcare agencies. *Journal of Nursing Administration, 29*(6), 23–29.

Tang, S., & Browne, A. J. (2008). "Race" matters: Racialization and egalitarian discourses involving Aboriginal people in the Canadian health care context. *Ethnicity & Health, 13*(2), 109–127.

Timmins, R. (2006). Critical practice in nursing care: analysis, action and reflexivity. *Nursing Standard, 20*(39), 39–54.

U.S. Department of Health and Human Services. (2001). *National standards for culturally and linguistically appropriate services in health care: Final report.* Washington, DC: Office of Minority Health.

UBC School of Nursing Undergraduate Curriculum. (2009). *Academic unit plan.* Retrieved from http://www.nursing.ubc.ca/about_us/Academic%20Unit%20Plan%202009.pdf

Varcoe, C. (2001). Abuse obscured: An ethnographic account of emergency nursing in relation to violence against women. *Canadian Journal of Nursing Research, 32*(4), 95–115.

Varcoe, C. (2008). Inequality, violence, and women's health. In B. S. Bolaria & H. Dickenson (Eds.). *Health, illness and health care in Canada* (4th ed., pp. 211–230). Toronto, ON: Nelson.

Varcoe, C., Hankivsky, O., & Morrow, M. (2007). Beyond gender matters: An introduction. In M. Morrow, O. Hankivsky, & C. Varcoe (Eds.), *Women's health in Canada: Critical theory, policy and practice* (pp. 3–30). Toronto, ON: University of Toronto Press.

Vissandjee, B., Thurston, W., Apale, A., & Nahar, K. (2007). Women's health at the intersection of gender and the experience of international migration. In M. Morrow, O. Hankivsky, & C. Varcoe (Eds.), *Women's health in Canada: Critical theory, policy and practice* (pp. 221–243). Toronto, ON: University of Toronto Press.

Waldram, J. B., Herring, D. A., & Young, T. K. (2006). *Aboriginal health in Canada: Historical, cultural, and epidemiological perspective* (2nd ed.). Toronto, ON: University of Toronto Press.

Waxler-Morrison, N., & Anderson, J. (2005). Introduction: The need for culturally sensitive health care. In N. Waxler-Morrison, J. M. Anderson, E. Richardson, & N. Chambers (Eds.), *Cross-cultural caring: A handbook for health professionals* (2nd ed., pp. 1–10). Vancouver, BC: UBC Press.

Wepa, D. (Ed.). (2005). *Cultural safety in Aotearoa New Zealand.* Auckland, NZ: Pearson New Zealand Limited.

Chapter 5

Anandarajah, G., & Hight, E. (2001). Spirituality and medical practice: Using the HOPE questions as a practical tool for spiritual assessment [Electronic version]. *American Family Physician, 63,* 81–89.

Anderson, J. M., & Reimer Kirkham, S. (1999). Discourses on health: A critical perspective. In H. Coward & P. Ratanakul (Eds.), *A cross-cultural dialogue on health care ethics* (pp. 47–67). Waterloo, ON: Wilfred Laurier University Press.

Canadian Institute of Wellbeing. (2009). *How are Canadians really doing?* Retrieved from http://www.ciw.ca/Libraries/Documents/FirstReportOfTheInstituteOfWellbeing.sflb.ashx

Ellison, C. W., & Paloutzian, R. F. (1982). *The spiritual well being scale.* Life Advance, Inc. Retrieved from http://www.lifeadvance.com/applications.htm

Hodge, D. R. (2001). Spiritual assessment: A review of major qualitative methods and a new framework for assessing spirituality. *Social Work, 46*(3), 8037–8046.

International Council of Nurses. (2005). *Fact sheet genetics and nursing.* Retrieved from http://www.icn.ch/matters_genetics.htm

McSherry, W., & Ross, L. (2001). Dilemmas of spiritual assessment: Considerations for nursing practice. *Journal of Advanced Nursing, 38*(5), 479–488.

Public Health Agency of Canada. (2003). *Healthy living unit: Helpful definitions.* Retrieved from http://www.phac-aspc.gc.ca/pau-uap/fitness/definitions.html

Roy, C., & Andrews, H. (1999). *The Roy adaptation model* (2nd ed.). Stamford, CT: Appleton & Lange.

Stoll, R. I. (1979). Guidelines for spiritual assessment. *American Journal of Nursing, 79*(9), 1574–1577.

Chapter 8

Ball, J. W., & Bindler, R. C. (2008). *Pediatric nursing: Caring for children* (4th ed.). Toronto, ON: Prentice Hall.

Canadian Paediatric Society & American Academy of Pediatrics. (2007). Prevention and management of pain in the neonate: An update—A joint statement with the American Academy of Pediatrics [Electronic version]. *Paediatric Child Health, 12*(2), 137–138.

Canadian Nurses Association. (2004). *Position statement: Providing culturally competent care.* Retrieved from http://www.cna-aiic.ca/CNA/documents/pdf/publications/PS73_Promoting_Culturally_Competent_Care_March_2004_e.pdf

Eliopoulos, C. (2005). *Gerontological nursing* (6th ed.). Philadelphia, PA: Lippincott.

Gilron, P., Watson, C., Cahill, & Moulin, D. (2006). Neuropathic pain: A practical guide for the clinician. *Canadian Medical Association Journal, 175*(3), 265–275.

McCaffery, M., & Pasero, C. (1999). *Pain: Clinical manual* (2nd ed.). St. Louis, MO: Mosby.

Melzack, R., & Wall, P. D. (1965). Pain mechanisms: A new theory. *Science, 150,* 971–979.

NANDA International. (2009). *Nursing diagnoses: Definitions and classification, 2009–2011.* Oxford, UK: Wiley-Blackwell.

Paice, J. A. (2002). Controlling pain. Understanding nociceptive pain. *Nursing, 32*(3), 74–75.

Chapter 9

Assessing the nutritional status of wound-care patients. (2008). *LPN, 4*(3), 23–26.

Dawson, B., & Favaloro, E.J. (2009). High rate of deficiency in the amino acids Tryptophan and Histidine in people with wounds: Implication for nutrient targeting in wound management—a pilot study. *Advances in Skin and Wound Care, 22*(2), 79–82

Fischbach, F., & Dunning, M.B. (2009). *A manual of laboratory and diagnostic tests* (8th ed.). Philadelphia, PA: Lippincott, Williams, & Wilkins.

Health Canada. (2002). *Nutrition for health: An agenda for action.* Retrieved from http://www.hc-sc.gc.ca/fn-an/nutrition/pol/nutrition_health_agenda-nutrition_virage_sante-eng.php

Health Canada. (2003a). *Canadian guidelines for body weight classification in adults.* Retrieved from http://www.hc-sc.gc.ca/fn-an/nutrition/weights-poids/guide-ld-adult/index-eng.php

Health Canada. (2003b). *Canadian guidelines for body weight classification in adults: Quick reference tool for professionals.* Retrieved from http://www.hc-sc.gc.ca/fn-an/nutrition/weights-poids/guide-ld-adult/cg_quick_ref-ldc_rapide_ref-eng.php

Health Canada. (2006). *Canadian community health survey: Cycle 2.2, nutrition (2004)—A guide to accessing and interpreting the data.* Retrieved from http://www.hc-sc.gc.ca/fn-an/alt_formats/hpfb-dgpsa/pdf/surveill/cchs-guide-escc-eng.pdf

Health Canada. (2007). *Eating Well with Canada's Food Guide.* Retrieved from http://www.hc-sc.gc.ca/fn-an/food-guide-aliment/index-eng.php

Hess, C. T. (2009). Monitoring laboratory values: Transferrin, C-reactive protein, erythrocyte sedimentation rate, and liver function. *Advances in Skin & Wound Care, 22*(2), 96.

Lee, C. M., Huxley, R. R., Wildman, R. P., & Woodard, M. (2008). Indices of abdominal obesity are better discriminators of cardiovascular risk factors than BMI: A meta-analysis. *Journal of Clinical Epidemiology, 61*(7) 646–653.

Manitoba Health. (1992). *Quality health care for Manitobans: The action plan.* Winnipeg: MB: Author.

NANDA International. (2009). *Nursing diagnoses: Definitions and classification, 2009–2011.* Oxford, UK: Wiley-Blackwell.

New Brunswick Government. (1990). *Health 2000: Toward a comprehensive health strategy.* Fredericton, NB: Author.

New Brunswick Government. (1993). *Public health service: Vision, mission, goals and objectives.* Fredericton, NB: Author.

Provincial Working Group on the Problems of Weight in Quebec. (2004). *Weight problems in Quebec: Getting mobilized.* Montreal, PC: ASPQ.

Safer, R., & Keenan, J. (2005). Health literacy: The gap between physicians and patients. *American Family Physician, 72*(3), 463–468.

Starky, S. (2005). *The obesity epidemic in Canada.* Retrieved from http://parl.gc.ca/information/library/prbpubs/prb0511-e.htm

Weiss, B. D., Mays, M. Z., Martz, W., Castro, K. M., DeWalt, D. A., Pignone, M. P., Mockbee, J., & Hale, F. A. (2005). Quick assessment of literacy in primary care: The newest vital sign. *Annals of Family Medicine, 3*(6), 514–522.

World Health Organization. (2000). *Obesity: Preventing and managing the global epidemic.* Retrieved from http://whqlibdoc.who.int/trs/WHO_TRS_894.pdf

Chapter 10

Brammer, L. M., Abrego, P., & Shostrum, E. (1993). *Therapeutic counseling and psychotherapy* (6th ed.). Upper Saddle River, NJ: Prentice Hall.

Carkhuff, R. R. (2000). *The art of helping in the 21st century.* Amherst, MA: Human Resources Development Press.

Cormier, L. S., Cormier, W. H., & Weiser, R. J. (1984). *Interviewing and helping, skills for health professionals.* Belmont, CA: Wadsworth.

Doenges, M. A., & Moorhouse, M. F. (1990). *Nursing diagnosis with interventions* (3rd ed.). Philadelphia, PA: F.A. Davis.

Gordon, M. (1990). Toward theory based diagnostic categories. *Nursing Diagnosis, 1*(1), 5–11.

Human Resources and Social Development Canada, the Public Health Agency of Canada, & Indian and Northern Affairs Canada. (2007). *The well-being of Canada's young children: Government of Canada report 2006.* Retrieved from http://www.socialunion.gc.ca/well_being/2007/en/chapter_5.shtml

Orem, D. E. (1991). *Nursing concepts and practice* (4th ed.). St. Louis, MO: Mosby.

Rogers, C. R. (1951). *Client-centered therapy.* Boston, MA: Houghton Mifflin.

Rogers, C. R. (1957). The necessary and sufficient conditions of therapeutic personality change. *Journal of Consulting Clinical Psychology, 21,* 95–103.

Chapter 11

NANDA International. (2009). *Nursing diagnoses: Definitions and classification, 2009–2011.* Oxford, UK: Wiley-Blackwell.

Chapter 12

NANDA International. (2009). *Nursing diagnoses: Definitions and classification, 2009–2011.* Oxford, UK: Wiley-Blackwell.

Chapter 13

NANDA International. (2009). *Nursing diagnoses: Definitions and classification, 2009–2011.* Oxford, UK: Wiley-Blackwell.

Chapter 14

NANDA International. (2009). *Nursing diagnoses: Definitions and classification, 2009–2011.* Oxford, UK: Wiley-Blackwell.

Chapter 15

NANDA International. (2009). *Nursing diagnoses: Definitions and classification, 2009–2011*. Oxford, UK: Wiley-Blackwell.

Chapter 16

Canadian Cancer Society. (2007). *October is breast cancer awareness month*. Retrieved from http://www.cancer.ca/Canada-wide/About%20us/Media%20centre/CW-Media%20releases/CW-2007/October%20is%20Breast%20Cancer%20Awareness%20Month.aspx?sc_lang=en

Canadian Cancer Society. (2009). *Breast cancer statistics*. Retrieved from http://www.cancer.ca/Canada-wide/About%20cancer/Cancer%20statistics/Stats%20at%20a%20glance/Breast%20cancer.aspx?sc_lang=en

Canadian Cancer Society. (2010). *Know your breasts*. Retrieved from http://www.cancer.ca/Canada-wide/Prevention/Knowing%20your%20body/Know%20your%20breasts.aspx?sc_lang=en

Jelinski, S., Maxwell, C., Onysko, J., & Bancej, C. (2005). The influence of breast self-examination on subsequent mammography participation. *American Journal of Public Health, 95*(3), 506–511.

NANDA International. (2009). *Nursing diagnoses: Definitions and classification, 2009–2011*. Oxford, UK: Wiley-Blackwell.

Society of Obstetricians and Gynaecologists of Canada. (2006). *SOGC committee opinion: Breast self-examination* (No. 181). Retrieved from http://www.sogc.org/guidelines/documents/181E-CO-August2006.pdf

Chapter 17

Canadian Women's Health Network. (2006). *Menopause and heart disease*. Retrieved from http://www.cwhn.ca/node/40802

Heart and Stroke Foundation. (2010). *Basic principles of physical activity*. Retrieved from http://www.heartandstroke.com/site/c.ikIQLcMWJtE/b.3483953/k.7D68/Basic_principles_of_physical_activity.htm?src=home

NANDA International. (2009). *Nursing diagnoses: Definitions and classification, 2009–2011*. Oxford, UK: Wiley-Blackwell.

Chapter 18

Canadian Cardiovascular Society. (2005). *Peripheral arterial disease*. Retrieved from http://www.ccs.ca/download/consensus_conference/consensus_conference_archives/CCFinalPre_CJC_Pub.pdf

Canadian Hypertension Education Program. (2009). *2009 CHEP recommendations for the management of hypertension*. Retrieved from http://hypertension.ca/downloads/chep/ids/docs/PDF/Complete_Recommendations_2009.pdf

NANDA International. (2009). *Nursing diagnoses: Definitions and classification, 2009–2011*. Oxford, UK: Wiley-Blackwell.

Chapter 19

NANDA International. (2009). *Nursing diagnoses: Definitions and classification, 2009–2011*. Oxford, UK: Wiley-Blackwell.

Chapter 20

NANDA International. (2009). *Nursing diagnoses: Definitions and classification, 2009–2011*. Oxford, UK: Wiley-Blackwell.

Chapter 21

NANDA International. (2009). Nursing diagnoses: *Definitions and classification, 2009–2011*. Oxford, UK: Wiley-Blackwell.

Chapter 22

Canadian Cancer Society. (2009). *Causes of cervical cancer*. Retrieved from http://www.cancer.ca/canada-wide/about%20cancer/types%20of%20cancer/causes%20of%20cervical%20cancer.aspx?sc_lang=en

NANDA International. (2009). *Nursing diagnoses: Definitions and classification, 2009–2011*. Oxford, UK: Wiley-Blackwell.

Chapter 23

NANDA International. (2009). *Nursing diagnoses: Definitions and classification, 2009–2011*. Oxford, UK: Wiley-Blackwell.

Chapter 24

NANDA International. (2009). *Nursing diagnoses: Definitions and classification, 2009–2011*. Oxford, UK: Wiley-Blackwell.

Chapter 25

Canadian Paediatric Society Nutrition and Gastroenterology Committee. (2005). Exclusive breastfeeding should continue to six months (reaffirmed February 2009) [Electronic version]. *Paediatrics and Child Health, 10*(3), 148.

Canadian Paediatric Society: Community Paediatrics Committee. (2009). Vision screening in infants, children and youth. *Paediatrics and Child Health, 14*(4), 246–248.

Dietitians of Canada, Canadian Paediatric Society, College of Family Physicians of Canada, and Community Health Nurses Association of Canada. (2010). *Promoting optimal monitoring of child growth in Canada*. Retrieved from http://www.cps.ca/english/statements/N/growth-charts-statement-FULL.pdf

Innis, S. M., Nelson, C. M., Wadsworth, L. D., MacLaren, I. A., & Lwanga, D. (1997). Incidence of iron-deficiency anaemia and depleted iron stores among nine-month-old infants in Vancouver, Canada. *Canadian Journal of Public Health, 88*, 80–84.

NANDA International. (2009). *Nursing diagnoses: Definitions and classification, 2009–2011*. Oxford, UK: Wiley-Blackwell.

Public Health Agency of Canada. (2007). *Immunizations schedules*. Retrieved from http://www.phac-aspc.gc.ca/im/is-cv/index-eng.php#a

Chapter 26

NANDA International. (2009). *Nursing diagnoses: Definitions and classification, 2009–2011*. Oxford, UK: Wiley-Blackwell.

Public Health Agency of Canada. (2004). *Physical abuse during pregnancy: Fact sheet*. Retrieved from http://www.phac-aspc.gc.ca/rhs-ssg/factshts/abuseprg-eng.php

Society of Obstetricians and Gynaecologists of Canada. (2001). *A guide for health professionals working with Aboriginal peoples*. Retrieved from www.sogc.org/guidelines/public/100E-PS3-January2001.pdf

Society of Obstetricians and Gynaecologists of Canada. (2003). *Policy statement: Diversity*. Retrieved from http://www.sogc.org/guidelines/public/140E-PS-Decembre2003.pdf

Chapter 27

Burke, M. M., & Walsh, M. B. (1997). *Gerontologic nursing* (2nd ed.). St. Louis, MO: Mosby.

Canadian Cancer Society. (2009). *Breast cancer in men*. Retrieved from http://www.cancer.ca/Canada-wide/About%20cancer/Types%20of%20cancer/Breast%20cancer%20in%20men.aspx?sc_lang=en

Canadian Diabetes Association. (2008). 2008 Clinical practice guidelines for the prevention and management of diabetes in Canada. *Canadian Journal of Diabetes, 32*(Supp. 1). Retrieved from http://www.diabetes.ca/for-professionals/resources/2008-cpg/

Canadian Hypertension Education Program. (2009). *Recommendations: 2009*. Retrieved from http://hypertension.ca/chep/recommendations-2009

Doerfler, E. (1999). Male erectile dysfunction: A guide for clinician management. *Journal of the American Academy of Nurse Practitioners, 11*(3), 117–123.

Ewing, J. (1984). Detecting alcoholism: The CAGE questionnaire. *Journal of the American Medical Association, 252*(14), 1905–1907.

Folstein, M., Folstein, S. E., & McHugh, P. R. (1975). Mini-mental state: A practical method for grading the cognitive state of patients for the clinician. *Journal of Psychiatric Research, 12*(3), 189–198.

Grodner, M., Long, S., & DeYoung, S. (2004). *Foundations and clinical applications of nutrition: A nursing approach.* St. Louis, MO: Mosby.

Health Canada. (2007). *Eating Well with Canada's Food Guide.* Retrieved from http://www.hc-sc.gc.ca/fn-an/food-guide-aliment/index-eng.php

Jensen, G., McGee, M., & Binkley, J. (2001). Nutrition in the elderly. *Gastroenterology Clinics of North America, 30*(2), 313–334.

Joaquin, A., & Gollapudi, S. (2001). Functional decline in aging and disease: A role for apoptosis. *Journal of the American Geriatrics Society, 49,* 1234–1240.

Lerman-Garber, I., Valivia Lopez, J., Flores Rebollar, A., Gomez Perez, F., Antonio Rull, J., & Hermosillo, A. (2000). Evidence of a linkage between neurocardiogenic dysfunction and reactive hypoglycemia. *La Revistade Investigacion Clinica, 52*(6), 603–610. (English translation)

Longo-Mbenza, B., Luila, E., Mbete, P., & Vita, E. (1999). Is hyperuricemia a risk factor of stroke and coronary heart disease among Africans? *International Journal of Cardiology, 71*(1), 17–22.

Miller, C. A. (2004). *Nursing for wellness in older adults: Theory and practice* (4th ed.). Philadelphia, PA: Lippincott Williams & Wilkins.

NANDA International. (2009). *Nursing diagnoses: Definitions and classification, 2009–2011.* Oxford, UK: Wiley-Blackwell.

Ni, H., Coriaty-Nelson, Z., Schiller, J., Cohen, R., & Barnes, P. (2004). *Early release of select estimates based on data from the January-September 2003 National Health Interview Survey.* National Center for Health Statistics. Retrieved from http://www.cdc.gov/nchs/nhis/about200403.htm

Perls, T., Kunkel, L., & Puca, A. (2002). The genetics of exceptional human longevity. *Journal of the American Geriatrics Society, 50*(2), 359–368.

Pfizer Inc. (2002). *The Pfizer global study of sexual attitudes and behaviors.* Retrieved from http://www.pfizer.ca/english/ newsroom/press%20releases/default.asp?s=1&year=2002& releaseID=70

Public Health Agency of Canada. (2002). *Prevention of unintentional injuries among seniors.* Retrieved from http://www.phac-aspc.gc.ca/seniors-aines/pubs/workshop_ healthyaging/pdf/injury_prevention_e.pdf

Public Health Agency of Canada. (2006). *Canadian immunization guide, Part 3: Recommended immunization, immunization of adults* (7th ed.). Retrieved from http://www.phac-aspc.gc.ca/publicat/cig-gci/p03-02-eng.php

Public Health Agency of Canada. (2008). *Seniors and diabetes.* Retrieved from http://www.phac-aspc.gc.ca/seniors-aines/publications/pro/healthy-sante/workshop-atelier/part2/index-eng.php

Statistics Canada. (2006a). *A portrait of seniors 2006 in Canada.* Retrieved from http://www.statcan.ca/english/freepub/89-519-XIE/89-519-XIE2006001.pdf

Statistics Canada. (2006b). *2006 Census: Population by home language, by province and territory and by census metropolitan area.* Retrieved from http://www12.statcan.ca/census-recensement/2006/dp-pd/hlt/97-555/T402-eng.cfm

Statistics Canada. (2010). *Aboriginal identity (8), sex (3) and age groups (12) for the population of Canada, provinces, territories, census metropolitan areas and census agglomerations, 2006 census—20% sample data.* Retrieved from http://www12.statcan.gc.ca/census-recensement/2006/dp-pd/tbt/Rp-eng.

Terry, L. C., & Halter, J. B. (1994). *Aging of the Endocrine System.* In W. R. Hazzard, E. L. Bierman, J. P. Blass, W. H. Ettinger, & J. B. Halter (Eds.), *Principles of geriatric medicine and gerontology* (3rd ed., pp. 791–806), New York, NY: McGraw Hill.

Photo Credits

Chapter 1

Case study: Lisa Peardon/Getty Images/Digital Vision.

Chapter 2

Case study: John Coletti/Getty Images—Photdisc.

Chapter 3

3.3: © Patrick J. Watson; **3.5**: Michael Newman/PhotoEdit; **3.6**: Tony Freeman/PhotoEdit; **Case study**: Thomas Barwick/Getty Images—Photodisc.

Chapter 4

4.1: James Smedley/First Light; **4.2**: Spencer Grant/Alamy; **4.3**: Erproductions/Blend/GetStock.com; **4.4**: Tannic Toohey/Toronto Star/First Light; **4.5**: Comstock Images/Thinkstock Photos; **Case study**: Caroline Woodham/Getty Images—Photodisc.

Chapter 5

Case study: Comstock/Corbis—Comstock Images Royalty Free.

Chapter 6

Table 6.1a: Nicole Harder; **Table 6.1e**: Serkan Savaseri/iStock Photo; **6.9a**: Clear View Stock/Shutterstock; **6.9b**: Nicole Harder; **6.11**: Nicole Harder; **Case study**: Getty Images Inc.—Rubberball Royalty Free.

Chapter 7

7.2: Images Source/Maxx Images; **7.3**: AJPhoto/Photo Researchers, Inc.; **7.4**: Avava/Shutterstock; **7.7 (top)**: Nicole Harder; **7.7 (bottom)**: PHANIE/Photo Researchers, Inc.; **Case study**: Ryan McVay/Getty Images—Photodisc.

Chapter 8

Case study: Photodisc Blue/Getty Images—Photodisc.

Chapter 9

9.5: Reprinted with permission from OMRON Healthcare, Inc.; **9.6**: BOD POD® Body Composition Tracking System. Reprinted with permission from Life Measurement, Inc.; **Table 9.4a–d**: Centers for Disease Control and Prevention (CDC); **Table 9-4e**: E.H. Gill/Custom Medical Stock Photo, Inc.; **Table 9-4f**: Centers for Disease Control and Prevention (CDC); **Table 9-4h**: Custom Medical Stock Photo, Inc.; **Table 9-4i**: Dr. M.A. Ansary/Photo Researchers; **Table 9-4j**: Centres for Disease Control and Prevention (CDC); **Table 9-4k**: O. Damika/Medical On-Line Ltd.; **Case study**: Getty Images/Digital Vision.

Chapter 10

Case study: Eduardo Jose Bernardino Photography/iStock Photo.

Chapter 11

11.3: © Patrick J. Watson; **11.4**: NMSB/Custom Medical Stock Photo, Inc.; **11.5**: Copyright © 1994, Carol H. Weiss. All rights reserved; **11.6**: © Patrick J. Watson; **11.9**: Zuber/Custom Medical Stock Photo, Inc.; **11.10**: Levy/Phototake NYC; **11.11**: Leonard Lessin/Peter Arnold; **11.12**: SPL/Photo Researchers, Inc.; **11.15**: Custom Medical Stock Photo, Inc.; **11.24**: Serkan Savaseri/iStock Photo; **11.26**: Logical Images/Custom Medical Stock Photo, Inc.; **11.29**: H.C. Robinson/Science Photo Library/Photo Researchers, Inc.; **11.30**: Custom Medical Stock Photo, Inc.; **11.31, 11.32, 11.33, 11.34**: Logical Images/Custom Medical Stock Photo Inc.; **11.53, 11.54**: Charles Stewart & Associates; **11.55**: Custom Medical Stock Photo, Inc.; **11.56**: P. Barber/Custom Medical Stock Photo Inc.; **11.57**: Custom Medical Stock Photo, Inc.; **11.58**: Logical Images/Custom Medical Stock Photo, Inc.; **11.59, 11.60**: Custom Medical Stock Photo, Inc.; **11.61**: SIU Bio Med/Custom Medical Stock Photo, Inc.; **11.62**: Logical Images/Custom Medical Stock Photo, Inc.; **11.63, 11.64**: NMSB/Custom Medical Stock Photo, Inc.; **11.65**: © Patrick J. Watson; **11.66**: National Archives and Records Administration; **11.67**: Edward H. Gill/Custom Medical Stock Photo, Inc.; **11.68**: NMSB/Custom Medical Stock Photo, Inc.; **11.69, 11.70**: Zeva Oelbaum/Peter Arnold, Inc.; **11.71**: Kenneth E. Greer/Visuals Unlimited; **11.72**: Phototake NYC; **11.73**: Visuals Unlimited; **11.74**: Courtesy of Elizabeth A. Abel, M.D., from the Leonard C. Winograd Memorial Slide Collection, Stanford Univeristy School of Medicine; **11.75**: Phototake NYC; **11.76**: Greenhill/Mediscan/Medical On-Line Ltd.; **11.77**: SPL/Photo Researchers, Inc.; **11.78**: NMSB/Custom Medical Stock Photo, Inc.; **11.79**: Courtesy of Dr. Hikka Helovuo, K.Kakkarainen, and K. Pannio. Oral Microbiol. Immuno. 8:75–79, (1993); **11.80**: NMSB/Custom Medical Stock Photo, Inc.; **11.81**: Dr. P. Marazzi/Photo Researchers, Inc.; **11.82, 11.83**: Logical Images/Custom Medical Stock Photo, Inc.; **11.84, 11.85**: Custom Medical Stock Photo, Inc.; **11.86**: Logical Images/Custom Medical Stock Photo, Inc.; **11.87**: Custom Medical Stock Photo, Inc.; **Case study**: Jess Alford/Getty Images—Photodisc.

Chapter 12

12.16: M.A. Ansary/Custom Medical Stock Photo, Inc.; **12.18**: © Dr. William H. Daughaday, University of California/Irvine. American Journal of Medicine (20) 1956. With permission of Excerpta Medica Inc.; **12.19**:NIH Phototake NYC; **12.20**: NMSB/Custom Medical Stock Photo, Inc. **12.21**: George Doyle/Thinkstock Photo; **12.24**: Streissguth, A.P., Clarren, S.K., & Jones, K.L. (1985, July). Natural history of the Fetal Alcohol Syndrom: A ten-year follow-up of eleven patients. *Lancet, 2*, 85–91; **12.25**: NMSB/Custom Medical Stock Photo, Inc.; **Case study**: C Squared Studios/Getty Images—Photodisc.

Chapter 13

13.2: Frre/Davis Photograph/Jupiter Images;**13.22**:Don Wong/Photo Researchers, Inc.; **13.41**: NMSB/Custom Medical Stock Photo, Inc.; **13.42**: © mediscan; **13.43**: Leonard Lessen/Peter Arnold, Inc.; **13.44**: Biophoto Associates/Science Source/Photo Researchers, Inc.; **13.45**: Custom Medical Stock Photo, Inc.; **13.46**: © Dorling Kindersley; **13.47**: Custom Medical Stock Photo, Inc.; **13.48**: M. English/Stockphoto.com/Medichrome/The Stock Shop, Inc.; **13.49**: Science Photo Library/Photo Researchers, Inc.; **13.50**: NMSB/Custom Medical Stock Photo, Inc.; **13.51**: Science Photo Library/Custom Medical Stock Photo, Inc.; **13.52**: National Eye Institute, National Institutes of Health; **13.53**:

Paul Parker/Photo Researchers, Inc.; **Case study**: Comstock/Think-stock Photo.

Chapter 14

14.14: Courtesy of Dr. Richard A. Bunkingham; **14.29**: Reproduced from Otolaryngology-Houston, at http://www.ghorayeb.com; **14.30**: Mediscan/Visuals Unlimited; **14.31**: Janet Hayes/Medical Images Inc.; **14.32**: Mediscan/Visuals Unlimited; **14.33**: Professor tony Wright/ Photo Researchers, Inc.; **14.34**: Medical On-Line Ltd.; **14.35**: Courtesy of Micomedics.com; **14.43**: Dr. P. Marazzi/Science Photo Library/ Custom Medical Stock Photo, Inc.; **14.44**: E.H. Gill/Custom Medical Stock Photo, Inc.; **14.45**: Barts Medical Library/Phototake NYC; **14.46**: Dr. R. Gottsegen/Peter Arnold, Inc.; **14.47**: E.H. Gill/Custom Medical Stock Photo, Inc.; **14.48**: Dr. P. Marazzi/Science Photo Library/Custom Medical Stock Photo, Inc.; **14.49**: E.H. Gill/Custom Medical Stock Photo, Inc.; **14.50**: Logical Images/Custom Medical Stock Photo, Inc.; **14.51**: O.J. Staats/Custom Medical Stock Photo, Inc.; **14.52**: Courtesy PD Dr. P. Itin, Kantonsspital Basel; **Case study**: David Fischer/Getty Images—Photodisc.

Chapter 15

Case study: James Woodson/Digital Vision/Thinkstock.

Chapter 16

16.9: CNRI/Phototake; **16.10**: Copyright © Carol H. Weiss. All rights reserved; **Case study**: Adam Crowley/Getty Images—Photodisc; **16.28**: John Radcliffe Hospital/Photo Researchers, Inc.; **16.29**: JPD/Custom Medical Stock Photo, Inc.; **Case study**: Adam Crowley/Getty Images—Photodisc.

Chapter 17

17.3, 17.4, 17.7: Todd A. Buck/Pearson Education; **17.16**: Nicole Harder; **17.17**: Reprinted with permission of the American Academy of Dermatology. All rights reserved; **Case study**: Ryan McVay/Getty Images—Photodisc.

Chapter 18

18.23: Dr. P. Marazzi/Science Photo Library/Photo Researchers, Inc.; **18.25**: P. Barber/Custom Medical Stock Photo, Inc.; **18.26**: Simon Fraser/RNC, Newcastle/Photo Researchers Inc.; **18.28**: Dr. P. Marazzi/ Photo Researchers Inc.; **18.29**: Shout Pictures/Custom Medical Stock Photo, Inc.; **18.30**: Dr. P. Marazzi/Photo Researchers, Inc.; **18.31**: O.J. Staats, MD/Custom Medical Stock Photo, Inc.; **Case study**: Getty Images/Digital Vision.

Chapter 19

19.7: Myrleen F. Cate/PhotoEdit; **19.23, 19.25, 19.26**: Nicole Harder; **Case study**: Paul Austring Photography/Getty Images.

Chapter 20

Case study: Ryan McVay/Getty Images—Photodisc.

Chapter 21

Table 21.2: From Van Wieringen et al.: *Growth Diagrams 1965*. Courtesy of Wolters-Noordhoff, the Netherlands; **21.20**: M. English/Custom Medical Stock Photo, Inc.; **21.21**: O.J. Staats/Custom Medical Stock Photo, Inc.; **21.22**: Centers for Disease Control and Prevention (CDC); **21.23**: Photo Researchers, Inc.; **21.34**: M. English/Custom Medical

Stock Photo, Inc.; **21.35a**: David M. Martin, M.D./Photo Researchers, Inc.; **21.35b**: M. English/Custom Medical Stock Photo, Inc.; **21.36**: Shout Pictures/Custom Medical Stock Photo, Inc.; **Case study**: Jason Stitt/ThinkStock.

Chapter 22

Table 22.1: From Van Wieringen et al.: *Growth Diagrams 1965*. Courtesy of Wolters-Noordhoff, the Netherlands; **22.6**: Michael English/Custom Medical Stock Photo, Inc.; **22.18**: Eye of Science/Photo Researchers, Inc.; **22.19**: Lester V. Bergman/Corbis/Bettmann; **22.20, 22.21, 22.22**: Centers for Disease Control and Prevention (CDC); **22.26**: © Gloria A. Bachmann, M.D., and Nicole S. Nevadunsky/UMDNJ Robert Wood Johnson Medical School; **22.27**: Custom Medical Stock Photo, Inc.; **22.28**: Centers for Disease Control and Prevention (CDC); **22.29**: NMSB/Custom Medical Stock Photo, Inc.; **Case study**: Getty Images, Inc.—Stockbyte.

Chapter 23

23.3, 23.5a, 23.5b: Todd A. Buck/Person Education; **23.15**: Judy Braginsky; **23.50**: Dr. P. Marazzi/Photo Researchers, Inc.; **23.51**: Princess Margaret Rose Orthopaedic Hospital, Edinburgh, Scotland/Science Photo Library/Photo Researchers, Inc.; **23.52**: © Dorling Kindersley; **23.54**: Medical On-Line Ltd.; **23.55**: Boyd Goldie/Medical On-Line Ltd.; **23.56**: Princess Margaret Rose Orthopaedic Hospital/Photo Researchers, Inc.; **23.58**: Medical On-Line Ltd.; **23.60**: Sue Ford/Photo Researchers, Inc.; **23.61**: © 1972–2004 American College of Rheumatology Clinical Slide Collection. Used with permission; **23.62**: Russ Kinne/Comstock Images; **23.63**: Princess Margaret Rose Orthopaedic Hospital/Photo Researchers, Inc.; **23.64**: NMSB/Custom Medical Stock Photo, Inc.; **23.65**: Biophoto Associates/Science Source/Photo Researchers, Inc.; **23.66**: Dr. P. Marazzi/Photo Researchers, Inc.; **23.67**: M. English/Custom Medical Stock Photo, Inc.; **23.68**: Medical On-Line; **Case study**: Ryan McVay/Getty Images—Photodisc.

Chapter 24

Case study: Ryan McVay/Getty Images—Photodisc.

Chapter 25

25.1: Gill/Custom Medical Stock Photo, Inc.; **25.3**: Dr. H.C. Robinson/ Photo Researchers, Inc.; **25.7**: From Van Wieringen et al.: *Growth Diagrams 1965*. Courtesy of Wolters-Noordhoff, the Netherlands; **25.15**: Science Photo Library/Photo Reserachers, Inc.; **25.16**: Custom Medical Stock Photo, Inc.; **25.20**: Custom Medical Stock Photo, Inc.; **Case study**: Getty Images/Digital Vision.

Chapter 26

26.1: Ian Hooten/Science Photo Library; **26.8d**: Logical Images/Custom Medical Stock Photo, Inc.; **26.11**: Photo courtesy of Techno-Aide; **Case study**: Stockdisc/Getty Images, Inc.—Stockdisc.

Chapter 27

Case study: Elke Van de Velde/Getty Images—Photodisc.

Index